BSAVA Manual of Canine and Feline Clinical Pathology
third edition

T0203138

Editors:

Elizabeth Villiers
BVSc FRCPath DipECVCP CertSAM CertVR MRCVS
Dick White Referrals, Veterinary Specialist Centre,
Station Farm, London Road, Six Mile Bottom,
Cambridgeshire CB8 0UH, UK

Jelena Ristić
BVetMed CertVC DSAM MRCVS
Axiom Veterinary Laboratories Ltd,
The Manor House, Brunel Road,
Newton Abbot, Devon TQ12 4PB, UK

Published by:

British Small Animal Veterinary Association
Woodrow House, 1 Telford Way,
Waterwells Business Park, Quedgeley,
Gloucester GL2 2AB

A Company Limited by Guarantee in England
Registered Company No. 2837793
Registered as a Charity

Figures 4.1, 6.3, 6.4, 6.8, 6.9, 6.11, 6.12, 6.13, 6.18, 8.1, 8.3, 8.7, 8.8, 8.10, 8.12, 8.13, 8.17, 8.21, 11.3, 11.8, 11.12, 12.3, 12.11, 12.16, 15.1, 15.2, 15.3, 15.9, 16.1, 16.7, 16.9, 16.12 and 17.13 were drawn by S.J. Elmhurst BA Hons (www.livingart.org.uk) and are printed with her permission.

A catalogue record for this book is available from the British Library.

ISBN 978 1 905319 63 3

The publishers, editors and contributors cannot take responsibility for information provided on dosages and methods of application of drugs mentioned or referred to in this publication. Details of this kind must be verified in each case by individual users from up to date literature published by the manufacturers or suppliers of those drugs. Veterinary surgeons are reminded that in each case they must follow all appropriate national legislation and regulations (for example, in the United Kingdom, the prescribing cascade) from time to time in force.

Printed in the UK by Cambrian Printers, Pontllanfraith NP12 2YA
Printed on ECF paper made from sustainable forests

15506PUBS21

Titles in the BSAVA Manuals series

Manual of Avian Practice: A Foundation Manual
Manual of Backyard Poultry Medicine and Surgery
Manual of Canine & Feline Abdominal Imaging
Manual of Canine & Feline Abdominal Surgery
Manual of Canine & Feline Advanced Veterinary Nursing
Manual of Canine & Feline Anaesthesia and Analgesia
Manual of Canine & Feline Behavioural Medicine
Manual of Canine & Feline Cardiorespiratory Medicine
Manual of Canine & Feline Clinical Pathology
Manual of Canine & Feline Dentistry and Oral Surgery
Manual of Canine & Feline Dermatology
Manual of Canine & Feline Emergency and Critical Care
Manual of Canine & Feline Endocrinology
Manual of Canine & Feline Endoscopy and Endosurgery
Manual of Canine & Feline Fracture Repair and Management
Manual of Canine & Feline Gastroenterology
Manual of Canine & Feline Haematology and Transfusion Medicine
Manual of Canine & Feline Head, Neck and Thoracic Surgery
Manual of Canine & Feline Musculoskeletal Disorders
Manual of Canine & Feline Musculoskeletal Imaging
Manual of Canine & Feline Nephrology and Urology
Manual of Canine & Feline Neurology
Manual of Canine & Feline Oncology
Manual of Canine & Feline Ophthalmology
Manual of Canine & Feline Radiography and Radiology: A Foundation Manual
Manual of Canine & Feline Rehabilitation, Supportive and Palliative Care: Case Studies in Patient Management
Manual of Canine & Feline Reproduction and Neonatology
Manual of Canine & Feline Shelter Medicine: Principles of Health and Welfare in a Multi-animal Environment
Manual of Canine & Feline Surgical Principles: A Foundation Manual
Manual of Canine & Feline Thoracic Imaging
Manual of Canine & Feline Ultrasonography
Manual of Canine & Feline Wound Management and Reconstruction
Manual of Canine Practice: A Foundation Manual
Manual of Exotic Pet and Wildlife Nursing
Manual of Exotic Pets: A Foundation Manual
Manual of Feline Practice: A Foundation Manual
Manual of Ornamental Fish
Manual of Practical Animal Care
Manual of Practical Veterinary Nursing
Manual of Psittacine Birds
Manual of Rabbit Medicine
Manual of Rabbit Surgery, Dentistry and Imaging
Manual of Raptors, Pigeons and Passerine Birds
Manual of Reptiles
Manual of Rodents and Ferrets
Manual of Small Animal Practice Management and Development
Manual of Wildlife Casualties

For further information on these and all BSAVA publications, please visit our website: **www.bsava.com**

Contents

Appendices

Contributors

Joy Archer
VMD MS PhD FRCPath, DipECVCP (hon) FRCVS
Department of Veterinary Medicine,
University of Cambridge,
Madingley Road,
Cambridge CB3 0ES, UK

Gad Baneth
DVM PhD DipECVCP
School of Veterinary Medicine,
Hebrew University,
P.O. Box 12,
Rehovot 76100, Israel

Rory Bell
MVB DSAM DipECVIM-CA FHEA MRCVS
Dick White Referrals,
Veterinary Specialist Centre,
Station Farm, London Road, Six Mile Bottom,
Cambridgeshire CB8 0UH, UK

Graham Bilbrough
MA VetMB CertVA MRCVS
IDEXX Europe B.V.,
Hoofddorp, Netherlands

Laura Blackwood
BVMS PhD MVM CertVR DipECVIM-CA (Onc) MRCVS
School of Veterinary Science,
University of Liverpool,
Leahurst Campus, Chester High Road,
Neston, Cheshire CH64 7TE, UK

Francesco Cian
DVM FRCPath DipECVCP MRCVS
Batt Laboratories,
University of Warwick Science Park,
Sir William Lyons Road, Coventry CV4 7EZ, UK

Lucy J. Davison
MA VetMB PhD DSAM DipECVIM-CA MRCVS
Department of Veterinary Medicine,
University of Cambridge,
Madingley Road,
Cambridge CB3 0ES, UK

Susan Dawson
BVMS PhD MRCVS
School of Veterinary Science,
University of Liverpool,
Leahurst Campus,
Chester High Road, Neston,
Cheshire CH64 7TE, UK

Emma Dewhurst
MA VetMB DipECVCP FRCPath MRCVS
IDEXX Laboratories Ltd,
Grange House, Sandbeck Way,
Wetherby, West Yorkshire LS22 7DN, UK

Gary C.W. England
BVetMed PhD DVetMed CertVA DipVR DipVRep DipECAR DipACT PFHEA FRCVS
School of Veterinary Medicine and Science,
University of Nottingham,
College Road, Sutton Bonington Campus,
Loughborough LE12 5RD, UK

Derek Flaherty
BVMS DVA DipECVAA MRCA FHEA MRCVS
School of Veterinary Medicine,
University of Glasgow,
Bearsden Road, Glasgow G61 1QH, UK

Kathleen P. Freeman
DVM BS MS PhD DipECVCP, FRCPath MRCVS
IDEXX Laboratories Ltd,
Grange House, Sandbeck Way,
Wetherby, West Yorkshire LS22 7DN, UK

Sarah L. Freeman
BVetMed PhD CertVA CertVR CertES DipECVS FHEA MRCVS
School of Veterinary Medicine and Science,
University of Nottingham,
College Road, Sutton Bonington Campus,
Loughborough, LE12 5RD, UK

Alexander J. German
BVSc PhD CertSAM DipECVIM-CA MRCVS
School of Veterinary Science,
University of Liverpool,
Leahurst Campus, Chester High Road,
Neston, Cheshire CH64 7TE, UK

Alex Gough
MA VetMB CertSAM CertVC PGCert MRCVS
Bath Veterinary Referrals,
Rosemary Lodge, Wellsway,
Bath BA2 5RL, UK

Peter A. Graham
BVMS PhD CertVR DipECVCP MRCVS
School of Veterinary Medicine and Science,
University of Nottingham,
College Road, Sutton Bonington Campus,
Loughborough LE12 5RD, UK

Edward J. Hall
MA VetMB PhD DipECVIM-CA MRCVS
School of Veterinary Sciences,
University of Bristol,
Langford House, Langford BS40 5DU, UK

Michael Herrtage
MA BVSc DVSc DVR DVD DSAM DipECVIM-CA DipECVDI MRCVS
Department of Veterinary Medicine,
University of Cambridge,
Madingley Road, Cambridge CB3 0ES, UK

Melanie Hezzell
MA VetMB PhD CertVDI CertVC MRCVS
Department of Clinical Studies,
School of Veterinary Medicine,
University of Pennsylvania,
Philadelphia, Pennsylvania, USA

Tim Jagger
BVM&S MSc FRCPath MRCVS
IDEXX Laboratories Ltd,
Grange House, Sandbeck Way, Wetherby,
West Yorkshire, LS22 7DN, UK

Gerard McLauchlan
BVMS DipECVIM-CA MRCVS FHEA
School of Veterinary Medicine,
University of Glasgow,
Bearsden Road, Glasgow G61 1QH, UK

Yvonne McGrotty
BVMS CertSAM DipECVIM-CA MRCVS
Veterinary Specialist Services,
Broadleys Veterinary Hospital,
Craig Leith Road, Stirling FK7 7LE, UK

Paola Monti
DVM FRCPath DipACVP (Clinical Pathology)
Dick White Referrals,
Veterinary Specialist Centre,
Station Farm, London Road, Six Mile Bottom,
Cambridgeshire CB8 0UH, UK

Carmel T. Mooney
MVB MPhil PhD DipECVIM-CA MRCVS
School of Veterinary Medicine,
University College Dublin,
Belfield, Dublin 4, Ireland

Tim Nuttall
BSc BVSc CertVD PhD Cbiol MSB MRCVS
Royal (Dick) School of Veterinary Studies,
University of Edinburgh,
Easter Bush Veterinary Centre, Roslin,
Midlothian EH25 9RG, UK

Natasha Olby
VetMB PhD DipACVIM (Neurology) MRCVS
Department of Clinical Sciences,
North Carolina State University,
College of Veterinary Medicine,
1060 William Moore Drive,
Raleigh, NC 27607, USA

Martina Piviani
DVM SPCAA MSc DipACVP (Clinical Pathology) MRCVS
School of Veterinary Science,
University of Liverpool,
Leahurst Campus, Chester High Road,
Neston, Cheshire CH64 7TE, UK

Alan Radford
BSc BVSc PhD MRCVS
School of Veterinary Science,
University of Liverpool,
Leahurst Campus, Chester High Road,
Neston, Cheshire CH64 7TE, UK

Ian Ramsey
BVSc PhD DSAM DipECVIM-CA FHEA MRCVS
School of Veterinary Medicine,
University of Glasgow,
Bearsden Road,
Glasgow G61 1QH, UK

Jelena Ristić
BVetMed DSAM CertVC MRCVS
Axiom Veterinary Laboratories Ltd,
The Manor House,
Brunel Road, Newton Abbot,
Devon TQ12 4PB, UK

Marco Russo
DVM PhD
Department of Veterinary Science and
Animal Productions,
University of Naples Federico II,
Italy

Niki Skeldon
MA VetMB DipECVCP FRCPath MRCVS
Axiom Veterinary Laboratories Ltd,
The Manor House,
Brunel Road, Newton Abbot,
Devon TQ12 4PB, UK

Barbara Skelly
MA VetMB PhD DipACVIM DipECVIM-CA MRCVS
Department of Veterinary Medicine,
University of Cambridge,
Madingley Road,
Cambridge CB3 0ES, UK

Laia Solano-Gallego
DVM PhD DipECVCP
Departament de Medicina i Cirurgia Animals,
Facultat de Veterinària,
Universitat Autònoma de Barcelona,
Spain

Tracy Stokol
BVSc PhD DipACVP
S1-058 Schurman Hall,
College of Veterinary Medicine,
Cornell University,
Upper Tower Road, Ithaca,
NY 14853-6401, USA

Harriet M. Syme
BSc BVetMed PhD FHEA DipACVIM DipECVIM-CA MRCVS
Department of Clinical Science and Services,
Royal Veterinary College,
Hawkshead Lane, North Mymms,
Hatfield, Hertfordshire AL9 7TA, UK

Elizabeth Villiers
BVSc FRCPath DipECVCP CertSAM CertVR MRCVS
Dick White Referrals,
Veterinary Specialist Centre,
Station Farm, London Road, Six Mile Bottom,
Cambridgeshire CB8 0UH, UK

Penny Watson
MA VetMD CertVR DSAM DipECVIM MRCVS
Department of Veterinary Medicine,
University of Cambridge,
Madingley Road,
Cambridge CB3 0ES, UK

Jon Wray
BVSc DSAM CertVC MRCVS
Dick White Referrals,
Veterinary Specialist Centre,
Station Farm, London Road, Six Mile Bottom,
Cambridgeshire CB8 0UH, UK

Foreword

In a world where standing still is tantamount to moving backwards, contemporary veterinarians rely on access to excellent diagnostic procedures and information. It's been sometime since we published the last *BSAVA Manual of Canine and Feline Clinical Pathology* and the BSAVA is now proud to publish this, the third edition. As we all know, without a good understanding of clinical pathology we simply can't function effectively, as the identification of disease is the platform from which our clinical care springs; this manual is a *sine qua non*.

I'm sure that all the clinicians who use this book in their day to day working lives will value its readily accessible yet robust science and that those who peruse it as a study or reference book, be they veterinarians, veterinary nurses or students, will devour the more comprehensive details at their leisure.

The authors and editors are to be congratulated for their endeavour and I'm extremely proud of them and of this essential manual.

Patricia Colville BVMS MBA MRCVS
BSAVA President 2015–16

Preface

It is hard to believe ten years have passed since publication of the second edition of the *BSAVA Manual of Canine and Feline Clinical Pathology*. It is only really in editing this edition that it has become apparent just how many advances in the field have been made over that time. For the busy practitioner there have been many improvements in the variety, reliability and cost effectiveness of in-house machinery. For the enthusiastic veterinary surgeon or client, techniques such as immunochemistry, polymerase chain reaction (PCR) and genetic testing have opened up new channels of definitive diagnosis.

It was decided to keep the format of the manual the same due to its previous success and its suitability for use in general practice. The first two chapters provide an introduction to the correct use of clinical pathology data and, with increasing awareness among the veterinary profession of evidence based medicine and clinical audit, provide a framework for correct test selection and interpretation. The sections on haematology have been updated to include new developments in technology and all the systems based chapters have been rewritten, incorporating the latest research. There are new chapters on cardiac disease and genetic disease reflecting advances in these areas and the popular format of case examples at the end of each chapter has been retained to allow readers to evaluate their own learning. The appendix section has been expanded to provide a quick reference for the practitioner who needs to find out the correct sample type in a hurry, or make an immediate interpretation of some results.

We have been fortunate that a team of highly qualified professionals agreed to write for the manual and would like to thank them all for their hard work and enthusiasm to share their knowledge. We would also like to thank the BSAVA publications team members who worked tirelessly to see the book through to completion.

We hope that as a team comprising one clinical pathologist and one practitioner we have been able to work with authors to ensure we share the most up-to-date information with our readers, but also in a way that is accessible to those in practice when time is of the essence. We really hope this manual will be as well received as the previous edition and prove useful to veterinary surgeons and nurses in practice, students and also contain the depth of information required for those with a more specific interest in clinical pathology.

Elizabeth Villiers and Jelena Ristić
February 2016

Chapter 1

In-house *versus* external testing

Graham Bilbrough

This chapter discusses the logical approach the veterinary surgeon (veterinarian) should take when deciding whether to perform diagnostic testing in-house or by submission to a reference laboratory. There are several factors to consider and it is unlikely that a practice will rely exclusively on one or the other, even for an individual patient. It is not a case of 'in' *versus* 'out'; rather, what is important is the approach to picking the right test at the right time.

Veterinary surgeons are impatient for laboratory results. To satisfy this impatience, commercial reference laboratories compete aggressively, with courier services and fast turnaround times, while the manufacturers of in-clinic analysers reduce patient-side run times to mere minutes. Everyone, it seems, is trying to get laboratory results sooner. But at what cost to quality?

Few would argue that there are sound clinical reasons for performing certain tests as quickly as possible, such as electrolyte levels, blood gases, some chemistries, haematology and coagulation tests. However, there are numerous cases where testing could wait several days without jeopardizing the patient's health. Indeed, the large majority of cases could be worked up using the complete range of options, using the veterinary surgeon's discretion as to what would be most appropriate given a wide range of factors.

A veterinary practice is all but obliged to have some, albeit minimal, in-clinic laboratory facilities. In the UK, the Royal College of Veterinary Surgeons (RCVS) organizes an initiative to set standards in veterinary practice to promote high quality care: the Practice Standards Scheme. Currently, the scheme is voluntary. The expectation is that every veterinary surgeon will have the facilities to perform certain basic diagnostic procedures at all times. The RCVS inspects and accredits practices, and the standards are updated on an annual basis (some examples are shown throughout the chapter). The requirements vary by practice type, with minimal stipulations for all practices ('Core Standards') and specific additional necessities for hospitals and emergency clinics.

However, just because a practice has an in-clinic laboratory, this does not remove the veterinary surgeon's discretion over whether to do a particular test in-clinic or at the reference laboratory.

Where to test?

When deciding where to perform a test, the veterinary surgeon is likely to have seven major types of influence:

- Medical factors
- Client preference
- Patient factors
- Practice management and economics
- Complexity of interpretation, specialist support and local knowledge
- Provision of dedicated in-clinic laboratory staff
- Provision for quality assurance.

Medical factors

The medical influences are probably the least controversial. For example, the need for serial evaluation of 'stat parameters' such as potassium (see Chapter 8) and lactate concentrations (see Chapter 9) over a period of hours means that measurement of these useful trends is only practicable when performed 'kennel side'. Arguing that parameters could be measured more accurately at the reference laboratory is irrelevant because the time delay would remove almost all the clinical utility.

When choosing an analyser for these serial measurements, the veterinary surgeon must be confident on two fronts: that the instrument provides sufficient precision to reveal any trend in a reasonable number of samples ('precision' is discussed in Chapter 2), and that they have the knowledge to interpret the results correctly.

Client preference

The client's influence on when to run a test should not be underestimated. At one commercial reference laboratory, the most commonly requested single test (as opposed to panels or profiles) marked as 'urgent' is feline total thyroxine (T4). Some might argue that if the submission form is marked 'suspect hyperthyroid' there is no medical reason why a T4 result is needed so promptly – it is raised arterial blood pressure, not T4, that will do harm if not corrected promptly!

However, clinicians have an excellent reason for wanting quick answers: client satisfaction. In the case of these urgent T4 requests, it is likely that the haematology and biochemistry have already been performed in-house and the T4 is required to complete the analysis. The veterinary surgeon simply wants to provide complete answers *and* client satisfaction. The quick T4 answer may also encourage long-term client loyalty, giving an edge in a competitive marketplace, and a healthy economic return for the practice.

However, client expectations can be managed and it would be wrong to assume that a pet owner would be unhappy to wait some hours longer for a test their veterinary surgeon had decided was better in the circumstances. Some practices allow the client to decide between paying a premium for immediate in-clinic testing – 'the value of now' – or to wait for a reference laboratory result. However, the client's anxiety and their limited understanding of test quality means that they cannot always be relied on to make a logical decision. It is the veterinary surgeon's role to give advice on this matter.

For practices offering a half-hour consultation or longer, it may be practicable to perform venepuncture, analysis and interpretation while the pet owner waits. This allows the results to be discussed, and potentially treatment supplied, in just one client visit.

Patient factors

As with human medicine, patient outcomes tend to be better when the patient can be treated at home and in a familiar environment. Therefore, while a reference laboratory test may be cheaper, a patient-side test with an immediate result can facilitate a faster return home. When making this patient-based decision, other considerations must also be taken into account: medical, client and practice management factors. An immediate answer will eliminate the inconvenience for the client in having to return at a later time. In addition, an immediate answer makes life easier for the veterinary surgeon, who otherwise would have to spend time trying to contact the client to report the results of the test.

Practice management and economics

Veterinary surgeons may want to utilize in-clinic analysers to increase practice income. Many companies have built their businesses around the fact that clients and clinicians want answers immediately, rather than having to wait, and that they are willing to pay more for a faster result.

Although the in-clinic laboratory is frequently a revenue-producing unit, it is incorrect to assume that it is always profitable. It will not be unless it is run thoughtfully and efficiently. What premium is justified for a faster answer? What is the most cost-effective way for the practice to achieve its clinical ambition?

Even after considering the cost of transportation to a reference laboratory, the economy-of-scale achieved at large facilities means that it is very unlikely to be cheaper to run the test in-clinic. An analyser running five samples per day cannot be as financially efficient as an analyser running 500, unless there is a compromise in quality.

For low-volume testing, it will almost never be possible to match the price paid at the reference laboratory. However, for medical reasons, or to increase client satisfaction, a practice may elect to accept a loss. For example, it may be hard to produce a favourable profit and loss statement for a coagulometer, but having one on site improves the standard of care for patients with rodenticide intoxication. For some practices, the relatively small price is worth paying.

When considering investing in any in-house analyser, all costs should be taken into account. For example, it is misleading to compare the cost of the consumables for a haematology analyser with the cost of performing a full blood count at a reference laboratory, where a trained haematologist thoroughly examines a blood smear. This is not meant to discount the many medical benefits of performing in-house haematology, but merely to suggest the need to include in the calculations the costs of staff time and training against the price of sending the blood film to an external laboratory.

For any new diagnostics, but particularly those with a large capital investment, such as in-clinic chemistry or haematology analysers, a business plan will be required. Instrument salespersons may promote a compelling case, by first establishing the cost currently being paid at the reference laboratory and the frequency of testing. This is used to calculate the revenue. After subtracting the lease cost and the reagent costs of the proposed equipment, the remainder is described as profit. This does not take into account the hidden costs of performing the test, such as quality processes and staff time and energy (Figure 1.1).

Alternatively, a business plan may be built around implementing a new testing programme, such as for wellness clinics or pre-anaesthetic testing. These can be successful if the calculation includes the correct number of veterinary surgeons committing to adopting the new strategy.

- The useful technical lifespan of most instrumentation, which should be viewed as 5–7 years
- Purchase or rental costs of the instruments
- Maintenance costs (planned and unexpected)
- Reagents for the paying tests, calibration, quality control (QC) and out-of-range samples
- Other consumables (e.g. pipette tips)
- Calibration and QC material – for low volume tests this may double (or more!) the cost of running the test
- Labour costs
- Training costs
- Cost of capital tied up in equipment and reagents
- Cost of electricity for the analysers and temperature control
- Waste disposal, including disposal of the analyser at the end of use

 1.1 Factors to consider when establishing the full cost of in-clinic testing.

Complexity of interpretation, specialist support and local knowledge

Specialists in veterinary pathology provide insight into a case that goes beyond the ability of the general practitioner. However, this expertise justifies a premium price, and the responsible veterinary surgeon, recognizing the complexity of the individual patient's dataset, must decide whether this is warranted or not.

When bringing any test in-clinic, it is incumbent on the veterinary surgeon to understand the statistics that describe the test's performance (Figure 1.2). For example, the manufacturers of many in-clinic assays are able to demonstrate an excellent correlation with the equivalent assay at the reference laboratory (there is a strong statistical relationship between the reported concentration from

- Understand the statistics that underpin the interpretation. For example:
  - How much variation can be expected from the analyser or the patient?
  - What is the sensitivity, specificity, positive predictive value (PPV) and negative predictive value (NPV) in the appropriate population? (see Chapter 2)
- Understand the impact of interfering substances, including haemolysis, lipaemia, icterus and medication
- Understand the reports (see Figure 1.5)
- Remain constantly sceptical, even with reference laboratory results
- Appreciate the importance of quality processes

1.2 Factors the user of a test must understand.

the two analysers) and yet the in-clinic assay may lack precision (meaning that if the sample is analysed repeatedly, there would be more variation in the in-clinic results). The presentation of the analyser comparison may hide clinically significant scatter in the results (Figure 1.3). It may still be clinically appropriate to use a relatively imprecise test to get the result faster, but you must know and understand this limitation when concluding whether a trend is present.

The clinician must understand the limitations of in-house analysers. Independent assessments of the performance of veterinary analysers, even those widely placed in practice, are surprisingly difficult to find. Many companies present performance data as a white paper or congress abstracts. Both of these provide some useful guidance, but neither should be considered equivalent to papers published in a peer-reviewed journal.

It is dangerous to assume that the results of 'simple looking' in-clinic tests or analysers will allow easy interpretation. For example, hand-held lactate analysers are popular in practice as a quick and cheap means of monitoring tissue perfusion: if oxygen delivery to the tissues is insufficient, blood lactate levels should increase. Furthermore, studies in dogs have demonstrated a strong statistical relationship between lactate levels and outcome both in cases of gastric dilatation–volvulus (GDV) and those presenting to an intensive care unit (ICU) in general (Stevenson *et al.*, 2007). Put simply, patients with a very high blood lactate concentration are likely to die. However, it is dangerous to use this prognostic indicator without consideration of the individual's disease. For a patient, rather than a population, if the cause of the poor tissue perfusion can be resolved, the prognosis might be good. Meanwhile, a downward trend in blood lactate concentration is encouraging. Knowing the underlying disease and how to interpret the inhouse results will help the veterinary surgeon and client decide how to proceed.

The veterinary surgeon should also be aware of the effect of interfering substances, particularly lipaemia, icterus and haemolysis, on the analyser in question (Figure 1.4). These substances are very commonly found in samples of blood from dogs and cats. It is incumbent on the clinician to understand all of the detail provided by the analyser, including any graphical output that may be produced (Figure 1.5).

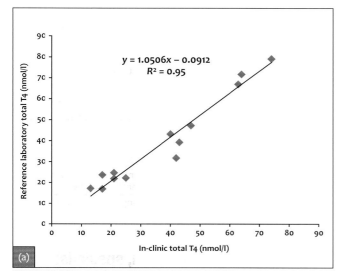

$$y = 1.0506x - 0.0912$$
$$R^2 = 0.95$$

	In-clinic T4 (nmol/l)	Reference laboratory T4 (nmol/l)
Run 1	64	72
Run 2	79	71
Run 3	53	74
Run 4	54	68
Run 5	72	67
Run 6	75	71
Average	66	71
Standard deviation (SD)	10	2
Coefficient of variation (CV) %	15	3

1.3 (a) Before purchasing an analyser for total T4, a practice performed a small comparison study using 13 feline samples analysed in clinic and at the reference laboratory. Some samples were drawn from cats with suspected hyperthyroidism and some from cats receiving medication for confirmed hyperthyroidism. There was excellent correlation (R^2 >0.9). (b) One sample was analysed six times on both analysers, with six separate aliquots being sent to the reference laboratory. The in-clinic assay was much less precise (see Chapter 2 for a detailed discussion of the coefficient of variation). This does not make the in-clinic analyser unacceptable; however, greater care must be taken when determining whether a trend is present. For example, it would be tempting to conclude that a cat receiving medication, in which the reported T4 concentration over time went from 79 to 53 nmol/l, was responding to the therapy. However, this result could be due to the relatively imprecise nature of the assay.

```
          VETSCAN VS2
      COMPREHENSIVE DIAGNOSTIC
09 JAN 2014                  16:33
SAMPLE TYPE:                   DOG
PATIENT ID:                    TAZ
ROTOR LOT NUMBER:          3285GB1
SERIAL NUMBER:         0000V07313
· · · · · · · · · · · · · · · · · · · · · · · ·
ALB      32        25-44      G/L
ALP      LIP       20-150     U/L
ALT      51        10-118     U/L
AMY      LIP       200-1200   U/L
TBIL     LIP       2-10       UMOL/L
BUN      4.5       2.5-8.9    MMOL/L
CA       LIP       2.15-2.95  MMOL/L
PHOS     1.41      0.94-2.13  MMOL/L
CRE      95        27-124     UMOL/L
GLU      5.9       3.3-6.1    MMOL/L
NA+      142       138-160    MMOL/L
K+       3.7       3.7-5.8    MMOL/L
TP       68        54-82      G/L
GLOB     36        23-52      G/L

QC       OK
HEM 2+      LIP 3+      ICT 0
```

1.4 Chemistry report from an in-clinic chemistry analyser. The presence of haemolysis and lipaemia is clearly indicated and the analytes that are severely affected are suppressed. The user of the in-clinic chemistry analyser should be aware of the influence of these interfering substances on their machine.

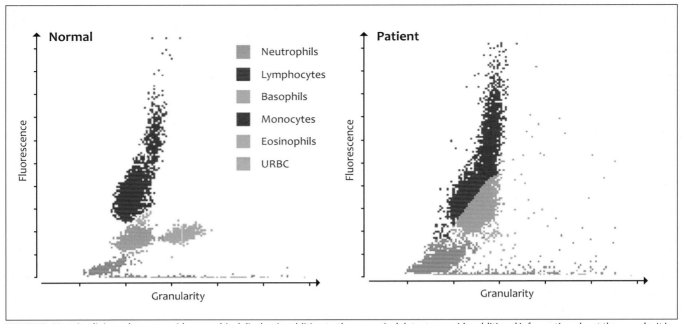

1.5 Most in-clinic analysers provide a graphical display, in addition to the numerical data, to provide additional information about the sample. It is important to appreciate these to gain full understanding. In this example of a 'white blood cell (WBC) dot plot' from an in-clinic haematology analyser, each dot represents a cell and each 'cloud' represents a subtype of white blood cell. The clouds are not cleanly separated, suggesting that a manual differential would be helpful. In this case, an immature population of neutrophils (e.g. 'bands') causes the neutrophil cloud (lilac) to extend further along the vertical axis, spreading over the lymphocyte and monocyte populations.

However, it would be wrong to assume that tests done at the reference laboratory are inherently better. Frequently, the statistics used to describe the performance of the assay are strikingly similar. Perhaps surprisingly, not all the tests offered at the external laboratory have been published and objectively reviewed. Furthermore, even the most reliable test cannot overcome the error introduced by an inappropriate sampling technique or handling. However, generally speaking, a reference laboratory comes with wise counsel from someone who understands the pitfalls for each test, and the operator has a meticulous approach to following detailed instructions from a standard operating procedure (SOP). Many reference laboratories offer 'non-interpreted profiles'. By selecting this cheaper option, the clinician assumes more of the responsibility for drawing meaningful conclusions from the results.

Provision of dedicated in-clinic laboratory staff

A major disadvantage of in-clinic laboratory testing is the issue of technical operator expertise. For many practices, the level of training required may not be affordable or available. This is probably the biggest determinant limiting the range of testing performed in clinic. Typically, the safety implications and corresponding mass of regulations for some areas of testing, for example microbiology, mean that most practices wisely decide to outsource this work to reference laboratories. Some larger veterinary practices employ a full-time laboratory technician to enable them to do more testing. The European School of Veterinary Postgraduate Studies (ESVPS) accredits a Nurse Certificate in Laboratory Techniques.

It is generally uneconomical to use veterinary staff for technical duties, and most of the testing will be the responsibility of the nursing staff. Obviously, staff duties must be organized to allow sufficient time for this work

and for maintaining the in-clinic laboratory. It is probably best to arrange for a single person to have primary responsibility for the laboratory work during normal office hours: the dedicated laboratory manager (Figure 1.6).

Provision for quality assurance

It is vital that appropriate quality control (QC) processes (see Chapter 2) are in place for all laboratories – including in-clinic laboratories – carrying out diagnostic work. However, 'quality' means different things to different

- Usually a veterinary nurse
- Must understand the basic laboratory technology
- Should have a willingness and enthusiasm for QC: a log should be kept detailing the internal and external schemes, problems encountered and actions taken
- Should have a mindset that seeks advice when confronted with uncertainty
- Is responsible for arranging delivery of samples to external laboratories and ensuring that the results are received and communicated to the client
- Ensures that all staff (including veterinary surgeons) receive basic training and are provided with written standard operating procedures (SOPs) that can be easily retrieved. Maintains training records
- Ensures that the data produced by the in-clinic laboratory is safely stored, including an off-site back-up
- (With assistance) provides written SOPs governing safety and waste, including COSHH risk assessments (see The veterinary laboratory and safety procedures below). Provides for regular reviews
- Maintains a fridge/freezer log (record of temperatures and action taken if a problem is detected)
- Maintains equipment (including microscope) calibration, maintenance and service records

1.6 The dedicated in-clinic laboratory manager. The RCVS Practice Standards Scheme states that: *All procedures must be undertaken by designated persons who are suitably trained in the tasks performed by them. A list of persons trained in handling laboratory specimens and in the risks of laboratory work must be kept.* COSHH = Control of Substances Hazardous to Health; QC = quality control.

people. In reference laboratories, the quality procedures typically involve analysis of samples with known concentrations several times during the day. Usually two QC materials are used, one in the normal range and one in the pathological range. Limits of acceptability are preset using very strict targets. If the results are outside these limits, the assay is recalibrated until the QC is deemed to be satisfactory. If this happens frequently, a documented troubleshooting process is instituted. Numerous statistical analyses are performed to track the performance of the assay over time.

An elaborate description of the QC programmes used in many references laboratories, particularly the statistical analysis used, is impenetrable for many general practitioners who are understandably busy with many other tasks. It is unreasonable to expect that the generalist will dedicate the time and money to match the reference laboratory. However, it is unacceptable for the general practitioner to ignore the issue or to take false reassurance from a programme that does not truly assess a test or analyser's performance.

The general practitioner should seek independent advice on their QC programmes. The supplier of the analyser has a potential conflict of interest because they will wish to emphasize ease of use, and their recommendations may be intentionally undemanding. The user should take particular care with terms such as 'electronic QC with every run' and 'internal quality control'; despite these being useful features, they do not provide testimony that all is well.

A low-volume, in-clinic laboratory cannot be excused from the onerous responsibility for ensuring quality, even if this entails analysing control samples with each and every patient sample. It is tempting for the clinic that only uses its analysers for rare emergency work to dismiss this consideration. However, by reserving the analysers for profoundly ill patients, when unexpected results are more likely, it becomes even harder to detect an analyser malfunction without proper QC. Indeed, it may be many months before the user becomes aware, and critically ill patients have the least tolerance for incorrect assessment. In some regions, there are local regulations requiring a practice to observe a quality programme, and the RCVS Practice Standards Scheme includes this matter in their inspection process.

A reasonable compromise of time and cost can be found, however. Each practice should have a designated person with responsibility for the quality programme. There should be repeated analysis of samples with known concentrations and review of the results for sudden or gradual shifts. A general principle is that when a QC check identifies a problem, only results obtained up to the last correct QC check can be considered valid. Sample analysis should be stopped until any problem is identified, corrected and the QC check has been passed. A QC programme should be a major consideration, not an afterthought. It is often badly done or absent in veterinary practice. Even when a programme is present, it is all too easy to forget the 'little analysers', such as the glucometer.

The RCVS Practice Standards Scheme states the following: *All practices: There must be suitable arrangements for quality control (QC) and assurance of automated practice laboratory tests. In addition to internal QC procedures, quality assurance by reference of internal samples to external laboratories or internal analysis of external samples must be routinely undertaken and results documented. The inspector will want to see the results of external quality* *assurance. The frequency of the external quality assurance should be related to the number of tests undertaken. It is expected that this will be at least quarterly.*

Selecting a reference laboratory

The veterinary surgeon must choose between in-clinic testing, a specialized veterinary laboratory and a human laboratory. Human laboratories can be immediately dismissed. The instrumentation, particularly for haematology, must be modified with species-specific parameters and algorithms. Likewise, veterinary-specific pathology support is not likely to be offered.

The geographical location of a veterinary practice and its proximity to a laboratory used to be an important determinant driving those in remote areas towards in-clinic analysis or human laboratories. However, veterinary reference laboratories are now being located in the hubs of international courier companies, meaning that a next-morning service is available to nearly every practice.

The major disadvantage of reference laboratories is the relatively fixed turnaround time dictated by the logistics of sample transportation. In addition, sample transportation is a major part of the cost incurred. However, there are many factors to consider when selecting an external laboratory service, not just price and turnaround time, despite their importance:

- Training and expertise of the clinical pathologist(s)
- Turnaround time for routine and esoteric testing
- Price and discount
- Species-specific testing and interpretation
- Telephone consultation
- Transfer of data to practice management software
- Laboratory accreditation.

Some commercial laboratories allow integration of reference laboratory and in-clinic results in a combined report, which provides a convenient review of all of the patient's data (Figure 1.7).

There is only one internationally recognized standard for testing laboratories that specifically demonstrates technical competence and the ability to generate technically valid results: BS EN ISO/IEC 17025:2005. Other standards are of relevance to the veterinary laboratory, but should not be taken as evidence that the organization has demonstrated the technical competence to provide valid and accurate data and results.

For example, International Organization for Standardization (ISO) 9001: 2000 is a general standard for quality management systems applicable to all organizations, irrespective of the service provided. Likewise, Good Laboratory Practice (GLP) is an accreditation system concerned with the organizational process and conditions under which laboratory studies are conducted. GLP compliance authorizes the laboratory to conduct safety and toxicity studies for regulatory authorities.

The RCVS Practice Standards Scheme for small animal practices states: *Where pathological samples are sent to external organisations, a suitable range of containers, envelopes and forms must be available. There must be an SOP for the post and packaging of pathological samples that complies with current packaging regulations.*

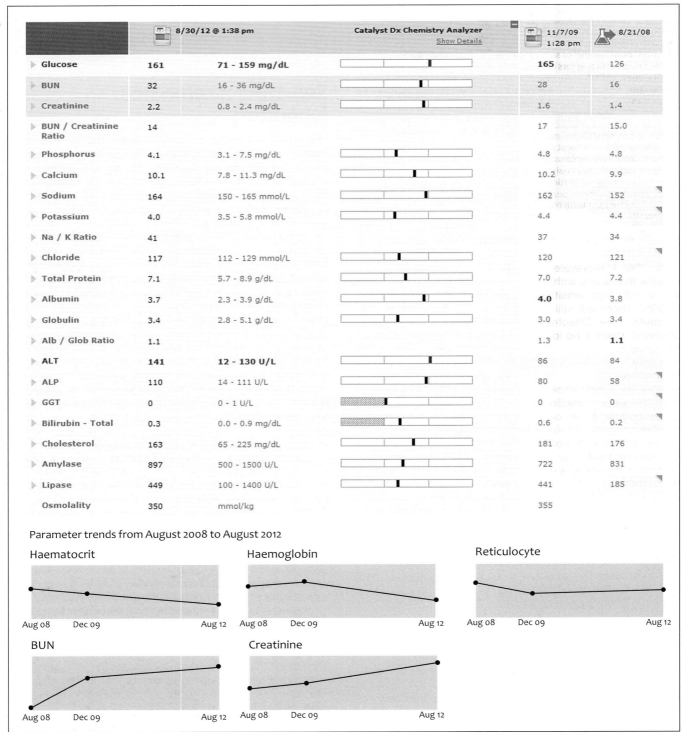

	8/30/12 @ 1:38 pm	Catalyst Dx Chemistry Analyzer Show Details		11/7/09 1:28 pm	8/21/08
Glucose	161	71 - 159 mg/dL		165	126
BUN	32	16 - 36 mg/dL		28	16
Creatinine	2.2	0.8 - 2.4 mg/dL		1.6	1.4
BUN / Creatinine Ratio	14			17	15.0
Phosphorus	4.1	3.1 - 7.5 mg/dL		4.8	4.8
Calcium	10.1	7.8 - 11.3 mg/dL		10.2	9.9
Sodium	164	150 - 165 mmol/L		162	152
Potassium	4.0	3.5 - 5.8 mmol/L		4.4	4.4
Na / K Ratio	41			37	34
Chloride	117	112 - 129 mmol/L		120	121
Total Protein	7.1	5.7 - 8.9 g/dL		7.0	7.2
Albumin	3.7	2.3 - 3.9 g/dL		4.0	3.8
Globulin	3.4	2.8 - 5.1 g/dL		3.0	3.4
Alb / Glob Ratio	1.1			1.3	1.1
ALT	141	12 - 130 U/L		86	84
ALP	110	14 - 111 U/L		80	58
GGT	0	0 - 1 U/L		0	0
Bilirubin - Total	0.3	0.0 - 0.9 mg/dL		0.6	0.2
Cholesterol	163	65 - 225 mg/dL		181	176
Amylase	897	500 - 1500 U/L		722	831
Lipase	449	100 - 1400 U/L		441	185
Osmolality	350	mmol/kg		355	

Parameter trends from August 2008 to August 2012

Haematocrit

Haemoglobin

Reticulocyte

BUN

Creatinine

1.7 Integration of reference laboratory and in-clinic results in a combined report allows for convenient review of all of the patient's data. However, for some parameters, if the testing is not performed consistently (e.g. on the same analyser and with the same sample handling) it may not be appropriate to draw conclusions from the trend in the results. Likewise, the user must understand the expected biological and analytical variation before deciding whether any change is clinically significant (see Chapter 2).

Bringing it all together: combining 'in' and 'out'

Reference laboratory testing and the in-clinic laboratory should be complementary, not competitive (Figure 1.8). For example, there are several testing options for feline leukaemia virus (FeLV; see Chapter 28), ranging from rela-tively cheap in-clinic immunoassays to more expensive reference laboratory testing. None of the options offers perfect sensitivity and specificity: false negatives and some false positives are inevitable. When testing for the virus in a population of cats with relatively few clinical signs, the prevalence of the virus will be very low, and consequently the predictive value of a positive test (PPV) will be poor.

Advantages of in-clinic testing

- The relatively rapid turnaround time in-house can allow immediate treatment and increase client satisfaction
- Faster results can command a premium price
- 'Insufficient sample' or suggested additional testing may be notified while the patient is still at the practice
- No pre-analytical errors associated with transportation – fresh is best!
- The quality of reference laboratories varies and this is only under your direct control when testing in clinic
- No cost of transportation
- Interesting and rewarding work for the practice staff

Advantages of reference laboratory testing

- Haste may result in an unacceptable deterioration of test quality
- Time to think – for most samples, a delay of even 48 hours is not critical. If the client is expecting near-immediate results, they may also expect a near-immediate explanation. Some delay allows time for contemplation and discussion with colleagues
- More sophisticated analysers and techniques
- A broader range of testing
- Experienced, trained personnel give better quality
- Facilities for long-term retention of samples (e.g. serum can be kept for years at –70 to –80°C)
- Practice nurses are able to dedicate more time to caring for patients

1.8 Advantages of in-house *versus* external laboratory testing.

In this low-prevalence group there is a logical sequence that starts with a low-cost in-house screening test with a very high sensitivity. Even if the specificity is close to 99%, there will still be more false positives than true positives (see Chapter 2). When a positive result is obtained, there is no logical reason to repeat the test with the same in-clinic device. If the instructions were followed correctly the first time, the result will not change. Furthermore, there is little to be gained by sending the sample to a reference laboratory if their immunoassay uses the same detection antibody. An initial false positive will probably have been due to cross-reactivity with another antigen, and therefore, it is likely to be repeated.

The appropriate confirmatory test is a test that uses a different methodology altogether, such as virus isolation. This does not imply a defect with the in-clinic test; rather, the purpose was to identify those cats where it was appropriate to invest in more costly testing. Consultative support

from the reference laboratory should help to integrate the in-clinic and reference laboratory testing.

Establishing a successful in-clinic laboratory requires planning (Figure 1.9) and financial investment. Despite the proliferation of practice laboratory facilities, almost all veterinary practices still use external laboratories for examination of pathological material. In general, external laboratories produce more accurate and reliable results for less money owing to their high throughput. However, these gains may be small and other factors might be more important.

Veterinary surgeons must consider many factors when selecting where to test (Figures 1.10 and 1.11). The decision-making process is relatively complex, and is made more so by the rapidly changing technologies and service options available. The clinician should maintain flexibility in the face of such uncertainty, avoiding long-term (>3 years) purchase or service agreements, and remain continuously open-minded to the possibility of changing.

Laboratory work should be performed in areas or rooms dedicated to that function. The following should be considered:

- Dedicated space, not a thoroughfare
- Non-slip, impervious flooring which can withstand repeated use of strong disinfectants
- Ample workspace with an impervious surface that can withstand repeated use of strong disinfectants
- Temperature-controlled environment (particularly important for some haematology analysers)
- Dust free, well ventilated
- Wash basin, preferably with elbow- or foot-operated taps
- An area where stains such as Diff-Quik® can be used and dried without making a mess in the laboratory
- Electrical sockets
- Access to the internet (a wired, rather than a WiFi, connection may be required)
- Good lighting
- A permanent place for the microscope where it can be used in comfort
- Convenient disposal of waste
- Gas supply if a Bunsen burner is being used
- Storage space for reagents at room temperature
- Fridge and freezer space for storage of reagents and samples (with temperature monitoring). Many suppliers recommend storage at –20°C and domestic freezers may not reach this temperature. Samples should be retained for use if further testing is required. Plasma and serum samples should be stored in a fridge (with monitored temperature), or preferably the freezer, for at least 7 days. Be aware that some analytes may degrade at refrigerator temperatures during this period
- Flammable solvents cupboard (if used on site)
- First-aid kit, eyewash, first-aid notice (detailing where to get help), accident log book
- Spillage kit, including gloves, paper towels, disinfectant, forceps for picking up broken glass and details of correct disposal
- Consider noise. Centrifuges, especially when incorrectly balanced, and some in-clinic analysers can be noisy. This is particularly problematic in small rooms with ceramic tiles, making for a stressful or unbearable working environment
- Facilities for off-site data back-up
- Storage for protective clothing. A clean, long-sleeved laboratory coat should be worn at all times in the laboratory. Disposable aprons, gloves and safety goggles should be available for use as dictated by SOPs
- Library space or computer for convenient access to SOPs, operator manuals, sample logs, etc.

1.9 Setting up an in-clinic laboratory. The RCVS Practice Standards Scheme states that: *Laboratory procedures must be performed in a clean and tidy area designated for that purpose. The designated area does not have to be a separate room; however, the designated area/bench must be clearly used only for laboratory purposes. The bench must be made of impervious materials and permit proper cleaning. There must be adequate facilities for washing of hands. There must be facilities for storage of specimens and reagents, including refrigeration and disposal of waste materials. Data must be stored safely in an easily retrievable form.*

- Has this test been validated for the species of interest? Be warned that 'validation' does not have specific criteria and it is for the user to decide whether the data provide sufficient evidence (see Figure 1.3)
- Has the test been demonstrated to work in the population of patients being tested? What are the positive or negative predictive value, sensitivity and specificity in the group of patients being tested (see Chapter 2)?
- Will having the results change how the patient is treated or help explain the situation to the client and predict the likely outcome?
- Will the analyser work with the appropriate sample types? For example, will this haematology analyser work with effusions as well as whole blood?
- Does the test cover the full dynamic range of interest? For example, one in-clinic bile acids assay will not report a concentration >30 µmol/l, resulting in a test that is useful to rule out hepatic dysfunction quickly, but is not suitable for making a diagnosis (see Chapter 12)

- Is it easy to use and robust? What is the hands-on time for maintenance and running the analyser?
- What footprint and workspace are required? At what temperature and humidity can the analyser operate? Is special ventilation required?
- Will the analyser transfer data to the practice management software? Is it bidirectional, in that test requests are received by the analyser and results are delivered from the analyser without leaving the consulting room?
- What are the storage requirements? What is the shelf-life?
- What are the health and safety implications? What are the requirements for disposal of waste?
- What support, both technical and with interpretation, can be expected from the company? What documentation is available?
- Do all the users agree? Any financial forecast will be valid only if it includes the correct prediction of use
- When, if ever, will the new test or analyser be profitable?

1.10 Before changing the practice policy for a certain type of test, it is important to consider whether the new methodology brings benefit to patients or the business. Many factors should be taken into account.

Parameter	Benefits of doing the work in clinic	Limitations of doing the work in clinic
Biochemistry	• Allows rapid, relatively broad assessment of internal organ function – may be important clinically and for customer satisfaction	• Limited or fixed selection of tests • For smaller practices, it may be hard to justify the financial investment without a concerted effort to use the analyser • For some patients, a reference laboratory would offer better value for money
Coagulation	• Sample quality deteriorates very rapidly • Any abnormality should be confirmed with repeat sampling and testing – far easier if the patient is still in the practice • Allows assessment, intervention and monitoring of therapy in a timely manner (e.g. rodenticide intoxication)	• The current in-clinic assessments (PT, aPTT, ACT, etc., see Chapter 6) offer a crude assessment of coagulation • Many small practices struggle to justify the financial investment
Cytology	• In-clinic cytology may provide a preliminary opinion while awaiting the report from a reference laboratory • For certain samples, such as skin scrapings, transportation to a laboratory can be problematic	• Practitioners may not be sufficiently trained to reach a conclusion confidently
Electrolytes and acid–base status	• Allows 'tailoring' of intravenous fluid therapy • Clinically significant trends may be apparent over hours • Abnormalities may require rapid intervention	
Endocrinology	• In some situations, it is logical to include T4 in the biochemistry panel; waiting for the endocrinology could compromise customer service • Canine Addison's disease can present as an emergency • Allows timely advice to breeders (progesterone)	• Limited range of tests • The lack of canine and feline QC material raises concern over quality. The majority of endocrine disorders do not require a rapid diagnosis • Many endocrinology panels benefit from expert interpretation
Haematology	• Sample quality deteriorates relatively rapidly • Clinically significant trends may be apparent over hours to days • Fast results may be particularly useful with critically ill patients and before surgery or chemotherapy	• Requires microscopic examination of the blood film by a trained member of staff • A manual WBC differential is also needed for some samples • The user must understand and use the graphical output from the analyser
Microbiology	• May allow earlier intervention with the appropriate antibiotic (this time advantage is being diminished by faster response times from the referral laboratories)	• Usually unable to identify the organism and perform accurate sensitivity testing (see Chapter 27) • Additional requirements for the handling of waste • Extensive staff training required
Serology	• Rapid identification of some infectious organisms • Cost-effective screening for common pathogens • Does not require investment in equipment (rapid, single-use test devices are available)	• Limited selection of tests • Shelf-life can be problematic • The user must understand the distinction between exposure and current infection
Urinalysis	• Relatively simple and requires little investment in equipment • A vital component of the preliminary patient evaluation – a delay here affects nearly all patients • Preferably, the analysis should be completed within 60 minutes	• Some important components, e.g. culture and sensitivity and cytology, may require submission to a reference laboratory

1.11 Review of the advantages and disadvantages of an in-clinic laboratory with respect to the area of testing offered. All offer the opportunity to increase the practice revenue and reduce the time-to-results. ACT = activated coagulation time; aPTT = activated partial thromboplastin time; PT = prothrombin time; QC = quality control; WBC = white blood cell.

The veterinary laboratory and safety procedures

Concerns related to health and safety have particular relevance to the laboratory and associated procedures. There are numerous regulations that govern safety in the laboratory, but before considering these it is important to start with common sense and good practice to define local rules that can be supplemented, where necessary, with details from the regulations.

All staff should be familiar with the local, general safety rules and should embrace them enthusiastically in order to reduce the risks they face. Copies of the local safety rules must be available to all staff and visitors entering the designated laboratory area. Suggestions for local rules for good laboratory practice include:

- Protective clothing should be worn at all times. Open-toed footwear is not permitted
- No food or drink should be consumed or stored in the laboratory area, including the refrigerator
- Smoking is not permitted
- Nothing is to be placed in the mouth e.g. pipettes, pens, pencils
- Cosmetics should not be applied in the laboratory
- Contact lenses should not be handled
- Hands must be washed frequently. In particular, they must be washed on entry and exit from the laboratory
- Any cuts and grazes must be covered with a waterproof dressing
- Visitors must be accompanied at all times
- Correct labelling of all substances is imperative
- The laboratory must be kept tidy at all times, especially the floor
- Worktops should be disinfected after each work session
- Instructions on equipment must be followed. Do not attempt to over-ride any safety mechanisms
- The SOPs must be read, understood and observed
- All spillages must be cleaned up immediately
- Waste must be disposed of correctly and in accordance with the SOP (Figure 1.12).

Every item within the laboratory should be considered in the light of the hazards it represents. However, the centrifuge seems to present a particular danger. It is not appropriate to use a centrifuge that can be opened while the rotor is still spinning. Care should be taken to balance the contents before use. If a breakage is suspected, the centrifuge should be stopped and left to rest for at least 30 minutes before opening, to allow any aerosols to settle. It should then be cleaned, decontaminated and disinfected in accordance with the manufacturer's recommendations.

The COSHH regulations (as defined in Control of Substances Hazardous to Health (COSHH), 2002; available at: http://www.hse.gov.uk/coshh/) govern the use of hazardous substances in the workplace in the UK. These regulations specifically require an assessment of the use of a substance and the employer to provide the necessary information and training for people exposed to hazardous substances.

The starting point for this is almost always the Material Safety Data Sheet (MSDS). The supplier of any test, reagent or analyser containing hazardous substances is obliged to provide an MSDS free of charge and in the appropriate local language. The practice should form a collection of these that are easily and quickly accessible in an emergency.

For the practice laboratory limited to haematology and biochemistry, the requirements are not particularly arduous and are similar to what is needed for other activities within the practice. The practice should be aware of the Collection and Disposal of Waste Regulations 1992. For the veterinary practice wishing to engage in microbiology or virology, there are additional requirements:

- Needles, blades, broken glass and other 'sharps' should be disposed of in the same manner as in the operating theatre, i.e. a rigid, securely closed container must be provided. A small benchtop container should be used to facilitate quick disposal of capillary tubes, coverslips and microscope slides
- Colour-coded waste bins (household waste in black bags, clinical waste in yellow bags) should be provided. The service provider may require that unbroken glass be placed in separate containers
- Bacteriological media and samples should be autoclaved, using a 'dirty autoclave' (i.e. not the one used for surgical instrumentation) before disposal as clinical waste
- Local regulations may provide other requirements. The appropriate containers should be conveniently placed for each category. The correct place for all waste generated should be specified in the SOPs for each test or analyser

1.12 Waste management.

The aim of COSHH is to identify risks associated with the use of individual products and to take action to reduce those risks. For each individual chemical, or group of chemicals, the risk assessment ('COSHH assessment') should contain information regarding the storage, spillage and disposal procedures and any specific first aid requirements. The risk assessments should be read by employees and be readily available at all times. Assessments must be reviewed at regular intervals. Each COSHH assessment should include:

- Identification and name of the activity
- Identification and list of hazardous substances
- Identification of route by which they are hazardous
- Protection required
- Means of disposal
- Assessment of risk.

The Health and Safety Executive (HSE) provides an up-to-date step-by-step guide to the COSHH assessment (available at: www.hse.gov.uk/pubns/books/HSG97.htm).

Health and safety at work is the responsibility of both the employer and the employee. Employers have a responsibility to protect their staff from hazards, but employees have a responsibility to take reasonable care of themselves and others. Employers, or the Practice Safety Officer, should ensure that staff understand and comply with the detailed contents of the practice Health and Safety Policy Document. All UK veterinary surgeons must comply with the Health and Safety at Work etc. Act 1974 and the Management of Health and Safety at Work Regulations 1999.

It is important that anybody working in the practice laboratory is either suitably trained or working under the close supervision of a trained person. The training must cover both technical proficiency and safe systems of work. It is the employer's duty to:

- Provide equipment which is free of risk
- Provide an environment that is free of risk
- Ensure that materials are used, moved and stored safely
- Ensure safe systems of work are implemented
- Provide the information and training necessary for health and safety

- Provide protective clothing (employees cannot be charged for this)
- Provide adequate first aid facilities
- Ensure that the appropriate safety signs are present and maintained
- Monitor and review safety procedures regularly.

Under the Health and Safety at Work etc. Act 1974, employers are required to have a policy setting out how they ensure that the risks to the health and safety of their employees, contractors and customers are kept as low as is reasonably practical. Where five or more people are employed, even if only temporarily, the policy must be set down in writing. The document should include a statement of intent as well as the organization and arrangements. It is considered to be good practice for all companies, even those with fewer than five employees, to have written procedures. The reader is referred to the Health and Safety Executive for detailed and up-to-date information (http://www.hse.gov.uk).

The Advisory Committee on Dangerous Pathogens produces guidelines that relate to the handling of specific pathogens (Advisory Committee on Dangerous Pathogens, 1995; for information, see: http://www.hse.gov.uk/aboutus/meetings/committees/acdp/). They are categorized into four groups, based upon their implications for human health. Some organisms of veterinary importance are included in Hazard Group 3 and must be handled in a safety cabinet. It is important to realize that the risk of handling individual samples is often not known. Primate and avian samples require particular caution.

The minimum first aid provision on any work site is a suitably stocked first aid box and an appointed person to take care of first aid issues. If it is considered that there is a significant risk of accidents then one or more staff should be trained in first aid techniques. The reader is referred to the First Aid Regulations 1981. The RCVS Practice Standards Scheme requires a risk assessment be completed and the documents to be readily available.

References and further reading

Flatland B, Freeman KP, Vap LM and Harr KE (2013) *ASVCP Guidelines: Quality Assurance for Point-of-Care Testing in Veterinary Medicine Version 1.0.* Available as a free-of-charge download from the website of the American Society of Veterinary Clinical Pathology (http://www.asvcp.org/pubs/qas/index.cfm)

Rishniw M, Pion PD and Maher T (2013) The quality of veterinary in-clinic and reference laboratory biochemical testing. *Veterinary Clinical Pathology* **41**, 92–109

Ristić J and Skeldon N (2011) Urinalysis in practice – an update. *In Practice* **33**, 12–19

Stevenson CK, Kidney BA, Duke T, Snead EC, Mainar-Jaime RC and Jackson ML (2007) Serial blood lactate concentrations in systemically ill dogs. *Veterinary Clinical Pathology* **36**, 234–239

Chapter 2

Quality assurance and interpretation of laboratory data

Paola Monti and Joy Archer

Laboratory test results form part of the database from which a clinical diagnosis may be made. History, clinical examination and ancillary tests (laboratory tests, radiographs, etc.) are interpreted in conjunction with each other to obtain the best possible diagnosis. Laboratory testing has an important role in the clinical work-up and monitoring of the therapy of veterinary patients. Hence, the care provided to patients is strongly dependent upon consistent and reliable laboratory data. Laboratory results should not be interpreted in isolation, but with an understanding of the laboratory methods used and the potential errors caused by inappropriate sample collection and handling.

Errors may be introduced into the diagnostic laboratory cycle at three main stages (Figure 2.1):

- **Pre-analytical:** inappropriate test request, patient preparation prior to sample collection or sample collection and handling; sample identification problems
- **Analytical:** equipment malfunction, interference, poor quality reagents and controls, poor quality control (QC) system

- **Post-analytical:** erroneous validation or interpretation of the results, delayed reporting to the clinician (excessive turnaround time).

In the last two decades, clinical laboratories have focused their attention on QC to minimize the number of errors that occur during the analytical process (analytical errors). This can be pursued by implementing routine internal checks and enrolling in external quality assessment programmes. However, recent surveys in human laboratory medicine have suggested that laboratory errors occur more frequently before or after the test has been performed (pre- and post-analytical errors).

Pre-analytical errors

Most errors affecting laboratory testing occur in the pre-analytical phase. Poor quality or inappropriate samples can lead to the generation of poor quality results. This can cause erroneous clinical interpretation, resulting in poor patient care.

According to the International Organization for Standardization (ISO) 15189 (2007) definition, the pre-analytical phase includes clinician request, preparation of the patient, collection of the sample and transportation to, and handling of, the sample in the laboratory, and ends when the analytical examination begins (Hawkins, 2012). Pre-analytical errors can be sub-classified as follows:

- Preparation of the patient prior to sampling, and patient variables
- Sample collection and handling
- Problems with identification.

Preparation of the patient prior to sampling and patient variables

The most common physiological changes or patient variables that can affect some test results are:

- Exercise or excitement/fear can cause changes in some haematology parameters due to the release of catecholamines. This leads to an increased neutrophil count and sometimes lymphocyte count due to their shift from the marginated to the circulating pool. These changes are referred to as physiological leucocytosis and are often observed in young cats
- Food consumption can affect biochemistry tests, in particular cholesterol, triglyceride, glucose and urea.

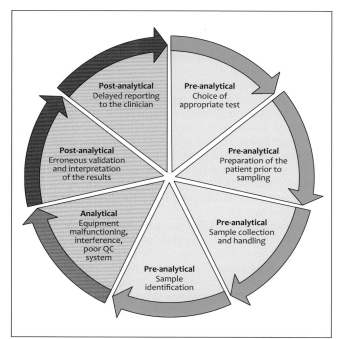

2.1 Laboratory cycle: pre-analytical, analytical and post-analytical phases with the most common areas where errors can occur. QC = quality control.

Additionally, a postprandial sample may be lipaemic and this can, depending on the analytical method, affect other biochemical tests, especially total protein, albumin (values are elevated) and electrolytes (values are lowered). Unless postprandial samples are required (e.g. for dynamic bile acid measurement) an overnight (12-hour) fast is preferred before general biochemical testing. Lipaemia may also interfere with the spectrophotometric assay for haemoglobin (Hb), resulting in falsely high Hb and mean corpuscular haemoglobin concentration (MCHC). Large lipid droplets may be falsely counted as leucocytes or platelets by some analysers (e.g. Cell-Dyn)

- If samples are to be collected for monitoring drug therapy (e.g. thyroid supplementation, digoxin levels, etc.), collection times can be important and should be timed to correspond with peak and trough drug levels; the times should be carefully recorded. Special tests, such as glucose tolerance tests and hormone stimulation tests, should have protocols defining test substance dosage and times of administration and sample collection. Times should be carefully recorded on the sample containers.

Additionally, there are some variables intrinsic to the patient that, if ignored, could lead to incorrect interpretation of the results. The more common patient variables are breed and age related (see examples later in the text).

Sample collection

Incorrect sample collection and handling can lead to an unsuitable sample for analysis, potentially leading to inaccurate results and an incorrect clinical decision.

The sampling technique is influenced by the testing required. For example, urine for microbiology testing should be collected aseptically by cystocentesis, while for routine urinalysis an uncontaminated voided sample collected into a clean container is often appropriate. Urine from the cage floor is unsuitable for any analysis.

The most common reasons why a sample may not be suitable for analysis are listed below.

- **Incorrect test requested:** when choosing a laboratory test, the clinician should consider the diagnostic accuracy and the predictive value of the test for identifying the suspected disease. For example, if hyperadrenocorticism is clinically suspected, measuring the urine cortisol to creatinine ratio would not be the test of choice because it is poorly specific although highly sensitive. This means that it is a good test to rule out hyperadrenocorticism, but better tests are available to confirm this disease (e.g. the adrenocorticotropic hormone (ACTH) stimulation test).
- **Haemolysed sample:** with blood collection for haematology, biochemistry and special tests, venepuncture should be performed rapidly and as atraumatically as possible to reduce the potential for haemolysis. Unless a vacutainer system is used for blood collection, the needle should be removed from the syringe before the blood is transferred *gently* to the tube to avoid damage to the cells and to minimize haemolysis. The parameters that are more affected by haemolysis are creatine kinase (CK), aspartate aminotransferase (AST), phosphate and total protein, although the effect varies depending on the method being used. The interference occurs because free

haemoglobin may absorb at the same wavelength as the coloured product of a reaction, or because the substance being measured is released from lysed red cells. Haemolysis falsely raises MCHC and lowers the packed cell volume (PCV) and the red cell count. In human laboratory medicine, haemolysis is the most common reason for sample rejection. Haemolysis is often caused by delayed sample separation, which can also lead to spurious elevations in potassium due to release from leucocytes and platelets. Blood replacement products prepared from bovine haemoglobin interfere with tests in a similar way to haemolysis (directly in a reaction or with colorimetric methods). The effects are dose dependent and persist for 48 hours or more after administration.

- **Clotted sample (micro and macro clots):** traumatic or delayed blood collection can cause platelet activation and secondary aggregation, leading to a spurious thrombocytopenia. The presence of micro or macro clots may also falsely decrease the white blood cell (WBC) count.
- **Under- or over-filling of blood tubes:** tubes should be filled to the correct volume and gently inverted to mix the blood with the pre-measured contents (e.g. ethylenediamine tetra-acetic acid (EDTA), sodium citrate, lithium heparin). It is important to collect an adequate volume of blood for the tests required, remembering that approximately 50–60% of the volume is plasma/serum. For routine haematology, the anticoagulant of choice is EDTA, potassium or sodium salt, because it preserves cell morphology. If the concentration of EDTA is excessive in relation to blood volume (tube under-filling), cells will shrink and falsely lower the PCV. EDTA tubes less than half full (>3.0 mg EDTA/ml blood) reduce the PCV by 5%. The calculated haematocrit (HCT) is unaffected because the red cells re-expand when they are mixed with the isotonic diluent used by the analyser. If liquid EDTA is used, this can add to the error by diluting the sample, thus further lowering cell counts. Conversely, insufficient EDTA in relation to blood will lead to clot formation. Small clots in the sample, which might be missed when visually inspecting the sample, can cause errors in machine-measured parameters, in particular the platelet count and white cell count. For the measurement of coagulation times, citrated plasma is used. The concentration of citrate in the sample affects the results, and maintaining a citrate to sample ratio of 1:9 is essential for an accurate result. If the tubes are under-filled, coagulation times will be falsely prolonged, while over-filling may lead to falsely shortened times. Sample handling is very important in haemostatic tests and is discussed in Chapter 6.
- **Contamination of the sample:** if a single sample is to be divided between several collecting tubes, it is good practice to collect it into a plain (serum) tube first, followed by tubes containing anticoagulant agents. This is to prevent possible contamination, especially with EDTA, which causes a false increase in potassium and a decrease in calcium, magnesium, CK and alkaline phosphatase (ALP). The Clinical and Laboratory Standards Institute (CLSI) has released a recommended order for collecting blood samples (Figure 2.2).

1. Culture tubes or serum tubes with no additive
2. Citrate tubes
3. Gel separator tubes and clot activator tubes
4. Heparin tubes
5. EDTA tubes
6. Other additive tubes (e.g. fluoride/oxalate)

2.2 Clinical and Laboratory Standards Institute (CLSI) guidelines for sample collection into blood tubes in order to avoid sample contamination. Blood should be placed into sample tubes in this order. EDTA = ethylenediamine tetra-acetic acid.

Sample handling

Once the sample has been collected into the correct tube, it should be processed promptly. For haematology, it is always best to make one or more blood films from an EDTA sample close to the time of collection and air-dry them. Although EDTA preserves cell morphology, changes begin to appear within hours, especially in white cells. Samples should be held in the refrigerator before shipping and/or analysing but blood films should not.

At the pre-analytical stage, the greatest numbers of errors for haematology tests are introduced by the ageing of the sample. For example, after 12 hours from collection, the mean cell volume (MCV) and HCT (calculated from the MCV and red blood cells (RBCs)) can significantly increase, and consequently the MCHC decreases.

Coagulation factors are degraded *in vitro* within hours of sampling. Hence, citrate plasma should be separated within 30 minutes from collection. Prothrombin time (PT) and activated partial thromboplastin time (aPTT) are stable for 48 hours in separated plasma at room temperature, but plasma should be frozen if a longer delay is anticipated (see Chapter 6).

Samples for measurement of ionized calcium and magnesium must also be handled carefully; serum should be separated quickly and stored anaerobically.

Samples for glucose determination need to be separated promptly or placed in fluoride/oxalate. Glucose decreases at a rate of 10% per hour if unseparated samples are held at room temperature. Separation of the sample shortly after collection should be preferred when possible because fluoride/oxalate may induce haemolysis.

Ammonia is another labile analyte that requires special handling and should be analysed immediately after sampling. Within hours at room temperature, ammonia concentration can increase up to 2–3 times.

Some endocrinology tests such as those for endogenous ACTH, parathyroid hormone (PTH) and renin require special handling. The samples should be collected in EDTA and the plasma separated immediately and promptly frozen. The sample should then be sent frozen to the reference laboratory.

Identification problems

Examples of problems with the identification of the sample are:

- Specimens not labelled or incorrectly labelled (e.g. blood tubes, cytology slides, etc.)
- Mismatch between the sample's label and the submission form
- Incorrect information provided on the submission form (e.g. incorrect species, breed, age; incomplete or wrong clinical history, etc.; Figure 2.3).

Each sample should be clearly labelled with patient identification and date of collection, and the time of

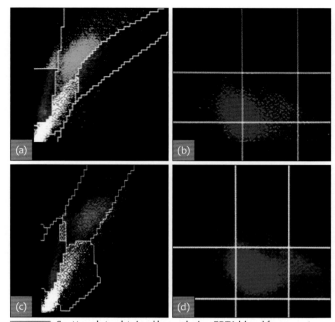

2.3 Scatter plots obtained by analysing EDTA blood from a cat with (a–b) canine settings and (c–d) feline settings. An EDTA blood sample from a cat was submitted to a reference laboratory for haematology analysis. This sample was accompanied by a submission form that stated that the animal was a dog. (a–b) The analyser (Advia® 120) scatter plots show the leucocyte and red cell scatter plots, respectively, that were obtained when the sample was analysed with the canine setting. (c–d) Leucocyte and red cell scatter plots obtained when the sample was analysed using the correct feline setting. Using the wrong setting caused an erroneous gating of the erythrocytes and leucocytes, leading to a falsely low mean cell volume (MCV), mean cell haemoglobin concentration (MCHC) and neutrophil count.

collection if relevant. Along with the samples, there should be a legible submission form which should indicate the tests requested, patient identification (name, number, species, age, breed and sex) and a brief history with clinical findings and information on any drug therapy or blood replacement products given.

Analytical errors

In the last two decades, advances in standardization, automation and technology have significantly decreased analytical errors, thus improving the reliability of laboratory results. Statistical QC activities have been introduced into the diagnostic laboratory to identify and subsequently correct analytical errors. These were first described by Levey and Jennings in 1950.

Analytical errors cannot be eliminated completely but only reduced. In order to guarantee reliable and clinically useful test results, the laboratory should set a total error that is allowable without compromising the quality of the results and the patient care. This is defined as *Total allowable error* (TEa) and is expressed as a percentage. The choice of the TEa is based on the clinical need for each test. In other words, the TEa is the maximum error allowed for a test in order to be able to describe medically important changes in test values. This is obtained based on the *clinical decision level* (TEa = [(clinical decision level − closest reference limit) x 100] / clinical decision level). The clinical decision level is a test value or a change of a test result that triggers additional clinical actions (e.g. further testing or treatment). Usually, the clinical decision level is set with a mutual agreement between the laboratory and clinicians.

Example

Knowing the canine potassium reference interval and clinical decision level in a specific laboratory, the TEa can be calculated as follows:

- Potassium reference interval: 3.4–5.6 mmol/l
- Potassium clinical decision level: 6.0 mmol/l

TEa = [(6.0 – 5.6) x 100]/6.0 = 6.6%

However, in veterinary medicine, it is not always easy to set clinical decision levels for each analyte, mostly owing to the variance in test results and changes related to different species, breeds, age, sex, etc.

An alternative to calculating the TEa on the basis of the clinical decision limit is to follow the guidelines recommended by the American Society of Veterinary Clinical Pathologists (ASVCP) and Clinical Laboratory Improvement Amendments (CLIA) (Figure 2.4). The ASVCP provides one or two TEa values for each analyte: one to be used when the analyte has a concentration close to the lower reference interval and one for a concentration near the higher reference interval. This is because the clinical importance of being able to detect a change in concentration at these two levels may be different. For example, for potassium it is more important to identify an increase rather than a decrease in concentration, so the TEa for the high concentration is smaller.

The performance of an analytical test is defined by the accuracy and precision of the analyser (see below).

The sum of these two variables gives the total calculated error (TEc). In order to estimate a 95% confidence interval for potential errors that may occur, the equation that is most commonly used for obtaining the total calculated error is: TEc = bias + 2CV (coefficient of variation). The laboratory should ensure that the TEc is kept below the predefined TEa, by defining QC and setting an internal quality control system.

Analytical accuracy and precision are inherent sources of variation in laboratory results and are defined below.

Accuracy (bias)

Accuracy is the degree of closeness of the measurements to the true value. This is a measure of the systematic error or bias (Figure 2.5).
Accuracy is obtained from the formula:

Accuracy = (mean $_{target}$ – mean $_{measured}$) x 100(%)

Precision (coefficient of variation)

Precision is the degree to which repeated measurements of the same sample under unchanged conditions give the same result. The closer these replicates are to each other, the more precise is the instrument or method. This is a measure of reproducibility or random error and is expressed as coefficient of variation (CV%). The coefficient of variation is obtained by dividing the standard deviation (SD) by the mean of the results (CV = SD/mean x 100%) (Figure 2.5).

Analyte	Low analyte value	Within RI	High analyte value	CLIA value
Total protein	10%	10%	10%	10%
Albumin	15%	15%	15%	10%
ALP	NCR	25% (20% desirable)	25% (20% desirable)	30%
ALT	NCR	25%	25%	20%
AST	NCR	30%	30%	20%
Bile acids	20%	20%	20%	Not found
GGT	NCR	20%	20%	15% (RCPA) 30% (CFX)
Total bilirubin	NCR	30% (25% desirable)	30% (25% desirable)	20%
Creatinine	20%	20%	20%	15%
Urea	15%	12%	12%	9%
Phosphorus	20%	15%	15%	10–23% (CAP)
Total calcium	10%	10%	10%	2% (BV) to 8% (CFX)
Sodium	5%	5%	5%	4 mmol/l
Chloride	5%	5%	5%	5%
Potassium	10%	5%	5%	0.5 mmol/l
Glucose	10%	20%	20%	6% low; 10% high
Amylase	NCR	25%	25%	30%
Cholesterol	20%	20%	20%	10%
Triglycerides	NCR	25%	25%	25%
CK	NCR	30%	30%	30%

2.4 American Society of Veterinary Clinical Pathologists (ASVCP) and Clinical Laboratory Improvement Amendments (CLIA) recommended TEa values for the most common chemistry tests. The low analyte values, within reference interval (RI) and high analyte values are TEa values recommended by the ASVCP, while the far right column refers to CLIA recommendations. The values vary depending on how near the value is to the clinical decision value (see text). ALP = alkaline phosphatase; ALT = alanine aminotransferase; AST = aspartate aminotransferase; BV = Spanish Society of Clinical Chemistry and Molecular Pathology (SEQC); CAP = College of American Pathologists Participant Summary (April 2004); CFX = Canadian Fixed Limits, The College of Physicians and Surgeons of Saskatchewan; CK = creatine kinase; GGT = gamma-glutamyl transferase; NCR = not clinically relevant; RCPA = Royal College of Pathologists of Australasia and the Australasian Clinical Biochemist Association Quality Assurance Program.
(Data from Harr et al., 2013)

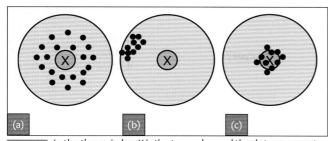

2.5 In the three circles, X is the true value and the dots represent results obtained from sequential analyses of the sample. (a) An accurate but imprecise method: the dots are widely but evenly distributed around the true value and the mean of all the values is equal to the true value. (b) A precise but inaccurate method: the dots are closely clustered together, showing good repeatability, but the results are consistently biased. (c) A method that is both accurate and precise: all the dots are close to the true values and are clustered closely together.

Sources of analytical error

There are different sources of analytical error, and being able to differentiate between systematic and random errors is helpful for identifying the cause of the problem.

Systematic errors may be caused by problems with the instrument or the calibration of the test, including:

- The instrument pipette is dispensing the wrong amount of sample or reagent
- Contamination of the reagents or calibrators (e.g. interfering substance)
- Unstable or incorrectly prepared reagents or calibrators.

Random errors are usually related to:

- Instability of the instrument (e.g. in response to changes in temperature of the laboratory environment)
- Inconsistency among different operators performing the test (how the samples or reagents are prepared, pipetting technique, etc.)
- Random problems with the analysis (e.g. a bubble in the sample causing the aspiration of the incorrect amount of specimen or reagent).

To minimize the analytical errors as much as possible, procedures should be followed in order to guarantee the best performance of the instruments and reagents, calibrators and controls used:

- Detailed records of equipment maintenance according to the manufacturer's instructions should be kept and any failures of performance addressed
- Reagents and materials for calibration and control should be inventoried with dates of receipt and lot and batch numbers
- Reagents etc. should be stored under the conditions recommended by the manufacturers and discarded when outdated
- When a new batch or lot of reagents/calibrators/ controls is started, its performance should be compared with the old batch and sample tests run in parallel to ensure that there are no significant changes in test performance.

Daily or more frequent checks on instrument and reagent performance are required to ensure correct analysis of patient samples. Manufacturers provide information on the expected performance of such materials. If the results obtained in the laboratory are outside these predetermined limits, patient samples should not be run until the cause has been addressed and corrected.

In addition, to minimize the imprecision caused by intraoperator differences, adequate training of the laboratory personnel and adoption of standard operating procedures (SOPs) are required.

Control and minimization of analytical error using quality control systems

There are two important QC systems in laboratory medicine:

- **Internal quality control:** to measure and monitor the precision and accuracy of the instrument (random and systematic errors)
- **External quality control programmes:** to measure and monitor the accuracy of the instrument (systematic error).

Internal quality control: The internal QC involves all the procedures used to monitor the laboratory operations continuously in order to guarantee that the performance of the instrument is good enough to produce reliable results. This can be performed by adopting a statistical QC programme able to detect errors that would invalidate patient results. This implies the use of daily checks to monitor that the results produced by the instrument remain reproducible and accurate.

Statistical QC consists of running one or more *quality control materials* (QCMs) for each analyte to monitor the performance of the analyser. The criteria that determine whether the QC results can be accepted or should be rejected (and consequently whether patient samples can be run or not) are expressed as *control rules*. The internal QC procedures primarily monitor the *bias* of data by using the QCMs and the *precision* of data by comparing multiple analyses of controls or samples.

Internal QC was first introduced by Levey and Jennings (1950), and was based on the assumption that multiple analyses of the same QCM and/or sample have a normal distribution (Gaussian distribution). This was then later developed by John Westgard (www.westgard.com), who developed a system of QC control rules (see below). The simplest of these is the 1_{2S} rule, which is commonly used as the rule for acceptance or rejection of an analytical run. This means that, if the result of one QCM (the figure '1' in the shorthand) is below or above the mean concentration of the QCM $\pm$ twice the standard deviation (SD; the '2_S' in the shorthand), the run should be rejected and patients' samples should not be tested. However, this rule has several disadvantages. First, it has a high rate of false rejection of approximately 1 out-of-control event every 20 runs, which equals a 5% rate of false rejection if only one control is used and 10% if two QCMs are analysed. This high rate of false rejection increases the amount of waste in terms of costs (control material and reagents) and time (delayed turnaround time). Additionally, the 1_{2S} rule is responsive only to random error and does not detect systematic errors.

Years later, Westgard investigated the performance of different control rules by using computer simulations. With these, he was able to calculate two probabilities of detecting error: the probability of false rejection (P_{fr}) and the probability of error detection (P_{ed}). In this regard, he recommends a P_{fr} <5% and a P_{ed} $\geq$90% (i.e. a 90%

chance of detecting a critical systematic shift that would cause a 5% risk of incorrect test results).

He also showed that QC procedures should usually consist of at least two control rules, one sensitive to random error and the other sensitive to systematic error. These rules are known as 'Westgard multirule control procedures' and have been introduced into the software of many instruments.

These rules can be visualized on Levey–Jennings control charts (Figure 2.6). These charts can be produced manually by plotting the daily QCM results, although most modern instrument software programs generate and store these charts and automatically perform statistical analysis of the data. Most charts are constructed to cover a period of 1 month or 30 days of data collection and analysis.

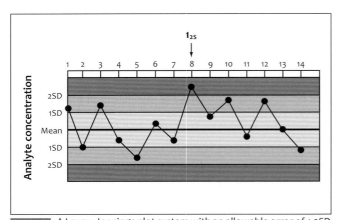

2.6 A Levey–Jennings plot system with an allowable error of ± 2SD from the mean (1_{2S}). The first seven values appear 'in control' and are close to the mean, evenly distributed either side of it. The eighth value is outside the control limits (as indicated by the arrow), but subsequent values are within control limits.

The most widely used Westgard rules are:

- The 1_{2S} rule (one control value exceeding mean ± 2SD) is an early warning for further testing using other control rules
- The 1_{3S} rule (one control value exceeding mean ± 3SD) is sensitive to random error (imprecision)
- The 2_{2S} rule (two consecutive values exceeding mean + 2SD or two consecutive values less than mean – 2SD) is sensitive to systematic error (bias)
- The R_{4S} rule rejects a run if one observation exceeds mean + 2SD and one observation is less than mean – 2SD within the same run. This rule can be applied when multiple QCMs are used, e.g. low and high QCM, but is sensitive to random error (imprecision)
- The 4_{1S} rule rejects a run if four consecutive control observations exceed mean + 1SD or are all less than mean – 1SD. This is sensitive to systematic error (bias)
- The 10X rule rejects a run if 10 consecutive control observations fall on one side of the mean. This is sensitive to systematic error (bias).

These rules help to classify the type of error into random or systematic error. Figure 2.7 shows a Levey–Jennings chart with several rules being violated. There are many control rules that can be used alone or in combination and various numbers of QCMs can be adopted for each analyte. The process of determining

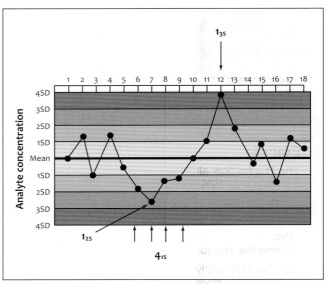

2.7 A Levey–Jennings plot using the Westgard Multirules system. The first five readings are 'in control'. Readings 6–9 all exceed 1SD on the same side of the mean, violating the 4_{1S} rule. This is an indicator of systematic error (bias). In addition, reading 7 violates the 1_{2S} rule. Following recalibration of the analyser, readings 10 and 11 are 'in control', but reading 12 exceeds 3SD, violating the 1_{3S} rule, reflecting random error. Troubleshooting revealed an error in the test procedure. Subsequent readings are 'in control'.

which control rules and how many QCMs should be used to achieve a high probability of error detection (P_{ed}) and a low probability of false rejection (P_{fr}) is called QC validation.

Specifically, the number of QCMs and the number and type of QC rules to be used to obtain the best P_{ed} and P_{fr} are obtained using complicated statistical models (whose description is beyond the scope of this chapter). Westgard has released a commercially available software package specifically designed for this purpose (EZ Rules statistic package). In general, the choice of the QC rules should take into account:

- The QC goals of the laboratory (TEa)
- The stability of the method of each test; different assays have different stability of reagents or calibrators that, if ignored, could introduce systematic errors in the results
- The performance of the instrument at different analyte concentrations near to the clinical decision points; the precision and accuracy of a test vary depending on the concentration of the analyte. Hence, it is important to determine whether the instrument is performing accurately at these concentrations.

It is important to consider that, every time there is a change in the performance of a method or the quality requirements, the type and number of control rules and the total quality control (TQC) strategy should be reassessed. Some large laboratories have recently adopted a more sophisticated control system called the Six Sigma Rules System, which was originally used for industrial manufacturing processes. Most veterinary laboratories however do not yet extend much beyond the control rules described above.

For every analyte that is measured in the laboratory, a specific QC procedure should be chosen in order to have the optimal compromise between the rate of error detection and false rejection.

PRACTICAL APPROACH TO 'IN-CLINIC' INTERNAL QC

1 Define the quality requirements (TEa) for each analyte: the TEa can be estimated from the clinical decision limit (see earlier in text) or may be extrapolated from the literature (e.g. ASVCP Guidelines, CLIA)

> ## Example
> The TEa for 'low albumin' value recommended by the ASVCP is 15%
>
> TEa = 15%

2 Evaluate the performance of the instrument and obtain the TEc for each analyte:

a. For each analyte, use two QCMs with concentrations similar to the clinical decision levels (e.g. low and high concentration) and analyse them every day for 5 days (in reference laboratories, 20 data points are used for this purpose)

> ## Example
> Albumin low QCM: manufacturer target value: 23 g/l
> Daily results (QCM run once daily for 5 days): 22, 23, 22, 21, 23 g/l

b. Calculate the instrument bias and CV using the QCM data obtained

> ## Example
> Mean = 22.2 g/l
>
> SD = 0.8 g/l
>
> **Bias** = (mean target – mean measured)/mean target x 100 = (23 – 22.2)/23 x 100 = 3.5%
>
> **CV** = (SD x 100)/mean = (0.8 x 100)/22.2 = 3.6%

c. Calculate the TEc by using the formula:
TEc = bias + 2CV

> ## Example
> TEc = bias (absolute number in %) + 2CV = 3.5% + (2 x 3.6) = 10.7%

d. The TEc is compared with the predefined TEa to deem the performance of the instrument to be adequate or not:
   - If TEc < TEa, the instrument performance is adequate
   - If TEc > TEa, the laboratory can:
     - Try to improve the performance of the analyser (e.g. more training for the operators, adjustments of the instrument, etc.)
     - Relax the initial quality requirements slightly, but only if there is room for additional error without compromising patient results
     - If no solution can be found, the instrument is not suitable for laboratory needs

> ## Example
> In this case the TEc (10.7%) < TEa (15%) and the instrument performance is considered adequate for the needs of this laboratory

3 Choose the number of QCMs to be run for each analyte for the daily internal QC procedure. Usually, for in-clinic laboratories, one or two levels of QCMs are sufficient. If possible, the QCMs should be chosen with concentrations similar to the clinical decision levels

Choose the QC rule(s) to be used to define the specific performance limits for a particular analyte. The choice of the QC rules (number and type) based on the P_{ed} and P_{fr} can be obtained by using specifically designed computer software or OPSpec charts (the description of these models is beyond the scope of this chapter and can be found on the Westgard website). For in-clinic laboratories, simple QC procedures are preferred such as the 1_{2S} rule (which may give rise to false rejections) and 1_{3S} rule. The latter may not detect all errors, so is more suitable for a test with good precision and accuracy and a higher TEa

4 For every QCM, prepare a *quality control chart* (e.g. Levey–Jennings chart). This can be started by using:

- The target mean and SD provided by the manufacturer of the QCMs
- Analysing the QCMs multiple times (at least 20 times) and then calculating the mean and SD. The use of in-house mean and SD is preferred because they adapt better to the instrument used. Once the mean for each QCM is known, the next step is to calculate decision limits. These limits are ± 1SD, ± 2SD and ± 3SD from the mean. These are drawn on the chart (see Figures 2.6 and 2.7)

5 Every day, before analysing patient samples, analyse the QCMs for each analyte and plot the result on the specific chart. By applying the adopted QC rule(s), accept or reject the run:

a. If the QCM data are within the ± 2SD or ± 3SD from the mean (depending on whether the QC rule in use is the 1_{2S} or 1_{3S}) then the run is accepted and the patient samples can be tested

b. If the QCM result exceeds the mean by ± 2SD or ± 3SD, the run is rejected. If this occurs, the source of error should be investigated. For example check whether:
   - An adequate amount of sample or reagent has been aspirated
   - There is any obvious problem with the instrument (e.g. leakage, tube blockage)
   - Reagents/calibrators/QCMs have expired
   - QCMs/reagents have been stored and reconstituted according to the manufacturers' guidelines
   - The operator performing the test has been sufficiently trained, and follows the SOP

c. If no obvious problems are found, repeat the QC. If this is accepted, analyse the patient samples. If this is rejected again, contact technical support for the instrument

External quality assessment: Most large veterinary laboratories participate in external QC programmes. The external quality assessment (EQA) is the process of controlling the accuracy of an analytical method by inter-laboratory comparison. In these programmes, an authorized agency prepares and sends sample materials to all the laboratories participating in the scheme. The laboratories analyse the samples and return the results to the agency. The agency then calculates the target values (consensus mean) and SDs. It also produces its own charts and statistics, the most important being the *standard deviation index* (SDI). The SDI shows the difference between the results of each laboratory and the consensus mean. These data are then sent back to the laboratories participating in the scheme. The simplest way to evaluate whether the EQA performance is acceptable is to verify that the results of the laboratory fall within ± 2SD from the consensus mean.

The most widely used external QC systems are based on human samples. These include the UK National External Quality Assessment Service (NEQAS) and the Randox International Quality Assessment Scheme (RIQAS) for haematology, biochemistry and endocrinology. A veterinary microbiology QC service is provided by the Animal Health Veterinary Laboratories Agency (AHVLA). A pilot EQA scheme for veterinary endocrinology has recently been set up by Dechra Specialist Laboratories in collaboration with the European Society of Veterinary Endocrinology (VEEEQAS or EVE-QAS).

Use of patient data in quality decisions: In human laboratories, QCMs are the primary samples used for the internal QC. Additionally, patient results can be used to supplement the QCMs, especially when the control products are very expensive or have a very short shelf life or when the QCM does not simulate the patient specimen accurately. For this purpose, samples from healthy subjects are usually used.

In veterinary laboratories, patient data are not easy to use for QC procedures, especially because the majority of samples are from sick animals. However, deviations from usual test result patterns can probably still be used to monitor performance. For example, a patient with very low calcium but no clinical signs attributable to hypocalcaemia would prompt a check on the assay performance.

Delta checks: A delta check is a flag (warning code) signalling a change in the patient's value for a test between one time and another. If the difference between two consecutive laboratory results exceeds a predefined limit, this should trigger further investigation to rule out an underlying error caused either by a pre-analytical or analytical error.

External accreditation services: Many large laboratories apply for accreditation to specific external agencies which provide assurance that the laboratory tests are performed and managed according to set standards. In the UK the major system is the United Kingdom Accreditation Service (UKAS), which follows international guidelines set down by the International Organization for Standardization (ISO) for laboratory performance.

Post-analytical errors

The ISO 15189 (2007) defines the post-analytical phase of all the procedures following the analysis of the sample, including formatting and interpretation of the result, authorization for release, and reporting and transmission of the results. Errors can occur as a result of reporting incorrect values or ascribing the results to the wrong patient (Hawkins, 2012). Occasionally the incorrect reference values for the species may be provided. However, the majority of errors at this stage are related to the interpretation of the results. Error may occur because the person interpreting the results is a third party and is incompletely informed (e.g. incomplete history, including drug therapy) or because the clinician in charge of the case is unaware of certain changes that can occur in laboratory tests in certain conditions.

Units of measurement

In many countries, laboratory test results are reported in SI units (Système International d'Unites), while in the USA they are still widely reported in conventional units (non-SI units) based on mass gravimetric measurements. A few non-SI units have been retained in other countries, either because of the complexity of converting them into SI units or because of their widespread use.

A litre (l) is the designated measure of volume. SI units report the concentration of constituents in terms of the numbers of dissolved molecules, measured in moles (with decimal units mol, mmol, μmol, pmol). A *mole* of a chemical contains the number of grams equivalent to its molecular weight. Conventional units report concentrations of constituents in terms of the dissolved mass in grams (g, mg, μg, pg).

SI units are not used for total protein, for example, because this is a complex of molecules of different molecular weights, therefore, it is usually reported as g/l. Albumin is also reported in g/l (although it could be reported in μmol/l), largely because total protein and albumin are considered together when test results are evaluated and used to determine the globulin concentration (globulin = total protein – albumin).

The SI unit of enzyme activity is the *katal*, which is defined as the amount of enzyme that will catalyse the transformation of 1 mole of substrate per second in an assay system. This is the reporting unit accepted by the IUPAC (International Union of Biochemistry), but not for clinical tests, and the international unit (IU) continues to be used. There is a constant relationship between katal and IU when measured under identical conditions: 1 katal = 60 million IU.

Some conversion factors are shown in Figure 2.8. A more complete conversion table can be found in Appendix 7. In addition, there are various conversion tools available online which can be useful, particularly for some of the more unusual analyses (for example http://www.globalrph.com/conv_si.htm).

Gravimetric unit conversion	SI unit
g/100 ml x 10	g/l
g/100 ml x $\dfrac{10}{\text{mol wt}}$	mol/l
pg/ml x $\dfrac{10^3}{\text{mol wt}}$	pmol/l
mEq/l x $\dfrac{1}{\text{valency}}$	lmol/l

2.8 Conversion factors from gravimetric units to SI units (see also Appendix 7).

Interpretation of test results

For sick patients, laboratory tests are used to help in the diagnosis of disease, or to monitor disease progression or the response to a treatment. In all cases, the results obtained by the laboratory are compared with species-specific reference intervals. However, when monitoring therapy or the course of a disease, useful information may be gained by comparing sequential laboratory results (e.g. before and after treatment).

For a correct interpretation of the laboratory data, it is essential to integrate the results with the patient history, physical examination, ancillary tests and the list of clinical differential diagnoses. The approaches in the interpretation of the laboratory results are:

- Comparison with predetermined reference values
- Comparison between two (or more) sequential results.

Comparison with predetermined reference intervals

A reference interval (RI) for a given analyte is a range of values expected to be found in healthy animals. This represents the interval between an upper and lower limit and commonly includes the central 95% of the values from the selected reference sample group, determined by statistical methods. Reference intervals may also be referred to as 'normal values', 'expected values' or, more commonly, as 'reference ranges'.

A 'reference range' is defined as the entire range of values (actual minimum to maximum measured values) obtained for a test on a reference sample group of healthy animals. The term 'normal value' should be avoided as this implies absence of disease, while sick patients may have some analytes that are within the reference intervals. Additionally, in some pathological conditions, finding some results within the RIs could be an indication of disease (e.g. a lymphocyte count within the RI in severely sick dogs may suggest an underlying hypoadrenocorticism; red cell parameters within RIs in a markedly dehydrated animal could mask an underlying anaemia).

Reference intervals may be classified as population-based or subject-based RIs. In the former, the RIs are obtained from a group of reference individuals selected (preferably randomly) from a reference population (see later). Subject-based RIs (or intra-individual RIs) are derived from sequential samples from a single individual.

The width of population based-RIs is wider than the width of subject-based RIs (Figure 2.9). Determining which type of RI is more appropriate for each analyte is very important when interpreting laboratory results. This is achieved by calculating the index of individuality for a given analyte, which is based on biological and analytical variation.

Biological variation and index of individuality

Biological variation (BV) is the random inherent variation of analytes around a homeostatic set point. The inherent oscillation of the analyte's concentration leads to a variation within each individual (within-subject BV or BV_I) and between animals (between-subject BV or BV_G) at any particular time point.

There are three types of biological variation:

- Variation over the lifespan (age): HCT, total protein, globulin, ALP, calcium, phosphate, CK

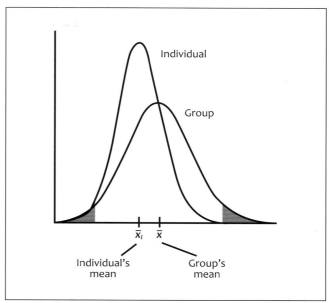

2.9 Illustration of the problems with population-based reference intervals (RIs) when applied to an individual. If the test of interest has marked individuality, a result may fall within the population-based RI even though it is too high for that individual.

- Predictable cyclical variation (daily, monthly, seasonal): cortisol, oestrogen, thyroxine
- Random variation: urea, creatinine.

Within-subject biological variation is represented by the mean coefficient of variation (CV) for consecutive values obtained from a single animal (CV_I). The between-subject biological variation is represented by the mean CV for values obtained from different individuals (CV_G). The CVs for commonly used analytes in dogs and cats are shown in Figure 2.10. The low CVs for electrolyte and protein levels reflect the regulation of these parameters within a small range in the body and the high precision of analytical tests for these parameters. Conversely, urea and creatinine have much higher CVs. Urea is affected by diet and creatinine is affected by muscle mass and exercise, and their levels are not so closely controlled in the body. Hormones have greater variability due to circadian rhythms and the test methods are not as accurate and precise as those for other biochemical tests.

Knowledge of the variation in CVs for different analytes is important when monitoring specific parameters. For example, in a dog with hypoadrenocorticism an increase in potassium of >3.3% (approximately 0.25–0.30 mmol/l) would reflect a 'real' increase and not be attributable to intra-patient biological variation or assay variation. However, a similar small increase in urea may simply reflect biological or assay variation, which could account for an oscillation of up to 19% from the homeostatic set point within one animal.

In 1974, the concept of index of individuality (II) was introduced in human laboratory medicine. The II is defined as the ratio between the intra-individual and between-individual BVs. The original equation included the analytical variation (CV_A) but this formula is often simplified to $II = CV_I/CV_G$.

As mentioned above, the II is used to investigate the utility of conventional population-based reference values compared with subject-based RIs. Analytes with $CV_I < CV_G$ have a low II and therefore have a marked individuality. This means that the variation that occurs in a

Analyte	CV$_G$ (%)	CV$_I$ (%)	CV$_A$ (%)	II
RBC	4.4	5.4	2.8	1.4
HCT	5.2	6.4	1.1	1.3
Hb	4.7	5.9	2.9	1.4
WBC	12.3	12.1	3.7	1.0
ALT	23.7	9.7	3.2	0.4
AST	10.9	11.4	3.3	1.1
ALP	34.4	8.6	1.7	0.3
Albumin	3.0	2.4	1.6	1.0
Total protein	3.1	2.6	1.1	0.9
Urea	35.1	16.1	3.8	0.5
Creatinine	12.9	14.6	2.9	1.2
Phosphorus	12.1	13.7	3.4	1.2
Cholesterol	15.1	7.3	3.0	0.5
Glucose	3.8	9.5	3.7	2.7
Potassium	3.6	3.3	0.1	0.9
aPTT	69.3	19.4	25.0	0.5
PT	4.6	1.4	2.0	0.8
(a) cPLI	49.5	193.8	8.4	3.9

Analyte	CV$_G$ (%)	CV$_I$ (%)
ALT	23.01	13.21
AST	14.97	14.65
ALP	33.72	12.45
Albumin	3.88	3.00
Total protein	13.95	8.31
Urea	15.54	10.43
Creatinine	11.43	5.97
Phosphorus	11.79	8.49
Cholesterol	22.35	10.74
Glucose	8.06	6.76
Potassium	4.91	3.63
Sodium	0.57	0.86
Chloride	1.16	1.17
Calcium	2.51	2.34
(b) Total bilirubin	94.31	87.46

2.10 (a) Data on biological variation (BV) and index of individuality (II) in dogs. (b) Data on biological variation (BV) in cats. BV values from other sources may vary. ALP = alkaline phosphatase; ALT = alanine aminotransferase; aPTT = activated partial thromboplastin time; AST = aspartate aminotransferase; cPLI = canine pancreatic lipase immunoreactivity; CV$_A$ = analytical variation; CV$_G$ = inter-subject BV; CV$_I$ = intra-subject BV; Hb = haemoglobin; HCT = haematocrit; PT = prothrombin time; RBC = red blood cells; WBC = white blood cells. (a, Adapted from Walton, 2012; b, Adapted from Baral et al., 2014)

single individual is smaller than the variation that occurs between different subjects. In dogs, examples of analytes with a marked individuality (low II) are ALP, alanine aminotransferase (ALT), cholesterol, thyroid-stimulating hormone (TSH) and coagulation times. For these tests, the use of population-based RIs is insensitive for detecting a change in the clinical status of the animal, and subject-based RIs or reference change values (RCVs – see below) would be preferred. In fact, in sick patients, these analytes may shift from their usual set point, but not enough to move the result outside the RIs (Figure 2.11). Conventionally, an analyte is considered markedly individual when its II is <0.6.

Conversely, for analytes with CV$_I$ >CV$_G$ (II >1.4), the use of population-based RIs is adequate (e.g. glucose, fructosamine, canine pancreatic lipase immunoreactivity). For those analytes with II lying between 0.6 and 1.4 (e.g. total protein, albumin), population-based RIs can be used, but with caution, and the interpretation of the results may be aided by using RCVs. Canine indexes of individuality are shown in Figure 2.10. Unfortunately, in laboratory medicine, obtaining subject-based RIs for each patient is impractical and unfeasible, and population-based RIs are commonly used independently from the II of the analytes. An alternative to having subject-based RIs when interpreting the result of a test with low II is the use of reference change values (see below).

Determination of the reference intervals

As discussed above, the reference interval is the most widely used medical decision-making tool. Hence, the quality of the RIs plays as important a role in result interpretation as the quality of the result itself. Because reference values are affected by pre-analytical and analytical variables, these stages should be subjected to rigorous QC before establishment of reference values.

In recent years, working groups of both the American and European Societies of Veterinary Clinical Pathology (ASVCP and ESVCP) have been preparing guidelines for establishing reference intervals *de novo*. These guidelines mirror the recommendations published by CLSI. In practice, it is often impossible for any single laboratory to perform these studies and alternative processes can be adopted, such as the transference of reference intervals. This is especially true in veterinary medicine because of the large number of species and breeds encompassed.

Definitions:

- **Reference individual:** a subject selected for testing based on stringent predefined inclusion and exclusion criteria.
- **Reference population:** the entire group of all selected reference individuals.
- **Reference sample group:** a subgroup of reference individuals, selected (preferably randomly) from the reference population that is used to determine the RIs.

Determination 'de novo' of the reference interval: Appropriate selection of the reference population to be used for the establishment of the RIs is essential. The reference population from which reference individuals are chosen should be predefined, and tight clinical parameters for 'healthy' must be established by defining the inclusion and exclusion criteria. Ideally, this population should be representative of the animals from whom samples are sent to the individual laboratory. In practice this is difficult to achieve. Bias may occur if a restricted group of animals is used, for example, values from a colony of young Beagle dogs or from cattery cats. The reference population should represent a general mix of breeds, sexes and ages, living in different environmental conditions. It is also important to consider the Veterinary Surgeons Act 1966 when establishing reference intervals. Collecting blood from healthy animals is not allowed for this purpose; however, excess blood from samples collected for the patient's benefit may be used, for example, surplus blood from pre-anaesthetic screens.

For the establishment of the RI, appropriate numbers of reference individuals should be randomly selected (reference sample group) from the reference population.

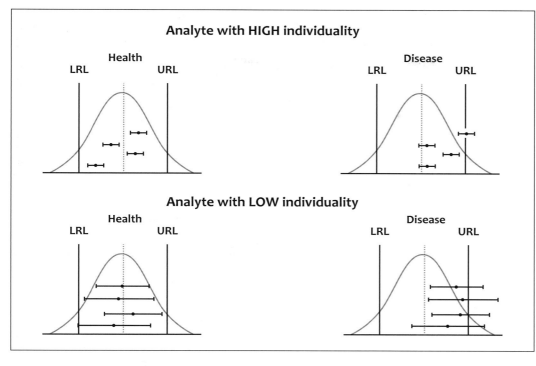

Analyte with HIGH individuality

Health

LRL   URL

Disease

LRL   URL

Analyte with LOW individuality

Health

LRL   URL

Disease

LRL   URL

2.11 Examples of two analytes with a high and a low index of individuality, respectively. The four horizontal bars represent the range of values in four individuals. In the case of high individuality, a significant change in the analyte concentration caused by the disease may be missed and the result may fall within the RI. In this case, the use of subject-based RIs or RCVs may be beneficial. LRL = lower reference limit; URL = upper reference limit.

The number of individuals needed for this purpose should be estimated based on the desired confidence interval (CI) of the RI. The CI reflects the probability that a reference limit derived from a sample group approximates the true reference limit from the entire reference population. Once the reference individuals have been selected, the values obtained from each of these animals are subjected to statistical analysis.

First, the data should be analysed for their distribution (normal distribution or not), preferably using graphical analysis (e.g. histograms; Figure 2.12) or by using goodness-of-fit statistical tests such as the Anderson–Darling test. This step also highlights potential outliers, which are reference values that do not belong to the underlying distribution. If these outliers are retained, they will widen the RIs, decreasing the sensitivity of the test.

The presence of outliers may be due to:

* Inclusion of non-healthy or non-representative subjects in the reference population
* Pre-analytical, analytical or post-analytical errors.

Unless these values are known to be the result of one of these possibilities, outliers should be retained. If not, after the outlier has been removed, retesting the remaining values for any additional outliers would be recommended. Specific statistical methods (e.g. Dixon's test and Horn's algorithm) can be adopted to identify outliers accurately.

Different statistical methods can be used to define the RIs, and the choice of test to be used depends on the number of reference subjects that are available and on the distribution of the results (Gaussian or not). The more data used, the more likely it is that the established RIs will accurately reflect the entire population. Conventionally, at least 120 healthy animals are required to produce reliable RIs, but as few as 40 subjects may be used if necessary.

If the values are normally distributed the reference intervals are established on the basis of the mean ± 2SD (Figure 2.13).

If the data do not have a Gaussian distribution, a non-parametric test is required. This consists of ranking values and using percentile limits. The value at the 97.5th percentile is the upper reference limit and the value at the

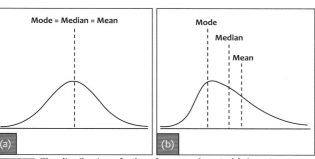

Mode = Median = Mean

Mode
Median
Mean

(a)   (b)

2.12 The distribution of values for an analyte. In (a) there is a Gaussian symmetrical distribution and the mean, median and mode are in the same central position. These data could be analysed by parametric methods, calculating the mean and 2SD to produce reference values. (b) The data points are not in a symmetrical distribution and the mode, median and mean are different. These data would be analysed by non-parametric methods (usually using percentiles) to produce reference values.

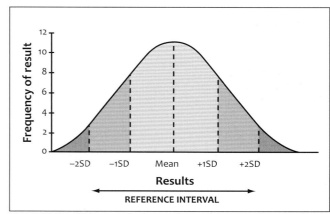

2.13 Establishment of reference intervals by using the central values with exclusion of the lowest and highest 2.5% of the reference values.

2.5th percentile is the lower reference limit. The values obtained from each reference individual are put into ascending order. If n is the number of samples, the position of the sample result lying on the 2.5th percentile is calculated using $(n + 1) \times 0.025$. The 97.5th percentile is calculated using $(n + 1) \times 0.975$. For example, if there are 78 dogs in the reference population the 2.5th percentile is calculated as $(78 + 1) \times 0.025 = 1.975$ (approximately 2). The samples are ranked in ascending order from 1 to 78. The value of the second result in the ascending series is the lower limit of the reference interval. The 97.5th percentile is $(78 + 1) \times 0.975 = 77$. The value of the 77th sample is the upper limit of the reference interval.

In both cases, the defined RIs represent 95% of the animals tested. Given this, it should be borne in mind that, using these methods, 5% of healthy animals would be classified as abnormal (2.5% below the limit for measured values and 2.5% above the limit for measured values). Therefore, for every 20 healthy animals there will be one animal with results outside the RI. For most tests and analytes this is acceptable, because truly diseased animals will be expected to have values far higher or lower than the RIs.

When evaluating a panel of test results from a single animal, there is a probability of $1 - 0.95^n$ (where n is the number of tests in the panel) that not all values will be within the set reference interval. Thus, for 20 results there is a 64% chance that one result will be 'abnormal' $[100 \times (1 - 0.95^{20})]$. This should be remembered when interpreting results from potentially clinically healthy animals for pre-anaesthetic screens or geriatric profiling.

A valuable aid in the statistical analysis of data for establishing the RIs is the use of the '*Reference Value Advisor*'. This is a set of macro instructions for Microsoft Excel™ that computes reference intervals using the standard and robust methods. This is available online for free download at http://www.biostat.envt.fr/spip/spip.php?article63.

Determination of the reference interval using patient data already analysed: The introduction and increased use of computer databases and laboratory information management systems (LIMs) have allowed stored patient data to be used to construct reference intervals. If a large proportion of the patient samples are from healthy individuals, computerized methods based on a combination of laboratory and diagnostic data can be used to select healthy patients to produce RIs. However, this approach does not guarantee that most of the data are derived from healthy subjects. Additionally, this type of data accumulation has inherently increased levels of error related to pre-analytical and analytical factors. For this reason, current guidelines do not endorse this method.

Transfer of reference intervals: This is another, more widely used and accepted, method to determine RIs. When new instrumentation or methods are introduced into a laboratory, reference intervals can be obtained from:

- An existing reference interval generated in the same laboratory on an old instrument or using a different method
- Values from another laboratory using the same instrument and/or method
- Values provided by the manufacturer.

When the method and instrument used are the same, RIs can be transferred directly. Otherwise a comparison of methods should be carried out. If a bias between the two methods or instruments is found, the reference limits may be adjusted using regression analysis.

Once the RIs have been transferred to a new instrument or method, these should be validated before being used in a clinical setting. A way to determine whether the RIs can be safely used is to measure the analyte(s) on 20 healthy animals and compare the results with the 95% CI provided. When ≤2 values exceed the interval, the RIs can be adopted. If 3 or 4 of the values lie outside the interval, an additional 20 healthy individuals can be tested and interpreted as above. If ≥3 are still outside the interval, the RIs should be rejected and new ones established.

It has to be noted that if the RIs to be transferred are inappropriately wide, this method will fail to identify unhealthy subjects accurately because there will be a greater chance that all samples will fall within the given interval.

Limitations of reference intervals

Most laboratories provide reference intervals that are based on a wide-ranging reference population. A narrower selection of healthy subjects partitioned into subgroups (e.g. age, breed, sex) would be ideal, but this is often impractical. If partitioned RIs are not available, it is important to be aware of the common deviations of specific subgroups from the ranges provided. A typical example is young animals, which have HCT, MCV, total protein, globulins, calcium, phosphorus and ALP values that differ from the adult concentrations. Likewise, certain hormone levels, electrolyte and protein values may vary outside the quoted values in pregnant (depending on the stage of gestation) and lactating animals. Specific breed-related differences should also be considered, including:

- Greyhounds and other sighthounds: higher HCT, RBC count, MCV, MCHC and Hb, higher creatinine and ALT; lower WBC, neutrophil and platelet counts, lower total calcium, total protein and globulin
- Japanese breed of dogs (e.g. Akitas, Chinese Shar Pei): microcytosis
- Cavalier King Charles Spaniels and Norfolk Terriers: macrothrombocytopenia.

Partitioned RIs based on age and some canine breeds have been published in the literature in the past few years. However, before adopting these RIs, they should be transferred and validated as described in the section above.

Interpretation of results by comparison between two sequential results

The comparison of two or more sequential laboratory results from the same patient is not as straightforward as it may seem. In fact, each result carries an inherent random variation so that the result is not a single number but a dispersion of numbers.

When two sequential results differ, their difference can be due to:

- An inherent source of variation: pre-analytical, analytical or biological variation
- Clinical improvement or deterioration of the patient.

A change in the condition of the patient is indicated when two consecutive results exceed a certain value known as the *reference change value* (RCV) (also called the significant change value) or, in other words, when the difference between the results is greater than the inherent variation of the test.

The inherent sources of variation of laboratory tests were described at the beginning of this chapter, when the pre-analytical (CV_P), analytical (CV_A) and biological variation (CV_I) were discussed. The total amount of inherent variation (CV_T) intrinsic in each laboratory result is given by the following formula: $CV_T = \sqrt{(CV_P^2 + CV_A^2 + CV_I^2)}$. Often, the pre-analytical variable is excluded from this equation when assuming that standardization of sample collection and handling and patient preparation has been adopted.

Due to the fact that the inherent variation is random, by definition this has a Gaussian distribution. As expected in a normal distribution, 99.7% of the values will fall within the range ± 3CV from the mean concentration, 95.5% within ± 2CV and 68.3 within ± 1CV. The multipliers 1, 2 and 3 are called *z-scores*. Therefore, every analytical value lies within ± Z x *total variation* with a probability appropriate to the z-score. When two consecutive results are compared, the total variation doubles. To be clinically relevant, the difference between two sequential results must be ≥ Z x $\sqrt{[2 \times (CV_A^2 + CV_I^2)]}$. This value represents the reference change value (RCV) and is expressed as a percentage.

When monitoring a patient, the use of RCVs is especially important for all those analytes that have a marked individuality and for which the population-based RIs are not sensitive enough. The main limitation of the use of RCVs in sick patients is that the biological variation (BV) data are often obtained from healthy animals and therefore may not truly mirror the BV of each analyte in the presence of disease. In fact, in human medicine there is evidence that the BV of some analytes is higher in diseased patients than in healthy subjects. As a consequence of this, the use of RCVs determined for healthy individuals to interpret sequential results from sick patients may cause a false positive interpretation of the results. Ideally, the BV of each disease-associated analyte should be estimated in patients with specific diseases.

Example

A 6-year-old, male neutered Jack Russell Terrier is presented with a history of protein-losing enteropathy.

Analyte	Day 1	Day 14
Albumin (g/l)	17	14

Clinical data

Analyte	CV_A	CV_I
Albumin	1.3%	2.4%

Laboratory analytical variation (CV_A) and biological variation (CV_I)

Question: Is the difference between the results obtained on day 1 and day 14 clinically significant or does this just reflect an inherent variation of the tests?

Answer: The albumin reference change value should be calculated. If the difference between the results on day 1 and day 14 is greater than the RCV, it would mean that the patient has deteriorated:

$RCV = Z \times \sqrt{[2 \times (CV_A^2 + CV_I^2)]}$

$Z = 2$ gives a probability of 95.5%
$Z = 3$ gives a probability of 99.7%   ▶

$$
\begin{aligned}
\text{Albumin RCV} &= 2 \times \sqrt{[2 \times (1.3^2 + 2.4^2)]} \\
&= (95.5\% \text{ probability}) \\
&= 7.7 \\[6pt]
&= 3 \times \sqrt{[2 \times (1.3^2 + 2.4^2)]} \\
&= (99.7\% \text{ probability}) \\
&= 11.58
\end{aligned}
$$

The difference between the albumin concentrations on day 1 and day 14 is 3 g/l, which expressed as a percentage is 17.6% (3/17 x 100).

This difference is higher than the RCV and therefore this change is significant and reflects a deterioration of the patient.

Clinical decision limits

When interpreting a laboratory result, the final clinical decision must take into consideration not only the RIs but also the clinical information and the clinical significance of a laboratory test. As discussed above, RIs representing the central 95% of the distribution of the values can be established. However, the final choice of the reference limits (cut-off values) should take account of the sensitivity and specificity required for a given test, especially where there is an overlap in the results from healthy and diseased patients.

This involves setting cut-off values that minimize the number of false negatives or false positives for a particular test. Cut-off values are determined using the concepts of sensitivity, specificity and predictive value, based on the distribution of test results from healthy animals, animals with the disease of interest and, in certain situations, a third group of animals with a different pathological condition.

For example, if one uses the urine cortisol:creatinine ratio for the diagnosis of hyperadrenocorticism and sets a *low* cut-off value, the test will have close to 100% diagnostic sensitivity (there will be very few false negative results) but a low specificity with many false positive results. This can be interpreted clinically to mean that if the test result is negative then it is highly likely to be a true negative and the animal does not have hyperadrenocorticism. However, there will be many false positive results and so other diagnostic tests, such as an ACTH stimulation test, would be required to confirm the presence of disease. If a *high* cut-off value is set, the specificity will be increased to close to 100% with very few false positive results but sensitivity will decrease and more false negatives will be generated.

In cases where tests are affected by more than one disease, setting cut-off limits becomes difficult. For example, amylase and lipase are excreted by the kidney. To obtain high specificity for the diagnosis of pancreatitis in an animal with renal compromise, a high cut-off limit for the pancreatic enzyme tests would have to be set and false negatives would be more likely. In general, cut-off limits are set at levels that produce the highest diagnostic efficiency for a particular disease.

The selection of the appropriate laboratory test should take into consideration the clinical performance characteristics of a test and the purpose of the selected test. If a test is used to screen for a disease of low prevalence in a healthy population, then it must be very sensitive (to identify a high proportion of affected animals), while specificity is less important (animals which test positive can be subjected to further, more specific tests). Screening tests also need to be safe and inexpensive. For tests that are used to confirm a diagnosis, specificity is more important (the test should not incorrectly identify non-diseased animals), especially if the consequences of a positive result are serious (e.g. chemotherapy, surgery or even euthanasia).

Clinical performance characteristics of a test

Based on the presence or absence of disease, test results can be classified into:

- **True positive (TP):** a result that correctly identifies a patient as having a specified disease
- **True negative (TN):** a result that correctly identifies a patient as not having a specified disease
- **False positive (FP):** a result that incorrectly identifies a patient as having a specified disease
- **False negative (FN):** a result that incorrectly identifies a patient as not having a specified disease.

Example

A population of 1000 dogs is tested for disease X. According to the gold standard test, 100 dogs are affected by the disease and 900 dogs are not (prevalence 10%) in case A; only 10 dogs are affected in case B whereas 990 are not affected (prevalence 1%). A new test for disease X is applied to this population and the results are as follows:

Case A

	Gold standard test		
	Dogs affected by disease X	Dogs not affected by disease X	
Dogs testing positive with new test	90 (TP)	45 (FP)	PPV = 67% (90/135)
Dogs testing negative with new test	10 (FN)	855 (TN)	NPV = 99% (855/865)
	SEN = 90% (90/100)	SPEC = 95% (855/900)	

Case B

	Gold standard test		
	Dogs affected by disease X	Dogs not affected by disease X	
Dogs testing positive with new test	9 (TP)	49 (FP)	PPV = 16% (9/58)
Dogs testing negative with new test	1 (FN)	941 (TN)	NPV = 99.9% (941/942)
	SEN = 90% (9/10)	SPEC = 95% (941/990)	

Using the ability (or inability) of a test to produce correct results, the clinical performance of each test can be calculated. The clinical performance of a test is described by the following: ▶

- **Diagnostic sensitivity (SEN):** the frequency of positive test results in animals that have the disease. The use of a test with a high diagnostic sensitivity is preferred when screening for the presence of a disease.
  SEN = TP/(TP + FN) x 100 = 90%
- **Diagnostic specificity (SPEC):** the frequency of negative test results in animals that do not have the disease. A highly specific test is used to confirm the presence of a disease.
  SPEC = TN/(TN + FP) x 100 = 95%
- **Positive predictive value (PPV):** probability that an animal with a positive test result has the disease; PPV = TP/(TP + FP) x 100 = 67%
- **Negative predictive value (NPV):** probability that an animal with a negative test result does not have the disease; NPV = TN/(TN + FN) x 100 = 99%
- **Prevalence:** estimate of the frequency of a disease in a population at a point in time.
  PREV = (TP + FN)/(TP + TN + FP + FN) = 10%

The above example shows how the prevalence is important in determining the predictive value of a test. While sensitivity and specificity reflect the *pre-test* probability of a test itself to correctly identify sick from healthy animals, the positive (and negative) predictive values represent a *post-test* probability that is determined by the amount of disease present in the population of interest. For a test with a diagnostic sensitivity and specificity of 95%, the predictive value of a positive test result (PPV) within a population with a disease prevalence of 50% is 95%. However, if the prevalence is only 5% then the predictive value of a positive test decreases to only 50%, causing the predictive value for the test to be no better than chance or flipping a coin.

Prevalence 50%, sensitivity and specificity 95%		
TP: 47.5%	FP: 2.5%	PPV = 47.5/50 x 100 = 95%
FN: 2.5%	TN: 47.5%	NPV = 47.7/50 x 100 = 95%

Prevalence 5%, sensitivity and specificity 95%		
TP: 4.75%	FP: 4.75%	PPV = 4.75/9.5 x 100 = 50%
FN: 0.25%	TN: 90.25%	NPV = 90.25/90.5 x 100 = 99.7%

A test that has reasonably high sensitivity and specificity and is a good diagnostic test in a population with a high probability of having the disease will, therefore, be very poor in a population where disease prevalence is very low, i.e. when used as a screening test in a healthy population. The typical example used to illustrate the PPV is the in-house assay (snap test enzyme-linked immunosorbent assay (ELISA)) for feline immunodeficiency virus (FIV). This test has a diagnostic specificity that is below 100% (i.e. false positive results may occur). This becomes extremely important in populations with a low prevalence of FIV, such as in the UK, where the reported prevalence of this infectious disease is <1%. Using an assay with diagnostic specificity of 95%, the PPV would be approximately 16%. So, every cat that tests positive should be retested with a 'gold standard assay' e.g. Western blotting or polymerase chain reaction (PCR). Conversely, if a cat that had a positive result with the test comes from a high-risk area (where the prevalence is higher), this result is more likely to be a true positive result.

Generally the aim is to maximize both sensitivity and specificity, but no test is 100% sensitive and 100% specific. As one is maximized, the other is decreased. In the diagnostic situation a test with 100% sensitivity may generate unacceptable numbers of false positive test results. Likewise, when a test is 100% specific it may generate unacceptable numbers of false negative results. In the clinical diagnosis of disease, other medical decision limits can be used, and where results have a numerical value (i.e. not just positive or negative), cut-off values can be selected to maximize the discriminatory power of the test (Figure 2.14).

Receiver-operating characteristic curve analysis

This can be used to show graphically the ability of a test to discriminate between diseased and healthy animals or to compare the efficiency of two tests in the diagnosis of a disease. To produce a receiver-operating characteristic (ROC) curve, sensitivity (true positive rate) is plotted against 1 – specificity (false positive rate). Different cut-off values can then be applied to generate the best values for decisions about diagnosis (Dawson-Saunders and Trapp, 2000). A perfect diagnostic test would have 100% sensitivity and 100% specificity and be close to the top left corner of the graph. A diagonal line (lower left corner to upper right corner) would indicate a useless test. The point on the

curve that is closest to the upper left corner is the cut-off value or decision limit that provides the greatest diagnostic accuracy (efficiency of the test) (Figure 2.15). The area under the curve (AUC) is a quantitative representation of the overall accuracy of the test and ranges between 0.5 and 1. The greater the AUC, the more accurate is the test in diagnosing the disease in question. Conventionally, values between 0.5 and 0.7 represent a test of low accuracy. If the AUC is >0.9, the test accuracy is high, while values in between (0.7–0.9) represent a test with moderate accuracy in the diagnosis of a specific disease.

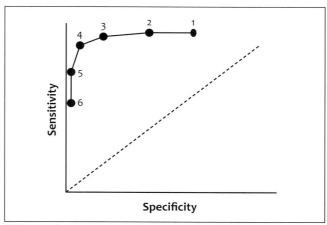

2.15 The receiver-operating characteristic (ROC) curve is a graphical representation of diagnostic sensitivity and specificity for a test at varying selected cut-off values, in this example numbered 1–6. Cut-off level 1 is the lowest cut-off plotted and gives a high sensitivity but low specificity. Cut-off level 6 is the highest cut-off plotted. The specificity is much higher (close to the y-axis) but the sensitivity is lower. Cut-off 4 has the best compromise of sensitivity and specificity, lying closest to the top left corner of the graph. A good test has values close to the upper left corner of the plot. Test results around the diagonal dotted line would indicate a useless test.

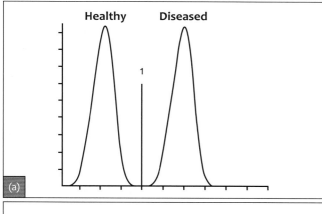

(a)

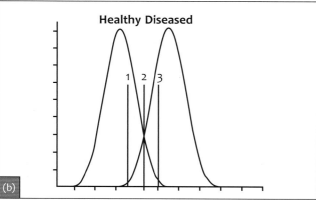

(b)

2.14 Demonstration of the problem of trying to establish cut-off points for any test between healthy individuals and diseased individuals. In (a) the test results from healthy animals do not overlap the test results from diseased animals and so there is a clear cut-off indicated by line 1. This test has 100% sensitivity and specificity. In (b) the test results from healthy animals overlap those from diseased animals. If the cut-off is set at line 1 the test is sensitive but not specific, because a high proportion of healthy animals will have results above the cut-off. Conversely, if the cut-off is set at line 3 the test becomes more specific (very few non-diseased animals have results above the cut-off), but is much less sensitive (a significant proportion of diseased animals have results below the cut-off. If line 2 is selected as the cut-off, the test has moderate sensitivity and specificity.

Example

The following contingency table represents the performance of the 'mitotic index' (MI) as a diagnostic test to predict the risk of death of a patient with an intermediate grade mast cell tumour (MCT). The MI cut-off value is set at 5 mitoses per high power field at 40× (≤5 equals a negative result; >5 equals a positive result). Based on the data in the table, calculate the sensitivity (SEN), specificity (SPEC), positive predictive value (PPV) and negative predictive value (NPV) of the test, assuming that 49 dogs were included in the study and 10 dogs died of their disease.

		Clinical outcome	
		Dogs that died of intermediate grade MCT	Dogs that did not die of intermediate grade MCT
Mitotic Index	Positive MI (MI >5)	6 (TP)	2 (FP)
	Negative MI (MI <5)	4 (FN)	37 (TN)

Results

SEN = TP/(TP + FN) x 100 = 6/(6 + 4) x 100 = 60%
SPEC = TN/(TN + FP) x 100 = 37/(37 + 2) x 100 = 95%
PPV = TP/(TP + FP) x 100 = 6/(6 + 2) x 100 = 75%
NPV = TN/(TN + FN) x 100 = 37/(37 + 4) x 100 = 90%

References and further reading

Baral RM, Dhand NK, Freeman KP, Krockenberger MB and Govendir M (2014) Biological variation and reference change values of feline plasma biochemistry analytes. *Journal of Feline Medicine and Surgery* **16(4)**, 317–325

Dawson-Saunders B and Trapp RG (2000) Evaluating diagnostic procedures. In: *Basic and Clinical Biostatistics, 3rd edn*, pp. 232–247. Appleton and Lange, Norwalk

Farr AJ and Freeman KP (2008) Quality control validation, application of sigma metrics, and performance comparison between two biochemistry analyzers in a commercial veterinary laboratory. *Journal of Veterinary Diagnostic Investigation* **20**, 536–544

Fraser CG (2001) *Biological Variation: from principles to practice*. AACC Press, Washington, DC

Friedrichs KR, Harr KE, Freeman KP *et al.* (2012) ASVCP reference interval guidelines: determination of *de novo* reference intervals in veterinary species and other related topics. *Veterinary Clinical Pathology* **41(4)**, 441–453

Harr KE, Flatland B, Nabity M and Freeman KP (2013) ASVCP guidelines: allowable total error guidelines for biochemistry. *Veterinary Clinical Pathology* **42(4)**, 424–436

Hawkins R (2012) Review article: managing the pre- and post-analytical phases of the total testing process. *Annals of Laboratory Medicine* **32(1)**, 5–16

Lester S, Harr KE, Rishniw M and Pion P (2013) Current quality assurance concepts and considerations for quality control of in-clinic biochemistry testing. *Journal of the American Veterinary Medical Association* **2(15)**, 182–192

Levey S and Jennings ER (1950) The use of control charts in the clinical laboratory. *American Journal of Clinical Pathology* **20(11)**, 1059–1066

Radford A and Dawson S (2005) Diagnosis of viral infections. In: *BSAVA Manual of Canine and Feline Clinical Pathology, 2nd edn*, ed. E Villiers and L Blackwood, pp. 410–423. BSAVA Publications, Gloucester

Rishniw M, Pion PD and Maher T (2012) The quality of veterinary in-clinic and reference laboratory biochemical testing. *Veterinary Clinical Pathology* **41(1)**, 92–109

Walton RM (2012) Subject-based reference values: biological variation, individuality, and reference change values. *Veterinary Clinical Pathology* **41(2)**, 175–181

Westgard JO (2000) *Basic Planning for Quality – Training in Analytical Quality Management for Healthcare Laboratories*. Westgard QC Publishing, Madison, WI

Useful websites

American Society for Veterinary Clinical Pathology
www.asvcp.org/pubs/index.cfm
Veterinary Biological Variation
http://vetbiologicalvariation.org
Westgard QC
www.westgard.com

Chapter 3

Introduction to haematology

Elizabeth Villiers

The complete blood count (CBC) is an integral part of the diagnostic investigation of any systemic disease process. It consists of two components:

- **Quantitative examination** of the cells, including: packed cell volume (PCV) or haematocrit (HCT), total red blood cell (RBC) count, haemoglobin (Hb) concentration, total white blood cell (WBC) count, differential WBC count, and platelet count. In addition, the red cell mean corpuscular volume (MCV), mean corpuscular haemoglobin (MCH) and mean corpuscular haemoglobin concentration (MCHC) are evaluated. Modern analysers also include the red cell distribution width (RDW), mean platelet volume and an automated reticulocyte count, and some provide reticulocyte parameters such as reticulocyte haemoglobin
- **Qualitative examination** of blood smears for changes in cellular morphology. This often provides very useful information which is not detected by the analyser, such as a left shift or toxic change in neutrophils, abnormal blast cells, platelet clumps (which lead to falsely low platelet counts) and red cell clumps which give clues to causes of anaemia such as spherocytes, Heinz bodies or red cell parasites.

Ideally a blood film should be examined as a routine part of the CBC. Indications for a blood film examination include:

- Anaemia: to assess for red cell regeneration and for a cause of anaemia
- Thrombocytopenia: to determine whether the count is genuine or false as a result of clumping; to assess for large platelets
- Neutrophilia or neutropenia: to assess for a left shift and/or toxic change
- Suspected sepsis in an animal with a normal neutrophil count: again to assess for left shift or toxic change
- Lymphocytosis: to assess for atypical morphology including the presence of blast cells
- When flags on the analyser report suggest that blood film examination would be useful.

Blood sampling

Jugular, rather than peripheral, vein venepuncture is recommended in order to minimize the potential for cell damage during blood sampling; 21 G needles are usually used in dogs, while 23 G needles are generally preferred in cats. However, smaller needles are more likely to cause cell damage and subsequent haemolysis. The phlebotomist should try to ensure a slick venepuncture technique, with minimal movement of the needle in and out of the vein, and should avoid excessive suction on the syringe during sampling. After the sample has been obtained, the needle is removed from the syringe and the sample is gently expressed into the appropriate anticoagulant tube. Ethylenediamine tetra-acetic acid (EDTA) is generally the anticoagulant of choice for haematology because cells are well preserved and smears stain well. However, with feline blood samples EDTA may contribute to the tendency for platelet clumping, resulting in falsely low automated platelet counts. Sodium citrate can be used as an alternative in this situation, although clumping may also occur with this anticoagulant. However, automated counts need to be corrected to allow for the dilution factor of citrate, which is 1 part citrate to 9 parts blood. Heparin is unsuitable for haematology because it results in poor leucocyte staining on blood films (although heparinized samples can be used to perform analyser counts).

The EDTA tube should be filled precisely to the level indicated. Under-filling, resulting in EDTA excess, may artefactually reduce red cell size and alter cell morphology. If liquid anticoagulant is being used, under-filling may also result in significant sample dilution. Over-filling may lead to clot formation. With small patients, 0.5 ml tubes can be useful. The sample should be mixed carefully by gently inverting it several times to ensure adequate distribution of the anticoagulant. The tube should not be shaken because this may cause haemolysis.

Blood smears should be made soon after obtaining the blood sample or cellular degeneration will impede interpretation (smears are made from anticoagulated blood). Cell morphology begins to deteriorate within 12 hours, so if blood is being mailed to an external laboratory, a blood smear should be made at the time of sampling (see below) and sent along with the EDTA sample. The EDTA sample should be kept in the fridge until it is dispatched.

Factors affecting sample quality
Presence of clots

Samples containing clots will have a falsely low platelet count (marked effect) and falsely low leucocyte count (mild to moderate effect, depending on the size of the clot). The red cell count and analyser HCT are falsely lowered although the spun PCV may be falsely increased or decreased. Prior to any analysis the sample should be checked for clots. This is best achieved by using a small wooden stick (an 'orange stick'), which is wiped around the inside of the tube and then removed and examined. Any clots in the sample should be scooped up by the stick (Figure 3.1).

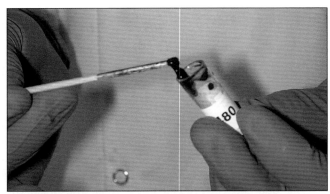

3.1 A blood clot in an EDTA sample is detected by wiping a wooden stick around the inner surface of the tube. Clotted samples should be discarded.

Haemolysis

Damage to the cells during or after sampling may lead to haemolysis (Figure 3.2a). This results in a falsely low RBC count and PCV (although the haemoglobin is not affected), and a falsely high MCHC and MCH. Causes of haemolysis include:

* Narrow gauge needle
* Excessive suction on the syringe
* Excessive agitation of the blood in the tube
* Prolonged storage
* Storage at high temperatures.

Haemolysis can also occur *in vivo* in the intravascular form of immune-mediated haemolytic anaemia (IMHA) as well as with other causes of haemolytic anaemia such as oxidative injuries.

Administration of haemoglobin solutions (e.g. Oxyglobin®) results in free haemoglobin in the plasma and

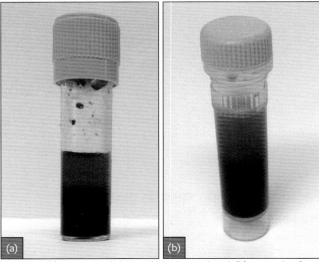

3.2 (a) A sample of plasma that is haemolysed. (b) A sample of plasma that is both haemolysed and lipaemic.

will therefore also lead to a false elevation in MCH and MCHC, because the total haemoglobin measured to calculate these parameters will include these solutions.

Lipaemia

This may be caused by insufficient fasting prior to sampling or may be due to various endocrinopathies, pancreatitis, proteinuria or familial hyperlipidaemia (see Chapter 15). Lipaemia leads to a falsely raised haemoglobin, which in turn leads to elevated MCH and MCHC (Figure 3.2b).

Presence of Heinz bodies

Large numbers of Heinz bodies, e.g. due to onion toxicity, can cause falsely high haemoglobin measurement, giving falsely high MCH and MCHC. Heinz bodies can also give spuriously high white cell counts or reticulocytes on some analysers.

Elevations in MCH and MCHC are generally spurious, because red cells cannot produce more than the normal concentration of haemoglobin. Therefore the sample should be assessed to determine the cause, by gross examination after centrifugation (to identify lipaemia and haemolysis) and by examination of a blood film to check for Heinz bodies. As discussed later, spherocytosis, eccentrocytosis and hyponatraemia can occasionally elevate the MCHC.

Sample ageing

Red cells undergo *in vitro* swelling which can be significant by 24 hours. This leads to a spurious increase in MCV and consequently in HCT, but does not affect the red cell count or haemoglobin measurement. The MCHC and MCH are falsely low (because these are calculated results – see below and Figure 3.6). Ageing also leads to deterioration in white cell morphology, as discussed above. It is important to specify the date of sampling, as well as providing a fresh blood film, when sending samples to an external laboratory.

Presence of autoagglutination

Severe autoagglutination can have a dramatic effect on automated counts because clumped red cells are counted incorrectly. Thus the red cell count and HCT (which is calculated from the red cell count) are falsely low, leading to falsely high MCH and MCHC. Aggregates of red cells are counted as one large red cell, giving a falsely high MCV. The haemoglobin measurement will not be affected by agglutination. Centrifugation of a microhaematocrit tube is required to give an accurate PCV (see below).

Basic quantification techniques

Packed cell volume

The manual PCV accurately reflects the red cell count as long as the mean volume of the red cells (MCV) is within reference limits. The PCV is readily measured using a microhaematocrit centrifuge. Blood in an EDTA tube should be well mixed and a microcapillary tube filled to about 65–75% by placing the haematocrit tube into the EDTA tube and tilting the latter. The base of the microhaematocrit tube is plugged with clay and it is then centrifuged for 5 minutes at high speed (12,500–15,000 rpm). When using a high-speed centrifuge, the sample is centrifuged for exactly 2 minutes at 15,800 rpm/13,700x*g* The red cells are packed at the bottom of the tube above the clay plug. The white cells form the buffy coat, which sits on top of the red cells and is seen as a grey/cream layer. The platelets lie at the top of the buffy coat and may be discernible as a thin, cream-coloured layer adjacent to the slightly greyer buffy coat. The plasma is found above the platelet layer (Figure 3.3). It is important to mix the sample carefully prior to loading the capillary tube, and to ensure that centrifugation speeds and times are adhered to in order to obtain accurate results.

In addition to the PCV, examination of the microhaematocrit tube provides other useful information. Gross examination of the plasma may detect icterus, haemolysis or lipaemia.

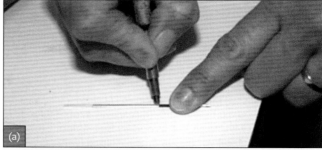

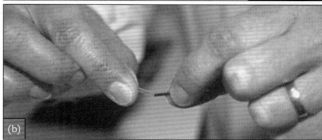

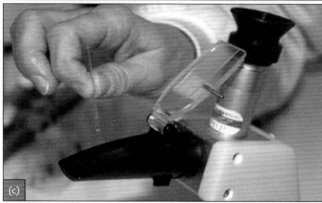

3.4 Measuring plasma protein using a refractometer. (a) The microhaematocrit tube is scored just above the buffy coat, using a diamond writer or razor blade. (b) The tube is broken at the scored line. (c) The plasma is expelled from the tube on to the refractometer prism by swiftly flicking the tube downwards towards the prism, taking care not to touch the prism with the tube. The prism cover is then replaced and the plasma protein read from the internal scale.

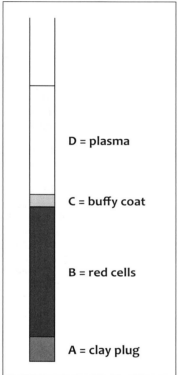

D = plasma

C = buffy coat

B = red cells

A = clay plug

3.3 Diagrammatic representation of a microhaematocrit tube following centrifugation. The PCV is calculated by dividing the length of the packed red cells (B) by the total length of the packed red cells, buffy coat and plasma (B + C + D), using either a sliding measuring device (haematocrit reader) or a microhaematocrit capillary tube reader.

Plasma protein

This can be measured using a refractometer (Figure 3.4). The microhaematocrit tube is scored and broken above the buffy coat. A drop of the plasma is expressed on to the prism and the protein value read from the scale. Plasma or total protein may also be measured using a biochemical analyser. Note that haemolysis, lipaemia and marked icterus falsely elevate plasma protein and may also interfere with the biochemical measurement.

Interpretation of PCV and plasma protein

Plasma protein and PCV should be interpreted together. In an anaemia caused by reduced production of red cells or haemolysis, the number of red cells falls while the volume of plasma present is unchanged and so the PCV is low. In contrast, acute haemorrhage results in loss of both red cells and plasma and therefore initially the PCV does not fall. Following the shift of interstitial fluid into the circulation, plasma volume expands and the PCV falls, reaching its nadir by 24 hours after the haemorrhage.

- **Low PCV with low plasma protein** suggests recent or ongoing haemorrhage. Plasma protein is being lost along with red cells. Internal haemorrhage may initially cause only a mild reduction in plasma proteins, following which proteins are rapidly reabsorbed and return to normal, while in external haemorrhage there is a more marked fall in plasma protein.
- **Low PCV with normal plasma protein** suggests the anaemia is due to haemolysis or reduced red cell production.
- **High PCV with high plasma protein** is seen with dehydration. Water lost from the body results in an increased concentration of both red cells and protein. However, these parameters provide only a crude estimate of an animal's hydration status.
- **High PCV with normal plasma protein** is unusual and suggests absolute polycythaemia or an increase in the number of red blood cells.
- **High plasma protein with low or normal PCV** is usually due to hyperglobulinaemia (see Chapter 7).

Automated cell counts

There is a choice of in-house haematology analysers, which fall into three groups: impedance analysers; flow cytometers; and quantitative buffy coat analysers.

- Impedance analysers include the VetScan HM 2 and HM 5 (Abaxis), Medonic CA620 (A. Menarini Diagnostics), Hemavet 950, 950LV and 1700 (Drew Scientific), Mythic 18 Vet (Woodley Equipment Ltd), scil Vet abc and scil Vet Focus 5 (scil Animal Care Company).
- In-house flow cytometric haematology analysers include the LaserCyte Dx® and ProCyte Dx® (Idexx), and the BC-5300Vet (A. Menarini Diagnostics).
- The QBC Vet Autoread™ (Idexx) works by quantitative buffy coat analysis.

Commercial laboratories typically use larger analysers which combine impedance and flow cytometry methods such as the Sysmex XT-2000iV® or the Advia® 120/2120 (Siemens).

Impedance cell counters

In these analysers a chamber containing an electrically conductive fluid is divided into two areas connected by a small aperture. An electric current is passed into this fluid and flows through the aperture. A stream of cells is directed towards the aperture; as cells pass through they interfere with the flow of current, creating a pulse (Figure 3.5). The pulse height is proportional to cell size; pulse frequency is proportional to cell number. The RBC count, MCV and platelet count are determined in diluted blood, platelets being distinguished from red cells by their smaller size. Haemoglobin (Hb) is measured spectrophotometrically after red cell lysis. Thus, for red cells the analyser measures RBC count, MCV and Hb. It then calculates the haematocrit (HCT), mean corpuscular haemoglobin (MCH) and mean corpuscular haemoglobin concentration (MCHC) using the formulae shown in Figure 3.6.

Given that the distinction between platelets and red cells is made on the basis of cell size, errors may occur when large platelets (macroplatelets or 'shift' platelets) are miscounted as small red cells or *vice versa*. This is more common in cats, because they have smaller red cells and often have variably sized platelets, and is also a significant problem in Cavalier King Charles Spaniels, which often

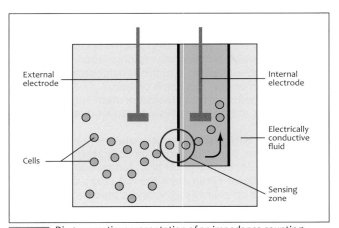

Calculation	Example
HCT (l/l) = MCV (fl) x RBC (x 10¹²/l)/1000	HCT = 69 x 6.23/1000 = 0.43 l/l
MCHC (g/dl) = Hb (g/dl)/HCT (l/l)	MCHC = 14.7/0.43 = 34 g/dl
MCH (pg) = Hb (g/dl) x 10/RBC (x 10¹²/l)	MCH = 14.7 x 10 / 6.23 = 23.6 pg

3.6 Erythrocyte indices used to calculate haematocrit (HCT), mean corpuscular haemoglobin (MCH) and mean corpuscular haemoglobin concentration (MCHC). In the example MCV = 69 fl, red blood cell (RBC) count = 6.23 x 10¹²/l and haemoglobin (Hb) = 14.7 g/dl.

have very large platelets. If very large numbers of macroplatelets are present this may falsely increase the RBC count and HCT and lower the MCV and platelet count (Figure 3.7). Conversely, if microcytic red cells are present, they may be miscounted as platelets, resulting in a falsely high platelet count.

Leucocytes are counted after lysing red blood cells. In some analysers cell-specific lysing solutions are used to produce a differential white cell count. In others the lysing agent results in shrinkage of the lymphocyte, monocyte and granulocyte nuclei at different rates, facilitating a three-part differential count. In general, impedance analysers have a relatively poor ability to differentiate the different white blood cells, when compared with flow cytometric analysers, and also cannot distinguish white blood cells from nucleated red blood cells. The differential becomes less reliable when abnormal cells are present, as in leukaemia or marked inflammatory reactions, and it is important to carry out a blood film examination and a manual differential in these situations. The white blood cell count must be corrected for the nucleated red blood cell count (see section on white cells).

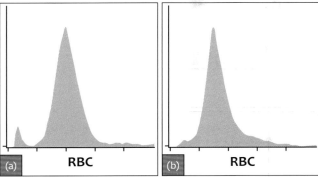

3.7 Histogram plots produced by the Cell-Dyn 3500 analyser showing separation of platelets and red cells on the basis of size. Plot (a), from a dog, shows good separation with a well defined peak of platelets to the left and red cells to the right. However on plot (b), from a cat, the two peaks are not well defined. The analyser gave a platelet count of 1481 x 10⁹/l. Inspection of the blood film suggested the count was much lower than this, with approximately 34 platelets per high power field, equivalent to a count of 510 x 10⁹/l. The MCV was low, and some of the microcytic red cells were being counted as platelets.

Flow cytometers

These analysers usually employ a combination of impedance technology and flow cytometry, and use additional stains to detect granulocytes and reticulocytes. The principle of flow cytometry involves the generation of a stream of single cells which is directed through a laser beam. When the cell encounters the laser beam, the laser light is scattered and several detectors measure scattered light at different angles. The amount of low angle or forward scatter correlates with cell size and the amount of high angle or side scatter correlates with cell granularity

3.5 Diagrammatic representation of an impedance counting chamber. Cells within an electrically conducting fluid pass through an aperture; in so doing they impede the flow of electricity through the aperture, creating a pulse.

External electrode

Internal electrode

Electrically conductive fluid

Cells

Sensing zone

or density. The LaserCyte® also measures the time of flight – the time taken for a cell to pass through the laser beam – to determine the cell volume. These analysers have a great advantage over impedance counting because not only size but also cell complexity/density is used to distinguish cell types. Platelets and red cells are more accurately distinguished; because red cells are packed with haemoglobin they are much denser than platelets. The Advia® 120 and 2120 differentiates types of leucocytes on the basis of their size, myeloperoxidase staining, granularity/complexity and susceptibility to a lysing reagent (basophils are resistant to lysis). The Sysmex XT and the ProCyte® use a fluorescent dye which stains RNA and DNA, as well as size and granularity, to differentiate leucocytes (Figure 3.8a). These analysers produce useful scatter plots to allow visual assessment of leucocyte populations, and can be helpful in the initial detection of a leukaemic population. However, leukaemic cells are often misclassified by an analyser, and therefore in cases of suspected leukaemia a blood film examination with a manual differential count is always required. The analyser typically generates flags prompting this (Figure 3.8b).

Flow cytometric analysers are very useful when evaluating cases of anaemia. Haemoglobin is measured after lysing an aliquot of red cells and then measuring the free haemoglobin spectrophotometrically. The Advia® 120/2120 generates red cell dot plots showing size on the x-axis and haemoglobin concentration on the y-axis; these plots are useful in detecting distinct cell populations including reticulocytes, microcytic hypochromic cells in iron-deficiency anaemia, and agglutinating cells (see Chapter 4). All flow cytometric haematology analysers generate an automated reticulocyte count, usually using fluorescent dyes which are optimized to stain RNA (see Figure 4.9), although new methylene blue is used by the LaserCyte®. In cats the automated reticulocyte count corresponds to the aggregate reticulocyte count and does not include punctate reticulocytes. The reference ranges for automated reticulocyte counts are generally higher than for manual reticulocyte counts and vary from one analyser to another, and therefore the reference range specific to the analyser should be used. The LaserCyte® has a negative bias when compared with the manual method (Moritz and Becker, 2010). The Advia® 120/2120 displays histograms showing reticulocyte size and haemoglobin content, and measures the reticulocyte haemoglobin content and the MCV of reticulocytes. These parameters are very useful in the detection of iron deficiency and in monitoring the response to iron supplementation (see Chapter 4).

Quantitative buffy coat (QBC) analysers

The QBC machines have largely been superseded by impedance or flow cytometers, but some are still in use. They rely on separation of red cells, granulocytes, monocytes/lymphocytes and platelets into various layers in a microhaematocrit tube containing the vital stain acridine orange, which is taken up by DNA, RNA and lipoprotein in the cells (Figure 3.9). The tube contains a cylindrical float that forces the cells to spread out in a thin layer between the float and the tube. After centrifugation, ultraviolet light is directed at the stained cells which then emit fluorescent light. Nucleated cells, which contain DNA, emit green fluorescence, while cells containing lipoprotein or RNA emit red light. The type and number of cells present is determined by measuring the relative amounts of green and red light. Small and large leucocytes are distinguished because more small cells 'fit' in a given length of the tube and so more light is emitted than from the same length of tube containing larger cells. The MCHC can be calculated because it is inversely correlated with the distance the float has sunk into the packed red cell layer. Hb is calculated from the PCV and MCHC. All calculated cell counts are based on the assumption that cell volumes are normal and, therefore, in disease states where cell volumes are altered (e.g. in leukaemia), inaccuracies may occur. The platelet count is determined from a platelet 'crit'. This has the advantage that it is not affected by the presence of large platelets (e.g. in Cavalier King Charles Spaniels) and so gives a better indication of the overall platelet mass. In theory this method should also provide superior counts in samples with platelet clumping, but this has not been found.

Optimizing in-clinic haematology

Careful adherence to quality control procedures and maintenance protocols is very important to optimize the performance of an in-clinic analyser (see Chapter 2). Prior to

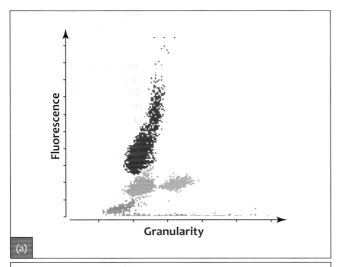

(a)

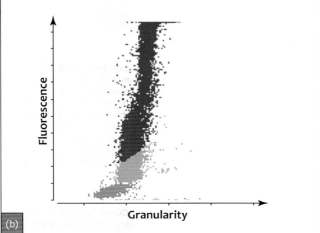

(b)

3.8 (a) Scatter plot from a normal dog obtained using the ProCyte Dx® analyser. Neutrophils are shown in lilac, monocytes in red, lymphocytes in blue, eosinophils in green and basophils in turquoise. (b) Scatter plot from a dog with leukaemia obtained using the ProCyte Dx® analyser. There is a marked increase in the number of white cells and an obviously abnormal dot plot presentation with overlapping 'clouds' (clusters), making misclassification highly likely. In such cases a blood film examination should be performed and reviewed by a cytologist.
(Courtesy of G Bilborough, Idexx)

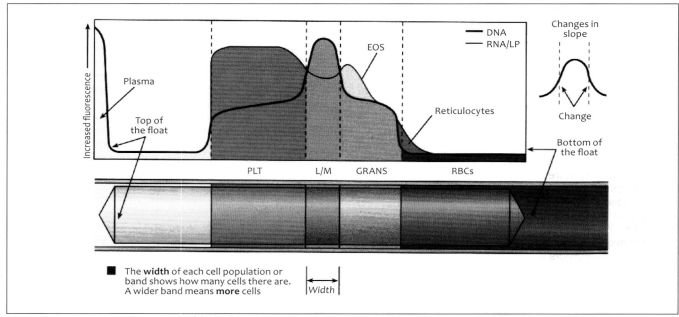

3.9 Diagrammatic representation of the buffy coat, expanded by a cylindrical float, and a histogram showing the amount of fluorescence emitted by DNA (in nucleated cells) and RNA/lipoprotein (in reticulocytes, platelets (PLT) and eosinophils (EOS)) in the various layers of the buffy coat. GRANS = granulocytes; L/M = lymphocytes and monocytes.
(Courtesy of Idexx Laboratories, Wetherby)

using any analyser the blood should be thoroughly mixed, ideally on a cell mixer or by carefully inverting the tube multiple times. Poor mixing is an important source of significant laboratory error, which could have marked effects on clinical decision-making. The sample should also be checked for clots using an orange stick as discussed above (see Figure 3.1).

Red blood cell parameters

The HCT, RBC count and Hb all give an indication of the red cell mass. As discussed above, HCT is a calculated value produced by the analyser and is usually expressed as l/l. It is equivalent to the PCV, which is usually expressed as a percentage, i.e. a HCT of 0.25 l/l is the same as a PCV of 25% although the manual PCV may be 2–3% different from the calculated HCT due to differences in methodology. All three parameters rise in dehydrated animals and fall in anaemic animals. In microcytic anaemia the reduction in HCT is more marked than that in the RBC count because the former is reduced further by the small cell size. Haemolysis falsely lowers the RBC count and HCT but Hb will not be affected because the already 'free' haemoglobin from the previously lysed cells will be measured along with Hb released from cells lysed in the analyser. Given that the MCHC and MCH are calculated by dividing Hb by the HCT and RBC count, respectively, these parameters are falsely elevated by haemolysis. They are also elevated by lipaemia because this spuriously elevates haemoglobin.

Red cell indices

Mean corpuscular volume

The MCV indicates the average size of the red cells. Increased MCV is seen in regenerative anaemia, along with decreased MCH and MCHC. Macrocytic anaemia may also be seen with a non-regenerative anaemia caused by myelodysplasia, which in cats may be associated with feline leukaemia virus (FeLV) infection. A hereditary macrocytosis of poodles leads to an elevated MCV without anaemia. Sample ageing results in red cell swelling and increased MCV. Autoagglutination leads to a spurious increase in MCV (see above). Non-regenerative anaemia is usually normocytic. Low MCV is seen in iron deficiency. These findings are discussed in detail in Chapter 4.

Red cell distribution width

The RDW describes the variability in erythrocyte size. It is a more sensitive indicator of altered red cell size than the MCV because, for the latter, a relatively large number of cells must have altered size before the *mean* value is altered. The RDW describes the entire population of red cells instead of one average value (Figure 3.10). The RDW is increased in cases of regenerative anaemia and with iron-deficiency anaemia, i.e. it increases when both large and small cells are present.

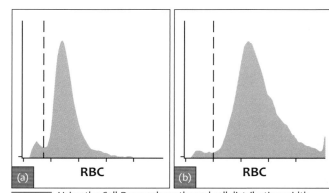

3.10 Using the Cell-Dyn analyser the red cell distribution width (RDW) is calculated from the frequency distribution plot of red cell size (size on x-axis, frequency on y-axis). The RDW is the coefficient of variation of red cell size and is expressed as a percentage. (a) Healthy dog (RDW = 15%). (b) A dog with a markedly regenerative anaemia (RDW = 25%): the red cell curve is much wider and extends further to the right, reflecting the numerous larger red cells present.

Mean corpuscular haemoglobin

The MCH is expressed in picograms (pg) and indicates the mean quantity (weight) of haemoglobin per average red cell. It does not take into account the volume of the red cell because it is calculated by dividing the Hb by the RBC count.

Mean corpuscular haemoglobin concentration

The MCHC indicates the mean concentration of haemoglobin per red cell. It is calculated by dividing the Hb by the HCT and, because the latter is affected by red cell size, MCHC is a more useful indicator of the amount of haemoglobin present in red cells. If a normal animal has an MCV towards the bottom of the normal range the MCH may be low, even though the cells contain a normal amount of haemoglobin relative to their size (smaller cells should have less total haemoglobin than large cells). The MCHC, which corrects for this variation in cell size, would be normal.

- Normal MCHC defines the red cells as normochromic and is seen in non-regenerative anaemia as well as in normal animals.
- Decreased MCHC is synonymous with hypochromasia and is seen in regenerative anaemia and iron deficiency.
- Raised MCHC is almost always spurious; it occurs as a result of haemolysis, lipaemia and Heinz body anaemia.
- Spherocytosis occasionally leads to increased MCHC because haemoglobin is concentrated into a smaller volume once the red cell membrane has been removed, but generally MCHC and MCV are within normal limits. Marked eccentrocytosis can occasionally cause an increased MCHC because haemoglobin is pushed into a smaller volume on one side of the cell while the two sides of the cell membrane fuse on the other side (see Chapter 4).
- Administration of Oxyglobin® leads to a marked increase in total haemoglobin, because both the haemoglobin solution and the patient's haemoglobin are included in the haemoglobin measurement and this in turn will spuriously elevate the MCH and MCHC.
- Hyponatraemia may cause a spurious elevation in MCHC and a low MCV. *In vivo* the red cells adjust to the hypo-osmolar environment by becoming more hypotonic. When these cells enter the analyser and are mixed with diluent, water diffuses out of the red cells into the more hypertonic diluent, creating microcytic hyperchromic red cells.

White cell counts

All haematology analysers can determine the total white cell count and this is usually expressed as cells x 10^9/l. Impedance analysers may give a three-part or five-part leucocyte differential count. QBC machines count neutrophils, eosinophils and mononuclear cells, but cannot distinguish lymphocytes and monocytes (these are counted together as mononuclear cells). Flow cytometric analysers give a full white cell differential count, i.e. the number and percentage of neutrophils, lymphocytes, eosinophils, monocytes and basophils are determined.

While the total WBC count is generally accurate, differential counts are not always accurate. Accuracy is lowest for QBC machines, intermediate for impedance analysers and highest for flow cytometers, but even the latter may generate erroneous results, and may misclassify band neutrophils as monocytes or monocytes as lymphocytes. Most analysers are unable to count basophils accurately. All are unable to distinguish band neutrophils from mature neutrophils, although the ProCyte® and Sysmex generate flags when bands are suspected. Nucleated red blood cells (nRBCs) are usually erroneously classified as lymphocytes although analysers may generate flags signalling their presence. On blood film examination nRBCs are usually counted as the number seen per 100 WBCs. The presence of nRBCs will have a significant effect on the white cell count when there are ≥10 nRBCs/100 WBCs, and the white cell count must be corrected using the formula:

$$\text{Corrected WBC} = \frac{(\text{measured WBC x 100})}{(100 + \text{number of nRBC/100WBC})}$$

Platelet counts

All analysers can perform a platelet count, although the accuracy of these counts is very variable depending on the analyser used. As discussed above, analyser error is more likely for cats because their small red cells can be falsely counted as platelets, or large platelets can be miscounted as small red cells. Significant laboratory error can also occur if platelets form clumps *in vitro*: platelets in clumps are not counted by the analyser and therefore lead to a falsely low count. This is a common laboratory error and is more likely to occur if the blood sampling procedure does not go smoothly; with cats it can even occur following atraumatic venepuncture, possibly owing to the effects of EDTA. Clumping may be reduced by sampling into sodium citrate tubes. Whenever a low platelet count is recorded by an analyser, a blood film should be examined: if platelet clumps are found at the tail of the smear (Figure 3.11) this is the likely cause of the apparent thrombocytopenia and a fresh blood sample is required to obtain an accurate platelet count. Macroplatelets or shift platelets are often present if there is an accelerated rate of thrombopoiesis and may be miscounted as small red cells (see above).

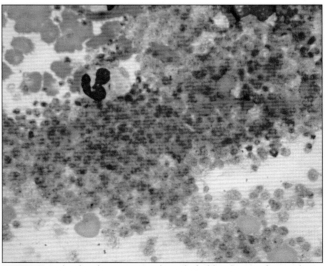

3.11 A platelet clump seen at the tail of a blood smear from a dog. Platelets are round with slightly grainy cytoplasm but no nucleus. (May–Grünwald–Giemsa stain; original magnification X1000)

Blood films

A blood smear should always be evaluated in conjunction with automated cell counts. This is required:

- To check the leucocyte differential count
- To assess cell morphology, e.g. polychromasia, anisocytosis, fragmented red cells, spherocytes, Heinz bodies, red cell parasites and nucleated red cells
- To assess white cell abnormalities, e.g. toxic neutrophils, left shifts, blast cells
- To assess platelet abnormalities, e.g. macroplatelets and platelet clumps.

Blood film examination is routinely performed in commercial laboratories, even where high tech quality controlled 'gold standard' analysers are being used. In the practice laboratory, where in-house analysers may provide less accurate leucocyte differential and platelet counts, blood film examination is perhaps even more important. Failure to perform blood film examination may result in frequent serious errors in clinical decision-making e.g. misdiagnosis of thrombocytopenia.

Preparation of blood films

Blood sample smears should be prepared soon after taking the blood sample. Polished glass slides with frosted ends are preferred because pencil can be used for easy labelling and will not wash off during staining. Slides should be handled by their edges/ends because grease from fingers can result in poor smearing. If in doubt the slide can be wiped clean using a tissue before use. The technique for smear preparation is shown in Figure 3.12.

Causes of poor quality smears are discussed and illustrated in Figures 3.13 and 3.14.

Stains

Several types of rapid 'dunking' kits (e.g. Diff-Quik®) are available. Hema-Gurr (BDH) is recommended by the author. These stains are more than adequate for in-house use. The kits have a three-stage staining procedure which incorporates a fixative pot (usually five dips), an orange/pink dye in the second pot (usually three dips) and a blue dye in the third pot (usually six dips). The intensity of the blue and orange staining can be altered by varying the number of dips in each pot and it is worth experimenting to determine the optimum staining procedure. Smears are dipped in buffered water to rinse them, and then air dried. It is helpful to add a coverslip because this greatly increases the clarity, especially for the 40X dry lens. One or two drops of immersion oil or mounting medium are placed on the slide and the coverslip slowly lowered on to the slide, avoiding the entrapment of air bubbles.

Film examination

A set procedure should be followed for blood film examination to ensure that all cell lines are examined properly. Initially the smear is checked for large platelet clumps (see Figure 3.11) by examining the feathered edge at low power (X10 or X40). The smear is then examined at higher power in the thin area near the feathered edge where the cells are evenly distributed in a monolayer (Figure 3.15). In this 'examination area' the red cells should not usually be touching one another. Do not examine cells at the feathered edge (distorted) or in thick areas of the smear

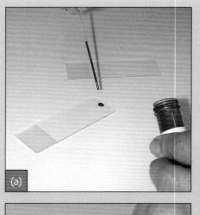
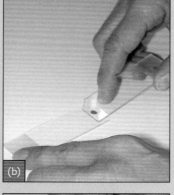
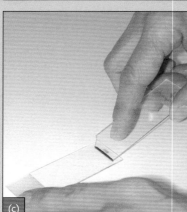
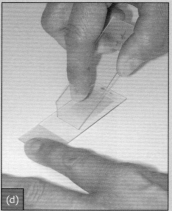
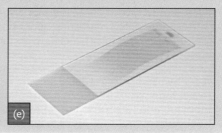

- A spreader slide is required to make the smear: this is narrower than the smear slide to avoid spreading the cells over the edge of the slide. Spreader slides can be made by breaking off a corner of a normal slide having first scored it with a blade or diamond writer. The spreader slide should be washed in water and dried regularly and should be replaced periodically as the edge can become roughened
- The blood sample is mixed carefully and then a sample harvested using a microhaematocrit tube. A drop of blood is placed on to the end of a slide (a)
- The spreader slide is held between the thumb and second finger, placing the index finger on top of the spreader when smearing (b)
- The spreader is placed at an angle of about 30 degrees in front of the blood spot and slid backwards until it comes into contact with the blood, which then rapidly spreads out along the spreader slide (c). The moment this occurs, the spreader is advanced forwards smoothly and quickly. As the smear is made a 'feathered edge' forms; do not lift the spreader slide until the feathered edge is completely formed (d)
- Ideally the smear should extend to approximately two-thirds of the length of the slide and should have a fairly square feathered edge (e)
- The smear should be allowed to fully air dry prior to staining

3.12 Preparation of blood films.

Problem	Cause	Solution
Smear too long (feathered edge has disappeared off the end) (Figure 3.14b)	Spreader speed too slow Low viscosity blood (i.e. anaemia) Excess blood applied to slide	More rapid spreader speed Apply smaller blood spot
Smear too short/thick (Figure 3.14d)	Spreader speed too fast High viscosity blood (i.e. high PCV)	Slower spreader speed
Feathered edge consists of long streaked tails (Figure 3.14a)	Uneven contact of spreader with slide Spreader has roughened edge	Apply even pressure using index finger on top of spreader Replace spreader
Smear has holes or gaps (Figure 3.14b)	Grease on slide Lipaemia	Clean slides before use
Smear thick at feathered edge end of film (Figure 3.14c)	Blood in front of the spreader	Ensure firm contact of spreader and slide when pulling spreader backwards towards blood spot

3.13 Causes and solutions for poor quality blood films.

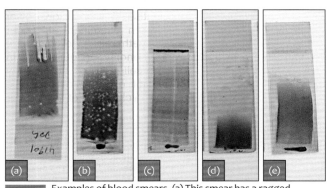

3.14 Examples of blood smears. (a) This smear has a ragged feathered edge due to uneven contact of the spreader with the slide, possibly because the spreader was dirty or roughened. (b) Holes in a smear, which may be due to grease on the slide or lipaemia. (c) This smear is too long because too much blood has been applied to the slide. Blood in front of the spreader has resulted in a dense line at the tail. (d) This smear is too short, possibly because insufficient blood was applied to the slide or the spreader was moved too rapidly. (e) A good smear with an even 'square' end.

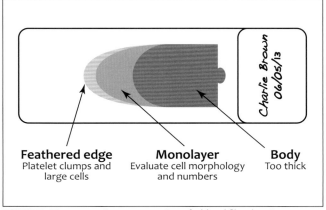

Feathered edge
Platelet clumps and large cells

Monolayer
Evaluate cell morphology and numbers

Body
Too thick

Charlie Brown 06/05/13

3.15 Diagrammatic representation of a blood film showing the feathered edge and the monolayer (where cells should be examined).
(Courtesy of P Monti)

where the cells are in clumps (cells do not lie flat in these areas). The red cells, white cells and platelets are examined in turn (Figure 3.16).

Examination of red cells

Evaluation of the red cells should include an assessment of colour, size and shape, and examination for inclusions. Red cells from dogs and cats are anucleate and stain pink. Canine red cells have a pale area in the centre of the cells (central pallor) which is not obvious in feline red cells. Canine red cells are larger (diameter 7 μm) than feline red cells (diameter 5.5 μm).

Anisocytosis refers to a variation in cell size. Some variation in cell size is normal in feline blood. Immature red cells (reticulocytes) are larger (macrocytic) than mature cells and also stain a blue–grey colour, which is described as polychromasia. Only small numbers (<1%) of immature red cells are seen in normal animals.

Poikilocytosis refers to altered red cell shape, e.g. due to the formation of acanthocytes or schistocytes. Red cell abnormalities are discussed in Chapter 4.

Examination of leucocytes

A differential white cell count is performed by counting leucocytes both at the edges and in the middle of the smear within the examination area; larger cells tend to be pushed to the edges of the smear, and smaller cells tend to be more concentrated in the middle. An example of a battlement meander method of counting is shown in Figure 3.17. A total of at least 100, preferably 200, cells should be counted. Nucleated red cells should be included and the corrected white cell count is calculated. The percentage of each cell type is then multiplied by the total white cell count to determine an absolute count for each cell type. White cell morphological abnormalities, such as toxic changes or atypical blast cells, should be noted (see Chapter 5).

Neutrophils are the predominant cell type, followed by lymphocytes. The ratio of neutrophils to lymphocytes is approximately 3.5:1 in the dog and 2:1 in the cat. Normal animals have only small numbers of eosinophils and monocytes and only very occasional to absent basophils.

Neutrophils: These are relatively large (approximately twice the diameter of a canine red cell, three times the diameter of a feline red cell) and have an elongated segmented nucleus with three to five lobes (Figure 3.16b). The cytoplasm is light blue–grey but the cytoplasmic granules present do not stain. Immature neutrophils, termed 'bands', are seen infrequently in health but increased numbers are present in inflammatory conditions. Band neutrophils have an elongated, often U-shaped, non-lobulated nucleus with parallel sides. Shallow indentations less than 50% of the width of the nucleus may be present. Toxic neutrophils are seen in severe inflammation, especially associated with bacterial infection, and are discussed in Chapter 5.

Monocytes: These are larger than neutrophils and have abundant sky-blue cytoplasm, often containing clear discrete vacuoles and sometimes fine pink dust-like granules (Figure 3.16c). The shape of the nucleus is very variable and can be round, kidney bean-shaped, lobulated, U-shaped or S-shaped. Monocytes with U-shaped nuclei may be difficult to distinguish from band neutrophils, especially those showing toxic change, but several differences aid identification, as shown in Figure 3.18.

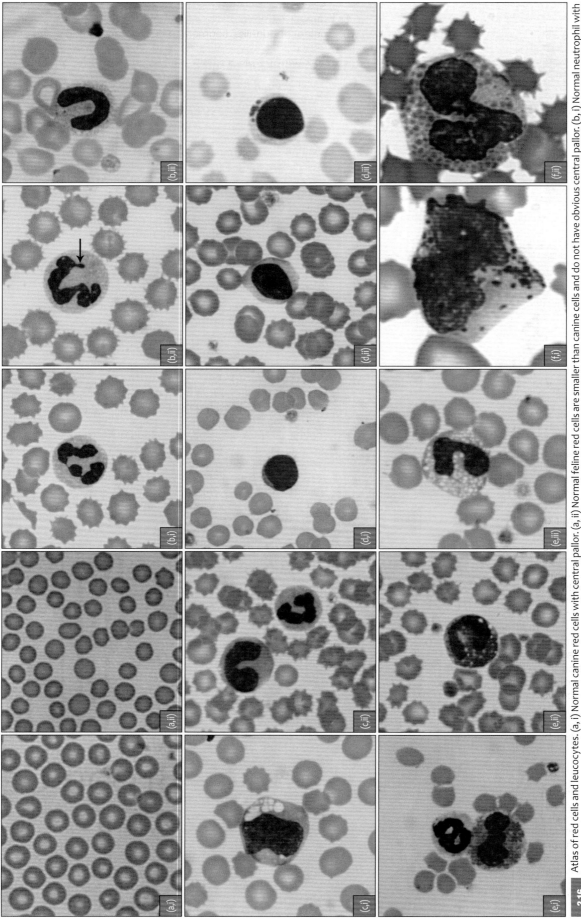

3.16 Atlas of red cells and leucocytes. (a, i) Normal canine red cells with central pallor. (a, ii) Normal feline red cells are smaller than canine cells and do not have obvious central pallor. (b, i) Normal neutrophil with segmented nucleus and light, clear cytoplasm. (b, ii) In females a proportion of neutrophils have a Barr body (arrowed), a small protuberance at one end of the nucleus which is the site of the X chromosome. (b, iii) Band neutrophil containing a nucleus with parallel sides (may have a shallow indentation). (c, i) Normal monocytes are larger than neutrophils, have variably shaped nuclei and basophilic cytoplasm containing several vacuoles. (c, ii) The monocyte nucleus (upper left) may be band-shaped but is wider than the neutrophil nucleus (lower right) and has more open, stippled chromatin. (d, i) Small lymphocyte with dense round nucleus and cytoplasm only visible at the top. (d, ii) Larger lymphocyte with more abundant cytoplasm. (d, iii) Large granular lymphocyte containing several large pink granules. (e, i) Feline eosinophil with rod-shaped cytoplasmic granules. The neutrophil above it is smaller and has clear cytoplasm. (e, ii) Canine eosinophil with larger round granules which are unevenly distributed in the cytoplasm. (e, iii) Eosinophil with vacuolated cytoplasm, from a Greyhound. (f, i) Canine basophil with an elongated ribbon-like nucleus and indistinct lilac granules. (f, ii) Feline basophil with lilac nucleus and purple granules. (a–e = May–Grünwald–Giemsa stain, f = Rapi-Diff® stain; original magnification X1000)

(f, Courtesy of L Blackwood)

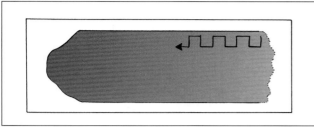

3.17 Battlement meander track for performing a differential white cell count.

Monocytes with U-shaped nuclei	Band neutrophils
Wider, larger nucleus with knob-shaped ends	Narrow nucleus
Open, stippled chromatin	Dense, condensed chromatin
Sky-blue to deeply basophilic cytoplasm	Pale grey cytoplasm Toxic bands may be slightly basophilic, but not as dark as monocytes
Cytoplasm often contains discrete vacuoles and sometimes contains fine, pink, dust-like granules	Cytoplasm non-vacuolated Toxic bands may be foamy (not discrete vacuoles) and contain distinct granules

3.18 Factors that aid in the differentiation of monocytes with U-shaped nuclei from band neutrophils.

Lymphocytes: These have a round nucleus with condensed, smudged chromatin and a narrow rim of basophilic cytoplasm (Figure 3.16d). Lymphocytes vary in size; small lymphocytes predominate, are slightly larger than canine red cells and have sparse cytoplasm which is not visible all the way round the nucleus. Medium-sized lymphocytes have a slightly larger nucleus and more abundant cytoplasm, often completely encircling the nucleus. Reactive lymphocytes are larger still, with a nucleus approximately 1.5 times the diameter of a canine red cell and abundant deeply basophilic cytoplasm, often with a darker tinge at the periphery. Occasional reactive lymphocytes may be seen in health, but these cells usually reflect antigenic stimulation. A few lymphocytes containing several prominent magenta/pink cytoplasmic granules on one side of the nucleus may be present. These are known as 'granular lymphocytes' or 'large granular lymphocytes'. Large lymphoid cells (large cells with one or more nucleoli) are not found on blood films from healthy animals but may be seen in small numbers following marked immune stimulation, along with reactive lymphocytes. More than occasional large lymphoid cells should raise suspicion of lymphoproliferative disease, especially when these are not accompanied by reactive lymphocytes.

Eosinophils: These are slightly larger than neutrophils, and are characterized by numerous prominent pink cytoplasmic granules (Figure 3.16e). In cats the granules are always abundant and are rod-shaped and uniform in size. In dogs the number and size of granules are very variable. Classically there are abundant small round granules, but there may be only small numbers of larger granules. The cytoplasm between the granules is light staining and may contain clear vacuoles. The eosinophils of Greyhounds have a vacuolated appearance because their granules do not stain (the vacuoles are actually non-staining granules). This phenomenon is occasionally seen in other breeds of dog. Eosinophil nuclei are often slightly larger than those of neutrophils and are lobulated but usually only have two to three lobes.

Basophils: These are rare in blood smears from normal animals. They are a similar size to eosinophils and have an elongated 'ribbon-like' segmented nucleus and variable numbers of cytoplasmic granules. In dogs these granules are sparse and dark purple; in cats they are abundant and pale lilac, sometimes with a few dark purple granules (Figure 3.16f).

Mast cells: These are not seen in the blood of healthy animals but may be seen in animals with severe inflammatory diseases such as peritonitis, pneumonia and pancreatitis, and with metastatic mast cell tumours. These are round cells with a round nucleus and moderate to abundant cytoplasm containing numerous purple granules.

Examination of platelets

Platelets are small round structures with no nucleus. They are one quarter to half the diameter of red cells with pink cytoplasm and fine granules. Platelet numbers can be estimated by counting the number of platelets seen per X1000 field (i.e. X10 eyepiece and X100 objective), having first determined that no platelet clumps are present. Five fields are counted and a mean value is calculated. The normal count is 10–30 platelets per X1000 field (Figure 3.19). Each platelet per X1000 field equates to *approximately* 15 x 10^9/l. Thus, if 10 platelets are seen per X1000 field, the platelet count is approximately 10 x 15 = 150 x 10^9/l. Animals with severe thrombocytopenia (<30 x 10^9/l) have only 0–3 platelets per field. The presence of large 'shift' platelets should be noted, because these may be an indicator of active thrombopoiesis, especially in dogs.

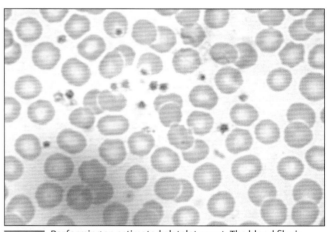

3.19 Performing an estimated platelet count. The blood film is examined using the X100 oil immersion lens in the examination area. The number of platelets per field is counted and a mean value for five fields is calculated. This value is multiplied by 15 to produce the count x 10^9/l.

References and further reading

Harvey JW (2012) Hematology procedures. In: *Veterinary Hematology. A Diagnostic Guide and Colour Atlas*, ed. JW Harvey, pp 11–32. Elsevier Saunders, St Louis

Moritz A and Becker M (2010) Automated hematology systems. In: *Schalms Veterinary Hematology, 6th edn*, ed. DJ Weiss and KJ Wardrop, pp 1054–1065. Lippincott, Williams and Wilkins, Philadelphia

Stockham SL and Scott MA (2012) Leucocytes. In: *Fundamentals of Veterinary Clinical Pathology, 2nd edn*, ed. SL Stockham and MA Scott, pp 53–106. Iowa State University Press, Ames

Stockham SL and Scott MA (2012) Erythrocytes. In: *Fundamentals of Veterinary Clinical Pathology, 2nd edn*, ed. SL Stockham and MA Scott, pp 107–222. Iowa State University Press, Ames

Welles EG (2012) Automated in-clinic hematology instruments for small animal practitioners: what is available, what can they really do, and how do I make a choice? *Veterinary Clinics of North America: Small Animal Practice* **42(1)**, 3–22

Chapter 4

Disorders of erythrocytes

Elizabeth Villiers

Erythrocyte disorders fall into two broad groups: anaemia and erythrocytosis (or polycythaemia). Anaemia may be due to reduced or defective red cell production, which results in non-regenerative anaemia, or increased red cell loss, which results in regenerative anaemia. Changes in red cell parameters, such as mean corpuscular volume (MCV) and mean corpuscular haemoglobin concentration (MCHC), reticulocyte count and morphological changes (e.g. presence or absence of polychromasia) aid in differentiating the causes of anaemia. To understand how these changes arise, it is necessary to review the process of erythropoiesis.

A review of erythropoiesis

Erythropoiesis takes place in the bone marrow, in islets around central macrophages known as nurse cells. These cells phagocytose extruded nuclear material, store iron as haemosiderin and supply iron for haemoglobin synthesis. The main regulator of erythropoiesis is erythropoietin (Epo), a glycoprotein produced in the kidney in response to renal tissue hypoxia. Some Epo is also produced by bone marrow macrophages and erythroid progenitors. Other hormones, such as thyroxine, growth hormone and corticosteroids, enhance the effect of erythropoietin. Certain cytokines released during inflammation, e.g. interleukin (IL) 1 and tumour necrosis factor, inhibit erythropoiesis.

- Pluripotent stem cells develop into early erythroid precursors, known as burst-forming units–erythroid (BFU-E), under the influence of IL-3.
- BFU-E divide and form colony-forming units–erythroid (CFU-E) which, in turn, divide and differentiate into rubriblasts (also known as proerythroblasts), under the influence of Epo as well as stem cell factor (SCF), insulin like growth factor 1 (IGF-1), glucocorticoids, IL-3 and IL-6.
- Rubriblasts develop into prorubricytes (early normoblasts) which, in turn, divide into basophilic and then polychromatic rubricytes (intermediate normoblasts) and then metarubricytes (late normoblasts) (Figures 4.1 and 4.2). As these divisions take place the cells progressively become smaller, and also accumulate increasing amounts of haemoglobin,

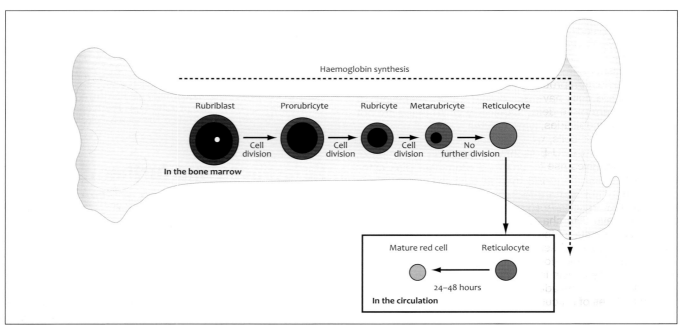

4.1 Erythropoiesis. The developing red cell precursors become progressively smaller and accumulate haemoglobin. They are released into the circulation as reticulocytes which then develop into mature red cells.

BSAVA Manual of Canine and Feline Clinical Pathology, 3rd edition. Edited by Elizabeth Villiers and Jelena Ristić. ©BSAVA 2016

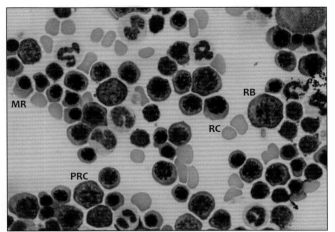

4.2 Stages of erythropoiesis shown on a bone marrow aspirate. MR = metarubricyte; PRC = prorubricyte; RB = rubriblast; RC = rubricyte. (Modified Wright–Giemsa stain; original magnification X1000)

which is synthesized within ribosomes in the cytoplasm. Cell divisions take place at the rubriblast stage through to the rubricyte stage, but metarubricytes are not capable of cell division. Each rubriblast gives rise to about 16 metarubricytes.
- In the metarubricyte stage the nucleus becomes progressively more condensed and is then extruded, and the reticulocyte is formed. The extruded nucleus is phagocytosed by the nurse macrophage.

Nuclear extrusion involves multiple molecular and cellular pathways but its precise control mechanism is poorly understood. It has been postulated that increasing haemoglobin content/concentration within erythroid precursors may be a negative regulator of cell division and may trigger nuclear extrusion. If haemoglobin synthesis is reduced or delayed, as in iron deficiency, the cells may undergo extra division(s), yielding smaller hypochromic cells. Conversely, when haemoglobin synthesis exceeds DNA synthesis, e.g. in the megaloblastic anaemia seen with feline leukaemia virus (FeLV) infection, the cell may skip a division and nuclear extrusion may occur early, yielding macrocytic cells. This relationship between haemoglobin concentration and cell division/nuclear extrusion seems plausible, but no mechanism for the connection between haemoglobin synthesis and erythroid proliferation has yet been established.

This enucleation process is unique to mammals, whose anucleated red cells have more capacity for haemoglobin storage and are more deformable, meaning they can pass though small capillaries, many of which have a smaller diameter than red cells, without being damaged. The maturation time from BFU-E to reticulocyte is 7–9 days and one rubriblast gives rise to approximately 16 reticulocytes. Reticulocytes remain in the bone marrow for 24–48 hours before being released into the circulation, where they reach full maturation after a further 24–48 hours and take on a biconcave disc shape. Some reticulocytes mature in the spleen. Reticulocytes are not capable of cell division but continue to synthesize haemoglobin until they reach maturation. They develop into mature erythrocytes when haemoglobin synthesis is completed and the cell size has reduced to that of the adult.

Key features of reticulocytes are:

- They are larger than mature red cells
- They contain less haemoglobin than mature red cells

- They contain numerous clumps of ribosomal RNA which impart a polychromatophilic (bluish-pink) colour to the cytoplasm on Romanowsky staining (Figure 4.3), stain as dark clumps with new methylene blue and can be detected by fluorescent stains in flow cytometric haematology analysers.

Mature erythrocytes circulate for approximately 110 days in the dog and 70 days in the cat. Senescent red cells are phagocytosed in the liver, spleen and bone marrow. As old cells are lost, they are replaced by reticulocytes released from the marrow and therefore small numbers of polychromatic cells or reticulocytes are seen on blood smears from normal dogs and cats.

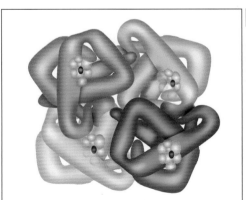

4.3 Blood film from a dog with regenerative anaemia due to blood loss. There is marked polychromasia (darker purple cells, bottom arrow). Target cells (codocytes) are present (top arrow); these have a wide area of central pallor within which there is a central circular density of haemoglobin. (May–Grünwald–Giemsa stain; original magnification X1000)

Normal erythropoiesis depends on normal haemoglobin synthesis and normal DNA synthesis. Haemoglobin consists of four interlinked globin chains (constructed from amino acids), each of which has a cleft containing a haem molecule. Haem consists of a protoporphyrin ring containing a central molecule of iron (Figure 4.4). The protoporphyrin ring is synthesized from the amino acid glycine and the Krebs cycle intermediate succinyl-CoA by a series of enzymatic reactions. Thus, the basic 'ingredients' of haemoglobin are amino acids and iron, and haemoglobin synthesis is impeded if there is protein deficiency (e.g. malnutrition) or iron deficiency (due to dietary deficiency or chronic external blood loss). Defective haemoglobin synthesis may also result from lead toxicity, owing to inhibition of some of the enzymatic reactions involved in protoporphyrin synthesis.

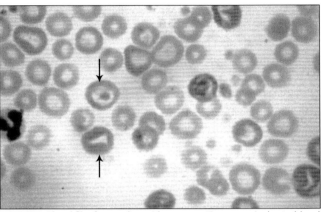

4.4 Diagrammatic representation of the structure of haemoglobin, with four haem rings connected by globin chains.

Anaemia

Anaemia is characterized by reduced numbers of erythrocytes, which on the complete blood count (CBC) manifests as a reduction in red blood cell (RBC) count, haemoglobin concentration (Hb) and haematocrit (HCT) as well as packed cell volume (PCV). HCT and PCV give the same information (the relative proportions of plasma and red cells by volume) but HCT is usually calculated from the RBC count and mean cell volume while PCV is determined after centrifugation.

There are many causes of anaemia; these all fall into one of two groups:

- Anaemia due to reduced red cell production which leads to non-regenerative anaemia
- Anaemia due to increased red cell loss which, after an initial lag phase of 3–5 days, leads to a regenerative anaemia. This may result from haemorrhage or haemolysis.

When anaemia is identified in a patient it is important to determine whether it is regenerative or non-regenerative because this helps to narrow down the differential diagnoses.

Characteristics of regenerative anaemia

A regenerative anaemia can be identified using several features:

- Red cell parameters MCHC and MCV
- Red cell cytograms
- Reticulocyte count
- Blood film morphology.

Red cell parameters

The bone marrow responds to red cell loss by increasing red cell production and, after an initial lag phase of 3–5 days, increased numbers of reticulocytes are released into the circulation. Since reticulocytes are larger than mature red cells, mean corpuscular volume (MCV) is increased, and because they have less haemoglobin than mature red cells, mean corpuscular haemoglobin concentration (MCHC) is reduced: the anaemia is *macrocytic* and *hypochromic*. However, MCV and MCHC are *mean* values and therefore, in a mildly regenerative anaemia, there may not be sufficient reticulocytes present to move the mean out of the normal range. The MCV and MCHC are not very sensitive markers of regeneration, and may be altered for other reasons, most notably delayed analysis – after 24 hours the MCV increases and the MCHC decreases as a result of *in vitro* swelling (Figures 4.5 and 4.6). The red cell distribution width (RDW, see Chapter 3) is a more sensitive indicator of a change in red cell size, because relatively small numbers of larger (or smaller) cells will increase (or decrease) this parameter.

Red cell cytograms

Impedance analysers produce a histogram showing red cell size on the *x*-axis and number on the *y*-axis. In healthy animals this shows a normal distribution while in regenerative anaemia a hump of larger cells is seen on the right of the curve, representing reticulocytes (Figure 4.7).

Flow cytometer cytograms on the Advia® 120 and 2120 are very helpful in evaluation of anaemia. The red cell cytogram shows cell size on the *y*-axis and haemoglobin concentration on the *x*-axis. A grid shows the location of normal cells. Reticulocytes appear in the upper left box corresponding to macrocytic and hypochromic cells (Figure 4.8).

Causes of altered MCV		Mechanism/other features
Increased MCV		
Regenerative anaemia		Increased circulating reticulocytes, which are larger
Feline leukaemia virus infection; myeloproliferative disease		During erythropoiesis there is delayed nuclear maturation alongside normal haemoglobin production, resulting in fewer cell divisions before the nucleus is extruded
Familial macrocytosis in Toy and Miniature Poodles (Schalm, 1976)		Increased nucleated red cells and Howell–Jolly bodies. Incidental finding. Pathogenesis unknown. No anaemia or clinical signs
Hereditary stomatocytosis in Alaskan Malamutes and Miniature Schnauzers (Fletch *et al.*, 1975; Brown *et al.*, 1994)		Stomatocytes are cup-shaped red cells that form when red cells take up excess sodium and water. Miniature Schnauzers are asymptomatic. Alaskan Malamutes have concurrent chondrodysplasia
Aged blood samples (>24 hours)		Red cell swelling *in vitro*
Autoagglutination		Clumps of red cells counted by analyser as one large red cell
Hyperosmolality (e.g. due to hypernatraemia)		When blood is mixed with analyser diluent, water moves into red cells leading to swelling
Decreased MCV		
Iron deficiency		During erythropoiesis there is a reduced rate of haemoglobin synthesis, so the nucleus is retained for longer. Extra cell divisions occur, resulting in formation of small red cells
Liver disease; portosystemic shunts		Cause unclear but likely to be due to abnormal iron metabolism. MCHC normal or mildly reduced. May also see mild anaemia
Anaemia of chronic inflammatory disease		Usually normocytic normochromic but may become microcytic if long-standing. Likely to be due to abnormal iron metabolism
Familial microcytosis in Akitas		Incidental finding
Hyponatraemia		When blood is mixed with analyser diluent, water moves out of hypotonic red cells into diluent causing red cells to shrink

4.5 Causes of altered mean corpuscular volume and their mechanisms.

Causes of altered MCHC	Mechanism/other features
Increased MCHC	
Intravascular haemolysis; haemolysis *in vitro*	Free haemoglobin (Hb) as well as Hb from cells is measured and this affects calculation of MCHC
Lipaemia; numerous Heinz bodies	Interference with spectrophotometric Hb assay
Marked spherocytosis	Haemoglobin concentrated into smaller volume
Marked eccentrocytosis	Haemoglobin pushed into smaller volume on one side of cell
Hyponatraemia	When blood is mixed with analyser diluent, water moves out of hypotonic red cells into diluent causing red cells to shrink
Decreased MCHC	
Regenerative anaemia	Increased circulating reticulocytes, which have less Hb. Not all regenerative anaemias have decreased MCHC
Iron deficiency	Reduced production of Hb
Aged blood samples (>24 hours)	Red cell swelling *in vitro* leads to increased HCT and consequent decreased calculated MCHC

4.6 Causes of altered mean corpuscular haemoglobin concentration and their mechanisms.

Reticulocyte counts

The traditional method of manually counting reticulocytes on methylene blue-stained blood films has largely been superseded by automated methods using flow cytometric haematology analysers. The ProCyte Dx®, Sysmex XT-2000iV® and Advia® analysers use a fluorescent dye which is taken up by the ribosomes in reticulocytes but not by the mature red cells. When laser light passes over a cell labelled with this dye, fluorescent light is emitted with a longer wavelength, which is detected and used to generate the reticulocyte count (Figure 4.9). In the Lasercyte Dx®, red cells are stained with new methylene blue, which stains the reticulocytes, increasing their granularity and resulting in an increase in side scatter of laser light.

The counts generated by these analysers correspond to the total reticulocyte count in the dog and the aggregate reticulocyte count in the cat (see below). Reference ranges differ slightly for each analyser, but in general the reference range is higher than for the manual method, owing to a slight positive bias (Lilliehöök and Tvedten, 2009; Serra *et al.*, 2012), although there is a negative bias for the LaserCyte Dx® compared with the manual and Advia® automated methods (Becker *et al.*, 2008).

Manual reticulocyte counts can be performed using supravital stains (which stain living cells), such as new methylene blue and brilliant cresyl green. These stain the

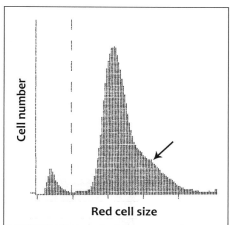

4.7 A histogram showing red cell size on the *x*-axis and cell number (*n*) on the *y*-axis, from a dog with regenerative anaemia. There is a 'hump' to the right of the main peak (arrowed) indicating increased numbers of large red cells.

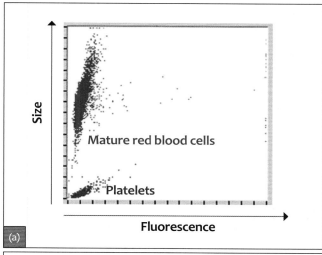

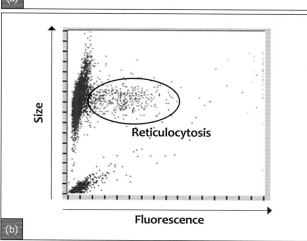

4.9 Scatter plot from a Procyte Dx® analyser showing the red cell plot from (a) a normal dog and (b) a dog with regenerative anaemia. The reticulocytes take up a dye which, on encountering laser light, emits fluorescent light. The platelet cloud (in blue) appears below the red cell cloud.
(Courtesy of G Bilborough, Idexx)

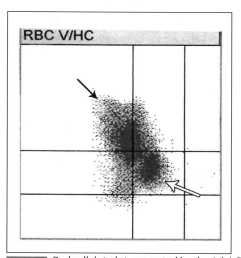

4.8 Red cell dot plot generated by the Advia® 120 analyser. Haemoglobin concentration is on the *x*-axis and cell size on the *y*-axis. Cells within the central box are normocytic and normochromic (white arrow). In regenerative anaemia a cloud of cells is found in the upper left box corresponding to macrocytic hypochromic cells (black arrow).

reticulum network of aggregated ribosomes, mitochondria and organelles present in immature cells. This reticulum network is lost as the red cell matures and therefore reticulocyte counts should be performed on fresh samples (preferably <6 hours old).

To perform a manual reticulocyte count:

1. Mix equal parts of blood (in ethylenediamine tetraacetic acid, EDTA) and a 0.5% solution of new methylene blue or brilliant cresyl green in normal saline.
2. Leave to stand at room temperature for 15–20 minutes.
3. Mix again.
4. Make a blood smear (see Chapter 3).
5. Scan the smear at low power first to check for an even distribution of reticulocytes. Occasionally, the reticulocytes are unevenly distributed and are preferentially pushed to the tail.
6. Evaluate the smear at high power (X100) in the monolayer region (examination area; see Chapter 3).
7. To perform the count, at least 300 cells, but preferably 1000 cells (mature red cells and aggregate reticulocytes), are counted and the percentage of reticulocytes is calculated.

In dogs, all reticulocytes are aggregate forms: these are larger than mature red cells and contain large clumps of aggregated ribosomes (Figure 4.10a). In cats there are two forms of reticulocyte: punctate and aggregate. Punctate reticulocytes are more mature than aggregate reticulocytes, are similar in size to mature red cells, and contain two to six fine dots of residual RNA (Figure 4.10b). Only aggregate reticulocytes should be included in the count (punctate reticulocytes are counted as mature red cells). Because there is a transition from the aggregate to the punctate stage, some cells may be difficult to classify.

Reticulocytes are absent or present only in small numbers (< approximately 80 x 10^9/l for dogs and <60 x 10^9/l for cats) in normal blood. Following acute haemorrhage or haemolysis, increased numbers of reticulocytes are not evident for at least 48 hours, with maximal production of canine reticulocytes and feline aggregate reticulocytes by 4–7 days. In cats, aggregate reticulocytes circulate for a short time (approximately 12 hours) before developing into punctate reticulocytes, which develop into mature red cells after 10 days. Aggregate reticulocytes are polychromatic on Romanowsky stains but punctate reticulocytes are not. Normal cats may have up to 10% punctate reticulocytes. Following an episode of red cell loss, punctate reticulocytes start to increase by 1 week, peak at around 2–3 weeks and then gradually decline. Thus, increased punctate reticulocytes indicate a regenerative response 2–4 weeks earlier, while increased aggregate reticulocytes indicate recent bone marrow stimulation. In mild anaemia the punctate count is useful because the aggregate reticulocytes are retained in the marrow until they mature into punctate reticulocytes.

In regenerative anaemia with a normally functioning bone marrow, the magnitude of the reticulocyte response should match the severity of the anaemia. For example, in a dog, mild anaemia and a PCV of 30% should lead to a slight increase in reticulocyte count (e.g. 100 x 10^9/l), while severe anaemia and a PCV of 15% should lead to a much higher reticulocyte count (e.g. 350 x 10^9/l). A guide for grading the severity of anaemia is shown in Figure 4.11. Haemolytic anaemia generally results in a more marked reticulocytosis than does haemorrhagic anaemia. Dogs have a more marked reticulocyte response to anaemia than cats.

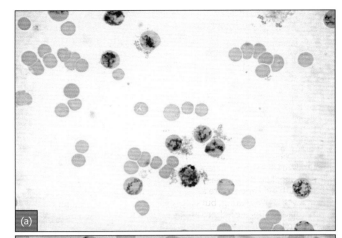

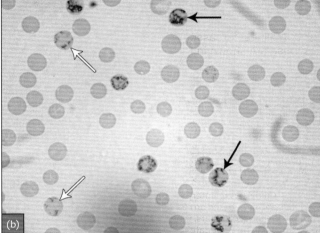

4.10 Appearance of reticulocytes on a blood film stained with new methylene blue. (a) In the dog, reticulocytes have numerous dark-staining aggregates. (b) In the cat, aggregate reticulocytes have large clumps of ribosomes (black arrows), while punctate reticulocytes have a few small inclusions (white arrows). (New methylene blue stain; original magnification X1000)

Severity of anaemia	Canine HCT (l/l)	Feline HCT (l/l)
Mild	0.30–0.37	0.20–0.27
Moderate	0.20–0.29	0.15–0.19
Severe	0.13–0.19	0.10–0.14
Very severe	<0.13	<0.10

4.11 A guide for grading the severity of anaemia using the haematocrit (HCT).

The reticulocyte count must be interpreted in the light of the degree of anaemia. It is preferable to use the absolute reticulocyte count, because this is not affected by variation in red cell number in the way that reticulocyte percentage is, as shown in Figure 4.12. Both the percentage and absolute count are generated by haematology analysers. For manual methods, the absolute count can be calculated as follows:

Absolute reticulocyte count (x 10^9/l) =
Observed % reticulocytes x RBC count (x 10^{12}/l) × 10

Example

A dog with a red cell count of 1.5 x 10^{12}/l and 15% reticulocytes:

Absolute reticulocyte count = 15 x 1.5 x 10 = 225 x 10^9/l

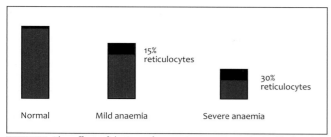

4.12 The effect of degree of anaemia on uncorrected reticulocyte percentage. The proportions of mature red cells and reticulocytes are shown schematically in red and black, respectively. The normal animal on the left has a low percentage of reticulocytes. In the animals with mild and severe anaemia, the same absolute number of reticulocytes is circulating, but the reticulocyte percentage is higher in severe anaemia because there are fewer mature cells. This gives a false impression that the severe anaemia is more regenerative than the mild anaemia.

Guidelines for assessing the degree of reticulocyte response are shown in Figure 4.13.

Degree of regeneration	Canine reticulocyte count (x 10⁹/l)	Feline reticulocyte count (x 10⁹/l)
Inadequate or no regeneration	<80	<60
Mild	80–150	60–100
Moderate	151–300	101–200
Marked	>300	>200

4.13 Guidelines for interpreting the reticulocyte response in dogs and cats, based on reticulocyte counts generated by flow cytometric analysers. In cats, the analyser reticulocyte count corresponds to the aggregate reticulocyte count on manual counting.

Identification of red cell regeneration on the blood film

On a blood film stained with a routine Romanowsky or rapid (e.g. Diff-Quik®) stain, the regenerative response manifests as polychromasia (increased numbers of poly-chromatic cells) and anisocytosis (variation in cell size) with macrocytosis (see Figure 4.3). The numbers of poly-chromatic cells and macrocytes per high power field should be assessed to gauge the regenerative response, as shown in Figure 4.14. The marrow response is propor-tional to the degree of anaemia; in severe anaemia the reticulocytes are released at an earlier stage, and the response may include basophilic rubricytes (which stain darker) and nucleated red cells. In cats, reticulocytes tend to remain in the marrow until they are only weakly polychromatophilic and therefore the degree of polychro-masia seen in a regenerative anaemia is less marked than for the dog.

Other features of regeneration seen on blood films include:

- Howell–Jolly bodies (remnants of nuclear material, most often seen in cats) (Figure 4.15)
- Target cells (see Figure 4.3) are frequently seen, but are not specific for regeneration. They may also be seen in renal and hepatic disorders, and hypochromic target cells are seen in iron deficiency (see below)
- Nucleated red cells (Figure 4.15)
- Basophilic stippling (due to aggregated ribosomes, appearing as small punctate inclusions) is *occasionally* seen in regeneration in small animals but is more often associated with lead poisoning.

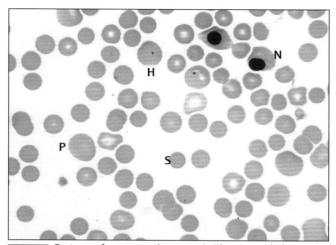

4.15 Features of a regenerative anaemia. There are polychromatic macrocytic red cells corresponding to reticulocytes (P), cells containing a Howell–Jolly body (H) and nucleated red cells (N). In this case the anaemia was due to immune-mediated haemolysis and there are numerous spherocytes (S). (Modified Wright's stain; original magnification X1000)

It is important to note that circulating nucleated red cells in the absence of polychromasia are not indicative of a regenerative response and may be seen with bone marrow disease (e.g. myeloproliferative disease) and with splenic disease (e.g. neoplasia), as well as in lead poisoning.

Polychromasia and increased reticulocytes are some-times seen *in the absence of anaemia*. This has been attri-buted to the effect of excitement/acute stress, when adrenaline (epinephrine) leads to splenic contraction and release of reticulocytes from the spleen into the general circulation. The effect is most marked in Greyhounds, because these dogs have large spleens and show a ten-dency to become stressed, but it can be seen in any dog, although it has not been described in cats. Another possible explanation is a compensated anaemia, in which red cell loss is being balanced by increased red cell production.

Grade	Polychromasia in dogs	Polychromasia in cats	Macrocytosis (dogs and cats)
Occasional	<1 cell/hpf	<1 cell every other hpf	Slightly larger cells, <1 cell/hpf
1+	1–2 cells/hpf	<1 cell/hpf	Slightly larger cells, 1–2 cells/hpf
2+	2–3 cells/hpf	1–2 cells/hpf	Slightly larger and larger still cells present, 3–5 cells/hpf
3+	4–8 cells/hpf	3–5 cells/hpf	Large cells present, 5–10 cells/hpf
4+	>8 cells/hpf	>5 cells/hpf	Large cells present, >10 hpf

4.14 A grading system for polychromasia and macrocytosis in dogs and cats. Occasional indicates no regeneration, 1+ and 2+ indicate mild regeneration, 3+ and 4+ indicate moderate and marked regeneration, respectively. This grading is subjective and will also depend on the thickness of the smear and the total number of cells per high power (X100) field (hpf). Grading systems may differ slightly among laboratories.

Characteristics of non-regenerative anaemia

In non-regenerative anaemia there is no increased release of reticulocytes from the bone marrow and the anaemia is normocytic and normochromic, with no increase in RDW. On a blood film, the red cells are uniform in size and polychromatic cells are rare (<1.5% of red cells or <1 per (X100) (hpf)). Immediately following red cell loss, anaemia appears non-regenerative, and an increase in circulating reticulocytes is not seen for 3–4 days.

Physiological response to anaemia

The release of oxygen from haemoglobin to the tissues is determined by the affinity of haemoglobin for oxygen. Lower affinity means that a higher proportion of the oxygen carried by haemoglobin is released to the tissues. Haemoglobin affinity is reduced in tissue hypoxia, because lactic acid released via anaerobic glycolysis leads to lowered pH in the microenvironment. In addition, haemoglobin affinity is regulated by 2,3-diphosphoglycerate (2,3-DPG), a compound found in high concentrations in red cells. Increased 2,3-DPG concentration leads to lowered affinity and hence greater delivery of oxygen to the tissues. The 2,3-DPG concentration increases in anaemia and in this way anaemic animals undergo a physiological adaptation to the anaemic state, maximizing the capacity of their reduced number of red cells to carry and deliver oxygen. Animals with chronic anaemia can compensate remarkably well and have relatively mild clinical signs for the degree of anaemia. In contrast, animals with acute anaemia, because they have not had time to adapt physiologically, have severe clinical signs associated with a relatively mild to moderate anaemia.

Blood loss anaemia

The clinical and clinicopathological pictures of acute and chronic haemorrhage differ in many respects and so are considered separately.

Acute haemorrhage

Acute haemorrhage may occur following trauma or surgery, or as a result of bleeding gastrointestinal ulcers or tumours, rupture of a vascular tumour (e.g. splenic haemangiosarcoma), coagulopathy (e.g. warfarin toxicity) or severe thrombocytopenia. Acute severe blood loss (up to 30–40% of blood volume, beyond which death is likely to occur) causes hypovolaemic shock with collapse, marked mucosal pallor, tachycardia and weak pulses (contrasting with the bounding pulses seen in animals with acute haemolysis). Immediately following acute haemorrhage the plasma protein and red cell parameters (including PCV) are normal because both red cells and plasma are lost in proportion. After about 4 hours, the PCV and plasma protein start to fall as blood volume is expanded by interstitial fluid moving into the circulation. Plasma protein usually falls first because splenic contraction may offset the fall in PCV. The PCV does not indicate the full magnitude of blood loss for at least 24 hours after the onset of haemorrhage.

Following **internal haemorrhage** up to approximately 65% of the red cells, as well as plasma proteins, are reabsorbed via the lymphatics over a few days, resulting in a rapid increase in PCV and plasma protein. Up to 80% of red cells are reabsorbed within 1–2 weeks. The remaining red cells are phagocytosed by macrophages and their iron is recycled. The anaemia resolves because of a combination of red cell reabsorption and bone marrow regeneration. The magnitude of the regenerative response may not be very marked if a large proportion of cells are reabsorbed.

In dogs, haemoabdomen is commonly associated with splenic haemangiosarcoma (accounting for 63.3% of cases of acute non-traumatic haemoabdomen in one study (Aronsohn et al., 2009), with the second most common cause being splenic haematoma (26.6% cases in that study), while coagulopathy appears to be an uncommon cause. Red cell fragmentation is sometimes seen with haemangiosarcoma, manifesting as circulating schistocytes, acanthocytes and keratocytes (Figure 4.16) although these cells are not specific for haemangiosarcoma and can also be seen with haemangioma, splenic torsion and disseminated intravascular coagulation (DIC) among others. The presence of schistocytes or anaemia should not be used as a marker of malignancy when splenic lesions are detected (Elders and Blackwood, 2003). Causes of red cell poikilocytosis are summarized in Figure 4.17.

In cats, non-traumatic haemoabdomen may occur with haemangiosarcoma, other tumours including hepatocellular carcinoma, coagulopathy and ruptured liver, which may occur in cats with amyloidosis (Culp et al., 2010).

If haemorrhage occurs into tissues rather than a body cavity, the red cells cannot be reabsorbed and are broken down by macrophages. Haemoglobin is broken down to bilirubin and therefore, in extensive tissue haemorrhage, serum bilirubin may be elevated until it is cleared by the liver. This combination of anaemia and jaundice could be confused with a haemolytic anaemia.

Following **external haemorrhage**, protein and red cells (and hence iron) are lost from the body and therefore recovery from anaemia depends totally on the bone marrow's response. This regenerative response is usually apparent in the peripheral blood after 3–4 days. The PCV rises quite rapidly and is usually low normal within 2–3 weeks of a single haemorrhagic episode. Plasma protein should return to normal after 5–7 days; persistently low protein beyond this time is suggestive of ongoing external blood loss.

Acute blood loss is usually associated with a neutrophilic leucocytosis with an increased number of band neutrophils, especially following haemorrhage into a body cavity. The presence of immature red cells and granulocytic

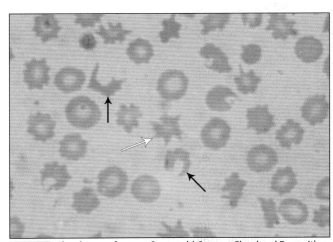

4.16 Blood smear from an 8-year-old German Shepherd Dog with a splenic mass, showing schistocytes (black arrows) and acanthocytes (white arrow). (Modified Wright's stain; original magnification X1000)

Poikilocyte	Appearance		Cause
Spherocyte		Small round cell, dense staining without central pallor	Immune-mediated haemolytic anaemia, snake bite, occasionally zinc toxicity, bee stings
Schistocytes		Fragmented red cells with pointed, irregular projections	DIC, haemangiosarcoma, splenic torsion, iron-deficiency anaemia, myelofibrosis, heart failure, doxorubicin toxicity, caval syndrome
Keratocyte		Spiculated red cell with two horn-like projections	Fragmentation due to DIC, haemangiosarcoma, vasculitis, caval syndrome
Acanthocyte/spur cell		Roundish but with irregular asymmetrical projections	Liver disease, haemangiosarcoma, DIC, lymphoma, glomerulonephritis, renal disease, internal haemorrhage
Echinocyte/crenated red cell		Round cell with small regular surface projections	Artefact seen in thick smears, snake bite, glomerulonephritis, uraemia, neoplasia, pyruvate kinase deficiency
Target cell/codocyte		Rim of haemoglobin surrounding pale area, with central 'button' of haemoglobin	Regenerative anaemia, renal, hepatic and lipid disorders
Ovalocytes and dacrocyte		Oval shaped and tear drop shaped	Myelofibrosis, neoplasia, possible artefact
Eccentrocyte		Clear area on one side of red cell bordered by membrane	Oxidative injury, e.g. zinc toxicity
Leptocyte		Large area of central pallor with thin rim of haemoglobin	Iron deficiency

4.17 Poikilocytes, their appearance and causes. DIC = disseminated intravascular coagulation.

precursors in the circulation is known as a leucoerythroblastic response and may also be seen in immune-mediated haemolytic anaemia (see Figure 5.6). Immediately following haemorrhage there may be a mild to moderate thrombocytopenia, reflecting increased consumption of platelets; this is usually rapidly followed by a rebound thrombocytosis with the production of large 'shift' platelets. Thrombocytopenia is often moderate or occasionally marked (<50 x 10^9/l) in dogs with haemoabdomen caused by haemangiosarcoma, and the platelet count and total solids are lower in dogs with haemangiosarcoma than in those with other splenic lesions (Hammond and Pesillo-Crosby, 2008).

In summary, the clinicopathological features of acute haemorrhage are:

- Anaemia: initially non-regenerative; after 3–4 days becomes regenerative. Acanthocytes may be seen with internal haemorrhage
- Low plasma proteins, returning to normal more quickly with internal haemorrhage
- Neutrophilia with left shift
- Thrombocytopenia then rebound thrombocytosis.

The cause or source of the haemorrhage may be obvious on clinical examination, or further investigations may be required. Depending on the clinical signs, coagulation tests (see Chapter 6), radiography, ultrasonography, and urine and faecal analysis may be indicated.

Chronic haemorrhage and iron-deficiency anaemia

Chronic haemorrhage results in chronic anaemia of insidious onset. The animal is able to adapt to the anaemic state and therefore shows relatively mild signs for the degree of anaemia. Chronic external haemorrhage initially leads to a regenerative anaemia but, as iron deficiency develops, the anaemia progressively becomes non-regenerative. Most body iron is found in haemoglobin (65%), and only small amounts of iron are found in myoglobin and enzymes, or attached to the transporter molecule transferrin (5%). The remainder is stored in various tissues as haemosiderin and ferritin; a small amount of ferritin is present in the plasma. Chronic external blood loss results in loss of haem iron. In response to the blood loss, iron stores are mobilized and utilized for erythropoiesis, but when these stores become depleted iron deficiency develops. Young animals become iron deficient following blood loss more quickly than adults because they have low iron stores, and the bone marrow has less capacity to increase the rate of haemopoiesis because it is very actively producing red cells to match the growth rate.

Iron deficiency results in inadequate haemoglobinization of red cells and the release of microcytic, hypochromic red cells into the circulation, with resultant low MCV and MCHC. MCV falls first; as iron becomes progressively depleted, MCHC then falls. The combination of microcytic and normocytic (present from prior to the onset of iron deficiency) red cells, leads to increased RDW. Persistent thrombocytosis is a common feature of chronic haemorrhage. Plasma proteins are lost along with red cells and, if blood loss is substantial, there is hypoproteinaemia with proportionately low albumin and globulin.

On the blood film the red cells do not always have a smaller diameter but are thin (flat) pale-staining cells termed leptocytes, which have a large area of central pallor and a thin rim of haemoglobin (Figure 4.18). Target cells (codocytes) and folded or fragmented red cells (schistocytes; see Figure 4.16) may be present.

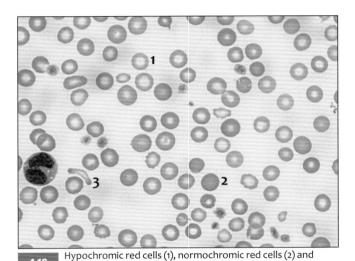

4.18 Hypochromic red cells (1), normochromic red cells (2) and fragmented red cells (3) from a dog with iron-deficiency anaemia. (Modified Wright's stain; original magnification X1000)

In summary, the clinicopathological features of chronic blood loss/iron-deficiency anaemia are:

- Microcytic hypochromic anaemia with hypochromic leptocytes seen on a blood film
- Low plasma protein with severe blood loss
- Thrombocytosis
- Reticulocyte count increased at first; it then falls as the animal becomes iron deficient.

Evaluation of the red cell scatter plot on the Advia® is helpful in identifying a microcytic hypochromic population, which is visible prior to the development of low MCV and high MCHC, as shown in Figure 4.19.

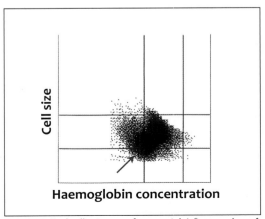

4.19 Red cell cytogram from an Advia® 120 analyser for a dog with iron-deficiency anaemia. There are two populations of cells: one is normocytic/normochromic (these cells were produced prior to the onset of iron deficiency) and one is microcytic/hypochromic (arrowed).

Measurement of reticulocyte haemoglobin content (CHr) and reticulocyte haemoglobin concentration are also very useful in the early detection of iron deficiency because these newly formed iron-deficient cells contain less haemoglobin than reticulocytes produced with normal iron stores. These parameters can be measured using the Advia® and Sysmex® analysers. A cut-off for CHr of <20.1 pg in dogs and <14.6 pg in cats using the Advia® provides a sensitive marker of early iron deficiency (Prins et al., 2009; Schaufer and Stokol, 2014). These parameters can also be used to monitor the response to treatment: if iron stores are normalized the reticulocyte haemoglobin will return to normal long before the MCV and MCHC normalize. CHr may be low in anaemia of chronic inflammatory disease although typically mild reductions are seen (see discussion on iron stores).

Once iron deficiency has been identified, this should prompt a search for external blood loss. Chronic external blood loss may result from blood loss into the gastrointestinal (GI), urogenital or respiratory tract, or from the skin surface (e.g. in severe flea infestation). GI bleeding is the most common cause of iron-deficiency anaemia in dogs and may be due to ulceration, parasitism, neoplasia or inflammatory bowel disease. Urogenital bleeding may be due to neoplasia, chronic infections/inflammatory conditions, haemorrhagic cystitis associated with cyclophosphamide or idiopathic renal haemorrhage. Respiratory tract bleeding may be due to nasal or pulmonary haemorrhage, most often caused by neoplasia. Blood can be coughed up and swallowed, thus mimicking GI haemorrhage. The source of bleeding may be evident from the clinical history (e.g. melaena, haematuria, lice or flea infestation). Otherwise, urinalysis and faecal occult blood tests should be carried out. The patient should be on a meat-free diet for at least 3 days before performing the faecal occult blood test, because myoglobin (present in meat) cross-reacts with haemoglobin in the test (white fish can be fed). Faecal analysis for endoparasitism and/or imaging (ultrasonography and contrast radiography) of the GI or urogenital tract may be useful in determining the site of blood loss.

Using iron stores to distinguish anaemia of chronic inflammatory disease and iron-deficiency anaemia

Anaemia of chronic inflammatory disease (AID; see later) usually leads to a mild to moderate normocytic normochromic non-regenerative anaemia, but occasionally leads to microcytic normochromic or microcytic hypochromic anaemia due to reduced iron availability. This can be confused with iron-deficiency anaemia. A severe microcytic hypochromic anaemia (PCV <20%) is almost certainly due to iron deficiency but, if the anaemia is mild or moderate, evaluation of iron stores is useful to distinguish iron-deficiency anaemia and AID (Figure 4.20). Iron stores may be assessed by measuring serum iron, total iron-binding capacity (TIBC), percentage transferrin saturation, bone marrow haemosiderin stores and serum ferritin.

Serum iron: Serum iron measures the total amount of iron bound to both transferrin and ferritin. However, the amount of ferritin–iron in serum is very small so serum iron generally reflects iron bound to transferrin. Iron within haemoglobin is not detected by this test. Serum iron concentration is low in iron-deficiency anaemia but may also be low in AID and with acute and chronic inflammatory reactions (owing to sequestration of iron within macrophages in the liver, spleen and marrow), and in dogs with portosystemic shunts.

Iron stores	Anaemia of chronic inflammatory disease	Iron-deficiency anaemia
Serum iron	Low or normal	Low
TIBC	Low or normal	Normal or sometimes high or low
Percentage transferrin saturation	Normal, high or low	Low
Ferritin	Increased or normal	Low
Stainable bone marrow iron in dogs	High	Low

4.20 Use of serum iron assays in animals with microcytic hypochromic anaemia to distinguish iron deficiency and chronic inflammatory disease. TIBC = total iron-binding capacity.

Total iron-binding capacity: TIBC is an indirect measurement of transferrin. The patient's serum sample is flooded with excess iron, which binds to all the available binding sites on transferrin. The unbound iron is then removed by chemical methods and the iron concentration in the remaining sample is evaluated. The amount of iron measured is proportional to the amount of transferrin present. TIBC is low or normal in AID, with severe liver disease (owing to reduced production of transferrin) and with protein-losing states such as protein-losing nephropathy, but it is normal or sometimes low or high in dogs and cats with iron-deficiency anaemia (it is elevated in most other species with iron deficiency).

Percentage transferrin saturation: This is calculated by dividing the serum iron concentration by the TIBC, and is an indicator of the percentage of transferrin binding sites which are occupied by iron. In normal animals this is approximately 33%; it is reduced in iron-deficiency anaemia but is variable in AID (Schaefer and Stokol, 2014).

Bone marrow haemosiderin stores: Haemosiderin stores can be assessed by staining a bone marrow aspirate with Prussian blue, where haemosiderin is seen as blue aggregates within macrophages. This is the most accurate method of assessing body iron stores in dogs, but is an invasive procedure. If there is stainable iron in the bone marrow, this rules out iron deficiency as a cause of the anaemia. Stainable iron is not present in the bone marrow of healthy cats and therefore feline marrow cannot be used to assess iron stores.

Ferritin: Ferritin concentrations in the serum correlate well with body iron stores and so are low in iron-deficiency anaemia. Since ferritin is an acute phase reactant it may be increased in AID although may be normal. Ferritin is also increased in haemolytic anaemia, histiocytic sarcoma and liver disease (Friedrichs et al., 2010). It is measured using species specific monoclonal antibodies which are not widely available.

Reticulocyte haemoglobin content: This parameter falls in iron deficiency (see above discussion on chronic blood loss) but may also fall in AID. In the former, CHr levels are typically <20.1 pg in dogs, while more modest reductions are seen in AID (Schaefer and Stokol, 2014). Typically in AID the low CHr is coupled with evidence of inflammation such as a leucocytosis and/or increased acute phase proteins.

Haemolytic anaemia

There are many causes of haemolysis, but the most important in dogs and cats are:

* Immune-mediated haemolytic anaemia (IMHA) (primary or secondary)
* Bacterial, protozoal and viral infections:
  * Haemoplasmas such as *Mycoplasma haemofelis*
  * Babesiosis
  * FeLV.
* Oxidative damage causing Heinz body/eccentrocyte anaemia
* Microangiopathic haemolytic anaemia, e.g. associated with haemangiosarcoma, splenic torsion, caval syndrome
* Inherited red cell defects
* Severe hypophosphataemia
* Envenomation due to snake bites and bee stings
* Erythrophagia associated with haemophagocytic histiocytic sarcoma and hepatosplenic T-cell lymphoma.

Haemolytic anaemia results in regenerative anaemia, although immune-mediated haemolytic anaemia may be non-regenerative (see Non-regenerative anaemia, later). The regenerative response in haemolytic anaemia is usually more marked than that seen following haemorrhage because iron is more readily utilizable. Depending on the cause, the red cells may be destroyed intra- or extravascularly, or both. In extravascular haemolysis, damaged red cells are phagocytosed by macrophages, mainly in the spleen and to some extent in the liver and bone marrow. The anaemia usually has an insidious onset (days to weeks) and may be mild to severe. In intravascular haemolysis, red cells are lysed within the circulation as a consequence of direct membrane damage. The anaemia is acute in onset (hours to days) and is severe. Free intravascular haemoglobin from lysed red cells immediately forms a complex with haptoglobin; this complex is cleared from the circulation by hepatocytes and macrophages, and within these cells haemoglobin is broken down to bilirubin. Accumulating haemoglobin–haptoglobin complexes results in haemoglobinaemia, which is observed as visibly haemolysed plasma. When the supply of haptoglobin becomes saturated, free haemoglobin accumulates in the plasma and haemoglobinaemia worsens. Free haemoglobin is able to pass through the glomerular barrier, resulting in haemoglobinuria and associated renal tubular damage.

Haemoglobinaemia can be detected by visual inspection of spun plasma or from analyser data. High mean corpuscular haemoglobin (MCH) and MCHC values are seen in the presence of haemoglobinaemia but also in sample lipaemia (see Figure 4.6). Free haemoglobin can be quantified on the Advia® and Sysmex® analysers by calculating the difference between the total and cellular haemoglobin values. Total haemoglobin is determined by a spectrophotometric method in which an aliquot of blood is lysed, and the liberated haemoglobin mixed with a chemical reagent leads to a colour change which is measured colorimetrically. Cellular haemoglobin measures only haemoglobin within red cells, by measuring laser light scatter.

Jaundice may be seen with both forms of haemolysis, if it is acute and/or severe. Haemoglobin is broken down within macrophages (and hepatocytes following intravascular haemolysis) to form unconjugated bilirubin, iron and amino acids. Iron and amino acids are recycled for future erythropoiesis. Unconjugated bilirubin is released from the macrophages and transported to the liver where it is taken up, conjugated and excreted in the bile. The rate-limiting step in this process is the excretion of conjugated bilirubin into bile. If this limit is exceeded, conjugated bilirubin backs up in hepatocytes and spills out into the circulation where it competes with unconjugated bilirubin for uptake by hepatocytes. Thus, both forms of bilirubin are increased in the plasma. Unconjugated bilirubin predominates at first but, with time, the proportion of conjugated bilirubin increases, and it may become the predominant form, especially if there is concurrent liver damage (e.g. due to hypoxia). The renal threshold for bilirubin excretion is low, especially in dogs, and so relatively minor increases in plasma bilirubin result in bilirubinuria. Thus, bilirubinuria is generally detected before tissue jaundice.

Immune-mediated haemolytic anaemia

IMHA is a common cause of haemolytic anaemia in dogs. It is more commonly seen in females and the Cocker Spaniel, English Springer Spaniel, Poodle, Old English Sheepdog, Irish Setter, Miniature Schnauzer and Collie are predisposed. The absence of dog erythrocyte antigen 7 has been reported to be associated with an increased risk of IMHA in Cocker Spaniels (Miller *et al.*, 2004). In dogs, 60–75% of cases are primary (idiopathic), and this is sometimes termed autoimmune haemolytic anaemia. IMHA may also be secondary to certain drugs (e.g. potentiated sulphonamides, cephalosporins, non-steroidal anti-inflammatory drugs), neoplasia, systemic lupus erythematosus and infections, such as babesiosis, ehrlichiosis, leishmaniosis, anaplasmosis or localized bacterial infections (e.g. subacute endocarditis). There are conflicting reports regarding the association of IMHA with vaccination but overall it is considered that, although vaccine-associated IMHA does occur, there is a low incidence (Duval and Giger, 1996; Gaskell *et al.*, 2002). In cats, primary IMHA is uncommon and accounted for only 4% of cases of feline anaemia in one study (Korman *et al.*, 2013). Secondary IMHA may be induced by haemotrophic *Mycoplasma* infections, FeLV infection, lymphoproliferative diseases and certain drugs. Neonatal isoerythrolysis and transfusion reactions are other examples of immune-mediated haemolysis and are discussed later.

Pathophysiology and laboratory findings: In IMHA the animal produces antibodies (most commonly IgG but sometimes IgM) directed against its own red cells. The most common presentation is of a moderate to severe anaemia resulting from extravascular haemolysis due to the presence of IgG on the surface of red cells, which is recognized by the Fc receptor on macrophages in the spleen and to a lesser extent in the liver. The entire cell may be phagocytosed or, if only part of the cell membrane is phagocytosed, the remaining cell contents are squeezed within a smaller surface area leading to spherocyte formation (Figure 4.21). Spherocytes are spherical in shape, and on blood films they appear smaller than normal red cells with darker/denser cytoplasm lacking central pallor (see Figures 4.17 and 4.22). Care should be taken to look in the examination area monolayer and avoid looking at the tail of the smear where cells are flattened and lose their normal central pallor, giving the false impression of spherocytes. Spherocytes are impossible to identify in feline blood because normal feline red cells have minimal or no central pallor. Spherocytes are less flexible than normal red cells and therefore become sequestered in the liver or spleen, leading to accelerated erythrophagocytosis. When seen in

moderate to large numbers (e.g. >10% of the cells, sometimes more than 50%) they are regarded as diagnostic for IMHA in dogs. However, small numbers of spherocytes may result from oxidative damage or fragmentation, or may not be significant, and do not provide evidence of IMHA. Spherocytes can also be seen with haemolytic anaemia caused by snake bites and bee stings. Rarely, zinc toxicity can lead to moderate or marked spherocytosis.

In severe cases, high levels of complement-fixing antibody (usually IgM) are present on the red cell surface, leading to severe membrane damage; extracellular water leaks into the cell leading to swelling and rupture within the circulation (Figure 4.23). Erythrocyte ghosts may be seen on the blood film as pale-staining 'empty' cells. The result is intravascular haemolysis, which leads to haemoglobinaemia and haemoglobinuria, and the anaemia is acute and severe.

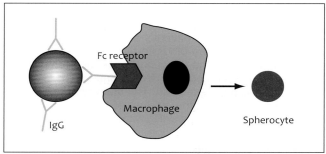

4.21 Extravascular haemolysis. Antibody Fc receptors on macrophages bind to the antibody on the red cell surface, leading to phagocytosis of the red cell. Phagocytosis of a portion of the red cell membrane leads to the formation of a spherocyte.

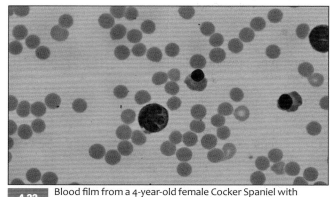

4.22 Blood film from a 4-year-old female Cocker Spaniel with immune-mediated haemolytic anaemia. Numerous spherocytes are seen, which are smaller and denser than normal red cells and lack central pallor. There are two nucleated red cells and two monocytes. (May–Grünwald–Giemsa stain; original magnification X1000)

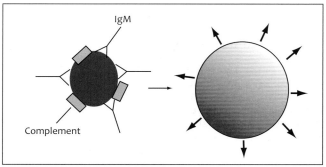

4.23 Intravascular haemolysis. Large amounts of antibody on the red cell surface lead to complement fixation, damage to the red cell membrane and movement of water into the cell, causing swelling and lysis.

Autoagglutination: If very high levels of antibody are present, individual antibodies can bind to more than one red cell, causing cells to clump together; this is autoagglutination. Cell clumps sequester in the spleen and liver, leading to accelerated removal and thus a higher rate of haemolysis. Autoagglutination may be seen grossly within the sample tube, or is detected by placing a few drops of blood on a glass slide and adding an equal volume of saline (which breaks up rouleaux). The slide is rocked gently and examined grossly before a coverslip is added for microscopic examination (Figure 4.24). Because autoagglutination may also develop as a non-specific finding, e.g. in association with neoplasia, inflammation, infection or organ failure, it is important to determine whether the agglutination persists after saline washing (Caviezel *et al.*, 2014). This test is performed as follows:

1. The EDTA sample is centrifuged for 5 minutes at 1000x*g* and the plasma removed.
2. The pellet of red cells is mixed with saline in a 1:4 ratio.
3. The tube is centrifuged for 5 minutes at 1000×*g*.
4. The supernatant is removed, leaving a red cell pellet.
5. Steps 2–4 are repeated two further times.
6. After removing the supernatant the cells are resuspended in a small amount of saline and examined macroscopically and microscopically.

Persistent agglutination provides evidence for IMHA. If the agglutination breaks up after washing it may not be significant, and a Coombs' test should be performed. There is no evidence that saline washing removes sufficient erythrocyte-bound antibody to render the Coombs' test falsely negative (Caviezel *et al.*, 2014).

In dogs, most cases of IMHA show extravascular haemolysis. The regenerative response is not seen for 3–4 days after the onset but then may be marked. Sometimes this form may present as a persistently non-regenerative anaemia because red cell precursors are phagocytosed before they are released from the bone marrow (see Non-regenerative anaemia, later). IMHA with intravascular haemolysis is less common and has a more acute presentation, sometimes with an apparent non-regenerative/'pre-regenerative' anaemia. Haemoglobinaemia and haemoglobinuria are seen in severe cases and are often transient. Haemoglobinuria is identified as circular 'droplets' of free haemoglobin which stain light green with new methylene blue. With both extravascular and intravascular forms jaundice is seen only in severe cases, although hyperbilirubinuria is common. Marked or persistent jaundice usually indicates concurrent hepatobiliary disease and has been shown to be a poor prognostic indicator. The features of these two forms are summarized in Figure 4.25.

In cats, IMHA typically leads to a moderate to severe anaemia. The anaemia may be regenerative, although a non-regenerative picture is seen more commonly (this form is discussed under causes of non-regenerative anaemia, later). Icterus is very variable. Autoagglutination is variably reported: in one study of 19 cats it was detected in all cases, although it persisted in only five cases after saline washing (Kohn *et al.*, 2006); in another study it was found in only 33% of cases (Korman *et al.*, 2013). In the latter study, autoagglutination was observed in almost half of the cases of infectious anaemia, e.g. those caused by feline leukaemia virus (FeLV), feline immunodeficiency virus (FIV), or combined FIV and *Haemoplasma* spp.

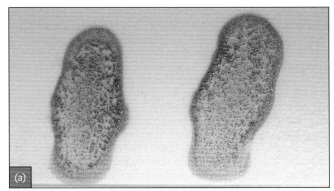

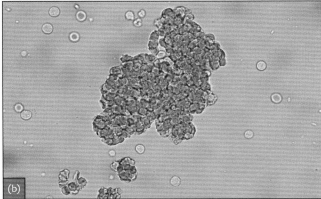

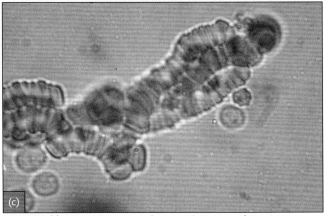

4.24 (a) Gross appearance of autoagglutination after mixing an equal volume of blood and saline on a slide. This should be confirmed by saline washing (see text) and examined microscopically. (b) Microscopic appearance of red cell agglutination with large irregular clumps of red cells. (Unstained cells; original magnification X400 with condenser lowered) (c) Rouleaux are long chains of stacks of red cells (Unstained cells; original magnification X400)

Intravascular haemolysis	Extravascular haemolysis
IgM mediated	IgG mediated
Acute onset	Subacute or more insidious onset
Severe anaemia	Mild to severe anaemia
Spherocytosis common, ghost cells may be seen	Spherocytosis common, ghost cells absent
Autoagglutination common	Autoagglutination less common
Haemoglobinaemia common	
Haemoglobinuria common	
May be jaundiced	Less commonly jaundiced
Guarded prognosis	More favourable prognosis

4.25 Features of the intravascular and extravascular forms of immune-mediated haemolytic anaemia.

Leucogram changes: In dogs with both forms of IMHA, a moderate to severe neutrophilia (which may exceed 50 x 10⁹/l) and monocytosis are common. There may be a marked left shift and toxic changes in the neutrophils and bands (see Chapter 5). The mechanism of this leucocytosis is unclear, but it may be a consequence of non-specific stimulation of the bone marrow, or secondary to the effects of complement which is increased owing to the immune-mediated disease. However, the leucocytosis may also be secondary to tissue necrosis caused by anaemic hypoxia (most frequently hepatic necrosis) or due to infarction caused by thromboembolism. There appears to be an association between the magnitude of the leucocytosis and the severity of necrosis (McManus and Craig, 2001). Necrosis results in release of various cytokines which stimulate granulopoiesis and release of neutrophils from the marrow.

In cats there may be a lymphocytosis and a mild monocytosis but neutrophilia is less common.

Coagulation abnormalities: Thrombocytopenia occurs in about 65% of cases of IMHA. It is severe (<50 × 10⁹/l) in fewer than 20% of patients, when it is associated with clinical signs such as petechial haemorrhages, epistaxis and melaena (Carr *et al.*, 2002). Thrombocytopenia may be due to consumption in a hypercoagulable state, which may progress to fulminant DIC and is associated with a poorer prognosis. Very severe thrombocytopenia (<15 × 10⁹/l) usually reflects concurrent immune-mediated thrombocytopenia and in a recent study of dogs with severe thrombocytopenia (presumed immune-mediated) and IMHA, but without DIC, the prognosis and outcome was similar to dogs with either disease alone. Overall, younger dogs were more likely to survive (Orcutt *et al.*, 2010).

Dogs with IMHA are frequently in a hypercoagulable state at the time of diagnosis and are at risk of DIC or thromboembolism (McCullough, 2003). Coagulation test abnormalities (elevations in activated partial thromboplastin time, prothrombin time and D-dimers) may be seen. Thromboelastography is useful for detecting a hypercoagulable state in dogs with IMHA (Sinnott and Otto, 2009).

Biochemical changes: Elevated liver enzymes may reflect hypoxic damage, as discussed above. Azotaemia may be prerenal, or may reflect haemoglobin-induced damage. Fibrinogen is frequently increased and hyperglobulinaemia is not uncommon.

Summary: The clinicopathological features of IMHA in dogs are:

- Moderate to severe anaemia, which is initially non-regenerative ('pre-regenerative')
- After 3–4 days the anaemia becomes regenerative: macrocytic hypochromic with marked polychromasia (3+ or 4+) reflecting marked reticulocytosis. Often the reticulocyte count is >350 x 10⁹/l. (Occasionally remains non-regenerative owing to intramedullary destruction of reticulocytes or erythroid precursors)
- Marked anisocytosis due to the presence of large reticulocytes and small spherocytes
- Spherocytes are usually seen (not always)
- Autoagglutination in severe cases, which should be confirmed with saline washing
- Mild, moderate or severe neutrophilia with left shift and sometimes toxic change
- Plasma proteins normal to slightly increased

- Bilirubin and liver enzymes may be elevated. Bilirubinuria is almost invariably present
- Haemoglobinaemia and haemoglobinuria may be present with intravascular haemolysis.

Confirmatory testing:

Coombs' test: The Coombs' test, or direct antibody test (DAT), is used to detect the presence of antibody and/or complement on the surface of red cells. Serial dilutions of Coombs' reagent, which contains species-specific polyvalent antiglobulin directed against IgM, IgG and complement, is incubated with the patient's washed red cells. Separate anti-IgG, -IgM and -complement antibodies can be used, although this does not increase the sensitivity of the test and they are not widely used (Overmann *et al.*, 2007). The antiglobulin binds with the antibodies/complement on the red cells, resulting in agglutination, which may be seen grossly as small specks of clumped cells suspended in the test well (Figure 4.26). A small amount of the suspension is placed on a microscope slide and examined at low power to confirm agglutination. The highest

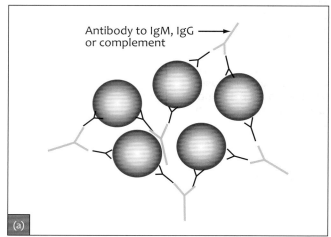

Antibody to IgM, IgG or complement

(a)

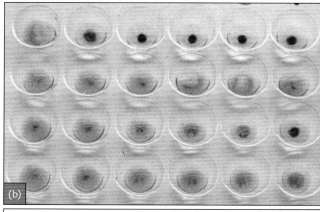

(b)

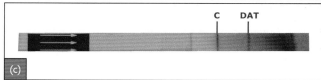

C   DAT

(c)

4.26 Coombs' test. (a) Antibody directed against IgM, IgG and complement is incubated with the patient's washed red cells. The antiglobulin binds to the antibodies/complement on the red cells, resulting in agglutination. (b) The test is performed on a microtitre plate, with progressively more dilute antiglobulin. In a positive test, small clumps of red cells remain suspended in the well; in a negative test the red cells sink to the bottom of the well, forming a button. (c) A positive DAT result using an immunochromatographic strip method.

dilution at which agglutination takes place is the recorded result. Serial dilutions are recommended to overcome the prozone effect, where a relative excess of antiglobulin in relation to red cell-bound IgG, IgM or complement leads to a failure to agglutinate.

There is no clear association between the titre and disease severity, although low-titre results are more commonly due to secondary rather than primary IMHA (Day, 2000) or may be seen in animals with diseases other than IMHA (Overmann et al., 2007). Other methods for the DAT have been validated for the dog: a capillary tube method, a gel tube method and an immunochromato-graphic strip method (Alvedia), where antibody-coated RBCs migrate and bind to a band impregnated with anti-globulin (Caviezel et al., 2014; Figure 4.26c). All of these techniques were found to correlate well with the traditional microtitre well test. The study found the DAT to be sensitive and specific in detecting IMHA, and anaemic dogs treated with immunosuppressive therapy had positive DAT results that remained positive after days to weeks of treatment. Thus, the DAT is recommended for anaemic dogs even when treatment has already been given. The study also showed that recent or previous transfusion does not appear to have an effect on the DAT, and that samples remained positive for up to 7 days post sampling when stored in the refrigerator, and therefore do not need to be tested immediately after sampling. However, other studies have shown lower sensitivity, which may vary depending on the antiglobulin used in the test. The sensitivity was reported to be 61% and 82% for two different antiglobulin reagents, with specificity of 100% and 95% (Overmann et al., 2007).

In summary, a diagnosis of IMHA is supported by one or more of the following:

- Autoagglutination, which persists after saline washing
- Marked spherocytosis
- Positive Coombs' test/DAT.

Other investigations: Given that IMHA may be secondary to neoplastic or infectious diseases, investigations should be performed to exclude or confirm an underlying cause. These tests should be tailored to the individual because blanket testing may be expensive and unrewarding.

In cats, FeLV testing and examination of smears for haemoplasma organisms, as well as polymerase chain reaction (PCR) testing (of EDTA samples) is useful. In dogs, blood film examination and PCR testing may be used to check for babesiosis and ehrlichiosis if there is a history of travel to an endemic area.

Screening radiographs may be useful to screen for underlying neoplasia. The antinuclear antibody (ANA) test is indicated if there are signs of multisystem involvement (e.g. glomerulonephritis, polyarthritis, polymyositis, immune-mediated skin disease) and systemic lupus erythematosus is suspected, but this is very rare and low false positive results can be seen as a result of many inflammatory conditions. Bone marrow analysis is useful if the anaemia is persistently non-regenerative, or where there is a suspicion of underlying lymphoproliferative disease.

Neonatal isoerythrolysis: This is seen in kittens with blood type A that are born to a type B mother. Type B cats have a naturally occurring high titre of anti-A antibodies, which in the lactating queen enter the colostrum and after suckling are absorbed into the kitten's bloodstream in the first 48 hours of life. Depending on the amount ingested, these antibodies cause severe haemolytic anaemia with

intravascular haemolysis, haemoglobinuria and icterus, and may lead to sudden death. Pre-breeding blood typing should be performed to prevent this disease by avoiding mating type A toms with type B queens.

Haemolytic anaemia associated with infections

Important infectious causes of haemolysis are FeLV (discussed under Non-regenerative anaemia), haemotrophic mycoplasmas and *Babesia* spp.

Haemotrophic **Mycoplasma** *infections in cats:* These are caused by a group of mycoplasmas which infect red cells by attaching to the cell membrane and causing haemolysis. This may occur as a primary disease or in combination with another disease process, such as FeLV or FIV infection, feline infectious peritonitis or toxoplasmosis. Four types of the bacterium have been identified:

- *M. haemofelis*
- *Candidatus* M. turicensis
- *Candidatus* M. haemominutum
- *Candidatus* M. haematoparvum-like.

These differ in their pathogenicity. Acute *M. haemofelis* infection can lead to severe haemolytic anaemia, although mild or moderate anaemia is seen in some cases. Young cats may be more likely to develop severe clinical disease. Infection with *Candidatus* M. turicensis rarely leads to anaemia, although a small drop in red cell parameters can occur, and anaemia has been rarely reported. Clinically affected cats often have concurrent disease or are immunocompromised and may be co-infected with other haemoplasma species. Likewise *Candidatus* M. haemominutum infection can cause a fall in red blood cell parameters, but anaemia does not develop except in cats with concurrent diseases, particularly FeLV infection, where *Candidatus* M. haemominutum may also play a role in inducing myeloproliferative disease (Tasker, 2010). There are no data on the pathogenicity of *Candidatus* M. haematoparvum-like, which has only been identified in North America.

These organisms attach themselves to the external surface of the red cell rather than passing into the cytoplasm, leading to mainly extravascular haemolysis. Attachment may also trigger formation of anti-erythrocyte antibodies, resulting in secondary IMHA. Following infection, cyclic episodes of parasitaemia, lasting 1–2 days, occur at roughly 6-day intervals. In cats infected with *M. haemofelis* or *Candidatus* M. turicensis the infection may clear spontaneously or with antibiotics, or a persistent carrier state may develop. The latter most commonly develops after *Candidatus* M. haemominutum infection. There is a potential for reactivation of infection in carrier cats, but this appears uncommon (Tasker, 2010).

Diagnosis: The anaemia caused by *M. haemofelis* is typically moderate to severe and regenerative but may be non-regenerative, reflecting concurrent disease (commonly FeLV infection). Leucocyte counts are variable, and platelets are usually normal. There may be autoagglutination and/or a positive Coombs' test if there is secondary IMHA. If samples are obtained during an episode of parasitaemia, pale purple small cocci or rods, singly or in chains, may be identified using the Romanowsky stains, although this is very insensitive for diagnosis and stain precipitate may give false positive results (Figure 4.27). Stain precipitate generally appears as clumps or dots of irregular size and shape, seen both within red cells and

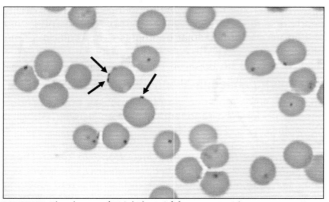

4.27 Blood smear (Wright's stain) from a cat with asymptomatic infection with *Candidatus* M. haemominutum. Arrows indicate individual organisms.
(Courtesy of S Tasker)

between cells. Filtering the stain immediately prior to use helps to reduce precipitation artefact. It is prudent either to make smears immediately after sampling with no anticoagulant, or to ensure that blood has been in EDTA for no more than 30 minutes prior to making smears, because EDTA may dislodge the organism from the red cell surface.

Given the low sensitivity of blood smear examination, the test of choice for this infection is real-time quantitative PCR, which allows the haemoplasmas to be differentiated and allows quantification of the amount of haemoplasma DNA. This is useful to indicate the significance of the infection and can be used to monitor response to therapy. In *M. haemofelis* infection, large and rapid fluctuations in DNA copy numbers can be seen over 2–3 days, which is now not thought to be due to tissue sequestration and may be due to rapid multiplication of organisms followed by rapid clearance from the blood and subsequent destruction. Cats can become PCR negative following antibiotic treatment and therefore it is important to take samples prior to starting therapy. PCR testing is useful to assess response to therapy: negative results are expected if treatment is effective. Testing every month for 2–3 months has been recommended (Tasker, 2010).

It is important to remember that a positive PCR result is not always significant, especially with *Candidatus* M. haemominutum and *Candidatus* M. turicensis.

Haemotrophic* Mycoplasma *infections in dogs: Haemoplasma infection is a rare cause of anaemia in dogs. Two species have been identified: *Mycoplasma haemocanis* and *Candidatus* M. haematoparvum. These only cause anaemia in immunocompromized dogs, e.g. dogs on chemotherapy or after splenectomy. Haemolytic anaemia in association with *M. haemocanis* infection has been described in a splenectomised dog in the UK (Hulme-Moir *et al.*, 2010). This dog had a moderate anaemia and thrombocytopenia, with organisms visible in 90% of the red cells. The proposed vector for transmission of infection is the brown dog tick *Rhipicephalus sanguineus* which is primarily a tick of southern Europe and warmer climates. As with cats, symptomatic carrier dogs infected with *Candidatus* M. haematoparvum and M. haemocanis have been reported. Diagnosis is by quantitative PCR.

Canine babesiosis: *Babesia* spp. are intracytoplasmic protozoan parasites that replicate by budding in the red cells. There are several different species, but in Europe,

the species that can infect dogs are *B. vogeli* and *B. canis* (which are large forms), and *B. microti*-like and *B. gibsoni* (which are small forms). The main vectors are *Rhipicephalus sanguineus*, which is found in Mediterranean regions, and *Dermacentor* spp., which are found in many European countries. Recently *Dermacentor reticulatus* has been reported in localized coastal regions in Wales, as well as the southwest and southeast of England (http://ecdc. europa.eu/en/healthtopics/vectors/vector-maps/Pages/VBORNET-maps-tick-species.aspx) and it is likely this tick will become more widespread. In addition, *B. gibsoni* was identified by PCR in 2.5% of *Ixodes* spp. ticks collected from dogs in the UK (Smith and Wall, 2013). In the UK, babesiosis is generally regarded as a disease affecting dogs that have travelled abroad, but there are low numbers of cases reported in dogs without a travel history, which is likely to reflect the change in tick distribution and tick infection. *Babesia gibsoni* may also be transmitted by biting and there is an increased incidence of this infection in Pit Bull Terriers reported in the United States.

Infection leads to both intravascular and extravascular haemolysis (and thus a regenerative anaemia) and, depending on the strain, can lead to moderate anaemia or marked anaemia with haemoglobinuria, haemoglobinaemia and jaundice. In addition, secondary complications, such as renal, hepatic, respiratory or central nervous system (CNS) dysfunction, can arise as a result of an excessive systemic inflammatory response. Thrombocytopenia is very common, as a result of either secondary immune-mediated thrombocytopenia or DIC. Secondary IMHA may also develop. Small strains tend to cause more severe disease than larger strains, with the exception of the large strain *B. rossi* (found in South Africa) which causes very severe disease. Dogs are sometimes co-infected with *Ehrlichia*. In the acute phase of infection, organisms may be seen on the blood film using Romanowsky stains. *B. canis* and *B. vogeli* appear as large pear-shaped organisms, usually in pairs (Figure 4.28). *B. gibsoni* are much smaller, circular bodies. Organisms are more often seen in capillary blood (e.g. from an ear prick) or on smears made from red cells just below the buffy coat. Smear examination may give false negative results. Serology may be negative in acute infection, while positive results may be due to past exposure rather than acute infection. Therefore, the test of choice is PCR (see chapter 29).

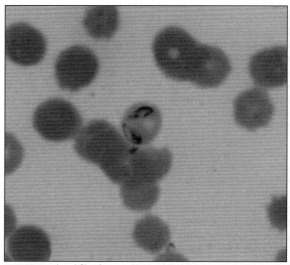

4.28 Blood film from a dog with babesiosis. Paired *Babesia canis* organisms are seen. (May–Grünwald–Giemsa stain; original magnification X1000)

Feline babesiosis: Babesiosis is rare in cats, and most reported cases are from Africa, especially South Africa where cats are affected by the small pathogenic *Babesia felis*. This may cause acute severe anaemia and jaundice but may also lead to a chronic subclinical infection. In the acute form there is a severe, regenerative anaemia and there may be a mildly elevated bilirubin although jaundice and fever are uncommon. There may be concurrent infections with haemoplasmas, FeLV and FIV. In the chronic form, cats may become asymptomatic carriers for years, and not succumb to disease unless they become immunocompromised (Ayoob *et al.*, 2010). Sporadic cases of infections with canine *Babesia* spp. occur in domestic cats in Europe and Israel, and *Babesia cati* has been described in India; these typically cause a mild disease (Hartman *et al.*, 2013). The parasites may be seen on blood films, but only when there is a high level of parasitaemia, and some species cannot be distinguished from *Cytauxzoon felis*. Diagnosis is made by PCR (see Chapter 29).

Haemolysis caused by oxidative damage

Oxygen is a potent oxidant because it can give rise to highly reactive derivatives, such as hydrogen peroxide and superoxide free radicals. Owing to the presence of oxygen within red cells, there is a constant low level of oxidant production. Oxidant damage within the cells is limited by several protective enzymes, such as reduced glutathione, superoxide dismutase and methaemoglobin reductase. When animals are exposed to oxidative toxins, these protective enzymes become overwhelmed and oxidative injury occurs. Oxidants can damage haemoglobin or red cells in three ways:

- Oxidation of the sulphydryl (–SH) groups on the globin chains in haemoglobin results in the formation of Heinz bodies (HBs), aggregates of precipitated haemoglobin attached to the inner erythrocyte membrane. Cats are more susceptible to HB formation because they have eight weak –SH groups on their haemoglobin compared with two in other species
- Direct damage to the red cell membrane results in haemolysis and the formation of eccentrocytes
- Oxidation of the ferrous iron (Fe^{2+}) to ferric iron (Fe^{3+}) in haem molecules results in the formation of methaemoglobin (metHb).

There are numerous substances reported to have caused oxidative damage in dogs and cats, including paracetamol (acetaminophen), onions and zinc. Oxidants may cause all three types of injury, or one type may predominate. For example, paracetamol leads to metHb and HB formation but not eccentrocytes. Consumption of onions leads to the formation of HBs and eccentrocytes in dogs, but not metHb. The reason for these differences is not known.

Heinz body haemolytic anaemia: HB formation has been associated with onion toxicity in both dogs and cats. The onions may be raw, cooked or dried. Onion powder in baby food is the most common source of onion causing toxicity in cats. Other causes of HB haemolytic anaemia include ingested paracetamol, zinc, garlic, naphthalene, application of benzocaine spray or cream to inflamed skin, injection of vitamin K (vitamin K3 and occasionally vitamin K1), and exposure to skunk spray. In cats, Heinz body anaemia can also develop in association with liver disease, especially hepatic lipidosis.

HBs damage red cells by reducing their deformability, leading to entrapment in the sinusoids of the spleen and subsequent extravascular haemolysis. In addition, depletion of –SH groups leads to altered membrane permeability, which can result in osmotic swelling of red cells and intravascular haemolysis. Thus, HB haemolytic anaemia is characterized by extravascular and sometimes intravascular haemolysis. There is a regenerative anaemia and often a neutrophilia and monocytosis. HBs are seen in a large proportion of the red cells as non-staining round bodies, usually protruding from the surface of the cell (Figure 4.29). HBs may interfere with the spectrophotometric assay for haemoglobin, resulting in a falsely high Hb (and hence MCHC), with low HCT and RBC count reflecting the true severity of the anaemia.

In cats, HB formation is not always associated with anaemia, and low to moderate numbers of HBs (in <10% of red cells) may be seen in cats with diabetes mellitus, hyperthyroidism and lymphoma, and after propofol administration. Propylene glycol can also cause HB formation in cats, and consequently this preservative is no longer used in commercial cat food. HB formation occurs more readily in cats owing to the structure of globin (eight –SH groups), and HBs are seen more frequently because the feline spleen does not contain sinusoids and therefore is not efficient at removing HBs from the red cell surface.

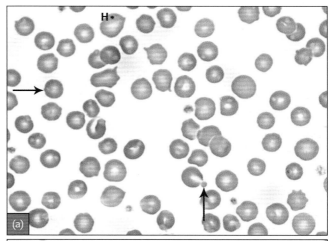

4.29 Blood films from a cat with hepatic lipidosis and anaemia. (a) There are frequent Heinz bodies (lighter-staining circular bodies) seen within and protruding from the surface of the red cells (arrowed). A Howell–Jolly body is labelled H. (Modified Wright's stain; original magnification X1000) (b) On a smear stained with new methylene blue, the Heinz bodies are obvious dark-staining round bodies. (Original magnification X1000)
(a, Courtesy of P Monti)

Oxidative injury leading to direct membrane damage:
Zinc and naphthalene (in mothballs) can cause severe membrane damage leading to intravascular haemolysis, with minimal or absent Heinz body or metHb formation, although zinc can also lead to HB formation. Membrane damage can also lead to the formation of eccentrocytes, which are red cells in which haemoglobin is displaced to one side of the cell leaving a pale 'empty' area on the other side (Figure 4.30). Again, these are less deformable than normal red cells and become entrapped in the spleen and removed by extravascular haemolysis. They are an indicator of severe oxidative injury.

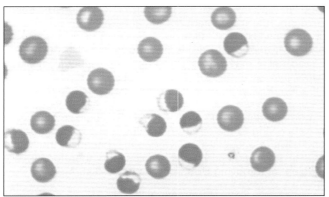

4.30 Blood film from a dog with zinc toxicity, showing large numbers of eccentrocytes with haemoglobin shifted to one side of the cell, leaving the other side clear. (Wright's stain; original magnification X1000)
(Courtesy of D DeNicola)

Oxidative injury leading to formation of methaemoglobin: In small animals, this is most commonly caused by paracetamol, especially in cats, where the toxic dose is very low (usually 50–60 mg/kg). This toxin causes the formation of metHb and HBs. HB formation leads to haemolysis, but the overriding clinical feature of paracetamol toxicity in cats is the hypoxia associated with metHb, which cannot take up oxygen. Blood appears chocolate-brown when 30–40% of total haemoglobin is in the form of metHb; death occurs when this level exceeds 80%. Methaemoglobinaemia can be readily detected by placing a drop of venous blood on white blotting paper; the spot of blood stays brown whereas normal venous blood would become oxygenated on exposure to air and the spot would turn red.

Haemolysis caused by mechanical damage: microangiopathic haemolytic anaemia

Red cells may become damaged as they pass through abnormal vessels within a vascular neoplasm, such as a haemangiosarcoma, or when passing through fibrin clots in the circulation in DIC. This may also be seen with splenic torsion and with portal vein hypoplasia. This mechanical damage results in the formation of schistocytes and/or acanthocytes which are subsequently phagocytosed in the spleen, leading to anaemia (see Figure 4.16). The anaemia is usually mild, unless there is concurrent haemorrhage (e.g. from a neoplasm).

Inherited red cell defects

Inherent metabolic defects, most frequently red cell enzyme deficiencies, have been reported in certain breeds. Such defects lead to membrane damage, with consequent haemolysis and anaemia.

Red cell pyruvate kinase deficiency: This occurs in Basenjis, Beagles, Dachshunds, West Highland White Terriers, Cairn Terriers, Labrador Retrievers and Pugs, and in many cat breeds including the Abyssinian, Somali and Domestic Shorthair. In dogs the anaemia is highly regenerative and moderate to severe, and there is progressive development of myelofibrosis and osteosclerosis, as well as liver failure leading to death between 1 and 5 years of age. Affected cats have a mild to moderate (sometimes intermittent) anaemia and may live to an advanced age. Genetic tests are available for many of these breeds, and these are constantly being updated. Genetic databases (including http://research.vet.upenn.edu/) list currently available genetic tests, which are constantly evolving (see Chapter 30).

Red cell phosphofructokinase (PFK) deficiency: This occurs in English Springer Spaniels, American Cocker Spaniels, Whippets and Wachtelhunds, as well as being reported in several mixed-breed dogs. The defect leads to energy depletion in red cells, causing low-grade red cell loss. There is a very marked regenerative response which may compensate completely for red cell loss, maintaining the PCV within the normal range. The defect also causes red cells to have marked alkaline fragility. Hyperventilation during strenuous exercise or excessive barking can lead to alkalosis and consequent intravascular haemolysis in these dogs; a haemolytic crisis associated with severe anaemia, jaundice and haemoglobinuria may ensue. PFK-deficient dogs may have a normal lifespan if alkalosis-inducing situations are avoided. Again, genetic tests are available.

Hypophosphataemia

Hypophosphataemia may arise in small animals following commencement of insulin therapy for diabetes mellitus and following tube-feeding of anorexic cats with hepatic lipidosis ('refeeding syndrome'), which may exacerbate the anaemia seen in this condition, associated with HB formation. Low phosphate concentrations cause depletion of adenosine triphosphate (ATP), increased red cell rigidity and haemolysis.

Envenomation

The venom of certain spiders, bees and wasps, and some snakes, including cobras and rattlesnakes, can cause direct haemolysis. Haemolytic anaemia with spherocytosis may occur after bee stings. Haemolysins in the venom may cause direct haemolysis while the spherocytes may be caused by a secondary IMHA.

Haemolytic anaemia associated with neoplasia

Two tumours associated with haemolytic anaemia are haemophagocytic histiocytic sarcoma and hepatosplenic T-cell lymphoma, both of which affect dogs.

The haemophagocytic form of histiocytic sarcoma is a malignant proliferation of histiocytic cells, which arise from splenic pulp and marrow macrophages. It affects Bernese Mountain Dogs, Golden Retrievers, Rottweilers and Labrador Retrievers, and occurs sporadically in other breeds. The tumour typically arises in the spleen, and may also involve the liver, lung and bone marrow. The neoplastic histiocytes are markedly erythrophagocytic, leading to a regenerative anaemia which is Coombs' negative. Other common findings include thrombocytopenia, hypoalbuminaemia and hypocholesterolaemia (Moore *et al.*, 2006). Diagnosis can be made by cytology and/or histology.

Hepatosplenic T-cell lymphoma usually arises in the liver and/or spleen without peripheral lymphadenopathy, although the bone marrow and lung may also be infiltrated. The neoplastic lymphoid cells have a characteristic appearance with an intermediate to large nucleus and moderate amounts of pale cytoplasm containing variable numbers of fine pink to magenta cytoplasmic granules. Erythrophagia occurs in some of the neoplastic lymphoid cells, but also in a secondary reactive proliferation of macrophages which develop within the tumour. There is a regenerative anaemia and commonly a thrombocytopenia, hypoalbuminaemia, and elevation in liver enzymes and bilirubin (Keller *et al.*, 2013). Again, diagnosis can be made by cytology and/or histology.

Non-regenerative anaemia

Non-regenerative anaemia may be due to primary bone marrow disease, secondary to underlying inflammatory or metabolic disease, or may be 'pre-regenerative', caused by acute red cell loss before the regenerative response has become established. The pre-regenerative anaemia will have developed acutely and the animal will show marked clinical signs, such as tachycardia, weakness and exercise intolerance, relative to the degree of anaemia. Conversely, truly non-regenerative anaemia develops gradually over weeks to months as a result of progressive loss of the already circulating red cells as they reach the end of their lifespan. The animal undergoes physiological adaptation to anaemia and shows relatively mild clinical signs for the degree of anaemia. Primary bone marrow disorders lead to moderate to severe anaemia, and depending on the cause there may be accompanying cytopenias affecting other cells, while anaemia of chronic disease leads to mild to moderate anaemia (PCV generally not less than 24% in dogs and 20% in cats) without other cytopenias.

Primary bone marrow disorders

Important causes of primary bone marrow disease are aplastic anaemia (aplastic pancytopenia), leukaemia, neoplasia, pure red cell aplasia, myelofibrosis, myelodysplastic syndrome (MDS) and FeLV infection. In addition to the sometimes severe anaemia, there may be depression of other cell lines and, depending on the cause, atypical circulating cells. Severe iron deficiency leads to non-regenerative anaemia and is discussed above.

Aplastic anaemia (aplastic pancytopenia): Aplastic anaemia results from damage to stem cells or the marrow microenvironment, leading to bone marrow failure and replacement with fat. The term aplastic anaemia is confusing because all cell lines are affected, not just the red cells. Marrow damage may be caused by infections, drugs, toxins or by immune-mediated mechanisms (this is the likely mechanism in idiopathic aplastic anaemia). In the acute form of the disease, destruction of progenitor and dividing cells leads to leucopenia/neutropenia and thrombocytopenia within 5 days and 8–10 days, respectively. Anaemia develops more gradually owing to the longer lifespan of the red cell. Bone marrow aspiration reveals a mix of fat cells, macrophages, endothelial cells, plasma cells, lymphocytes and mast cells. Depending on the cause, the bone marrow may recover and be repopulated, usually within 3 weeks of the original marrow injury, or the disease may progress to the chronic form. In the chronic form the stem cell damage is irreversible, and the red marrow is replaced by fat, leading to neutropenia, thrombocytopenia and moderate to severe anaemia. Causes of aplastic anaemia are summarized in Figure 4.31.

Drugs	Infections	Idiopathic
• Oestrogen (dogs) • Phenylbutazone (dogs) • Trimethroprim–sulphadiazine (dogs) • Albendazole (dogs and cats) • Fenbendazole (dogs) • Griseofulvin (cats) • Azathioprine (dogs) • Meclofenamic acid (dogs) • Quinidine (dogs)	• Parvovirus • Ehrlichiosis • Sepsis • FeLV	• Possible immune-mediated mechanism

4.31 Causes of aplastic anaemia.

Oestrogen toxicity: The dog is very susceptible to the myelotoxic effects of oestrogen, when given for urinary incontinence or used after mismating to prevent pregnancy, or when released from a testicular tumour (either Sertoli cell tumour or interstitial cell tumour) or, rarely, an ovarian tumour. Toxicity can be due to an overdose of administered oestrogen, but may also occur as an idiosyncratic reaction to a therapeutic dose. In the first 2–3 weeks there is a neutrophilia, often marked with a left shift, and a thrombocytopenia. The latter may lead to spontaneous bleeding and associated anaemia. This initial neutrophilia is followed by neutropenia and continuing thrombocytopenia, and a non-regenerative anaemia develops. Clinical signs relate to thrombocytopenia (petechial haemorrhages, melaena, etc.) and neutropenia (pyrexia and sepsis), as well as the anaemia (lethargy and pallor). There may also be signs of feminization in males with testicular neoplasms. The mechanism of oestrogen toxicity is not fully understood, but it is thought to be due to an oestrogen-induced production of a myelopoiesis-inhibitory factor (Sontas *et al.*, 2009). Bone marrow damage may be irreversible, or the condition may resolve following a long recovery period and supportive care with bone marrow stimulants including lithium carbonate.

Pure red cell aplasia and non-regenerative IMHA: These conditions affect both dogs and cats and are characterized by immune-mediated destruction of red cell precursors in the bone marrow, leading to severe non-regenerative anaemia. Other cell lines are usually unaffected although there may be a concurrent neutropenia (more commonly seen in cats) or a thrombocytopenia. This is a common cause of severe non-regenerative anaemia in the cat and appears to be more common than regenerative IMHA in this species.

In pure red cell aplasia (PRCA), there is depletion of the entire red cell series due to selective destruction of the early erythroid precursors. Bone marrow aspiration reveals a complete absence of erythroid cells, or very small numbers of rubriblasts and prorubricytes (the earliest precursors). In non-regenerative IMHA (NRIMHA), red cell destruction takes place at a later stage, and therefore the bone marrow contains increased numbers of erythroid precursors up to the point of destruction. Two forms are recognized: one with a maturation arrest at the level of the erythroid precursor being targeted (commonly metarubricytes are depleted); and a second with erythroid hyperplasia and complete maturation of the erythroid series (Figure 4.32). In the latter the target of destruction is presumably the reticulocyte stage. In both PRCA and NRIMHA the granulocytic and platelet precursors are usually present in normal to increased numbers, although occasionally there may be secondary dysplastic changes in these cell lines giving rise to ineffective production, and hence neutropenia or thrombocytopenia. Plasma cells are commonly increased in dogs, while in cats there may be a marked increase in small lymphocytes, which can constitute up to 56% of total marrow cells and on histology are seen in aggregates (Weiss, 2008). Spherocytes are sometimes seen in dogs, and the Coombs' test is positive in some cases, although often with a low titre. Iron stores are normal to increased. Immunosuppressive therapy (as for IMHA) is often effective although the response to treatment tends to be delayed.

Secondary PRCA occurs in association with human recombinant erythropoietin therapy or parvovirus infection, and in cats infected with FeLV subgroup C. FeLV-induced PRCA is progressive, invariably fatal, and does not lead to increased numbers of lymphocytes in the bone marrow.

time (neutrophils and platelets) become depleted first. Anaemia develops more slowly, and may not have developed at the time of first presentation in very acute cases. A similar picture may develop in dogs with stage V lymphoma when the marrow becomes infiltrated with neoplastic lymphoid cells (Figure 4.33). In chronic leukaemia, the neoplastic cells undergo differentiation within the bone marrow and the neoplastic infiltrate develops more slowly. Bone marrow suppression is much less marked and may be confined to a mild to moderate, non-regenerative anaemia, sometimes with a mild thrombocytopenia.

Disseminated histiocytic sarcoma may infiltrate the bone marrow and lead to a non-regenerative anaemia as well as thrombocytopenia, attributable to a combination of marrow crowding and cytophagia. Neutrophil numbers are typically normal or mildly raised. The erythrophagocytic form leads to a regenerative anaemia and is discussed above under haemolytic anaemia. Other tumours, such as mammary carcinomas and mast cell tumours, can occasionally metastasize to the bone marrow.

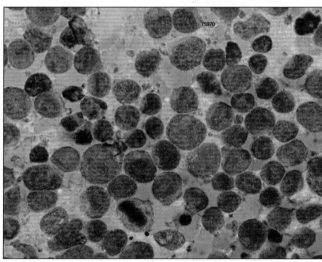

4.33 Bone marrow aspirate from a dog with stage V lymphoma. There is a predominance of large lymphoid cells with only occasional myeloid and erythroid precursors. (Modified Wright–Giemsa stain; original magnification X1000)

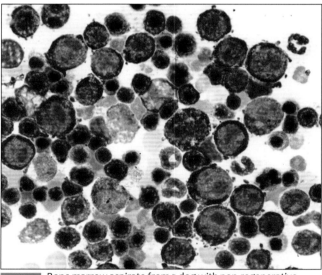

4.32 Bone marrow aspirate from a dog with non-regenerative IMHA showing marked erythroid hyperplasia. There is a marked predominance of erythroid precursors at all stages of maturation with only occasional myeloid cells. (Modified Wright–Giemsa stain; original magnification X1000)

Bone marrow neoplasia: This includes leukaemia, lymphoma, disseminated histiocytic sarcoma and metastatic neoplasia, and commonly leads to a combination of cytopenias, rather than isolated anaemia.

Leukaemia is characterized by neoplastic transformation of haemopoietic precursor cells of one cell line in the bone marrow, leading to clonal expansion of the affected cell line and, usually, release of large numbers of neoplastic cells into the circulation (see Chapter 5). The bone marrow becomes crowded out by the neoplastic cells, leading to suppression of normal haemopoiesis. The neoplastic cells compete for nutrients and also may release inhibitory substances, all adding to the suppression. The result is anaemia, neutropenia and thrombocytopenia, together with circulating atypical (leukaemic) cells. In acute leukaemia, in which the cells do not undergo differentiation but remain at a primitive blast stage, the neoplastic infiltrate develops rapidly and those cell lines with the shortest circulating

Myelofibrosis: Myelofibrosis is characterized by proliferation of fibroblasts and deposition of reticulin and collagen fibres in the haemopoietic spaces. This frequently causes a non-regenerative anaemia, often without leucopenia and thrombocytopenia, although these may be present in advanced cases. Fibrosis is usually secondary to an underlying cause, such as IMHA, pure red cell aplasia, neoplasia (within or outside the bone marrow), toxic marrow damage, e.g. due to phenobarbital, and the inherited red cell defect pyruvate kinase deficiency. Bone marrow aspiration yields a dry tap (blood with occasional individual haemopoietic precursors), and the diagnosis is made from the core biopsy sample, where fibrous tissue is seen extending throughout the haemopoietic spaces. Haemopoietic precursors are seen between the fibrosed areas and these areas may be hyper- or hypocellular (Figure 4.34). A severe anaemia and hypocellular marrow are associated with a poor prognosis. Idiopathic (primary) myelofibrosis appears to be very rare in small animals. This is a myeloproliferative disease involving megakaryocytes and granulocytes in which neoplastic cells release growth factors that stimulate fibrosis.

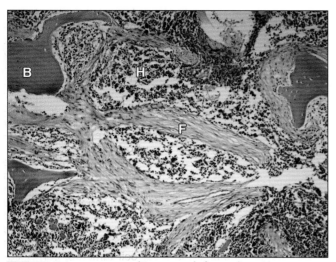

4.34 Bone marrow core biopsy sample from a dog with myelofibrosis. There is trabecular bone (B) with haemopoietic spaces containing haemopoietic tissue (H) and streaming fibrous tissue (F). (Haematoxylin and eosin stain; original magnification X200)

Myelodysplastic syndrome: Primary myelodysplastic syndrome (MDS) results from mutations in haemopoietic stem cells that lead to ineffective haemopoiesis, dysplasia and premature cell death in one or more cell lines. This leads to cytopenias, sometimes confined to anaemia, but often bi- or pancytopenia. The bone marrow is hypercellular, but early precursors do not develop normally into their mature counterparts and exhibit abnormal morphology. Dysplastic features include asynchronous nuclear/cytoplasmic development with immature nuclei and mature cytoplasm, altered granularity, giant nuclei, ring-shaped nuclei in granulocyte precursors, fragmented nuclei and multinucleation. There may be increased numbers of blast cells, but these do not exceed 20%.

There are various subtypes of MDS, which vary in severity and disease progression. MDS–refractory anaemia leads to anaemia only, and can have an indolent course, often showing good response to erythropoietin therapy. MDS–excessive blasts is characterized by a higher proportion of blasts in the bone marrow (5–20%) and leads to bi- or pancytopenia. The prognosis for this form is very poor and survival times range from days to months. Death frequently results from sepsis as a result of neutropenia. This form may progress to acute myeloid leukaemia (AML) (Weiss, 2005). In cats, the disease may be triggered by FeLV, leading to a macrocytic non-regenerative anaemia. Secondary myelodysplasia is often termed dysmyelopoiesis, which may be triggered by underlying diseases such as IMHA and lymphoma and may lead to a similar haematological picture, but is reversible if the underlying disease process is successfully treated.

Non-regenerative anaemia associated with feline viral infections

Historically, FeLV was a common cause of anaemia due to a variety of mechanisms including leukaemia, myelodysplasia, aplastic anaemia, secondary PRCA and IMHA and FeLV-related immunosuppression leading to anaemia of chronic disease. However, as the prevalence of this virus has declined, it has become a less frequent cause of anaemia, and was identified in only 4.1% of anaemic cats in one study (Korman *et al.*, 2013). In that study, FIV was present in 4.8% of cases; feline infectious peritonitis (FIP) was diagnosed in 9.4% of cases, and the severity of anaemia varied from mild to very severe within this group.

Anaemia due to nutritional deficiencies

Iron deficiency is the most common nutritional deficiency and is discussed above under chronic blood loss. Severe malnutrition may also cause anaemia, owing to combined deficiency of protein, energy, B vitamins and minerals. Deficiency in folate or cobalamin (vitamin B12) may cause anaemia because these vitamins are required for DNA synthesis. The effect of deficiency on erythropoiesis is that nuclear maturation lags behind cytoplasmic maturation, and the red cell precursor divides fewer times than usual before the nucleus is extruded. The result is the formation of large red blood cells which contain a normal amount of haemoglobin (macrocytic normochromic anaemia).

Deficiencies of these vitamins are unusual in dogs and cats, but cobalamin deficiency occurs as an autosomal recessive disorder in Giant Schnauzers, Border Collies, Shar Peis and Australian Shepherds, as a result of defective ileal absorption. Affected puppies may have a mild to moderate non-regenerative anaemia (normocytic, but with increased RDW and some macrocytic cells present on the blood film) and also neutropenia (again due to defective DNA synthesis). Platelet numbers are usually normal. All these abnormalities resolve following parenteral supplementation with cobalamin. Cobalamin deficiency may occur in cats with exocrine pancreatic insufficiency and severe ileal disease, although this does not always lead to anaemia. Folate-deficiency anaemia is very uncommon, despite widespread use of drugs that cause folate depletion, such as phenobarbital.

Anaemia secondary to inflammatory or metabolic disease

Non-regenerative anaemia commonly results from a disease outside the bone marrow. Such diseases can be broadly categorized into anaemia of inflammatory disease (AID), anaemia of chronic renal failure and anaemia secondary to endocrine disease.

Anaemia of inflammatory disease: This is often termed anaemia of chronic (inflammatory) disease, although anaemia may develop quite quickly (within 10 days) in association with many inflammatory disorders, e.g. chronic infection, tissue trauma or tissue necrosis associated with malignant neoplasms. Several factors contribute to the development of anaemia.

- There is increased production of hepcidin, a hormone produced mainly in the liver which decreases the bioavailability of iron by limiting dietary absorption and mobilization from iron stores. Hepcidin is an acute phase protein and therefore increases in both acute and chronic systemic inflammation as a result of increased levels of IL-1 and IL-6. Low iron bioavailability leads to reduced erythropoiesis.
- Shortened red cell survival, possibly due to increased oxidative damage or binding of immunoglobulin to red cell membranes, leading to increased clearance by macrophages.
- Blunted release of, and response to, erythropoietin, probably due to the effect of cytokines, such as IL-1 and tumour necrosis factor, which are released in inflammation.

The anaemia is usually normocytic and normochromic, although occasionally it is microcytic and hypochromic (owing to relative iron deficiency), in which case evaluation of iron stores is useful to distinguish this from true iron deficiency (see Figure 4.20). There is often an inflammatory leucogram, and acute phase proteins as well as globulins may be elevated.

Anaemia secondary to renal failure: Chronic renal failure causes decreased production of erythropoietin, leading to decreased erythropoiesis, which results in normocytic normochromic non-regenerative anaemia. Other factors contributing to the anaemia include haemorrhage, due to gastric ulceration, and reduction in red cell lifespan, due to uraemic toxins. Unlike other secondary anaemias, the anaemia of renal failure can be severe and cause significant clinical signs.

Anaemia secondary to endocrine disease: Both cortisol and thyroxine enhance the effects of erythropoietin, therefore, deficiencies in these hormones lead to anaemia. Mild anaemia is often seen in hypothyroidism, and can be considered a physiological adaptation to lowered metabolic rate. Mild to moderate anaemia frequently occurs in dogs with hypoadrenocorticism, although this may be masked by haemoconcentration. GI haemorrhage may occur, in which case a more severe anaemia is seen.

Bone marrow sampling

The bone marrow should be evaluated in animals with non-regenerative anaemia, once it has been established that the anaemia is truly non-regenerative rather than pre-regenerative, and when underlying causes of secondary anaemia have been ruled out. Renal failure is the main secondary cause of severe non-regenerative anaemia (PCV <20% in dogs, <18% in cats) while AID and endocrine disease are unlikely to cause such severe anaemia. Bone marrow may be examined by obtaining either a bone marrow aspirate or a core biopsy sample. Aspirates provide superior cellular detail while core biopsy samples allow evaluation of cellularity and the presence of fibrous tissue. Often an aspirate and core sample are taken simultaneously as the samples provide complementary information. Other indications for bone marrow sampling are given in Chapter 5.

Depending on the site of aspiration, the bone marrow aspirate and core biopsy samples can be obtained under general anaesthesia or with sedation and local anaesthesia. The proximal humerus is generally the preferred site, although general anaesthesia will be required for appropriate positioning of the patient and because the procedure is painful. Where there is a contraindication to general anaesthesia, the iliac crest can be used with a combination of sedation, analgesia and local anaesthesia. The trochanteric fossa and tibial crest are other possible sites.

A high-quality bone marrow needle with stylet is required. The main choice is between the locked stylet (Jamshidi type), where the stylet cannot be pushed back during insertion, and the non-locking stylet (Klima and Rosenthal needles), where care has to be taken to keep the stylet in position during insertion. The Jamshidi can be used to obtain both aspirates and core samples, while the Klima is only used for aspirates. Spinal needles are not suitable. The size of needle should be appropriate to the patient and the site being aspirated, as shown in Figure 4.35. Other equipment required includes microscope slides, a scalpel blade, lidocaine, sterile gloves and drape,

Animal weight	Suggested Jamshidi needle (G)
Cats Dogs <5 kg	16–18
Dogs 5–15 kg	15–16
Dogs 15–30 kg	13–15
Dogs 30–50 kg	11–13
Dogs >50 kg	8

4.35 A guide to the size of Jamshidi needles used in bone marrow aspiration and biopsy.

a 20 ml syringe and sterile anticoagulant. Citrate, phosphate, dextrose and adenine (CPDA) collected from a blood transfusion bag is preferable, although a solution of EDTA prepared from a blood collection tube is adequate. The EDTA solution is prepared by filling an EDTA tube to the line with sterile saline. Ten or so microscope slides are placed ready for the sample, leaning on a near vertical slope, e.g. against a sandbag. Further slides are required for making smears and are positioned nearby.

Procedure for sampling from the greater tubercle of the humerus:

1. The patient is anaesthetized and placed in lateral recumbency. This should be right lateral recumbency for a right-handed operator and left lateral recumbency for a left-handed operator.
2. The area over the shoulder joint is clipped and surgically prepared.
3. An assistant flexes the elbow and shoulder joints and rotates the elbow inwards towards the body wall, such that the shoulder joint is turned outwards. The spine of the scapula and the distal end of the acromium are palpated. The next bony prominence distal to this is the greater tubercle of the humerus, which is the site for the aspirate.
4. Local anaesthetic, e.g. 2% lidocaine, is instilled (0.25 ml in cats and up to 1–2 ml in dogs) into the area, first into the subcutaneous tissues using a 23 G needle. The needle is advanced down to the surface of the greater tubercle and lidocaine is injected into the periosteum by applying pressure on the needle and syringe.
5. A small skin incision is made using a scalpel blade over the distal end of the greater tubercle.
6. The Jamshidi needle is primed with the anticoagulant solution. The stylet is withdrawn from the needle and, with the 20 ml syringe, anticoagulant is flushed through the needle and the syringe emptied. The stylet is replaced and locked in place.
7. The Jamshidi needle is held in the palm of the hand using a pistol grip, with the heel of the needle in the palm of the hand and the needle supported by the index finger.
8. The needle is inserted into the greater tubercle parallel to the long axis of the humerus, aiming for the point of the elbow. It may be difficult to get a purchase in the bone, but with repeated twisting of the needle to and fro with firm pressure the needle tip enters the bone cortex. Further firm pressure is applied while rotating the needle to and fro to advance the needle. Similarly, firm counterpressure needs to be applied by an assistant to stop the animal being pushed off the table.
9. Once it is in the medullary cavity the needle should feel firmly lodged and it should not be possible to wobble the needle from side to side. Indeed the animal could be lifted off the table by raising the needle.

10. The stylet is removed and the 20 ml syringe attached. The syringe is then firmly aspirated by pulling sharply on the plunger 2–3 times, applying around 15 ml of suction each time and holding the barrel of the syringe firmly (Figure 4.36a). Bone marrow (thick bloody material) should appear in the syringe. Once marrow appears, further aspiration should not be attempted because this could result in haemodilution.

11. The syringe is removed, leaving the Jamshidi needle in place, and marrow is quickly transferred to glass slides before it clots.

12. A drop of marrow is placed at the top of each of the tilted glass slides. Blood runs down to the base of the slides, leaving marrow spicules on the slides. Squash smears are made by placing a second slide flat over the first slide at right angles to it (flattening spicules), and then drawing the second slide quickly and smoothly over the first slide (Figure 4.36b,c).

13. Before allowing the patient to recover from anaesthesia, one or two slides should be stained with a Diff-Quik® stain kit to check that marrow spicules have been harvested. Spicules appear as densely stained blue areas, but it is preferable to check under the microscope that the samples are of diagnostic quality and not excessively haemodiluted (Figure 4.37).

14. A core biopsy sample can then be obtained by advancing the needle a further 2–3 cm down the humeral shaft without the stylet in place. Once advanced, the needle is moved sideways quickly in different directions or rotated repeatedly in the same direction, to ensure that the core is sectioned at its base.

15. The needle is then withdrawn. The core is pushed out of the needle by placing a blunt probe in the needle tip end and pushing the core sample out of the handle end (this is because the needle is tapered, and wider at the handle end).

16. Impression smears can be made by rolling the core down a glass slide, before placing it in formalin for histopathological analysis.

17. A sterile dressing is placed and opioid analgesia given for 4–6 hours after the procedure.

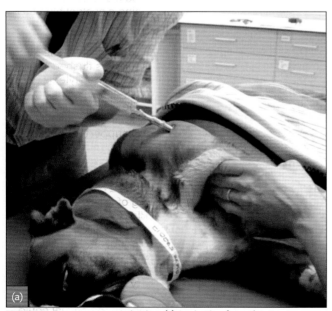

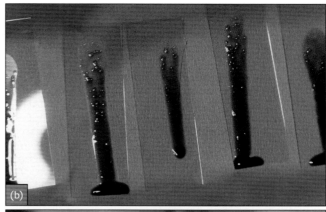

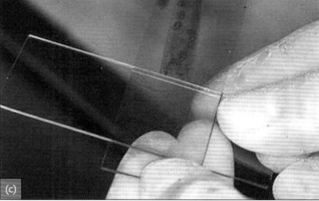

4.36 Bone marrow aspiration. (a) Aspiration from the greater tubercle of the humerus. (continues) ▶

4.36 (continued) Bone marrow aspiration. (b) Drops of marrow are placed at the top of the tilted slide, allowing blood to run off to the bottom of the slide but retaining the spicules. (c) Smears are made by placing a second slide over the first, thus spreading the spicules, and then smoothly drawing the slides apart.

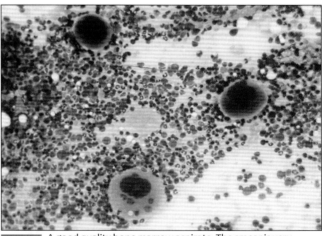

4.37 A good quality bone marrow aspirate. The smear is very cellular and cells have spread into a monolayer without clotting. Three megakaryocytes are present, with large multilobulated nuclei. (May–Grünwald–Giemsa stain; original magnification X1000)

If attempts at marrow aspiration are unsuccessful, this may be the result of poor technique or the presence of myelofibrosis or myelophthisis. Aspiration can be attempted at another site such as the other greater tubercle or iliac crest. If repeated aspirates are unsuccessful a core biopsy sample should be taken. An impression smear of the core can be made by rolling the core on to a glass slide. Lysine-coated slides may harvest more cells than standard slides.

Erythrocytosis

Erythrocytosis (also referred to as polycythaemia) is characterized by an increase in the red cell count, haemoglobin concentration and PCV. It can be classified as relative or absolute. Absolute erythrocytosis is categorized as primary (true) or secondary. *Relative erythrocytosis* is caused by disturbances in fluid balance resulting in dehydration. The total red cell mass remains normal but the decrease in plasma volume results in an increase in the total plasma protein concentration.

Animals with erythrocytosis may have red mucous membranes and congested retinal blood vessels. The hyperviscosity may lead to polyuria and polydipsia (PU/PD), weakness, ataxia and, in severe cases, seizures or visual disturbances.

Primary erythrocytosis

Primary erythrocytosis, also known as polycythaemia rubra vera, is a chronic myeloproliferative disease characterized by clonal proliferation of erythroid precursor cells with maturation and differentiation into morphologically normal red blood cells. This proliferation is not controlled by normal feedback mechanisms and is not driven by erythropoietin. Indeed, erythropoietin levels are usually low or undetectable as a result of negative feedback.

Secondary erythrocytosis

This occurs in response to increased erythropoietin secretion, which may be an *appropriate* compensatory response to chronic hypoxia due to:

- Chronic pulmonary disease
- Right to left cardiovascular shunting, e.g. patent ductus arteriosus, tetralogy of Fallot
- Living at high altitude
- Persistent methaemoglobinaemia.

Alternatively, the increased levels of erythropoietin may be present without systemic hypoxia, termed *inappropriate* secondary erythrocytosis. This has been reported in conjunction with renal tumours (carcinoma, adenocarcinoma, fibrosarcoma and lymphoma) and is thought to be the result of local hypoxia within the kidney or secretion of erythropoietin by the tumour. Benign renal cysts and hydronephrosis have also been suggested as causes of inappropriate secondary erythrocytosis. Extrarenal neoplasia is uncommonly associated with erythrocytosis, but in dogs has been reported with caecal leiomyosarcoma, schwannoma and nasal fibrosarcoma (Durno *et al.*, 2011). In the cat, most cases of erythrocytosis are primary. Secondary erythrocytosis is much less common, and is usually in response to hypoxia although there are a few reports in association with renal adenocarcinoma (Klainbart *et al.*, 2008). Mild erythrocytosis may occur with hyperthyroidism and hyperadrenocorticism but does not cause clinical signs.

Differentiating causes of erythrocytosis

In relative erythrocytosis, clinical examination usually reveals signs of dehydration. In addition, total protein, urea and creatinine are usually elevated. The PCV returns to normal once the dehydration is corrected.

If relative erythrocytosis can be ruled out, causes of secondary erythrocytosis should be investigated. The history and physical examination may provide vital clues, e.g. a heart murmur or renal mass. Thoracic radiographs and echocardiography are used to assess the cardio-pulmonary system. Arterial blood gases are useful in assessing hypoxia, and renal ultrasonography is used to detect renal neoplasia.

If no secondary cause is identified a presumptive diagnosis of primary erythrocytosis is made. Bone marrow aspiration is not helpful in distinguishing primary and secondary erythrocytosis because in both cases erythroid hyperplasia is present, but the red cells and their precursors are morphologically normal. Measurement of erythropoietin is helpful: erythropoietin is low or low normal in primary erythrocytosis and is usually elevated in secondary erythrocytosis, in particular in animals with renal tumours. However, erythropoietin is not always elevated in secondary erythrocytosis and may be normal in animals with primary erythrocytosis, thus, erythropoietin concentrations should never replace a thorough clinical and laboratory evaluation.

Blood typing

Rapid in-house tests are available for typing of canine and feline blood. These tests are used prior to blood transfusion and, in cats, can be used prior to mating to avoid neonatal isoerythrolysis.

In cats the major blood type system is the AB system, in which there are three blood types: A (most common); B (uncommon); and AB (very rare). Type A is common in the Domestic Shorthair. Type B is common in the British Shorthair and to a lesser extent the Cornish and Devon Rex and Birman breeds, and type AB is very rare although the prevalence varies in different geographical regions. All type B cats have high titres of naturally occurring anti-A isoantibodies. If a type B cat receives a type A blood transfusion a severe life-threatening or fatal transfusion reaction will take place. A proportion of type A cats have naturally occurring anti-B isoantibodies; these lead to mild/delayed transfusion reactions when such a cat is given type B blood. Transfusion reactions can be prevented by ensuring the donor and recipient are of the same blood type using in-house test cards which rely on agglutination for detection (Rapid Vet-H® (feline)) or immunochromatographic tests (Alvedia and RapidVet-H IC®).

Dogs have at least seven blood group systems, termed dog erythrocyte antigens (DEA), although there is no DEA 2 blood group. Canine red cells are either positive or negative for a given blood type, and an individual may be positive for several groups. Commercial blood typing tests are available only for DEA 1, which is the most potent stimulator of isoantibody production. As with cats, both agglutination methods and immunochromatographic methods are available. The DEA 1 group is now thought to be a single blood group which is variably expressed in a continuum from weak to moderate to strongly positive, rather than comprising two or three blood types (previously known as DEA 1.1, 1.2 and 1.3). This explains why weak reactions are sometimes seen when using immunochromatographic tests such as the Alvedia cartridge test. Weakly positive donors should be regarded as DEA 1 positive although it is prudent to give weakly positive recipients DEA 1 negative blood (Acierno *et al.*, 2014).

Blood typing, cross-matching and transfusion are discussed in detail in the *BSAVA Manual of Canine and Feline Haematology and Transfusion Medicine*.

Case examples

CASE 1

SIGNALMENT

5-year-old male Bernese Mountain Dog.

HISTORY

The dog has a history of weakness, exercise intolerance and anaemia. On examination the mucous membranes are very pale and there is splenomegaly.

CLINICAL PATHOLOGY DATA

Haematology	Result	Reference interval
Haemoglobin (g/dl)	**3.1**	12.0–18.0
RBC (x 10¹²/l)	**1.19**	5.5–8.5
HCT (l/l)	**0.11**	0.37–0.55
MCV (fl)	**89.0**	60.0–77.0
MCHC (g/dl)	**29.4**	30.0–38.0
MCH (pg)	**26.1**	19.5–25.5
RDW (%)	**22.6**	12.0–14.9
Reticulocytes (x 10⁹/l)	**338**	<80
Nucleated red cells (x 10⁹/l)	**1.6**	0
WBC (x 10⁹/l)	**17.4**	6.0–15.0
Neutrophils (x 10⁹/l)	**13.22**	3.0–11.5
Lymphocytes (x 10⁹/l)	1.39	1.0–4.8
Monocytes (x 10⁹/l)	**2.43**	0.2–1.4
Eosinophils (x 10⁹/l)	0.35	0.1–1.2
Basophils (x 10⁹/l)	0.00	0.0–0.1
Platelets (x 10⁹/l)	**96**	200–500

Abnormal results are in **bold**.

Film comment: red cells show marked anisocytosis and polychromasia. Leucocyte morphology normal. Platelet numbers appear consistent with count, no clumping seen. Some large platelets.

Biochemistry	Result	Reference interval
Total protein (g/l)	**49**	54–77
Albumin (g/l)	**23**	25–40
Globulin (g/l)	26	23–45
Urea (mmol/l)	**12.5**	2.5–7.4
Creatinine (µmol/l)	87	40–145
Glucose (mmol/l)	**8.3**	3.3–5.8
ALT (IU/l)	24	13–88
ALP (IU/l)	104	14–105
Bilirubin (µmol/l)	**27**	0–16
Calcium (mmol/l)	2.1	2.1–2.8
Phosphate (mmol/l)	1.4	0.6–1.4
Cholesterol (mmol/l)	4.5	3.8–7.0
Triglyceride (mmol/l)	0.4	0.4–1.2

Abnormal results are in **bold**.

WHAT ABNORMALITIES ARE PRESENT AND WHAT ARE THE DIFFERENTIALS?

Haematology shows a severe anaemia with a strong regenerative response (high reticulocyte count, polychromasia and anisocytosis with a high red cell distribution width, numerous nucleated red cells). There is a moderate thrombocytopenia and a mild established inflammatory response. There is a mild elevation in bilirubin, a low total protein and albumin and mild elevation in urea and glucose.

Possible causes for regenerative anaemia are haemorrhage and haemolysis. Anaemia with concurrent low proteins and thrombocytopenia may suggest haemorrhage, e.g. due to a bleeding splenic lesion such as haemangiosarcoma (especially with the splenomegaly), or may be unrelated to the spleen, e.g. GI blood loss. The elevated urea might suggest GI bleeding, although elevated urea could also be prerenal as a result of dehydration or hypovolaemia. Low total protein and albumin can also be seen in erythrophagocytic histiocytic sarcoma, which would be an important consideration in this breed.

The combination of anaemia and elevated bilirubin suggests haemolysis. This could be immune-mediated (although no spherocytes were seen), or could be associated with erythrophagocytic histiocytic sarcoma, babesiosis (no history of travel in this case) and oxidative damage (no Heinz bodies or eccentrocytes noted on the blood film). The normal liver enzymes suggest the elevated bilirubin is not intra- or post-hepatic. The hyperglycaemia is likely to be due to stress.

The moderate thrombocytopenia may be immune-mediated, due to DIC, haemorrhage, splenic sequestration (given the reported splenomegaly) and bone marrow disease. Ehrlichiosis and babesiosis would be considerations if there were a history of travel.

Given the breed and the splenomegaly, erythrophagocytic histiocytic sarcoma of the spleen was the prime consideration. This would cause anaemia due to erythrophagia (i.e. extravascular haemolysis) and consequent elevation in bilirubin, as well as low albumin, and could cause thrombocytopenia due to DIC, splenic sequestration, secondary immune-mediated thrombocytopenia (IMT) or a combination of these.

WHAT FURTHER INVESTIGATIONS WOULD YOU PERFORM?

- Coagulation times.
- Abdominal ultrasonography and potentially fine-needle aspiration of spleen or any enlarged lymph nodes
- Coombs' test.

FURTHER RESULTS

Coagulation times were normal, excluding DIC, and a Coombs' test was negative. Ultrasound examination revealed generalized splenomegaly with a heterogeneous appearance, but no other abnormalities. Ultrasound-guided aspirates of the spleen revealed a population of macrophages and histiocytic cells phagocytosing red

→ CASE 1 CONTINUED

cells. The phagocytic cells did not exhibit marked criteria of malignancy, but this can be the case in the erythrophagocytic form of histiocytic sarcoma, in which the cells can be difficult to distinguish from macrophages. Hence the differentials were IMHA or erythrophagocytic histiocytic sarcoma.

FURTHER FOLLOW-UP

After a blood transfusion a splenectomy was performed and liver biopsy samples and a bone marrow aspirate obtained. Histology of the spleen showed moderate to

large numbers of macrophages/histiocytic cells containing phagocytosed red cells, but again these cells did not show marked criteria of malignancy. Similar cells were seen in the liver within hepatic sinusoids, and small numbers were seen in the bone marrow. In order to obtain a definitive diagnosis, immunohistochemistry was performed. The phagocytic cells stained with CD11d and CD18, which confirmed the diagnosis of erythrophagocytic histiocytic sarcoma involving the spleen, liver and bone marrow. Treatment was initiated with lomustine but there was a poor response, with progressive anaemia resulting in euthanasia 2 months after the initial presentation.

CASE 2

SIGNALMENT

10-year-old male neutered Border Collie.

HISTORY

Sudden onset of severe weakness and dark red–brown urine over a 2-day period. On examination he is very pale with tachycardia and a haemic murmur but no other abnormalities.

CLINICAL PATHOLOGY DATA

Haematology	Result	Reference interval
Total haemoglobin (g/dl)	3.7	12.0–18.0
Cellular haemoglobin (g/dl)	2.3	12.0–18.0
RBC (x 10^{12}/l)	1.11	5.5–8.5
HCT (l/l)	0.09	0.37–0.55
MCV (fl)	77.3	60.0–77.0
MCHC (g/dl)	27.4 [a]	30.0–38.0
MCH (pg)	21.1 [a]	19.5–25.5
RDW (%)	16.8	12.0–14.9
Nucleated red cells (x 10^9/l)	4.3	0
WBC (x 10^9/l)	33.0	6.0–15.0
Neutrophils (x 10^9/l)	28.01	3.0–11.5
Band neutrophils (x 10^9/l)	1.32	<0.5
Lymphocytes (x 10^9/l)	1.93	1.0–4.8
Monocytes (x 10^9/l)	1.65	0.2–1.4
Eosinophils (x 10^9/l)	0.05	0.1–1.2
Basophils (x 10^9/l)	0.00	0.0–0.1
Platelets (x 10^9/l)	284	200–500

[a] Values calculated using cellular haemoglobin. Abnormal results are in **bold**.

WHAT ARE THE SIGNIFICANT ABNORMALITIES? WHY ARE THE TWO HAEMOGLOBIN MEASUREMENTS DIFFERENT AND HOW COULD THIS EXPLAIN THE APPEARANCE OF THE URINE?

There is very severe anaemia, which is macrocytic, hypochromic with an increased RDW suggesting regeneration. The total haemoglobin is higher than the

cellular haemoglobin which suggests intravascular haemolysis – the total haemoglobin includes any free in the plasma as well as that in the red cells, while the cellular haemoglobin is measured on the basis of the light scatter generated by the red cells. Intravascular haemolysis will cause haemoglobinuria, which could explain the discoloured urine.

There is a significant neutrophilia with a left shift and mild monocytosis indicating an acute inflammatory response.

DESCRIBE THE ABNORMALITIES PRESENT IN FIGURE 4.38. CAN YOU IDENTIFY A CAUSE FOR THE ANAEMIA? WHAT FURTHER TESTS ARE INDICATED?

There are numerous spherocytes (labelled 1), there are red cell ghosts reflecting intravascular haemolysis (labelled 2) and there is evidence of red cell regeneration with polychromasia (labelled 3). The leucocytes show toxicity with basophilic cytoplasm. The marked spherocytosis is consistent with IMHA, and the red cell ghosts, haemolysed plasma and suspected haemoglobinuria suggest intravascular haemolysis, concurring with the acute history.

Further tests should include:

- Coombs' test
- Biochemistry screen
- Coagulation screen
- Urinalysis
- Imaging to rule out an underlying trigger.

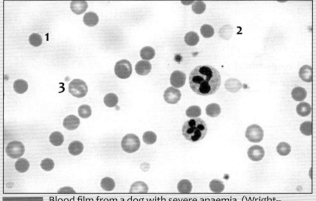

4.38 Blood film from a dog with severe anaemia. (Wright–Giemsa stain; original magnification X1000) →

→ CASE 2 CONTINUED

FURTHER RESULTS

Coombs' test positive at 1 in 128.
Plasma moderately haemolysed.

Urinalysis	Result
Appearance	Dark red–brown
Dipstick	4+ blood/Hb. Other dipstick tests difficult to interpret owing to discoloration
Specific gravity	1.025
Sediment	No red cells or white cells seen, a moderate amount of brownish particulate debris

Biochemistry	Result	Reference interval
Total protein (g/l)	68	54–77
Albumin (g/l)	34	25–40
Globulin (g/l)	34	23–45
Urea (mmol/l)	6.8	2.5–7.4
Creatinine (μmol/l)	124	40–145
Glucose (mmol/l)	**6.2**	3.3–5.8
ALT (IU/l)	**345**	13–88
ALP (IU/l)	**462**	14–105
Bilirubin (μmol/l)	**20**	0–16
Calcium (mmol/l)	2.6	2.1–2.8
Phosphate (mmol/l)	1.2	0.6–1.4

Abnormal results are in **bold**.

Coagulation screen	Result	Reference interval
Prothrombin time (seconds)	12	7–12
aPTT (seconds)	**37**	15–25
D-dimers	**500–1000**	<250

Abnormal results are in **bold**.

SUMMARIZE THESE FINDINGS AND THEIR SIGNIFICANCE

The positive Coombs' test with high titre together with spherocytes is consistent with IMHA.

Urinalysis confirms the suspicion of haemoglobinuria: red cells are absent and the brownish-red particulate material is free haemoglobin.

Elevated liver enzymes may be due to hypoxia or possibly thrombus formation, leading to ischaemic damage. Elevated bilirubin is more likely to be prehepatic, due to haemolysis. There is no azotaemia (renal tubular damage can be a sequel of haemoglobinuria).

The coagulation screen shows a prolonged activated partial thromboplastin time (aPTT) and elevated D-dimers, which in the context of the other clinical findings suggest a prothrombotic state or early DIC, which is quite commonly seen in IMHA, especially with intravascular haemolysis.

Thoracic radiography and abdominal ultrasonography were unremarkable; no secondary cause for IMHA was detected.

The dog was treated with a transfusion of packed cells, azathioprine and immunosuppressive doses of prednisolone. Initially there was a poor response but after a week the red cell parameters began to improve and the coagulation abnormalities resolved.

CASE 3

SIGNALMENT

7-year-old female neutered Springer Spaniel.

HISTORY

3-week history of progressive exercise intolerance, weakness and lethargy. On clinical examination she is pale but reasonably bright and alert and there are no other abnormalities.

CLINICAL PATHOLOGY DATA

Haematology	Result	Reference interval
Haemoglobin (g/dl)	**3.1**	12.0–18.0
RBC (x 10¹²/l)	**1.34**	5.5–8.5
HCT (l/l)	**0.10**	0.37–0.55
MCV (fl)	74.0	60.0–77.0
MCHC (g/dl)	31.0	30.0–38.0
MCH (pg)	23.1	19.5–25.5
RDW (%)	**17**	12.0–14.9
Reticulocytes (x 10⁹/l)	11	<80
WBC (x 10⁹/l)	13.07	6.0–15.0 ▶

Abnormal results are in **bold**.

Haematology *continued*	Result	Reference interval
Neutrophils (x 10⁹/l)	9.74	3.0–11.5
Lymphocytes (x 10⁹/l)	**0.90**	1.0–4.8
Monocytes (x 10⁹/l)	**1.94**	0.2–1.4
Eosinophils (x 10⁹/l)	**0.08**	0.1–1.2
Platelets (x 10⁹/l)	394	200–500

Abnormal results are in **bold**.

Biochemistry	Result	Reference interval
Total protein (g/l)	56	54–77
Albumin (g/l)	29	25–40
Globulin (g/l)	27	23–45
Urea (mmol/l)	6.0	2.5–7.4
Creatinine (μmol/l)	50	40–145
Glucose (mmol/l)	5.6	3.3–5.8
ALT (IU/l)	**192**	13–88
ALP (IU/l)	**334**	14–105
Bilirubin (μmol/l)	4	0–16
Calcium (mmol/l)	2.3	2.1–2.8
Phosphate (mmol/l)	1.4	0.6–1.4

Abnormal results are in **bold**.

→ **CASE 3 CONTINUED**

SUMMARIZE THE ABNORMALITIES. ARE THERE ANY SIGNIFICANT BLOOD FILM FINDINGS? WHAT FURTHER TESTS WOULD YOU DO?

There is a very severe non-regenerative anaemia (normocytic, normochromic with a low reticulocyte count). Given the duration of the clinical signs this appears genuinely non-regenerative rather than pre-regenerative, and the dog is coping quite well clinically suggesting a gradual onset. There is a stress leucogram.

The blood film shows normochromic red cells with no polychromasia (Figure 4.39). There are a few oval or tear drop-shaped cells, an acanthocyte and some red cells with an irregular shape suggesting fragmentation. These changes are sometimes seen in myelofibrosis. The red cell poikilocytosis may explain the increased RDW.

The biochemistry shows mildly elevated liver enzymes which are not likely to be significant and may be due to hypoxia. There is no evidence of renal failure.

To investigate this anaemia further, a bone marrow aspirate and core sample were obtained, after treatment with packed red cells which raised the HCT to 0.22 l/l.

The bone marrow aspiration was unsuccessful and only a small amount of bloody fluid was obtained without any marrow spicules. The core biopsy sample showed extensive fibrosis with approximately 50% of the haemopoietic space occupied by fibrous tissue. There was abundant haemosiderin, normal numbers of

megakaryocytes and a reduced myeloid:erythroid ratio (i.e. more erythroid than myeloid precursors present).

The diagnosis was myelofibrosis. There were no abnormal megakaryocytes or myeloid cells to suggest primary idiopathic myelofibrosis and the disease was pre-sumed to be secondary. The underlying trigger was not identified, but non-regenerative IMHA is often suspected in such cases and treatment with immunosuppressive therapy was commenced. There was a poor initial response with a fall in red cell parameters to pre-transfusion levels within 3 weeks and the owner then declined further treatment.

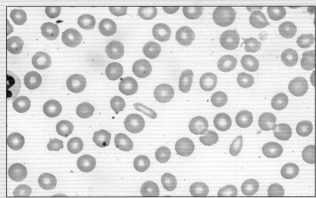

4.39 Blood film from a dog with severe non-regenerative anaemia. (Wright–Giemsa stain; original magnification X1000)

CASE 4

SIGNALMENT

11-year-old female neutered Domestic Shorthair cat.

HISTORY

3-month history of diarrhoea, progressive weakness and lethargy. On examination she is pale but there are no other abnormalities.

CLINICAL PATHOLOGY DATA

Haematology	Result	Reference interval
Haemoglobin (g/dl)	**5.0**	8.5–15.3
RBC (x 10¹²/l)	**6.84**	5.8–11.6
HCT (l/l)	**0.17**	0.27–0.46
MCV (fl)	**24.1**	36.9–54.9
MCHC (g/dl)	30.1	26.2–35.9
MCH (pg)	**7.3**	11.3–17.2
RDW (%)	**27.8**	13.8–18.1
Reticulocytes (x 10⁹/l)	**79**	<60
WBC (x 10⁹/l)	10.58	5.5–19.5
Neutrophils (x 10⁹/l)	6.71	2.5–12.5
Lymphocytes (x 10⁹/l)	2.35	1.5–7.0	▶

Abnormal results are in **bold**.

Haematology *continued*	Result	Reference interval
Monocytes (x 10⁹/l)	0.24	0.2–1.2
Eosinophils (x 10⁹/l)	1.28	0.1–1.2
Platelets (x 10⁹/l)	**218**	250–800

Abnormal results are in **bold**.

Film comment: moderate numbers of hypochromic red cells, moderate numbers of keratocytes and schistocytes. Numerous platelet clumps.

WHAT ABNORMALITIES ARE PRESENT AND WHAT IS THE LIKELY CAUSE?

There is a moderate microcytic, slightly regenerative anaemia with low MCH and hypochromic cells seen on the blood film, which is suggestive of iron deficiency due to external GI blood loss. The red cell fragmentation is a common feature of iron deficiency because the thin floppy red cells are liable to fragmentation damage. Increased RDW is due to the presence of small and normal-sized red cells (the latter were produced prior to the onset of iron deficiency) and also due to red cell fragmentation. MCH typically falls before MCHC in iron deficiency. The platelet count is falsely low owing to clumping.

→ **CASE 4 CONTINUED**

WHAT FURTHER TESTS COULD BE PERFORMED?

- Evaluation for a source of external blood loss, which could include faecal occult blood testing and urine analysis.
- Abdominal imaging.
- Evaluation of iron status would be useful: evaluating the reticulocyte haemoglobin, serum iron and total ion binding capacity.

Iron status	Result	Reference interval
Reticulocyte haemoglobin (pg)	**11.9**	14.6–19.0
Serum iron (μmol/l)	**4.5**	12–37
TIBC (μmol/l)	**71**	19–37

Abnormal results are in **bold**.

FURTHER RESULTS

- Urine analysis was unremarkable with no evidence of haematuria.
- Abdominal imaging showed a thickened area of small intestine with loss of layering.

The low reticulocyte haemoglobin content gives an early indication of developing iron deficiency. Serum iron is low, but this is also possible in inflammatory diseases. However, the elevated TIBC is supportive of iron deficiency (TIBC is low or normal in inflammation).

Faecal occult blood was not evaluated in this case because of the delay necessary to feed a suitable diet prior to sampling. Since urinary tract blood loss had been excluded and in view of the thickened area of intestine, GI blood loss was considered the likely cause. Following a transfusion, thoracic radiography was performed and no metastases were detected. An exploratory coeliotomy was performed and a jejunal mass was resected. Histopathology revealed an adenocarcinoma.

References and further reading

Acierno M, Raj K and Giger U (2014) DEA 1 expression on dog erythrocytes analyzed by immunochromatographic and flow cytometric techniques. *Journal of Veterinary Internal Medicine* **28**, 592–598

Aronsohn MG, Dubiel B, Roberts B *et al.* (2009) Prognosis for acute non-traumatic hemoperitoneum in the dog: a retrospective analysis of 60 cases (2003–2006) *Journal of the American Animal Hospital Association* **45**, 72–77

Ayoob AL, Prittie J and Hackner SG (2010) Feline babesiosis. *Journal of Veterinary Emergency and Critical Care* **20**, 90–97

Becker M, Moritz A and Giger U (2008) Comparative clinical study of canine and feline total blood cell count results with seven in-clinic and two commercial laboratory hematology analyzers. *Veterinary Clinical Pathology* **37**, 373–384

Brown DE, Weiser MG, Thrall MA *et al.* (1994) Erythrocyte indices and volume distribution in a dog with stomatocytosis. *Veterinary Pathology* **31(2)**, 247–250

Carr AP, Panciera DL and Kidd L (2002) Prognostic factors for mortality and thromboembolism in canine immune-mediated hemolytic anemia: a retrospective study of 72 dogs. *Journal of Veterinary Internal Medicine* **16**, 504–509

Caviezel LL, Raj K and Giger U (2014) Comparison of 4 direct Coombs' test methods with polyclonal antiglobulins in anaemic and non-anaemic dogs for in-clinic or laboratory use. *Journal of Veterinary Internal Medicine* **28**, 583–591

Culp WTN, Weisse C, Kellogg ME *et al.* (2010) Spontaneous hemoperitoneum in cats: 65 cases (1994–2006). *Journal of the American Veterinary Medical Association* **236**, 978–982

Day MJ (2000) Immune-mediated haemolytic anaemia. In: *Schalms Veterinary Haematology, 5th edn*, ed. BF Feldman, JG Zinkl and NC Jain, pp. 799–806. Lippincott, Williams and Wilkins, Philadelphia

Day MJ and Kohn B (2012) *BSAVA Manual of Canine and Feline Haematology and Transfusion Medicine, 2nd edn*. BSAVA Publications, Gloucester

Durno AS, Webb JA, Gauthier MJ and Bienzle D (2011) Polycythemia and inappropriate erythropoietin concentrations in two dogs with renal T-cell lymphoma. *Journal of the American Animal Hospital Association* **47**, 122–128

Duval D and Giger U (1996) Vaccine associated immune-mediated haemolytic anaemia in the dog. *Journal of Veterinary Internal Medicine* **10**, 290–295

Elders R and Blackwood L (2003) Haematological parameters in benign and malignant canine splenic diseases. *Proceedings of the American College of Veterinary Internal Medicine 2003*, p. 932

Fletch SM, Pinkerton PH and Brueckner PJ (1975) The Alaskan Malamute chondrodysplasia (dwarfism – anemia) syndrome: in review. *Journal of American Animal Hospital Association* **11**, 353–361

Friedrichs KR, Thomas C, Plier M *et al.* (2010) Evaluation of serum ferritin as a tumour marker for canine histiocytic sarcoma. *Journal of Veterinary Internal Medicine* **24**, 904–911

Gaskell RM, Gettinby G, Graham SJ *et al.* (2002) *Veterinary Products Committee Working Group on Feline and Canine Vaccination: Final report to the VPC*. DEFRA Publications, London

Goggs R, Boag AK and Chan DL (2008) Concurrent immune-mediated haemolytic anaemia and severe thrombocytopenia in 21 dogs. *Veterinary Record* **163(11)**, 323–327

Hammond TN and Pesillo-Crosby SA (2008) Prevalence of hemangiosarcoma in anemic dogs with a splenic mass and hemoperitoneum requiring a transfusion: 71 cases (2003–2005). *Journal of the American Veterinary Medical Association* **232**, 553–558

Hartman K, Addie D, Belak S *et al.* (2013) Babesiosis in cats. ABCD guidelines on prevention and management. *Journal of Feline Medicine and Surgery* **15**, 643–646

Hulme-Moir KL, Barker EN, Stonelake A, Helps CR and Tasker S (2010) Use of real-time polymerase chain reaction to monitor antibiotic therapy in a dog with naturally acquired *Mycoplasma haemocanis* infection. *Journal of Veterinary Diagnostic Investigation* **22**, 582–587

Keller SM, Vernau W, Hodjes J *et al.* (2013) Hepatosplenic and hepatocytotropic T-cell lymphoma: two distinct types of T-cell lymphoma in dogs. *Veterinary Pathology* **50**, 281–290

Klainbart S, Segev G, Loeb E *et al.* (2008) Resolution of renal adenocarcinoma-induced secondary inappropriate polycythaemia after nephrectomy in two cats. *Journal of Feline Medicine and Surgery* **10**, 264–268

Kohn K, Weingart C, Eckmann V *et al.* (2006) Primary immune mediated haemolytic anaemia in 19 cats: diagnosis, therapy and outcome (1998–2004). *Journal of Veterinary Internal Medicine* **20**, 159–166

Korman RM, Hetzel N, Knowles TG *et al.* (2013) A retrospective study of 180 anaemic cats: features, aetiologies and survival data. *Journal of Feline Medicine and Surgery* **15**, 81–90

Lilliehöök I and Tvedten H (2009) Validation of the Sysmex XT-2000iV hematology system for dogs, cats, and horses. I. Erythrocytes, platelets, and total leukocyte counts. *Veterinary Clinical Pathology* **38**, 163–174

McCullough S (2003) Immune-mediated haemolytic anaemia: understanding the nemesis. *Veterinary Clinics of North America: Small Animal Practice* **33**, 1295–1315

McManus P and Craig LE (2001) Correlation between leucocytosis and necropsy findings in dogs with immune-mediated haemolytic anaemia: 34 cases (1994–1999). *Journal of the American Veterinary Medical* Association **218**, 1308–1313

Miller SA, Hohenhaus AE and Hale AS (2004) Case controlled study of blood-type, breed, sex and bacteremia in dogs with immune-mediated haemolytic anaemia. *Journal of the American Veterinary Medical* Association **224**, 232–235

Moore PF, Affolter VK and Vernau W (2006) Canine hemophagocytic histiocytic sarcoma: A proliferative disorder of CD11d+ macrophages. *Veterinary Pathology* **43**, 632–645

Orcutt ES, Lee JA and Bianco D (2010) Immune-mediated hemolytic anemia and severe thrombocytopenia in dogs: 12 cases (2001–2008). *Journal of Veterinary Emergency and Critical Care* **20**, 338–345

Overmann JA, Sharkey LC, Weiss DJ and Borjesson DL (2007) Performance of 2 microtiter canine Coombs' tests. *Veterinary Clinical Pathology* **36**, 179–183

Prins M, van Leeuwen MW and Teske E (2009) Stability and reproducibility of ADVIA 120-measured red blood cell and platelet parameters in dogs, cats, and horses, and the use of reticulocyte haemoglobin content (CH(R)) in the diagnosis of iron deficiency. *Tijdschrift voor Diergeneeskunde* **134**, 272–278

Schaefer DMW and Stokol T (2015) The utility of reticulocyte indices in distinguishing iron-deficiency anaemia from anaemia of inflammatory disease, portosystemic shunting, and breed-associated microcytosis in dogs. *Veterinary Clinical Pathology* **44(1)**, 109–119

Schalm OJ (1976) Erythrocytic macrocytosis in miniature and toy poodles. *Canine Practice* **3**, 55–57

Serra M, Freeman KP, Campora C and Sacchini F (2012) Establishment of canine hematology reference intervals for the Sysmex XT-2000iV hematology analyzer using a blood donor database. *Veterinary Clinical Pathology* **41**, 207–215

Sinnott VB and Otto CM (2009) Use of thromboelastography in dogs with immune-mediated hemolytic anemia: 39 cases (2000–2008). *Journal of Veterinary Emergency and Critical Care* **19(5)**, 484–488

Smith FD and Wall LE (2013) Prevalence of *Babesia* and *Anaplasma* in ticks infesting dogs in Great Britain. *Veterinary Parasitology* **198**, 18–23

Sontas HS, Dokuzeylu B, Turna O *et al.* (2009) Oestrogen-induced myelotoxicity in dogs: A review. *Canadian Veterinary Journal* **50**, 1054–1058

Tasker S (2010) Haemotropic mycoplasmas: what's the real significance in cats? *Journal of Feline Medicine and Surgery* **12**, 369–381

Weiss DJ (2005) Recognition and classification of dysmyelopoiesis in the dog: A review. *Journal of Veterinary Internal Medicine* **19(2)**, 147–154

Weiss DJ (2008) Bone marrow pathology in dogs and cats with non-regenerative immune-mediated haemolytic anaemia and pure red cell aplasia. *Journal of Comparative Pathology* **138**, 46–53

Useful websites

European Centre for Disease Prevention and Control
ecdc.europa.eu/en/healthtopics/vectors/vector-maps/Pages/VBORNET-maps-tick-species.aspx

Chapter 5

Disorders of leucocytes

Laura Blackwood

Leucocytes (white blood cells) include granulocytes (neutrophils, eosinophils and basophils) and mononuclear cells (monocytes and lymphocytes). Leucocytes are vital for host defence, and for initiation and control of inflammation and immunity. Neutrophils, macrophages and natural killer (NK) cells (specialized lymphoid cells) provide the innate immune response, which is the first line of defence against an invading pathogen and does not involve immunological memory. Lymphoid cells orchestrate the adaptive or acquired immune response, activated by the inflammation induced by any pathogen that gets past the innate response. The adaptive immune response develops immunological memory.

In addition to being effector cells (carrying out functions), leucocytes play important regulatory roles in haemopoiesis, inflammation and immunity. Although generally protective of the host tissue, leucocytes are also involved in host-harmful inflammation, allergic and immune-mediated disease.

Normal leucocyte production is illustrated in Figure 5.1, and an overview of erythropoiesis is given in Chapter 4. The haemopoietic cells in the bone marrow can be

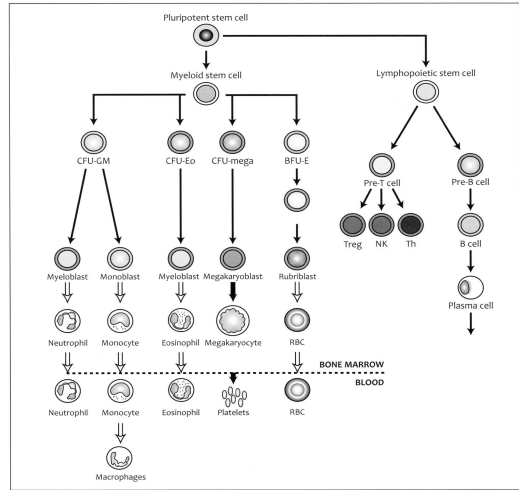

5.1 Haemopoiesis. BFU-E = burst-forming unit – erythroid; CFU-Eo = colony-forming unit – eosinophil; CFU-GM = colony-forming unit – granulocyte–monocyte; CFU-mega = colony-forming unit – megakaryocyte; NK = natural killer cell; RBC = red blood cell; Th = T helper cell; Treg = regulatory T cell.

divided into three groups: pluripotent stem cells; differentiating progenitor cells; and fully functional mature blood cells. Pluripotent stem cells are capable of self-renewal. As cells become committed to a certain cell lineage, their ability to proliferate is reduced and eventually lost. Thus, the marrow has a pyramidal structure, in which one stem cell gives rise to many daughter cells (see Figure 5.1). Specific information concerning production of all cell lines in dogs and cats is lacking, so some information in this chapter is drawn from information available for other mammalian species. The factors controlling granulopoiesis are less well defined than those controlling erythropoiesis.

Assessment of leucocytes

Assessment of white blood cells requires total and differential white cell counts (determined using blood samples taken into ethylenediamine tetra-acetic acid (EDTA)) and blood smear examination (see Chapters 2 and 3). A fresh blood smear should be submitted to the laboratory with every EDTA blood sample, because artefactual changes in cells occur in vitro within hours of sampling. There are some limitations when using in-house analysers: most produce reliable total white blood cell (WBC) counts and neutrophil counts, but differential and platelet counts are generally less reliable (Papasouliotis et al., 2006; Wengler-Riggenbach et al., 2006; Welles et al., 2009; Bauer et al., 2012; Goldman et al., 2012). They do not detect band neutrophils or toxic change, and differentials are less accurate for low numbers of cells and when there is neutropenia. Most analysers count nucleated red blood cells (RBCs) as white blood cells, although flow cytometry analysers may generate flags when nucleated red cells are present. Platelet counts should be verified by smear examination, and automated analysers do not always provide accurate platelet counts for cats (see Chapters 4 and 6). Ideally, machine-generated differential counts should be verified by a manual 200-cell differential count, and in every case a blood smear should be evaluated for morphological abnormalities.

Buffy coat smears (where a smear is made of the buffy coat only, after centrifugation) allow very large numbers of white blood cells to be examined rapidly: these are useful in identifying low numbers of aberrant cells or intracellular organisms where only a small proportion of leucocytes are affected.

Reference intervals

Reference intervals derived from available 'normal' populations are seldom truly demographically appropriate for the individual patient. Ideally age-, breed- and sex-matched animals with similar backgrounds and environments, and from the same geographical area, should be used (see Chapter 2) but this is clearly impractical. The reference interval provided by the laboratory carrying out the analysis should always be used.

Age- and breed-related changes

Leucocyte counts in infant and juvenile cats and dogs differ from those in adults, and this reflects the new challenges they face. Changes are also apparent in dams: total WBC counts are increased during pregnancy and lactation, and return to normal after weaning. Kittens have

a normal leucogram at birth, but by 3–4 months of age neutrophil and lymphocyte counts considerably exceed the adult range. These return to the adult range by 5–6 months of age.

Most of the age related data for dogs are based on laboratory Beagles; in these dogs band neutrophils may be above the reference range for the first few days of life but are within the adult range by 7–10 days (Shafrine et al., 1973). Lymphocytosis is a common finding, and dogs less than 6 months of age typically have lymphocyte counts between 2 and 10 x 10^9/l. Total WBC counts have also been assessed in a group of Beagles and Labrador Retrievers: total leucocyte counts were higher at 3–8 weeks of age than at any later lifestage, and remained elevated above adult values until 4 months of age (Harper et al., 2003). In this group, total WBC counts tended to decrease from 2 years of age, and WBC counts in dogs under 5 years old were significantly greater than for those over 5 years (Harper et al., 2003). For the young (<1 year) and the old (>8 years) there were also significant differences in total count between the two breeds, with Beagles having higher counts, especially as puppies. Thus, ranges based on laboratory Beagles may not reflect normality in other breeds.

Other breed-related physiological (rather than pathological) leucocyte abnormalities have been identified. Sighthounds, including Lurchers, tend to have lower WBC counts than other breeds. Breed-specific reference intervals are available for Greyhounds (Campora et al., 2011; Lefebvre, 2011) but cannot be applied to all sighthounds (Uhríková et al., 2013). Importantly, the lower limit of the neutrophil reference interval for Greyhounds ranges from 2.1 to 2.6 x 10^9/l for most analysers (Zaldívar-López et al., 2011), which would be neutropenic if non-Greyhound reference intervals were used. Belgian Tervuren dogs in the USA have been documented to have lower neutrophil, monocyte and lymphocyte counts than other dogs (Greenfield et al., 2000), although a study failed to show such physiological leucopenia in Tervurens in their home country (Gommeren et al., 2004). The latter study also supported a decrease in total WBC count with ageing, as found in Labradors and Beagles. There is also evidence of reduced neutrophil function in elderly Beagles (>8 years) (Hall et al., 2010).

Senior cats (>10 years of age) have been shown to have lower total WBC counts, lower lymphocyte and lower eosinophil counts than younger adults (Campbell et al., 2004).

Morphological variations in leucocytes are also breed-related. For example, Greyhounds have abnormal eosinophils, whose granules do not stain and appear as numerous clear cytoplasmic vacuoles, but these dogs have no related disease problems. Similarly, Birman cats show atypical neutrophil granulation that is not associated with neutrophil dysfunction.

Granulocytes

Granulopoiesis is the process by which granulocytes are produced. The CFU-C (so called because it was first described in colony-forming units in culture) is the multipotent stem cell for the granulocyte series. These stem cells are morphologically similar to small lymphocytes. In the presence of colony-stimulating factors (CSFs) they proliferate and differentiate into the cells of the granulocyte–monocyte lineages. The CFU-GM (granulocyte–monocyte colony-forming unit) has been identified as the particular CFU-C progenitor that gives rise to both granulocytes and monocytes.

G-CSF (granulocyte colony-stimulating factor) and GM-CSF (granulocyte–monocyte colony-stimulating factor) are the specific CSFs involved in granulopoiesis. There are probably CSFs for each cell lineage. In addition to CSFs, macrophages, activated lymphocytes and endothelial cells produce local factors (mainly cytokines, including interleukin (IL)-2, IL-1, stem cell factor or kit ligand, IL-6 and IL-11) that stimulate granulopoiesis. Regulation of production is partly achieved by a negative feedback effect, mediated by inhibitory substances from mature neutrophils and prostaglandin E from macrophages, unless there is continued stimulation of granulocyte release.

The first morphologically recognizable granulocyte is the myeloblast. These cells differentiate through progranulocyte, myelocyte, metamyelocyte and band forms to become mature granulocytes (Figure 5.2). The capacity for cell division is lost at the metamyelocyte stage, by which time 16–32 myelocytes have arisen from each myeloblast.

Neutrophils

The neutrophil, or polymorphonuclear (PMN) leucocyte (Figure 5.3), is approximately 10–15 μm in diameter (about 1.5–2 canine red cells) and has a nucleus divided into three to five lobes by indentations. The nucleus has dark purple-staining clumped chromatin. The cytoplasm contains microbicidal and enzymatic granules important to its function, but these are either indiscernible or only faintly

visible as eosinophilic granules against the pale pink cytoplasm on Romanowsky stains. Barr bodies (see Figure 3.16bii) are protrusions of the nucleus that are present in females and represent the inactive X chromosome. They are of no clinical significance.

Neutrophils exist in the body in three major pools (Figure 5.4):

* Bone marrow
* Blood
* Tissue.

The bone marrow pool consists of the mitotic (dividing) pool, the maturation pool and the storage pool. In normal animals the storage pool of mature neutrophils harbours 5–7 days' worth of neutrophils. Release from the bone marrow is mediated by various factors, including complement 5a, tumour necrosis factors α and β, G-CSF and GM-CSF. Only when the demand is great, and the storage pool is depleted, are immature neutrophils released from the maturation pool, and band forms or more immature cells (see Figure 5.3) enter the circulation. In the circulation, the neutrophils form two pools, the circulating and marginating pools. The marginating pool consists of cells stuck to or rolling along the endothelium of small blood vessels. Blood samples only harvest cells from the circulating pool, and movement of cells between the marginating and circulating pools can affect counts. In dogs, roughly half the neutrophils exist in each pool, but in cats the marginating pool is three times greater than the circulating pool.

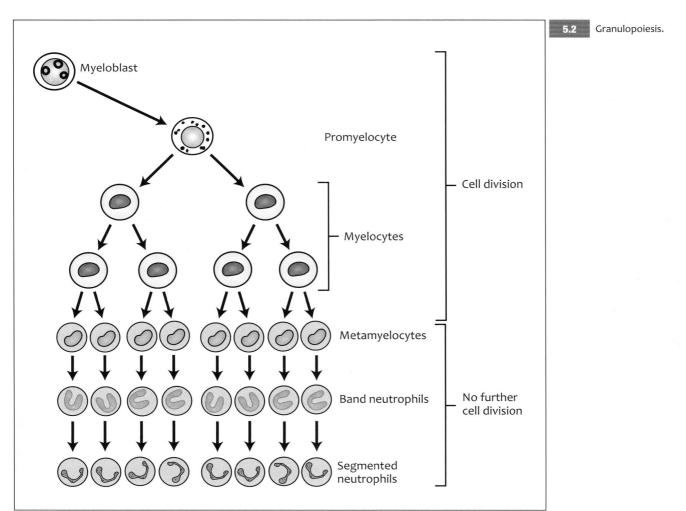

5.2 Granulopoiesis.

Myeloblast

Promyelocyte

Myelocytes

Metamyelocytes

Band neutrophils

Segmented neutrophils

Cell division

No further cell division

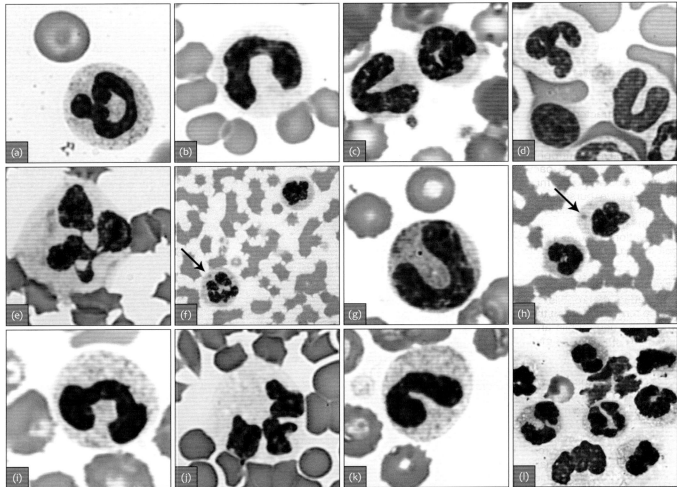

5.3 Neutrophils, characterized by a segmented nucleus with three to five lobes. (a) Normal neutrophil from a dog. (b–d) Band neutrophils, with U-shaped nuclei lacking segmentation. In (c) the band cell is to the left of a poorly preserved segmented neutrophil. (e–f) Hypersegmented neutrophils (feline). There is also pyknotic change. In (f) the neutrophil on the right has a condensed nucleus while the one on the left is hypersegmented; blue Döhle bodies are also evident (arrowed). In both (e) and (f) there is red cell crenation, supporting *in vitro* change due to an aged sample. These changes make appreciation of toxic change difficult. (g–k) Toxic changes in band and mature neutrophils. In (g) there is nuclear swelling, chromatin clumping, cytoplasmic basophilia and faint granulation. In (h) there is nuclear swelling, cytoplasmic basophilia and a Döhle body (arrowed). In (j) there is a swollen nucleus, with slightly clumped chromatin, and faint vacuolation. In (k) nuclear swelling, chromatin clumping and cytoplasmic basophilia are seen. (l) Degenerate neutrophils, with nuclear swelling, eosinophilia and lysis. Degenerative changes occur in neutrophils in the tissues and these changes are almost never seen in the circulation. (May–Grünwald–Giemsa stain (except (b, l) Rapi-Diff II® stain); original magnification X1000 (except (f, h) X400))

5.4 The major neutrophil pools of the body.

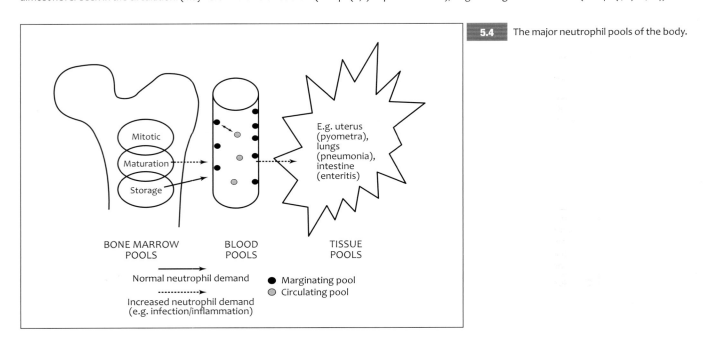

The circulating half-life of neutrophils in dogs and cats is only 6–12 hours, and counts can change rapidly in disease states. Even in the normal animal, the total neutrophil pool is replaced 1–2.5 times daily. Neutrophils leaving the circulation are lost across mucosal surfaces or phagocytosed in the liver and spleen. In the normal animal, there is no appreciable tissue pool, although large numbers of neutrophils may accumulate in tissues in disease, when they are attracted into tissue by various cytokines and chemokines. Neutrophils in normal tissues survive only 1–4 days, and survival is shortened in disease.

In disease, neutrophils can phagocytose organisms and kill or inactivate bacteria, yeasts, fungi or parasites (using lysosomal enzymes, microbicidal substances and the 'oxidative burst'). Neutrophils also help to eliminate infected and transformed cells, and modulate the immune and inflammatory responses, and are also involved in coagulation. Neutrophil numbers and distribution alter rapidly in disease states.

Neutrophil shifts

Circulating neutrophils may show left and right shifts. These terms arise from the side of the cell counter/page on which the neutrophils are recorded: band neutrophils are recorded to the left of mature neutrophils, so an increased number of immature cells gives a left shift.

Left shift: This occurs when the storage pool is depleted and there is continued demand for neutrophils, which is met by the release of immature neutrophils (predominantly band forms) from the maturation pool. If disease is severe or protracted, metamyelocytes and earlier precursors may also appear. Band neutrophils are of similar size to mature cells but have a minimally indented (suggested <50% of the width) U-shaped nucleus with almost parallel sides (see Figure 5.3b–d). Clinical pathologists are variably strict in their definition of a band neutrophil and how deep nuclear indentations can be before the neutrophil is mature, and this results in different normal reference intervals for band forms. The nuclei of band forms stain less heavily than those of mature neutrophils, as the chromatin is less condensed.

Left shifts may be either regenerative or degenerative:

- In a *regenerative* left shift, there are increased band neutrophils and there is a neutrophilia in which mature neutrophils exceed bands. A neutrophilia with a declining left shift may reflect declining tissue demand or accelerated bone marrow production meeting demand, and can be a good prognostic indicator
- In a *degenerative* left shift, there is a low or normal leucocyte count and band cells exceed mature neutrophils. This suggests that the bone marrow is unable to maintain adequate neutrophil numbers to meet the increased demand. A degenerative left shift is a poor prognostic indicator (Burton *et al.*, 2013).

There is no universally accepted value for what constitutes a significant left shift, but >1 × 10^9/l band neutrophils is often used. An increase in band neutrophils reflects an active inflammatory response, which could be due to infection, immune-mediated disease, tissue damage/necrosis or neoplasia; band cells are not pathognomonic for bacterial infection (see below). (In animals with Pelger–Huët anomaly, band neutrophils are released into the circulation and a left shift is not indicative of an increased inflammatory response.)

Right shift: This occurs when there is reduced egress from the circulation, most often mediated by endogenous cortisol or exogenous corticosteroids. A mature neutrophilia results, though this may be indistinguishable from other types of mature neutrophilia unless morphological changes occur. Hypersegmentation and pyknosis represent normal ageing change but neutrophils usually exit the circulation before these changes are evident; these changes may be seen in a right shift. Both changes may also occur *in vitro*, and are common artefacts (see Figure 5.3e–f). However, the presence of such cells in a fresh blood smear suggests extended neutrophil transit time. Hypersegmented neutrophils have more than five lobes in the nucleus.

Neutrophilia

The most common causes of neutrophilia are summarized in Figure 5.5.

Cause	Associated conditions	Mechanism of neutrophilia	Recognition factors
Physiological neutrophilia	Emotional distress Fear Vigorous exercise	Redistribution of neutrophils from marginating to circulating pools	No left shift Concurrent abnormalities • Lymphocytosis (cats especially) • Hyperglycaemia
Stress/steroid response	Hyperadrenocorticism Exogenous corticosteroids	Increased release of neutrophils from storage pool Shift from marginating to circulating pool Prolonged circulation time	No left shift Concurrent abnormalities (dogs) • Monocytosis • Lymphopenia • Eosinopenia • Elevated alkaline phosphatase Concurrent abnormalities (cats) • Lymphopenia • Eosinopenia
Acute inflammatory response	Bacterial infections Other infections Immune-mediated disease Neoplasia Tissue necrosis	Increased demand in response to pathogens and inflammation	May feature • Left shift • Toxic change Superimposed stress haemogram
Other (rare)	Chronic granulocytic leukaemia Neutrophil dysfunction	See Figure 5.7	See Figure 5.7

5.5 Common causes of neutrophilia in dogs and cats.

Physiological neutrophilia: This is especially common in cats, and can simply be a result of the stress of blood sampling. Emotional distress or fear results in release of adrenaline (epinephrine), and neutrophils redistribute from the marginating to the circulating pools. There is no left shift. Vigorous exercise also produces a similar response, most commonly in young dogs. Physiological neutrophilia may be accompanied by lymphocytosis (which is often greater in magnitude than the neutrophilia in cats) and/or hyperglycaemia, and is transient (20 minutes).

Stress/steroid-induced neutrophilia: Endogenous cortisol or exogenous corticosteroids produce a mature neutrophilia, mainly as a result of increased release of neutrophils from the storage pool, and also, to a lesser extent, due to a shift of cells from the marginating to the circulating pool, and reduced endothelial adherence resulting in prolonged circulation time (a true right shift). There is usually no left shift. Counts in dogs tend to be in the range $15–25 \times 10^9/l$ but may occasionally be as high as $40 \times 10^9/l$. Increases in cats are less marked and the total WBC count does not usually exceed $20 \times 10^9/l$ (but may occasionally be as high as $30 \times 10^9/l$). Other steroid-associated abnormalities may be present: in dogs, monocytosis, lymphopenia and eosinopenia, and biochemical changes (markedly elevated alkaline phosphatase (ALP) with moderately elevated alanine transaminase (ALT)) are typical; in cats, monocytosis is not common and lymphopenia and eosinopenia may be the only other abnormalities, because there is no steroid-induced alkaline phosphatase.

Acute inflammatory response: Neutrophilia due to inflammation is seen in a wide range of disease processes, and may feature a left shift. The left shift may be regenerative or degenerative, depending on the demand for neutrophils and the marrow's ability to meet demand. In the face of increased demand, marrow transit time may be reduced and the neutrophils (mature and immature) may show toxic change (see below). Although bacterial infections are a very common cause of an acute inflammatory response, immune-mediated diseases and neoplasia are also frequent causes. In immune-mediated haemolytic anaemia (IMHA), a marked neutrophilia with a left shift is common. This is thought to be due to non-specific effects of marrow hyperactivity in response to the anaemia, endogenous steroid production and systemic inflammatory response secondary to tissue hypoxia and thrombosis. If the left shift is profound and accompanied by a strongly regenerative anaemia with circulating nucleated red blood cells (normoblastosis), this is called a leucoerythroblastic blood picture (Figure 5.6; see also Chapter 4). In many animals with an acute inflammatory response there is a superimposed stress haemogram, and eosinopenia and lymphopenia are common.

Toxic change

Toxic change refers to the morphological abnormalities (see Figure 5.3g–k) seen in neutrophils in severe inflammatory disease, especially severe bacterial infections, and in IMHA. These changes occur in the bone marrow prior to release and are associated with enhanced neutrophil turnover and reduced maturation time, as a result of intense stimulation of granulopoiesis. Some drugs and toxins can cause similar morphological changes, and some of the features of toxic change can develop in stored samples.

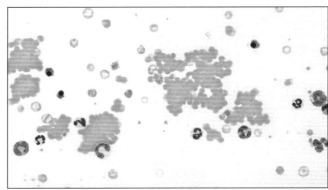

5.6 A leucoerythroblastic blood picture in a dog with immune-mediated haemolytic anaemia. There is red cell agglutination, and most of the red cells that have agglutinated are spherocytes. There is a strongly regenerative red cell response, with reticulocytes and normoblasts, and a similarly regenerative myeloid response, with band neutrophils and also band-like monocytes. (May–Grünwald–Giemsa stain; original magnification X400)

Toxic changes include:

- Increased cytoplasmic basophilia, as a result of increased residual cytoplasmic RNA
- Cytoplasmic vacuolation due to loss of granule and membrane integrity during disturbed maturation. (Vacuolation can develop as an artefact in stored samples)
- Döhle bodies: these are grey–blue intracytoplasmic inclusions representing aggregates of cytoplasmic reticulum. Döhle bodies are found in normal cats and are not considered to reflect toxic change unless they are frequent and prominent. (Döhle bodies can develop as an artefact in stored samples)
- Toxic granulation due to retention of acid mucopolysaccharides in primary granules (which stain with Romanowsky stains, unlike the secondary granules usually present in normal neutrophils)
- Giant neutrophils
- Nuclear swelling
- Doughnut nuclei.

Degenerative changes

Degenerative changes occur in neutrophils in the tissues rather than in the circulation, as a result of endotoxin exposure; they include nuclear swelling, chromatin dissociation and nuclear eosinophilia (see Figure 5.3l). These changes are more often appreciated in tissue and fluid samples, and are only rarely seen in the circulation in bacteraemia septicaemia.

Extreme neutrophilia

Markedly elevated neutrophil counts are seen in a wide variety of disease situations, and have been associated with poor prognosis in both dogs and cats. Extreme neutrophilias where there is a marked left shift have been described as leukaemoid reactions, because of the presence of immature cells. This term is misleading, and either extreme neutrophilia or extreme neutrophilic leucocytosis is preferred. The absolute numbers that constitute an extreme neutrophilia are controversial, but a total WBC count $>50 \times 10^9/l$, with >50% neutrophils, has been suggested for dogs and cats (Lucroy and Madewell, 1999, 2001). The causes of extreme neutrophilia are summarized in Figure 5.7. All diseases that can cause extreme neutrophilias can also cause less marked neutrophilia.

Cause	Examples of disease processes	Mechanism of neutrophilia	Recognition factors
Severe localized pyogenic infections	Pyometra Pyothorax Peritonitis Abscess	Extreme demand for neutrophils as disease process not controlled	Compatible clinical signs and imaging findings Toxic change in neutrophils Significant left shift
Other infectious diseases	Parasitic infections (dirofilariasis) Rickettsial infections (*Ehrlichia*, *Hepatozoon*) Fungal infections	Extreme demand for neutrophils as disease process not controlled	Compatible clinical signs Imaging, cytological, serological and polymerase chain reaction (PCR) findings
Immune-mediated disease	Immune-mediated haemolytic anaemia (IMHA) Immune-mediated thrombocytopenia (IMTP) Immune-mediated polyarthritis (IMPA)	Non-specific stimulation of granulopoieisis (IMHA, IMTP) Response to inflammation Tissue necrosis due to hypoxia (IMHA), thrombosis	Compatible clinical signs and laboratory findings: • IMHA: markedly regenerative anaemia, spherocytosis, possibly autoagglutination or positive direct antibody or Coombs' test (see Chapter 4) • IMTP: profound thrombocytopenia • IMPA: appropriate joint fluid cytology (see Chapter 23)
Neoplasia	Any solid tumour	Tissue necrosis in large mass lesions Possible production of colony stimulating factors by the tumour	Compatible clinical signs ± imaging (mass lesion)
Tissue necrosis	Trauma Infection Neoplasia Vascular occlusion (torsions, thrombosis, tumour emboli)	Response to inflammation at site of necrosis	Clinical signs and imaging findings of primary disease
Chronic granulocytic leukaemia		Neoplastic transformation of committed mature granulocyte	Left shift Aberrant cells Thrombocytopenia Extramedullary granulopoiesis in multiple sites
Neutrophil dysfunction	Leucocyte adhesion deficiency (Irish Setters)	Continued demand for neutrophils as pathogens not eliminated due to neutrophil dysfunction	Breed Demonstrable neutrophil dysfunction Positive genetic testing (homozygous for causative mutation)

5.7 Causes of extreme neutrophilia in dogs and cats.

Neutropenia

Neutropenia is generally a result of:

* Overwhelming demand and increased migration from circulation to tissues
* Decreased survival of cells
* Reduced or ineffective granulopoiesis.

Overwhelming demand is most common in severe bacterial infections, such as pyometra, peritonitis or pyothorax. In these cases, toxic change and a degenerative left shift are common, and there are compatible clinical signs. Reduced granulopoiesis is due either to bone marrow disease or to drug toxicity (cytotoxic drug-related myelosuppression or idiosyncratic drug reactions), and other cell lines may be affected. There is also a fourth, less common, type of neutropenia caused by shift from the circulating to marginating pool due to increased expression of adhesion molecules on the neutrophil surface. This is a transient cause of neutropenia in the first minutes to hours of endotoxic or anaphylactic shock. The causes of neutropenia, and features that help differentiate them, are summarized in Figure 5.8.

Collies have two inherited forms of neutropenia. Trapped neutrophil syndrome is an autosomal recessive condition of Border Collies reported in the UK, USA, Japan, Australia, New Zealand and Europe. These dogs have a mutation in the canine vesicle sorting protein (VPS) 13B gene. Genetic testing is now available in several countries, and carriers appear to be relatively frequent (Shearman and Wilton, 2011; Schnelle and Barger, 2012;

Mason et al., 2014). Finally, canine cyclic haemopoiesis is an autosomal recessive disorder of grey collies resulting in cyclic fluctuations in neutrophil, eosinophil, platelet and reticulocyte counts. It is caused by mutations in the gene encoding adapter protein complex 3, which is responsible for trafficking proteins to lysozymes, but which also has a role in feedback inhibition in normal haemopoeisis: this is disrupted and cyclic neutropenia results.

Neutrophil dysfunction

Hereditary neutrophil dysfunction has been reported in Irish Setters and crosses, who may suffer from canine leucocyte adhesion deficiency, an autosomal recessive defect resulting in reduced neutrophil function due to decreased expression of adhesion molecules CD11 and CD18. Genetic testing is available. Inherited neutrophil dysfunction has also been reported in other breeds: Weimaraners (oxidative metabolic disorder) and Dobermanns (defect in bacterial cell killing).

Chédiak–Higashi syndrome is an inherited autosomal recessive disorder of the microtubules and granules in leucocytes and other cells, reported in smoke-blue Persian cats with yellow–green irises. Haematologically, abnormally large eosinophilic granules are seen in neutrophils and eosinophils. Affected cats have bleeding tendencies due to platelet dysfunction. They have low to normal neutrophil counts, and the neutrophils show impaired chemotaxis and bacterial cell killing.

Many disease states including neoplasia are recognized causes of neutrophil dysfunction in humans. Acquired neutrophil dysfunction is probably quite common in small

Cause	Examples of disease process	Mechanism of neutropenia	Recognition factors
Peracute bacterial infections	Endotoxic or septic shock Peritonitis Pyometra Aspiration pneumonia Acute salmonellosis	Overwhelming demand/decreased survival	Left shift (may be degenerative) Toxic change Appropriate clinical signs
Extreme pyrexia	Heat stroke Septic shock	Overwhelming demand/decreased survival due to systemic inflammatory response	Appropriate clinical signs
Initial period of endotoxic or anaphylactic shock		Shift from circulating to marginating pool	Transient (minutes to hours) May resolve or neutropenia may persist due to increased demand if endotoxaemic
Retroviral infection	Feline leukaemia virus (FeLV) Feline immunodeficiency virus (FIV)	Reduced or ineffective granulopoiesis FeLV: maturation arrest, possible immune-mediated aetiology in some cases, myelodysplastic syndromes and leukaemias FIV: disturbance of myeloid progenitor growth	Appropriate virological results (see Chapter 28) FeLV: other haematological abnormalities common (especially anaemia (non-regenerative, possibly macrocytic), occasional pancytopenia). Neutropenia may be transient, persistent or cyclical FIV: non-regenerative anaemia, lymphopenia common Neutropenia often mild and transient in clinical cases
Parvovirus infection	Feline panleucopenia virus Canine parvovirus	Increased consumption (endotoxaemia, gastrointestinal disease) Viral cytotoxicity to haemopoietic stem cells Ineffective neutrophil production	Compatible history and clinical signs Profound degenerative left shift with early and aberrant precursors Canine parvovirus faecal enzyme-linked immunosorbent assay (ELISA) or polymerase chain reaction (PCR) positive (dog; see Chapter 28)
Myelodysplastic (MDS) disease	MDS refractory cytopenia	Ineffective granulopoiesis	Non-specific clinical signs Other cytopenias (often anaemia, especially cats) Bone marrow evaluation shows >10% of the cells in one or more bone marrow cell lines are dysplastic: cells are morphologically abnormal, maturation may appear disorderly Blasts are <20% Progression to myeloid leukaemia May be associated with FeLV infection
Leukaemia	Acute lymphoblastic leukaemia (ALL), acute myeloid leukaemia (AML) (less severe neutropenia with chronic leukaemias)	Reduced/ineffective granulopoiesis due to marrow infiltration by tumour cells	Non-specific clinical signs Pyrexia, sepsis, petechial haemorrhages, disseminated intravascular coagulation, paraneoplastic syndromes Thrombocytopenia Mild anaemia Circulating abnormal cells (usually in large numbers) Bone marrow infiltrate (>20% neoplastic blast cells for AML, 40% for ALL: often the marrow is virtually ablated by tumour cells)
Myelophthisis	Leukaemia (see above) Metastatic neoplasia Myelofibrosis/osteopetrosis Occasionally granulomatous disease	Reduced/ineffective granulopoiesis due to marrow infiltration by non-haemopoietic or leukaemic cells	Signs of underlying disease Non-specific clinical signs Other cytopenias Bone marrow required for diagnosis (NB myelofibrosis in dogs is characterized by a non-regenerative anaemia and significant other cytopenias are uncommon. Myelofibrosis in cats may be associated with FeLV infection, and in these cases neutropenia is common)
Cytotoxic drug therapy	Virtually all cytotoxic agents (L-asparaginase not myelosuppressive)	Targeting of cytotoxic effect to rapidly dividing cells in the marrow	History of recent cytotoxic drug administration Pyrexia, clinical signs of sepsis Possibly thrombocytopenia Left shift and toxic change as recover Usually occurs 5–10 days after drug administration and resolves in 24–72 hours
Idiosyncratic drug reactions	Oestrogen Chloramphenicol Phenobarbital Phenylbutazone Cephalosporins Azathioprine in cats Thiamazole (methimazole) (cats) Many others (trimethoprim–sulphas; TMP:S)	Toxicity to progenitor and committed cells at any level Immune-mediated component suspected in many drugs	Oestrogen toxicity produces initial neutrophilia, then neutropenia, thrombocytopenia and anaemia Others may affect only neutrophils or cause pancytopenia (aplastic anaemia) May be reversible or irreversible (TMP:S more commonly associated with immune-mediated thrombocytopenia (IMTP) or immune-mediated haemolytic anaemia (IMHA)

5.8 Causes of neutropenia in dogs and cats. (continues) ▶

Cause	Examples of disease process	Mechanism of neutropenia	Recognition factors
Chédiak–Higashi (rare)	Autosomal recessive disorder in Persian cats	Impaired release of neutrophils from the marrow Other factors	Breed Hypopigmentation of skin, hair, eyes Neutrophils, eosinophils and basophils contain large pink to purple granules Increased susceptibility to bacterial infections (neutrophil dysfunction) Platelet dysfunction leading to bleeding tendency
Trapped neutrophil syndrome in Border Collies (rare)	Autosomal recessive disorder in Border Collies	Mutation in the canine vesicle sorting protein (VPS) 13B gene	Breed Susceptibility to infections from young age Pyrexia, neutropenia, musculoskeletal signs Positive genetic test (homozygous for mutation)
Cyclic haemopoiesis in grey collies (rare)	Autosomal recessive, grey collies	Mutations in the adapter protein complex 3 gene affecting feedback inhibition in normal haemopoeisis	Breed Susceptibility to infections from young age Other white cell, platelet and reticulocyte counts also fluctuate cyclically Rebound neutrophilia after 2–4 days of neutropenia
Immune-mediated neutropenia (rare)		Idiosyncratic drug reaction Primary immune-mediated destruction Secondary immune-mediated destruction	No other cytopenias Demonstrable anti-neutrophil antibodies (flow cytometry) (Response to steroids)
Hereditary neutropenia (rare)		Giant Schnauzers, Border Collie, Shar-Pei and Australian Shepherd: selective malabsorption of vitamin B12 and resultant neutropenia	Age and breed; family history Giant Schnauzers: concurrent anaemia (Giant Schnauzers may also be predisposed to immune-mediated neutropenia, often with concurrent thrombocytopenia)

5.8 (continued) Causes of neutropenia in dogs and cats.

animals, but seldom recognized. However, reduced neutrophil function has been shown in sepsis, diabetes mellitus, chronic kidney disease, neoplasia (carcinomas and sarcomas) and leishmaniosis in dogs (Andreasen and Roth, 2000; Webb *et al.*, 2007; LeBlanc *et al.*, 2010; Hostetter, 2012; Almeida *et al.*, 2013; Silva *et al.*, 2013). Defective chemotaxis and reduced bacterial killing have been reported in cats with feline leukaemia virus (FeLV) infection, and defective chemotaxis in feline infectious peritonitis. Lastly, drug administration can affect neutrophil function. Glucocorticoids result in impaired neutrophil function in humans and recent experimental work in healthy dogs showed reduced neutrophil function after high-dose methylprednisolone succinate treatment.

Other hereditary neutrophil abnormalities

Pelger–Huët anomaly is an autosomal dominant inherited disorder reported in Domestic Shorthair cats and in dogs. The homozygous form is lethal, and in heterozygotes granulocytes fail to lobulate from band to segmented forms, so there is a persistent left shift, although these band-shaped nuclei have mature chromatin. These unsegmented neutrophils appear to have normal function. Megakaryocytes are also hyposegmented. Birman cat neutrophil granulation is another inherited anomaly with no apparent immunodeficiency.

Cytoplasmic inclusions

The cytoplasm of neutrophils may contain abnormal granules, vacuoles, organisms and various other inclusions, not of all which are associated with disease states.

Döhle bodies and toxic granulation are associated with toxic change (see above and Figure 5.3). The neutrophils of Birman cats may contain similar granules, which are more azurophilic, but are normal in this breed. Both dogs and cats with genetic defects in mucopolysaccharide metabolism resulting in lysosomal storage diseases may have coarse red granules in their neutrophils (and large abnormal basophil granules).

Cytoplasmic vacuolation may develop in neutrophils in EDTA; these vacuoles are clear and few in number, and are not as pronounced or 'foamy' as those seen in toxic change (see Figure 5.3). Vacuolation has been associated with high doses of chloramphenicol and phenylbutazone, and subtle vacuolation may be seen in cholesteryl ester storage disease.

Infectious agents are sometimes seen within neutrophils: these include *Ehrlichia ewingii*, *Anaplasma phagocytophilum*, *Histoplasma capsulatum*, *Hepatozoon canis* and *Leishmania donovani* (see Chapter 29). However, the sensitivity of microscopic detection for diagnosis is generally (very) low. It is very unusual to see bacteria within circulating neutrophils, except in a septicaemic crisis.

Canine distemper inclusions may be seen in dogs either following vaccination or after natural infection: these are homogeneously pink–magenta roundish structures.

Haemosiderin granules have been observed in the neutrophils of dogs following blood transfusion; their significance is unknown.

Eosinophils

The eosinophil is a striking cell, slightly larger than a neutrophil, with a segmented nucleus with only two or three lobes and coarse eosinophilic cytoplasmic granules. In the dog, these granules are round and variably sized, and numbers are very variable: occasionally, only one or two very large granules are seen within a cell (Figure 5.9). In the cat, the small rod-shaped orange–pink granules are very numerous and uniform (Figure 5.9). These granules contain an arsenal of preformed toxins. Background cytoplasm is lightly basophilic.

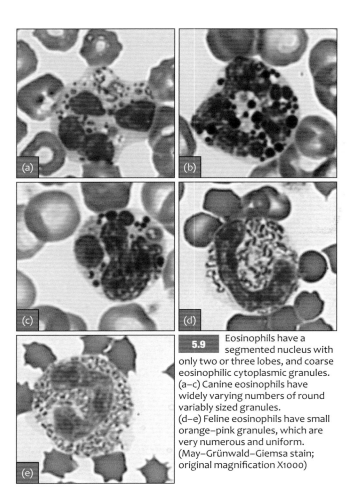

Causes	Disease process
Parasitic	• **Ectoparasites** • Pulmonary (*Aelurostrongylus*, *Angiostrongylus*) • Heartworm (dirofilariasis) • Enteric (*Giardia*, coccidia, ascarids)
Allergic	• **Feline asthma (cats)** • **Eosinophilic bronchopneumopathy (dogs)** • **Flea allergic dermatitis** • **Eosinophilic granuloma complex (cats)** • **Atopy (dogs)** • **Food hypersensitivity**
Inflammatory	• **Inflammatory bowel disease (eosinophilic enteritis)** • **Eosinophilic myositis** • Panosteitis • Focal inflammation • Lower urinary tract disease (cats) • Rhinitis/sinusitis • Eosinophilic granuloma complex • Steatitis
Neoplastic	• **Mast cell tumour (disseminated/intestinal)** • Lymphoma • Myeloproliferative disease (eosinophilic leukaemia, hypereosinophilic syndrome (cats)) • Miscellaneous tumours
Infectious	• Feline panleucopenia virus • Feline infectious peritonitis • Toxoplasmosis • Upper respiratory tract infection • Pyometra
Miscellaneous	• **Hypoadrenocorticism (dogs)** • Chronic renal failure (cats) • Cardiac disease (cats) • Immune-mediated skin disease • Other

5.9 Eosinophils have a segmented nucleus with only two or three lobes, and coarse eosinophilic cytoplasmic granules. (a–c) Canine eosinophils have widely varying numbers of round variably sized granules. (d–e) Feline eosinophils have small orange–pink granules, which are very numerous and uniform. (May–Grünwald–Giemsa stain; original magnification X1000)

5.10 Causes of eosinophilia in cats and dogs. The more frequent causes are shown in **bold**.

Eosinophils are important defenders against parasites, particularly helminths, and mediate inflammatory reactions. Additionally, they are often the effector cell of host tissue damage in allergic disease. Like neutrophils, they have a marrow storage pool and a short circulating half-life, but, unlike neutrophils, there is a large tissue pool of eosinophils in normal animals. They congregate in the loose connective tissues of organs vulnerable to entry by pathogens: the skin, the respiratory tract and the gastro-intestinal tract. Because eosinophils normally represent only a small percentage of the circulating granulocytes, a 500-cell differential count is recommended for accurate determination of numbers, but this is rarely carried out.

Eosinophilia

There are very many potential causes of eosinophilia, particularly in cats: these are summarized in Figure 5.10. As eosinophils are really tissue cells, local eosinophilic inflammation is not always accompanied by circulating eosinophilia. In addition, the degree of eosinophilia is variable, and is not indicative of the disease process. Paraneoplastic eosinophilias are particularly common in cats, and may be associated with many tumours, including lymphoma. This is reported in feline, canine (and human) intestinal T-cell lymphomas, and is mediated by excessive production of the cytokine IL-5 by the neoplastic T cells (Barrs *et al.*, 2002; Cave *et al.*, 2004; Marchetti *et al.*, 2005). In some diseases, there may be tissue infiltration as well as eosinophilia, and a resultant hypereosinophilic syndrome. There is also a case report of a cat with intestinal T-cell lymphoma and concurrent hypereosinophilic syndrome (see below).

Hypereosinophilic syndrome (HES) is characterized by a persistent, marked, predominantly mature eosinophilia and eosinophilic infiltration of multiple tissues. Most cases are idiopathic, with no underlying cause, and idiopathic HES is uncommon in cats and extremely rare in dogs, though Rottweilers are over-represented. In cats, bone marrow, lymph node and small intestine are major sites of infiltration. Diagnosis relies upon exclusion of the causes of secondary eosinophilia and/or eosinophilic infiltration, particularly paraneoplastic eosinophilia in lymphoma and other tumours. Although the prognosis for HES is guarded, individual cases can respond to treatment (prednisolone and hydroxurea/hydroxycarbamide) and there may be a role for ciclosporin. Differentiation of idiopathic HES in cats from chronic eosinophilic leukaemia (CEL) is difficult, if not impossible, as both are characterized by eosinophilic hyperplasia in the bone marrow and eosinophilic infiltration of other organs. It has been suggested that abnormal eosinophil precursor morphology, higher numbers of circulating myeloblasts and concurrent anaemia suggest CEL. In any case, the prognosis is generally guarded for both, and they may represent variants of the same disease. It is controversial whether eosinophilic leukaemia occurs in the dog.

Eosinopenia

Eosinopenia is a relative term because many reference intervals extend to zero, but it may be seen in acute infections, in response to corticosteroids and as part of the stress leucogram. Corticosteroids inhibit eosinophil release from bone marrow and also promote sequestration of eosinophils in tissues.

Basophils

The basophil is larger than the neutrophil (similar to the eosinophil and monocyte) with a long mildly lobulated ribbon-like nucleus. In the dog, unevenly scattered dark purplish cytoplasmic granules are seen against a pale grey–blue cytoplasm (Figure 5.11). In the cat, the round to oval granules are much denser and tend to pack the cell: these stain less intensely with Romanowsky stains and appear pale grey–lavender with a pink to orange tint (Figure 5.11).

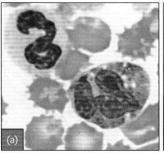
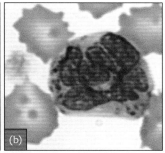
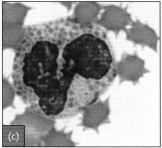

5.11 Basophils. (a) Canine basophil and neutrophil. The basophil (on the right) is larger than the neutrophil and has a long mildly lobulated ribbon-like nucleus. (b) Canine basophil with unevenly scattered dark purplish cytoplasmic granules against a pale grey–blue cytoplasm. (c) Feline basophil, showing much more densely packed oval grey–lavender granules. (May–Grünwald–Giemsa stain; original magnification X1000)

Basophils are involved in allergic disease and in the immune response to some parasites. Basophils also participate with eosinophils in inflammatory reactions, and they may also have roles in delayed hypersensitivity, haemostasis and lipolysis. Like neutrophils and eosinophils, they have a marrow storage pool and a short circulating half-life. In tissues, they may survive up to 2 weeks. Automated analysers do not recognize basophils reliably, and a manual differential count is likely to be more useful. However, because basophils normally represent only a tiny percentage of the granulocytes, accurate counts can only be determined by counting several hundred cells. Toluidine blue or histamine immunocytochemical stains help identify these cells.

Basophilia tends to echo eosinophilia, and is most often due to allergic disease or parasitism; it is occasionally seen in inflammatory haemograms. *Dirofilaria immitis* infection is an important cause in endemic areas (infection is reported in the USA, parts of Canada, Alaska, South America, southern Europe, Australasia and the Middle East).

Basophilia may also be seen in animals with mast cell neoplasia; it is a common finding in humans with leukaemia and myeloproliferative disorders and is reported in dogs with thrombocythaemia (see Chapter 6). Basophilic leukaemia has been reported in cats and dogs, and may be associated with hyperhistaminaemia.

Basopenia is rarely appreciated, but can be caused by corticosteroids.

Mast cells

Mast cells are not seen in the circulation in healthy animals but may be seen infrequently in inflammatory or neoplastic conditions. They are round cells with a central round to oval nucleus, which may stain pale blue, but is often at least partially obscured by the variably sized, red to purple granules in the cytoplasm (Figure 5.12). Mast cells are essentially tissue cells, and have important roles in allergic and other inflammatory responses, where they interact with other leucocytes. If present in the circulation, termed mastocythaemia, mast cells on a blood smear tend to accumulate at the feathered edge, because they are large cells.

Circulating mast cells are not pathognomonic of mast cell tumours in either dogs or cats. Low numbers of circulating mast cells may be seen in dogs with a variety of non-neoplastic and neoplastic conditions, and are often found in inflammatory conditions, accompanying an inflammatory leucogram. Circulating mast cells in cats are most often seen with mast cell tumours or lymphoma (Piviani *et al.*, 2013), but can be seen with other conditions. Low numbers of circulating mast cells may be overlooked if a buffy coat smear is not examined.

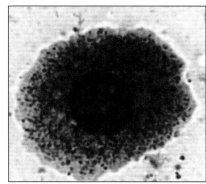

5.12 Canine mast cell. This is a round cell with a central round to oval nucleus, partially obscured by the variably sized red to lilac and purple granules in the cytoplasm. (Rapi-Diff II® stain; original magnification X1000)

Mononuclear cells

Monocytes

The monocyte appears larger than a neutrophil; although the cells are similar in size, in a smear the monocyte adheres more to the glass and becomes more flattened. It has a variably shaped nucleus (round, oval, bean to dumbbell, bi- or multilobed) with reticular or lacy chromatin. The cytoplasm is relatively abundant and blue–grey in colour with a ground glass appearance and occasional fine pink/magenta granules (canine monocytes are more granular than feline) (Figure 5.13). Vacuolation in blood samples is usually an *in vitro* change but can also reflect increased phagocytic activity. The cells may have rather irregular cytoplasmic boundaries and appear round or slightly angular, or even have small projections or pseudopodia. It can be difficult to differentiate a toxic band neutrophil from a monocyte: monocytes that have band-shaped nuclei usually have rounded knob- or dumbbell-shaped ends (Figure 5.13h).

The monocyte is the circulating precursor of the macrophage, and circulates for only a short time (approximately 8 hours in the cat) before migrating into the tissues, or sometimes returning to the marrow under steady-state conditions. There is no storage pool of monocytes, but in the dog there are probably marginating and circulating pools. The tissue pool is sizeable (and there are probably monocyte/macrophage precursors in tissue), and resident macrophages in normal tissue have a very

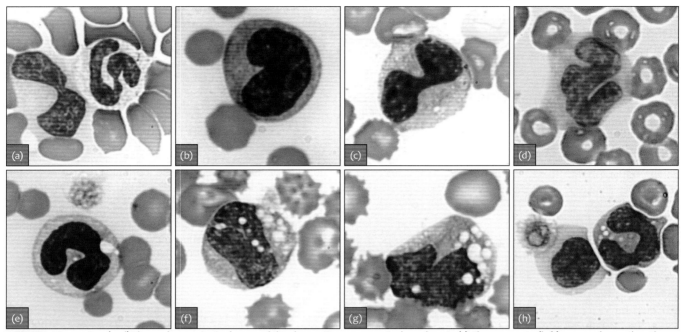

5.13 Monocytes. (a–d) The nucleus varies in shape and the chromatin appears reticular or lacy. In (a), the monocyte (left) appears larger than the neutrophil. (e–h) Vacuolation in blood samples is usually an *in vitro* change but can also reflect increased phagocytic activity. In (h) a medium-sized lymphocyte (left) is beside a monocyte with a band-shaped nucleus with rounded ends. ((a, c, f, g) Rapi-Diff II® stain, (b, d, e, h) May–Grünwald–Giemsa stain; original magnification X1000)

long lifespan (up to years), while those recruited by chemo-attractants in inflammation and disease are much shorter lived. Macrophages, along with neutrophils and natural killer cells, are the first line of defence in the innate immune response. They present antigen to lymphocytes to initiate the adaptive immune response, and secrete cytokines and chemical mediators of inflammation. Monocytes/macrophages also phagocytose pathogens, dead or infected cells, cells coated with antibodies and foreign material. Macrophages within the bone marrow provide an essential supporting role for haemopoiesis. Monocytes/macrophages are essential for life, and, together with specialized macrophages in some tissues, form the mononuclear phagocyte system (MPS).

Monocytosis is traditionally associated with chronic inflammation and may accompany neutrophilia in these cases. However, monocytosis may also be seen in acute inflammatory responses and overall is an inconsistent finding in inflammatory diseases. It is common in immune-mediated disease and in disease processes where there is tissue necrosis, e.g. where there is a large solid tumour or tumours with areas that have outgrown the blood supply, and may be seen in dogs with bacteraemia. Occasionally, monocytosis may be seen in neutropenic animals, when it is believed to be a 'compensatory' response, and a rebound monocytosis is common in animals recovering from neutropenia. Monocytosis is also part of a stress leucogram, but is not always present in dogs and is not generally observed in cats. Finally, monocytosis may be seen in monocytic or myelomonocytic leukaemias, where counts are likely to exceed the normal range greatly. Causes of monocytosis are summarized in Figure 5.14.

Cause	Associated conditions	Comment	Recognition factors
Acute inflammation	Trauma, IMHA, other immune-mediated diseases	Inconsistent finding	Clinical signs of the primary disease Neutrophilia (may feature left shift, toxic change) Superimposed stress haemogram
Stress/steroid response	Hyperadrenocorticism Exogenous corticosteroids Many others	Inconsistent finding in dogs, not generally observed in cats	Concurrent abnormalities (dogs): • Neutrophilia (no left shift) • Lymphopenia • Eosinopenia • Sometimes elevated alkaline phosphatase
Chronic inflammation	Infection Malignancy Pyogranulomatous inflammation Internal haemorrhage Tissue necrosis	Inconsistent finding	Clinical signs of the primary disease (Neutrophilia)
Compensatory	Secondary to neutropenia	Can occur after drug-induced myelosuppression	Clinical signs of the primary disease Neutropenia/previous neutropenia
Leukaemia	Monocytic or myelomonocytic leukaemia		Very high cell counts, circulating atypical cells Concurrent cytopenias

5.14 Causes of monocytosis in cats and dogs. IMHA = immune-mediated haemolytic anaemia.

Lymphocytes

Lymphopoiesis

Most lymphopoiesis occurs in the secondary or peripheral lymphoid tissues (lymph nodes, lymphoid follicles in tonsils, Peyer's patches, spleen, etc.) in response to antigenic stimulation. There are no lymphoid germinal centres in normal marrow, and lymphoid cells make up only 5% or less of the marrow haemopoietic cells in dogs, although in cats they may constitute up to 15% of haemopoietic cells. Primitive lymphocytes (pre-T cells) migrate from the bone marrow and undergo development in the thymic cortex (and some other peripheral lymphoid sites) into T cells. Pre-B cells develop into B cells in the marrow, then migrate to the peripheral lymphoid tissues. Immunologically, T cells are defined by the surface expression of a T-cell receptor complex called CD3, while B cells express a B-cell receptor complex called CD79a. These two complexes, and many other cell surface markers, are used to identify T and B cell tumours by immunohistochemistry and flow cytometry (see below).

Both T and B lymphocytes become activated on exposure to appropriately presented antigens. Various subsets of T cells have been identified:

- T helper cells (Th, CD4+) mediate cell-mediated immunity and humoral immunity. Th cells are vital to the process by which activated B lymphocytes undergo transformation to large lymphoid cells, then plasma cells, which produce antigen-specific immunoglobulin
- Regulatory T cells (Treg, CD25+; another group of CD4+ cells) are generally immunosuppressive T cells required for maintenance of self-tolerance and control of immune function. Activation of these cells is thought to be part of the pathogenesis during feline immunodeficiency virus infection (Vahlenkamp et al., 2004)
- Cytotoxic T cells (CD8+ cells) and natural killer (NK) cells (morphologically large granular lymphocytes) mediate cell killing.

The pathways of cell activation and regulation are highly coordinated, and activated T cells orchestrate the antigen-specific immune response through a complex web of intercellular signals and interactions. Much lymphocyte production occurs in the periphery in response to these signals.

Distribution

Most of the lymphocytes in the circulation are small lymphocytes. These cells have densely staining round to slightly oval/indented nuclei and very scant pale blue cytoplasm, which appears to extend only partway round the nucleus (Figure 5.15). The nuclei have smudged chromatin and no nucleoli. A few slightly larger (up to about the size of a neutrophil) medium lymphocytes, with more cytoplasm, are also a normal finding, and occasionally cells containing a few reddish granules are seen. Reactive lymphocytes may be larger and have increased amounts of intensely basophilic cytoplasm. Atypical and malignant large lymphoid cells may be seen in lymphoproliferative diseases: features of malignancy are discussed in Chapter 21 and illustrated in Figure 5.15.

Blood acts as a transport system for lymphocyte redistribution and recirculation, but only 5% of the total body lymphocyte pool is circulating in the blood. This does not mean that lymphocytes are static cells in the tissues; unlike other cells they re-enter the circulation after migrating into the peripheral lymphoid tissues. There is a

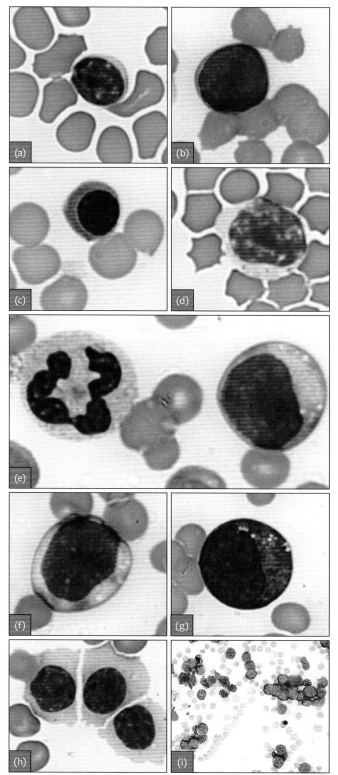

5.15 Lymphocytes. (a) Normal canine small lymphocyte, with very scant blue cytoplasm that appears to extend only partway round the nucleus. (b) Normal feline small lymphocyte, larger than a red blood cell. Note the absence of nucleoli. (c) Rubricyte (nucleated red blood cell). This is NOT lymphoid and is smaller, with an eccentrically placed nucleus and clumped chromatin. (d–f) Medium lymphocytes may be up to about the size of a neutrophil; occasionally the cells contain a few reddish granules. (g) Large reactive lymphocyte with increased amounts of intensely basophilic cytoplasm. (h) Large atypical neoplastic cells from a case of lymphoid leukaemia. (i) Large lymphoid cells showing features of malignancy: cytoplasmic basophilia, coarse nuclear chromatin, prominent nucleoli and nuclear moulding. (May–Grünwald–Giemsa stain; original magnification (a–h) X1000, (i) X400)

continuous recirculation of lymphoid cells throughout the body. Lymphoid cells drain from tissues (via afferent lymphatics) to the regional lymph nodes, then (via efferent lymphatics) enter the thoracic duct. The lymphoid cells enter the circulation via the thoracic duct, and leave the circulation in response to adhesion factors expressed in vascular endothelium. This recirculation and a continued ability to perform mitosis are unique features of lymphoid cells. The circulating lymphocytes consist of a mix of T cells, B cells and NK cells but, in normal animals, most are long-lived recirculating memory T cells.

Lymphocytosis

Although increased proliferation of lymphocytes is common in lymph nodes during the response to antigen, this seldom causes lymphocytosis, although a few reactive lymphocytes may be seen in the circulation. Lymphocytosis is often physiological, mediated by adrenaline release (especially in cats); counts may be >20 x 10^9/l. Young dogs and cats tend to have higher lymphocyte counts than adult animals. Lymphocytosis may also occur transiently after vaccination, or prolonged immune stimulation. It is also relatively common in cats with IMHA or pure red cell aplasia. In lymphoproliferative diseases, either lymphocytosis or lymphopenia may be seen; in lymphoma, lymphopenia is more common. Thymoma may be associated with lymphocytosis. Mild lymphocytosis, or a normal lymphocyte count despite medical stress, is a common finding in canine hypoadrenocorticism. Causes of lymphocytosis are summarized in Figure 5.16.

Lymphopenia

Lymphopenia is most commonly seen as a result of exogenous or endogenous corticosteroids, which cause a shift of lymphocytes from the circulation, and also lymphocytolysis. This is a common feature of the stress haemogram. However, in acute inflammation, lymphopenia may not simply be a 'stress' response but may result from increased margination of lymphocytes to the site of inflammation and to lymph nodes, coupled with reduced migration out of lymph nodes. Lymphopenia is also a feature of the acute phase of many viral infections, and may be seen in sepsis or endotoxaemia. Loss of lymph, e.g. in chylothorax or lymphangiectasia, can depress circulating lymphocyte numbers. More canine and feline lymphoma patients show lymphopenia than lymphocytosis; this may reflect either

Cause	Associated conditions	Comment	Recognition factors
Lymphocytosis			
Physiological	Emotional distress, fear, vigorous exercise	May be marked, especially in cats	Neutrophilia with no left shift Hyperglycaemia
Reactive	Young animals Transiently after vaccination Any prolonged immune stimulation Hyperthyroidism Non-regenerative IMHA (cats) Lymphocytic cholangitis (cats)		Age, history Clinical signs of the primary disease
'Reverse' stress leucogram	Hypoadrenocorticism	Mild lymphocytosis (or normal lymphocyte count) in sick animal	Absence of stress leucogram: normal neutrophil count in sick animal Electrolyte abnormalities (hyperkalaemia, hyponatraemia, mild to moderate hypercalcaemia) Hypoglycaemia Azotaemia
Neoplastic disease	Lymphoma ALL, CLL (Thymoma)	Most lymphoma patients have lymphopenia (stress)	Clinical signs of the primary disease Very high cell counts, circulating atypical cells in ALL High lymphocyte count in CLL Concurrent cytopenias in leukaemia
Lymphopenia			
Stress/steroid response	Hyperadrenocorticism Exogenous corticosteroids Many (including lymphoma)		Concurrent abnormalities – dogs: • Neutrophilia (no left shift) • (Monocytosis) • Eosinopenia • Elevated alkaline phosphatase Concurrent abnormalities – cats: • Neutrophilia (no left shift) • Eosinopenia
Acute inflammatory response/acute phase of infections	Any acute inflammatory response Viral infection Sepsis/endotoxaemia	Probably several mechanisms: reduced migration from lymph nodes, increased margination to affected tissues	Clinical signs of the primary disease Neutrophilia (stress haemogram, acute inflammatory haemogram)
Loss	Chylothorax Lymphangiectasia		Clinical signs of the primary disease
Decreased production	Immunosuppressive drug therapy Feline immunodeficiency virus infection (Myelophthisis) (Thiamazole/methimazole)		History (Concurrent cytopenias in myelophthisis)
Obstruction of lymph flow	Inflammation Neoplasia	Lymphopenia common in lymphoma, stress and possibly obstruction to flow	Clinical signs of the primary disease

5.16 Causes of lymphocytosis and lymphopenia in cats and dogs. ALL = acute lymphoblastic leukaemia; CLL = chronic lymphocytic leukaemia; IMHA = immune-mediated haemolytic anaemia.

stress or blockage of normal lymphatic flow and failure of cells to reach the circulation. Immunosuppressive drug therapy reduces circulating lymphocyte numbers. Rarely, animals with primary immunodeficiencies may be lymphopenic (but counts may also be normal). Severe combined immunodeficiency syndrome with profound lymphopenia has been reported in Jack Russell Terriers, and an X-linked form in male Welsh Corgis and Bassett Hounds. Causes of lymphopenia are summarized in Figure 5.16.

Reactive lymphocytes

Reactive lymphocytes are antigenically stimulated lymphocytes that are occasionally seen in the circulation in a very wide range of conditions. They may be large, and their nuclei have clumped chromatin (but no prominent nucleoli) and a scalloped outline. These cells have increased amounts of intensely basophilic cytoplasm and may have a perinuclear Golgi zone (see Figure 5.15g). It can be difficult to distinguish very reactive lymphoid cells from neoplastic cells (seen in leukaemia/lymphoma). In a reactive population, atypical cells are seen in small numbers and there is evidence of transition from normal, to mildly reactive, to more markedly reactive. Reactive lymphocytes often accompany an inflammatory response with neutrophilia, sometimes with a left shift, and may be seen more commonly in young animals.

Abnormal lymphocytes

The presence of circulating abnormal cells is much more suggestive of lymphoproliferative disease than any change in lymphocyte count. The features associated with malignancy are discussed in Chapter 21 and illustrated in Figure 5.15. The terms 'overspill leukaemia' and 'leukaemic phase of lymphoma' are sometimes used to describe increased or aberrant lymphoid cells in the circulation of patients with lymphoma; these terms are misleading, because these patients do not have leukaemia. In lymphoma, abnormal lymphoid cells on blood smear examination may reflect either escape of cells from neoplastic peripheral lymphoid tissue into the circulation (so-called 'overspill') or bone marrow involvement.

Leukaemias

Lymphoproliferative disorders include lymphoma, lymphoid leukaemias and plasma cell myeloma (discussed in Chapter 7), while myeloproliferative disorders encompass myeloid, monocytic, megakaryocytic and erythroid leukaemias (i.e. all non-lymphoid leukaemias) and myelodysplastic syndromes. Leukaemia is a neoplastic condition of the bone marrow, in which neoplastic cells arising from either lymphoid or non-lymphoid haemopoietic stem cells, or their progeny, undergo clonal expansion, with or without cellular differentiation. Frequently, the leukaemic cells are released into the peripheral blood, often in large numbers, and they may also infiltrate other organs, such as the liver, spleen and peripheral lymph nodes. Leukaemia causes clinical signs by four main mechanisms:

- Failure of normal haemopoiesis leading to cytopenias
- Organ dysfunction due to infiltration by leukaemic cells
- Hyperviscosity due to very high circulating numbers of aberrant cells
- Paraneoplastic syndromes (mainly in chronic lymphocytic leukaemia, CLL).

Leukaemia may be acute or chronic, but acute is more common. Acute leukaemias occur when neoplastic transformation occurs at the stem cell/committed blast stage, and the malignant cells have little differentiation potential. The neoplastic cells are poorly differentiated, and proliferate rapidly and in an uncontrolled manner, with arrested or defective maturation. The clinical course is rapid, and clinical signs are severe. Marrow infiltration due to uncontrolled proliferation of tumour cells results in crowding of normal marrow elements, competition for nutrients, failure of marrow to elaborate stimulatory factors and the build-up of inhibitory factors released by the neoplastic cells. As a result of this, normal blood cell production is reduced. The first manifestation of this is usually neutropenia, because neutrophils have a half-life of hours in the circulation, and a storage pool in the marrow which will provide a supply for about 5 days. Platelets are also short-lived, so concurrent thrombocytopenia is common, and some patients show thrombocytopenia first. Red cells have a long circulating lifespan, so anaemia develops later as pre-existing cells maintain levels for longer. The haemopoietic consequences of leukaemia, and clinical consequences of these, are summarized in Figure 5.17.

Chronic leukaemias occur when the neoplastic transformation occurs in either a stem cell or later cell but the progeny retain a strong tendency to differentiate. Although proliferation is uncontrolled, the cells are morphologically well differentiated (but often are functionally abnormal). These conditions generally have an insidious onset of less severe clinical signs, and less profound cytopenias, but may still present acutely.

Haematological features suggestive of leukaemia	Clinical manifestations
Neutropenia	Sepsis
Thrombocytopenia	Petechial and ecchymotic haemorrhages Melaena, epistaxis
Leucocytosis	Possibly hyperviscosity syndrome: • Bleeding diatheses • Ocular changes • Neurological signs • Polyuria/polydipsia • Thromboembolic disease

5.17 Haematological features of leukaemia and the clinical consequences of these abnormalities.

Acute leukaemia

Acute lymphoblastic leukaemia (ALL) is more common than acute myeloid leukaemia (AML) in both the dog and the cat. In either type, animals present with acute-onset lethargy, malaise, anorexia and weakness. Clinical signs include pallor, hepatosplenomegaly, mild lymphadenopathy, pyrexia, shifting lameness and, occasionally, central nervous system signs. Marked neutropenia and thrombocytopenia are common and there are usually abnormal cells in the circulation, resulting in raised cell counts: if counts are very high, hyperviscosity may result. However, in some cases cell counts are not raised and occasionally no blasts are seen (this occurs more frequently with AML). Bone marrow aspirates show neoplastic blast cells, and often the marrow is virtually ablated by these cells, resulting in depletion of megakaryocytes and both erythroid and myeloid series (including the storage pool) (Figure 5.18).

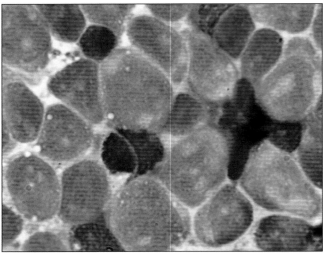

5.18 Bone marrow aspirate from a dog with acute lymphoblastic leukaemia. The marrow has been ablated by tumour cells, and virtually no normal haemopoietic cells are seen. In this field, there are densely packed large neoplastic blast cells. These cells show features of malignancy (stippled chromatin, pleomorphic nucleoli, cytoplasmic basophilia and nuclear moulding). (Wright-Giemsa stain; original magnification X1000)

The diagnosis of leukaemia is generally straightforward when concurrent haematology and bone marrow are examined, although typing can be difficult. The main cytological differential diagnosis for acute leukaemia is bone marrow in the acute stages of repopulation, for example after chemotherapeutic drug administration or parvovirus infection; in these cases, the diagnosis is usually clear. It can be difficult to differentiate ALL from stage V lymphoma with bone marrow involvement, and the criteria are summarized in Figure 5.19.

Ideally, immunophenotyping is carried out by flow cytometry (blood, or marrow in EDTA if the cell counts are low) to identify whether the tumour is myeloid or lymphoid, and to subtype the cell of origin further in some cases. Where this is not available, immunocytochemistry/immunohistochemistry (smears or biopsy samples) can be used, but generally only lymphoid markers are widely available.

The biochemical changes seen in acute leukaemias may reflect organ infiltration (e.g. raised liver enzymes) or hyperviscosity (azotaemia). Artefactual hyperkalaemia and hypoglycaemia are common, particularly in patients with high cell counts, owing to release of potassium from tumour cells and glucose consumption by tumour cells *in vitro*. Hypercalcaemia and hypergammaglobulinaemia are possible in ALL.

Lymphoma with bone marrow involvement
• Massive lymphadenopathy • Mild or no cytopenia • May not be systemically ill • Lower number of circulating neoplastic cells • Morphology variable • CD34 negative
Acute lymphoblastic leukaemia
• Mild to moderate lymphadenopathy • Severe cytopenias • Usually systemically ill • Higher number of circulating neoplastic cells • Morphologically primitive blasts • CD34 positive (usually)

5.19 Criteria to assist differentiation of lymphoma with bone marrow involvement from acute lymphoblastic leukaemia.

Chronic leukaemia

Chronic lymphocytic leukaemia

Chronic lymphocytic leukaemia (CLL) usually affects middle-aged to old dogs, and there may be a male predisposition. It is very rare in cats. Animals present with vague signs, which may wax and wane, commonly:

- Anorexia
- Lethargy
- Polyuria and polydipsia
- Mild hepatosplenomegaly
- Lymphadenopathy
- Pallor and pyrexia.

Lymphocytosis (6 to >100 x 10^9/l) is seen, with a population of morphologically normal mature lymphocytes, and mild cytopenias (particularly anaemia and thrombocytopenia).

Diagnosis requires exclusion of other causes of lymphocytosis, haematology and aspiration or biopsy of bone marrow, though in a small proportion of these cases (especially large granular leukaemias) disease may originate in the spleen. Bone marrow examination is recommended, and demonstrates increased numbers of small lymphocytes (>30% of nucleated cells in the bone marrow); either apparently normal or mildly decreased erythroid and myeloid activity is commonly seen. Immunophenotyping by flow cytometry and polymerase chain reaction (PCR) for antigen receptor rearrangements (PARR) analysis may be useful in confirming the diagnosis (see below; Avery, 2012). Dogs with CLL may have hypercalcaemia or monoclonal gammopathies.

Chronic granulocytic leukaemia

Chronic granulocytic leukaemia (CGL) is rare and difficult to diagnose. Clinical signs are vague, with lethargy, inappetence and weight loss over an insidious course. There may be hepatosplenomegaly. Haematology shows a massive mature neutrophilia, and bone marrow aspirates typically show marked myeloid hyperplasia with no obvious atypical features, and therefore do not differentiate CGL from a reactive neutrophilia. Diagnosis relies on elimination of other causes of neutrophilia/granulocytosis. A BCR–ABL chromosomal translocation has been identified in canine chronic monocytic leukaemia (CML) (Cruz Cardona *et al.*, 2011), analogous to the Philadelphia chromosome abnormality seen in humans.

Myelodysplastic syndromes

Primary myelodysplastic syndromes (MDS) are challenging to diagnose, and rely on examination of a bone marrow aspirate, and concurrent haematology, by an experienced clinical pathologist. The hallmark of MDS is ineffective haemopoiesis with disturbed maturation. On marrow examination, more than 10% of the cells in one or more bone marrow cells lines are dysplastic: the cells are morphologically abnormal and maturation may appear disorderly. However, blast percentages are lower than 20%. This is a heterogeneous group of conditions and in some circumstances may represent a preleukaemic state (in particular preceding AML). Haematological features include non-regenerative anaemia (which is occasionally macrocytic), neutropenia, thrombocytopenia and occasionally monocytosis.

Myelodysplasia may occur secondary to immune-mediated disease, lymphoma, drug administration, myelofibrosis and heavy metal toxicity. This is sometimes termed secondary dysmyelopoiesis.

Myelofibrosis

Myelofibrosis involves an increase in collagen and other fibrous elements in the marrow matrix (see Figure 4.34). It is thought to be a secondary reactive marrow response that can be associated with many diseases, especially immune-mediated haematological disease such as IMHA, but often the initiating cause is unknown. Myelofibrosis is also associated with some myeloid leukaemias, and is common in cats with MDS or AML, where the primary disease dominates presentation. FeLV infection or exposure may play a role. Idiosyncratic drug reactions may also initiate myelofibrosis in both species. It is thought that in many cases, irrespective of initiating cause, the secondary reactive response is immune mediated.

In humans, myelofibrosis is also often a secondary reactive change, but it can occur as a primary disease called idiopathic myelofibrosis. This is a myeloproliferative disease involving megakaryocytes and myeloid precursors, which produce cytokines stimulating the production of fibrous tissue. This appears to be very rare in small animals.

Dogs with myelofibrosis usually present with non-regenerative anaemia, without other cytopenias, although infrequently there is also leucopenia. Patients present when the anaemia becomes severe, weeks to months after the initiating insult, which is seldom identified. The diagnosis can only be confirmed on core biopsy of the bone marrow.

Beyond the haemogram: other evaluations of leucocytes

Bone marrow aspiration

Bone marrow evaluation is required to diagnose and sub-type myelodysplastic and leukaemic diseases, and is very useful in many disease situations (Figure 5.20).

In normal marrow, the myeloid to erythroid ratio is approximately 0.75–1.5:1 in dogs, and 1–4:1 in cats. Myeloid hyperplasia, and an increase in this ratio, will be seen in any inflammatory response. Where there is an ongoing demand for neutrophils, depletion of the storage pool may be evident, and there may be toxic change. Sampling of bone marrow and sample handling are discussed in Chapter 4.

- (Persistent) neutropenia
- Thrombocytopenia
- Pancytopenia
- Abnormal/immature lymphocytes or granulocytes in the circulation
- Inexplicably high numbers of any cell line in the circulation
- Non-regenerative anaemia
- Lymphoma
- Hyperproteinaemia
- Hypercalcaemia of unknown origin
- Pyrexia of unknown origin
- Suspected systemic infections with *Ehrlichia*, *Leishmania* or fungi
- (Detection of feline leukaemia virus in discordant cats)

5.20 Indications for bone marrow sampling in cats and dogs.

Immunophenotyping of leucocytes

Immunophenotyping is the determination of cell type by the identification of cell surface markers using antibodies. In canine lymphoma, immunophenotyping is of prognostic significance because, in general, T-cell tumours carry a poorer prognosis. The morphological subtype, based on cytological evaluation, may also prove to be of prognostic relevance (Ponce *et al.*, 2004), and there are also established clinical prognostic indicators. Immunophenotyping may have a role in prognostication and treatment selection in leukaemias: morphological or cytochemical differentiation of acute lymphoid and myeloid leukaemias is often difficult or impossible. Immunophenotyping not only gives a cell lineage, but also, in some cases, can suggest the stage of maturation arrest and clonal expansion, because some cell surface markers are expressed during restricted phases of cell development.

Immunophenotyping of haemolymphatic cells relies on detection of cell surface markers, which are usually assigned CD (clusters of differentiation) numbers. There are more than 150 CDs assigned in human medicine, but only relatively few currently have defined roles in leucocyte disorders in small animals: selected important CDs are summarized in Figure 5.21. In many laboratories, samples are initially screened for CD3 and CD79a to confirm lymphoid origin and identify T- or B-cell lineage. However, some lymphoid tumours are negative for CD3 and CD79a while some are dually positive for CD3 and CD79a; the use of a panel of antibodies will often help determine the cell of origin.

Immunophenotyping may be carried out by immunocytology or immunohistology (Figure 5.22), or by flow cytometry (Figure 5.23). Immunochemical techniques often work best on unfixed tissues/smears but it is best to consult the laboratory for submission requirements; for example, lysine-coated slides may be required for immunocytochemistry on fine-needle aspirates. Immunocytochemical stains for myeloid cells are not widely available.

Flow cytometry

Flow cytometry (FC) is a generic technology that counts and measures multiple characteristics of individual particles in a flow stream; the technology is used by many automated haematology analysers (see Chapter 3). In immunological FC, the cells to be investigated are labelled with one or more fluorochrome-labelled antibodies (fluorochromes are coloured dyes that accept light energy at a given wavelength and re-emit it at a higher wavelength). A stream of labelled cells is then directed through a laser beam; the amount of fluorescence and the light scatter patterns are recorded and analysed by a computer to produce histograms and dot plots from which the cell types present can be identified. Further information can be found at www.hmds.org.uk/cytometry.html. FC can be used in a variety of clinical situations:

- To immunophenotype lympho- and myeloproliferative diseases, where it detects specific marked antigens on the surface of the cells
- To confirm immune-mediated disease (especially immune-mediated thrombocytopenia), where it detects antibodies bound to target cells (not currently available in the UK)
- For the detection of minimal residual disease in lymphoproliferative disease (not currently well established for small animals).

Antigen detected	Specificity
Antibodies commonly used in flow cytometry for dogs	
T-cell markers:	
CD3	All T cells
CD4	T helper cells
CD5	All T cells
CD8	Cytotoxic T cells
B-cell markers:	
CD21	B cells (mature)
CD79a	B cells (from B-cell precursors through to mature cells)
Surface IgM	B cells
Surface IgG	B cells
Myeloid markers:	
CD14	Monocytes and their precursors
Myeloperoxidase	Neutrophils and their precursors
MAC 387	Neutrophils and monocytes, and their precursors
CD11b	Granulocytes, monocytes, subset of lymphocytes
CD41	Platelets and their precursors
CD61	Platelets and their precursors
Other:	
CD45	All leucocytes
CD34	Stem cells (expressed in acute leukaemia)
MHCII	B cells, T cells, monocytes, macrophages
Antibodies commonly used in flow cytometry in cats	
T-cell markers:	
CD4	T helper cells
CD5	All T cells
CD8	Cytotoxic T cells
B-cell markers:	
CD21	B cells (mature)
Myeloid markers:	
CD14	Monocytes and their precursors
	Myeloperoxidase neutrophils and their precursors
Antibodies commonly used for immunohistochemistry/immunocytochemistry	
T-cell markers:	
CD3 and CD5 (dogs and cats)	All T cells
B-cell markers:	
CD79a (dogs and cats)	B cells (from precursors through to mature cells)
CD20 (dogs and cats)	B cells (from precursors through to mature cells)
Pax 5 (dogs)	B cells (from precursors through to mature cells)

5.21 Antibodies commonly used in flow cytometry for immunophenotyping lymphoma and leukaemia, and in immunohistochemistry/immunocytochemistry. CD = cluster of differentiation; Ig = immunoglobulin; MHC = major histocompatibility complex.

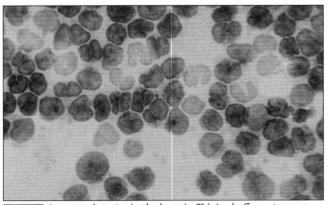

5.22 Immunophenotyping leukaemia. This is a buffy coat smear, from a dog with leukaemia, stained with anti-CD3 antibodies. The brown staining is a positive result, indicating that this is a tumour of T-cell origin.
(Courtesy of E Villiers)

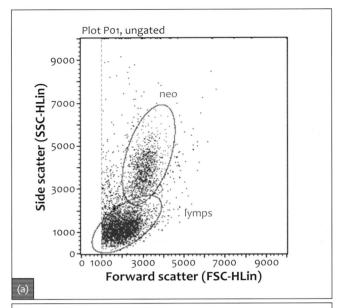
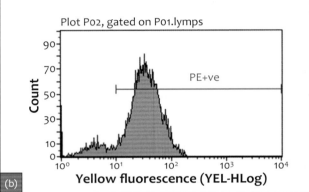

5.23 (a) A scatter plot obtained from a blood sample from a dog with acute lymphoblastic leukaemia. Cell size is on the x-axis and granularity/complexity on the y-axis. The cells in the red gate are atypical lymphoid cells, those in the blue gate are neutrophils (labelled lymps and neo, respectively). (b) Histogram showing staining of the lymphoid cells with CD79a. The fluorescence is shown on the x-axis and cell number on the y-axis. The vast majority of the lymphoid cells stain with CD79a, which is conjugated to phycoerythrin (PE +ve), indicating a B-cell leukaemia.

In the UK, FC is available at the University of Cambridge and Dick White Referrals (see http://www.cimr.cam.ac.uk/about/facilities/cytometry and http://www.dwrdiagnostics.com/tests-and-profiles/flow-cytometry.aspx, for submission requirements for blood and bone marrow).

Polymerase chain reaction

PCR tests for infectious organisms may be useful in cases where arthropod-borne infections are suspected (see Chapter 29). PCR can also be used to assess clonality in suspected lymphoproliferative disease.

PCR for antigen receptor rearrangements (PARR)

This test uses EDTA blood samples or lymph node aspirates, and is available in several centres in both the USA (including Colorado State University, North Carolina State University, University of California–Davis, and Michigan State University) and Europe (including TDDS Ltd, University of Cambridge and Genefast); general and submission information can be found on the appropriate websites (e.g. http://csu-cvmbs.colostate.edu/academics/ mip/ci-lab/Pages/PARR-FAQs.aspx). In veterinary medicine the term PARR refers to a specialized PCR that amplifies either the immunoglobulin gene (from B cells) or the T-cell receptor gene (from T cells), and detects either a single gene produced from clonal populations of neoplastic cells, or many different products in a reactive process. Thus the main use is to distinguish reactive (polyclonal) lymphocytes from neoplastic (monoclonal) lymphocytes where there is lymphadenopathy or lymphocytosis. Sensitivity is good, but false negatives occur (i.e. not all tumours are recognized), and some tumours show clonal rearrangements of both T- and B-cell markers. False positives can occur in infectious disease (e.g. ehrlichiosis). In addition, PARR should not be relied upon as the sole determinant of immunophenotype (T- or B-cell lineage) and is also unreliable in differentiating lymphoid from myeloid tumours in cytologically ambiguous cases (where FC is more appropriate).

PARR is used on EDTA blood samples to detect microscopic residual disease in human patients with leukaemia or lymphoma, and particular genetic derangements specific to neoplastic cells in the individual tumour can be detected. This technique has been reported in canine lymphoma patients, although its clinical value has not been proven (Keller *et al.*, 2004; Lana *et al.*, 2006; Williams *et al.*, 2008). Finally, PARR (using DNA from a biopsy sample or fine-needle aspirate) may be useful in differentiating feline intestinal lymphoma from inflammatory bowel diseases, though this is a controversial area.

Cytochemical tests

The main role of cytochemical stains was in the classification of acute myeloid leukaemias, using a panel of stains to overcome the lack of sensitivity and specificity of individual stains (Figure 5.24). However, immunophenotyping is superior and, as more antibodies have become available, the use of cytochemical stains has reduced, and tests are not readily available. In human medicine, classification of leukaemia integrates clinical information, cell morphology, cytochemistry, immunophenotyping, cytogenetic and molecular genetic diagnostic techniques. In companion animals, often only clinical information, cell morphology and immunophenotyping are used.

Functional tests

Leucocyte functional testing is not commonly carried out in clinical veterinary medicine, and there are few readily available tests, though there are data from immunotoxicology testing in experimental dogs and from clinical research. B-cell function can be crudely assessed by quantifying immunoglobulins (Ig)G, IgA and IgM, but it is important to have age-matched reference ranges or controls. Deficiencies in T-cell responses can be identified by assessing the response to stimulation in a lymphocyte stimulation (or blastogenesis) assay.

Neutrophil dysfunction may involve abnormalities in any of the steps in neutrophil activity (adherence, chemotaxis and migration, phagocytosis, cytotoxicity), and ideally all steps should be assessed. There are currently no commercially available tests of neutrophil function for small animals. However, a variety of assays have been carried out experimentally, including neutrophil adherence, chemotaxis, migration and bacterial cell killing tests in dogs with infectious diseases, chronic kidney disease, sepsis, diabetes mellitus and neoplasia (Andreasen and Roth, 2000; Webb *et al.*, 2007; LeBlanc *et al.*, 2010; Hostetter, 2012; Almeida *et al.*, 2013; Silva *et al.*, 2013).

Cytochemical stain	Lymphoid leukaemia	Myeloid leukaemia	Monocytic leukaemia
Peroxidase	Negative	Positive (variable number of cells, but >3%); may be negative in cats	Negative or weakly positive in dogs; negative in cats
Alkaline phosphatase	Negative	Positive (some cells)	Negative
Lipase	Negative	Negative	Positive
Chloroacetate esterase (CAE) (specific esterase)	Usually negative	Positive	Negative
Alpha naphthyl butyrate esterase (NBE) (non-specific esterase)	Negative (or focal staining)	Negative	Positive
Sudan black	Negative	Positive	Positive in dogs; negative in cats

5.24 Cytochemical tests for leukaemia, and typical staining characteristics. Lymphoid cells generally do not stain with cytochemical stains (and are more readily identified by immunophenotyping), but are occasionally positive with alkaline phosphatase or alpha naphthyl butyrate esterase. However, negative staining does not indicate a lymphoid neoplasm because myeloid neoplasms may also stain negatively. Results can be difficult to interpret, and the use of a screening panel makes successful identification more likely, for example by picking up markers of both myeloid and monocytic cells in myelomonocytic leukaemia.

Case examples

CASE 1

SIGNALMENT

6-year-old female neutered crossbreed.

HISTORY

A diagnosis of idiopathic epilepsy was made 3 months previously and treated with phenobarbital. There was a 2-week history of exercise intolerance, then inappetance and polydipsia/polyuria for the last few days. Clinical examination revealed mild pyrexia (39.3°C), and palpable hepatosplenomegaly.

CLINICAL PATHOLOGY DATA

Haematology	Results	Reference interval
RBC (x 10¹²/l)	**3.58**	5.5–8.0
Haematocrit (l/l)	**0.25**	0.37–0.55
Haemoglobin (g/dl)	**8.24**	12.6–19.4
MCV (fl)	69.5	62.0–70.0
MCHC (g/dl)	33.0	33.0–36.0
Reticulocytes (%)	**1.8**	0.0–1
Reticulocyte count (x 10⁹/l)	**64**	<60
WBC (x 10⁹/l)	**0.77**	6.7–18.5
Neutrophils (band) (x 10⁹/l)	0.03	0.0–0.3
Neutrophils (segmented) (x 10⁹/l)	**0.18**	3.6–12.5
Lymphocytes (x 10⁹/l)	**0.31**	0.7–6.0
Monocytes (x 10⁹/l)	0.21	0.1–1.70
Eosinophils (x 10⁹/l)	**<0.01**	0.1–1.80
Basophils (x 10⁹/l)	<0.01	Rare
Platelets (x 10⁹/l)	**100**	150–400

Abnormal results are in **bold**.

Film comment: possible rouleaux/autoagglutination. No platelet clumps.

Biochemistry	Results	Reference interval
Total protein (g/l)	66	57–78
Albumin (g/l)	**21**	23–31
Globulin (g/l)	**45**	27–40
ALP (IU/l)	**452**	0–100
ALT (IU/l)	27	7–50
Sodium (mmol/l)	146	140–153
Potassium (mmol/l)	4.7	3.8–5.3
Chloride (mmol/l)	112	99–115
Calcium (mmol/l)	2.5	2.2–2.7
Phosphate (mmol/l)	1.23	0.80–2.0
Glucose (mmol/l)	**6.5**	3.5–5.5
Urea (mmol/l)	4.1	3.5–6.0
Creatinine (µmol/l)	42	20–110
Cholesterol (mmol/l)	**10.6**	3.2–6.5
Bilirubin (µmol/l)	2.1	0–20

Abnormal results are in **bold**.

WHAT ABNORMALITIES ARE PRESENT?

Haematology

- Moderate, essentially non-regenerative anaemia.
- Profound neutropenia.
- Moderate thrombocytopenia.
- Lymphopenia.
- Eosinopenia.
- Possible autoagglutination/rouleax.

Biochemistry

- Mild hypoalbuminaemia.
- Elevated cholesterol.
- Moderately elevated (4.5x) ALP.
- Very mildly elevated glucose.

HOW WOULD YOU INTERPRET THESE RESULTS AND WHAT ARE THE LIKELY DIFFERENTIAL DIAGNOSES?

There is a pancytopenia (anaemia, leucopenia, thrombocytopenia), suggesting failure of bone marrow to produce sufficient blood cells. Given the dog's history, this may be due to an idiosyncratic reaction to phenobarbital. Other less likely differentials are leukaemia, myelophthisis or possibly myelodysplasia. There is no history of exposure to exogenous oestrogens.

The degree of anaemia is mild compared with the degree of neutropenia and thrombocytopenia. There is no evidence of regeneration (despite the 2 week history of exercise intolerance). The possible agglutination raises the possibility of (non-regenerative) immune-mediated haemolytic anaemia but there are no other supporting features. Non-regenerative anaemia is usually due to marrow disease. The anaemia here is too severe to be simply anaemia of chronic disease/inflammatory disease.

The lymphopenia is likely to be a stress response, although margination of lymphocytes to sites of inflammatory response may also contribute.

The mild hypoalbuminaemia may be part of an acute phase response in this pyrexic, neutropenic patient. It could also reflect a protein-losing nephropathy, third space loss or loss due to hemorrhage (with loss of globulin but insufficient to reduce an elevated globulin to subnormal). Severe liver disease is less likely with the normal ALT (unless end-stage) and elevated globulin. The slightly elevated globulin probably reflects an inflammatory response.

The moderately elevated ALP is likely to be phenobarbital induced and the very mildly elevated glucose is most probably stress related. The elevated cholesterol may reflect failure to fast, prior to sampling (hyperadrenocorticism and hypothyroidism have not been excluded; pancreatitis, chloestasis or protein-losing nephropathy are less likely, diabetes mellitus is excluded).

WHAT FURTHER TESTS WOULD YOU RECOMMEND?

- Bone marrow aspiration and core biopsy.
- Ultrasonography and fine-needle aspiration of spleen and/or liver.

→ CASE 1 CONTINUED

- Urinalysis (including protein:creatinine ratio).
- Possibly in-saline agglutination (to identify true agglutination) and a Coombs' test.

OUTCOME

Bone marrow aspirates were of low cellularity but revealed relative granulocyte hyperplasia, normal maturation of erythroid and myeloid series and megakaryocyte hypoplasia. There was no evidence of a neoplastic infiltrate. Later core biopsy specimens confirmed there was no evidence of myelofibrosis or myelonecrosis.

Abdominal ultrasonography revealed heptomegaly with hypoechoic change, and splenomegaly with normal echogenicity. Liver aspirate revealed only normal hepatocytes. Urinalysis was unremarkable apart from an equivocal urine specific gravity (USG = 1.023) and there was no proteinuria.

Both in-saline agglutination and Coombs test (carried out because of the suspicion of agglutination) were negative.

Broad spectrum antibiotic therapy and supportive care were given. Therapy with levetiracetam was started and phenobarbital withdrawn. Within 10 days the anaemia and thrombocytopenia had resolved, and the neutrophil count increased to 1.6 x 10⁹/l. Within 1 month all values were within reference intervals.

Phenobarbital is (infrequently) associated with blood dyscrasias in dogs, which occurs as an idiosyncratic drug reaction. Typical abnormalities are a thrombocytopenia, neutropenia or anaemia, or combinations of these, and in some cases bone marrow evaluation shows necrosis or myelofibrosis. In most cases, patients respond to appropriate supportive care and drug discontinuation, unless there is advanced myelofibrosis. However, rapid withdrawal of phenobarbital can cause recurrence of seizures.

CASE 2A

SIGNALMENT

7-year-old female entire Border Collie.

HISTORY

Presented with a 1-week history of lethargy and anorexia. On clinical examination, mucous membranes were very pale. The dog was tachycardic (140 beats per minute) and tachypnoeic (56 breathes per minute) at rest.

CLINICAL PATHOLOGY DATA

Haematology	Results	Reference interval
RBC (x 10¹²/l)	**1.44**	5.5–8.0
Haematocrit (l/l)	**0.09**	0.37–0.55
Haemoglobin (g/dl)	**3.52**	12.6–19.4
MCV (fl)	63.8	62.0–70.0
MCH (pg)	24.4	22.0–25.0
MCHC (g/dl)	38.3	33.0–36.0
Reticulocytes (%)	**50**	0.0–1
Reticulocyte count (x 10⁹/l)	**720**	<60
WBC (x 10⁹/l)	**26.4**	6.7–18.5
Metamyelocytes (x 10⁹/l)	**1.1**	0
Neutrophils (band) (x 10⁹/l)	**7.4**	0.0–0.3
Neutrophils (segmented) (x 10⁹/l)	**13.0**	3.6–12.5
Lymphocytes (x 10⁹/l)	2.9	0.7–6.0
Monocytes (x 10⁹/l)	0.26	0.1–1.70
Eosinophils (x 10⁹/l)	0.26	0.1–1.80
Basophils (x 10⁹/l)	<0.01	Rare
Nucleated red cells (x 10⁹/l)	**1.1**	0
Platelets (x 10⁹/l)	310	150–400

Abnormal results are in **bold**.

Film comment: large numbers of spherocytes, marked anisocytosis and polychromasia.

Biochemistry	Results	Reference interval
Total protein (g/l)	60	57.0–78.0
Albumin (g/l)	25	23.0–31.0
Globulin (g/l)	35	27.0–40.0
ALP (IU/l)	**224**	0–100
ALT (IU/l)	17	7–50
Sodium (mmol/l)	144	140–153
Potassium (mmol/l)	4.8	3.8–5.3
Chloride	111	99–115
Calcium (mmol/l)	2.4	2.2–2.7
Phosphate (mmol/l)	1.6	0.8–2.0
Glucose (mmol/l)	**6.8**	3.5–5.5
Urea (mmol/l)	**6.2**	3.5–6.0
Creatinine (μmol/l)	50.6	20–110
Cholesterol (mmol/l)	**13.9**	3.2–6.5
Bilirubin (μmol/l)	5.3	0–20

Abnormal results are in **bold**.

WHAT ABNORMALITIES ARE PRESENT?

Haematology

- Severe, markedly regenerative anaemia.
- Slightly elevated mean corpuscular haemoglobin concentration (MCHC).
- Neutrophilia with a mild increase in mature forms, and severe left shift (including metamyelocytes).
- Nucleated red blood cells.
- Spherocytes on film examination.

Biochemistry

- Moderately elevated alkaline phosphatase (2.25x).
- Slight hyperglycaemia.
- Elevated cholesterol.
- Marginal elevation in urea.

→ **CASE 2A CONTINUED**

HOW WOULD YOU INTERPRET THESE RESULTS AND WHAT ARE THE LIKELY DIFFERENTIAL DIAGNOSES?

The main differentials for regenerative anaemia are haemorrhage or haemolysis. Acute haemorrhage resulting in this level of anaemia would be fatal; chronic haemorrhage would be expected to result in iron-deficiency anaemia. The presence of spherocytes in large numbers is strongly supportive of immune-mediated haemolysis. The small increase in MCHC is likely to be artefactual due to the presence of free haemoglobin in the plasma. The strong reticulocyte response is accompanied by premature release of nucleated red blood cells. These nucleated cells contribute to the total WBC count as they are counted with the nucleated leucocytes.

The neutrophilia with a very marked left shift suggests an acute inflammatory response, reflecting massive demand in response to systemic inflammation and also a non-specific stimulation of the marrow during strong erythroid activity (endogenous steroid production may also contribute). This is common in IMHA, whether primary or secondary to an inflammatory underlying cause (e.g. bacterial cholangitis).

This combination of a marked left shifted neutrophilia and a very regenerative red cell response is a leukoerythroblastic blood picture.

The moderate elevation in alkaline phosphatase is a non-specific finding and may reflect cholestasis or a reactive hepatopathy. The normal ALT is unusual in a dog with this degree of anaemia and the mild hyperglycaemia probably reflects stress.

Elevated cholesterol may be postprandial if the patient was not fasted, and this would also explain the very slight elevation in urea. Endocrine causes seem less likely. Subclinical pancreatitis and cholestasis are other possible causes. Protein-losing nephropathy is unlikely given the normal albumin.

WHAT FURTHER TESTS WOULD YOU RECOMMEND?

- Thoracic and abdominal imaging to rule out initiating comorbidities.
- In-saline agglutination and, if negative, a Coombs' test.

OUTCOME

Thoracic radiographs revealed no abnormalities, and abdominal ultrasonography showed no changes (including no organomegaly or lymphadenopathy).

Saline agglutination was negative: a Coombs' test was not carried out, but a presumptive diagnosis of IMHA was made.

The dog was treated with prednisolone and azathioprine and with supportive care (including Oxyglobin®). She responded well although there were some partial relapses: she was weaned off treatment after 13 months.

CASE 2B

SIGNALMENT

9-year-old female Border Collie (later presentation of dog in Case 2A)

HISTORY

Weaned off treatment for immune-mediated haemolytic anaemia after 13 months (with prednisolone and azathioprine) 4 months ago; presented for routine follow up check. No significant clinical findings.

CLINICAL PATHOLOGY DATA

Haematology	Results	Reference interval
RBC (x 10¹²/l)	5.86	5.5–8.0
Haematocrit (l/l)	0.40	0.37–0.55
Haemoglobin (g/dl)	13.4	12.6–19.4
MCV (fl)	67.5	62.0–70.0
MCH (pg)	22.9	22.0–25.0
MCHC (g/dl)	33.8	33.0–36.0
Reticulocytes (%)	3	0.0–1
Reticulocyte count (x 10⁹/l)	**175.8**	<60
WBC (x 10⁹/l)	**2.87**	6.7–18.5
Neutrophils (band) (x 10⁹/l)	0.22	0.0–0.3
Neutrophils (segmented) (x 10⁹/l)	**0.7**	3.6–12.5

Abnormal results are in **bold**.

Haematology *continued*	Results	Reference interval
Lymphocytes (x 10⁹/l)	1.3	0.7–6.0
Monocytes (x 10⁹/l)	0.28	0.1–1.70
Eosinophils (x 10⁹/l)	0.28	0.1–1.80
Basophils (x 10⁹/l)	<0.01	Rare
Platelets (x 10⁹/l)	322	150–400

Abnormal results are in **bold**.

Film comment: mild polychromasia.

WHAT ABNORMALITIES ARE PRESENT?

Haematology

- Moderate reticulocytosis with normal haematocrit.
- Marked neutropenia.

HOW WOULD YOU INTERPRET THESE RESULTS AND WHAT ARE THE LIKELY DIFFERENTIAL DIAGNOSES?

The moderate reticulocytosis in the face of a normal haematocrit may reflect increased red cell destruction and replacement in poorly controlled IMHA, or early relapse. Alternatively, it may be an appropriate response to undetected blood loss. Transient reticulocytosis can also be seen following excitement/fear when adrenaline causes the release of reticulocytes from the spleen.

The differentials for the marked neutropenia include consumption (although the lack of clinical signs makes

→ CASE 2B CONTINUED

this unlikely, and there is no significant or degenerative left shift or toxic change); myelodysplasia, leukaemia or myelophthisis (but there are no other cytopenias or circulating abnormal cells); drug reaction (but no recent drug administration); or idiopathic immune-mediated neutropenia.

WHAT FURTHER TESTS WOULD YOU RECOMMEND?

* Thoracic and abdominal imaging to rule out underlying consumptive cause.
* Bone marrow aspiration.

OUTCOME

Thoracic radiographs revealed only mild interstitial change compatible with age, and abdominal ultrasonography showed mild hepatomegaly with generalized hypoechoic changes compatible with steroid hepatopathy.

Bone marrow aspirates showed normal cellularity with active granulopoiesis, and normal erythropoiesis and thrombopoiesis. The granulocytic series was very active with, subjectively, an increased proportion of earlier precursors, especially myelocytes and metamyelocytes. However, these were progressing through to bands and neutrophils.

Based on these results, differentials were immune-mediated neutropenia or consumptive neutropenia, which was thought unlikely given the clinical presentation, imaging findings and lack of left shift and toxic change on haematology. The dog was treated with immunosuppressive doses of corticosteroids and the neutrophil count normalized within a week. She was weaned off treatment 4 months later. She subsequently relapsed with IMHA, after a season, restarted therapy and was spayed.

CASE 3

SIGNALMENT

8-year-old female neutered crossbreed dog.

HISTORY

Being treated with vinblastine and prednisolone as part of multimodality therapy for a recurrent subcutaneous mast cell tumour of the dorsum. The owner reported the dog was normal at home, and urinating and defecating normally. Clinical examination revealed only slight, residual subcutaneous thickening at the tumour site. Routine haematology testing was performed prior to continuing chemotherapy.

CLINICAL PATHOLOGY DATA

Haematology	Results	Reference interval
RBC (x 10¹²/l)	5.99	5.4–8.0
Haematocrit (l/l)	0.45	0.35–0.55
Haemoglobin (g/dl)	15.0	12.0–18.0
MCV (fl)	**76.7**	65.0–75.0
MCH (pg)	**25.1**	19.5–24.5
MCHC (g/dl)	32.7	32.0–37.0
Reticulocytes (%)	0.5	0.0–1
WBC (x 10⁹/l)	**18.73**	6.0–18.0
Neutrophils (band) (x 10⁹/l)	**1.5**	0.0–0.3
Neutrophils (segmented) (x 10⁹/l)	**16**	3.0–12.0
Lymphocytes (x 10⁹/l)	**0.94**	1.0–3.8
Monocytes (x 10⁹/l)	0.56	0–1.20
Eosinophils (x 10⁹/l)	**<0.01**	0.1–1.30
Basophils (x 10⁹/l)	0	Rare
Platelets (x 10⁹/l)	364	150–400

Abnormal results are in **bold**.

Film comment: no morphological abnormalities.

WHAT ABNORMALITIES ARE PRESENT?

Haematology

* Mild neutrophilia with left shift.
* Mild lymphopenia.

HOW WOULD YOU INTERPRET THESE RESULTS AND WHAT ARE THE LIKELY DIFFERENTIAL DIAGNOSES?

Neutrophilia with a left shift reflects an acute inflammatory response. This may occur in response to infection, immune-mediated disease, neoplasia or tissue necrosis. A mild neutrophilia and left shift can also be seen as transient 'rebound' effect on recovery from chemotherapy induced myelosuppression. Neutrophilia due to a stress response or the prescribed corticosteroids may be superimposed. Lymphopenia is most likely part of a stress haemogram.

WHAT FURTHER TESTS WOULD YOU RECOMMEND?

In the absence of any clinical indicators of acute inflammation, urine testing was recommended as occult urinary tract infections are not uncommon in patients on immunosuppressive therapy:

* Urinalysis
* Urine culture and sensitivity (cystocentesis sample).

RESULTS OF FURTHER TESTS

Urinalysis	Results
pH	6.5
Protein	+
Glucose	–ve
Ketones	–ve
Urobilinogen	–ve

→ **CASE 3 CONTINUED**

Urinalysis *continued*	Results
Bilirubin	+
Blood	+
Haemoglobin	–ve
Specific gravity (use refractometer)	1.033
Sediment examination	Occasional fat globules. No white blood cells or bacteria seen
Protein:creatinine ratio	0.13

The absence of abnormalities on routine urinalysis does not rule out urinary tract infection, and dogs on immunosuppressive therapy, particularly corticosteroids, often do not have an active urine sediment when they have urinary tract infections. Culture is more sensitive for the presence of bacteriuria than sediment examination so was performed in this case.

Urine culture revealed a heavy growth of *Proteus mirabilis*, which was sensitive to enrofloxacin.

OUTCOME

The dog received a 3-week course of enrofloxacin and culture was subsequently negative. Occult urinary tract infections are relatively common in immunosuppressed patients (particularly those on long-term therapy for oncological and dermatological conditions) and some authors recommend intermittent cystocentesis, urinalysis and culture in all cases.

CASE 4

SIGNALMENT

1.5-year-old female Akita.

HISTORY

Presented as an emergency out-of-hours with a 2-week history of intermittent vomiting and diarrhoea, restlessness and tachypnoea. On clinical examination, the dog was reasonably bright and alert but constantly panting. Abdominal palpation suggested possible hepatomegaly and fluid-filled intestines. There was saliva staining on the paws.

CLINICAL PATHOLOGY DATA (IN-HOUSE ANALYSERS)

Haematology	Results	Reference interval
RBC (x 10^{12}/l)	6.8	5.6–8.9
Haematocrit (l/l)	0.39	0.37–0.62
Haemoglobin (g/dl)	**12.9**	13.1–20.5
MCV (fl)	**56.6**	61.6–73.5
MCH (pg)	**18.9**	21.2–25.9
MCHC (g/dl)	33.3	32.0–37.9
Reticulocytes (%)	0.9	
Reticulocyte count (x 10^9/l)	62.2	10–110
WBC (x 10^9/l)	11.17	5.05–16.76
Neutrophils (x 10^9/l)	4.61	2.95–11.64
Lymphocytes (x 10^9/l)	3.20	1.05–5.10
Monocytes (x 10^9/l)	0.48	0.16–1.12
Eosinophils (x 10^9/l)	**2.82**	0.06–1.23
Basophils (x 10^9/l)	0.06	0–0.10
Platelets (x 10^9/l)	**143**	148–484

Abnormal results are in **bold**.

Film comment: manual differential confirms eosinophilia (count 2.4 x 10^9/l). Platelet numbers appear adequate. Microcytosis but no anisocytosis.

Biochemistry	Results	Reference interval
Total protein (g/l)	77	52–82
Albumin (g/l)	29	23–40
Globulin (g/l)	**48**	25–45
ALP (IU/l)	40	23–212
ALT (IU/l)	65	10–100
Sodium (mmol/l)	**161**	144–160
Potassium (mmol/l)	4.1	3.5–5.8
Chloride (mmol/l)	122	109–122
Calcium (mmol/l)	2.7	2.0–3.0
Phosphate (mmol/l)	1.3	0.8–2.2
Glucose (mmol/l)	4.8	4.1–7.9
Urea (mmol/l)	4.5	2.5–9.6
Creatinine (µmol/l)	95	44–159
Cholesterol (mmol/l)	**2.6**	2.8–8.3
Bilirubin (µmol/l)	5.0	0–15

Abnormal results are in **bold**.

WHAT ABNORMALITIES ARE PRESENT?

Haematology

- Mildly reduced haemoglobin.
- Reduced mean corpuscular volume (MCV) and mean corpuscular haemoglobin (MCH) (microcytosis on film).
- Eosinophilia.
- (Marginal thrombocytopenia on machine count.)

Biochemistry

- Mild hyperglobulinaemia.
- Low cholesterol.
- (Marginal elevation in sodium.)

HOW WOULD YOU INTERPRET THESE RESULTS AND WHAT ARE THE LIKELY DIFFERENTIAL DIAGNOSES?

The microcytosis and low MCH is likely to be breed related, and results in a haemoglobin level just below the reference interval for 'normal' breeds.

→

→ CASE 4 CONTINUED

There is a moderate eosinophilia. Taking into account the presenting history, important differentials are: hypoadrenocorticism; parasites (enteric, pulmonary, ectoparasites); eosinophilic bronchopneumonopathy; eosinophilic enteropathy or inflammatory bowel disease; or less likely neoplasia (lymphoma or mast cell tumour). Given the possible involvement of multiple organs, hypereosinophilic syndrome is a differential, although counts are often higher.

The lack of any features of a stress haemogram (and normal glucose) further supports hypoadrenocorticism. There are no supportive electrolyte changes on biochemistry but a corticosteroid-only deficiency is also possible.

Mild hypergammaglobulinaemia may result from mild hypovolaemia (supported by the marginal elevation in sodium), or as part of an inflammatory response. Low cholesterol in a young dog is most often seen in portosystemic shunts but this is unlikely in this case given the history and other clinicopathological findings. Low cholesterol can also be seen in protein-losing enteropathy or severe liver disease.

WHAT FURTHER TESTS WOULD YOU RECOMMEND?

- Adrenocorticotropic hormone (ACTH) stimulation test.
- Thoracic and abdominal imaging and fine-needle aspiration of abnormal organs.
- Faecal analysis for parasites.
- Possibly bronchoalveolar lavage.
- Possibly gastrointestinal (GI) endoscopy and biopsy.
- (Bile acid stimulation test.)

RESULTS OF FURTHER TESTS

ACTH stimulation test		Result	Reference interval
Serum cortisol (nmol/l)	0 hour	54	50–250
	1 hour	430	150–550

Thoracic radiographs showed a mild to moderate pulmonary interstitial pattern, and mild bronchial pattern. Abdominal ultrasonography showed moderate hepatomegaly but normal echogenicity and echotexture. There was mild enlargement of all abdominal lymph nodes examined. There were no changes in intestinal thickness or layering. A small volume of fluid was present.

Cytology of fine-needle aspirates from the liver showed normal hepatocytes and numerous cytologically normal eosinophils. Aspirates from the medial iliac nodes were non-diagnostic.

The abdominal fluid was a modified transudate with predominantly eosinophils. The owner declined further investigations beyond imaging and the ACTH stimulation test.

OUTCOME

The dog received fenbendazole while the owners considered whether they wished to undertake further investigations. On presentation 10 days later, the owners reported a complete resolution of signs. The dog was clinically normal and the eosinophilia had resolved. It is most likely that migrating enteric parasites (and possibly Angiostrongylus) were the cause of her clinical signs and eosinophilia. There has been no recurrence of clinical signs.

CASE 5

SIGNALMENT

4-year-old female neutered crossbreed dog.

HISTORY

Diagnosed with multicentric lymphoma 4 months ago, and receiving CHOP chemotherapy. In complete remission at the last visit, 5 days previously, when she received a bolus dose of cyclophosphamide. Presented as an emergency with a 48-hour history of lethargy, inappetance, vocalization and apparent distress. Clinically, she was depressed with a low head carriage (head and/or neck pain) and was reluctant to walk. The submandibular lymph nodes were moderately enlarged. She was not pyrexic. Haematology was performed and, in view of the neck pain, a cerebrospinal fluid (CSF) tap was performed as well.

CLINICAL PATHOLOGY DATA

Haematology	Results	Reference interval
RBC (x 10¹²/l)	**5.02**	5.4–8.0
Haematocrit (l/l)	0.36	0.35–0.55
Haemoglobin (g/dl)	12.1	12.0–18.0
MCV (fl)	71.7	65.0–75.0
MCH (pg)	24.2	19.5–24.5
MCHC (g/dl)	33.7	32.0–37.0
Reticulocytes (%)	0.4	0.0–1
WBC (x 10⁹/l)	**2.14**	6.0 – 18.0
Neutrophils (band) (x 10⁹/l)	<0.01	0.0–0.3
Neutrophils (segmented) (x 10⁹/l)	**1.30**	3.0–12.0
Lymphocytes (x 10⁹/l)	**0.65**	1.0–3.8
Monocytes (x 10⁹/l)	0.06	0–1.20
Eosinophils (x 10⁹/l)	**<0.01**	0.1–1.30
Basophils (x 10⁹/l)	<0.01	Rare
Platelets (x 10⁹/l)	256	150–400

Abnormal results are in **bold**.

Film comment: neutrophils show toxic change.

→ CASE 5 CONTINUED

CSF tap		
Fluid analysis	Results	Reference interval
RBC (x 10¹²/l)	**10**	0 (but some often seen)
WBC (/µl)	**236**	0–6
Neutrophils (%)	31	
Lymphocytes (%)	40	
Large mononuclear cells (%)	25	
Eosinophils (%)	4	
Protein (g/l)	**0.81**	<0.30 g/l

Abnormal results are in **bold**.

CSF cytology: the sample is hypercellular with well preserved cells in a clear background. Nucleated cells consist of a mixed population of lymphocytes, neutrophils and large mononuclear cells. Neutrophils are non-degenerate. Lymphocytes are mixed: they include small lymphocytes but also large lymphoid cells. These have medium-sized and round and eccentric nuclei and have moderately abundant lightly basophilic cytoplasm. Large mononuclear cells are monocytes and they have variably shaped nuclei. Some of these are round to oval, others are bean-shaped or convoluted. The cytoplasm is moderate to abundant and lightly basophilic. No infectious agents are seen.

WHAT ABNORMALITIES ARE PRESENT?

Haematology

- Moderate neutropenia with toxic change.
- Lymphopenia.
- (Slightly low RBC count with normal haemoglobin and haematocrit: not considered significant.)

CSF

- Increased protein.
- Mixed pleocytosis. Given this and the mixed lymphoid population itself, it is more supportive of a reactive rather than neoplastic population, although lymphoma infiltration is still possible.

HOW WOULD YOU INTERPRET THESE RESULTS AND WHAT ARE THE LIKELY DIFFERENTIAL DIAGNOSES?

The neutropenia is most likely due to cyclophosphamide administration 5 days ago. Toxic change reflects enhanced turnover as the marrow attempts to meet demand.

Differentials for the increased CSF protein and mixed pleocytosis include granulomatous meningoencephalitis (GME), viral or protozoal diseases, neoplasia (lymphoma), ischaemia and other causes.

WHAT FURTHER TESTS WOULD YOU RECOMMEND?

- Flow cytometry or PARR on CSF to confirm if reactive or neoplastic.
- Serology or PCR for *Neospora* and toxoplasmosis.

RESULTS OF FURTHER TESTS

There was insufficient sample for flow cytometry.

PARR results

- BCR clonality: monoclonal.
- TCR clonality: polyclonal.

A clonal expansion of the BCR is consistent with a neoplastic B-cell population present in the CSF. Central nervous system (CNS) involvement in lymphoma.

Neospora antibody titre was <100, consistent with a negative result. *Toxoplasma* IgG antibody titre was 100, consistent with exposure to *Toxoplasma*, but *Toxoplasma* IgM antibody titre was <20 and therefore not consistent with current infection (but suggestive of past exposure).

OUTCOME

The patient received L-asparaginase and then, once the neutropenia had resolved, rescue therapy with lomustine, procarbazine and prednisolone, then dexamethasone, melphalan, actinomycin and cytosine. She was euthanased approximately 10 weeks after presenting with CNS signs due to progressive disease.

References and further reading

Almeida FM, Narciso LG, Bosco AM *et al.* (2013) Neutrophil dysfunction varies with the stage of canine visceral leishmaniosis. *Veterinary Parasitology* **196**, 6–12

Andreasen CB and Roth JA (2000) Neutrophil function abnormalities. In: *Schalm's Veterinary Hematology*, ed. BF Feldman *et al.*, pp. 356–365. Lippencott Williams & Wilkins, Baltimore

Avery AC (2012) Molecular diagnostics of hematologic malignancies in small animals. *Veterinary Clinics of North America: Small Animal Practice* **42**, 97–110

Barrs VR, Beatty JA, McCandlish IA and Kipar A (2002) Hypereosinophilic paraneoplastic syndrome in a cat with intestinal T cell lymphosarcoma. *Journal of Small Animal Practice* **43**, 401–405

Bauer NB, Nakagawa J, Dunker C, Failing K and Moritz A (2012) Evaluation of the impedance analyzer PocH-100iV Diff for analysis of canine and feline blood. *Veterinary Clinical Pathology* **41**, 194–206

Burton AG, Harris LA, Owens SD and Jandrey KE (2013) The prognostic utility of degenerative left shifts in dogs. *Journal of Veterinary Internal Medicine* **27**, 1517–1522

Campbell DJ, Rawlings JM, Koelsch S, Wallace J, Strain JJ and Hannigan BM (2004) Age-related differences in parameters of feline immune status. *Veterinary Immunology and Immunopathology* **100**, 73–80

Campora C, Freeman KP, Lewis FI, Gibson G, Sacchini F and Sanchez-Vazquez MJ (2011) Determination of haematological reference intervals in healthy adult greyhounds. *Journal of Small Animal Practice* **52**, 301–309

Cave TA, Gault EA and Argyle DJ (2004) Feline epitheliotropic T-cell lymphoma with paraneoplastic eosinophilia – immunochemotherapy with vinblastine and human recombinant interferon α2b. *Veterinary and Comparative Oncology* **2**, 91–97

Cruz Cardona JA, Milner R, Alleman AR *et al.* (2011) BCR–ABL translocation in a dog with chronic monocytic leukemia. *Veterinary Clinical Pathology* **40**, 40–47

Goldmann F, Bauer N and Moritz A (2012) Evaluation of the IDEXX ProCyte Dx analyzer for dogs and cats compared to the Siemens ADVIA 2120 and manual differential. *Comparative Clinical Pathology* **23**, 1–14

Gommeren KWG, Daminet S, Vanholen L, Vandenberghe A and Duchateau L (2004) Prevalence of physiologic leucopenia in the Tervuren and the Groenendael in Flanders. In: *Scientific Proceedings, BSAVA 47th Annual Congress*, Birmingham, p. 566

Greenfield CL, Messick JB, Solter PF and Schaeffer DJ (2000) Results of hematologic analyses and prevalence of physiologic leukopenia in Belgian Tervuren dogs. *Journal of the American Veterinary Medical Association* **216**, 866–871

Hall JA, Chinn RM, Vorachek WR, Gorman ME and Jewell DE (2010) Aged Beagle dogs have decreased neutrophil phagocytosis and neutrophil-related gene expression compared to younger dogs. *Veterinary Immunology and Immunopathology* **137**, 130–135

Harper EJ, Hackett RM, Wikinson J and Heaton PR (2003) Age-related variations in hematologic and plasma biochemical test results in Beagles and Labrador Retrievers. *Journal of the American Veterinary Medical Association* **223**, 1436–1442

Harvey JW (2012) Evaluation of leukocyte disorders. In: *Veterinary Haematology: A Diagnostic Guide and Colour Atlas*, ed. JW Harvey, pp. 122–176. Elsevier Saunders, Missouri

Hostette SJ (2012) Neutrophil function in small animals. *Veterinary Clinics of North America: Small Animal Practice* **42**, 157–171

Jones RF and Paris R (1963) The Greyhound eosinophil. *Journal of Small Animal Practice* **4**(Suppl), 29–33

Keller RL, Avery AC, Burnett RC, Walton JA and Olver CS (2004) Detection of neoplastic lymphocytes in peripheral blood of dogs with lymphoma by polymerase chain reaction for antigen receptor gene rearrangement. *Veterinary Clinical Pathology* **3**, 144–149

Keller SM, Keller BC, Grest P, Börger CT and Guscetti F (2007) Validation of tissue microarrays for immunohistochemical analyses of canine lymphomas. *Journal of Veterinary Diagnostic Investigation* **19**, 652–659

Kheiri SA, MacKerrell T, Bonagura VR, Fuchs A and Billett HH (1998) Flow cytometry with or without cytochemistry for the diagnosis of acute leukaemias. *Cytometry* **34**, 82–86

Lana SE, Jackson TL, Burnett RC, Morley PS and Avery AC (2006) Utility of polymerase chain reaction for analysis of antigen receptor rearrangement in staging and predicting prognosis in dogs with lymphoma. *Journal of Veterinary Internal Medicine* **20**, 329–334

LeBlanc CJ, LeBlanc AK, Jones MM, Bartges JW and Kania SA (2010) Evaluation of peripheral blood neutrophil function in tumor-bearing dogs. *Veterinary Clinical Pathology* **39**, 157–163

Lefebvre HP (2011) Greyhound-specific reference intervals: a good start to a long race. *Veterinary Clinical Pathology* **40**, 405–406

Lucroy MD and Madewell BR (1999) Clinical outcome and associated diseases in dogs with leukocytosis and neutrophilia: 118 cases (1996–1998). *Journal of the American Veterinary Medical Association* **214**, 805–807

Lucroy MD and Madewell BR (2001) Clinical outcome and diseases associated with extreme neutrophilic leukocytosis in cats: 104 cases (1991–1999). *Journal of the American Veterinary Medical Association* **218**, 736–739

Marchetti V, Benetti C, Citi S and Taccini V (2005) Paraneoplastic hypereosinophilia in a dog with intestinal T-cell lymphoma. *Veterinary Clinical Pathology* **34**, 259–263

Mason SL, Jepson R, Maltman M and Batchelor DJ (2014) Presentation and management of trapped neutrophil syndrome (TNS) in UK Border Collies. *Journal of Small Animal Practice* **55(1)**, 57–60

Papasouliotis K, Cue S, Crawford E, Pinches M, Dumont M and Burley K (2006) Comparison of white blood cell differential percentages determined by the in-house LaserCyte hematology analyzer and a manual method. *Veterinary Clinical Pathology* **35**, 295–302

Piviani M, Walton RM and Patel RT (2013) Significance of mastocytemia in cats. *Veterinary Clinical Pathology* **42**, 4–10

Ponce F, Magnol JP, Ledieu D *et al.* (2004) Prognostic significance of morphological subtypes in canine malignant lymphomas during chemotherapy. *The Veterinary Journal* **167**, 158–166

Schnelle AN and Barger AM (2012) Neutropenia in dogs and cats: causes and consequences. *Veterinary Clinics of North America: Small Animal Practice* **42**, 111–122

Shafrine M, Munn SL, Rosenblatt LS, Bulgin MS and Wilson FD (1973) Hematologic changes to 60 days of age in clinically normal Beagles. *Laboratory Animal Science* **23**, 894–898

Shearman JR and Wilton AN (2011) A canine model of Cohen syndrome: trapped neutrophil syndrome. *BMC Genomics* **12**, 258

Silva ACRA, de Almeida BFM, Soeiro CS, Ferreira WL, de Lima VMF and Ciarlini PC (2013) Oxidative stress, superoxide production, and apoptosis of neutrophils in dogs with chronic kidney disease. *Canadian Journal of Veterinary Research* **77**, 136–141

Uhríková I, Lačňáková A, Tandlerová K *et al.* (2013) Haematological and biochemical variations among eight sighthound breeds. *Australian Veterinary Journal* **91**, 452–459

Vahlenkamp TW, Tompkins MB and Tompkins WA (2004) Feline immunodeficiency virus infection phenotypically and functionally activates immunosuppressive CD4+CD25+ T regulatory cells. *Journal of Immunology* **172**, 4752–4761

Webb C, McCord K and Dow S (2007) Neutrophil function in septic dogs. *Journal of Veterinary Internal Medicine* **21**, 982–989

Welles EG, Hall AS and Carpenter DM (2009) Canine complete blood counts: a comparison of four in-office instruments with the ADVIA 120 and manual differential counts. *Veterinary Clinical Pathology* **38**, 20–29

Wengler-Riggenbach B, Hässig M, Hofmann-Lehmann R and Lutz H (2006) Evaluation of the LaserCyte: an in-house hematology analyzer for dogs and cats. *Comparative Clinical Pathology* **15**, 117–129

Williams MJ, Avery AC, Lana SE, Hillers KR, Bachand AM and Avery PR (2008) Canine lymphoproliferative disease characterized by lymphocytosis: immunophenotypic markers of prognosis. *Journal of Veterinary Internal Medicine* **22**, 596–601

Zaldívar-López S, Marín LM, Iazbik MC, Westendorf-Stingle N, Hensley S and Couto CG (2011) Clinical pathology of Greyhounds and other sighthounds. *Veterinary Clinical Pathology* **40**, 414–425

Chapter 6

Disorders of haemostasis

Tracy Stokol

Haemostasis is a simple word that means 'stop bleeding'. Yet the simplicity of the word belies the incredible complexity of a process whereby an array of cells and proteins intimately interact in a finely tuned and balanced system, first to form a fibrin clot then to dissolve the clot to restore vessel patency. Deficiencies or abnormalities in either haemostatic cells or proteins disrupt the delicate harmony and tip the balance towards inadequate clot formation, which leads to excessive haemorrhage, or its converse, accelerated clot formation or thrombosis (see also the *BSAVA Manual of Canine and Feline Haematology and Transfusion Medicine*). Clinically, excessive haemorrhage is far easier to recognize than thrombosis and most available diagnostic tests of haemostasis are geared towards detecting deficiencies that result in inadequate clot formation and haemorrhage. It is only recently that the diagnostic emphasis has shifted towards recognition of hypercoagulable states, i.e. conditions that promote thrombosis. Aside from maintaining vascular integrity, the haemostatic system also functions in innate immunity, with activated coagulation factors stimulating inflammatory responses, and fibrin and platelets trapping and clearing infectious agents. Although these responses can be protective, they can also contribute to disease pathogenesis when in excess (e.g. a vicious cycle can be set up when inflammation activates haemostasis and then haemostatic proteins fuel the fire).

Overview of haemostasis

The important players in haemostasis are cells, particularly platelets, and various proteins, including coagulation factors (Figure 6.1). Indeed, physiological haemostasis proceeds on and is restricted to the surface of cells; this is now called the cell-based model of haemostasis (Smith, 2009). Haemostasis does not occur under steady-state conditions because the intact endothelium acts as a barrier preventing circulating platelets and coagulation factors from interacting with procoagulant proteins in the extracellular matrix. The most important triggers for haemostasis are tissue factor (TF or coagulation factor III) and extracellular matrix proteins, such as collagen. Once the endothelial barrier is disrupted, these proteins are exposed and activate the haemostatic system. For ease of understanding, haemostasis can be conceptually separated into three stages, each of which has its specific interactive network of cells and proteins (Figure 6.2):

- Primary haemostasis: formation of the platelet plug
- Secondary haemostasis: formation of fibrin
- Fibrinolysis: dissolution of the fibrin clot.

However, these stages do not occur sequentially, but can be activated simultaneously and proceed concurrently *in vivo*. The degree of vessel injury, nature of the injured vessel, and a complex interplay between activating and inhibitory forces dictate which stage dominates, in a temporal and spatial manner. For instance, immediately on vessel injury procoagulant forces dominate over fibrinolysis, whereas once the vessel injury begins to seal, fibrinolytic forces take over. Superficial injuries to small vessels (as occurs in oral vessels exposed daily to the trauma of eating) only trigger platelet activation and platelet plug formation, which are sufficient to repair the injury. However, deeper injury to larger vessels, such as the impact of weight-bearing on vessels supplying joints, requires fibrin formation to solidify the platelet plug and seal off the injured vessel. There are also crucial links between each of these stages. For instance, activated platelets are the cellular surface on which secondary haemostasis proceeds. They also release intracellular constituents, such as polyphosphates and coagulation factors, which promote clotting and inhibit fibrinolysis. Thrombin, the pivotal enzymatic product of secondary haemostasis, activates platelets and simultaneously inhibits fibrinolysis, to prevent the clot from being broken down as it is being formed. The complex interplay between the stages yields a haemostatic pendulum, which sways between procoagulant forces and clot formation

Function	Proteins (not an exhaustive list)
Adhesive (bind to cells)	Collagen, von Willebrand factor, fibrinogen
Enzymes	Activated coagulation factors: FXIIa, XIa, Xa, IXa, IIa (thrombin)
Cofactors (amplify enzyme activity)	Tissue factor, FVa, FVIIIa, vitamin K (required for binding of factors to phosphatidylserine-expressing membranes)
Platelet agonists	ADP, thromboxane A_2, thrombin
Crosslinking agent	Factor XIIIa
Inhibitors	Tissue factor pathway inhibitor, antithrombin, protein C, protein S

6.1 Functional roles of haemostatic proteins. ADP = adenosine diphosphate.

Stage	Endpoint	Cells	Proteins: facilitators	Proteins: inhibitors
Primary haemostasis	Platelet plug	Platelets	von Willebrand factor, collagen, fibrinogen	ADPase[a], prostacyclin[a], nitric oxide[a]
Secondary haemostasis	Fibrin	**Initiation:** fibroblasts **Progression:** platelets	**Initiation:** tissue factor, FVII **Progression:** thrombin, intrinsic (FXI down) and common (FX down) pathway factors	**Initiation:** tissue factor pathway inhibitor[a] (TFPI) **Progression:** antithrombin[b] (potentiated by heparin), protein C[b] (activated by thrombin binding to thrombomodulin), protein S[b] (cofactor for protein C and TFPI), non-specific protease inhibitors[b] (e.g. α_2-macroglobulin)
Fibrinolysis	Vessel patency	Endothelial cells	Plasminogen, tissue plasminogen activator	Thrombin-activatable fibrinolytic inhibitor[b] (TAFI), antiplasmin[b], plasminogen activator inhibitor-1[a]

6.2 Important cellular and protein players in haemostasis. [a] Produced by endothelial cells. [b] Produced by the liver. ADP = adenosine diphosphate.

and anticoagulant forces or clot dissolution. The direction of the pendulum depends on the activating and inhibitory forces that govern each process. Initially, coagulation is favoured, permitting formation of a stable thrombus. Fibrinolysis then dominates, promoting thrombus dissolution and restoration of vessel patency (Figure 6.3).

Primary haemostasis

- **Definition:** formation of the platelet plug.
- **Cellular constituents:**
  - *Platelets:* form the plug
  - *Endothelial cells:* source of von Willebrand factor (vWf).
- **Protein constituents:**
  - *Extracellular matrix proteins (principally collagen):* bind the platelet receptors, $\alpha_4\beta_1$ and glycoprotein (GP) VI, on unactivated platelets
  - *vWf:* binds to the platelet receptor GPIb–IX–V complex on unactivated platelets. Acts as a 'glue' to attach platelets to exposed matrix proteins. Produced in endothelial cells and stored in Weibel–Palade bodies; stores are released on vessel injury (creating high localized concentrations). Although vWf is a plasma protein, endothelial cells preferentially release vWf into the subendothelial matrix, and hence matrix-bound vWf can be thought of as 'functional' vWf
  - *Fibrinogen:* binds the fibrinogen receptor (GPIIb/IIIa) on activated platelets and bridges adjacent platelets, forming the platelet plug.
- **Sequence of events** (Figure 6.4):
  - *Platelet adhesion:* unactivated platelets bind to exposed subendothelial matrix proteins, collagen and vWf, through specific surface receptors (see above)
  - *Platelet activation:* once platelets bind, they become activated, initiate metabolic pathways and undergo structural changes. Agonists are released (adenosine diphosphate (ADP), thromboxane A_2) which recruit and activate circulating non-adherent platelets to the site of injury:
    - Shape change: increases the platelet surface area
    - Release reaction: release of **preformed** cytoplasmic granules, which contain platelet agonists (ADP), polyphosphates, stored coagulation factors (e.g. factor V or FV) and adhesive proteins (P selectin)
    - Membrane (arachidonic acid) metabolism: surface membrane phospholipids are metabolized into potent platelet agonists (thromboxane A_2) and proinflammatory lipids

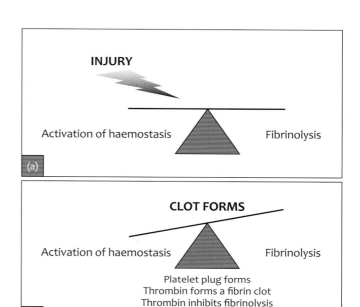

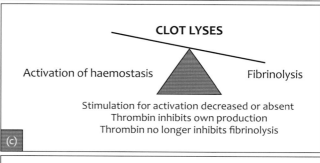

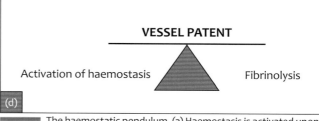

6.3 The haemostatic pendulum. (a) Haemostasis is activated upon blood vessel injury. (b) This swings the pendulum in favour of procoagulant forces. Exposure of procoagulant extracellular matrix proteins and tissue factor initiates platelet plug formation and thrombin generation, respectively. Thrombin forms the fibrin clot, which is enmeshed with the platelet plug. At the same time, thrombin inhibits fibrinolysis, preventing clot breakdown. (c) Once the clot has formed and the vessel heals, the stimulus for thrombin generation decreases, thrombin begins to inhibit its own production and no longer inhibits fibrinolysis, swinging the pendulum in favour of fibrinolysis. (d) Lysis of the clot restores vessel patency and the original status quo.

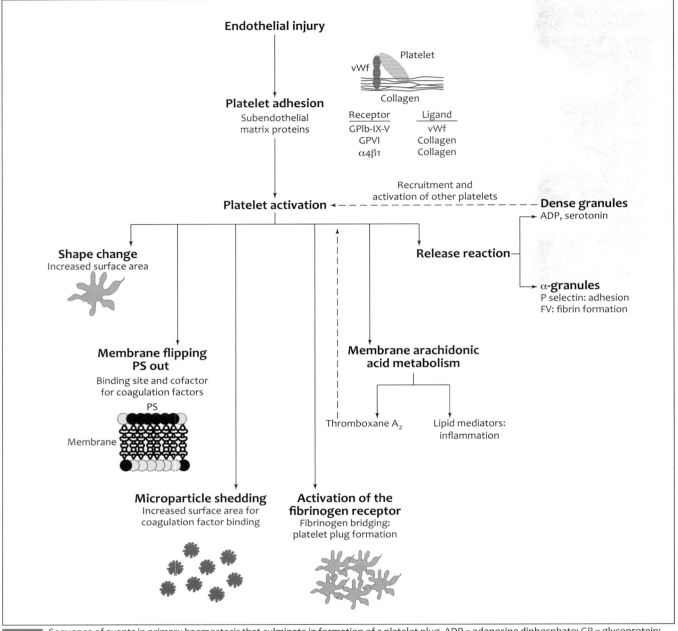

6.4 Sequence of events in primary haemostasis that culminate in formation of a platelet plug. ADP = adenosine diphosphate; GP = glycoprotein; PS = phosphatidylserine; vWF = Willebrand factor.

- Membrane flipping and microvesiculation: the negatively charged phospholipid phosphatidylserine (PS, previously known as platelet factor 3) is flipped to the outer platelet membrane. This provides a binding surface for activated coagulation factor complex assembly. Small PS-enriched membrane microparticles are released and increase the platelet surface area on which fibrin can be formed
- Activation of the fibrinogen receptor, the integrin GPIIb/IIIa: this is switched from 'inactive' to 'active' mode and binds fibrinogen.
- *Platelet aggregation (plug formation):* this is mediated by fibrinogen bridging adjacent platelets via GPIIb/IIIa.
- **Inhibitors:** The endothelial cell is the source of physiological platelet inhibitors (see Figure 6.2).

Pharmacological inhibitors affect:
- *Arachidonic acid metabolism:* aspirin (irreversibly) and non-steroidal anti-inflammatory drugs (NSAIDs, reversibly) inhibit cyclo-oxgenase, which is needed for thromboxane A_2 production
- *ADP agonist activity:* clopidogrel is an ADP receptor antagonist.
- **Clinical manifestations of primary haemostatic defects:**
  - *Decreased number or function:* platelet plug formation is inadequate with any defect in primary haemostasis. This usually manifests as haemorrhage from small blood vessels subjected to daily minor trauma, e.g. those supplying mucosal surfaces (e.g. epistaxis, haematuria) (Figure 6.5). Haemorrhage can be spontaneous with severe thrombocytopenia or induced by trauma or surgery

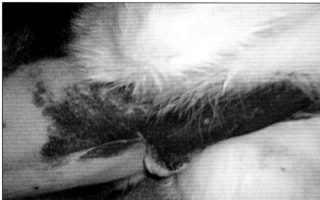

6.6 Severe preputial and abdominal ecchymoses after castration of a German Shepherd Dog with Scott syndrome. Scott syndrome is caused by an inherited defect in platelet membrane flipping, i.e. activated platelets do not exteriorize phosphatidylserine and do not support fibrin formation. Note that such ecchymoses are **not** specific for disorders of primary haemostasis but can be seen with defects of secondary haemostasis and fibrinolysis.
(Courtesy of Dr M Brooks, Comparative Coagulation Laboratory, Cornell University)

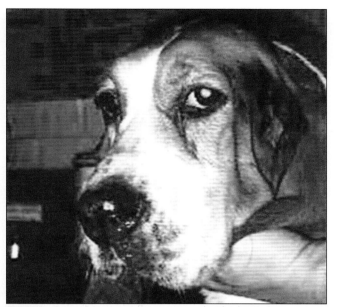

6.5 Epistaxis in a young Bassett Hound with inherited thrombopathia, which is due to a mutation in calcium diacylglycerol guanine nucleotide exchange factor-1 (CalDAG–GEF1) in platelets. This is a signalling protein that is important for activation of the fibrinogen receptor on platelets, and the mutation results in an absence of platelet aggregation in response to ADP and collagen. Epistaxis can be seen in any disorder of primary haemostasis but is not typical of disorders of secondary haemostasis.
(Courtesy of Dr M Brooks, Comparative Coagulation Laboratory, Cornell University)

with milder defects. Since platelets plug small holes in vessels, thrombocytopenia or abnormal platelet function (thrombopathia) can result in pinpoint mucosal or cutaneous haemorrhages (petechiae). Petechiae are not usually seen in von Willebrand's disease (vWD), due to decreased or defective vWf. Ecchymoses and purpura can also occur, particularly after trauma or surgery (Figure 6.6) or with severe defects

- *Increased number or function:* platelet hyperreactivity and increased vWf concentrations contribute to hypercoagulability, i.e. are risk factors for thrombosis, but are unlikely to induce thrombosis alone. Thrombocytosis in animals is not usually associated with abnormal thrombotic events.

- **Tests of primary haemostasis** (Figure 6.7; see below for more detail)**:**
  - *Screening tests:* platelet count, buccal mucosal bleeding time (BMBT), platelet function analyser testing
  - *Specific tests (available to practitioners):* von Willebrand factor antigen (vWf:Ag), genetic testing for vWD and defined inherited thrombopathias (e.g. calcium diacylglycerol guanine nucleotide exchange factor-1 (CalDAG–GEF1) defect in Bassett Hounds and Eskimo Spitz, GPIIb/IIIa deficiency or Glanzman's thrombasthenia in Otterhounds and Pyrenean Mountain Dogs
  - *Non-routine specialized testing (not readily available):* flow cytometric tests for platelet activation (P selectin expression), platelet function in primary haemostasis (aggregation, release reaction), procoagulant activity (PS exteriorization, microparticle quantification, thrombin generation assays), platelet-associated antibodies, reticulated platelets.

Primary haemostasis

- *Screening*
  - Buccal mucosal bleeding time[a]: vWD, thrombopathia, thrombocytopenia
  - Platelet function analysis (PFA): vWD, thrombopathia, thrombocytopenia
- *Specific*
  - Platelet number: count[a], crit
  - Platelet function: adhesion, aggregation, activation, procoagulant activity, genetic testing[a] (breed specific)
  - vWD: vWf:Ag[a], vWf activity (collagen binding assay, aggregation), multimeric assay (vWf structure), genetic testing[a] (breed specific)
  - Biopsy[a]: vascular disorders

Secondary haemostasis

- *Extrinsic pathway*
  - Screening: prothrombin time[a]
  - Specific: FVIIa activity[a]
- *Intrinsic pathway*
  - Screening: activated coagulation time[a], activated partial thromboplastin time[a]
  - Specific: factor activities[a] (FXIIa, FXIa, FIXa, FVIIIa), genetic testing[a] (breed specific)
- *Common pathway*
  - Screening: fibrinogen concentration[a], thrombin clot time[a]
  - Specific: factor activities (FXa[a], FVa[a], FXIIIa)
- *Multiple pathways*
  - Screening: proteins induced by vitamin K absence/antagonism[a], anticoagulant rodenticide screens
- *Inhibitors*: antithrombin activity[a], protein C activity[a], protein S, thrombin–antithrombin complexes (indicates thrombin generation or hypercoagulability)

Fibrinolysis

- *Screening*: fibrin(ogen) degradation products (FDP)[a], D-dimer[a]
- *Specific*: plasminogen, tissue plasminogen activator, plasmin
- *Inhibitors*: plasminogen activator inhibitor-1, plasmin–antiplasmin complexes

Global haemostasis

- Viscoelastic methods[a], thrombin generation assays, clot signature profiles

6.7 Tests for the diagnosis of haemostatic disorders. [a]Tests available to the veterinary practitioner, either in-house or through referral laboratories. vWD = von Willebrand's disease; vWf:Ag = von Willebrand factor antigen.

Secondary haemostasis

- **Definition:** formation of fibrin by coagulation factors on the surface of activated platelets. *Synonym:* coagulation (i.e. fibrin clot formation). The key event is the generation of thrombin by activated coagulation factors, which assemble as potent enzymatic complexes on negatively charged membrane surfaces, provided by inside-out flipping of PS. Thrombin generation occurs through sequential phases: initiation, amplification and propagation. Thrombin is required for both fibrin formation **and** inhibition of fibrinolysis, which is essential for the fibrin clot to form properly (see Figure 6.3).
- **Cellular constituents:**
  - *Fibroblasts:* initiation
  - *Platelets:* amplification and propagation. Platelets have multifactorial roles in secondary haemostasis. They are the main cellular source of PS. They release stored coagulation factors (taken up from plasma) and polyphosphates, which accelerate thrombin generation and retard fibrinolysis. Thrombin is a potent platelet agonist and activates them further
  - *Leucocytes, erythrocytes:* these can provide PS surfaces and are probably involved in fibrin formation to a greater extent than currently appreciated.
- **Protein constituents:**
  - *All coagulation factors:* these have been conveniently grouped into sequential pathways called the coagulation cascade. This cascade was based on coagulation assays, which were triggered by surface contact or TF (Figure 6.8). However, these pathways do not represent how fibrin formation proceeds *in vitro*. Activated factors are designated by the postscript 'a':
    - Extrinsic: this starts with TF, which binds FVII and requires calcium (Ca^{2+}) and PS
    - Intrinsic: this starts with surface contact, which activates FXII. FXIIa then activates FXI, which then activates FIX, with FVIIIa being an essential cofactor for FIX. This pathway also requires Ca^{2+} and PS
    - Common: this starts with FX, which can be activated by TF–FVIIa–PS–Ca^{2+} of the extrinsic pathway ('extrinsic tenase') or FIXa–FVIIIa–PS–Ca^{2+} of the intrinsic pathway ('intrinsic tenase'). FXa forms a 'prothrombinase' complex with FVa, PS and Ca^{2+} and cleaves prothrombin to thrombin. Thrombin then converts fibrinogen to fibrin. Factor XIII is activated by thrombin and crosslinks fibrin. Calcium and PS are required.
  - *Vitamin K:* essential cofactor for the enzyme that modifies specific coagulation factors (FII, FVII, FIX, FX) and inhibitors (protein C, protein S), allowing them to bind to PS. If the factors do not bind to PS, they cannot participate efficiently in fibrin formation or inhibition.
- **Sequence of events *in vivo*** (Figure 6.9):
  - *Initiation of thrombin generation via the extrinsic pathway:* TF, which is constitutively expressed on extravascular fibroblasts, binds to its enzymatic partner in plasma, FVII. The TF–FVIIa complex or 'extrinsic tenase' activates factor X, and then a prothrombinase complex consisting of TF–FVIIa–FX produces a small amount of thrombin on the fibroblast surface. The TF–FVII complex can also

activate FIX of the intrinsic pathway directly ('alternative pathway')
- *Amplification of thrombin generation via intrinsic and common pathways:* thrombin production moves from fibroblasts to platelets, which are in the vicinity (having bound to exposed extracellular matrix proteins). The small amount of thrombin generated by TF–FVIIa–FXa is insufficient to form fibrin or inhibit fibrinolysis, however thrombin then amplifies its own production via activation of FXI (intrinsic pathway) and the cofactors FV and FVIII. FXIa helps form the potent FIXa–FVIIIa 'intrinsic tenase' complex on platelets, which is supplemented by FIXa produced by the TF–FVIIa complex. Note that FXII has no role in this process
- *Propagation of thrombin generation on platelet surfaces:* the PS surface of activated platelets provides binding sites for coagulation factors, promotes their assembly into complexes, enhances their activity and protects them from inhibition. Platelets also release stored FV, which provides high local concentrations of this cofactor for FXa. All this helps produce large amounts of thrombin ('thrombin burst') by the 'prothrombinase' complex (platelet-bound FXa–FVa)

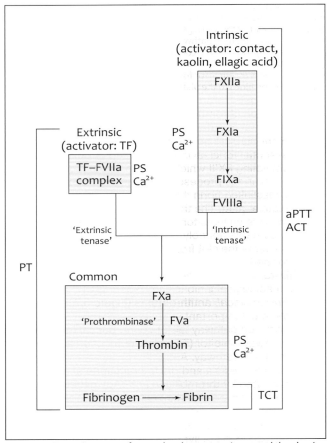

6.8 Screening tests of secondary haemostasis created the classic model of the coagulation cascade, whereby fibrin formation can be initiated by surface contact activation of FXII in the intrinsic pathway or with exogenous tissue factor (TF, in the form of brain thromboplastin) in the extrinsic pathway. However, contact or FXIIa does not activate secondary haemostasis and FXII has no role in fibrin formation under physiological conditions *in vivo*. This is exemplified by cats with FXII deficiency, which do not show clinical signs of abnormal haemorrhage. ACT = activated coagulation time; aPTT = activated partial thromboplastin time; Ca^{2+} = calcium ions; PS = phosphatidylserine; PT = prothrombin time; TCT = thrombin clot time.

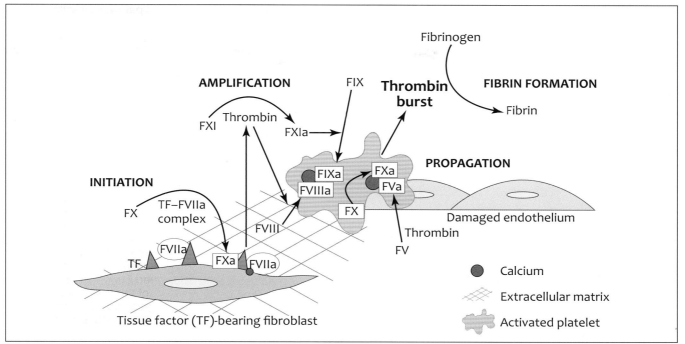

6.9 Sequence of events in secondary haemostasis. **Initiation:** on endothelial injury, plasma FVII binds to tissue factor (TF) on subendothelial fibroblasts. Once bound to TF, FVII autoactivates and the TF–FVII complex forms the 'extrinsic tenase', which activates FX on fibroblast membranes. The extrinsic pathway is rapidly inhibited by tissue factor pathway inhibitor and produces only a small amount of thrombin. **Amplification:** the small amount of thrombin generated by the extrinsic pathway amplifies its own production by activating FXI of the intrinsic pathway and FVIII and FV, the intrinsic and common pathway cofactors. FXIa then activates FIX, which forms a potent 'intrinsic tenase' complex with FVIIIa on the platelet surface. FIX produced by the TF–FVIIa complex (alternative pathway) supplements the 'intrinsic' tenase (not shown). **Propagation:** the phosphatidylserine (PS)-enriched surfaces of activated platelets help amplify and propagate thrombin generation, producing a 'thrombin burst'. **Fibrin formation:** the thrombin burst is essential for forming crosslinked fibrin from fibrinogen (and also for concurrently inhibiting fibrinolysis). The formed fibrin closely intercalates and binds to the platelet plug, forming a stable fibrin clot. Note that calcium and PS-expressing surfaces are crucial for fibrin formation.

- *Fibrin formation by thrombin:* the thrombin burst is essential for cleaving fibrinogen to soluble fibrin and activating FXIII which then crosslinks the soluble fibrin (in the process forming the D-dimer epitope). Crosslinked fibrin then binds to and stabilizes the platelet plug. The thrombin burst is also needed to activate an inhibitor of fibrinolysis, called thrombin-activatable fibrinolytic inhibitor (TAFI), which prevents the clot from being broken down as it is formed.
- **Inhibitors:** there are both physiological and pharmacological inhibitors of secondary haemostasis:
  - *Physiological:* antithrombin (AT) and protein C are the most important inhibitors of intrinsic and common pathway factors, whereas tissue factor pathway inhibitor (TFPI) is the main inhibitor of the extrinsic pathway. Antithrombin's main inhibitory targets are FXa and thrombin. Protein C is actually activated by thrombin, after it binds to a receptor on endothelial cells, thrombomodulin. Protein S is a cofactor that supports the inhibitory action of protein C and TFPI. All of these inhibitors are produced in the liver
  - *Pharmacological:* the most commonly used pharmacological inhibitors of secondary haemostasis are unfractionated and low molecular weight heparin, which potentiate the action of AT; and warfarin, which inhibits the recycling of vitamin K, resulting in a relative vitamin K deficiency.
- **Clinical manifestations:**
  - *Decreased number or function:* since fibrin is required to stabilize the platelet plug, decreased

fibrin formation from coagulation factor or vitamin K deficiency results in bleeding from larger vessels. This manifests as haematomas (in skin, muscle or subcutaneous tissue) and haemorrhage into body cavities (haemarthrosis, haemoperitoneum, etc.), which can be spontaneous (Figure 6.10). As for defects in primary haemostasis, traumatic or surgery-induced haemorrhage can occur, and this does not discriminate between abnormalities in primary or secondary haemostasis. Deficiencies of inhibitors can also lead to thrombosis
  - *Hypercoagulability:* this is defined as excessive generation of thrombin and is caused by aberrant activation of secondary haemostasis, usually by TF (e.g. massive endothelial injury, aberrant intravascular expression of TF on monocytes or cancer cells) combined with a lack of adequate inhibition. Animals in hypercoagulable states are at risk of or may already be developing microvascular thrombi. High concentrations of some coagulation factors, such as fibrinogen and FVIII, may contribute to a hypercoagulable state, but alone will not result in thrombosis. Loss or decreased production of inhibitors, such as AT or protein C, may also result in hypercoagulability or thrombosis. Thrombosis is very difficult to recognize clinically. This is because thrombi frequently occur in internal small vessels, thrombotic sequelae of hypoxic injury to vital organs may be masked by other diseases, and there is a paucity of sensitive and specific diagnostic or imaging tests for thrombi.

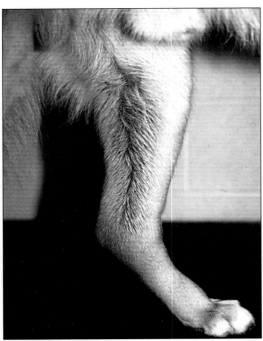

6.10 Spontaneous severe ecchymoses on the inner leg of a German Shepherd Dog with haemophilia A (<1% factor VIII coagulant activity). This extensive spontaneous haemorrhage is more typical of disorders of secondary haemostasis than primary haemostasis.
(Courtesy of Dr M Brooks, Comparative Coagulation Laboratory, Cornell University)

- **Tests of secondary haemostasis** (see Figure 6.7 and below for more detail):
  - *Screening tests:* prothrombin time (PT), activated partial thromboplastin time (aPTT), activated coagulation time (ACT), thrombin clot time (TCT), fibrinogen concentration
  - *Specific tests (available to practitioners):* individual coagulation factor activities
  - *Tests for inhibitors:* antithrombin activity, protein C activity, therapeutic heparin monitoring (anti-FXa activity, aPTT prolongation), anticoagulant rodenticide testing
  - *Non-routine specialized testing (not readily available):* coagulation factor inhibitors (anti-phospholipid antibodies etc), fibrinogen antigen, thrombin–antithrombin (TAT) complexes.

Fibrinolysis

- **Definition:** dissolution of the fibrin clot by the fibrinolytic enzyme, plasmin.
- **Cellular constituents:**
  - *Endothelial cells:* source of tissue plasminogen activator (tPA).
- **Protein constituents:**
  - *Tissue plasminogen activator:* released from injured endothelial cells and converts plasminogen to plasmin. Activity is greatly enhanced when plasminogen is bound to fibrin, which helps localize and restrict fibrinolysis to the clot
  - *Plasminogen:* precursor of plasmin. Produced in the liver. Binds to fibrin, localizing fibrinolysis
  - *Factor XIIa/kallikrein complex:* both of these enzymes are weak plasminogen activators
  - *Bradykinin:* produced by FXIIa/kallikrein complex-mediated cleavage of high molecular weight kininogen. Most potent inducer of tPA release from endothelial cells. Thus, FXII is not involved in fibrin formation under physiological conditions but, instead, is involved in fibrin breakdown.
- **Sequence of events** (Figure 6.11):
  - *Generation of plasmin:* tissue plasminogen activator (tPA) is released from endothelial cells upon vessel injury or bradykinin stimulation. It cleaves plasminogen to plasmin within the local environment of the fibrin clot, to which plasminogen is bound. This restricts plasmin activity to fibrin. Plasmin is a non-specific protease and, if not restricted to the fibrin clot, would cleave other proteins
  - *Liberation of degradation products:* plasmin cleaves fibrinogen, soluble fibrin and crosslinked fibrin. Cleavage of fibrinogen or soluble fibrin (generated by the action of thrombin on fibrinogen) yields similar degradation products, called fibrin(ogen) degradation products (FDP). None of these products have crosslinks. In contrast, plasmin cleavage of crosslinked fibrin yields different degradation products, called X-oligomers (X for crosslinked), the smallest of which is the neo-antigen D-dimer. These degradation products are used as laboratory markers of fibrinolysis (Figure 6.12).
- **Inhibitors:** Fibrinolytic inhibitors are rarely used therapeutically. This is because it is difficult conclusively to identify hyperfibrinolysis as a cause of

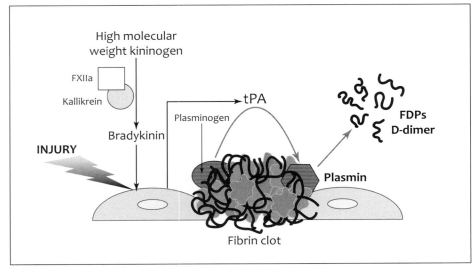

6.11 Fibrinolysis is triggered when injured endothelial cells release tissue plasminogen activator (tPA), which then cleaves plasminogen (which is tightly bound to fibrin) to plasmin. Plasmin lyses fibrin into degradation products (FDPs, D-dimer). The FXIIa/kallikrein complex converts high molecular weight kininogen into bradykinin, which is a potent stimulus of tPA release. Kallikrein and FXIIa can also act as weak plasminogen activators (not shown).

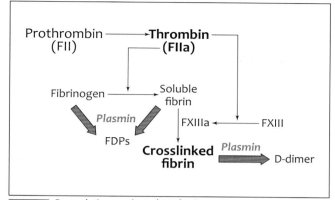

6.12 Degradation products (FDPs) released from plasmin-mediated cleavage of fibrinogen or fibrin. Classic FDPs (measured in serum or plasma) are released when plasmin cleaves fibrinogen or soluble fibrin. In contrast, crosslinked degradation products are released when plasmin cleaves crosslinked fibrin; the smallest crosslinked product is D-dimer. Since crosslinking requires thrombin to activate FXIII and create the D-dimer neo-epitope, D-dimer is specific for crosslinked fibrinolysis. In contrast, FDPs can be yielded by plasmin-mediated cleavage of fibrinogen without thrombin being present.

excessive haemorrhage in dogs and cats (mainly owing to the lack of sensitive and specific assays for fibrinolysis):

- *Physiological:* thrombin-activatable fibrinolytic inhibitor, plasminogen activator inhibitor-1 (PAI-1) and antiplasmin
- *Pharmacological:* tranexanemic acid and ε-aminocaproic acid (see below for therapeutic uses of the latter drug).
- **Clinical manifestations:**
  - *Defective fibrinolysis:* this is usually due to excess inhibition by PAI-1, rather than decreased concentrations or dysfunction of tPA or plasmin. This is most frequently seen in human patients with sepsis-induced disseminated intravascular coagulation (DIC) and results in thrombosis. A recent study has identified decreased fibrinolysis in dogs with diseases associated with thrombosis (systemic inflammation, protein-losing nephropathy, hyperadrenocorticism, diabetes mellitus; Spodsberg *et al.*, 2013), suggesting that defective fibrinolysis may contribute to thrombosis (although no direct association was made between decreased fibrinolysis and documented thrombi)
  - *Excessive fibrinolysis:* this is usually a consequence of DIC and is attributed to excess plasmin generation, which rapidly destroys fibrin clots leading to haemorrhage. Dogs have far more active fibrinolytic enzymes than humans, which may explain why DIC usually manifests as bleeding *versus* thrombosis in this species. A syndrome of delayed (36–48 hours) postsurgical bleeding in Greyhounds may also be due to excessive fibrinolysis (Marin *et al.*, 2012).
- **Tests of fibrinolysis** (see Figure 6.7 and below for more details):
  - *Screening tests:* fibrin(ogen) degradation products (plasma, serum), D-dimer (plasma)
  - *Specific tests (available to practitioners):* none
  - *Tests for inhibitors (not readily available):* plasminogen activator inhibitor-1, antiplasmin
  - *Non-routine specialized testing (not readily available):* plasminogen, tPA, plasmin–antiplasmin complexes, tPA-modified thromboelastography.

Diagnostic assays for haemostasis

This section will focus primarily on screening assays, with information provided on global haemostasis testing, specifically viscoelastic-based clot detection, thromboelastography (TEG) or thromboelastometry (TEM), which is making its way into the clinic. The most commonly used screening assays for the diagnostic evaluation of an animal demonstrating excessive haemorrhage are a platelet count (which is mandatory for all bleeding patients) and standard coagulation assays, usually the prothrombin time (PT) and activated partial thromboplastin time (aPTT) at a bare minimum, which can be performed in sequence or in parallel. The results of these tests dictate the need for further or more specific diagnostic testing or may prompt additional assays (Figure 6.13). The choice of assays (screening or otherwise) should also be guided by knowledge of the patient (age, breed, sex, access to anticoagulant rodenticides, clinical suspicion of *Angiostrongylus vasorum*, type of bleeding signs, presence of underlying disease, etc.).

If assay results are still not fruitful and the animal is still suspected of having a haemostatic disorder, more complex or specialized testing is required, and referral of the patient to a haemostasis specialist could be considered. Referral of the actual patient *versus* samples collected from the patient is recommended because some testing requires the use of fresh platelets from the patient and cannot be done on stored or shipped samples, e.g. platelet function assays. Tests for inhibitors or fibrinolytic end products are not usually included in routine screening assays but are included in DIC panels offered by some laboratories. Most haemostatic screening assays are designed to detect abnormalities that result in haemorrhage. They are less or not useful for detecting hypercoagulability or thrombosis. Unfortunately, we lack tests that can reliably detect hypercoagulability, which still remains a diagnosis based on a high clinical index of suspicion and known disease or drug associations. Once thrombi have formed, or a large enough Doppler ultrasonography can be used to assess blood flow in vessels and make a presumptive diagnosis of a thrombus.

Blood sample collection

Blood for haemostasis testing is generally collected into two tubes.

- **Ethylenediamine tetra-acetic acid (EDTA):**
  - *Primary haemostasis:* platelet count, vWf:Ag, genetic testing
  - *Fibrinolysis:* D-dimer, although separated citrate plasma is the preferred sample for testing.
- **Citrate:**
  - *Primary haemostasis:* vWf antigen, platelet function analyser testing
  - *Secondary haemostasis:* coagulation screening assays, specific factor activity assays
  - *Inhibitors:* antithrombin activity, protein C activity, therapeutic heparin monitoring
  - *Fibrinolysis:* FDPs, D-dimer
  - *Global haemostasis:* viscoelastic-based clot detection.

It cannot be overemphasized that blood must be collected and handled properly to ensure accurate haemostasis test results (Figure 6.14). Coagulation factors are

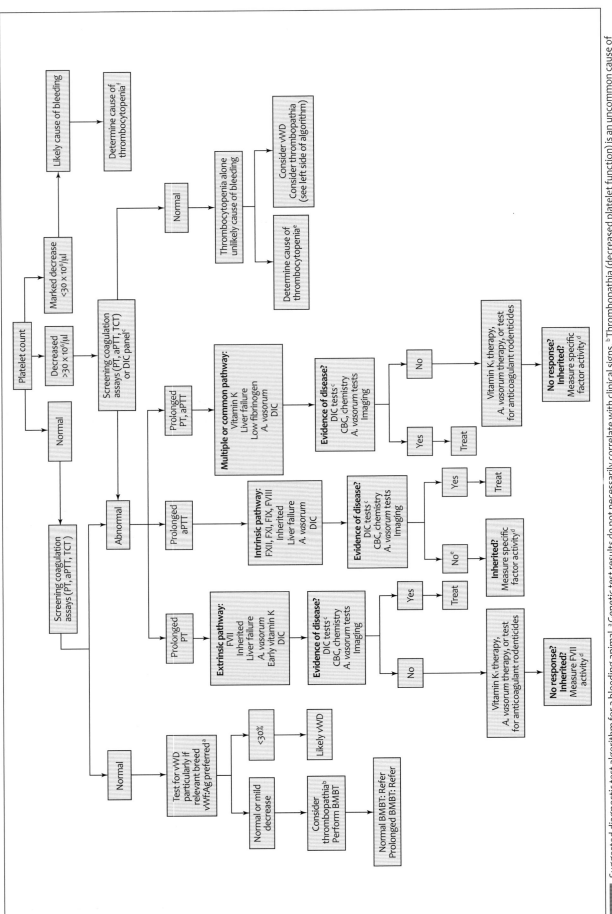

6.13 Suggested diagnostic test algorithm for a bleeding animal. [a] Genetic test results do not necessarily correlate with clinical signs. [b] Thrombopathia (decreased platelet function) is an uncommon cause of haemorrhage, but can be inherited or secondary to drugs (e.g. aspirin) or disease (e.g. uraemia). A complete medical history, including drug administration or exposure to toxins, is imperative for bleeding animals. [c] Disseminated intravascular coagulation (DIC) panels vary, but usually include FDP/D-dimer, fibrinogen and antithrombin activity along with screening assays. NB If there is a high clinical suspicion of DIC (sick animal with underlying predisposing disease, e.g. bacterial sepsis), consider concurrent DIC panel and platelet count (versus sequential testing as illustrated). [d] If a specific diagnosis has not been obtained, consider referral of the patient. [e] If diagnostic tests are not helpful, still consider empirical treatment for Angiostrongylus vasorum in endemic areas. [f] See section on thrombocytopenia. aPTT = activated partial thromboplastin time; BMBT = buccal mucosal bleeding time; CBC = complete blood count; PT = prothrombin time; TCT = thrombin clot time; vWD = von Willebrand's disease; vWf:Ag = von Willebrand factor antigen.

- Samples should be collected directly into tubes or syringes containing citrate (if using the syringe method, the citrate can be withdrawn from vacutainer or non-vacutainer tubes; a 5 ml collection tube contains 0.5 ml of citrate)
- Ideally, use a short butterfly catheter and a syringe pre-filled with the correct volume of citrate (3.2 or 3.8%). For example, to collect 3 ml of blood, place 0.3 ml of citrate into a 3 ml syringe and collect to the 3 ml mark (2.7 ml of blood). To collect 5 ml of blood, place 0.5 ml of citrate into a 5 ml syringe and collect to the 5 ml mark (i.e. 4.5 ml of blood). Collection of 5 ml of blood is ideal because this provides plenty of plasma for diagnostic assays, but 3 ml of blood is sufficient for screening assays. Place blood into a non-anticoagulant tube and mix by inversion with subsequent righting of the tube (minimum 3 times)
- If a citrate vacutainer is preferred, use a butterfly catheter with a needle at both ends and let the vacuum withdraw the appropriate amount of blood. Invert the tube during sample collection (if possible) or promptly once the vacuum draw is complete. Some vacutainers may slightly under-fill with blood (or veins can collapse with the vacuum), and therefore the syringe method is preferred
- Collection of blood into a syringe containing no anticoagulant and then into a vacuum or non-vacuum citrate tube is not recommended, but if these are the only available tubes (and contain insufficient citrate to draw into a syringe, or no liquid citrate is available), then the first few ml of blood should be discarded to minimize the effect of contact activation or tissue factor contamination of the sample (which will have a variable effect on clotting times)
- Clean venepuncture – preferably from a large peripheral vein with a 21 or 22 G needle or short butterfly catheter (long butterfly catheters may activate clotting)
- Constant steady blood flow during venepuncture and filling of vacutainer tube or syringe
- Correct filling of citrate vacutainer or pre-filled syringe: under- or over-filling can prolong or shorten coagulation times (under-filling is more of a problem)
- Adequate mixing of blood with anticoagulant: invert the tubes several times (minimum of three complete inversions)
- Minimize frothing, shearing, haemolysis – do not force blood through needles, do not shake tubes
- Centrifuge sample promptly and separate plasma from cells
- Ship cooled plasma (on ice) to reach laboratory within 24 hours
- Delay in submission >24 hours: freeze sample in a dedicated (not frost-free) freezer and submit on dry ice

6.14 Guidelines for sample collection and handling of citrate tubes for haemostasis testing.

readily activated by poor venepuncture (contamination of the sample with perivascular TF) and coagulation factors are not stable in stored samples, particularly whole blood. Whenever possible, blood should be collected from a resting, quiet animal. Known stressors, such as surgical trauma or drugs, can influence test results, hindering interpretation. For example, increases in D-dimer and fibrinogen can occur as a consequence of surgery-induced fibrinolysis and inflammation, respectively. If an animal bleeds excessively during a surgical procedure, however, perioperative sample collection will be necessary. In such cases, abnormal results of screening assays should reflect the cause of haemorrhage rather than being a consequence of surgery (surgery alone does not affect screening coagulation test results, such as the PT or aPTT).

There are several different ways to collect blood for haemostasis testing, and controversy exists regarding the optimum method of collection (vacutainer *versus* syringe; discard or don't discard the first few millilitres). Collection of blood into a syringe that is pre-filled with the correct amount of citrate (1 part citrate to 9 parts blood) is recommended (see online video, Comparative Coagulation Laboratory at Cornell University website: https://ahdc.vet. cornell.edu/sects/Coag/). This method allows tailoring of the collected blood volume to the patient, in contrast to the use of vacutainer tubes, which require a specific volume of blood and create more turbulent blood flow. If clean venepuncture is performed, it is not necessary to discard the first 3 ml of blood.

It also cannot be overemphasized that results of haemostasis tests should **never** be interpreted in isolation. They should **always** be interpreted in the context of the patient (clinical signs, historical details, signalment). Artefactual changes can and do occur, and can yield misleading results. If the results do not make sense they should be questioned. Treat the patient, not the laboratory data.

Diagnostic assays for primary haemostasis

Platelets

Platelet counts: Platelet counts are the first step in haemostasis testing and are considered mandatory for any patient presenting with clinical signs potentially attributable to a haemostatic disorder (see Figure 6.13). They can be performed by several methods; however, each has limitations (Figure 6.15). Any count provided should be verified by checking the EDTA tube for clots (by visual assessment and by twirling two wooden orange sticks in the sample to detect microclots), examining a blood smear for platelet clumps and performing a platelet estimate (Figure 6.16). In general, platelet clumps decrease the count, although clumps may falsely increase the count in automated buffy coat analysers (Figure 6.15).

Smooth venepuncture will minimize platelet clumping, but there will always be patients whose platelets clump regardless of collection technique. The reasons for platelet clumping in such individual patients are unknown, but it is possible that these animals have activated platelets *in vivo*. Clumping occurs readily in cats regardless of the collection procedure. There are also EDTA-dependent antibodies, which cause platelet aggregation in the presence of EDTA. This phenomenon is quite rare and has only been reported in dogs. Collection of blood into citrate anticoagulant may offset this problem and yield more accurate platelet counts; however, this practice should not be performed routinely because platelet counts in dogs are consistently lower in blood samples anticoagulated in citrate compared with EDTA. Regardless of the cause of clumping, a general rule of thumb is that, in the presence of clumps, the platelet count should be considered a minimum number and the 'real' count is likely to be much higher. Sometimes, the platelet clumping is so severe that even a platelet estimate cannot be performed because all the platelets are within clumps. Mild to moderate thrombocytopenia may be missed in such samples.

Medical decision limits: These have been extrapolated from human medicine (based on transfusion threshold guidelines from the British Committee for Standards in Haematology) and may not be applicable to animals. In addition, these limits are based on level III/IV evidence (i.e. case reports, anecdotal data, expert opinion):

- $<10 \times 10^9/l$: at risk of spontaneous haemorrhage
- $10–30 \times 10^9/l$: likely to be at risk of spontaneous haemorrhage
- $<50 \times 10^9/l$: at risk of surgical or trauma-induced haemorrhage.

Spontaneous or induced haemorrhage may occur at higher counts than indicated above if there are concurrent

Method	Requirement	Limitations
Manual	• Microscope with X100 oil immersion • Counting chamber (haemocytometer) • Dilution chamber (e.g. Thrombo-TIC®, Bioanalytic • Skilled technician • Alternative: estimate from blood smear (1 platelet/X100 oil immersion field = 15 x 10⁹/l in dogs and 15–20 x 10⁹/l in cats)	• Requires training and technical skill • Subjective identification of platelets • Most imprecise method (variable between and within observers) • Difficult to distinguish platelets from debris or cytoplasmic fragments from other cells • Count or estimate falsely decreased by platelet clumps
Automated: buffy coat	• Specific equipment (e.g. VetAutoread™ Haematology Analyser)	• Less accurate than other automated counting methods • Count falsely increased by platelet clumps
Automated: impedance	• Specific equipment (e.g. Cell-Dyn 3500, Sysmex® XT-2000iV, VetScan HM5, Hemavet 950, ProCyte Dx®) • Skilled technician	• Requires training and technical skill • Difficult to distinguish platelets from small red blood cells (RBCs), RBC and other cell fragments, debris • Does not count large platelets if above counting threshold (analyser dependent) • Count falsely decreased by platelet clumps
Automated: optical or laser	• Specific equipment (e.g. Sysmex XT-2000iV, Advia® 120 or 2120) • Skilled technician	• Requires training and technical skill • Difficult to distinguish platelets from small RBCs, RBC and other cell fragments (including haemolysed RBC), debris • May not count large platelets if above counting threshold (analyser dependent) • Count falsely decreased by platelet clumps

6.15 Platelet counting methods.

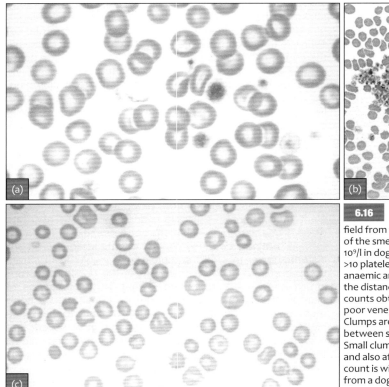

6.16 (a) Platelet numbers can be estimated from the **monolayer** of a good quality blood smear (usually a distance of one X10 objective field from the feathered edge of the blood smear, moving towards the body of the smear). Approximately 1 platelet/X100 oil immersion field (OIF) = 15 x 10⁹/l in dogs and 15–20 x 10⁹/l in cats. Healthy dogs and cats typically have >10 platelets/OIF (>150 x 10⁹/l). A monolayer may not be present in very anaemic animals. In this case, a platelet estimate should be performed at the distance indicated above. (b) Platelet clumps decrease the platelet counts obtained by most methods. These are usually a consequence of poor venepuncture technique in dogs, but are often unavoidable in cats. Clumps are typically seen at the feathered edge; the number and size vary between samples and between blood smears made from the same sample. Small clumps can also be seen throughout the body of the smear (arrowed) and also affect the platelet count. It should not be assumed that the platelet count is within reference intervals if clumps are present. (c) Blood smear from a dog with severe immune-mediated thrombocytopenia; no platelets are seen in the monolayer (and no clumps were detected).

defects in platelet function, secondary haemostasis or fibrinolysis. Furthermore, the actual count does not always correlate with clinical signs of bleeding, because not all animals with severe thrombocytopenia (<30 × 10⁹/l) will bleed excessively. Recent studies suggest that haemorrhage in thrombocytopenic animals may be caused by concurrent tissue inflammation.

Mean platelet volume (MPV): Impedance and optical-based automated analysers provide the MPV (in femtolitres, fl), which can be useful. During active thrombopoiesis, larger platelets than normal are produced. These can be observed in blood smears and, if in sufficient number, will

increase the MPV above reference intervals. Large platelets are generally presumed to be young platelets; however, large size is not synonymous with immature or young platelets. Large platelets can also be seen under the following conditions:

• Sample storage (artefact): platelets activate and swell with storage, particularly at 4°C; the preferred temperature of storage for EDTA blood for complete blood counts (CBCs)
• Platelet clumping (artefact): smaller clumps that fall within the counting size threshold are 'seen' as single large platelets by most automated analysers

- 'Normal' finding: healthy non-thrombocytopenic cats
- Inherited defect in platelet production: β1-tubulin defect in Cavalier King Charles Spaniels, Norfolk and Cairn Terriers and other breeds (Boudreaux M; http://www. vetmed.auburn.edu/faculty/pathobiology-faculty/ boudreaux#.UpENRZGxPZp)
- Bone marrow neoplasia (abnormal production): myelodysplastic syndrome, acute myeloid leukaemia.

Platelet crit: The platelet crit (%) is a result provided by some automated haematology analysers that measure MPV and platelet number (and is the product of these two results) or buffy coat-based analysers (which measure the platelet crit directly in the tubes). However, this result is not usually reported as part of a routine CBC. Studies have shown that Cavalier King Charles Spaniels with inherited macrothrombocytopenia have a normal platelet crit, because the large size of their platelets 'compensates' for the mild to moderate thrombocytopenia. This may explain the lack of bleeding tendencies in these dogs, because they have a normal 'mass' of platelets. It is likely that storage and platelet clumping will falsely increase the platelet crit for the same reasons as MPV (see above).

von Willebrand factor

von Willebrand factor antigen (vWf:Ag): Measurement of vWf:Ag is performed to diagnose von Willebrand's disease (vWD), which is caused by a deficiency of, or abnormality in, vWf. The test is called an antigen test because vWf protein is detected using antibodies raised against human or canine vWf in enzyme-linked immunosorbent assays (ELISAs). This test can be used to diagnose vWD in any animal and is cheaper than genetic-based tests for vWD, which are only available for select breeds of dogs. Also, antigen levels do correlate somewhat with clinical signs, so it is still the recommended test for determining whether bleeding signs can be attributed to vWD (see Figure 6.13). NB vWf used to be called FVIII-related antigen, but this term is obsolete.

- **Result interpretation:** vWf:Ag results are expressed as a percentage or unit value of a species-specific standard plasma pool, which is designated as 100% or 100 IU/dl:
  - >70% (>70 IU/dl): probably does not have vWD (however, genetic testing has shown that some dogs with high values are heterozygous for a vWf mutation)
  - 50–70% (50–70 IU/dl): animal may or may not have vWD, but should not clinically bleed
  - <50% (<50 IU/dl): likely to have vWD (genetic testing has shown that some dogs with low values do not have the breed-specific mutation for vWD; this may be due to false decreases in vWf:Ag – see below)
  - <35% (<35 IU/dl): likely to have vWD and is at risk of bleeding due to vWD (however, not all animals with vWf:Ag concentrations below this value will bleed excessively).
- **Non-disease variables affecting results:** false decreases and increases in vWf:Ag concentrations can be seen if samples are not collected or stored properly. For shipping internationally, citrate plasma samples should be frozen and submitted on dry ice to prevent uncontrolled thawing (vWf:Ag is stable for several months frozen, but only for 24 hours if maintained at 4°C, even if stored as separated plasma).

von Willebrand factor structure and function: Collagen-binding assays (testing the ability of vWf to bind collagen *in vitro*) and multimeric analysis are specialized tests used to identify vWD variants with reduced functional protein, e.g. type II.

Genetic tests: Tests for the breed-specific vWf gene mutation are available for select breeds, e.g. Scottish Terrier, Dobermann, Manchester Terrier, Dutch Kooiker Dogs (see www.vetgen.com, www.vetnostic.com, www.genomia.cz, www.laboklin.co.uk, University of Utrecht) and can be performed on blood samples (collected into any anticoagulant) or cheek swabs. DNA samples are stable for airmail shipping. Genetic tests are best used for carrier detection in breeding programmes (because vWf:Ag concentrations overlap in carrier and unaffected dogs). Genetic tests do not provide information about vWf:Ag concentrations (which can be predictive of clinical bleeding) and are more expensive and less readily available than vWf:Ag assays.

Global screening assays of primary haemostasis

Buccal mucosal bleeding time (BMBT): This is a global test of primary haemostasis but is not specific for a particular disorder. A shallow cut is made in the everted upper buccal mucosa (kept in place by a light gauze tie, taking care not to over-tighten it and restrict the circulation) with a dedicated device (e.g. Simplate II, Organon Teknika). The time required for cessation of bleeding is recorded by blotting just below the cut. The device produces a cut of standard length and depth, shallow enough to be sealed by the platelet plug and not requiring fibrin (secondary haemostasis). Therefore, it specifically tests primary haemostasis and is normal in dogs with inherited disorders of secondary haemostasis (haemophilia A or B) or those given warfarin. This test should be performed by a skilled operator to maximize reproducibility. The BMBT is most commonly used as an in-house screening test in a bleeding animal if other screening tests are normal (see Figure 6.13) or as a pre-surgical test, particularly in dogs with inherited disorders of primary haemostasis (such as vWD) or in predisposed breeds. However, there is no conclusive evidence that the BMBT is predictive of surgical haemorrhage in human or canine patients. The BMBT should not be performed in severely thrombocytopenic dogs (it provides no additional diagnostic information and may initiate haemorrhage).

- **Result interpretation:**
  - *Healthy animals:*
    - Dogs: 1.7–3.3 minutes in restrained unsedated or unanaesthetized dogs; up to 4.2 minutes in anaesthetized or sedated dogs
    - Cats (anaesthetized): <3.3 minutes
  - *Abnormal values (BMBT longer than the above limits):*
    - Moderate thrombocytopenia ($<75 \times 10^9$/l)
    - Thrombopathias: inherited (e.g. Chédiak–Higashi syndrome in cats) or acquired (e.g. aspirin mildly prolongs the BMBT; BMBT is prolonged in some dogs with azotaemia)
    - vWD: will only detect severe defects, i.e. vWf:Ag <20% (cannot distinguish between dogs with and without vWD). This test should be avoided in dogs with suspected type II and type III vWD owing to the severity of the haemostatic defect (induced bleeding may be difficult to stop or control).

- **Variables affecting results:** there is high intra- and inter-observer variation, with small factors such as the degree of pressure placed on the mucosa when using the device (higher pressure increases cut depth), tightness of the gauze used to tie back the mucosa (vessel engorgement will exacerbate bleeding) and technique (touching the cut with the blotting paper will impair plug formation) affecting test results. Anaemia and hypofibrinogenaemia may also prolong the BMBT.

Platelet function analysers: Analysers have been developed specifically to screen for disorders in primary haemostasis. The analyser most commonly used for this purpose is the PFA-100® (Siemens), which has mostly been used in dogs. Citrate-anticoagulated blood is drawn into a flow channel across a membrane impregnated with platelet agonists. When platelets contact the membrane, they become activated, then aggregate and form a plug across the membrane, resulting in decreased blood flow that is detected by the analyser. Results are expressed as the time taken for the platelets to seal ('close') the membrane and stop blood flow, or closure time. There are two available membranes, which contain collagen and either ADP or adrenaline (epinephrine) as agonists. As a screening tool, this method is preferred to the BMBT for non-anaemic dogs because it is standardized and less subject to operator error and variability. Closure times are normal in dogs with anticoagulant rodenticide toxicosis, supporting the specificity of the test for primary haemostasis.

- **Result interpretation:**
  - *Reference intervals:*
    - Dogs:
      - Collagen/ADP: <105 seconds (preferred agonist for dogs)
      - Collagen/adrenaline: most healthy dogs have closure times of <250 seconds, but some healthy dogs can have closure times >300 seconds. The long closure times are likely to be due to the weak agonist activity of adrenaline in this species.
    - Cats with collagen/ADP: 43–176 seconds.
  - *Abnormal values:*
    - Moderate thrombocytopenia (<100 × 10^9/l) with collagen/ADP. Note that there is weak to no correlation between platelet counts and collagen/ADP closure time (dogs with severe thrombocytopenia can have only mildly prolonged closure times)
    - Drug-associated thrombopathias: closure times with collagen/ADP do not change substantially in the presence of anti-platelet drugs (aspirin and NSAIDs), whereas they are significantly prolonged with collagen/adrenaline. However, many treated dogs have normal closure times with collagen/adrenaline, indicating that this is a poor technique for monitoring the effects of anti-platelet agents
    - vWD: will only detect severe defects, i.e. vWf:Ag <25% with collagen/ADP (i.e. cannot distinguish between dogs with and without vWD)
    - Inherited thrombopathia: platelet aggregation defects (in response to ADP) are anticipated to prolong closure times, but no studies have been done in such dogs to confirm this.
- **Variables affecting results:**
  - Haematocrit (HCT): anaemia (HCT <0.33 l/l) will falsely prolong collagen/ADP closure times, and therefore prolonged times may not be informative in anaemic patients (which limits the usefulness of the test). Conversely, higher HCT (e.g. Greyhounds) may yield shorter closure times
  - Citrate concentration (3.2 or 3.8%): closure times with collagen/ADP are shorter in 3.2% citrate (which may be due to the higher HCT in this citrate concentration), although this is unlikely to be clinically relevant.

Diagnostic assays for secondary haemostasis

Screening assays

Screening tests of secondary haemostasis are based on trigger reagents, which cause a fibrin clot to form in the sample in the presence of phospholipid and calcium (see Figure 6.8). The clot is then detected by various means (visual, optical, mechanical). As indicated previously, these tests are configured to detect deficiencies of factors that result in defective clot formation and are insensitive to accelerated clot formation (hypercoagulability). The most commonly used screening assays are the PT and aPTT, with the activated clotting time (ACT) being available as a point-of-care test. Some laboratories also include fibrinogen concentration and a TCT as screening tests for secondary haemostasis. Combinations of test results are used to identify coagulation factor deficiencies and dictate the need for further testing (see Figures 6.7, 6.8 and 6.17). As for platelet counting, different reagents and methods have their own strengths and weaknesses.

Ideally, all clotting assays should be optimized to detect factor deficiencies, but this is really only done by a handful of referral laboratories, particularly those with expertise in haemostasis testing. In particular, testing should be done by a veterinary laboratory because animal plasma clots far quicker than human plasma and erroneous results may be obtained if clot formation is missed. These tests can also be performed in-house. Reference intervals should still be established and/or samples from control animals tested with patients to verify results; control data can then be used to establish intervals. These in-house analysers may not be sensitive to mild factor deficiencies; if the results do not match the clinical signs, sample referral to a specialized testing laboratory is advised. Because coagulation tests are not created equal and results from one instrument or method cannot be extrapolated readily to another, it is best to be completely familiar with the method used for testing and be aware of its limitations. There is also no consensus on result interpretation, e.g. percentage change over a control sample run simultaneously, percentage change or absolute increase above upper reference limit, or the degree of change that is actionable. Haemostasis tests do show marked individuality, which means that the variation in results obtained repeatedly from a single healthy animal is less than the variation in results between animals. This suggests that comparison of results to population-based reference intervals may not be the best method of interpretation, i.e. population-based intervals may be too broad for coagulation tests and may not detect small changes that are abnormal for that individual animal (that exceed the expected individual variation in test results but are within the population-based reference interval).

Activated coagulation time (ACT):

- **Tests:** intrinsic and common pathways (see Figure 6.8).
- **Trigger:** contact with a negatively charged surface, which activates FXII.
- **Sample:** whole blood collected into an ACT tube, which contains a clot activator. Various commercial tubes are available with different activators, e.g. diatomaceous earth, a combination of celine–kaolin–glass beads (MAX-ACT™, Helena Biosciences). There are also cartridges for hand-held point-of-care devices that contain clot activators for ACT measurement, such as kaolin and celite. Requires endogenous calcium and phospholipid from the patient's platelets to drive the reaction.
- **Test requirements:** prewarm tube and perform at 37°C (preferably in a heating block or warm water, but the armpit is a good surrogate).
- **Clot detection:** visual clot formation. After addition of blood, the tube is gently inverted until a visible clot forms.
- **Reported reference intervals:** these intervals are specific for individual tubes and activators. Intervals are only available for diatomaceous earth activator tubes and MAX-ACT™ tubes. There are no published studies on the validity of the ACT cartridges in dogs or cats.
  - *Dogs:* 60–90 seconds (diatomaceous earth activator), 55–80 seconds (MAX-ACT™; See *et al.*, 2009).
  - *Cats:* <165 seconds (diatomaceous earth activator), 55–85 seconds (MAX-ACT™; See *et al.*, 2009).
- **Abnormal (prolonged) results:** this test is less sensitive to factor deficiencies, requiring <10% of normal activity of intrinsic and common pathway factors. Mild factor deficiencies will be missed.
  - *Anticoagulant rodenticide toxicity:* this usually results in marked deficiencies of active factors. If toxicosis is suspected, testing for vitamin K_1 epoxide to vitamin K_1 ratios can be done, or the animal could be treated empirically with vitamin K_1 (see Figure 6.13).
  - *DIC:* if factor deficiencies are severe.
  - *Inherited defects:* In intrinsic or common pathways (e.g. haemophilia A or B), if severe.
  - *Severe thrombocytopenia (<10 x 10⁹/l):* will mildly prolong the ACT (lack of phospholipid).

Prothrombin time (PT):

- **Tests:** extrinsic and common pathways (see Figure 6.8).
- **Trigger:** exogenous TF (from animal brain or recombinant protein).
- **Sample:** citrated plasma.
- **Test requirements:** see Figure 6.14.
- **Clot detection:** visual, optical or mechanical methods. Clotting is triggered by TF in the presence of exogenous calcium. A source of exogenous phospholipid is also added, removing the requirement for the patient's platelets.
- **Reported reference intervals:** vary among laboratories. The data below are from the Comparative Coagulation Laboratory at Cornell University, in which the PT reagent is diluted to optimize sensitivity:
  - *Dogs:* 11–16 seconds
  - *Cats:* 15–20 seconds.
- **Abnormal (prolonged) results** (see Figures 6.13 and 6.17):
  - *Vitamin K deficiency/antagonism:* anticoagulant rodenticides, synthetic liver failure, cholestatic liver disease, drugs that interfere with vitamin K metabolism. Factor VII has the shortest half-life of all vitamin K-dependent factors; therefore the PT can be prolonged earlier than the aPTT. However, most animals with anticoagulant rodenticide toxicosis have prolongations in PT and aPTT at presentation. Can be used to monitor treatment with vitamin K_1
  - *Heparin therapy:* can be used for monitoring treatment with unfractionated but not low molecular weight heparin. Target level is 1.5–2× baseline
  - *DIC:* less sensitive than the aPTT in dogs with DIC
  - *Angiostrongylus vasorum:* not a consistent finding with this parasite
  - *Synthetic liver failure:* most coagulation factors (except for FVIII) are produced in the liver
  - *Hypofibrinogenaemia:* since fibrinogen is the endpoint of all clotting-based assays, a low fibrinogen alone (<0.75 g/l in dogs and <0.50 g/l in cats) will prolong the PT and aPTT. Low fibrinogen is usually due to DIC or synthetic liver failure

Test result			Defect in secondary haemostasis	Associated diseases or drugs[a]
PT	aPTT	TCT		
↑	N	N	Extrinsic pathway: FVII	Inherited, vitamin K absence or antagonism (e.g. rodenticides, cholestasis, warfarin therapy), *Angiostrongylus vasorum* (unusual in natural infection), synthetic liver failure, DIC
N	↑	N	Intrinsic pathway: FXII, FXI, FIX, FVIII	Inherited, vitamin K absence or antagonism, *Angiostrongylus vasorum* (unusual in natural infection), liver failure, DIC
N	N	↑	Fibrinogen conversion to fibrin	Hypo/dysfibrinogenaemia (e.g. inherited), heparin therapy, monoclonal gammopathy (e.g. multiple myeloma)
↑	↑	N	Common pathway: FX, FII, FV. Defects in multiple pathways	Inherited. Vitamin K absence or antagonism, *Angiostrongylus vasorum* (unusual in natural infection), liver failure, DIC
↑	↑	↑	Fibrinogen conversion to fibrin. Defects in multiple pathways	Severe hypofibrinogenaemia (e.g. liver failure, inherited, DIC), excessive heparin therapy. *Angiostrongylus vasorum*, liver failure, DIC

6.17 Combinations of abnormal screening haemostasis test results, with related defects in secondary haemostasis and potential associated diseases. [a] This list is not exhaustive. aPTT = activated partial thromboplastin time; DIC = disseminated intravascular coagulation; N = normal; PT = prothrombin time; TCT = thrombin clot time.

- *Inherited FVII deficiency:* TF is never deficient *in vivo*; aPTT will be normal (see Figures 6.8 and 6.17)
- *False changes with poor sample collection:* Under-dilution and activation of clotting during collection may prolong the PT.

Activated partial thromboplastin time (aPTT):

- **Tests:** intrinsic and common pathways (see Figure 6.8).
- **Trigger:** contact activators, e.g. kaolin, ellagic acid.
- **Sample:** citrated plasma.
- **Test requirements:** see Figure 6.14.
- **Clot detection:** visual, optical or mechanical methods. Clotting is triggered by the contact activator, which activates FXII in the presence of exogenous calcium. A source of exogenous phospholipid is also added, removing the requirement for the patient's platelets.
- **Reported reference intervals:** vary among laboratories. The data below are from the Comparative Coagulation Laboratory at Cornell University:
  - *Dogs:* 10–17 seconds
  - *Cats:* 15–19 seconds.
- **Abnormal (prolonged) results** (see Figures 6.13 and 6.17):
  - *Vitamin K deficiency/antagonism:* see comment for PT above
  - *Heparin therapy:* see comment for PT above
  - *Synthetic liver failure:* decreased production
  - *DIC:* more likely to be prolonged than the PT in dogs with DIC. May be less sensitive than the PT to DIC in cats
  - *Angiostrongylus vasorum:* not a consistent finding with this parasite
  - *Hypofibrinogenaemia:* see comment for PT above
  - *Inherited deficiency in FXII, FXI, FIX, FVIII:* haemophilia A (FVIII deficiency) and Hageman trait (FXII deficiency) are the most common defects in dogs and cats, respectively. Cats with Hageman trait are usually asymptomatic. PT will be normal (see Figures 6.8 and 6.17)
  - *False increases with poor sample collection:* under-dilution and activation of clotting during collection will prolong the aPTT (more sensitive than the PT to *in vitro* factor activation).

Thrombin clot time (TCT):

- **Tests:** fibrinogen being converted to fibrin.
- **Trigger:** thrombin.
- **Sample:** citrated plasma.
- **Test requirements:** see Figure 6.14.
- **Clot detection:** visual, optical or mechanical methods. Clotting is triggered by exogenous thrombin, which converts fibrinogen to fibrin in the presence of exogenous calcium.
- **Reported reference intervals:** vary among laboratories. The data below are from the Comparative Coagulation Laboratory at Cornell University:
  - *Dogs:* 5–9 seconds
  - *Cats:* 5–8 seconds.
- **Abnormal (prolonged) results** (see Figure 6.17):
  - *Hypofibrinogenaemia or afibrinogenaemia:* most common cause is DIC or synthetic liver failure. There are rare reports of inherited afibrinogenaemia
  - *Dysfibrinogenaemia:* abnormal fibrinogen that cannot be converted to crosslinked fibrin. This is rare but has been reported in liver disease in humans
  - *Endogenous thrombin inhibitors:* heparin therapy

- *Endogenous inhibitors of fibrin polymerization:* high concentrations of FDPs or monoclonal globulins (e.g. multiple myeloma).

Fibrinogen concentration: Fibrinogen is produced in the liver and its production is stimulated in response to inflammation as part of the acute phase response. Therefore, fibrinogen concentrations in disorders such as DIC reflect the balance between consumption (in excess clotting) and production (because inflammation is one of the main instigators of DIC in animals).

- **Method of measurement:** two methods are used:
  - *Modification of the TCT:* this is done in citrated plasma. To eliminate the effect of inhibitors, an inhibitor of thrombin is added and the reagent is diluted. Thrombin is then added and the time to clot formation is measured. The clotting time is then dependent on the amount of fibrinogen; this is converted to a fibrinogen concentration (g/l) by comparing the patient's clotting time with a standard curve derived from purified fibrinogen. Sensitivity is highest when species-specific purified fibrinogen is used for the curve
  - *Heat precipitation:* this is done in EDTA-anticoagulated blood. The fibrinogen concentration is equivalent to the difference in plasma protein (as measured by a refractometer) before and after heating plasma to 56°C (which precipitates fibrinogen). The test is crude and insensitive (detects changes as high as 1.0 g/l, which is also the lowest measurable value) and is not recommended for use in small animals.
- **Reported reference intervals:** vary among laboratories. The data below are from the Comparative Coagulation Laboratory at Cornell University, which uses the TCT clotting method and species-specific fibrinogen to generate the standard curve:
  - *Dogs:* 1.47–4.79 g/l
  - *Cats:* 0.76–2.7 g/l.
- **Test interpretation:**
  - *Low concentrations:*
    - Synthetic liver failure (decreased production)
    - DIC (consumption)
    - Inherited disorders (rare).
  - *High concentrations:*
    - Inflammation (positive acute phase response).

Specific assays of secondary haemostasis

Coagulation factor activity: Individual factor assays are performed to determine the underlying defect responsible for abnormal screening coagulation tests (see above and Figure 6.13). The assays are modifications of the screening assays, where the ability of patient plasma to correct the prolonged clotting times of specific factor-deficient plasma is determined. Results are expressed as a percentage of the activity of a standard plasma pool, which is assigned a value of 100%. An inability to correct the prolonged time indicates a deficiency of that factor. Typically, single factor deficiencies with factor activities <25–30% of pooled plasma, which is designated as 100%, can cause haemorrhage, but if multiple factor deficiencies exist, milder reductions (30–50% factor activity) may yield clinical signs.

Tests for anticoagulant rodenticide toxicosis: Vitamin K (in the reduced form) is an essential cofactor for the hepatocellular enzyme γ-glutamyl carboxylase. This enzyme adds carboxyl groups (–COOH) to glutamic acid residues in coagulation factors II, VII, IX and X, which is required for these factors to bind to PS. Thus, non-carboxylated factors are 'inactive'. During the carboxylation reaction, vitamin K is oxidized to vitamin K epoxide and is reverted back to its reduced form by vitamin K_1 epoxide reductase. The latter enzyme is inhibited by anticoagulant rodenticides, which prevent vitamin K being in the reduced form needed to support the carboxylase reaction. Therefore, the vitamin K-dependent coagulation factors are not activated and cannot participate efficiently in fibrin formation, resulting in spontaneous haemorrhage.

Anticoagulant rodenticide toxicosis results in prolongation of all screening haemostasis assays (PT, aPTT and ACT) because extrinsic (FVII), common (FX, FII) and intrinsic (FIX) pathway factors are inactive. Because FVII has the shortest half-life of these factors, experimental studies have shown that the PT becomes prolonged earlier than the aPTT, but in natural cases both assays are usually prolonged. The PT may be used to monitor response to treatment with vitamin K_1. However, these screening assays are not specific for anticoagulant rodenticide toxicity (see Figures 6.13 and 6.17). To confirm a diagnosis of anticoagulant rodenticide toxicosis, direct detection of the toxins using chemical screening is the gold standard (e.g. high-performance liquid chromatography, HPLC; Waddell et al., 2012). Unfortunately, this is expensive and not readily available.

Alternatively, vitamin K_1 epoxide to vitamin K_1 ratios, which are increased with anticoagulant toxicosis, can be measured to confirm the diagnosis (e.g. at the Nutristasis Laboratory., St Thomas' Hospital, London). The protein-induced vitamin K absence (PIVKA) assay used to be in vogue for the diagnosis of potential vitamin K-responsive haemostatic abnormalities, such as liver disease in cats and anticoagulant rodenticide toxicity. However, this is a modified screening test that is most sensitive to FX deficiency and is not specific for vitamin K absence or antagonism, being prolonged in DIC and inherited deficiencies of any vitamin K-dependent factor. This test has fallen out of favour and has been supplanted (by some investigators) with direct measurement of FVIIa activity as a surrogate marker for vitamin K deficiency.

Antithrombin activity and therapeutic monitoring for heparin: Antithrombin (AT) is produced in the liver and is an important endogenous anticoagulant, inhibiting the activity of most activated coagulation factors, although its greatest inhibitory effect is against thrombin or FXa. Its activity is enhanced by heparin (hence its use as an anticoagulant), which is provided *in vivo* by heparin-like glycosaminoglycans on the surface of endothelial cells. When thrombin is generated *in vivo* by an activated haemostatic system, AT binds thrombin to form thrombin–antithrombin complexes (TAT), which are cleared by the liver. High concentrations of TAT indicate excessive generation of thrombin or hypercoagulability, but this assay is expensive and only performed in research settings. AT is a small protein and can be lost with protein-losing diseases, along with albumin.

- **Method of AT activity measurement:** AT-mediated inhibition of thrombin or FXa in citrated plasma is measured. The assay system includes heparin (to promote full AT activity) and a chromogenic substrate that is cleaved by thrombin or FXa. Since AT inhibits these enzymes, a high AT concentration will result in greater enzyme inhibition and less substrate cleavage,

so the AT concentration is inversely proportional to the residual factor activity. The result is expressed as a percentage of a species-specific standard pool, designated as 100%. By excluding heparin from the assay, AT activity assays can be used for therapeutic monitoring of heparin. This is usually done with FXa as the inhibitory target and the results are expressed as FXa inhibitory units (in IU/ml).

- **AT activity interpretation:**
  - *Reference intervals:* vary among laboratories. The data below are from the Comparative Coagulation Laboratory at Cornell University:
    - Dogs: 65–145%
    - Cats: 75–110%.
  - *Decreased activity:* low AT activity is rare in cats. Activity in dogs <50% is associated with an increased risk of thrombosis:
    - Synthetic liver failure (decreased production)
    - DIC (consumption with subsequent formation of TAT complexes): along with increased D-dimer, low AT activity is one of the most sensitive indicators of DIC in dogs. Low AT activity is not a consistent feature of DIC in cats
    - Protein-losing enteropathy or nephropathy (loss)
    - Inflammation: negative acute phase protein in dogs (there is some suggestion that AT increases in cats with inflammation, i.e. acts as a positive acute phase protein)
    - Drugs: L-asparaginase (decreased production).
- **Therapeutic heparin monitoring (measurement of anti-FXa activity):** unlike clotting times, AT activity can be used to monitor treatment with both unfractionated and low molecular weight heparin:
  - *Target value:* 0.35–0.7 IU/ml for unfractionated heparin and 0.5–1.0 IU/ml for low molecular weight heparin. This is based on human studies; data specific for companion animals are not available.

Protein C activity: Protein C, a vitamin K-dependent enzyme, is produced in the liver. Protein C is activated when thrombin binds to thrombomodulin on endothelial cells and inhibits the 'intrinsic tenase' and prothrombinase cofactors, FVIIIa and FVa, respectively. Inhibition of these cofactors markedly decreases activity of the complexes, slowing thrombin generation. Activity of protein C is enhanced by free protein S (also vitamin K dependent). In addition to its anticoagulant properties, protein C is profibrinolytic (inactivates PAI-1) and anti-inflammatory. Its anti-inflammatory actions are mediated indirectly by inhibition of thrombin (which stimulates inflammation by binding to thrombin receptors on endothelial cells and monocytes) and directly by activating cell signalling pathways after binding to the protein C receptor on endothelial cells.

- **Method of measurement:** protein C-mediated cleavage of a specific chromogenic substrate.
- **Protein C activity interpretation:**
  - *Reference intervals:* vary among laboratories. The data below are from the Comparative Coagulation Laboratory at Cornell University:
    - Dogs: 75–135%
    - Cats: 65–120%.
  - *Decreased activity:* this applies mostly to dogs. Less information is available for cats. Low protein C activity can predispose an animal to thrombosis or inflammation:
    - Liver disease: low protein C activity can be seen in synthetic liver failure, extrahepatic bile duct

obstruction (possibly due to vitamin K deficiency) and portosystemic shunts in dogs. Similarly, cats with various liver diseases (inflammation, neoplasia, lipidosis) have low protein C activity. Shunts directly affect protein C activity independently of liver synthetic ability. Low protein C activity is seen in up to 88% of dogs with congenital or acquired shunts, but is not a feature of microvascular dysplasia in dogs
  – DIC (consumption and decreased activation)
  – Vitamin K deficiency/antagonism
  – Inflammation and sepsis: due to decreased activation (downregulation of thrombomodulin, decreased free protein S).

Diagnostic assays for fibrinolysis

Tests for fibrinolysis are generally restricted to FDPs and D-dimer, because other assays, such as measurements of plasminogen, tPA and PAI-1, are not readily available or routinely offered by diagnostic laboratories. Tissue plasminogen activator-triggered fibrinolysis of clots formed with viscoelastographic testing has been recently used to evaluate fibrinolytic potential in dogs with disorders associated with thrombosis (Spodsberg *et al.*, 2013; see below). This technique shows promise in detecting disorders of fibrinolysis; however, further studies are needed. D-dimer assays have mostly supplanted FDP assays, because D-dimer is considered more specific for fibrinolysis (see Figure 6.11). D-dimer assays are readily performed in-house or with automated methods on citrated plasma. Therefore, only the D-dimer assay will be discussed here.

D-dimer

D-dimer is a new antigen (neo-antigen) that is produced when FXIIIa crosslinks soluble fibrin. Cleavage of cross-linked fibrin by a proteolytic enzyme, such as plasmin, exposes this neo-epitope, which can then be detected using immunological assays. Thus, D-dimer indicates both generation of thrombin (to produce soluble fibrin and activate FXIIIa) and plasmin. D-dimer can be measured in body cavity fluids (peritoneal fluid, cerebrospinal fluid) as a marker of localized fibrinolysis.

- **Method of measurement:** D-dimer is detected with anti-human D-dimer monoclonal antibodies using semi-quantitative point-of-care latex agglutination or colorimetric card filtration kits and quantitative immunoturbidometric reagents on automated analysers. Because some, but not all, antibodies detect a protein in canine and feline plasma (presumably D-dimer), it is important to use a method validated in animals. D-dimer can be measured in EDTA- or citrate-anticoagulated plasma; concentrations are slightly lower in EDTA, but this is not clinically relevant.
- **D-dimer interpretation:**
  - *Reported reference intervals:* vary among laboratories. The data below are from the Comparative Coagulation Laboratory at Cornell University (which uses an immunoturbidometric assay):
    – Dogs and cats: <0.250 mg/l. NB Some healthy dogs may have higher concentrations.
  - *High concentrations:* D-dimer requires thrombin generation for its production, and therefore increased D-dimer concentration is considered a marker of hypercoagulability:

  – False increases: haemolysed samples stored for 48 hours or more at room temperature (associated with *in vitro* clot formation)
  – Physiological fibrinolysis: wound healing, post-surgery
  – Pathological conditions:
    – Internal haemorrhage
    – Any cause of thrombosis (including DIC) or thromboembolism (including pulmonary thromboembolism, e.g. sepsis, neoplasia). The highest D-dimer concentrations (>1.0 mg/l) are seen in animals with DIC or thromboembolism, and experimental studies show this is the first test to become abnormal in experimental endotoxaemia in dogs. D-dimer concentration and AT activity are the most sensitive tests for the diagnosis of DIC in dogs; however, D-dimer does not appear to be as useful in cats. For unknown reasons, many cats with aortic thromboembolism do not have high D-dimers
    – Sick animals with no clinical or laboratory evidence of DIC: D-dimer concentrations are increased in cats and dogs with many diseases, e.g. inflammatory, non-inflammatory (lipidosis) and neoplastic hepatopathies in cats, congestive heart failure and extrahepatic bile duct obstruction in dogs. Although the highest D-dimer concentrations are seen in animals with thrombosis or thromboembolic disease, there is overlap in D-dimer concentrations between clinically ill animals with and without DIC. Indeed, D-dimer can be increased in some animals without any clinical or histological evidence of thrombosis and may be the only abnormal haemostatic test result in some dogs. In these cases, it is difficult to explain or know what to do about the high D-dimer result. In some patients, high D-dimer may reflect the action of non-plasmin proteases on fibrin, e.g. neutrophil or bacterial proteases. Although the high D-dimer concentrations could reflect underlying hypercoagulablity or small thrombi in such patients, this ambiguity limits the diagnostic usefulness of the test. This emphasizes that D-dimer should not be part of routine screening assays (because there are likely to be many high or difficult to explain results) but should be reserved for patients suspected to have DIC, thrombosis or hypercoagulability. D-dimer results should never be interpreted in isolation, but together with the other haemostatic test results.

Global tests of haemostasis

Cells, such as platelets, play crucial roles in fibrin formation; however, these cells are excluded from standard clotting assays because these are performed on platelet-poor plasma (except for the ACT). Furthermore, screening coagulation assays are insensitive to hypercoagulable states, being optimized to detect decreased and not accelerated clot formation. There has been a recent resurgence of interest in methods that incorporate cells and assess all components of haemostasis simultaneously (global haemostasis). These techniques, including viscoelastic clot detection and fluorogenic monitoring of thrombin generation, are being increasingly used in veterinary medicine. Currently, thrombin generation assays are restricted to research settings; however, viscoelastic techniques are becoming more commonplace, particularly in emergency or critical care facilities, and will be discussed here.

Viscoelastic clot detection: thromboelastography and thromboelastometry

In traditional clotting assays, the time taken for fibrin strands to form in platelet-poor plasma samples is measured after addition of an activator. These tests provide no information about the dynamics of fibrin formation or breakdown, or the contribution of cells to this process. In contrast, viscoelastic-based clot detection methods are performed on whole blood and measure the viscous and elastic properties of fibrin as it forms, using optical or mechanical sensors. These methods provide information on the onset and rate of fibrin formation, the strength of the formed clot, and fibrinolysis (Figure 6.18).

Depending on the analyser, the technique is called thromboelastometry (ROTEM®) or thromboelastography (TEG®; Sonoclot®). In the past few years, there has been an explosion of articles on viscoelastic clot detection, with several excellent reviews (Koi and Borjesson, 2010; McMichael and Smith, 2011). This method is mostly being used to detect hyper- and hypocoagulable states in animals in research and clinical settings. Recently, tPA-activated TEG has been used to assess decreased fibrinolysis in dogs with clinical evidence of thrombosis, suggesting that this modified TEG may be a useful assay for fibrinolytic disorders.

A major disadvantage is that these tests must be performed rapidly after sample collection and they are expensive, restricting widespread use. Furthermore, they are of questionable use as a diagnostic tool, particularly in anaemic animals, and there is little concrete evidence showing that test results substantially affect patient care or improve outcomes. As currently used, the data obtained from these methods do not specifically identify the nature of the defect in haemostasis (e.g. they cannot distinguish hypocoagulability due to platelet function defects from other causes of hypocoagulability). Thus, viscoelastic-based testing is not recommended as a screening tool in animals with excessive bleeding but normal platelet counts or screening coagulation tests (e.g. to confirm thrombopathia or vWD). Indeed no abnormalities are observed in TEG® tracings in canine whole blood in the presence of the platelet inhibitors abciximab (a GPIIb/IIIa inhibitor) or acetylsalicylic acid, suggesting that tracings may be normal in animals with vWD and thrombocytopathia. However, there are no published studies to support or refute this. In human medicine, these tests are used to dictate transfusion therapy during surgical procedures (e.g. cardiopulmonary bypass) and to monitor the response to transfusions in such settings, rather than as a diagnostic tool.

- **Sample type:** citrate-anticoagulated blood. Can be performed on non-anticoagulated blood; however, this requires immediate patient-side testing, which is not feasible.
- **Method:** whole blood is placed into a cup into which a probe (torsion wire or optical sensor) is inserted. Calcium, with or without a specific activator, is added and movement is initiated in either the cup (TEG®) or

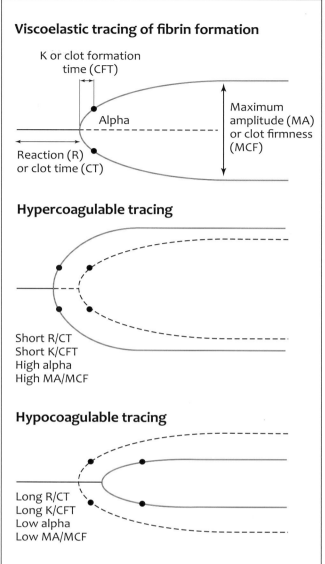

Viscoelastic tracing of fibrin formation

K or clot formation time (CFT)

Alpha

Maximum amplitude (MA) or clot firmness (MCF)

Reaction (R) or clot time (CT)

Hypercoagulable tracing

Short R/CT
Short K/CFT
High alpha
High MA/MCF

Hypocoagulable tracing

Long R/CT
Long K/CFT
Low alpha
Low MA/MCF

6.18 Representative thromboelastographic tracings and data generated with the analyser (TEG®) in a normal (upper image), hypercoagulable (middle image) and hypocoagulable sample. For the hyper- and hypocoagulable tracings, the dotted line is a superimposed normal tracing. The most frequently used data from the analyser include the time for fibrin to start forming or reaction time (R), rate of fibrin formation (K and alpha) and the strength of the fibrin clot or maximum amplitude (MA). (NB Coagulability index and fibrinolytic results are not shown.) Similar tracings are obtained using thrombelastometry, although different terminology is used (clot *versus* reaction time, clot formation time *versus* K and maximal clot firmness *versus* amplitude).

probe (ROTEM®), such that the cup and probe move relative to each other. The most commonly used activators are human recombinant TF and kaolin or ellagic acid. As fibrin strands form between the cup and probe, they resist (decrease) the rotation occurring between the cup and the probe. The rotation of the cup or probe is converted into a fibrin generation curve or tracing (Figure 6.18).

Large amounts of data are generated, including the time to onset of fibrin formation (reaction or clot time), the rate of fibrin formation (K or clot formation time and the alpha angle), and clot strength (maximum amplitude or clot firmness). These values can be incorporated into an equation to yield an overall coagulability index. If allowed to proceed, the clot lyses within the cup and various fibrinolytic results (e.g. percentage lysis at 30 or 60 minutes) are obtained. Most investigators have used clot formation kinetic *versus* fibrinolytic data. Results obtained with TF or kaolin/ellagic acid as activators are analogous to a cell-enriched PT and aPTT, respectively.

Unfortunately, owing to a lack of standardization of methods (different analysers, activators, concentration of activators, timing of analysis after sample collection) and interpretation (notably, test results used to define hypercoagulability), it is difficult to compare results across studies. Furthermore, there are many variables that affect the test results (see below), particularly HCT, and viscoelastic techniques may not yield accurate or useful information on *in vivo* coagulation status in anaemic or polycythaemic animals. Viscoelastic testing does show promise for detecting disorders of fibrinolysis. Fibrinolytic potential can be assessed after the addition of exogenous recombinant tPA to the sample. Doses of tPA have been optimized for native, TF-, or kaolin-activated canine blood, such that fibrinolysis is stimulated without affecting clot formation (Spodsberg *et al.*, 2013). In this study, the percent lysis of the clot at 30 or 60 minutes was decreased in several dogs (between 50–70%) with prothrombotic disorders, e.g. systemic inflammatory response syndrome or protein-losing enteropathy, suggesting that they had decreased fibrinolysis. However, this was not associated with documented thrombosis and there was overlap in fibrinolytic results in diseased and healthy dogs. Furthermore, the assay showed a high degree of analytical variation (the coefficients of variation ranged from 7 to 115%, particularly for native blood or when no activator was added to stimulate clot formation), which may limit the diagnostic utility of this assay. Thus, the clinical relevance of decreased fibrinolysis is uncertain and this single study does not support the use of anti-fibrinolytics in dogs with these disorders.

- **Result interpretation:**
  - *Hypocoagulability:* decreased onset (long reaction or clot time), slow rate (prolonged K or clot formation time, low alpha), and decreased clot strength (maximum amplitude (MA) or clot firmness) alone or in combination indicate defective clot formation (see Figure 6.18). Since abnormalities in coagulation factors and platelets affect these test results to varying degrees, the resultant changes can provide clues as to the nature of the underlying defect and possibly dictate therapy, although no guidelines have been established for this purpose. For instance, a prolonged reaction time indicates coagulation factor deficiencies, whereas a decreased MA could represent defective platelet aggregation or decreased fibrinogen. Dogs with inherited intrinsic pathway deficiencies, e.g. haemophilia A, have normal thromboelastographic results when TF is used as an activator (as they would have a normal PT). Severe thrombocytopenia (<30 × 10^9 platelets/l) may result in hypocoagulable tracings (decreased alpha and MA, high K) and viscoelastic techniques may not be informative of other haemostatic defects in such patients
  - *Hypercoagulability:* rapid onset (short reaction or clot time) and rate (short K or clot formation time, high alpha) of fibrin formation and increased clot strength (maximum amplitude or clot firmness) alone or in combination indicate increased fibrin formation (see Figure 6.18). These results have been used in a plethora of studies to diagnose hypercoagulability in animals. Unfortunately, there is no consensus or standard definition of hypercoagulability and the most common abnormal result, increased clot strength, is strongly influenced by fibrinogen, i.e. a high fibrinogen alone will increase clot strength and result in hypercoagulable tracings. It is highly unlikely that all animals with hyperfibrinogenaemia are truly hypercoagulable

  - *Fibrinolytic disorders:* viscoelastographic testing provides results for the percentage of clot lysis at 30 and 60 minutes after clot formation. Addition of tPA will accelerate lysis of the formed fibrin clot and, to some extent, standardize this endpoint. Decreased percentage clot lysis indicates that more of the clot is left at these times, which could be due to inhibition or inadequate stimulation of fibrinolysis. This could predispose animals to thrombosis; however, the assay does not provide clues to the cause of these changes. Potentially, increased percentage clot lysis could support accelerated fibrinolysis as a cause of excessive haemorrhage; however, normal dogs can have as high as 80–90% lysis at 30 and 60 minutes. It is possible that accelerated fibrinolysis (i.e. less time to achieve a set amount of fibrinolysis, such as 50%) may yield more information on hyperfibrinolytic conditions than percentage clot lysis at defined endpoints.

- **Factors affecting results of clot formation:** these factors do not appear to influence fibrinolytic measurements; however, the strength of clot formation will affect fibrinolysis (dense fibrin fibrils are more resistant to fibrinolysis than thinner fibrils):
  - *Timing of analysis after sample collection:* this must be standardized because activation of whole blood occurs *in vitro*. Reference intervals have been established for set times after sample collection (30 minutes, 2 hours) and are only valid for those times
  - *HCT:* this has a substantial impact on results (with the exception of reaction/clot time), with hypercoagulable and hypocoagulable tracings seen in anaemic patients (HCT <30%) and animals with high HCT (e.g. Greyhounds), respectively. This is thought to be an artefact of the system rather than reflecting real *in vivo* changes
  - *Blood viscosity:* *in vitro* studies suggest that blood viscosity may alter tracings (e.g. decreased viscosity may result in hypercoagulability)
  - *Contact activation:* the cup itself can activate fibrin formation *in vitro* through contact activation of FXII. Contact activation is accelerated with storage of the sample and influences clotting times, especially if low concentrations of TF or calcium alone are used as activators.

Disorders of haemostasis

Haemostatic disorders can be inherited (Figure 6.19) or acquired and are recognized clinically by excessive haemorrhage. Inherited disorders predisposing animals to thrombosis (decreased anticoagulants, defective fibrinolysis) are rare and it is difficult to recognize thrombosis clinically, leading to under-recognition of acquired prothrombotic diseases. With regard to disorders characterized by excessive haemorrhage, the history, signalment and clinical signs can guide a clinician as to the likely

Condition	Defect	Breeds	Helpful diagnostic tests
Primary haemostasis			
Thrombocytopenia	β1-tubulin	CKCS, Norfolk and Cairn Terrier, others (see text)	Gene defect, persistent macrothrombocytopenia in an asymptomatic animal
Glanzmann's thrombasthenia Thrombopathia Unknown thrombopathia	GPIIb/IIIa (fibrinogen receptor) CalDAG–GEF1 catalytic domain ADP receptor (P2Y12) ?Signalling defects	Pyrenean Mountain Dog, Otterhound Bassett Hound, Eskimo Spitz, Landseer Greater Swiss Mountain Dog Boxer, mixed breeds	↑ BMBT, absent aggregation to agonists, ↓ clot retraction, ↓ GPIIb/IIIa, gene defect ↑ BMBT, absent aggregation to ADP and collagen, ↓ aggregation to thrombin, gene defect Absent aggregation to ADP, gene defect ↑ BMBT, ↓ aggregation
Storage pool deficiency Chédiak–Higashi syndrome	?Dense granule defect Dense granule defect	American Cocker Spaniel Persian	↑ BMBT, ↓ release reaction ↑ BMBT, ↓ aggregation, inclusions in leucocytes
Scott syndrome	Defective platelet PS exposure	German Shepherd Dog	↓ Platelet procoagulant activity (↓ PS, ↓ thrombin generation on activation)
vWD	Deficiency (type I or III) or abnormality (type II) in vWf	Type I: many; Type II: GWHP, GSHP; Type III: Scottish Terrier and others (see text)	↓ vWf:Ag (<50%), ±↑ BMBT, genetic defect
Secondary haemostasis			
Haemophilia A	FVIII deficiency, sex-linked	Many dogs and cats	↑ aPTT, ±↑ ACT, ↓FVIII activity (<25–30%)
Haemophilia B	FIX deficiency, sex-linked	Many dogs, British Shorthair, Siamese, DSH	↑ aPTT, ±↑ ACT, ↓ FIX activity (<20%), genetic defect
Haemophilia C	FXI deficiency, autosomal	German Shepherd Dog, Kerry Blue Terrier, Pyrenean Mountain Dog	↑ aPTT, ±↑ ACT, ↓ FXI activity
Factor X deficiency	Autosomal	Boxer, American Cocker Spaniel, Jack Russell Terrier, DSH	↑ aPTT, ↑ PT, ±↑ ACT, ↓ FX activity
Factor VII deficiency	Autosomal	Beagle, Alaskan Malamute	↑ PT, ↓ FVII activity
Hageman trait	FXII deficiency	Poodles, cats	↑ aPTT, ±↑ ACT, ↓ FXII activity, asymptomatic (no bleeding)
Vitamin K-dependent factors (FII, FVII, FIX, FX)	Defect in γ-glutamyl carboxylase enzyme	Devon Rex	↑ aPTT, ↑ PT, ±↑ ACT, ↑ PIVKA, responsive to high-dose vitamin K

6.19 Inherited disorders of haemostasis. Unless indicated, animals present with clinical signs of haemorrhage that are related to the underlying disorder (e.g. mucosal haemorrhage in primary haemostatic disorders and body cavity haemorrhage in secondary haemostatic disorders). ACT = activated clotting time; ADP = adenosine diphosphate; aPTT = activated partial thromboplastin time; BMBT = buccal mucosal bleeding time; CalDAG–GEF1 = calcium diacylglycerol guanine exchange factor-1; CKCS = Cavalier King Charles Spaniel; DSH = Domestic Shorthair; GSHP = German Shorthaired Pointer; GWHP = German Wirehaired Pointer; PIVKA = protein-induced vitamin K absence; PS = phosphatidylserine; PT = prothrombin time; vWF = von Willebrand factor; vWF:Ag = von Willebrand factor antigen; VWD = von Willebrand's disease.

underlying disorder. For instance, disorders of primary haemostasis are characterized by mucosal haemorrhage. Small bleeds (petechiae, purpura) should alert a clinician to an underlying thrombocytopenia or thrombopathia. Secondary haemostasis disorders yield larger bleeds, for example, haematomas and intracavity bleeding. Thus, a thorough history (travel, exposure to toxins, drug treatment) and clinical examination (assessment of the skin and all mucosal surfaces for haemorrhage) are mandatory in bleeding animals. Ancillary diagnostic testing (e.g. CBC, biochemical panels, radiographic and ultrasonographic examination) may be indicated in individual animals, particularly those that are sick, to confirm or rule out underlying disease as a cause for the haemostatic disorder. Inherited defects should be suspected in young animals, especially those that are clinically healthy, are of a predisposed breed, demonstrate recurrent bleeding episodes, or have a known family history. Acquired disorders affect animals of any age, but are more common in older animals, as a consequence of underlying diseases.

Disorders of primary haemostasis

As indicated above, these are characterized by mucosal haemorrhage and small bleeds, including petechiae and purpura. Ecchymoses and traumatic or surgery-induced haemorrhage can also occur, with clinical signs depending on the severity of the defect. The most common disorders of primary haemostasis are acquired thrombocytopenia, for which there are many causes (Figure 6.20) and inherited vWD (see Figure 6.19).

Disorders of platelet number

Platelets are produced in the bone marrow from megakaryocytes by a process of cytoplasmic fragmentation, which requires major changes in the megakaryocyte membrane and cytoskeletal system, including actin and tubulin. Platelet production is driven primarily by thrombopoietin, which is produced in the liver, kidney and bone marrow stromal cells. Thrombopoietin stimulates platelet production by binding to a specific thrombopoietin receptor (the product of the *mpl* gene) on megakaryocytes. Once bound, downstream signalling involves janus activated kinase-2 (JAK2) and stat proteins, and stimulates megakaryocyte production and differentiation. Once within the circulation, platelets have a half-life of approximately 6 days in dogs. Up to one-third of platelets may be temporarily 'sequestered' in the spleen in rabbits and humans (and presumably in other species); therefore splenomegaly of any cause may result in mild to moderate thrombocytopenia (Figure 6.20) and splenic contraction (e.g. secondary to adrenaline) may result in a mild thrombocytosis. Effete platelets are removed by the mononuclear–macrophage

Mechanism	Degree[a]
• **Decreased production** • *Immune-mediated*: dog > cat • *Infectious agents*: rickettsial (e.g. *Erhlichia canis*), viruses (e.g. feline leukemia virus, canine distemper, parvovirus) • *Drugs*: cytotoxicity (e.g. oestrogen, chemotherapeutic agents) or immune-mediated (e.g. azathioprine, sulphonamides) • *Neoplasia*: crowding out of normal cells (myelophthisis), competition for nutrients, altered microenvironment, immune-mediated, defective production (e.g. acute leukaemia, myelodysplastic syndrome, multiple myeloma) • *Bone marrow necrosis*: secondary to drugs, hypoxic injury, neoplasia, toxins	Mild to severe (usually moderate to severe)
• **Increased clearance** • *Immune-mediated* (also called destruction): – Primary: isolated thrombocytopenia (common; dog > cat), part of a systemic process (e.g. systemic lupus erythematosus, rare) – Secondary (common): infectious agents (e.g. *Anaplasma*, *Ehrlichia*, Rocky Mountain spotted fever, *Borrelia*, *Babesia*, *Leishmania*, distemper), neoplasia (e.g. lymphoma in dogs), drugs (e.g. sulphonamides in dogs, methimazole and propylthiouracil in cats), transfusion-related • *Activation with subsequent aggregation* (also called consumption): – This can occur in animals with or without clinical or laboratory evidence of DIC. Drugs (protamine sulphate), snake venoms, inflammation (heat stroke, pancreatitis, vasculitis), infectious agents (bacterial sepsis, feline infectious coronavirus, *Angiostrongylus vasorum*, *Babesia*), neoplasia (e.g. haemangiosarcoma)	Moderate to severe (usually severe) Mild to moderate (can be severe, but infrequent) Mild to moderate (infrequently severe)
• **Sequestration/redistribution** • Splenomegaly of any cause (e.g. vascular engorgement, altered blood flow due to infiltrates, sedative or anaesthetic agents, hypothermia) • Pulmonary circulation – secondary to sepsis, endotoxaemia	Mild to moderate Transient (unlikely to see clinically)
• **Loss** • Massive severe haemorrhage, e.g. trauma, anticoagulant rodenticide toxicity	Mild to moderate

6.20 Mechanisms and degrees of acquired thrombocytopenia. [a] Mild = 100–200 × 10⁹/l; moderate = 30–100 × 10⁹/l; severe = <30 × 10⁹/l. DIC = disseminated intravascular coagulation.

system, primarily in the spleen. Adhesive interactions in the pulmonary circulation secondary to sepsis can also result in a mild to moderate thrombocytopenia; however, this is usually too transient to be clinically evident and other mechanisms of thrombocytopenia (e.g. DIC) are more likely to be operative in these conditions.

- **Thrombocytopenia:** this can be inherited or acquired, but the latter is far more common. As indicated earlier, the alarm level (the patient is at risk of bleeding) is a platelet count <30 × 10⁹/l.
  - *Inherited:* inherited macrothrombocytopenia, due to a mutation in the gene encoding β1-tubulin, has been documented in several dog breeds, notably the Cavalier King Charles Spaniel and Norfolk and Cairn Terriers, but also other breeds (e.g. Labrador Retriever, poodles, Chihauhau, Shih Tzu, Maltese, Jack Russell Terrier; see http://www.vetmed.auburn.edu/faculty/pathobiology-faculty/boudreaux#.UpENRZGxPZp). The tubulin mutation results in defective fragmentation of the megakaryocyte cytoplasm, producing decreased numbers of large platelets. In Cavalier King Charles Spaniels and Norfolk Terriers, platelet counts obtained using impedance- or laser-based or manual methods range from as low as 30 × 10⁹/l to 150 × 10⁹/l, but affected dogs are usually asymptomatic and have normal platelet crits (owing to increased platelet size). Greyhounds have lower platelet counts than other dog breeds (ranging from 80 to 295 × 10⁹/l), for unknown reasons. Since inherited thrombocytopenia is not usually severe in affected breeds, a severe reduction in platelet count should raise suspicion of a pathological cause, particularly in a bleeding animal.
  - *Acquired:* this can be seen in various disorders and can occur through several mechanisms, including decreased production, premature destruction (usually via immune-mediated mechanisms), consumption due to activation/aggregation secondary to DIC and non-DIC causes, sequestration and loss. The degree of reduction in platelet count can be helpful in preliminarily distinguishing between these mechanisms (Figure 6.20). Sequestration and loss are the least likely causes of thrombocytopenia.
- *Immune-mediated thrombocytopenia (ITP):* this can be primary or secondary to infectious diseases (e.g. rickettsial or viral infections) or neoplasia. A high prevalence of primary ITP is found in Cocker Spaniels, Poodles, German Shepherd Dogs and Old English Sheepdogs, suggesting a genetic predisposition to ITP in these breeds. Animals typically present with mucosal haemorrhage, petechiae, purpura and ecchymoses. Platelet counts are usually <30 × 10⁹/l (see Figure 6.16). Routine coagulation screening tests (PT, aPTT, TCT) are within reference intervals, although the ACT may be mildly prolonged because it relies on platelet phospholipid for clot formation.
- **Thrombocytosis:** this is due to acquired causes and is secondary to increased platelet production rather than decreased clearance. Platelet production is usually dependent on thrombopoietin; however, it can be thrombopoietin-independent in haemopoietic neoplasia affecting megakaryocytes, e.g. essential thrombocythaemia. Extreme thrombocytosis (platelet counts >1000 × 10⁹/l) due to essential thrombocythaemia is associated with either haemorrhage or thrombosis in human patients. Similar associations have not been made in companion animals, and most animals with thrombocytosis are apparently asymptomatic. Causes of thrombocytosis include:

- *Drugs:* these can cause splenic contraction, e.g. adrenaline, or increased platelet production, e.g. vincristine (due to defective microtubule function) and corticosteroids (mechanism unknown)
- *Reactive (cytokine-driven):* inflammatory cytokines such as interleukins (IL)-1, -6 and -11 drive thrombopoiesis indirectly by stimulating thrombopoietin production. This is a common cause (probably the most common cause) of thrombocytosis in sick animals and can occur secondary to inflammation, gastrointestinal disease or neoplasia
- *Iron deficiency:* thrombocytosis can accompany iron-deficiency anaemia, although the mechanism for the thrombocytosis is unknown
- *Megakaryocytic neoplasia:* mutations in the thrombopoietin receptor or downstream signalling pathway of this receptor are causes of essential thrombocythaemia in humans. Indeed, a specific mutation in JAK2 is the most common cause of this chronic myeloid leukaemia (the kinase is constitutively active and does not require thrombopoietin for activation). Such mutations have not been identified in companion animals with this neoplasm; however, it is exceedingly rare in both dogs and cats.

Disorders of platelet function

Abnormalities in any aspect of platelet function (adhesion, aggregation, release reaction, PS exposure) can result in defective platelet plug formation and manifest as excessive haemorrhage. These conditions are called thrombopathia and can be inherited (see Figure 6.19) or acquired, secondary to underlying disease (liver, kidney, neoplasia, infectious agents, DIC) or drugs (aspirin, NSAIDs). Drugs known to interfere with platelet function, such as aspirin (which inhibits function for the lifespan of the platelet, i.e. approximately 6 days), should be avoided in animals with proven or suspected haemostatic defects. Thrombopathias are uncommon, but may be underdiagnosed owing to lack of available testing (diagnosis requires specific analysers or tests, most of which are unavailable to the general practitioner; see Figure 6.7). Thrombopathias should be suspected in an animal with clinical signs attributable to defects in primary haemostasis, but with a normal (or mildly to moderately reduced) platelet count and vWf:Ag concentration. A BMBT may confirm a thrombopathia, but is a subjective, difficult to standardize test and may be normal in rare disorders of primary haemostasis (e.g. Scott syndrome; see Figure 6.19). Platelets can also be hyperfunctional as a result of underlying disease (Wiinberg *et al.*, 2012), predisposing to thrombosis, but this is not frequently recognized clinically.

von Willebrand's disease

vWD is the most common inherited disorder of haemostasis in dogs and is due to deficient or abnormal vWf. vWD is infrequently diagnosed in cats. It is inherited as an autosomal dominant trait and is readily diagnosed by measurement of vWf:Ag concentrations, although tests for the genetic mutation in vWf are available for selected breeds and are recommended for breeding purposes. Clinical signs usually manifest at a young age (excessive bleeding with teething or at spaying or neutering) and are most apparent in animals with severe decreases in vWf:Ag

(<15%, severe type I or type III) or dysfunctional vWf (type II). As noted before, petechial haemorrhages are not seen in vWD. There is no definitive proof that vWD is an acquired disorder in animals.

- **Type I vWD:** Decreased vWf with normal multimeric structure. Most common type – highly prevalent in Dobermanns (60%), Manchester Terriers, Airedale Terriers and Rottweilers. Due to a splice site defect in the vWf gene. Some, but not all, breeds display clinical signs (dogs with vWf:Ag concentrations <35% are at risk of haemorrhage and will have prolonged BMBT if vWf:Ag is <20%).
- **Type II vWD:** Decreased vWf with abnormal structure (loss of more functional high molecular weight multimers). German Wirehaired and Shorthaired Pointers. More clinically severe owing to decreased function of vWf (vWf:Ag concentrations are decreased but not usually <20%).
- **Type III vWD:** Most severe type, with absolute vWf deficiency (vWf:Ag <1%). Scottish Terriers, Shetland Sheepdogs, Chesapeake Bay Retrievers and Dutch Kooiker Dogs.

As discussed previously, a BMBT test is not recommended in dogs with suspected type II and type III vWD owing to the risk of severe haemorrhage.

Disorders of secondary haemostasis

These most frequently manifest as excessive haemorrhage due to coagulation factor deficiencies, although some deficiencies (notably FXII) are asymptomatic. Factor deficiencies result in large bleeds (haematomas) in subcutaneous tissues and haemorrhage into body cavities, joints or the central nervous system. Depending on the severity of the defect, haemorrhage can be spontaneous or induced by trauma or surgery. The most common disorder of secondary haemostasis is anticoagulant rodenticide toxicosis, whereas haemophilia A (FVIII deficiency, see Figure 6.19) and Hageman trait (FXII deficiency) are the most common inherited disorders of secondary haemostasis in dogs and cats, respectively. Only the more common symptomatic defects will be discussed further. Coagulation factor deficiencies are identified by prolonged screening coagulation assays (PT, aPTT, TCT); the combination of assay abnormalities provides clues as to the underlying defect (see Figures 6.13 and 6.17). High concentrations of some coagulation factors, including fibrinogen and FVIII, are risk factors for thrombosis in humans and rodent models; however, similar associations have not been made in dogs and cats.

Haemophilia A and B

These are both sex-linked disorders (males are affected; dams are obligate carriers unless the mutation is *de novo*) and have been diagnosed in many dog breeds, but rarely in cats. Haemophilia A is most prevalent in German Shepherd Dogs. Dogs present at a young age with haematomas, bleeding after surgery and recurring joint lameness (due to haemarthrosis). Haemophilia A and B will prolong the aPTT (but not the PT) and are confirmed by specific factor testing (see Figure 6.19). Depending on method and reagent, mild haemophilia A may be missed because only mild increases in aPTT are seen. The ACT is insensitive and should not be used for diagnosis. The worst clinical signs are seen with severe deficiency (<1% FVIII/FIX activity), with more subtle signs seen in dogs with mild (5–25%) or moderate (1–5%) deficiencies. The genetic defect has been identified in specific breeds and genetic testing would be useful in eliminating female carriers from the breeding pool and reducing disease prevalence.

Anticoagulant rodenticide toxicosis and other causes of vitamin K deficiency

Vitamin K is an essential cofactor for the activation of coagulation factors II, VII, IX and X. Anticoagulant rodenticides inhibit recycling of vitamin K by specifically inhibiting the enzyme vitamin K_1 epoxide reductase. When this enzyme is inhibited, the vitamin K epoxide cannot be converted into vitamin K, resulting in a relative vitamin K deficiency. Inactive factors cannot participate in clot formation, resulting in excessive haemorrhage, which is usually spontaneous and can be quite severe. Classic laboratory results are a prolonged PT and aPTT (see Figures 6.13 and 6.17), although the ACT can also be a reliable screening test because the coagulation deficiencies are so severe. Given that FVII is presumed to have the shortest half-life of all the coagulation factors in dogs, prolongation of the PT may precede prolongation of the aPTT. Hence the PT is considered a more sensitive test for detection of vitamin K antagonism by anticoagulant rodenticides and for monitoring response to therapy with vitamin K_1. Previous studies have shown that the PT is generally prolonged 2–3 days after intoxication or after cessation of vitamin K_1 therapy if the toxin is still present in the animal.

Mild toxicosis may be missed with all these screening assays, although it is doubtful that such dogs would suffer severe bleeds. Measurement of FVII activity could be performed; however, like all these tests, it is not specific for anticoagulant rodenticide toxicoses, being decreased with inherited FVII deficiency, DIC and synthetic liver disease. Testing for the actual toxin with specific chemical screens (e.g. HPLC) is the gold standard for diagnosis (Waddell et al., 2012), but this is not frequently performed owing to low availability and high cost. An alternative is measurement of the vitamin K_1 epoxide to vitamin K_1 ratio, which is a more readily available test because it is performed at human hospitals. Given that anticoagulant rodenticides inhibit the vitamin K_1 epoxide reductase, vitamin K_1 epoxide accumulates, resulting in a high vitamin K_1 epoxide to vitamin K_1 ratio. Increases in the epoxide:vitamin K_1 ratio are seen within 8 days of experimental toxicosis. Although useful for diagnosis, the epoxide:vitamin K_1 ratio is not recommended for monitoring treatment responses (Mount and Kass, 1989). Some animals have a mild to moderate thrombocytopenia (mechanism unclear) and, when they bleed internally, can have high D-dimer. Thus laboratory test results may mimic DIC; however, affected animals usually lack an underlying disease that could trigger DIC (Waddell et al., 2012).

Vitamin K deficiency also occurs with cholestatic liver disease (vitamin K is fat soluble, and bile salts are required for fat and vitamin K absorption), fat malabsorption (e.g. exocrine pancreatic insufficiency) and with some drugs (e.g. sulfaquinoxolone). Inherited defects in the γ-carboxylase enzyme have been identified in Devon Rex cats (see Figure 6.19). All such disorders respond to supplementation with vitamin K_1 (high doses are required for Devon Rex cats); however, this can take several hours to have an effect on clinical signs. If an immediate response is required in an animal with life-threatening haemorrhage, transfusion with plasma (fresh frozen, frozen plasma, cryosupernatant) is needed. Transfusion with whole blood is best avoided so as not to sensitize the animal to erythrocyte antigens and which could lead to future transfusion reactions.

Most first-generation anticoagulant rodenticides, e.g. warfarin, have a short half-life (approximately 15 hours), and thus treatment should be given for at least 1 week if animals are intoxicated with these compounds. However, second-generation anticoagulant rodenticides, e.g. brodifacoum, or first-generation indandiones, e.g. diphacinone, have longer half-lives (up to 6 days) and require vitamin K_1 therapy for up to 4–6 weeks. Since the nature of the ingested compound is frequently unknown, it is best to treat animals suspected of having rodenticide toxicosis for a minimum of 4–6 weeks, which is expensive. If this is not possible, a shorter duration of vitamin K_1 therapy could be considered, with measurement of the PT within 2–3 days of cessation of treatment. However, this is not recommended because animals may clinically bleed again during this time.

Disorders of fibrinolysis

Owing to the lack of specific diagnostic tests, fibrinolytic disorders are not frequently recognized in small animal patients. Inherited disorders of fibrinolysis have not been reported in dogs and cats. The main disorder associated with abnormalities in fibrinolysis is DIC (see below). It also appears that the delayed (36–48 hours) bleeding tendency associated with surgery in Greyhounds may be related to increased fibrinolysis because significantly fewer dogs treated with an inhibitor of fibrinolysis, ε-aminocaproic acid, showed postoperative haemorrhage after elective spaying or castration (Marin et al., 2012).

Disorders of global haemostasis

This encompasses disorders in which there are abnormalities in several aspects of haemostasis, including those asso-ciated with thrombosis, of which DIC is the most common and important (and will be the focus of this section).

Thrombosis

Virchow's triad of endothelial injury, blood flow abnormalities (particularly stasis) and hypercoagulability is still thought to represent the three main mechanisms of thrombosis, although there is likely to be overlap between them. Hypercoagulability refers to a haemostatic state that is shifted towards procoagulant forces and is defined by excess thrombin generation, indicating activation of secondary haemostasis. Hyperfunctional or activated platelets, deficiency of anticoagulant proteins (e.g. AT, protein C) and insufficient fibrinolysis may all contribute to a hypercoagulable state. Since thrombosis is not an inevitable consequence of hypercoagulability, it should be thought of as a 'pre-' or 'prothrombotic' state that puts a patient at risk of thrombosis. What tips the balance from this prothrombotic state into actual thrombosis is unknown. Currently, there is a lack of sensitive and specific diagnostic assays for hypercoagulability. The promise of global haemostatic testing with viscoelastic methods has not been borne out, with accumulating evidence that these test results are not reflective of in vivo haemostasis. We still have some way to go before we can truly identify animals at risk of thrombosis and know how to prevent it adequately.

Disseminated intravascular coagulation

When anything and everything that can go wrong with haemostasis does go wrong, DIC is the result. DIC is characterized by abnormal activation of haemostasis, with subsequent generation of excess thrombin, and lack of spatial and temporal control, such that haemostasis is not restricted to one site and occurs throughout the microvasculature, forming many small thrombi. This is the thrombotic phenotype of DIC or 'non-overt' DIC and, in human patients, is exacerbated by concurrent inhibition of fibrinolysis. This phase of DIC is difficult to diagnose, because screening tests of haemostasis are usually within reference intervals, thrombi are difficult to detect using standard imaging methods, and there are few available tests for excess thrombin generation, the key finding of this phase.

The formation of microvascular thrombi eventually consumes platelets, coagulation factors and inhibitors, resulting in abnormal bleeding. Haemorrhage is exacerbated by excess generation of plasmin (stimulation of fibrinolysis), which also cleaves and inactivates coagulation factors, compounding deficiencies. This is called the fibrinolytic phenotype of DIC or 'overt' DIC and is diagnosed by the typical laboratory abnormalities associated with DIC (see below). Although haemorrhage is the most apparent clinical manifestation of DIC, microthrombi have far more serious sequelae, due to the effects of hypoxic injury on end-organ function. It is usually end-organ injury or failure that results in the demise of the patient, and DIC should be thought of first as a thrombotic syndrome and second as a haemorrhagic one. Which phase of DIC dominates depends on the initiating cause and species. Dogs have robust fibrinolysis so the haemorrhagic phenotype of DIC dominates. In contrast, haemorrhage is uncommon in cats with this disorder, suggesting that they may be more like humans and suffer from the thrombotic phenotype of DIC. The disease is, therefore, far more difficult to diagnose in cats.

DIC is **never** a primary disease, but is always initiated by another disease. The most common diseases associated with DIC are moderate to severe inflammation (see Figure 6.20), endothelial injury, neoplasia and bacterial sepsis. *Angiostrongylus vasorum*, a nematode found in the pulmonary circulation, also triggers a DIC-like syndrome in some affected dogs (see below). These diseases probably trigger DIC via the exposure of large amounts of extravascular TF (massive endothelial injury) or aberrant intravascular TF expression on monocytes (induced by bacterial lipopolysaccharide, inflammatory cytokines) or cancer cells (constitutive expression). Procoagulant (PS- and/or TF-expressing) microparticles are released from platelets, monocytes and dying cells, which disseminate throughout the circulation, amplifying thrombin generation as they go. This is coupled by inadequate inhibition, as a result of the downregulation and inactivation of inhibitors (usually a consequence of the primary disease process). As indicated previously, with DIC induced by bacterial sepsis, a self-perpetuating cycle between inflammation and haemostasis activation can be established, making it very difficult to treat DIC in this setting (successful resolution of sepsis will not resolve the haemostatic dysfunction). The reader is referred to recent reviews for additional information on DIC (Stokol, 2010; Ralph and Brainard, 2012).

- **Diagnosis:** regardless of the phase of DIC, documentation of the initiating underlying disease is crucial. Not only is this necessary for diagnosis, but successful treatment of the primary disease is usually required for complete resolution of the syndrome. There is no single pathognomonic test for DIC; the diagnosis requires documentation of a constellation of test abnormalities, usually in all aspects of haemostasis (primary, secondary, fibrinolysis, inhibition). Thus, DIC panels that address all aspects are recommended.
  - *Overt or thrombohaemorrhagic DIC:* this occurs more frequently and is more readily diagnosed in dogs than cats. This phase is characterized by deficiencies of haemostatic cells and proteins and clinical signs of excessive haemorrhage.
    - Primary haemostasis: thrombocytopenia. This is a highly sensitive test; indeed it is difficult to diagnose overt DIC in the absence of thrombocytopenia or a low normal platelet count in dogs. Platelet counts do not appear to be very useful in cats with DIC, owing to difficulties in obtaining accurate counts in this species.
    - Secondary haemostasis: prolonged PT and/or aPTT. In dogs, the aPTT is more sensitive than the PT (more frequently prolonged). In cats, the converse may be true. The ACT will be prolonged with severe factor deficiencies but should not be relied upon for diagnosis of DIC. Hypofibrinogenaemia or high concentrations of FDPs may prolong the TCT, but because fibrinogen concentrations are frequently high (the initiating disease stimulates production) or normal (reflecting a balance of production and consumption), these are insensitive tests for DIC.
    - Fibrinolysis: high D-dimer concentrations are a highly sensitive test for the diagnosis of DIC (more so than the PT or aPTT) in dogs. D-dimer does not appear as sensitive in cats.
    - Lack of inhibitors: low AT and protein C activity can be seen in dogs with DIC, and low AT activity has a similar high sensitivity to D-dimer for diagnosis of DIC in dogs. Low AT activity is not a common finding in cats with DIC.
    - Supportive findings: red blood cell fragmentation (schistocytes, acanthocytes, keratocytes), presumably secondary to 'shearing' through microvascular thrombi, is not specific for DIC, particularly in cats, and is also insensitive.
  - *Non-overt or thrombotic DIC:* documentation of excessive thrombin generation is paramount to diagnosing this phase of DIC. The most specific test involves measurement of high concentrations of TAT complexes; however, this is not readily available. D-dimer is an indirect marker of thrombin formation and is the next best test but, unfortunately, this is not specific for DIC. Screening haemostasis assays, including platelet counts, are frequently normal on single testing. Currently, the best way to diagnose this stage of DIC is to have a high clinical index of suspicion and document worsening haemostasis results (decreasing platelet count and AT, increasing PT/aPTT and D-dimer) on sequential testing (24–48 hours apart) in at-risk patients.
- **Treatment**: this is highly controversial and clinician dependent. Treatment of the initiating disorder is mandatory. Anticoagulant treatment is recommended for human patients with non-overt DIC, whereas replacement of platelets and coagulation factors is recommended for human patients with overt DIC. In both phases of DIC, supplementation of inhibitors, which have anti-inflammatory as well as anticoagulant properties, may be helpful, but these can only be administered through plasma transfusions in animals. Readers are referred to human medical texts for further recommendations.

Angiostrongylus vasorum

Infections with this nematode parasite are associated with haemostatic dysfunction, particularly excessive haemorrhage, which is readily recognized clinically. The disease is endemic in continental Europe, the southwest of England, Ireland and Wales, but cases are being reported in Scotland and the north of England. Dogs are infected after ingestion of third-stage larvae in intermediate (snails or slugs) or paratenic (frog) hosts. Adult worms are located in the heart (right ventricle) and pulmonary artery, and clinical signs are mostly referable to the respiratory system, particularly coughing, dyspnoea, tachypnoea and gagging, and/or coagulopathy. Young dogs are frequently affected (probably due to indiscriminate eating habits). Haemorrhage is usually associated with the respiratory tract (epistaxis, haemoptysis), but dogs can also suffer from petechiae, ecchymoses, sublingual and episcleral haemorrhage, subcutaneous haematomas, haemarthrosis, and excessive bleeding after surgery or from wounds. Intracavity bleeds also occur and can result in death of the animal from exsanguination. Haemorrhage into the brain and spinal cord can precipitate neurological signs (seizures, ataxia, behavioural changes, paresis, paralysis).

Although haemorrhage typifies the clinical manifestation of nematode infection, chronic arterial thrombi are observed in many pulmonary vessels. Some larger thrombi can contain adult worms and larvae. Haemorrhage has been largely attributed to a DIC-like syndrome, with a mild to moderate thrombocytopenia and prolonged aPTT and/or PT being observed after experimental infection of dogs with high numbers of infective larvae. High concentrations of D-dimer (or FDPs) are seen in dogs with natural infections. The presence of fibrin thrombi in vessels distant from the pulmonary vasculature (e.g. portal veins) supports the existence of a systemic thrombohaemorrhagic disorder in infected dogs. Haemorrhage can also result from direct vessel rupture.

The mechanism by which the parasites cause haemostatic dysfunction is unknown; however, the worms are thought to irritate the endothelium mechanically. This irritation probably induces an inflammatory response (vasculitis is observed histologically in tissues from infected dogs), which triggers thrombin generation through both intrinsic (FXII) and extrinsic (TF) pathways, resulting in pathological thrombosis. Subsequent activation or consumption of coagulation factors and platelets could cause the abnormal haemostatic test results.

The diagnosis of A. vasorum infection can be achieved through detection of the first-stage (L1) larvae in faeces using a modified Baermann technique. However, this test is insensitive (testing samples from three separate days can increase sensitivity) and larvae from other nematodes, such as Filaroides spp., can confound test interpretation. Newer molecular and serological diagnostic tests have become available, including polymerase chain reaction (PCR)-based techniques (which can be performed on blood or faeces) and an enzyme-linked immunosorbent assay (ELISA) for parasite antigen. These tests are more sensitive and specific than faecal larval identification. A point-of-care antigen spot test is now available for diagnosis of A. vasorum (Angio Detect™, IDEXX); independent validation of the test is yet to be reported. The worms or larvae can occasionally also be detected in cytological smears of lung aspirates and bronchoalveolar lavages; however, such procedures may be contraindicated in a severely dyspnoeic animal. Testing for the worm is recommended for dogs presenting with typical signalment and clinical signs, particularly in endemic areas.

The laboratory findings of thrombocytopenia, eosinophilia and hyperglobulinaemia on screening clinical pathological testing should also raise suspicion of A. vasorum infection, and empirical treatment with anthelmintics (e.g. moxidectin, milbemycin oxime, fenbendazole) should be considered in dogs with suspected infection. It should be noted that screening CBC, biochemical and haemostasis tests may be normal in infected dogs, and laboratory evidence of haemostatic dysfunction does not correlate with clinical signs. The reader is referred to an excellent review on this nematode (Helm et al., 2010).

Case examples

CASE 1

SIGNALMENT

1.5-year-old male neutered German Shepherd Dog.

HISTORY

Developed severe spontaneous epistaxis when 8 months old, which resolved after transfusion of whole blood. At 1.5 years of age, developed severe bruising after neutering. Results of a CBC, including platelet count, and chemistry profile were within reference intervals and no abnormalities were noted on physical examination. Haemostasis screening test results are given below.

HAEMOSTASIS TEST RESULTS

Test	Result	Reference interval
aPTT (s)	14	10–17
PT (s)	11	11–16
TCT (s)	5	5–9
BMBT (min)	2.8	1.7–3.3

BASED ON SIGNALMENT, HISTORY AND CLINICAL SIGNS, IS THE DISORDER LIKELY TO BE INHERITED OR ACQUIRED, AND WHICH PATHWAY OF HAEMOSTASIS IS LIKELY TO BE INVOLVED?

This is a young, apparently otherwise healthy dog that has already demonstrated two episodes of excessive haemorrhage. Recurrent bleeding in a young animal with no evidence of underlying disease supports an inherited

→ CASE 1 CONTINUED

disorder. Since surgery-induced haemorrhage can occur with defects in any pathway of haemostasis, the informative clinical sign is spontaneous epistaxis, which points towards an abnormality in primary haemostasis. The most commonly reported haemostatic defects in German Shepherd Dogs are haemophilia A (FVIII deficiency) and vWD; however, the screening haemostasis results do not support either diagnosis. The aPTT would be expected to be prolonged with haemophilia A and the BMBT with vWD, particularly if vWf:Ag concentrations were low enough to induce spontaneous haemorrhage.

BASED ON THE RESULTS OF THE SCREENING HAEMOSTASIS ASSAYS, WHAT DISORDER IS SUSPECTED AND HOW COULD THIS DIAGNOSIS BE CONFIRMED?

German Shepherd Dogs also suffer from the rare autosomal inherited disorder called Scott syndrome, which is due to a defect in platelet membrane flipping. Affected dogs do not exteriorize PS and their platelets do not efficiently support fibrin formation. Since there is no requirement for platelet PS in screening coagulation assays (PT, aPTT, TCT), these tests will be normal in this syndrome. Also, PS has no role in platelet plug formation, so the BMBT will also be normal. Even though platelets are required for clot formation in the ACT, PS can be provided by other surfaces, so the ACT is also normal in affected dogs and would not be helpful as a screening tool. Similarly, platelet function analysis and viscoelastic methods are normal in Scott syndrome.

The only way to confirm this diagnosis is to demonstrate that the platelets lack procoagulant activity, i.e. do not exteriorize PS on activation with platelet agonists. This is most readily accomplished using a flow cytometry-based test that detects PS on the surface of activated platelets. Since screening assays are normal in affected dogs, this syndrome remained undiagnosed until the advent of tests that relied upon PS exposure. This was first accomplished with a global haemostasis test called the clot signature analyser, which showed defective clot formation in whole blood and was subsequently confirmed with platelet procoagulant tests. A causative mutation has been detected (Brooks M, personal communication) and will hopefully lead to a genetic test.

Surgery- and trauma-induced haemorrhage is the most common clinical sign in affected dogs. It is interesting that, although the defect is one of fibrin formation (or secondary haemostasis), it usually manifests as mucosal haemorrhage, particularly from the nose, which is a feature of defects in primary haemostasis. Notably, petechiae are not seen in affected dogs (because this requires platelet plug formation only) (Jandry et al., 2012). An alternative diagnosis to Scott syndrome is an inherited defect in fibrinolysis (which would also result in normal results in the above screening assays); however, this has not been reported in dogs to date. (Excessive fibrinolysis may, however, explain the delayed postoperative haemorrhage seen in some Greyhounds (Marin et al., 2012), as indicated earlier.)

HOW SHOULD THIS DISORDER BE TREATED?

Transfusion therapy with products that contain fresh platelets is required to treat or prevent bleeding episodes. Platelet transfusions are ideal but are less readily available than whole blood transfusions, which come with all the attendant risks along with a poor success rate (several blood transfusions are required to stop haemorrhage). Indeed, in this case, the dog was pretreated with whole blood prior to castration and still developed extensive haemorrhage in the inguinal area after the procedure. Haemorrhage can be quite severe and intractable in some dogs. This dog developed severe epistaxis at 7 years of age, which only ceased after emergency sphenopalatine artery embolization.

CASE 2

SIGNALMENT

9-year-old male neutered Weimaraner.

HISTORY

Presented with lethargy for 3 days, followed by an acute onset of recumbency. There was no known exposure to toxins, the dog was not on any drugs and had not travelled recently. The dog did have unsupervised outdoor access. On examination, the dog was hypothermic, with pale mucous membranes and a palpable abdominal fluid wave. Extensive bruising was noted on the right side of the abdomen. The referring veterinary surgeon (veterinarian) had given the dog a whole blood transfusion prior to referral. Abdominal ultrasonography confirmed an abdominal effusion and a right-sided abdominal wall mass. Radiography revealed an additional right retroperitoneal mass. The CBC results are provided below. Biochemical panel results were unremarkable. Cytological findings on an aspirate of abdominal fluid were consistent with a haemorrhagic effusion (fluid packed cell volume of 37% with erythrophagia and absence of platelets). Results from a haemostasis panel are also given below.

PERTINENT CLINICAL PATHOLOGY DATA

Haematology	Result	Reference interval
HCT (l/l)	**0.24**	0.41–0.60
Reticulocytes (%)	**3.8**	0.2–1.5
Absolute reticulocytes (x 10⁹/l)	**125**	11–95
Nucleated red cells (per 100 WBC)	**2**	0–1
WBC (x 10⁹/l)	**14.9**	5.7–14.2
Segmented neutrophils (x 10⁹/l)	**12.1**	2.7–9.4
Band neutrophils (x 10⁹/l)	0	0–0.1

Abnormal results are in **bold**.

→ **CASE 2 CONTINUED**

Haematology *continued*	Result	Reference interval
Lymphocytes (x 10⁹/l)	0.7	0.9–4.7
Platelets (x 10⁹/l)	60[a]	179–483
MPV (fl)	16.0	8.4–13.2
Platelet smear estimate	Low	

[a]Platelet clumps noted on smear. Any count provided should be
considered a minimum count.

Haemostasis test	Result	Reference interval
aPTT (s)	22	10–17
PT (s)	30	11–16
TCT (s)	6	5–9
Fibrinogen (g/l)	7.85	1.5–4.5
AT activity (%)	77	65–145
D-dimer (mg/l)	2.88	0.03–0.25

Abnormal results are in **bold**.

BASED ON SIGNALMENT, HISTORY AND CLINICAL SIGNS, IS THE DISORDER LIKELY TO BE INHERITED OR ACQUIRED, AND WHICH PATHWAY OF HAEMOSTASIS IS LIKELY TO BE INVOLVED?

Since this is an older dog, with no prior history of bleeding, the disorder is likely to be acquired. Intracavity haemorrhage, such as the documented haemorrhagic effusion, is characteristic of a disorder of secondary haemostasis. The extensive, severe, apparently spontaneous ecchymoses are also more characteristic of a severe disorder of secondary haemostasis, but are not specific for this.

BASED ON THE RESULTS OF THE SCREENING HAEMOSTASIS ASSAYS, WHAT DISORDER IS SUSPECTED AND WHY?

Screening haemostasis assays indicate abnormalities in primary haemostasis (thrombocytopenia), and secondary haemostasis (prolonged PT and aPTT) with evidence of fibrinolysis (high D-dimer). The thrombocytopenia alone does not explain the signs of haemorrhage (the high MPV is not informative in this case because it could be an artefact of platelet clumping). The high fibrinogen indicates an inflammatory response (fibrinogen is a positive acute phase protein) and this result, with the normal AT activity and absence of liver test abnormalities on the biochemical panel, argues against synthetic liver failure. Note that the changes in the leucogram could indicate a corticosteroid response (or 'stress' leucogram) or inflammation.

The main differential diagnoses for these haemostasis results are anticoagulant rodenticide toxicosis, *Angiostrongylus vasorum* infection and DIC. The first diagnosis is favoured because the PT is more prolonged than the aPTT and the AT activity is not low (the aPTT is usually more sensitive than the PT in dogs with DIC and the AT is quite sensitive, but no test is 100% sensitive).

Although the PT and aPTT can be this prolonged with naturally occurring *A. vasorum* infection, the abdominal masses described would be unusual and the dog lacked respiratory signs related to the parasite. These results also do not rule out DIC secondary to cancer such as haemangiosarcoma, particularly with the apparent abdominal masses (although the mass locations described would be unusual for haemangiosarcoma).

HOW COULD THIS DIAGNOSIS BE CONFIRMED?

Anticoagulant rodenticide toxicity can be confirmed by measurement of the vitamin K_1 epoxide to vitamin K_1 ratio (see text) or by rodenticide screening for specific toxins in blood. Alternatively, trial therapy with vitamin K_1 could be instituted, with resolution of clinical signs supporting a diagnosis of toxicosis. Testing for *A. vasorum* would be worthwhile in areas endemic for this parasite. There is no specific test to confirm DIC; however, a primary disease would need to be identified in this dog (an initiating disease is an absolute prerequisite for DIC diagnosis). Measurement of FVII activity would not be helpful because this could be decreased in both conditions (from lack of activation with rodenticides and consumption during clotting or cleavage by plasmin in DIC).

A rodenticide screening test with HPLC was performed on the dog and 10 parts per billion of brodifacoum was detected, confirming rodenticide toxicity in this case. The dog was treated with fresh frozen plasma and vitamin K_1. The PT and aPTT normalized within 2 days of hospitalization and the dog was discharged with a 30-day course of vitamin K_1. The abdominal masses were not investigated further, but were suspected to be haematomas.

Anticoagulant rodenticides result in a haemorrhagic diathesis due to a relative deficiency of vitamin K, which prevents adequate activation of factors II, VII, IX and X. Mild to moderate thrombocytopenia can be seen in dogs with anticoagulant rodenticide toxicosis, although the mechanisms are unclear (possible loss with acute severe haemorrhage, a consequence of blood transfusions, activation/consumption). D-dimer is frequently increased secondary to internal haemorrhage (extravascular fibrinolysis) and results can be quite high (Waddell *et al.*, 2012), as seen in this dog. The internal haemorrhage is also the cause of the dog's moderate regenerative anaemia. Thus, laboratory findings with rodenticide toxicosis can mimic DIC, and differentiating between these disorders is imperative. In this case, neoplasia-induced DIC was possible based on the older age of the animal and the presence of abdominal masses; however, the latter were likely to be haematomas. If the rodenticide screening tests were negative and the dog's haemostatic dysfunction did not respond to vitamin K_1 therapy, vigorous pursuit of an underlying disease would have been essential in this dog (assuming negative test results for *A. vasorum*), and a diagnosis of DIC would have been favoured. Empirical treatment for *A. vasorum* could also be offered even if diagnostic tests for this parasite were negative, particularly in endemic areas.

CASE 3

SIGNALMENT

11-year-old male neutered Siberian Husky.

HISTORY

4-day history of anorexia, lethargy, vomiting and increased respiratory effort. 1-day history of pasty diarrhoea. Treated with potentiated clavulanic acid by the referring veterinary surgeon. On physical examination, the dog was depressed and febrile with purple mucous membranes and a normal capillary refill time. The abdomen was tense on palpation and ecchymoses were noted on the ventral neck. An alveolar pattern in the left cranial lung lobe and a mottled enlarged pancreas surrounded by hyperechoic tissue with hypoechoic liver nodules were identified on radiographic and ultrasonographic examination of the thorax and abdomen, respectively. Pertinent results from a CBC, full biochemical test results, and results of a haemostasis panel are shown below.

PERTINENT CLINICAL PATHOLOGY DATA

Haematology	Result	Reference interval
HCT (l/l)	0.45	0.41–0.60
WBC (x 10⁹/l)	**20.5**	5.7–14.2
Segmented neutrophils (x 10⁹/l)	7.6	2.7–9.4
Band neutrophils (x 10⁹/l)	**10.0**	0–0.1
Monocytes (x 10⁹/l)	**1.2**	0.1–1.0
Platelets (x 10⁹/l)	**45**	179–483
MPV (fl)	11.4	8.4–13.2
Platelet smear estimate	Low	
WBC morphology	Marked toxic change	

Biochemistry	Result	Reference interval
Sodium (mmol/l)	149	142–151
Potassium (mmol/l)	4.2	3.9–5.3
Chloride (mmol/l)	117	107–117
Bicarbonate (mmol/l)	18	15–25
Anion gap (mmol/l)	18	13–25
Urea nitrogen (mmol/l)	4.6	2.9–10.7
Creatinine (µmol/l)	70.7	44.9–114.2
Calcium (mmol/l)	2.3	2.3–2.9
Phosphate (mmol/l)	1.7	0.9–1.7
Magnesium (mmol/l)	0.6	0.6–0.8
Total protein (g/l)	56	56–71
Albumin (g/l)	**29**	31–41
Globulin (g/l)	27	19–36
A:G ratio	1.1	0.9–1.9
Glucose (mmol/l)	5.8	3.3–6.7
ALT (IU/l)	**247**	25–106
AST (IU/l)	**891**	16–50 ▶

Abnormal results are in **bold**.

Biochemistry *continued*	Resort	Reference interval
ALP (IU/l)	**644**	12–122
Total bilirubin (µmol/l)	3.4	0–5.1
Amylase (IU/l)	**5382**	286–1124
Creatine kinase (IU/l)	240	58–241
Pancreatic lipase (µg/l)	**1000**	<200
Serum lipase testing was not performed		

Haemostasis test	Result	Reference interval
aPTT (s)	**20**	10–17
PT (s)	14	11–16
TCT (s)	8	5–9
Fibrinogen (g/l)	**6.5**	1.5–4.5
AT activity (%)	**56**	65–145
D-dimer (mg/l)	**1.5**	0.03–0.25

Abnormal results are in **bold**.

BASED ON SIGNALMENT, HISTORY AND CLINICAL SIGNS, IS THE DISORDER LIKELY TO BE INHERITED OR ACQUIRED, AND WHICH PATHWAY OF HAEMOSTASIS IS LIKELY TO BE INVOLVED?

This is likely to be an acquired disorder because this is an older dog, with no prior history of bleeding, and the dog is sick, with evidence of systemic inflammation (inflammatory leucogram characterized by a degenerative left shift with toxic change and mild monocytosis, high fibrinogen, hypoalbuminaemia), pulmonary disease (on radiographic examination), liver injury (high transaminases), possible cholestasis or corticosteroid excess (high alkaline phosphatase) and pancreatitis (high amylase and pancreatic lipase and supportive ultrasonographic examination findings). Neck ecchymoses do not pinpoint which haemostatic pathway is affected, because this can occur with a defect in any pathway, including fibrinolysis.

BASED ON THE RESULTS OF THE SCREENING HAEMOSTASIS ASSAYS, WHAT DISORDER IS SUSPECTED AND WHY?

Screening haemostasis assays indicate abnormalities in primary haemostasis (moderate thrombocytopenia) and secondary haemostasis (prolonged aPTT) with evidence of fibrinolysis (high D-dimer) and consumption or decreased production of inhibitors (low AT activity). The thrombocytopenia alone does not explain the haemorrhage, but an acquired thrombopathia (from high FDPs) could be occurring concurrently (although the TCT is normal, suggesting that FDPs are not high enough to interfere with fibrin polymerization). The primary differential diagnosis is overt DIC (haemorrhagic phenotype), because the dog has a disease process that can initiate DIC (severe inflammation due to pancreatitis, and possible pneumonia and cholangiohepatitis), is demonstrating signs of excessive (and spontaneous) haemorrhage and has evidence of platelet, coagulation factor and inhibitor consumption and fibrinolysis. Hepatic synthetic failure could result in some of these abnormalities, including prolonged aPTT and AT (decreased production) and high

→ CASE 3 CONTINUED

D-dimer (decreased clearance) (Kavanagh *et al.*, 2012). However, decreased fibrinogen and a prolonged PT would be expected as well. It can be difficult to differentiate between DIC and liver failure, because haemostasis results may be similar. Although haemorrhage is the clinical sign indicating a haemostatic disorder, thrombosis is probably occurring and contributing to the organ dysfunction (liver injury, dyspnoea) in this case.

HOW COULD THIS DOG BE TREATED?

The dog should be treated for pancreatitis and likely sepsis, but there is no consensus on specific treatment for DIC and treatment recommendations are based on opinion and not solid evidence. Considering that the dog is in the haemorrhagic overt phase of DIC, administration of fresh frozen plasma to provide coagulation factors and inhibitors is probably indicated (the platelet count is not critically low). These are unlikely to 'fuel the fire' as previously believed and may be crucial for preventing serious bleeds. However, the dog is also currently thrombosing, and anticoagulant therapy aimed at limiting thrombin generation (the key and defining event in DIC) should be initiated, such as heparin therapy. Unfortunately, there is a paucity of data showing therapeutic efficacy of anticoagulants and treatment of DIC is going to remain empirical and on a case-by-case basis. This dog was treated with intravenous fluids, antibiotics, antiemetics and anti-diarrhoeal medication, along with plasma transfusions and heparin. Unfortunately, the dog continued to deteriorate and was euthanased.

References and further reading

Day MJ and Kohn B (2012) *BSAVA Manual of Canine and Feline Haematology and Transfusion Medicine, 2nd edn*, ed. MJ Day and B Kohn. BSAVA Publications, Gloucester

Helm JR, Morgan ER, Jackson MW, Wotton P and Bell R (2010) Canine angiostrongylosis: an emerging disease in Europe. *Journal of Veterinary Emergency and Critical Care* **20**, 98–109

Jandry KE, Norris JW, Tucker M and Brooks MB (2012) Clinical characterisation of platelet procoagulant deficiency (Scott syndrome). *Journal of Veterinary Internal Medicine* **26**, 1402–1407

Kavanagh C, Shaw S and Webster CRL (2012) Coagulation in hepatobiliary disease. *Journal of Veterinary Emergency and Critical Care* **21**, 589–604

Koi A and Borjesson DL (2010) Application of thromboelastography/thromboelastometry in veterinary medicine. *Veterinary Clinical Pathology* **39**, 405–416

Marin LM, Iazbic MC, Zaldivar-Lopez S, Guillaumin J, McLoughlin MA and Couto CG (2012) Epsilon aminocaproic acid for the prevention of delayed postoperative bleeding in retired racing greyhounds undergoing gonadectomy. *Veterinary Surgery* **41**, 594–603

McMichael MA and Smith S (2011) Viscoelastic coagulation testing: technology, applications and limitations. *Veterinary Clinical Pathology* **40**, 140–153

Mount ME and Kass PH (1989) Diagnostic importance of vitamin K1 and its epoxide measured in serum of dogs exposed to an anticoagulant rodenticide. *American Journal of Veterinary Research* **50**, 1704–1709

Ralph AG and Brainard BM (2012) Update on disseminated intravascular coagulation: When to consider it, when to expect it and when to treat it. *Topics in Companion Animal Medicine* **27**, 65–72

See AM, Swindells KL, Sharman MJ *et al.* (2009) Activated coagulation times in normal dogs and cats using MAX-ACT™ tubes. *Australian Veterinary Journal* **87**, 292–295

Smith S (2009) The cell-based model of coagulation. *Journal of Veterinary Emergency and Critical Care* **19**, 3–10

Spodsberg EH, Wiinberg B, Jessen LR, Marschner CB and Kristensen AT (2013) Endogenous fibrinolytic potential in tissue-plasminogen-activator-modifed thromboelastography analysis is significantly decreased in dogs suffering from diseases predisposed to thrombosis. *Veterinary Clinical Pathology* **42**, 281–290

Stokol T (2010) Disseminated intravascular coagulation. In: *Schalm's Veterinary Hematology, 6th edn*, ed. DJ Weiss and KJ Wardrop, pp. 679–688. Wiley-Blackwell, Ames, IA

Waddell LS, Poppenga RH and Drobatz KJ (2012) Anticoagulant rodenticide screening in dogs: 123 cases (1996–2003). *Journal of the American Veterinary Medical Assocation* **242**, 516–521

Wiinberg B, Jessen LR, Tarnow I and Kristensen AT (2012) Diagnosis and treatment of platelet hyperactivity in relation to thrombosis in dogs and cats. *Journal of Veterinary Emergency and Critical Care* **22**, 42–58

Useful websites

Boudreaux M
http://www.vetmed.auburn.edu/faculty/pathobiology-faculty/boudreaux#.UpENRZGxPZp

Comparative Coagulation Laboratory at Cornell University
https://ahdc.vet.cornell.edu/sects/Coag/

eClinPath, an online textbook on Clinical Pathology at Cornell University: http://eclinpath.com

Chapter 7

Disorders of plasma proteins

Yvonne McGrotty, Rory Bell and Gerard McLauchlan

Plasma protein abnormalities are associated with a wide variety of disease processes and are a significant biochemical finding in both dogs and cats. The *plasma* proteins are comprised of albumin, globulin and fibrinogen fractions. Measurement of *serum* proteins excludes fibrinogen, which is involved in blood clotting, and so serum values are approximately 5% lower than plasma protein levels. Adult reference ranges are shown in Figure 7.1; results should always be interpreted using a laboratory's own reference ranges. Reference ranges for juvenile animals are lower than those of adults.

Proteins	Dogs (g/l)	Cats (g/l)
Total protein	50–78	60–85
Albumin	29–36	26–36
Globulin	28–42	27–45
Fibrinogen	2–4	2–4

7.1 Adult serum and plasma protein reference ranges from Glasgow University Diagnostic Services. Reference ranges will vary for different laboratories.

Albumin

Albumin is a large osmotically active protein with an average molecular weight of 69,000 daltons and a half-life of between 17 and 19 days. Almost 75% of colloid oncotic pressure is attributed to albumin. Any decrease in albumin concentration can result in a significant decrease in oncotic pressure, with a resultant fluid shift from the intravascular space into the interstitium. This causes hypotension, oedema (subcutaneous, pulmonary) and body cavity effusions (pleural effusion, ascites). Increases in albumin concentration are usually a result of dehydration and haemoconcentration.

Globulin

Globulins have molecular weights ranging from 90,000 daltons (β_1-globulin) to 156,000 daltons (γ-globulin). In addition to providing oncotic support and drug transport, the main components of the globulin fraction are the immunoglobulins (IgG, IgM, IgA and IgE), which are produced by lymphoid tissue in response to antigenic stimulation. The globulin fractions can be separated by serum protein electrophoresis (SPE).

Fibrinogen

Fibrinogen is converted to insoluble fibrin during the coagulation cascade, leading to the formation of a stable blood clot. Increased levels of fibrinogen signify non-specific inflammation while reduced levels can result from severe hepatic insufficiency, disseminated intravascular coagulation or, rarely, a congenital deficiency (factor I deficiency). The presence of a clot within the sample or the use of lithium heparin as an anticoagulant will lead to falsely reduced fibrinogen levels.

Methods of measuring protein

Total protein is measured by spectrophotometry or the Biuret method. The Biuret method uses a reagent composed of copper ions at an alkaline pH. A violet-coloured complex is formed when serum or plasma are mixed with the reagent. The intensity of the violet colour is proportional to the number of peptide bonds present and so is also proportional to the amount of total protein present. The amount of protein is then quantified using spectrophotometric methods.

An estimate of protein concentration can be obtained using a refractometer, which measures total solids. This method can only be used with clear, non-lipaemic serum, because several factors falsely increase refractometer measurements of total solids:

- Haemolysis
- Lipaemia
- Synthetic colloids (including haemoglobin-based oxygen-carrying solutions and tetrastarches such as Voluven®)
- Severe hyperglycaemia
- Azotaemia
- Hypernatraemia
- Hyperchloraemia
- Hyperbilirubinaemia.

Spectrophotometric methods of total protein measurement will be falsely increased by haemolysis and lipaemia and may be increased by hyperbilirubinaemia with some analysers.

Albumin concentration can be determined by binding to bromocresol green (BCG) dye. The resulting coloured solution is then measured spectrophotometrically. Globulin concentration is determined by subtracting the albumin concentration from the total protein measurement. A more accurate determination of the globulin fraction is obtained by electrophoresis. Fibrinogen can be measured by either heat precipitation (Figure 7.2) or the Von Clauss method; the latter method evaluates the time taken for a fibrin clot to form after adding thrombin to citrate plasma, although it is not widely available. The heat precipitation process is not sufficiently accurate to detect decreased fibrinogen and so cannot be used in the assessment of disseminated intravascular coagulation (DIC) or fibrinogen deficiency.

Fill two haematocrit tubes with heparinized blood (tubes A and B)

1. Heat one tube to 56–58°C for three minutes (B)
2. Centrifuge tubes A and B in a microhaematocrit centrifuge
3. Measure total solids in each of the tubes using a refractometer
4. Calculate the amount of fibrinogen according to the following formula:

Fibrinogen measurement = Total solids of tube A (g/l) − Total solids of tube B (g/l)

7.2 Measurement of fibrinogen by heat precipitation.

Serum protein electrophoresis

One-dimensional (1D) serum protein electrophoresis (SPE) can be used to separate different protein fractions using the cellulose acetate, agarose gel or capillary zone method. Electrophoresis is defined as the migration of ions under the influence of an electrical field. The most common clinical application of SPE is to evaluate animals with marked hyperglobulinaemia and to distinguish monoclonal and polyclonal gammopathies. Studies have looked at establishing normal reference intervals for the various protein fractions in dogs (Fayos *et al.*, 2005). Factors other than disease can lead to alterations in the electrophoretogram: these include breed, age, hormonal status and nutrition (Eckersall, 2008).

Cellulose acetate or agarose gel method

Serum or plasma, in an alkaline environment, is placed on an agarose gel or cellulose acetate strip in an electrical field. The individual protein fractions migrate towards the anode at different speeds, based on their electrical charge, shape and mass. Albumin migrates the furthest because it is a small anionic molecule. The trace is then stained using an organic stain that non-covalently binds to proteins (e.g. Ponceau S) and is subsequently scanned by a densitometer. The intensity of the staining is illustrated as an electrophoretic trace; the darkest band (indicating high levels of protein) results in the highest peak on the trace. Each peak can reflect the staining of a single protein (e.g. albumin) or multiple proteins. Electrophoresis using cellulose acetate separates proteins into between five and nine protein bands, while the agarose gel method can separate the proteins into 10 to 15 bands. Cellulose acetate electrophoresis is considered to be more accurate than agarose methods.

Capillary zone method

Capillary zone electrophoresis has now become more commonplace as it has a faster turnaround time and is fully automated. The results are considered to be more accurate than those of other methods. The capillary zone method involves electrophoresis of samples within very narrow-bore silica tubes. A high voltage is applied across the capillary tube and the proteins within the capillary tube migrate along its length at different rates. The separated molecules pass via a viewing window towards the cathode, where they are detected by an ultraviolet monitor, which then transmits a signal to a computer.

Interpretation of electrophoretic traces

Electrophoretic traces from normal animals produce a tall narrow albumin spike at one end and three globulin fractions: α-globulins, β-globulins and γ-globulins. Canine and feline α-globulins and β-globulins are further subdivided into α_1, α_2, β_1 and β_2 subfractions. The immunoglobulins (IgG, IgM, IgE and IgA) are the main components of the globulin fraction and are primarily located in the β and γ sections of the SPE. Figure 7.3 illustrates an agarose gel electrophoretic trace from a normal dog. If plasma is used instead of serum, a large fibrinogen peak will be present between the β- and γ-fractions which can obscure the immunoglobulin fraction and make interpretation difficult. Figure 7.4 lists the main proteins present in the three globulin fractions.

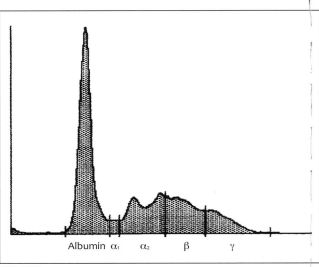

7.3 Serum protein electrophoresis trace from a healthy dog.

Alpha-globulins (α-globulins)
• α_1 antitrypsin
• α_1 acid glycoprotein
• α_2 macroglobulin
• Ceruloplasmin
• Protein C
• Haptoglobin
• α_1-lipoproteins
Beta-globulins (β-globulins)
• Fibrinogen
• Complement
• C-reactive protein
• Ferritin
• Transferrin
• β-lipoproteins
• IgA
• IgM
Gamma-globulins (γ-globulins)
• IgE
• IgG
• C-reactive protein

7.4 Constituents of the α-globulins, β-globulins and γ-globulins.

Following 1D SPE, immunoelectrophoresis can be performed to further classify the increased serum proteins, most commonly using antibodies to identify the immunoglobulins present. Antibody is placed in a trough alongside the zone of electrophoresis and allowed to diffuse passively through the gel. Precipitation occurs if the antibody (e.g. anti-IgM) binds with the relevant antigen (e.g. IgM). Immunoelectrophoresis also aids in determining whether a hyperglobulinaemia is polyclonal or monoclonal (see Hyperglobulinaemia below).

Recent developments

More recently, two-dimensional (2D) polyacrylamide gel electrophoresis (PAGE) has been used in combination with mass spectrometry to classify both the human and canine proteomes further. This technique has allowed identification of many additional proteins in the globulin subclass, including serpin peptidase inhibitor and kininogen-1, which can be elevated in canine lymphoma (Atherton *et al.*, 2013a). It is possible, therefore, that widespread application of 2D PAGE may provide further information about the changes in serum proteins in different disease processes in veterinary patients.

Functions of plasma proteins

The plasma proteins have a wide variety of functions including maintenance of oncotic pressure, blood buffering, coagulation and transport of hormones and drugs.

- **Oncotic pressure:** capillary walls are relatively impermeable to the large osmotically active plasma proteins. The net effect is the movement of water into the intravascular space, and this is known as oncotic pressure. Approximately 75% of colloid oncotic pressure is attributed to albumin.
- **Blood buffering:** buffers donate or accept hydrogen ions in order to minimize a change in the blood pH. Bicarbonate is the most important blood buffer, but the plasma proteins provide approximately 20% of the blood buffering capacity (see Chapter 9). Albumin plays a greater role than globulin.
- **Hormone transport:** thyroxine, reproductive hormones and a wide variety of other hormones are bound to the plasma proteins in the circulation.
- **Drug transport:** numerous drugs including non-steroidal anti-inflammatory drugs (NSAIDs), thiopentone and furosemide are highly protein bound.
- **Coagulation:** secondary haemostasis involves the conversion of soluble fibrinogen to insoluble fibrin by the action of thrombin.
- **Acute phase response:** acute phase proteins are produced by the liver in response to inflammation and serve to assist healing and limit tissue damage.

Hyperproteinaemia

Hyperproteinaemia results from hyperalbuminaemia, hyperglobulinaemia or both in combination. Hyperglobulinaemia is more common. Hyperproteinaemia can be relative (secondary to dehydration) or absolute in nature.

Hyperalbuminaemia

Increases in serum albumin concentration are seen secondary to haemoconcentration and are therefore accompanied by other haematological and clinical indicators of dehydration (e.g. increased packed cell volume, tachycardia and increased urine specific gravity). Hyperalbuminaemia has also been reported occasionally in dogs with hyperadrenocorticism although the mechanisms of this are unclear. Artefactual hyperalbuminaemia secondary to lipaemia can be seen when spectrophotometric methods are used. There has been a single case report of a hepatocellular carcinoma resulting in hyperalbuminaemia as a paraneoplastic process in a dog (Cooper *et al.*, 2009).

Hyperglobulinaemia

Increased globulin concentrations occur with several neoplastic, infectious and inflammatory diseases (e.g. canine pyoderma, feline gingivitis/stomatitis). Antigen presentation results in increased immunoglobulin production. In many cases this hyperglobulinaemia is mild and generally not further classified. More severe hyperglobulinaemia is classified as either a monoclonal or polyclonal gammopathy by performing SPE. In addition to the quantification of protein fractions, SPE can also produce useful diagnostic information. Since the immunoglobulins constitute the main part of the fraction it is likely that small to moderate increases in α fractions (see above) will not result in a detectable increase in total globulins, but would be detected using SPE (Atherton *et al.*, 2013b).

Monoclonal and polyclonal gammopathies

Polyclonal gammopathies are much more commonly detected than monoclonal gammopathies in dogs and cats (Taylor *et al.*, 2010; Tappin *et al.*, 2011). The polyclonal response is due to multiple immunoglobulins being produced as a result of clonal expansion of several plasma cell lineages (plasma cells being the cells that produce immunoglobulins) (Figure 7.5). Polyclonal gammopathies are generally associated with a chronic inflammatory/infectious or immune-mediated aetiology, although they have also been documented in neoplasia and chronic hepatopathies. Polyclonal gammopathies are characterized by broad-based peaks, seen mainly in the β and γ regions of the electrophoretogram. Restricted polyclonal gammopathies (also known as oligoclonal gammopathies) have been reported in cases of ehrlichiosis, leishmaniosis and feline infectious peritonitis (FIP). This occurs when a number of different immunoglobulins migrate to a narrow band on the electrophoretogram and produce a narrow band spike (most commonly in the γ region) superimposed on a broad polyclonal base. Differentiating a monoclonal gammopathy from a restricted polyclonal gammopathy can be difficult and requires immunoelectrophoresis to be performed using antibodies against different portions of the immunoglobulin, i.e. light chains (anti-kappa and anti-lambda antibody). In a monoclonal response only one precipitate will form; however, in a restricted polyclonal gammopathy both antibodies will form arcs (Figure 7.6). For example, the monoclonal gammopathy documented in a patient with dirofilariasis was found to be IgA mediated (De Caprariis *et al.*, 2009), whereas most of the monoclonal gammopathies previously reported in canine ehrlichiosis have been reclassified as restricted polyclonal gammopathies that primarily consisted of IgG and IgM/IgA. Restricted

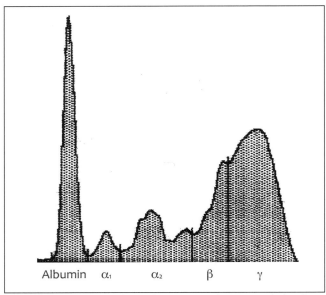

7.5 Serum protein electrophoresis trace showing a polyclonal response typical of an inflammatory or infectious hyperglobulinaemia. Note the broad-based peaks in the β and γ regions of the trace.

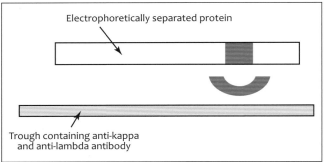

7.6 Immunoelectrophoresis being used to differentiate a monoclonal gammopathy from a restricted polyclonal gammopathy. Anti-kappa and anti-lambda antibodies are loaded into the trough; following incubation these diffuse through the gel. An arc of precipitation forms where the antibody binds to the patient's globulin. In this case a single precipitation arc has formed, indicating a monoclonal gammopathy.

polyclonal gammopathies will also produce both kappa and lambda light chains in the urine.

Monoclonal gammopathies (also called paraprotein-aemias) are indicated by a tall, narrow 'spike' on the electrophoretogram, which results from clonal proliferation of a single plasma cell (B lymphocyte) line. They occur with a heterogeneous group of canine diseases (Figure 7.7). There is often a simultaneous reduction in the production of other globulins. Monoclonal spikes are most commonly seen in the γ/β region but can, rarely, occur in the α region of the electrophoretogram, possibly as a result of the formation of immunoglobulins with altered charge by neoplastic cells (Tappin et al., 2011; Atherton et al., 2013a). A monoclonal gammopathy indicates synthesis of a homogenous immunoglobulin or a portion of it (i.e. a heavy/light chain subunit) as a result of clonal B lymphocyte proliferation. Monoclonal gammopathies are most commonly associated with a lymphoproliferative neoplastic process in dogs and cats but have also been reported in various infectious/inflammatory diseases including leishmaniosis, ehrlichiosis and dirofilariasis (Giraudel et al., 2002; Yarim

- Multiple myeloma
- Waldenströms macroglobulinaemia
- Lymphoma
- Extramedullary plasmacytoma
- Chronic lymphocytic leukaemia
- Monoclonal gammopathy of undetermined significance
- Ehrlichiosis *
- Leishmaniosis *
- Plasmacytic gastroenterocolitis *
- Dirofilariasis
- Primary hyperparathyroidism

7.7 Conditions associated with monoclonal gammopathies in dogs. *Indicates may actually be a restricted polyclonal gammopathy.

et al., 2007; De Caprariis et al., 2009), plasmacytic gastroenterocolitis, chronic pyoderma and primary hyperparathyroidism (Diehl et al., 1992; Burkhard et al., 1995; Benchekroun et al., 2009). However, these apparent monoclonal gammopathies may have been restricted polyclonal gammopathies. Idiopathic monoclonal gammopathies have been reported in both canine and human studies.

Alpha-globulins: As well as the proteins listed in Figure 7.4, further work has identified additional proteins that make up the α-globulin region, including apolipoprotein A1 and vitamin D binding protein (Atherton et al., 2013b). Since the α-globulin group contains the acute phase proteins (APPs) α_1 lipoprotein, α_2 macroglobulin and haptoglobin it is not surprising that this fraction is increased in inflammatory/infectious conditions (Ceron et al., 2005; Tappin et al., 2011). It has also been shown to be increased in various neoplasias and endocrine disease (Tappin et al., 2011). Recent work examined the SPE profiles of dogs with lymphoma; while the majority had a normal serum globulin level, the SPE profile commonly revealed a spike in the α_2 fraction that was thought to represent an increase in haptoglobin as part of the acute phase response (Figure 7.8; Atherton et al., 2013a).

Beta-globulins: The β-globulin fraction includes transferrin, lipoproteins, complement and immunoglobulins (in particular IgM and IgA, as well as Bence–Jones proteins). Previous reports have shown this fraction to be increased in inflammatory, infectious, immune-mediated, neoplastic and hepatic diseases (Tappin et al., 2011). A monoclonal β spike has been documented in feline lymphoma (Gerou-Ferriani et al., 2011).

Gamma-globulins: The γ-globulin fraction is composed of the immunoglobulins (in particular IgG and IgE) and the acute phase protein C-reactive protein (CRP). Increases in the γ-globulin fraction of the electrophoretogram can be seen in inflammatory, infectious or neoplastic disease states. Decreases in the γ-globulin fraction have been documented in immunodeficiencies and some endocrine disorders.

Bence–Jones proteinuria/light chain proteinuria: Plasma cell tumours typically overproduce a single type of immunoglobulin or component of immunoglobulin called the M component/M protein, or paraprotein (although biclonal gammopathies have been reported). A monomorphic population of light chains, Bence–Jones (BJ) proteins have been reported in almost all conditions causing monoclonal gammopathies. They are particularly prevalent in cases of multiple myeloma (MM); they have been reported to occur in between 25 and 40% of cases of canine MM and 17% of

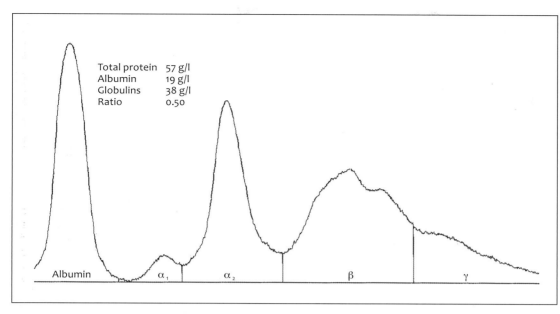

Total protein 57 g/l
Albumin 19 g/l
Globulins 38 g/l
Ratio 0.50

Albumin α_1 α_2 β γ

7.8 Serum protein electrophoresis trace from a Boxer with an intervertebral disc herniation. The total globulin was within normal limits; however, there was a peak in the α-globulins, probably indicating an acute phase response with an increase in haptoglobin.

feline MM. Light chain components have a low molecular weight and are freely filtered by the glomerulus, where they form protein precipitates which appear in the urine. These precipitates can result in renal tubular damage and subsequent progressive azotaemia and renal failure. Standard urine dipsticks are not able to detect BJ proteinuria and so other methods must be used by laboratories. Previously the heat precipitation method was favoured; however, it has been superseded by more sensitive methods such as urine electrophoresis/immunoelectrophoresis (Gentilini *et al.*, 2005). See Chapter 10 for information on urine protein electrophoresis.

Solitary plasma cell tumours: Cutaneous, gastrointestinal and solitary osseous plasma cell tumours, along with plasma cell tumours at other extramedullary sites, may all uncommonly be associated with hyperglobulinaemia. Progression of solitary osseous plasma cell tumours to multiple myeloma has been reported in both dogs and cats. Generally these tumours can be considered benign; however, the intestinal form is more aggressive and early metastatic spread to local lymph nodes may be seen.

Monoclonal gammopathy of unknown significance (MGUS): MGUS has been reported in both human and, rarely, veterinary medicine. It is not associated with osteolysis, bone marrow infiltration or BJ proteinuria. In humans around 16% of patients with MGUS will progress to develop multiple myeloma.

Multiple myeloma: Multiple myeloma (MM) is a systemic proliferation of malignant plasma cells (or precursors) which arise as a clone of a single cell; it usually involves multiple bone marrow sites. MM accounts for <1% of canine malignancies; however, it accounts for 8% of haemopoietic tumours and 3.6% of bone tumours. There is no sex predilection and the average age of affected dogs is 8 years. In one study German Shepherd Dogs were over-represented (Mateus *et al.*, 1986). The reported incidence rate of feline MM is significantly lower (0.012% of feline malignancies) and the presentation differs in that feline cases are more commonly associated with extramedullary involvement and less likely to have bone marrow infiltration and bony lysis (Mellor *et al.*, 2006).

Clinical signs commonly associated with MM include bone disease, bleeding diathesis, hyperviscosity syndrome, renal disease, hypercalcaemia, susceptibility to infection, cytopenias and cardiac disease; these occur secondarily to either high circulating levels of paraprotein, organ/bone infiltration and damage, or both. Multiple myeloma should be high on the differential list for any dog presenting with a monoclonal gammopathy. In the dog, a diagnosis of multiple myeloma can be made if a case fulfils at least three of the four following criteria.

- **Plasma cell infiltration of the bone marrow:** in cases of MM the bone marrow normally consists of >30% malignant plasma cells, seen in clusters. The degree of differentiation ranges from cells that can resemble normal plasma cells to very large, anaplasmic round cells with a high mitotic index (Figure 7.9). In some instances aspirates from multiple locations may be required in order to document this infiltration. Under general anaesthesia it is possible to obtain fine-needle aspirates from lytic bone lesions; however, care should be taken as there is a risk of pathological fracture. Fine-needle aspirates can also be obtained from the ribs (entry via the costochrondal junction) under sedation. Infectious causes of plasma cell infiltration of the bone marrow such as *Leishmania* and *Ehrlichia* should be excluded via a combination of surveying for antibodies (serology) and detection of DNA (polymerase chain reaction).
- **Monoclonal gammopathy:** monoclonal gammopathies (Figure 7.10) in dogs with MM are comprised of either IgG or IgA in equal prevalence; however, in cats the ratio of IgG to IgA monoclonal gammopathy is around 5:1. Biclonal gammopathies can also be seen. Non-secretory MM has been reported rarely in dogs.
- **Bony lytic lesions:** generally associated with a punch-hole (or moth-eaten) appearance, these lesions are most commonly reported on the spinous processes of the vertebrae, ribs, pelvic bones and the distal/proximal long bones. Osteolytic lesions are reported in up to 60% of canine cases, but occur far less commonly (8%) in cats with MM (Mellor *et al.*, 2006).
- **Bence–Jones proteinuria:** see above.

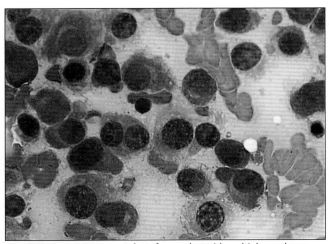

7.9 Bone marrow cytology from a dog with multiple myeloma. Note the large, occasionally binucleate plasma cells with only occasional red cell precursors. (Modified Wright's stain; original magnification X1000)

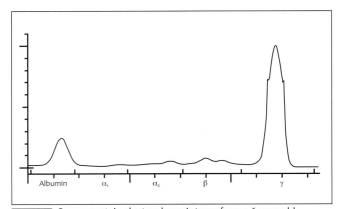

7.10 Serum protein electrophoresis trace from a 6-year-old neutered male terrier cross diagnosed with multiple myeloma. There is a monoclonal spike in the γ region of the electrophoretogram. (Courtesy of Claire Crompton, CTDS Lab)

Cats may have a different presentation, and the term myeloma-related disorder (MRD) is therefore used in this species. Affected cats have a monoclonal or biclonal gammopathy, commonly display extramedullary involvement (e.g. liver, spleen), uncommonly have radiographically detectable lytic bone lesions and have bone marrow involvement in <50% of cases (Mellor *et al.*, 2006).

Hypercalcaemia is reported as a paraneoplastic syndrome in 20% of canine MM and is thought to be due to either osteolysis, increased protein-bound calcium or, rarely, increased parathyroid hormone related protein (PTHrP). In cases where renal function is compromised this may worsen the hypercalcaemia. Recent work has identified hypercalcaemia in around 10% of cases (Mellor *et al.*, 2006).

Waldenström's macroglobulinaemia: Waldenström's macroglobulinaemia (WM) is a rare lymphoproliferative neoplasia of dogs, cats and humans. The World Health Organization (WHO) classifies WM as a lymphoplasmacytic lymphoma. It is a proliferation of lymphoplasmacytoid cells with a small percentage of plasma cells; however, the morphology can range from predominantly lymphocytic to lymphoplasmacytoid to overt plasma cell. WM leads to an IgM monoclonal gammopathy (rather than one composed of IgG or IgA as seen in MM) and

because this is a large molecule, hyperviscosity syndrome is commonly seen. The tumour normally involves the bone marrow and sometimes the liver or spleen, but not the peripheral blood. Dogs with WM may have alterations in their clotting pathways (Gentilini *et al.*, 2005; Jaillardon and Fournel-Fleury, 2011); however, clinical signs of haemorrhage are less common (Vail 2007; Jaillardon and Fournel-Fleury, 2011). The typical lytic bone lesions seen in MM are rarely reported in cases of WM (Gentilini *et al.*, 2005) and hypercalcaemia is not seen in WM.

Proteinuria is relatively common in dogs with paraproteinaemia and it is thought that this is due to a combination of glomerular deposition of immunoglobulins and hyperviscosity syndrome. BJ proteinuria (light chain M component) was generally considered less common in cases of WM than in MM; however, that may have been due to previously reported cases of WM being diagnosed by heat precipitation, which is a less sensitive method of detecting BJ proteins.

Hyperviscosity syndrome: Hyperviscosity syndrome (HVS) has been seen in approximately 20% of cases of canine MM and historically was thought to be less common in cats with MM. The magnitude of the viscosity change depends on the type, size, shape and concentration of the paraprotein in the blood. It generally occurs when particularly high levels of IgA/IgG occur or where IgM is the paraprotein, owing to the increased molecular weight of this immunoglobulin (e.g. in WM). Hyperviscosity can also occur with excess circulating erythroid or myeloid cells in diseases such as polycythaemia vera and leukaemia.

Clinical signs reported with HVS include bleeding diathesis, neurological abnormalities (depression, seizures and coma), ophthalmic abnormalities (retinal haemorrhage or dilated retinal vessels) and cardiomyopathies due to increased circulatory workload. The clinical signs are due to sludging of blood in small vessels, hypoxia and coagulation abnormalities. Bleeding diathesis (gingival bleeding and epistaxis are common manifestations) can occur as a result of the paraprotein interfering with coagulation by inhibiting platelet aggregation and the release of platelet factors, causing absorption of minor clotting proteins or resulting in a functional decrease in calcium. Around 50% of dogs with MM will have prolongation in either the prothrombin time (PT) or partial thromboplastin time (aPTT).

A viscometer can be used to measure serum viscosity, and there are many reported reference ranges but values >2 centipoise (cp) are suspicious for HVS (many animals have values >5 cp).

Hypoproteinaemia

Hypoproteinaemia is caused by increased losses, decreased production, decreased absorption or increased catabolism of plasma proteins. Albumin and globulin may be reduced contemporaneously (e.g. in haemorrhage) or selective reductions of either albumin or globulin may occur independently.

Hypoalbuminaemia

Hypoalbuminaemia can occur either independently of hypoglobulinaemia or in conjunction with hypoglobulinaemia. It is important to evaluate globulin levels concurrently. If levels of both albumin and globulin are decreased, protein-losing enteropathy, haemorrhage, dermal protein losses and dilution are the most likely differentials (Figure 7.11). In cases with septic peritonitis, severe hypoalbuminaemia is common; globulins are often also decreased. Hypoalbuminaemia results from either increased loss or decreased production of albumin and should always be considered a significant finding, especially if persistent and severe (Figure 7.12). Severe hypoalbuminaemia (<15 g/l) is likely to be associated with increased risk of effusion formation, though precise values vary because there are other factors involved in effusion formation; for example, there is a higher risk if portal vein pressures are increased in a patient with hypoalbuminaemia.

The acute phase response generally leads to only a mild and transient hypoalbuminaemia; this occurs when the liver switches off production of albumin (a negative acute phase protein) temporarily in favour of producing positive acute phase proteins such as CRP or haptoglobin. In such cases, other markers of inflammation will usually also be present, e.g. neutrophilia or hyperglobulinaemia.

It is important to remember that juvenile animals will have a lower reference range for albumin than mature animals and this should be taken into consideration when interpreting results from young patients. Protein levels are low at birth, increase following colostrum absorption, then decrease again over the following 5 weeks as colostrum is metabolized. Adult ranges for protein levels are generally reached by 6–12 months of age. The protein levels increase towards the adult reference range over this timescale as a result of normal immune stimulation and improved liver function and intestinal absorption. Both albumin and globulin levels tend to decrease slightly with advanced age.

Protein-losing enteropathy Haemorrhage Dermal loss Dilutional hypoproteinaemia	Globulins usually decreased
Protein-losing nephropathy	Globulins not affected
Liver dysfunction	Globulins normal or increased
Third spacing	Globulins low, normal or increased
Negative acute phase response	Globulins may be increased

7.11 Conditions associated with hypoalbuminaemia and the expected effects on globulin levels.

1. Obtain full history
2. Perform thorough clinical examination
3. Evaluate albumin and globulin levels concurrently
4. Perform urinalysis including urine protein to creatinine ratio (UPCR) on urine sample to exclude urinary protein losses. Concurrent sediment examination is required to interpret UPCR
5. Perform bile acid stimulation test to exclude liver dysfunction
6. Imaging (assessing for any free body cavity fluid)
7. Investigate further for enteric protein losses if protein-losing nephropathy and liver dysfunction have been excluded (e.g. folate/cobalamin/α_1 protease inhibitor/intestinal biopsy)

7.12 Logical diagnostic approach to the hypoalbuminaemic patient.

Increased losses

Protein-losing enteropathy (PLE): PLE includes a spectrum of intestinal diseases which result in increased intestinal permeability or defects in lymphatic drainage and result in excessive protein loss into the gut. Albumin may be lost prior to loss of globulins and concurrent hypocholesterolaemia is generally noted. The presence of canine α_1 protease inhibitor in faeces can be used as an early screening test to detect gastrointestinal protein loss before significant hypoproteinaemia occurs (see Chapter 13).

Infiltrative bowel disease encompasses both inflammatory and neoplastic mucosal infiltrates. Inflammatory bowel disease (IBD) is classified on the basis of the predominant cell type identified on intestinal biopsy samples (e.g. lymphocytic–plasmacytic, eosinophilic, neutrophilic, granulomatous). Histology is required to confirm the diagnosis. IBD can be primary (idiopathic) or secondary to other gastrointestinal disorders (e.g. *Giardia*, *Campylobacter* infection). A diagnosis of idiopathic IBD requires all other secondary causes to have been excluded.

Neoplastic intestinal infiltrates can also lead to protein loss. The differentiation between lymphocytic–plasmacytic IBD and intestinal lymphoma can be difficult on endoscopic biopsy samples, and generally full thickness specimens are preferable. However, there may be an increased risk of wound dehiscence in patients with severe hypoalbuminaemia.

Lymphangiectasia: Intestinal lymphangiectasia (IL) is rare in cats, but more common in dogs, and can be either primary or secondary. Primary IL is a rare congenital disorder in which malformation of the lymphatic vessels results in obstructed lymphatic flow. Secondary intestinal lymphangiectasia occurs when lymphatic drainage becomes obstructed, as a consequence either of neoplasia or inflammation within the intestinal wall, or of increased central venous pressure (e.g. with congestive heart failure or pericardial disease). The lacteals within the intestinal villi dilate as lymphatic pressures rise, and leak lymph into the intestinal lumen. Lymph is a protein-rich fluid also containing chylomicrons and lymphocytes. IL results in diarrhoea, weight loss and hypoalbuminaemia. Ascites may develop secondary to severe hypoalbuminaemia. Patients with IL may also have hypocholesterolaemia and lymphopenia, in addition to panhypoproteinaemia. Yorkshire Terriers, Norwegian Lundehunds and Soft Coated Wheaten Terriers appear to be predisposed to IL.

Protein-losing nephropathy (PLN): Primary glomerular diseases such as glomerulonephritis and amyloidosis lead to a selective loss of albumin into the urine. The glomerulus should act as a charge- and size-selective filter which retains large molecules such as proteins, but in the diseased state albumin and molecules of a similar size, such as antithrombin, are lost into the urine. Hypoalbuminaemia is often severe in cases of PLN. Globulins are unaffected owing to their larger size. The urine protein to creatinine ratio (UPCR) is used to quantify urinary protein loss but will give falsely increased results in the presence of an active sediment (e.g. gross haematuria, pyuria; see Chapter 10). Urine electrophoresis can be performed to confirm that the protein being lost into the urine is indeed albumin. PLN may lead to development of nephrotic syndrome, and blood cholesterol levels may be increased.

Dermal protein loss: Severe inflammatory and exudative skin disease, especially burns, may lead to significant protein loss in the exudates.

Whole blood loss: Both albumin and globulin will be lost in equal proportion as a result of haemorrhage; however, in the peracute setting, proteins may be unaffected until extravascular fluid moves intravascularly and a dilutional effect occurs. Reductions in protein levels will become apparent around 2–3 hours after an acute bleeding episode. Red blood cell parameters would also be expected to decrease in patients with haemorrhage, but this may be offset by splenic contraction initially.

Septic peritonitis: Septic peritonitis can lead to quite profound hypoalbuminaemia as a result of third spacing. Hypoalbuminaemia is attributed to massive protein loss into the peritoneal fluid due to peritoneal inflammation. Globulins are generally also decreased, but occasionally can remain within range. In addition, it is likely that a patient presenting with septic peritonitis will have additional clinicopathological changes, including a neutrophilia or neutropenia with a left shift and toxic change, electrolyte disorders and increased liver enzymes.

Decreased production

Severe hepatic dysfunction: The liver is the source of albumin production, so in cases of severe hepatic dysfunction albumin production will decrease, resulting in hypoalbuminaemia. Other changes indicative of hepatic dysfunction would also be expected, e.g. prolongation of clotting times, decreased urea levels. Globulin levels are generally unaffected, or may be increased as a result of inflammation. Alanine transaminase (ALT) and alkaline phosphatase (ALP) are not always significantly increased in patients with chronic hepatic disease. A bile acid stimulation test is required to evaluate hepatic function further (see Chapter 12).

Acute phase response: Typically the acute phase response will result in mild hypoalbuminaemia. This will be discussed in more detail later in the chapter.

Cachexia/malabsorption/maldigestion: Hypoalbuminaemia can also occur following severe starvation or malnutrition.

Sequestration and dilution

- Body cavity effusions.
- Third spacing into body cavity effusions, e.g. bacterial peritonitis, can lead to significant hypoalbuminaemia.
- Over-hydration with intravenous fluids.
- Congestive heart failure results in fluid retention which causes a dilutional hypoproteinaemia. In addition, proteins may be lost into ascitic or pleural fluids. Intestinal oedema may also lead to intestinal protein malabsorption.

Hypoglobulinaemia

Hypoglobulinaemia can occur with concurrent hypoalbuminaemia or independently, and may be due to increased losses or decreased production of globulins. Both inherited and acquired diseases can result in hypoglobulinaemia. Decreased levels of α- and β-globulins are not considered significant; SPE is necessary to determine which globulin fraction is affected. The most important cause of selective hypoglobulinaemia is immunoglobulin deficiency, in which defective production leads to decreased γ-globulins. Single radial immunodiffusion (SRID) techniques can be used to quantify the individual immunoglobulins. In this method an agarose gel is impregnated with an antibody raised against the immunoglobulin of interest (Figure 7.13). Wells are cut into the gel and the test sera and a set of known concentrations of the immunoglobulin are added. During 24 hours of incubation, immunoglobulin diffuses from the well and forms a complex with the antibody, resulting in a ring of precipitation. The diameter of the ring is proportional to the concentration of immunoglobulin present. The immunoglobulin concentration of the test samples can then be calculated by plotting the value against a standard curve.

There are some breed-specific variations in reference ranges for globulins, with Greyhounds having a lower reference range than other breeds (Steiss *et al.*, 2002).

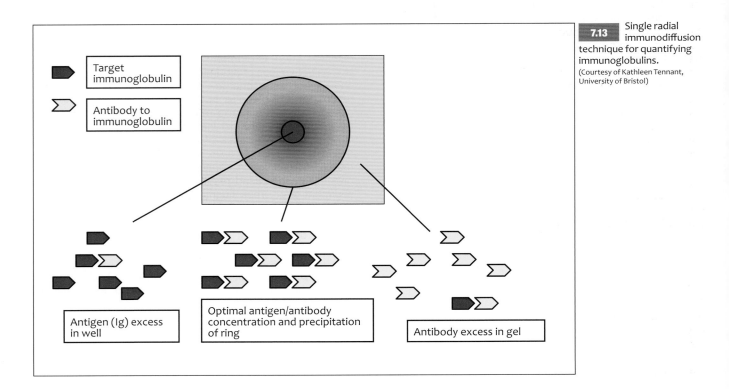

7.13 Single radial immunodiffusion technique for quantifying immunoglobulins.
(Courtesy of Kathleen Tennant, University of Bristol)

Target immunoglobulin

Antibody to immunoglobulin

Antigen (Ig) excess in well

Optimal antigen/antibody concentration and precipitation of ring

Antibody excess in gel

Immature dogs and cats may have decreased IgG levels until their immune system matures at around 6 months of age, and until then they may be more susceptible to respiratory tract infections. Maternally derived IgG transferred via colostrum to the neonate prevents endogenous production of IgG until around 12–15 weeks of age, so congenital immunodeficiencies are not detected until around this age.

Increased globulin losses

Decreases in all globulin fractions (α, β and γ) may be present with PLE, severe exudative skin disease, peritonitis or blood loss. In the aforementioned situations, albumin is lost contemporaneously, leading to panhypoproteinaemia. PLN and other causes of hypoalbuminaemia are less likely to result in a reduction in globulin levels (see Figure 7.11).

Decreased globulin production

Specific genetic primary immunodeficiencies with resultant hypoglobulinaemia have been reported in several breeds of dog, but are relatively rare. Clinical signs are generally detected once maternally derived immunity has been lost at around 12–15 weeks of age. These animals present with signs of chronic recurrent infections, illness following live vaccine administration and infections at multiple sites. Measurement of immunoglobulins using the SRID technique is useful in these patients.

Immunoglobulin (Ig)A deficiency has been reported in Shar Peis, German Shepherd Dogs and Beagles. These animals typically present with recurrent infections of the respiratory tract, urinary tract or skin infections. Some Dobermanns have been documented as having a selective IgM deficiency but this is typically asymptomatic as long as other classes of immunoglobulins are not also decreased (Plechner, 1979).

Serum IgG deficiency (and sometimes IgM and IgA) has been reported in Weimaraners (Day et al., 1997). These dogs present with recurrent infections, left-shifted neutrophilia and a poor response to treatment of infections.

A more severe X-linked combined immunodeficiency (X-SCID) has been reported in Bassett Hounds and Cardigan Corgis (Pullen et al., 1997). These animals present with a variety of bacterial or viral infections after loss of maternal immunity at around 12–15 weeks of age. In these dogs, low levels of IgG and IgA have been documented along with lymphopenia (see Chapter 5). These animals typically succumb to infections and die at a young age. A similar immunodeficiency, with an autosomal recessive inheritance, has been documented in Jack Russell Terriers.

Lethal acrodermatitis of English Bull Terriers is an autosomal recessive condition, associated with IgA deficiency; it results in cutaneous hyperkeratosis, respiratory and skin infections and stunted growth. Plasma zinc levels are decreased in affected animals.

Acute phase proteins

Acute phase proteins (APPs) are produced rapidly as part of the acute phase response that may occur following any type of tissue injury. The acute phase response also results in a wide variety of metabolic, endocrinological and immunological changes such as fever, enhanced leucocyte activity, increased cortisol concentrations, decreased thyroxine concentrations and an overall shift towards catabolism.

Individually, APPs have a wide variety of often poorly understood roles, but collectively they modulate the body's innate immune response to tissue injury. Acute phase proteins are produced very rapidly following tissue injury, in large quantities. Measurement of circulating concentrations can therefore be a sensitive marker of inflammation, although it is not specific. An increase in APP concentrations may be up to six times more sensitive a marker of inflammation than an increase in white cell count.

Acute phase proteins production is triggered by pro-inflammatory cytokines such as interleukin (IL)-1, IL-6 and tumour necrosis factor (TNF)-α. These cytokines are produced principally by monocytes and macrophages. It was previously thought that APP production was exclusive to hepatocytes, but other cell lines (e.g. lymphocytes, myocytes, adipocytes) can also participate in APP production, although hepatocytes retain a central role. In terms of their response to tissue injury, APPs can be divided into three main categories (Figure 7.14).

Major APPs have a low resting circulating concentration that can increase rapidly (often within 24–48 hours) and dramatically (5–50-fold increase) following tissue injury. Following resolution of that injury, concentrations will decline, equally precipitously, towards baseline. The moderate APPs are so called because their concentrations increase relatively slowly (within 4–7 days) and to a lesser extent (often not exceeding a 2–10-fold increase) following injury, with a correspondingly gradual return to baseline following resolution of injury (minor APPs also exist, but because their concentrations usually only double in response to inflammation, they are not frequently measured in clinical medicine). A final category of APP, negative APPs, are so called because their concentrations decline following tissue injury and then gradually return towards baseline once that injury has resolved. The APPs and their behaviour are species specific; the more commonly measured APPs in dogs and cats are shown in Figure 7.15.

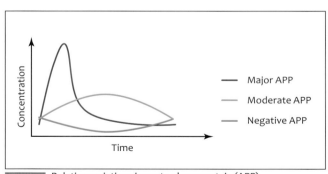

7.14 Relative variations in acute phase protein (APP) concentrations in response to an inflammatory stimulus.

Species	Major APP	Moderate APP	Negative APP
Dog	C-reactive protein (CRP) Serum amyloid A (SAA)	Haptoglobin (Hp) α₁ acid glycoprotein (AGP) Ceruloplasmin (Cp)	Albumin Transferrin
Cat	Serum amyloid A (SAA) α₁ acid glycoprotein (AGP)	Haptoglobin (Hp)	Albumin Transferrin

7.15 Commonly measured acute phase proteins (APPs) in dogs and cats.

Assay methodology

It is important to note that reference ranges for any specific APP may vary depending on the specific assay used.

Measurement of CRP is generally via immunoassay using species-specific antibodies, and several formats are available such as enzyme-linked immunosorbent assays (ELISAs), latex agglutination tests and immunoturbidimetric assays. Time-resolved fluorometric assays are also available. Recently, several cage-side assay kits have become available. These assays are either fully quantitative or simply indicate whether circulating CRP concentrations are increased above the reference range or not. Several of these assays have been validated for use in dogs.

Canine and feline serum amyloid A (SAA) is usually measured via ELISA using species-specific antibodies. The structure of SAA appears to be quite highly conserved across different mammalian species, and because of this, immunoassays (ELISA and immunoturbidimetric assays) have been developed that measure canine and feline SAA using monoclonal anti-human SAA antibodies. Assays using polyclonal antiserum against canine SAA have also been used to measure feline SAA.

The α_1 acid glycoprotein is usually measured via a radial immunodiffusion method using species-specific antiserum. This assay usually results in a delay because it takes 24–48 hours for diffusion to be complete before the results can be read. An immunoturbidimetric assay has been developed and offers a more rapid turnaround.

Haptoglobin (Hp) is most commonly measured via spectrophotometric assays based on haptoglobin's affinity for haemoglobin. The Hp concentration can then be measured, based either on the alteration of the absorbance capacity of haemoglobin induced by the binding of Hp or on preservation of peroxidase activities at an acidic pH. Immunoassays based on the rate of precipitation of antigen–antibody complexes have also been developed but are less commonly used.

Ceruloplasmin is not as frequently measured as the other APPs described here, and interpretation of assay results is complicated by the lack of commercially available reference materials. Assays based on the oxidation of different compounds have been described.

Albumin, the most commonly measured negative APP, is usually measured via the bromocresol green assay, while transferrin concentrations can be assayed using immunoassay. However, given that transferrin's major biological action concerns the binding and transport of iron in the bloodstream, it is more commonly assayed by measuring serum total iron-binding capacity.

Although the effect of storage and anticoagulant use on canine APP measurement appears to be relatively minor, haemolysis, lipaemia and hyperbilirubinaemia can give falsely decreased measurements of CRP and Hp when samples are analysed via some ELISA and colorimetric assays, but not when samples are run using time-resolved immunofluorometric assays.

APPs in canine medicine

Relative to feline medicine, more is known about the acute phase response in the dog. Our current knowledge of the canine acute phase response can be considered under four broad categories:

- Non-inflammatory variables affecting APPs
- The use of APPs to diagnose and differentiate between disease states
- The use of APPs to monitor disease
- APPs as prognostic indicators.

Effect of non-inflammatory variables on APP concentrations

Canine haptoglobin (Hp) is particularly sensitive to corticosteroids and elevated levels of Hp are found both after treatment with corticosteroids and during spontaneously occurring hyperadrenocorticism (HAC). Hp concentrations are therefore of little use in monitoring inflammatory disease in dogs on corticosteroid therapy because steroid treatment will interfere with interpretation. Although concurrent HAC or exogenous glucocorticoid treatment appears to blunt the magnitude of CRP elevation in dogs with severe inflammatory disease, CRP concentrations do appear to remain a useful indicator of an inflammatory response in these patients. Given that endogenous or exogenous corticosteroids can increase neutrophil counts in the peripheral circulation, CRP concentrations may be useful in differentiating between a stress- or corticosteroid-induced and an inflammatory leucogram.

Concentrations of Hp and SAA decrease in response to treatment of spontaneously occurring hyperadrenocorticism in dogs, while concentrations of CRP do not change. The alteration in APP concentrations following treatment does not, however, appear to give additional information when compared with conventional monitoring using adrenocorticotropic hormone (ACTH) stimulation testing (Arteaga et al., 2010). In this study, dogs with pituitary-dependent HAC were treated with trilostane and although there was a significant decline in Hp concentrations following treatment, Hp concentrations in the treated group remained above the reference range. When compared with ACTH stimulation testing, a cut-off value of 4.8 g/l was moderately informative of clinical control (sensitivity 73%, specificity 91%) but could not replace the utility of ACTH stimulating testing in assessing the response to trilostane treatment.

Several other physiological states (pregnancy and age) and breed associations have been found to influence APP concentrations. Prolonged exercise may also increase APP concentrations. It is likely that physiological influences contribute, at least in part, to the wide interindividual variation seen in the acute phase response among dogs with otherwise similar disease conditions.

Use of APPs to diagnose and discriminate among various disease states

APP concentrations are reliably increased in dogs with a wide variety of inflammatory disease states. In contrast to the situation in humans, where APPs and in particular CRP have been extensively used to discriminate among disease states, relatively little work has been done with dogs in this regard. Circulating concentrations of APPs, principally CRP, have been utilized for example to distinguish between dogs with steroid-responsive meningitis–arteritis (SRMA) and other forms of neurological disease (Bathen-Noethen et al., 2008) and between bitches with cystic endometrial hyperplasia and those with pyometra (Fransson et al., 2004). Other studies have shown a very wide interindividual variation in APP concentrations among dogs with otherwise very similar disease states (Chan et al., 2009; Whittemore et al., 2011) and this interindividual variation generally creates a broad overlap between groups of dogs with different diseases. This makes it difficult to apply cut-off values of APP concentrations that allow reliable differentiation of disease states.

It is possible that measuring local production of APPs, for example in body cavity effusions, might be more useful than assessing circulating concentrations. Concentrations of CRP in the cerebrospinal fluid (CSF) tend to be higher in dogs with SRMA than in dogs with other types of neurological disease, such as central nervous system (CNS) neoplasia and intervertebral disc disease. In dogs with body cavity effusions, effusion CRP concentrations may be higher in protein-rich than in protein-poor transudates (Parra *et al.*, 2006).

Use of APPs to monitor various disease states

A progressive decline in APP concentrations has been associated with, and used to monitor, the therapeutic response in dogs with a variety of infectious diseases (e.g. babesiosis, leishmaniosis, spirocercosis and parvovirus enteritis), or other inflammatory diseases such as immune-mediated polyarthritis, immune-mediated haemolytic anaemia, IBD, acute pancreatitis and lymphoma. A fall in APP concentrations following an initial postsurgical elevation has also been observed in dogs recovering successfully from surgical procedures such as hemilaminectomy and ovariohysterectomy. One potential advantage of using APPs to monitor disease activity is that they represent a relatively inexpensive, non-invasive way of quantifying inflammation, and may therefore replace, at least in part, the need for more expensive invasive tests. One example of this approach has been documented in dogs with SRMA.

Attention has also focused on the potential use of APPs as markers of remission or relapse of SRMA because conventional monitoring of this disease depends largely on CSF collection and analysis, an expensive and invasive procedure. Serum concentrations of CRP decline in parallel with CSF nucleated cell counts in response to prednisolone therapy and, in patients that discontinue therapy following successful treatment, CRP and SAA concentrations fall to within the reference range (Lowrie *et al.*, 2009b). Concentrations of CRP and SAA within the CSF also decline following treatment but changes are not as marked as those seen in serum (Lowrie *et al.*, 2009a). In patients that suffer a relapse of SRMA, serum CRP and SAA concentrations appear to be increased, even though inflammatory cell infiltrates in the CSF are often absent (Lowrie *et al.*, 2009a). Serum Hp concentrations remained unaltered during therapy, reflecting the influence glucocorticoids have on Hp concentrations. Hp concentrations declined in successfully treated dogs once glucocorticoid therapy was withdrawn (Lowrie *et al.*, 2009b).

What is notable is that, despite high interindividual variability in APP concentrations among patients with otherwise similar disease states, dogs that respond to therapy tend to have a progressive decline in APP concentrations. This illustrates one of the principles guiding interpretation of APPs in an individual: the change of concentrations of APPs over time is usually of greater significance than absolute concentrations measured at a single point in time. Patients whose inflammatory disease responds to therapy tend to have a corresponding decrease in APP concentrations.

It is, however, important to be aware of the lack of specificity of APPs for any particular disease process when using these proteins to monitor a patient's response to therapy. An increase in APP concentrations simply indicates the presence of inflammation; it does not indicate where, or the nature of the inflammatory focus. A patient may have multiple foci of inflammation, all of which can potentially contribute to a measured increase in APP concentrations. The clinician must always be aware of these potentially confounding variables when interpreting APP profiles in an individual patient.

It is also important to note the extreme sensitivity of CRP in detecting any type of tissue damage. It is certainly possible for non-significant tissue damage to elicit a small increase in major APP concentrations, and this degree of damage may be below the limit of detection afforded by a clinical examination. This is of clinical relevance in terms of how we interpret APP concentrations; specifically that a small (1.5–2-fold) increase in concentration of a major APP may not *necessarily* reflect clinically significant disease. As with any diagnostic test, APP concentrations should be interpreted in light of the overall clinical picture, rather than in isolation.

Although absolute concentrations of APPs are perhaps less useful as a marker of disease activity than evaluating a change in circulating concentrations over time, a recent test (the canine lymphoma blood test (cLBT; Avacta Group plc)) utilizes an algorithm incorporating circulating concentrations of CRP and Hp with patient variables such as age, gender and presence of lymphadenopathy. This test produces a score that indicates the response of canine lymphoma to chemotherapy, with low scores corresponding to remission and higher scores indicating a relapse. A recent study showed that high scores documented at the time of diagnosis were associated with a shorter survival, and also showed that scores increase in advance of relapse detected on palpation/imaging. This suggests that the test could be used to provide an early marker of relapse in dogs in remission following chemotherapy (Alexandrakis *et al.*, 2014).

APPs as prognostic indicators

In human medicine, patients with very high APP concentrations on admission or those whose APP concentrations fail to decline following therapy tend to have a poor outcome in terms of increasing morbidity and mortality.

In canine medicine, the wide degree of interindividual variation in APP concentrations in patients with otherwise similar diseases appears adversely to affect the prognostic significance of an APP profile recorded at a single time point. The majority of canine studies have shown no correlation between APP concentrations measured on admission and outcome (Chan *et al.*, 2009; Whittemore *et al.*, 2011). Several studies have shown that, in dogs with various diseases, a progressive change in APP concentrations over time, rather than the APP concentration measured on admission, has been associated with outcome. This has been illustrated in dogs with a range of specific diseases such as systemic inflammatory response syndrome (SIRS; Gebhardt *et al.*, 2009), acute abdomen (Galezowski *et al.*, 2009), acute pancreatitis (Mansfield *et al.*, 2008), postoperative recovery following pyometra (Dabrowski *et al.*, 2009) and parvovirus enteritis (McClure *et al.*, 2010). In those studies, all of which measured CRP concentrations, dogs with a favourable outcome tended to have significantly greater decreases in CRP concentrations over time than groups of dogs that showed increased morbidity or mortality. Many dogs with a poor outcome had CRP concentrations that remained unchanged or increased over time.

APPs in feline medicine

There have been fewer investigations of the feline acute phase response than for the canine response, and our understanding of the behaviour of APPs in cats is correspondingly more limited. As mentioned above, SAA and α_1 acid glycoprotein (AGP) function as major APPs while Hp is a minor APP in cats. A study of cats with various inflammatory diseases, including abscesses, pyothorax and fat necrosis, showed that while AGP was increased in 100% of cats examined and Hp increased in 93%, leucocytosis was only found in 76%. This provided some evidence of the increased sensitivity of APPs over a traditional leucogram in detecting inflammation or infection (Ottenjann et al., 2006). Determination of SAA concentrations may be particularly useful in cats because it has been shown to be the most rapidly responding APP when compared with AGP, CRP and Hp in a variety of inflammatory and infectious conditions. CRP concentrations do not change significantly in response to infection or inflammation, reflecting the lack of utility of this APP in cats.

Existing clinical knowledge of the acute phase response in cats can be considered under the following categories:

- Non-inflammatory variables affecting APPs
- The use of APPs to diagnose and differentiate among disease states
- The use of APPs to monitor disease and as prognostic indicators.

Non-inflammatory variables affecting APP concentrations

One study (Kann et al., 2012) showed that SAA, AGP and Hp concentrations were higher in older cats and SAA concentrations also appeared to be higher in female cats, which suggests that signalment may affect resting APP concentrations in cats. Korman et al. (2012) showed that feline immunodeficiency virus (FIV) infection may affect APP production in response to Mycoplasma spp. infection, and it is therefore possible that retroviral infection may affect the acute phase response to other disease states.

Use of APPs to diagnose and differentiate among disease states

Concentrations of APPs have been most extensively studied in cats as potential markers for feline infectious peritonitis (FIP). The measurement of AGP in feline serum and peritoneal fluid has become a recognized test for the identification of FIP. It is important to note that inflammatory conditions other than FIP, including enteric coronavirus infection, can also cause elevations in AGP concentrations. Allowing for the effect of other inflammatory diseases on AGP concentrations, one study (Paltrinieri et al., 2007) demonstrated that when there is a high clinical suspicion of FIP based on the patient history and clinical examination, a moderate elevation in AGP (1.5–2 mg/ml) can discriminate cats with FIP from those with other diseases. However, in cats where there is a low index of suspicion of FIP, a high concentration of circulating AGP (>3 mg/ml) is necessary to support a diagnosis of FIP. Although evaluating circulating concentrations of AGP does not replace the utility of polymerase chain reaction (PCR) testing of effusions or histopathology and immunohistochemistry on biopsy specimens in definitively diagnosing FIP, AGP does represent a non-invasive and inexpensive means of supporting the interpretation of other test results in reaching this challenging diagnosis (see Chapter 28).

Elevated concentrations of AGP have also been reported in tumour-bearing cats, but there does not appear to be a significant difference in AGP concentrations among cats with sarcomas, carcinomas or round cell tumours. Circulating concentrations of AGP are also increased in cats with lymphoma, but in contrast to reports of APP responses in dogs with lymphoma, concentrations of AGP in cats with lymphoma do not appear to alter according to remission status. Concentrations of AGP on initial diagnosis do not appear to correlate with survival times or response to chemotherapy.

Circulating concentrations of APPs, specifically AGP, SAA and Hp, have been studied in cats infected with mycoplasmas. Infections involving Mycoplasma haemofelis appear to induce greater elevations in APP concentrations than infections with the less pathogenic Candidatus Mycoplasma haemominutum (Korman et al., 2012).

Use of APPs to monitor disease and as prognostic indicators

At present, there is a paucity of knowledge regarding the potential utility of APPs in feline medicine as a means of monitoring disease activity or affording a prognosis. A single case report (Tamamoto et al., 2009) documented a good association between SAA concentrations and recovery or recurrence of disease in a cat with pancreatitis, and it is possible that APPs can function as a means of monitoring disease activity in cats as they do in dogs.

Summary

APPs have been shown to have some utilities in small animal medicine. They are sensitive, but non-specific, markers of inflammation, can be used to monitor response to treatment and may have some prognostic significance. It is likely that over time these proteins will become an integral part of routine biochemical profiles.

Guidelines for interpretation and use of APPs in clinical practice

- **APPs are extremely sensitive markers of inflammation:** even relatively small foci of inflammation can cause an increase in circulating APP concentrations. Therefore, a small (1.5–2-fold) increase in circulating concentrations of major APPs may not always be clinically significant.
- **APPs are extremely non-specific:** an increase in APP concentrations will indicate that inflammation is present, but does not indicate the location of the inflammatory focus. Multiple foci of inflammation (which may not necessarily be related) can contribute to a total measured increase in circulating concentrations of APPs. For example, a dog may have an increase in APP concentrations due to a combination of periodontal disease and a subcutaneous abscess. It is vital to perform a thorough clinical examination in all patients with an increased APP concentration in order to determine what lesion(s) are causing the increase.
- **A decline in APP concentrations may indicate a response to treatment:** repeatedly measuring APP concentrations may allow an objective measurement of therapeutic response. This might be of value where other means of objectively monitoring response to treatment involve invasive and/or expensive tests (e.g. arthrocentesis, CSF analysis) or where the nature and location of the underlying disease is uncertain (e.g. trial therapy for fever of unknown origin with antibiotics or anti-inflammatories). It is important to note that knowledge of the acute phase response in specific

disease states is incomplete. In some instances, following an apparent clinical response to treatment, APP concentrations may remain *mildly* increased. This may be due to persisting subclinical inflammation from the disease under treatment, *or* the presence of concurrent, potentially unrelated inflammatory foci. Again, this indicates the need to interpret APP concentrations in the light of a thorough clinical

examination. APP concentrations within the reference range suggest disease remission at the time of sampling, but do not predict ongoing remission or relapse. Further monitoring of APP concentrations, along with a thorough clinical examination, is recommended following discontinuation of treatment, as a subsequent increase in APP concentrations may indicate relapse prior to the emergence of clinical signs.

Case examples

CASE 1

SIGNALMENT

8-year-old female neutered Boxer.

HISTORY

Lethargy, periocular non-pruritic alopecia, recurrent bilateral epistaxis and generalized mild peripheral lymphadenopathy.

CLINICAL PATHOLOGY DATA

Haematology	Result	Reference interval
RBC (x 10⁹/l)	**4.8**	5.5–8.5
Hb (g/l)	**10.0**	12.0–18.0
HCT (l/l)	**0.30**	0.37–0.55
MCV (fl)	72	60–77
MCH (pg)	22.5	19.5–24.5
MCHC (g/dl)	34	31.0–37.0
Reticulocytes (%)	0	0–0.5
WBC (x 10⁹/l)	**20.9**	6–17.1
Neutrophils (x 10⁹/l)	**16.5**	3–11.5
Lymphocytes (x 10⁹/l)	**0.90**	1–4.8
Monocytes (x 10⁹/l)	**3.5**	0.15–1.5
Eosinophils (x 10⁹/l)	0.0	0–1.3
Basophils (x 10⁹/l)	0.0	0–0.2
Platelets (x 10⁹/l)	280	200–500

Abnormal results are in **bold**.

Film comment: normocytic, normochromic erythrocytes. Mature neutrophilia with no left shift or toxic change.

Biochemistry	Result	Reference interval
Sodium (mmol/l)	152	146–155
Potassium (mmol/l)	4.4	4.1–5.3
Chloride (mmol/l)	112	107–115
Glucose (mmol/l)	5.2	3.4–5.3
Urea (mmol/l)	6.2	3–9.1
Creatinine (μmol/l)	112	98–163
Calcium (mmol/l)	2.45	2.13–2.7

Abnormal results are in **bold**.

Biochemistry *continued*	Result	Reference interval
Inorganic phosphate (mmol/l)	1.45	0.8–2.0
Total protein (g/l)	**105**	49–71
Albumin (g/l)	**23**	28–39
Globulin (g/l)	**82**	21–41
ALT (IU/l)	**250**	13–88
ALP (IU/l)	176	19–285
Total bilirubin (μmol/l)	1.6	0–2.4

Abnormal results are in **bold**.

WHAT ABNORMALITIES ARE PRESENT?

Haematology

- Mild normocytic, normochromic, non-regenerative anaemia.
- Leucocytosis – mature neutrophilia and monocytosis.

Biochemistry

- Moderate hypoalbuminaemia.
- Marked hyperglobulinaemia.
- Moderate increase in ALT indicative of hepatocellular damage.

HOW WOULD YOU INTERPRET THESE RESULTS AND WHAT ARE YOUR DIFFERENTIAL DIAGNOSES?

Haematology

There is a mild non-regenerative anaemia (as indicated by the reticulocyte count). This could be due to chronic disease (where cytokine activity depresses erythroid production), bone marrow suppression/infiltration or recent blood loss from epistaxis. There is a moderate neutrophilia which can be seen with an inflammatory, infectious, immune-mediated or neoplastic process. The lack of left shift or toxic change makes a septic process less likely. The combination of neutrophilia, monocytosis, lymphopenia and eosinopenia can be seen in a stress leucogram. The monocytosis generally indicates a chronic inflammatory/infectious state.

Biochemistry

A moderate increase in ALT indicates hepatocellular damage. Differentiating a primary from secondary hepatopathy cannot be done at this stage without further investigations.

→ CASE 1 CONTINUED

There is a moderate hypoalbuminaemia which could indicate either a protein-losing nephropathy, protein-losing enteropathy, third spacing of fluid or a lack of production due to impaired liver function. The history of epistaxis means blood loss could be contributing to the hypoalbuminaemia. A reduction in albumin of this magnitude could also be seen in a systemic inflammatory response and may be seen in association with hyperglobulinaemia.

There is a marked hyperglobulinaemia which can be seen in a range of conditions causing monoclonal gammopathies (most commonly neoplastic conditions such as multiple myeloma) or polyclonal gammopathies (various inflammatory, infectious or immune-mediated diseases). Haemoconcentration seems unlikely because the haematocrit (HCT) is low.

DIFFERENTIAL DIAGNOSES

- Multiple myeloma.
- Leishmaniosis.
- Inflammatory/infectious hepatic disease.
- Lymphoma.
- Ehrlichiosis.

WHAT FURTHER INVESTIGATIONS WOULD YOU CONSIDER?

Serum protein electrophoresis to define the hyperglobulinaemia and determine whether there is a monoclonal or polyclonal response. A monoclonal response would be more consistent with a neoplastic aetiology (most likely multiple myeloma), whereas a polyclonal gammopathy would be more consistent with an inflammatory or infectious aetiology (although a monoclonal/oligoclonal gammopathy has been reported with leishmaniosis and ehrlichiosis).

Urinalysis including protein:creatinine ratio to exclude a protein-losing nephropathy and an assay for Bence–Jones proteins, which are present in up to 40% of canine multiple myelomas. Hypersthenuria would indicate haemoconcentration which could contribute to the hyperproteinaemia.

A clotting profile should be performed to investigate the epistaxis. Normal platelet count and clotting times would indicate that the epistaxis was secondary to either platelet dysfunction (could be assessed with a buccal mucosal bleeding time), hyperviscosity syndrome or intranasal pathology.

Bone marrow aspiration could be considered after SPE to help reach a definitive diagnosis. Survey radiographs to assess for the presence of lytic bony lesions associated with multiple myeloma could also be considered. Fine-needle aspiration of the peripheral lymph nodes could be performed to determine whether a neoplastic, infectious or inflammatory process was present.

Serum protein electrophoresis was performed (Figure 7.16).

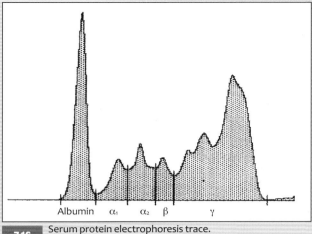

7.16 Serum protein electrophoresis trace. (Courtesy of Jo Morris, University of Glasgow)

IS THIS A MONOCLONCAL OR POLYCLONAL GAMMOPATHY? WHAT ARE THE DIFFERENTIALS FOR THIS?

Results of further tests

- SPE showed a polyclonal response (β- and γ-globulins) indicating an inflammatory/infectious aetiology of the hyperproteinaemia.
- Bone marrow aspiration (performed under sedation from the costochondral junction) showed normal erythroid, myeloid and platelet lineages with no neoplastic cells identified. Cytological examination of the bone marrow also identified amastigotes, which provided a definitive diagnosis of leishmaniosis.
- Serology for *Leishmania* was positive with a high titre of 1:640.
- Urinalysis showed a mild increase in UPCR (1.2) and was negative for Bence–Jones proteins.
- Clotting profile was within normal limits, and therefore the epistaxis was presumed secondary to hyperviscosity syndrome or platelet dysfunction.

CASE OUTCOME

After discussing the zoonotic potential of *Leishmania* spp. (which is low) with the owner, the decision was made to treat with a combination of meglumine antimoniate at a dose of 100 mg/kg s.c. q24h and allopurinol at a dose of 10–15 mg/kg orally q12h. The epistaxis resolved in 5 days, as did the lymphadenopathy. After 4 weeks, repeat biochemistry documented a resolution of the elevated liver parameters and a normal serum albumin and globulin. At this point the meglumine antimoniate was stopped and the allopurinol continued for a further 6 months with no evidence of clinical relapse.

Many treated dogs respond clinically but *Leishmania* cannot be eliminated from the body with drugs. The combination of antimony and allopurinol has been shown to be superior to allopurinol alone. A vaccine is available which offers a degree of protection from infection.

CASE 2

SIGNALMENT

8-year-old female neutered Jack Russell Terrier.

HISTORY

3-week history of vomiting, diarrhoea, lethargy, anorexia and weight loss.

CLINICAL PATHOLOGY DATA

Haematology	Result	Reference interval
RBC (x 10^{12}/l)	**4.4**	5.5–8.5
Packed cell volume (l/l)	**0.31**	0.39–0.55
Hb (g/dl)	**10.5**	12.0–18.0
MCV (fl)	71.1	60.0–77.0
MCHC (g/dl)	33.5	32.0–36.0
Reticulocytes (%)	0.0	0.0–0.5
WBC (x 10^9/l)	**28.5**	6.0–15.0
Neutrophils (segmented) (x 10^9/l)	**20.81**	3.60–12.00
Band neutrophils (x 10^9/l)	**0.57**	0.00–0.04
Lymphocytes (x 10^9/l)	2.85	0.70–4.80
Monocytes (x 10^9/l)	**1.71**	0.00–1.50
Eosinophils (x 10^9/l)	0.0	0.0–1.0
Basophils (x 10^9/l)	0.0	0.0–0.2
Atypical mononuclear cells (x 10^9/l)	2.57	
Platelets (x 10^9/l)	**126**	200–500

Abnormal results are in **bold**.

Film comment: red blood cells are normocytic, normochromic. Platelet clumping was not present. Band neutrophils present, but no evidence of toxic changes. Atypical mononuclear cells were identified. These were 1.5–2 times the size of a red blood cell with a round nucleus and basophilic cytoplasm, possibly reactive lymphocytes.

Biochemistry	Result	Reference interval
Total protein (g/l)	**30**	58–73
Albumin (g/l)	**12**	26–35
Globulin (g/l)	18	18–37
ALP (IU/l)	47	20–60
ALT (IU/l)	59	15–60
Creatinine (µmol/l)	37	30–90
Urea (mmol/l)	6	1.7–7.4
Glucose (mmol/l)	4	3.0–5.0
Calcium (mmol/l)	**1.71**	2.30–3.00
Phosphate (mmol/l)	1.2	0.90–1.20
Sodium (mmol/l)	146	139–154
Potassium (mmol/l)	**2.9**	3.6–5.6
Cholesterol	**3.0**	3.8–7.0

Abnormal results are in **bold**.

WHAT ABNORMALITIES ARE PRESENT?

Haematology

- Mild normocytic, normochromic anaemia.
- Leucocytosis which is due to a neutrophilia with a mild left shift.
- Mild monocytosis.
- Mild thrombocytopenia.
- Atypical mononuclear cells.

Biochemistry

- Severe hypoalbuminaemia.
- Low normal globulin.
- Hypocalcaemia.
- Hypokalaemia.
- Hypocholesterolaemia.

HOW WOULD YOU INTERPRET THESE RESULTS AND WHAT ARE THE LIKELY DIFFERENTIAL DIAGNOSES?

The haematology shows a neutrophilia with a left shift, indicating an inflammatory response. Mild non-regenerative anaemia may result from any chronic disease, bone marrow disease or acute blood loss (with insufficient time for the bone marrow to respond). Thrombocytopenia occurs owing to decreased production (bone marrow disease), increased destruction (immune-mediated thrombocytopenia), disseminated intravascular coagulation or loss (blood loss) of platelets.

A mild monocytosis in conjunction with neutrophilia is consistent with a stress leucogram, which is often present in sick animals (although stress does not typically lead to a left shift). The presence of atypical mononuclear cells is suspicious of an underlying neoplastic disorder, but may also be a response to a severe inflammatory process (if the cells are reactive lymphocytes).

The biochemical changes are dominated by severe hypoalbuminaemia with concurrent low normal globulin. Hypoalbuminaemia with low normal or decreased globulins may be due to:

- Protein loss:
  - Protein-losing enteropathy (globulins are typically low)
  - Protein-losing nephropathy (globulin concentration usually normal)
  - Haemorrhage (PCV decreased and globulins low)
  - Effusions (globulins may be low normal).
- Decreased production of protein:
  - Severe liver insufficiency
  - Malabsorption
  - Maldigestion
  - Congestive heart failure
  - Starvation.

Calcium is highly protein bound; therefore, hypoalbuminaemia will result in a decreased serum calcium concentration. An ionized calcium concentration will determine whether the biologically active calcium fraction is decreased. Hypokalaemia occurs as a result of decreased intake (e.g. anorexia) or increased losses (e.g. renal failure, diarrhoea). Severe hypokalaemia can cause profound weakness, paralytic intestinal ileus and cardiac arrhythmias.

→ CASE 2 CONTINUED

The biochemical and haematological abnormalities are suggestive of a protein-losing enteropathy and this correlates with the clinical signs. Severe inflammatory bowel disease, alimentary lymphosarcoma and lymphangiectasia are all possible differential diagnoses.

WHAT FURTHER TESTS WOULD YOU RECOMMEND?

- **Urinalysis:** to exclude protein loss via the urine (including urine protein:creatinine ratio and sediment examination), although low/low normal globulin makes PLN less likely in this case.
- **Bile acid function test:** to exclude severe hepatic insufficiency as the cause of hypoalbuminaemia.
- **Abdominal ultrasonography:** to assess gastrointestinal wall thickness and architecture. Mesenteric lymph node size can also be assessed; if enlarged, fine-needle aspirates can be obtained.
- **Thoracocentesis/abdominocentesis:** if clinical signs indicate the presence of a body cavity effusion, centesis should be performed to determine protein content and cytology of the fluid.

- **Gastrointestinal biopsy:** endoscopic or full-thickness biopsy samples are necessary to determine the underlying cause of a PLE. Severe hypoalbuminaemia may impair wound healing and increase the risk of surgical wound dehiscence following full-thickness biopsy. Endoscopic biopsy is safer in such cases, but only superficial tissue is obtained and therefore pathological changes in deeper layers of the intestinal wall may be missed.

CASE OUTCOME

The small intestinal wall was diffusely thickened on ultrasonography, and local mesenteric lymph nodes were enlarged. Endoscopic biopsy samples were collected and revealed a moderate to marked infiltrate of lymphocytes and plasma cells into the lamina propria of the small intestine, consistent with lymphoplasmacytic inflammatory bowel disease. The dog was treated with immunosuppressive doses of prednisolone combined with metronidazole and a hypoallergenic diet. The dog improved clinically and biochemically, but albumin levels did not return to the reference range.

CASE 3

SIGNALMENT

4-year-old male neutered Boxer cross.

HISTORY

Presented with a 2-week history of intermittent pyrexia and lethargy. The dog had a left-sided perineal hernia diagnosed 8 months previously; this had been managed conservatively with stool softeners, had not progressed over that time and was not causing dyschezia. He had undergone a dental procedure 1 month previously from which he had made an uneventful recovery.

On clinical examination rectal temperature was 39.8°C. A grade II/VI left-sided systolic murmur was audible with a point of maximal intensity over the cardiac apex. This murmur had not been recognized previously.

CLINICAL PATHOLOGY DATA

Haematology	Result	Reference interval
RBC (x 10⁹/l)	**4.1**	5.5–8.5
Hb (g/l)	**11**	12.0–18.0
HCT (l/l)	**0.32**	0.37–0.55
MCV (fl)	68	60–77
MCH (pg)	20.2	19.5–24.5
MCHC (g/dl)	32.2	31.0–37.0
Reticulocytes (%)	0	0–0.5
WBC (x 10⁹/l)	**28.35**	6–17.1
Neutrophils (x 10⁹/l)	**24.05**	3–11.5
Band neutrophils	**1.40**	<0.2

Abnormal results are in **bold**.

Haematology *continued*	Result	Reference interval
Lymphocytes (x 10⁹/l)	**0.90**	1–4.8
Monocytes (x 10⁹/l)	**2.50**	0.15–1.5
Eosinophils (x 10⁹/l)	0.0	0–1.3
Basophils (x 10⁹/l)	0.0	0–0.2
Platelets (x 10⁹/l)	350	200–500

Abnormal results are in **bold**.

Biochemistry	Result	Reference interval
Sodium (mmol/l)	149	146–155
Potassium (mmol/l)	4.8	4.1–5.3
Chloride (mmol/l)	110	107–115
Glucose (mmol/l)	4.4	3.4–5.3
Urea (mmol/l)	4.6	3–9.1
Creatinine (μmol/l)	100	98–163
Calcium (mmol/l)	2.19	2.13–2.7
Inorganic phosphate (mmol/l)	0.9	0.8–2.0
Total protein (g/l)	61	49–71
Albumin (g/l)	**25**	28–39
Globulin (g/l)	36	21–41
ALT (IU/l)	67	13–88
ALP (IU/l)	210	19–285
Total bilirubin (μmol/l)	1.2	<10
C-reactive protein (mg/l)	**134**	<10
Haptoglobin (g/l)	**26**	<3

Abnormal results are in **bold**.

→ CASE 3 CONTINUED

WHAT ABNORMALITIES ARE PRESENT?

- Mild non-regenerative anaemia.
- Neutrophilic leucocytosis with mild left shift.
- Monocytosis.
- Mild hypoalbuminaemia.
- Marked elevations of acute phase proteins.

HOW WOULD YOU INTERPRET THESE ABNORMALITIES?

- The neutrophilic and monocytic leucocytosis would be consistent with inflammation. The monocytosis would suggest that this inflammation has been present for some time and the left shift implies that this leucogram represents a response to inflammation rather than stress alone.
- The mild non-regenerative anaemia is likely to be due to inflammatory disease, in light of the elevation in APPs and the inflammatory leucogram.
- APP concentrations were initially measured to detect and quantify any inflammatory response. The marked elevation in APPs is consistent with an inflammatory focus, but does not indicate the location or the nature of the inflammatory focus. Hypoalbuminaemia would also be non-specifically consistent with inflammation because albumin is a negative APP; however, other causes of hypoalbuminaemia (urine loss, gastrointestinal loss and third space loss) could not be excluded. Hepatic failure would be unlikely given the lack of other supporting biochemical evidence.

WHAT ARE YOUR DIFFERENTIALS AND WHICH DIAGNOSTIC TESTS WOULD YOU CONSIDER NEXT?

- The history of a recent dental procedure and examination findings of a previously unrecognized cardiac murmur could suggest endocarditis and therefore echocardiography should be performed.
- The patient should be screened for evidence of inflammatory disease, bearing in mind that neoplastic, infectious and immune-mediated disease are all possibilities. In the absence of any localizing signs, thoracic and abdominal radiographs, ultrasonography, urinalysis with culture and blood culture would all be reasonable tests.
- Particularly if the dog had a history of tick exposure, screening for tick-borne infection (e.g. *Ehrlichia*, *Borrelia*, *Anaplasma*) should be considered. *Bartonella* would be another consideration.

FURTHER TEST RESULTS

- Echocardiography showed vegetative lesions adherent to the mitral valve resulting in mitral regurgitation, which together with the fever in a medium-sized dog supported a diagnosis of bacterial endocarditis.
- The dog was screened for other septic foci; thoracic radiographs and abdominal ultrasonography and urinalysis were unremarkable. Blood and urine cultures were negative as was a PCR for *Bartonella* spp. Up to 70% of blood cultures can be negative in dogs with endocarditis, and this means that the choice of antimicrobials is empirical.

- Antibiosis was commenced using drugs (amoxicillin–clavulanate (co-amoxiclav) and enrofloxacin) effective against organisms likely to be involved in a bacterial endocarditis. The pyrexia resolved within 3 days of commencing therapy and the patient was much brighter.

HOW WOULD YOU MONITOR THIS DOG'S RESPONSE TO TREATMENT?

- Repeatedly monitoring acute phase protein concentrations may yield useful information.
- Having excluded other potential causes of inflammation, endocarditis is the most likely cause for the increase in APP concentrations.
- A major challenge in treating endocarditis lies in monitoring the response to therapy; valvular vegetations can persist even if the lesions themselves become sterile and it is therefore difficult to determine how long antibiotic treatment should be continued.
- If the increase in APPs was indeed due to the endocarditis, the concentrations of APPs should decline towards normal as the endocarditis resolves.
- There was a slight concern that the ongoing perineal herniation might be contributing to the increase in APPs; it was therefore important to take account of this when using APP concentrations to monitor the dog's condition.

INITIAL FOLLOW-UP

- **Day 7:** the pyrexia had abated and the dog was reportedly much better. The mitral murmur was still present.
- **Week 6:** neutrophil counts declined to within the reference range (Figure 7.17); however, concentrations of Hp and particularly CRP were still increased. Antibiotic therapy was continued.
- **Week 12:** echocardiography showed lessened but persistent valvular lesions. Concentrations of CRP

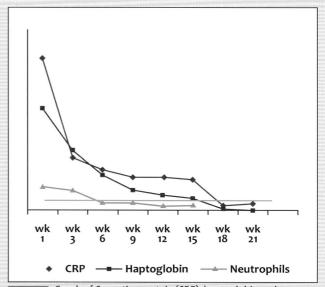

7.17 Graph of C-reactive protein (CRP), haptoglobin and neutrophil counts over time. Values are expressed as multiples of the upper limit of the normal range (denoted by the solid line).

→ **CASE 3 CONTINUED**

and Hp, which had previously declined precipitously, were plateauing and CRP remained approximately four times normal, indicating an ongoing inflammatory response. At this point, the perineal hernia and cardiac murmur were both still present and unchanged in nature. The rest of the clinical examination was unremarkable and the dog remained very bright.

HOW WOULD YOU INTERPRET THIS ACUTE PHASE PROFILE IN LIGHT OF THE PATIENT'S CONDITION AND WHAT MIGHT YOU DO NEXT TO MANAGE THIS PATIENT?

- It is not certain whether the ongoing inflammatory response was due to active endocarditis or inflammation emanating from herniated and potentially compromised bowel wall. This reflects the non-specific nature of the acute phase response. Repeated physical examinations had failed to yield any evidence of inflammatory foci other than at those two sites.
- At this point, the options available are either to continue antimicrobial therapy or to intervene surgically to correct the herniation.

FURTHER FOLLOW-UP

- **Week 15:** herniorrhapy was performed because of concerns that bacterial translocation through compromised bowel wall might be responsible for the ongoing inflammatory response and endocarditis as evidenced by persistently elevated APP concentrations. Postoperative recovery was unremarkable. Histological evaluation of the herniated bowel showed mild inflammatory changes within the mucosa.
- **Week 18:** APPs were within normal limits. Interestingly, echocardiography documented complete resolution of the valvular lesions at that point. Antibiosis was stopped.
- **Week 21:** repeat APP profiles confirmed the absence of any inflammatory disease.

It is possible that the herniated bowel was contributing to the total measured increase in APP concentrations. It was very important to monitor APP concentrations following discontinuation of antibiotic therapy to detect any subsequent increase that might have served as an early indicator of relapsing or persistent endocardial infection.

This case illustrates how APPs can be used to document the resolution of inflammatory disease and thus, in the absence of any other reliable disease markers, may help guide therapeutic interventions.

References and further reading

Alexandrakis I, Tuli R, Ractliffe SC et al. (2014) Utility of a multiple serum biomarker test to monitor remission status and relapse in dogs with lymphoma undergoing treatment with chemotherapy. *Veterinary and Comparative Oncology.* DOI: 10.1111/vco. 12123

Arteaga A, Dhand NK, McCann T et al. (2010) Monitoring the response of canine hyperadrenocorticism to trilostane treatment by assessment of acute phase protein concentrations. *Journal of Small Animal Practice* 51, 204–209

Atherton MJ, Braceland M, Fontaine S et al. (2013a) Changes in the serum proteome of canine lymphoma identified by electrophoresis and mass spectrometry. *The Veterinary Journal* 3, 320–324

Atherton MJ, Braceland M, Harvie J et al. (2013b) Characterisation of the normal canine serum proteome using a novel electrophoretic technique combined with mass spectrometry. *The Veterinary Journal* 3, 315–319

Bathen-Noethen A, Carlson R, Menzel D, Mischke R and Tipold A (2008). Concentrations of acute phase proteins in dogs with steroid responsive meningitis arteritis. *Journal of Veterinary Internal Medicine* 22, 1149–1156

Bell T, Butler K, Sill H, Stickle J, Ramos-Vara J and Dark M (2002) Autosomal recessive severe combined immunodeficiency of Jack Russell Terriers. *Journal of Veterinary Diagnostic Investigation* 14, 194–204

Benchekroun G, Desmyter A, Hidalgo A et al. (2009) Primary hyperparathyroidism and monoclonal gammopathy in a dog. *Journal of Veterinary Internal Medicine* 23, 211–214

Burkhard MJ, Meyers DJ, Rosychuk RA, O'Neil SP and Schultheiss PC (1995) Monoclonal gammopathy in a dog with chronic pyoderma. *Journal of Veterinary Internal Medicine* 9, 357–360

Bush BM (1991) *Interpretation of Laboratory Results for Small Animal Clinicians, 1st edn.* Blackwell Science Ltd., Oxford

Ceron JJ, Eckrsall PD and Martinez-Subiela M (2005) Acute phase proteins in dogs and cats: current knowledge and future perspectives. *Veterinary Clinical Pathology* 34, 85–99

Chan DL, Rozanski EA and Freeman LM (2009) Relationship among plasma amino acids, C-reactive protein, illness severity and outcome in critically ill dogs. *Journal of Veterinary Internal Medicine* 23, 559–563

Cooper SE, Wellman ML and Carsillo ME (2009) Hyperalbuminaemia associated with hepatocellular carcinoma in a dog. *Veterinary Clinical Pathology* 38, 516–520

Dabrowski R, Kostro K, Lisiecka U, Szczubial M and Krakowski L (2009) Usefulness of C-reactive protein, serum amyloid A component and haptoglobin determinations in bitches with pyometra for monitoring early post ovariohysterectomy complications. *Theriogenology* 72, 471–476

Day M, Power C, Oleshko J and Rose M (1997) Low serum immunoglobulin concentrations in related Weimaraner dogs. *Journal of Small Animal Practice* 38, 311–315

De Caprariis D, Sasanelli M, Paradies P, Otranto D and Lia R (2009) Monoclonal gammopathy associated with heartworm disease in a dog. *Journal of the American Animal Hospital Association* 45, 296–300

Diehl KJ, Lappin MR, Jones RL and Cayatte S (1992) Monoclonal gammopathy in a dog with plasmacytic gastroenterocolitis. *Journal of the American Animal Hospital Association* 201, 1233–1236

Eckersall PD (2008) Proteins, proteomics and the dysproteinemias. In: *Clinical Biochemistry of Domestic Animals, 6th edn.* Academic Press, San Diego

Eckersall PD and Bell R (2010) Acute phase proteins: Biomarkers of infection and inflammation in veterinary medicine. *Veterinary Journal* 185, 23–27

Fayos M, Couto CC, Iazbik MC and Wellman ML (2005) Serum protein electrophoresis in retired racing greyhounds. *Veterinary Clinical Pathology* 34, 397–400

Fransson BA, Karlstam EK, Bergstrom A et al. (2004) C-reactive protein in the differentiation of pyometra from cystic endometrial hyperplasia/mucometra in dogs. *Journal of the American Animal Hospital Association* 40, 391–399

Galezowski AM, Snead EC, Kidney BA and Jackson ML (2010) C-reactive protein as a prognostic indicator in dogs with acute abdomen syndrome. *Journal of Veterinary Diagnostic Investigation* 22, 395–401

Gebhardt C, Hirschberger J, Rau S et al. (2009) Use of C-reactive protein to predict outcome in dogs with systemic inflammatory response syndrome or sepsis. *Journal of Veterinary Emergency and Critical Care* 19, 450–458

Gentilini F, Calzolari C, Buonacucina A, Di Tommaso M, Militerno G and Famigli Bergamini P (2005) Different biological behaviour of Walderstrom's macroglobulinemia in two dogs. *Veterinary and Comparative Oncology* 3, 87–89

Gerou-Ferriani M, McBrearty AR, Burchmore RJ, Jayawardena KGI, Eckersall PD and Morris JS (2011) Agarose gel serum electrophoresis in cats with and without lymphoma and preliminary results of tandem mass fingerprinting analysis. *Veterinary Clinical Pathology* 40, 159–173

Giori L, Giordano A, Giudice C, Grieco V and Paltrinieri S (2011) Performance of different diagnostic tests for feline infectious peritonitis in challenging clinical cases. *Journal of Small Animal Practice* 52(3), 152–157

Giraudel JM, Pages JP and Guelfi JF (2002) Monoclonal gammopathies in the dog: A retrospective study of 18 cases (1986–1999) and literature review. *Journal of the American Animal Hospital Association* 38, 135–147

Griebsch C, Arendt G, Raila J, Schweigert FJ and Kohn B (2009) C-reactive protein concentrations in dogs with primary immune mediated hemolytic anemia. *Veterinary Clinical Pathology* 38(4), 421–425

Jaillardon L and Fournel-Fleury C (2011) Waldenström's macroglobulinaemia in a dog with bleeding diathesis. *Veterinary Clinical Pathology* 40, 351–355

Kann RK, Seddon JM, Henning J and Meers J (2012) Acute phase proteins in healthy and sick cats. *Research in Veterinary Science* 93(2), 649–654

Korman RM, Ceron JJ, Knowles TG, Barker EM, Eckersall PD and Tasker S (2012) Acute phase response to *Mycoplasma haemofelis* and 'Candidatus

Mycoplasma haemominutum' infection in FIV-infected and non-FIV-infected cats. *Veterinary Journal* **193(2)**, 433–438

Lowrie M, Penderis J, Eckersall PD, McLaughlin M, Mellor D and Anderson TJ (2009a) The role of acute phase proteins in diagnosis and management of steroid-responsive meningitis arteritis in dogs. *Veterinary Journal* **182**, 125–130

Lowrie M, Penderis J, McLaughlin M, Eckersall PD and Anderson TJ (2009b) Steroid responsive meningitis–arteritis: a prospective study of potential disease markers, prednisolone treatment, and long-term outcome in 20 dogs (2006–2008). *Journal of Veterinary Internal Medicine* **23**, 862–870

Mansfield CS, James FE and Robertson ID (2008) Development of a clinical severity index for dogs with acute pancreatitis. *Journal of the American Veterinary Medical Association* **233**, 936–944

Mateus RE, Leifer CE, MacEwen EG and Hurvitz AI (1986) Prognostic factors for multiple myeloma in the dog. *Journal of the American Veterinary Medicine Association* **11**, 1288–1292

McClure V, van Schoor W, Goddard A *et al.* (2010) Serial C-reactive protein concentrations as a predictor of outcome in puppies infected with parvovirus. *Proceedings ECVIM-CA 20th Annual Congress,* p. 242

McGrotty YL and Knottenbelt CM (2002) Significance of plasma protein abnormalities in dogs and cats. *In Practice* **24(9)**, 512–517

Mellor PJ, Haugland S, Murphy S *et al.* (2006) Myeloma related disorders in cats commonly presented as extramedullary neoplasms in contrast to myelomas in human patients: 24 cases with clinical follow up. *Journal of Veterinary Internal Medicine* **20**, 1376–1383

Ottenjann M, Weingart C, Arndt G and Kohn B (2006). Characterization of the anemia of inflammatory disease in cats with abscesses, pyothorax, or fat necrosis. *Journal of Veterinary Internal Medicine* **20**, 1143–115

Paltrinieri S, Giordano A, Tranquillo V and Guazzetti S (2007) Critical assessment of the diagnostic value of feline α_1-acid glycoprotein for feline infectious peritonitis using the likelihood ratios approach. *Journal of Veterinary Diagnostic Investigation* **19**, 266–272

Parra MD, Papasouliotos K and Ceron JJ (2006) Concentrations of C-reactive protein in effusions in dogs. *Veterinary Record* **158**, 753–757

Patel RT, French AF and McManus PM (2005) Multiple myeloma in 16 cats: a retrospective study. *Veterinary Clinical Pathology* **34**, 341–352

Plechner A (1979) IgM deficiency in two Dobermann Pinschers. *Modern Veterinary Practice* **60**, 150

Pullen R, Somberg R, Felsburg P and Herthorn P (1997) X-linked severe combined immunodeficiency in a family of Cardigan Welsh Corgis. *Journal of the American Animal Hospital Association* **33**, 494–499

Rivas A, Tintle L, Agentieri D *et al.* (1995) A primary immunodeficiency syndrome in Shar Pei dogs. *Clinical Immunology and Immunopathology* **74**, 243–251

Steiss J, Brewer W, Welles E and Wright J (2002) Haematological and serum biochemical reference values in retired racing Greyhounds. *Compendium on Continuing Education for the Practicing Veterinarian* **22**, 243–248

Stockham SL and Scott MA (2002) Proteins. In: *Fundamentals of Veterinary Clinical Pathology,* pp. 251–276. Iowa State Press, Ames, IA

Tamamoto T, Ohno K, Ohmi A, Seki I and Tsujimoto H (2009) Time course monitoring of serum amyloid A in a cat with pancreatitis. *Veterinary Clinical Pathology* **38**, 83–86

Tappin SW, Taylor SS, Tasker S, Dodkin SJ, Papasouliotis K and Murphy KF (2011) Serum protein electrophoresis in 147 dogs. *The Veterinary Record* **168**, 456–462

Taylor SS, Tappin SW, Dodkin SJ, Papasouliotis K, Casamian-Sorrosal D and Tasker S (2010) Serum protein electrophoresis in 155 cats. *Journal of Feline Medicine and Surgery* **12**, 643–653

Vail DM (2007) Plasma cell neoplasms In: *Small Animal Clinical Oncology, 4th edn.* WB Saunders, Philadelphia

Whittemore JC, Marcum BA, Mawby DI, Coleman MV, Hacket TB and Lappin MR (2011) Associations among albuminuria, C-reactive protein concentrations, survival predictor index scores, and survival in 78 critically ill dogs. *Journal of Veterinary Internal Medicine* **25(4)**, 818–824

Willard MD, Tvedten H and Turnwald GH (1994) *Small Animal Clinical Diagnosis by Laboratory Methods, 2nd edn.* WB Saunders, Philadelphia

Yarim GF, Nisbet C and Oncel T (2007) Serum protein alterations in dogs naturally infected with *Toxoplasma gondii. Parasitology Research* **101**, 1197–1202

Chapter 8

Electrolyte imbalances

Barbara Skelly

The major electrolytes in the body are potassium, sodium, calcium and magnesium. Electrolyte concentrations are closely controlled by the action of multiple hormones and by the kidneys. Derangements affect many body organs including the nervous system and cardiac and skeletal muscle. Major imbalances can cause severe clinical signs and death. Imbalances of these electrolytes will be dealt with individually.

Measurement of electrolyte concentrations in serum and plasma

Sodium and potassium concentrations

Many techniques are available to measure electrolytes but most central laboratories and point-of-care testing (POCT) devices use the ion-selective electrode (ISE) method. Indirect ISE devices use diluted plasma (or serum) samples, and the results are generally comparable to those of flame photometry (the gold standard, but now little used, method). Direct ISE devices (usually used for POCT) use whole (undiluted) blood samples; these measurements are not equivalent to those results obtained by the flame photometry or indirect ISE methods but are usually made comparable by the application of an intra-device algorithm. Spectrophotometric measurement methods that are used in some laboratory equipment designed for use in veterinary practice environments are inferior and prone to giving less accurate results.

Variables such as haemolysis, fibrin clots within the specimen, inadequate mixing of the specimen with anticoagulant and varying the ratio of blood sample to anticoagulant can all significantly affect POCT results. Other factors that have an effect on accuracy include contamination of blood samples by inadvertent contact with ethylenediamine tetra-acetic acid (EDTA) and the use of expired or incorrectly stored cartridges.

Chloride concentrations

Chloride can be measured in serum or plasma samples using spectrophotometric and colorimetric methods and by using ISEs. Cells should be separated from plasma after blood has been exposed to air to avoid alterations in the distribution of chloride between cells and plasma due to changes in blood pH.

Lipaemia, hyperbilirubinaemia and haemoglobinaemia can artificially raise the chloride concentration when colorimetric methods are used. ISEs are the most prone to interference from bromide ions in animals being treated with potassium bromide, which gives a falsely increased chloride concentration.

Disorders of potassium homeostasis

Distribution of potassium in the body

Potassium is primarily intracellular in location and is maintained in this compartment by the sodium/potassium adenosine triphosphatase (ATPase) pump that transports three sodium ions out of the cell for the exchange of two potassium ions. The result of this pumping mechanism is that the serum concentration of potassium is low (3.5–5.8 mmol/l in dogs and 3.6–4.5 mmol/l in cats), while the intracellular potassium concentration is high (140–150 mmol/l in both species).

How is potassium balance maintained?

Potassium is ingested in food, and concentrations are controlled mainly through renal excretion. Aldosterone mediates the balance of loss or uptake of potassium in the distal nephron, depending on plasma concentration. Both hyper- and hypokalaemia have profound effects on the heart. Hyperkalaemia leads to bradycardia, atrial standstill and ventricular escape, while hypokalaemia can predispose to tachyarrhythmias.

The factors influencing the development of hyper- or hypokalaemia are summarized in Figure 8.1 and are discussed in the following sections.

Hyperkalaemia

Hyperkalaemia may be due to failure of renal excretion or redistribution of potassium out of cells into the extracellular fluid. Hyperkalaemia may also arise from laboratory error (Figure 8.2).

Hyperkalaemia due to laboratory or interpretative error

Elevated numbers of platelets (thrombocytosis) and leucocytes can release their intracellular potassium *in vitro*,

BSAVA Manual of Canine and Feline Clinical Pathology, 3rd edition. Edited by Elizabeth Villiers and Jelena Ristić. ©BSAVA 2016

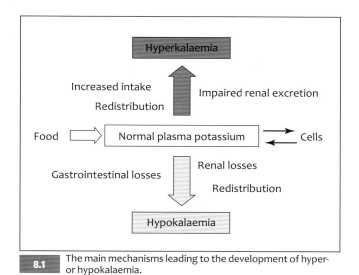

8.1 The main mechanisms leading to the development of hyper- or hypokalaemia.

Laboratory, sampling or interpretative error
• Haemolysed blood sample, particularly in susceptible breeds, e.g. Akitas • Thrombocytosis • Massive leucocytosis (>100 x 10⁻⁹ cells/l) • EDTA contamination of blood samples

Increased potassium from exogenous sources
• Increased dietary intake or supplementation (unlikely when renal function normal) • *Intravenous fluid therapy containing potassium salts*

Reduced potassium excretion
• *Anuric or oliguric renal failure* • *Urinary outflow obstruction* • *Urinary bladder rupture* • *Hypoadrenocorticism* • Pseudohypoadrenocorticism (gastrointestinal disease, trichuriasis, perforated duodenal ulcer) • Pleural effusion with repeated drainage • Primary hypoaldosteronism • Drug therapy: potassium-sparing diuretics, e.g. spironolactone • Angiotensin converting enzyme inhibitors • Non-steroidal anti-inflammatory agents lower renin secretion and impair angiotensin II-mediated aldosterone secretion. The consequent fall in aldosterone reduces urinary potassium excretion

Potassium redistribution – movement from cells into extracellular fluid
• *Metabolic acidosis – caused by an inorganic acid* • Insulin deficiency in diabetic ketoacidosis • Hyperosmolality • Massive tissue destruction e.g. tumour lysis syndrome • Beta-adrenergic blockade • Digitalis toxicity

8.2 The differential diagnosis of hyperkalaemia. The most common differentials are shown in *italics*.

especially in clotted serum samples, with resultant hyperkalaemia. A haemolysed blood sample may have an increased potassium concentration, although, because red cells have a low intracellular potassium concentration, the increase observed may reflect the lysis of other cell lines. Red cells of Akitas, however, have unusually high intracellular potassium and red cell lysis thus produces a more dramatic effect. Spurious hyperkalaemia is particularly seen in samples that have been analysed ≥1 day after collection (e.g. samples posted to external laboratories) when the serum or plasma has not been separated from the cells.

EDTA contamination of blood samples: If the syringe tip touches the inside of an EDTA tube it may become contaminated with potassium EDTA so that when the remaining sample is expelled into the serum/heparin tube, the sample itself becomes contaminated. This results in the combination of marked hyperkalaemia, hypocalcaemia (calcium is chelated by the EDTA) and also a low alkaline phosphatase (ALP).

Hyperkalaemia due to failure of renal excretion

Failure of renal excretion, either due to renal failure or because of urinary tract obstruction, is probably the most common cause, while hypoadrenocorticism, although less common, tends to result in a more pronounced hyperkalaemia.

Renal failure as a cause of hyperkalaemia: For renal failure to cause hyperkalaemia there must be a significant reduction in urine production, i.e. either anuric or oliguric renal failure, usually due to acute renal failure (caused by toxic or ischaemic damage), or when chronic renal failure reaches the end-stage. Serum potassium rises because a fall in the glomerular filtration rate (GFR) reduces distal tubular flow and, as a consequence, reduces potassium excretion.

Urinary tract obstruction: Urinary tract obstruction is most commonly a consequence of feline lower urinary tract disease in a male cat, although it can occur in either cats or dogs in association with multiple aetiologies. If there is complete obstruction to urine outflow the potassium concentrations rise rapidly and dramatically owing to a sudden marked reduction in GFR, with resultant reduced potassium excretion. Metabolic acidosis also develops and this exacerbates the hyperkalaemia as a result of a shift of potassium out of cells into the interstitium and plasma in exchange for hydrogen ions. In addition to hyperkalaemia, azotaemia, hyperphosphataemia and hypocalcaemia are commonly present.

Urinary tract rupture: Urinary tract rupture is most commonly caused by abdominal trauma. Urine, which contains a high concentration of potassium, is not voided but spills into the abdomen and is then re-absorbed into the systemic circulation down a concentration gradient with a subsequent rise in plasma potassium. Sodium diffuses from the blood into the free urine in the abdominal cavity and the resultant hyponatraemia triggers aldosterone release. Aldosterone mediates the retention of sodium and increases urinary potassium loss which, in these circumstances, exacerbates the increase in serum potassium because the urine is not being excreted.

The measurement of high levels of creatinine in an abdominal tap exceeding the serum level, can suggest that urinary tract rupture has occurred (see Chapter 22).

Hypoadrenocorticism: Hypoadrenocorticism (Addison's disease) is caused by diminished release of cortisol and aldosterone due to the probable immune-mediated destruction of the adrenal cortex (see Chapter 18). Low levels of aldosterone lead to decreased sodium resorption and reduced potassium excretion in the distal nephron. This usually results in a marked elevation in serum potassium coupled with hyponatraemia and hypochloraemia, and hence a marked reduction in the sodium:potassium ratio (<24). However, a small proportion of cases do not have electrolyte abnormalities (Sadek and Schaer, 1996).

An adrenocorticotropic hormone (ACTH) stimulation test provides the definitive diagnosis, with cortisol levels usually being undetectable pre- and post-ACTH (see Chapter 18).

There is a single case report of hyperreninaemic hypoaldosteronism in which a dog presented with electrolyte abnormalities but a normal ACTH stimulation test. In this case renin was measured to prove that aldosterone was low in the face of high renin and that aldosterone production and release were therefore impaired. This, however, is an extremely rare presentation in dogs and has not been reported in cats (Lobetti, 1998). Similarly, hyporeninaemic hypoaldosteronism has been reported recently, again as a single case report. In this scenario it is speculated that chronic volume expansion and damage to the juxtaglomerular apparatus leads to a decrease in the appropriate release of renin, and hyperkalaemia again results (Kreissler and Langston, 2011).

Hyperkalaemia due to potassium redistribution

The mechanisms of potassium redistribution are summarized in Figure 8.3.

Acid–base disturbances: The accumulation of a cation (positively charged ion) in the extracellular fluid (ECF)/plasma will result in either a shift of anions (negatively charged ions) into the ECF or a shift of a second cation out of the ECF into cells. Hydrogen ions from strong acids such as hydrochloric acid are able to displace potassium from cells, resulting in hyperkalaemia. This occurs because chloride, the major extracellular anion, cannot follow H^+ ions into cells. Organic acids such as lactic acid or ketoacids do not provoke this movement of potassium, or do so to a limited extent, presumably because their associated anions follow them to an intracellular location more easily. The hyperkalaemia of diabetic ketoacidosis occurs via a different mechanism (solvent drag) whereby water movement out of cells,

prompted by extracellular hyperosmolality, draws potassium into the extracellular fluid. Respiratory acidosis does not appear to provoke potassium redistribution and the reasons for this are unclear.

Pseudohypoadrenocorticism: This has been described in dogs with *Trichuris vulpis* infestation as well as other primary gastrointestinal diseases (DiBartola *et al.*, 1985; Graves *et al.*, 1994). In these cases animals have diarrhoea with hyperkalaemia and hyponatraemia, although aldosterone levels are usually found to be normal or high. Fluid sequestration into body cavities or into the pericardial sac may also cause electrolyte abnormalities that mimic hypoadrenocorticism (Willard *et al.*, 1991). The mechanisms for these forms of pseudohypoadrenocorticism are complex and involve:

- Hypovolaemia inducing antidiuretic hormone (ADH) release and water retention
- A reduction in tubular fluid flow to the distal tubule due to decreased GFR, leading to reduced potassium excretion
- Repeated drainage of effusions leading to total body sodium loss
- Patient thirst, leading to increased water intake
- Hypovolaemic acidosis due to bicarbonate loss, leading to potassium redistribution into the extracellular compartment.

The net result is a dilution of extracellular sodium and an increase in extracellular potassium.

Massive tissue breakdown: The three most frequently encountered causes leading to hyperkalaemia are:

- Tumour lysis syndrome following chemotherapy in the face of a large tumour burden e.g. lymphoma; there is accompanying hyperphosphataemia and hypocalcaemia
- Reperfusion injury following aortic thromboembolic disease in cats. In these cases there may be concurrent increases in aspartate aminotransferase (AST) and creatine kinase (CK)
- Severe trauma; there may be other biochemical changes depending on the nature of the trauma.

In all cases, hyperkalaemia is the result of the release of massive amounts of intracellular potassium into the circulation.

Miscellaneous causes of hyperkalaemia

Drug therapy: Angiotensin converting enzyme (ACE) inhibitors are probably the most commonly used class of drug that causes hyperkalaemia by inhibition of angiotensin-mediated aldosterone release. As they are frequently used in conjunction with loop diuretics, which lower potassium, this effect is often not discernible in cardiac patients.

Hypokalaemia

The causes of hypokalaemia are summarized in Figure 8.4 and the most common causes are discussed below.

Decreased intake

Anorexia is probably the most common cause of hypokalaemia in small animal practice because food supplies the body's potassium needs.

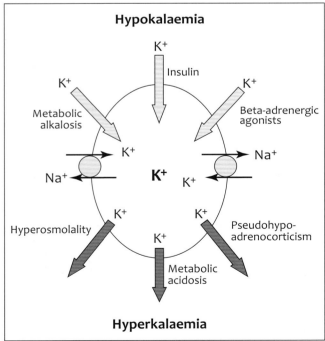

8.3 Factors affecting potassium movement into and out of the cell (represented by an oval in this diagram). The $Na^+/K^+/ATPase$ pump mediates the movement of potassium into the cell whereas outward movement is caused by solvent drag or by displacement of potassium by other cations.

Decreased intake
• Anorexia
• Fluid therapy using K⁺-free fluids

Increased loss
• Gastrointestinal losses: *vomiting and diarrhoea*
• Urinary losses:
• *Chronic renal failure*
• *Post-obstructive diuresis*
• *Polyuria*
• Renal tubular acidosis
• Hyperadrenocorticism
• Hyperaldosteronism
• Hypomagnesaemia
• Metabolic acidosis e.g. diabetic ketoacidosis
• Drug therapy:
– Penicillin
– *Loop and thiazide diuretics*
– Mineralocorticoid excess

Potassium redistribution – movement into cells from extracellular fluid
• Alkalaemia
• Elevated insulin levels/exogenous insulin administration
• Beta-adrenergic agonist administration
• Hypothermia
• Hypokalaemic myopathy of Burmese cats

8.4 The differential diagnosis of hypokalaemia. The most common differentials are shown in *italics*.

Iatrogenic causes: Fluid therapy using potassium-free fluids (0.9% NaCl) or low-potassium fluids (Hartmann's solution) can lead to hypokalaemia, particularly in those animals that have concurrent anorexia. Similarly, fluids containing glucose, or insulin therapy, will cause the serum/plasma potassium concentration to drop as potassium moves into cells from the extracellular fluid (see Figure 8.2).

Increased loss of potassium

Gastrointestinal disease: Vomiting or diarrhoea, or the two combined, can lead to clinically significant hypokalaemia. Vomiting of gastric contents leads to metabolic alkalosis and subsequent enhanced renal potassium excretion. The important mechanisms are summarized as follows:

- Potassium, along with sodium, chloride and hydrogen ions, is lost in vomitus
- Volume contraction stimulates aldosterone release and retention of sodium, with concurrent potassium loss
- Metabolic alkalosis promotes movement of potassium into cells from the extracellular fluid in exchange for H⁺.

Gastrointestinal disease losses are exacerbated by a reduced oral potassium intake due to anorexia or inappetence.

Chronic renal failure: Cats with chronic renal failure are much more likely to be hypokalaemic than dogs, and the syndrome of muscle weakness associated with potassium depletion is primarily a feline problem. Although it is commonly encountered, the mechanism behind the hypokalaemia is not well understood and is probably multifactorial, involving both increased urinary and gastrointestinal losses as well as reduced absorption. An improvement in renal function occurs following potassium supplementation, and there is a decline in renal function seen in cats fed a potassium-restricted diet (DiBartola *et al.*, 1993).

Hyperaldosteronism and hyperadrenocorticism: Aldosterone is synthesized and released normally in response to activation of the renin–angiotensin–aldosterone system (RAAS) in conditions such as hypovolaemia and congestive heart failure. Therefore, in these conditions, although aldosterone concentrations will be high, renin will be elevated concurrently: so-called high-renin hyperaldosteronism. This is a normal physiological response to counter volume changes and such patients are not hypokalaemic. When there is an adrenal tumour synthesizing aldosterone autonomously this is done in the absence of renin and is called low-renin hyperaldosteronism (known as Conn's syndrome in human medicine). Hypokalaemia due to low-renin hyperaldosteronism is seen rarely in dogs but may be more common in cats. Hypokalaemia develops owing to excessive urinary excretion of potassium. Animals with this syndrome also have systemic arterial hypertension due to sodium retention and volume expansion. It is unusual for there to be a significant concurrent hypernatraemia because although sodium is retained, water moves with it and expands the circulating fluid volume. However, a mild hypernatraemia is seen in some cases.

Clinical signs of low-renin hyperaldosteronism include muscle weakness manifesting as plantigrade locomotion, cervical ventroflexion and collapse, mydriasis, hyphaema, retinal detachment and blindness. An abdominal mass may be palpable and there may also be signs of skin fragility, particularly if the adrenal tumour is also secreting cortisol or progesterone. The heart may be affected and there may be a systolic murmur and arrhythmias. These signs are due to a combination of arterial hypertension and also the profibrotic properties of high aldosterone concentrations.

Definitive diagnosis relies on demonstrating an elevated aldosterone concentration in the face of low or normal renin concentrations. The ratio of plasma aldosterone to plasma renin activity is the best screening test for this disease (Djajadiningrat-Laanen *et al.*, 2011). However, a presumptive diagnosis may be made in cats presenting with appropriate clinical signs and an adrenal mass that is secreting aldosterone.

Hypokalaemia with normal sodium levels or hypernatraemia can also occur in hyperadrenocorticism when excess cortisol acts as an agonist for the aldosterone receptor. This effect is usually blocked by the rapid conversion of cortisol to cortisone in the kidney, but can be seen when adrenal tumours produce excessive amounts of cortisol that exceed the maximum rate of this conversion.

Drug-associated hypokalaemia: Loop diuretics such as furosemide and thiazide diuretics commonly cause hypokalaemia. For patients with congestive heart failure who require chronic furosemide therapy, spironolactone, a potassium-sparing diuretic, is often used in combination to offset the hypokalaemia induced by furosemide. Dogs and cats that are receiving digoxin must be monitored particularly closely because hypokalaemia potentiates digoxin toxicity and predisposes to arrhythmia development.

Hypokalaemia caused by potassium shift into cells

Just as metabolic acidosis causes potassium to move out of cells, so the converse, alkalaemia, can cause potassium to move into cells (see Figure 8.3). This effect is, however, much less pronounced than with acidosis and is rarely a cause of clinically significant hypokalaemia (see also the section below on Diabetes mellitus). Beta-adrenergic agonists, e.g. dobutamine, can induce an intracellular movement of potassium, though this effect is seen mainly when overdose occurs.

Hypokalaemic myopathy of Burmese cats: Burmese cats may develop intermittent spontaneously improving weakness, with an age of onset of 2–6 months. Affected cats have generalized muscle weakness, walk with a stiff gait and have ventroflexion of the head (Figure 8.5). Exertion may precipitate tremors and collapse. Serum potassium is usually below 3.0 mmol/l and CK is often elevated. Diagnosis is by exclusion of other known causes and by proving that the fractional excretion of potassium is normal, i.e. appropriately decreased, in a potassium-depleted animal (less than 5%).

Hyperthyroidism: Hypokalaemia has been reported as a rare consequence of hyperthyroidism in cats and is speculated to be either secondary to polyuria, causing potassium wasting, or due to potassium shift into cells.

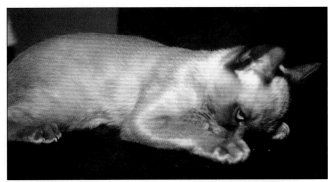

| 8.5 | Young Burmese cat showing generalized weakness and cervical ventroflexion due to hypokalaemic myopathy. |

(Courtesy of ME Herrtage, University of Cambridge)

Diabetes mellitus: a cause of both hyper- and hypokalaemia

Uncontrolled or ketoacidotic diabetic patients may present with normal or low potassium levels or may be hyperkalaemic, although most have whole-body potassium depletion due to polyuria (osmotic diuresis). Several mechanisms are involved, including serum hyperosmolality and insulin deficiency. In addition, ketones such as acetoacetate and β-hydroxybutyrate act as non-absorbable anions in the urine, trapping cations so that potassium excretion is enhanced. Once insulin therapy is started, this drives potassium to an intracellular location, leaving the animal hypokalaemic, and the whole-body potassium deficit becomes apparent. Once fluid therapy for management of a ketoacidotic crisis is underway, potassium monitoring is vital in order to avoid potentially severe hypokalaemia.

Causes of abnormalities in the sodium:potassium ratio

Although hypoadrenocorticism is the most common cause of a low sodium:potassium ratio, particularly when the ratio is <15, there are other causes that should be considered as differential diagnoses (Figure 8.6). Primary renal and parasitic or non-parasitic gastrointestinal diseases most commonly lead to significant reductions in the

- Hypoadrenocorticism
- Primary gastrointestinal disease – including *Trichuris vulpis* or *Toxocara canis* infestation
- Pleural, peritoneal or pericardial effusion
- Renal failure
- Heart failure
- Pancreatitis
- Diabetic ketoacidosis
- Urinary tract rupture
- Urinary bladder incarceration in perineal hernia
- Pyometra
- Neoplastic disease
- Late gestation pregnancy (Schaer *et al.*, 2001)

| 8.6 | The differential diagnosis of a low sodium:potassium ratio. |

sodium:potassium ratio. Differentiation of these diseases from true hypoadrenocorticism requires a basal cortisol assay or ideally an ACTH stimulation test (see Chapter 18) which, in most cases, will show elevated cortisol levels as a reflection of ongoing disease rather than cortisol suppression. The mechanisms leading to pseudohypoadrenocorticism were discussed earlier in this chapter (see Hyperkalaemia).

Disorders of sodium homeostasis

The role of sodium in the body

Sodium is primarily responsible for providing the means with which water is retained or lost through the action of the kidneys. Under normal conditions the sodium, and therefore the water, content of the body is maintained within a narrow range. This balance is upset by either:

- Loss of sodium and water (volume depletion)
- Loss of water alone (dehydration).

In cats and dogs normal serum sodium concentrations range between 135 and 155 mmol/l.

Sodium is the major cation present in the extracellular fluid and is responsible for the preservation of electroneutrality. Each sodium ion is balanced with an appropriate anion. Chloride makes up two-thirds of the total concentration of anions in the extracellular fluid, with bicarbonate the next most prevalent.

Regulation of plasma sodium

Plasma sodium levels are controlled by the regulation of blood volume and plasma osmolality via the following mechanisms:

- Activation of the renin–angiotensin–aldosterone system (RAAS)
- Release of antidiuretic hormone (ADH).

Reduced blood volume results in activation of the RAAS leading to the formation of angiotensin II and release of aldosterone (Figure 8.7). Angiotensin II causes increased sympathetic tone and therefore increased blood pressure, and increased absorption of sodium, chloride and water in the proximal tubule of the kidney. Aldosterone causes increased resorption of sodium in exchange for potassium in the distal tubule.

Volume reduction and *effective* volume reduction, as found in congestive heart failure, also trigger release of ADH via stimulation of carotid sinus baroreceptors (Figure 8.7). However, these volume receptors are much less sensitive and, unlike the RAAS, are activated only after a substantial decrease in circulating volume. These changes are reversed if there is an expansion of circulating volume.

Plasma osmolality

Plasma osmolality is a reflection of the number of osmotically active particles of solute, measured in mosmol/kg, and is regulated by ADH and the thirst mechanism (Figure 8.8). Changes in plasma osmolality, principally caused by changes in sodium concentration, are detected by osmoreceptors in the hypothalamus. Increased osmolality leads to activation of the thirst mechanism and ADH release from the neurohypophysis of the pituitary gland. ADH acts at the renal collecting ducts to increase the reabsorption of water.

The maintenance of normal osmolality involves the gain or loss of *water* while the maintenance of circulating volume involves the gain or loss of *sodium*. When volume depletion is severe, even if osmolality is low, ADH release and the thirst mechanism are activated, leading to dilutional hyponatraemia (see later).

Hypernatraemia
Clinical signs of hypernatraemia

In animals where the hypernatraemia is secondary to volume depletion, the early clinical signs reflect hypovolaemia. When the plasma sodium concentration increases, plasma osmolality increases. This creates an osmotic gradient that favours water movement out of cells and cellular dehydration, which is detrimental to the cells of the nervous system. This movement of water out of cells leads to rupture of cerebral vessels and focal haemorrhage. Clinical signs include lethargy, weakness, vocalization, muscle rigidity, twitching, seizures and coma; signs similar to those associated with hyponatraemia. Again, the severity of the clinical signs depends on the rate at which the hypernatraemia develops as well as the magnitude of the sodium concentration.

Causes of hypernatraemia

For an animal to become hypernatraemic it must either lose water in excess of sodium or have an increased sodium intake, either orally or through parenteral routes, e.g. intravenous fluid therapy. The differential diagnoses of hypernatraemia are listed in Figure 8.9.

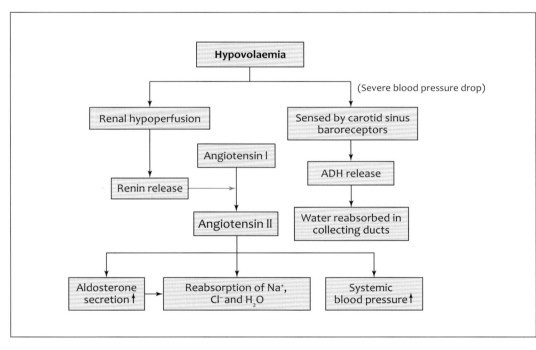

8.7 Activation of the renin–angiotensin system leading to aldosterone secretion and an increase in systemic blood pressure. When there is a significant drop in blood pressure, antidiuretic hormone (ADH) release is also stimulated.

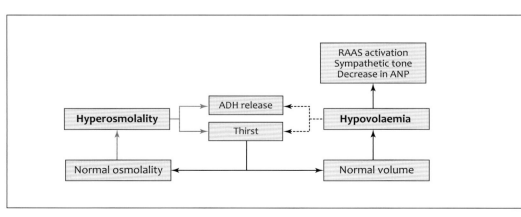

8.8 The relationship between osmoregulation and volume regulation. Although hyperosmolality is the primary stimulus for antidiuretic hormone (ADH) release and increase in thirst, severe hypovolaemia can also stimulate the same mechanisms. ANP = atrial natriuretic peptide; RAAS = renin–angiotensin–aldosterone system.

Hypernatraemia with water loss in excess of sodium

• Hypotonic fluid loss:
   • *Gastrointestinal disease – vomiting and/or diarrhoea*
   • Renal failure
   • Diabetes mellitus
   • Diuretic therapy
• Loss of pure water:
   • Central diabetes insipidus
   • *Nephrogenic diabetes insipidus*
   • Primary adipsia
   • Heatstroke
   • Pyrexia
   • Burns or extensive degloving injury
   • Water deprivation

Hypernatraemia caused by excessive sodium gain
• Increased salt ingestion • Hypertonic intravenous fluid therapy • Intravenous sodium bicarbonate • Hyperaldosteronism • Hyperadrenocorticism

8.9 The differential diagnosis of hypernatraemia. The most common differentials are shown in *italics*.

Hypernatraemia with water loss in excess of sodium

Hypotonic fluid loss: When water is lost in excess of sodium, for example in vomitus or diarrhoeal fluids, hypovolaemia and whole-body sodium depletion may occur in the face of hypernatraemia. Movement of hypotonic fluid into a body cavity (ascites or pleural effusion) or other third spaces can occasionally lead to hypernatraemia, although this is not a common finding. Renal hypotonic losses can occur secondary to the use of diuretics, osmotic diuresis (e.g. glucosuria) or post-obstructive diuresis. Hypovolaemia due to hypotonic fluid loss is the most common cause of hypernatraemia because the diseases underlying the electrolyte imbalance are so frequently encountered.

Central diabetes insipidus: Central diabetes insipidus is an uncommon condition in which there is a complete or partial absence of the production and release of ADH in response to increased plasma osmolality or to volume depletion. It can be congenital or acquired secondary to trauma, neoplasia, pituitary cysts, inflammation or pituitary malformation. Affected animals are unable to concentrate their urine and produce large quantities of very dilute urine (urine specific gravity typically <1.005). Polydipsia occurs secondarily to try to maintain adequate water balance. Hypernatraemia results when pure water loss exceeds intake. Diagnosis of this condition relies on the water deprivation test or modified water deprivation test and the response to exogenously administered synthetic ADH (1-desamino-8-D-arginine vasopressin, DDAVP; see Chapter 10).

Nephrogenic diabetes insipidus (NDI): Congenital nephrogenic diabetes insipidus is extremely rare, while acquired NDI is a relatively common consequence of many systemic diseases, e.g. hyperadrenocorticism, hypoadrenocorticism, hepatic disease, hypercalcaemia and diseases in which there is a septic focus such as pyometra. Although ADH is produced and released in response to hyperosmolality, the kidney is unable to respond adequately. The congenital form of this disease is difficult to confirm and is a diagnosis of exclusion (Luzius *et al.*, 1992).

Primary adipsia (essential hypernatraemia): Primary adipsia is a rare condition defined by a defect in the central thirst mechanism caused by malfunction of the osmoreceptors of the hypothalamus. Consequently, ADH secretion from the hypothalamus fails to occur in response to increased plasma osmolality but can occur when volume is depleted (Jeffery *et al.*, 2003). This condition is usually congenital but there have been reports of acquired forms in older animals secondary to inflammatory disease (Mackay and Curtis, 1999). Plasma sodium levels are typically >170 mmol/l and overt neurological signs are often present although animals are not volume depleted.

Heatstroke, pyrexia, burns or extensive degloving injury: This group of conditions is characterized by free water loss through the skin as a consequence of skin deficits caused by traumatic injury or the increase in water evaporation from the skin and respiratory tract as an animal attempts to lower its body temperature.

Water deprivation: This may occur in animals that are either unable or unwilling, due to illness, to drink water. Disorientated geriatric patients or those with neurological disease may become water deprived and should be assisted in drinking accordingly.

Hypernatraemia caused by excessive sodium gain

Increased salt ingestion, hypertonic intravenous fluid therapy, intravenous sodium bicarbonate: When the whole-body sodium load increases, serum osmolality rises and ADH release is stimulated. This leads to hypervolaemia because of water retention. It is not common for hypernatraemia to result from excessive salt intake (Khanna *et al.*, 1997) but it can happen secondary to the ingestion of sea water, the ingestion of home-made children's modelling dough, following the use of sodium phosphate enemas and as a consequence of intravenous fluid therapy using hypertonic saline or large doses of sodium bicarbonate (Goldkamp and Schaer, 2007; Kasai and King, 2009).

Why the brain is vulnerable to hypernatraemia

The delicate vasculature of the brain is particularly vulnerable to damage caused by the osmotic movement of water either into or out of neural cells. When there is hypernatraemia the water moves out of neural cells, and cell shrinkage leads to subarachnoid and subcortical haemorrhages, vascular tearing, haematoma formation, venous thrombosis, infarction and neurological damage (Adrogue and Madias, 2000).

Acute *versus* chronic hypernatraemia with hypervolaemia must be treated differently because this has an impact on treatment response. If salt ingestion is acutely observed (<4 hours ago) then rapid correction of hypernatraemia is possible. This is because idiogenic organic osmoles have not had a chance to form within the central nervous system (see Figure 8.10). Later, idiogenic osmoles will have formed and these provide protection to the brain from cellular dehydration so that rapid fluid administration will lead to movement of water into neural cells and consequent oedema. In these more chronic cases a reduction of sodium of <1–2 mmol/l/h is recommended (Pouzot *et al.*, 2007).

Hyperaldosteronism and hyperadrenocorticism: Hypernatraemia can occur secondary to aldosterone or cortisol excess produced by secretory tumours of the adrenal gland. This is discussed in more detail in the section on hypokalaemia and occurs infrequently.

Hyponatraemia

Clinical signs

Clinical signs are generally not observed at all until the plasma sodium concentration falls below 125 mmol/l. If there is a rapid decrease in sodium and of plasma osmolality then water can move into the brain rapidly and cerebral oedema develops (Figure 8.10), resulting in lethargy, weakness, nausea, vomiting, incoordination and seizures. If hyponatraemia develops gradually, the clinical signs are few and less severe: the brain is protected from becoming oedematous by the movement of organic osmotically active molecules (osmolytes) and potassium ions out of the cells, thus ensuring that the intracellular osmolality decreases with the extracellular osmolality.

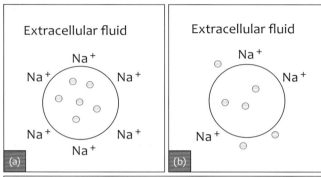

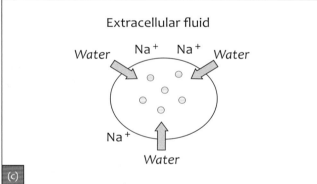

8.10 The cellular adaptation to hyponatraemia in the nervous system. (a) Cells within the nervous system are protected from dehydration by the presence of idiogenic organic osmoles (shown as small circles). (b) When hyponatraemia develops slowly, re-equilibration can occur and osmotic balance is maintained. However, when hyponatraemia develops rapidly, the intracellular space is hyperosmolar with respect to the extracellular fluid, water moves into the cells and cerebral oedema develops (c).

Causes of hyponatraemia

Hyponatraemia may be due to excess loss of sodium or gain of water or a combination of both (Figure 8.11).

Spurious hyponatraemia

Pseudohyponatraemia refers to the falsely low sodium concentrations measured in plasma when significant hyperproteinaemia or hyperlipidaemia is present. Normally, the volume of plasma occupied by proteins and lipoproteins is a small fraction (<5%) of total plasma volume, but in severe hyperproteinaemia or hyperlipidaemia, the volume occupied is large enough to change the concentration of plasma constituents that exist almost exclusively in the aqueous fraction, such as sodium. Some analytical methods, such as direct ISE devices, do not require the

Sodium loss
• *Gastrointestinal signs, e.g. vomiting and diarrhoea*
• Third-spacing of fluid: • Pleural effusion, e.g. chylothorax or lung lobe torsion   • Peritoneal effusion, e.g. septic or non-septic peritonitis, ruptured bladder
• *Hypoadrenocorticism*
• Diuretic administration

Volume overload
• Congestive heart failure
• Nephrotic syndrome
• Liver disease
• Advanced renal disease

Hyponatraemia with normovolaemia
• Inappropriate fluid therapy, e.g. administration of hypotonic fluids
• Psychogenic polydipsia
• Inappropriate ADH secretion
• Hypothyroid myxoedematous coma
• Exercise-associated hyponatraemia

Hyponatraemia due to increase in plasma osmolality
• *Diabetes mellitus*
• Mannitol administration

Pseudo-hyponatraemia
• Hyperlipidaemia
• Hyperproteinaemia

8.11 The differential diagnosis of hyponatraemia. The most common differentials are shown in *italics*.

volume of the sample to be known and therefore are not affected by lipid or protein in the blood (see Chapter 15).

Hyponatraemia due to sodium loss

Hypoadrenocorticism: The most common cause of hyponatraemia due to sodium loss is hypoadrenocorticism. Aldosterone mediates sodium uptake and potassium loss in the distal tubule, so the combination of hyponatraemia with hyperkalaemia provides the classic electrolyte profile for hypoadrenocorticism. In this case, although there is volume depletion, the urine specific gravity and osmolality are inappropriately low. An ACTH stimulation test will provide confirmation, as described previously.

Sodium loss with volume depletion due to gastrointestinal, renal or third space loss: Animals may become hyponatraemic when they are volume depleted as a consequence of loss of electrolytes concurrent to their loss of water (Figure 8.12). This can happen when water is lost through the gastrointestinal (GI) tract or when fluid moves into a third space, e.g. the pleural or peritoneal cavity, or when renal losses have occurred. Although fluid losses, particularly through the GI tract, are usually hypotonic in nature, the subsequent physiological responses (increase in ADH release, increase in thirst, decrease in renal water excretion) serve to dilute the plasma via an increase in water intake and water retention. In volume-depleted animals the urine specific gravity will be appropriately increased as free water excretion is decreased.

Diuretic administration: Animals receiving treatment particularly with thiazide diuretics, and to a lesser extent with loop diuretics, are commonly mildly hyponatraemic. Severe hyponatraemia is unusual, though idiosyncratic reactions can occur. Thiazide diuretics can produce a situation whereby sodium and potassium are lost in excess of water. Electrolyte monitoring is important for animals receiving chronic diuretic therapy.

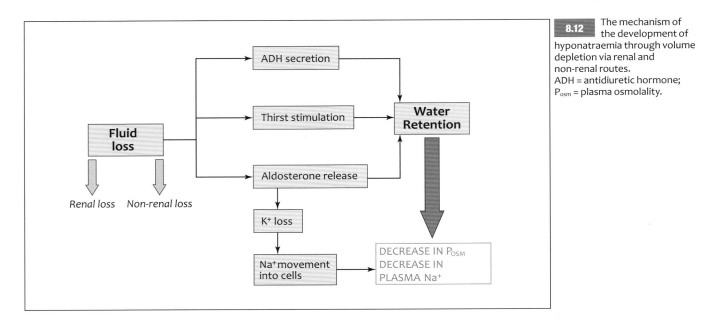

8.12 The mechanism of the development of hyponatraemia through volume depletion via renal and non-renal routes.
ADH = antidiuretic hormone; P_{osm} = plasma osmolality.

Hyponatraemia due to volume overload

Congestive heart failure (CHF), hepatic failure, nephrotic syndrome and end-stage renal failure: The common feature in these conditions is volume expansion in the face of a perceived, but not true, hypovolaemia. Hyponatraemia results from decreased sodium concentration in an expanded volume. Total body stores of sodium are generally increased.

In *CHF*, as cardiac output falls, renal perfusion and consequently GFR decrease. This increases the proximal tubule's ability to reabsorb sodium and water and decreases the tubular flow to more distal sites where tubular fluid would then be diluted to allow water to be excreted. The renin–angiotensin system is rapidly activated and ADH release is precipitated through the stimulation of baroreceptors in the arterial circulation. Volume overload on the venous side of the circulation, though sensed by baroreceptors in the left atrium, fails to prevent ADH release. What is perceived is a volume deficit, though what has really occurred is a redistribution of volume and a decrease in effective volume (i.e. the volume effectively involved in tissue perfusion).

In *nephrotic syndrome* or where there is *hepatic cirrhosis*, similar volume redistribution occurs. Reduced plasma protein levels result in reduced plasma oncotic pressure so that water moves into extravascular locations and volume depletion leads again to ADH release. Other mechanisms also contribute to a reduction in circulating volume. In hepatic disease, portal hypertension leads to the development of ascites, while arteriovenous shunting reduces the perceived circulating volume. Nephrotic syndrome presents a complex picture in which volume expansion and oedema develop as a result of sodium retention that is governed by mechanisms other than the renin–angiotensin system (Brown *et al.*, 1982).

In advanced renal failure polydipsia can lead to an excessive water load that the poorly functioning kidneys find difficult to excrete. This results in volume expansion and dilutional hyponatraemia.

Hyponatraemia with normovolaemia

Hypotonic fluid administration: Hypotonic fluids are classified as those that result in a net water gain and include fluids such as 5% dextrose. When 5% dextrose is infused, the sugar is rapidly taken up by cells, leaving an addition of water to the circulation. Much of the water is also redistributed between body compartments so that the circulation is not appreciably expanded. The net result is that the induction of natriuresis leads to hyponatraemia in the face of normovolaemia.

Psychogenic polydipsia: Psychogenic polydipsia is usually described in large-breed dogs and can be related to a particularly disruptive episode in the dog's life. The syndrome is classified as a behavioural problem in that there is no deficiency of ADH synthesis, release and function but the normal control of thirst is over-ruled. As the daily water consumption increases, water excretion also increases, along with renal sodium excretion. Thus both the plasma and urine osmolalities are low. A water deprivation test or modified water deprivation test (designed to correct medullary washout) can identify most cases and can differentiate between psychogenic polydipsia and diabetes insipidus (see Chapter 10).

Syndrome of inappropriate ADH secretion: Inappropriate ADH release, or potentiation of the effects of ADH, is rarely identified in veterinary patients although it is widely recognized in human medicine. One report describes the syndrome of inappropriate ADH secretion occurring in conjunction with granulomatous meningoencephalitis in a dog (Brofman *et al.*, 2003). This syndrome has also been reported in association with heartworm, hypothalamic tumours and congenital hydrocephalus (Shiel *et al.*, 2009). To recognize this syndrome, five criteria must be met (Baylis, 2003):

* Hyponatraemia
* Natriuresis (this may be identified through measurement of the urinary fractional excretion of sodium, as discussed in Chapter 11)
* Urine osmolality > plasma osmolality
* Absence of oedema and volume depletion
* Normal renal and adrenal function.

Hypothyroid myxoedematous coma: Hypothyroid myxoedema may lead to hyponatraemia through ADH release, mediated by a reduction in cardiac output and GFR, and a movement of water from the intravascular compartment into the interstitium. Hyponatraemia results from a dilutional effect while normal volume is maintained.

Hyponatraemia due to increased plasma osmolality

This effect is most commonly seen in animals with hyperglycaemia and increased plasma osmolality due to diabetes mellitus, or those that have received mannitol. Movement of water out of cells by osmosis expands the extracellular volume, consequently lowering the plasma sodium concentration.

Disorders of chloride homeostasis

Hyperchloraemia

Given that chloride exists in the body as an anion to balance sodium as a cation, many of the conditions that lead to hypernatraemia also lead to hyperchloraemia; for example, hyperchloraemia may occur due to:

- Increased intake, either iatrogenic (fluid therapy) or accidental (salt poisoning; see section on Hypernatraemia)
- Decreased excretion (renal failure).

The following situations would be likely to lead to hyperchloraemia *without* concurrent hypernatraemia:

- Increased loss of bicarbonate in the gut due to diarrhoea leading to non-ion gap metabolic acidosis (see Chapter 9)
- Chronic respiratory alkalosis (see Chapter 9)
- Chloride containing therapy (e.g. KCl as a fluid supplement)
- Total parenteral nutrition, because some forms have high levels of cationic amino acids that release chloride.

Animals that are hyperchloraemic but normonatraemic are usually acidotic and clinical signs reflect the acid–base balance rather than the hyperchloraemia *per se*.

Pseudohyperchloraemia

Pseudohyperchloraemia can occur in dogs receiving potassium bromide therapy for epilepsy. Bromide, in common with other halides, is measured using most of the methods used to measure chloride but this is particularly true when using ISEs.

Hypochloraemia

Hypochloraemia may arise along with hyponatraemia (see above). Hypochloraemia with normal sodium levels usually suggests the presence of alkalosis (excess bicarbonate results in a reduction in chloride to maintain electroneutrality) and the clinical signs shown are also secondary to the acid–base disturbance. The most common cause of a metabolic alkalosis and hypochloraemia in small animal practice is the vomiting of stomach contents. Other causes of hypochloraemia include:

- Diuretics such as thiazides or loop diuretics (e.g. furosemide)
- Any drugs or types of fluid therapy that contain proportionately more sodium than chloride, e.g. penicillins and sodium bicarbonate, though this latter effect is rarely seen at commonly used dosages
- Hyperadrenocorticism, because steroid hormones increase sodium reabsorption and renal chloride loss.

Disorders of magnesium homeostasis

Measuring serum magnesium

Only a small fraction (about 1%) of total body magnesium is present in serum. Like calcium, the physiologically active form of magnesium is the ionized form that makes up about 55% of the total. Few laboratories offer ionized magnesium measurement so total serum levels are generally used. The drawbacks to this include:

- Variation in total magnesium levels with hyper- and hypoalbuminaemia (like calcium, although to a lesser degree because less magnesium is protein bound by comparison)
- Poor representation of total body magnesium status through serum measurement
- The occurrence of normal serum magnesium in the face of whole-body hypomagnesaemia.

The reference range for total magnesium concentration is 0.59–0.86 mmol/l for dogs and 0.74–1.20 mmol/l for cats (Department of Clinical Pathology, Cambridge Veterinary School). Published values for both total and ionized magnesium are variable so it is preferable to refer to the reference range for the laboratory used.

The importance of magnesium in the body and the consequences of imbalances

Magnesium exists in the body in an intracellular location and, after potassium, is the second most abundant intracellular cation. Magnesium is a critical cofactor for the functioning of the sodium/potassium ATPase pump and thus has an important role in the partitioning of sodium and potassium into their extra- and intracellular compartments, respectively. Magnesium is absorbed through the gut and is excreted by the kidneys, but no hormone has been found to have a role in regulating the concentration of magnesium in the blood.

The clinical signs of magnesium imbalance have a major impact on the cardiovascular system and the neuromuscular system. There is little published data or experience in the management of magnesium disorders in veterinary patients, though there is considerable interest in this electrolyte in critical care patients.

Hypermagnesaemia

Hypermagnesaemia is a rare disorder, and the main cause in veterinary medicine is renal failure, where the rate of magnesium excretion falls in parallel with the decline in GFR. This situation is similar to the development of hyperkalaemia in renal failure. Other less common causes of hypermagnesaemia include iatrogenic overdose, although cats and dogs seem more resistant to the clinical signs associated with this than humans.

Clinical signs of hypermagnesaemia are not obvious unless the serum concentration is severely elevated. Electrocardiographic changes include prolongation of the PR interval and widening of the QRS complex. This can progress to complete atrioventricular block and asystole. Neuromuscular signs include myotactic hyporeflexia and, in extreme cases, muscle paralysis (Martin, 1998).

Hypomagnesaemia

Many of the conditions that result in hypokalaemia will also cause hypomagnesaemia. Causes of hypomagnesaemia include:

- Gastrointestinal loss
- Anorexia
- Renal tubular disease
- Hypercalcaemia
- Glucosuria
- Drug administration (diuretics, digoxin, cisplatin, ciclosporin)
- Endocrine disease (hyperthyroidism, hypoparathyroidism)
- Redistribution induced by insulin or catecholamines.

Magnesium supplementation can be useful in the management of arrhythmias caused or exacerbated by hypokalaemia (see section on Hypokalaemia) and can decrease the sensitivity of the heart to digoxin-induced arrhythmias. These arrhythmias may be difficult to control without magnesium as well as potassium supplementation because magnesium is required for efficient functioning of the Na$^+$/K$^+$ ATPase pump. Neuromuscular signs also occur when there is concurrent hypokalaemia or hypocalcaemia, and include muscle weakness, muscle fasciculations, ataxia or seizures.

In metabolic disorders such as diabetic ketoacidosis, magnesium depletion may exist alongside hypokalaemia that is refractory to potassium supplementation unless magnesium is administered simultaneously (Dhupa and Proulx, 1998). Similarly, in human critical care patients hypomagnesaemia has been identified frequently as either a primary electrolyte disorder or as part of a complex disorder alongside hypokalaemia.

Disorders of calcium homeostasis

Calcium imbalance remains one of the most interesting of biochemical abnormalities to investigate because hypercalcaemia and hypocalcaemia can be associated with a diverse range of conditions. Calcium is found in three forms in plasma: ionized; protein bound (chiefly to albumin); and chelated to lactate, citrate or bicarbonate. Bone acts as a reservoir for calcium, releasing it or storing it as required. An understanding of the control of calcium homeostasis is pivotal to working out the aetiology of the change in calcium for each individual. Figure 8.13 summarizes the basics of calcium homeostasis. The important, and measurable, hormones involved in calcium homeostasis are listed below.

- **Parathyroid hormone (PTH):** this hormone is synthesized and released by the chief cells in the four parathyroid glands associated with or embedded within the thyroid gland. PTH is released when the calcium-sensing receptor (expressed in parathyroid and renal tissue) senses that calcium concentration in plasma has decreased. The target organs are the kidneys, where renal uptake is stimulated, and bone, where osteoclastic activity is stimulated and skeletal calcium liberated. PTH also increases gut uptake of calcium via its effect on vitamin D metabolism (see below). Increased calcium leads to a fall in PTH.
- **Parathyroid hormone related peptide (PTHrP):** PTHrP has a physiological role in calcium homeostasis in the fetus. After birth, PTHrP is very low in healthy animals, but increased levels have been implicated in

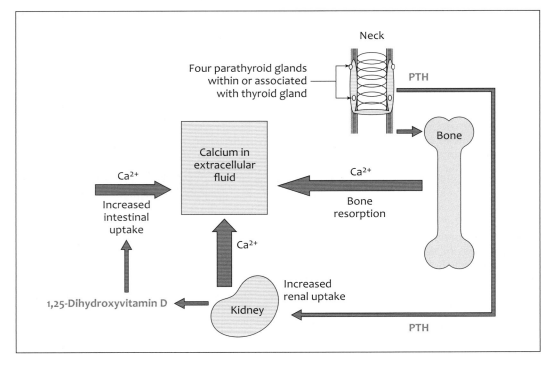

8.13 The basics of calcium homeostasis. The important hormones are parathyroid hormone (PTH) and 1,25-dihydroxyvitamin D.

the aetiology of humoral hypercalcaemia of malignancy (HHM) (Wysolmerski and Broadus, 1994). PTHrP has the same physiological effects as PTH. The measurement of PTHrP has become part of the diagnostic work-up for hypercalcaemia, particularly when neoplasia is suspected.

- **1,25-Dihydroxyvitamin D:** cholecalciferol is the basic vitamin D, which is hydroxylated once by the liver to produce 25-hydroxycholecalciferol (25(OH)-vitamin D, calcidiol). This is not a closely regulated step and produces a pool of vitamin D ready for activation to 1,25-dihydroxyvitamin D (1,25(OH)$_2$-cholecalciferol, calcitriol). This step *is* regulated and occurs in the kidney, prompted by increased PTH release, via alpha hydroxylase and reduced by an increased concentration of phosphate. 25(OH)-cholecalciferol can also be catabolized by 24-hydroxylation, after which it is removed from the circulation.
- **Calcitonin:** a peptide synthesized by the C cells of the thyroid gland. This hormone causes hypocalcaemia and has a role in limiting postprandial hypercalcaemia. Though calcitonin can counteract the effects of excessive PTH, its role is relatively minor.

Laboratory investigation of disorders of calcium homeostasis

Measurement of calcium

Although the measurement of total calcium can provide information about whether a disturbance of calcium homeostasis is present, it is ionized calcium that is more useful and easier to interpret in such cases. Figure 8.14 details the sample-associated factors to be taken into account when calcium is measured.

Ionized calcium is measured using an analyser that has an ISE. Differences between analysers exist, and reference ranges will differ depending on the laboratory involved, but the reference range will frequently be 1.20–1.45 mmol/l. Cage-side analysers that use whole blood to measure iCa are often found to underestimate the calcium concentration when measured in serum so reference ranges supplied for these instruments may vary. Care must be taken with sample handling because exposing the blood sample to air will cause an increase in pH due to the loss of CO_2, which will decrease ionized calcium. Samples should therefore be taken anaerobically, sealed from air exposure and analysed quickly to obtain accurate results. Separated serum or plasma stored anaerobically is, however, stable.

Sample associated variables	Serum or plasma calcium measurements
Factors associated with sample anticoagulant	Oxalate, citrate and EDTA should not be used because they bind calcium
Haemolysis	May falsely increase [tCa] and [iCa]
Hyperbilirubinaemia	May falsely decrease [tCa] and [iCa] but is analyser dependent
Dilution	Do not dilute samples for iCa measurement because it renders the measurement inaccurate
Age	Dogs and cats <6 months of age have higher serum calcium concentrations related to bone growth[a]

8.14 The sample-associated variables to be considered when measuring calcium in serum or plasma. [a]The age at which this effect is seen varies according to the age at which the dog reaches skeletal maturity and therefore may be much higher in giant-breed dogs. iCa = ionized calcium; tCa = total calcium.

Heparin binds calcium and can also affect results. Each unit of heparin added per ml of blood will decrease ionized calcium by 0.01 mmol/l and therefore care must be taken not to over- or under-fill heparin tubes.

Other biochemical parameters

Hypercalcaemia may exist without any other significant biochemical abnormalities. However, as hypercalcaemia can cause renal damage and renal insufficiency can cause hypercalcaemia, differentiating which came first can be diagnostically challenging. Urea and creatinine levels may be elevated along with phosphate concentrations as a consequence of pre-existing renal damage or prerenal factors, or may reflect ongoing renal damage due to elevated calcium concentrations. As an example, the changes associated with primary hyperparathyroidism with secondary prerenal azotaemia or renal failure can mimic those of primary renal disease with secondary PTH elevation and hypercalcaemia (Figure 8.15).

Parameter	PHPT	Secondary renal hyperparathyroidism
Total calcium	↑	↑ or normal or ↓
Ionized calcium	↑	↓ or normal
Phosphate	↓	↑
PTH	↑	↑ or high normal
PTHrP	Normal	Normal or ↑[a]

8.15 Differentiating primary hyperparathyroidism (PHPT) from chronic renal disease with secondary hyperparathyroidism. [a]The level of parathyroid hormone related peptide (PTHrP) may be elevated in renal disease because of a reduction in renal excretion of this molecule. PTH = parathyroid hormone.

Measurement of PTH

PTH is found in the blood as both intact hormone and carboxy-terminal fragments that are the result of hormone degradation. To measure PTH concentration, the intact hormone must be measured (amino acids 1–84), because it is only this portion that is biologically active. Currently, enzyme-linked immunosorbent assay (ELISA) is the predominant method used to measure PTH in the UK. A canine-specific ELISA, which has also been validated for cats, is available, although some laboratories have validated human-specific PTH testing kits for use in the dog and cat. Testing methods change rapidly as new methods are developed but it is important that the method chosen has been validated for the appropriate species. Samples of EDTA plasma are preferred for PTH measurement; it must be remembered that PTH is a labile hormone and that samples require specific handling involving immediate plasma separation and freezing. The laboratory providing the test will often provide information and freezer packs for sample submission. The reference interval for PTH is approximately 20–65 pg/ml in the dog and <25 pg/ml in the cat but may differ depending on the laboratory and assay used.

Measurement of PTHrP

PTHrP is measured by two-site immunoradiometric assay (IRMA) and by N-terminal radioimmunoassay (RIA). There are several circulating forms of PTHrP that have biological activity, including intact PTHrP (amino acids 1–141), an N-terminal fragment (1–36) and an N-terminal plus mid-region fragment (1–86). The roles of the different forms are not completely understood. Like PTH, PTHrP is not stable and is measured preferentially in plasma, using EDTA as an anticoagulant (similar sample handling is required as for PTH). The reference level for PTHrP is generally <0.5 pmol/l in both dogs and cats.

Measurement of vitamin D

Previously, vitamin D measurements were only available through human hospital services. Now, however, vitamin D (25-hydroxycholecalciferol and 1,25-dihydroxycholecalciferol) can be measured in cats and dogs through veterinary specialist laboratories.

Measurement of calcitonin

This is not routinely measured in cases where there is dysregulation of calcium and no assays are currently offered.

Hypercalcaemia

Clinical signs of hypercalcaemia

The clinical signs vary depending on the magnitude and duration of the hypercalcaemia. A mild to moderate hypercalcaemia is usually well tolerated, particularly if it has developed slowly over months. Conversely, severe hypercalcaemia (>3.8 mmol/l) will produce more obvious clinical signs. Rapidly changing calcium concentrations will always be more keenly noticed by a pet owner. Signs include:

- Polyuria and polydipsia (due to ADH inhibition)
- Lethargy and depression
- Exercise intolerance and muscle weakness
- Inappetence, anorexia, vomiting, constipation and diarrhoea
- Dental pain
- Cardiac arrhythmias (rare).

Hypercalcaemia is a cause of renal tubular damage, particularly when there is concurrent hyperphosphataemia. Calculating the calcium/phosphate product and using the value to predict the degree of renal risk to an individual is not recommended and *all* hypercalcaemic patients must be considered at risk of renal damage, although patients with primary hyperparathyroidism are considered to be at a lower risk than those with hypercalcaemia of malignancy.

A hypercalcaemic animal loses its ability to concentrate urine as a result of ADH antagonism, and may be hyposthenuric, isosthenuric or weakly hypersthenuric. The animal may also be azotaemic and this may either be due to a prerenal azotaemia caused by water loss in the face of poor concentrating ability, or it may reflect true renal damage. It is difficult, in these circumstances, to make judgements on whether the kidneys have sustained significant damage, and important prognostic decisions should not be based on the presence or degree of azotaemia until the hypercalcaemia has been resolved and fluid balance corrected.

Causes of hypercalcaemia

The most common causes of hypercalcaemia and the mechanisms leading to an increase in calcium concentration are listed in Figure 8.16. An algorithm for the work-up of hypercalcaemia is shown in Figure 8.17.

Malignancy: Lymphoma (dogs and cats) and anal sac adenocarcinoma (dogs) are probably the most common types of neoplasia to be associated with hypercalcaemia; however, the list also includes tumours as diverse as thymoma, pulmonary carcinoma, multiple myeloma and malignant melanoma. The mechanisms of malignancy-associated hypercalcaemia in people generally fall into three categories: humoral hypercalcaemia due to secreted factors (such as PTHrP); local osteolysis due to tumour invasion of bone; and absorptive hypercalcaemia due to excess vitamin D. Of these, the first mechanism is probably the most common and, when the factor is PTHrP, the most easily characterized. However, it must be remembered that PTHrP does not mediate all cases of malignancy-related hypercalcaemia, and finding a low PTHrP does not rule out malignancy as an inciting cause. If hypercalcaemia of malignancy is driven by PTHrP, a high total and ionized calcium would be expected alongside low or low normal phosphate. Where renal damage or pre-existing renal disease is present, phosphate may be elevated concurrently and the animal may be azotaemic.

Primary hyperparathyroidism: Primary hyperparathyroidism (PHPT) is an uncommon disease in dogs and is rare in cats but must still be considered as a possible cause of hypercalcaemia, particularly in an older, relatively asymptomatic dog. PHPT develops when one or more of the parathyroid glands begin to function autonomously. Hyperparathyroidism is defined by hypercalcaemia in the face of inappropriately high concentrations of PTH (either above or within the reference interval).

In dogs, the Keeshond is the only breed in which PHPT is known to be inherited. The mode of inheritance was investigated by Goldstein *et al.* (2007) and by Skelly and Franklin (2007). Keeshonds have an autosomal dominant form of PHPT that has partial, age-dependent penetrance. This means that a Keeshond need only have one copy of the mutated allele to develop the disease, and those dogs carrying the mutation will go on to develop the disease if they live long enough. A genetic test is available for PHPT in the Keeshond but the mutation and the identity of the gene involved have not yet been published and the validity of the test is seemingly unproven. The test is available from Cornell University (https://ahdc.vet.cornell.edu/Sects/Molec/PHPTtesting.cfm).

Ultrasonography of the ventral neck is the most useful imaging modality when investigating parathyroid adenomas, with 90–95% positively identified by experienced imagers (Figure 8.18). The surgical appearance of a parathyroid nodule is shown in Figure 8.19.

Chronic renal failure: Chronic renal failure (CRF) is associated with phosphate retention caused by a decrease in renal phosphate excretion. Ionized calcium tends to fall as a consequence to allow the calcium/phosphate product to remain constant (the law of mass action). Rising phosphate inhibits 1-alpha hydroxylase, the enzyme that activates 25(OH)-vitamin D to 1,25(OH)$_2$-vitamin D, and calcium absorption through the gut is not enabled. In addition, the declining renal function means that ultimately 1-alpha hydroxylase production starts to fall (see Chapter 11 for further discussion of calcium metabolism in CRF). The results are that:

- Calcium balance shifts towards hypocalcaemia
- PTH production and secretion increase (*renal secondary hyperparathyroidism*).

Classification	Disease	tCa, iCa, PO$_4$	PTH	PTHrP	Vitamin D
Parathyroid gland overactivity	Primary hyperparathyroidism (parathyroid adenoma or hyperplasia, adenocarcinoma)	Mediated by elevated PTH tCa and iCa both elevated PO$_4$ low or low normal	PTH elevated	Normal	Normal though 1,25-dihydroxy-vitamin D may be elevated
	Chronic renal failure[a]	tCa may be mildly elevated due to increased complexed calcium (not via PTH) iCa usually normal but can be low or occasionally elevated PO$_4$ elevated	PTH elevated to counter effects of PO$_4$ suppression of vitamin D production	PTHrP may be elevated owing to reduced renal excretion	Normal to low owing to PO$_4$ inhibition of active vitamin D production
Parathyroid independent	Malignancy (lymphoma, anal sac adenocarcinoma, other carcinomas, thymoma, multiple myeloma, metastatic or primary bone neoplasia)	tCa and iCa elevated, PO$_4$ may be low or normal in PTHrP-driven hypercalcaemia, or elevated in metastatic or primary bone neoplasia	PTH normal or low	PTHrP may be elevated Not all tumours associated with hypercalcaemia produce PTHrP	
Vitamin D dependent	Iatrogenic (cod liver oil supplementation, etc) Plants (calcitriol glycosides found in nightshade, jessamine and other plants) Rodenticide toxicity (cholecalciferol) Anti-psoriasis creams (calcipotriol and calcipotriene)	tCa and iCa elevated PO$_4$ normal or elevated	Low PTH	Low PTHrP	Vitamin D may be measurably elevated depending on which form has been ingested
Granulomatous disease – dependent on local vitamin D production	Panniculitis Blastomycosis (rare in UK) Granulomatous lymphadenitis (steroid-responsive) Other granulomatous disease		PTH expected to be low	Elevated PTHrP in some cases (Fradkin et al., 2001)	Can be difficult to characterize owing to unknown aetiology of hypercalcaemia. Sometimes elevated vitamin D is implicated (Boag et al., 2005; Mellanby et al., 2006; LeBlanc et al., 2008)
Mechanism unknown	Hypoadrenocorticism (Addison's disease) Feline idiopathic hypercalcaemia (FIH)	Associated with no measurable changes in key molecules Total and ionized calcium increased	PTH lower half of reference range (Schenck et al., 2004)		

8.16 The differential diagnosis of hypercalcaemia and the mechanisms leading to an increase in calcium. [a] Chronic renal failure has been included here although it rarely causes hypercalcaemia. Parathyroid gland involvement occurs to counter the negative effects of phosphate on vitamin D production. iCa = ionized calcium; PO$_4$ = phosphate; PTH = parathyroid hormone; PTHrP = parathyroid hormone related peptide; tCa = total calcium.

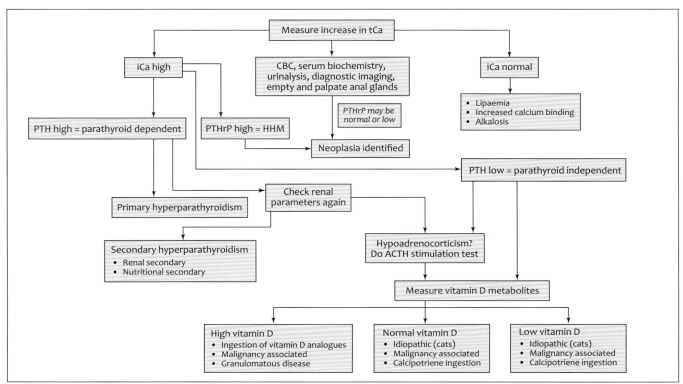

8.17 Algorithm illustrating the work-up of hypercalcaemia. ACTH = adrenocorticotropic hormone; CBC = complete blood count; iCa = ionized calcium; HHM = humoral hypercalcaemia of malignancy; PTH = parathyroid hormone; PTHrP = parathyroid hormone related peptide; tCa = total calcium.

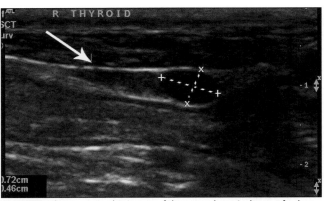

8.18 Ultrasonographic image of the ventral cervical area of a dog with primary hyperparathyroidism. A hypoechoic nodule (delineated by dotted lines) can be seen within the thyroid tissue (arrowed).

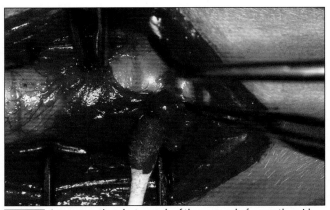

8.19 Intraoperative photograph of the removal of a parathyroid adenoma. The thyroid gland (dark red tissue) is visible overlying the trachea with a smaller, paler parathyroid gland associated (touching the cotton bud).
(Courtesy of E Friend)

This may initially correct the hypocalcaemia, but hyper-, normo- and hypocalcaemic states are possible in animals with chronic renal failure. Thus, renal failure is a condition in which calcium homeostasis is disrupted with consequences that may differ markedly among individuals.

When animals are found to be hypercalcaemic and in renal failure there is a poor correlation between total and ionized calcium, so it is important to assess the ionized calcium. Many animals with renal failure have elevated PTH levels, elevated total calcium but normal to low ionized calcium concentrations. More calcium is present in complexed form in these cases. Ionized hypercalcaemia occurs in the minority of cases of renal failure (9% in a study of 490 dogs; Schenck and Chew, 2005) but when it does occur there is a risk that it will worsen renal disease. In a small number of animals with CRF, PTH secretion becomes excessive as the set point for PTH changes (the parathyroid glands become less responsive to inhibition by elevated ionized calcium concentrations). This results in animals with CRF having both elevated ionized and total calcium concentrations alongside markedly elevated PTH levels. This situation is difficult to distinguish from primary hyperparathyroidism although more than one parathyroid gland would be expected to be enlarged and, in the face of severe renal compromise, phosphate concentrations would be elevated.

Hypoadrenocorticism and hyperadrenocorticism: The effects of steroids on calcium homeostasis are variable and difficult to understand mechanistically. A proportion of dogs (30%) with hypoadrenocorticism are concurrently hypercalcaemic, and hypercalcaemia has a cardioprotective role to prevent extreme bradycardia at high potassium concentrations (Peterson *et al.*, 1996; Gow *et al.*, 2009). The mechanism for hypercalcaemia is not mediated by PTH, PTHrP or vitamin D. Although frequently described as mild (total calcium <3.3 mmol/l), in this author's experience hypercalcaemia in hypoadrenocorticoid patients can be severe (total calcium >3.8 mmol/l), although it is completely reversible with appropriate treatment. Hypercalcaemia can also be a sign that patient stabilization is poor because it is the first electrolyte to show abnormalities in some patients (those patients that presented *initially* with hypercalcaemia).

Overproduction of steroid hormones can also disrupt calcium homeostasis and has been termed adrenal secondary hyperparathyroidism (Ramsey *et al.*, 2005). Most animals are normocalcaemic but occasionally mild hypercalcaemia can be documented.

Idiopathic feline hypercalcaemia: Unlike in dogs, where adequate investigation will almost always find a cause, hypercalcaemia in cats is frequently termed idiopathic. Idiopathic feline hypercalcaemia (IFH) was first recognized in the USA in the early 1990s (Midkiff *et al.*, 2000) but has subsequently been identified in the UK and other countries. Clinical signs range from subclinical disease, to weakness, weight loss and poor appetite. Cats can experience a benign disease course with several years of apparently clinically insignificant raised serum calcium, but some will progress to develop renal failure as a result of the condition (Midkiff *et al.*, 2000; Chew and Schenck, 2009). Serum phosphate is within the normal range in cats that do not have concurrent renal compromise. Urine specific gravity may also show good concentrating ability in the face of hypercalcaemia unless kidney function is impaired. Although IFH cases have been investigated using the standard diagnostic tests available (PTH, PTHrP, vitamin D) the syndrome remains elusive and the mechanism behind the calcium elevation unclear (Schenck *et al.*, 2004).

Vitamin D intoxication: The use of psoriasis creams containing vitamin D derivatives can lead to severe intoxication in dogs that ingest these creams either acutely, or who lick their owner's skin when they have been applied. Diagnosis is based on appropriate clinical pathological changes (total and ionized hypercalcaemia and hyperphosphataemia) resulting from increased gut absorption of calcium and particularly where there has been known exposure or access (see Case examples).

Another infrequently encountered example of hypercalcaemia caused by excess vitamin D can occur when owners supplement their dogs with cod liver oil or other vitamin D-rich supplements. Vitamin D-containing rodenticides, although less common than coumarin-based rodenticides, can cause intoxication and hypercalcaemia.

Granulomatous disease: The mechanism through which hypercalcaemia occurs in granulomatous disease is unclear but it is speculated that macrophages produce 1,25-dihydroxyvitamin D through a process of autonomous 1-alpha hydroxylase activity. This excess vitamin D can be measured within the circulation to assist with diagnosis. In humans this is a rare phenomenon, and the same is true in dogs (Mellanby *et al.*, 2006). It has been associated with fungal infections (e.g. blastomycosis, coccidioidomycosis), nodular panniculitis and granulomatous lymphadenitis in dogs. Three dogs were reported to be hypercalcaemic in association with *Angiostrongylus vasorum* infection and one was shown to have an elevated vitamin D metabolite concentration (Boag *et al.*, 2005). Cats have been reported to be hypercalcaemic in association with histoplasmosis, blastomycosis, cryptococcosis, actinomycosis, nocardiosis and atypical mycobacterial infections.

Hypocalcaemia

Clinical signs of hypocalcaemia

Mild hypocalcaemia is usually asymptomatic but when hypocalcaemia becomes severe (iCa <0.8 mmol/l, tCa <1.6–1.8 mmol/l) or when calcium concentrations have dropped precipitously, the following can be seen:

- Nervousness, panting, vocalization
- Focal muscle twitching
- Facial rubbing
- Muscle cramps, stiffness, tetany
- Seizures
- Elevated rectal temperature
- Cataract
- Tachyarrhythmias (rare).

All these clinical signs are induced or worsened by exercise and stress.

Causes of hypocalcaemia

The causes of, and mechanisms for, the development of hypocalcaemia are listed in Figure 8.20. An algorithm for the investigation of hypocalcaemia is shown in Figure 8.21.

One of the most common causes of hypocalcaemia is hypoalbuminaemia. This causes a decrease in total calcium but not ionized calcium, emphasizing the importance of measuring both, or concurrently checking albumin if ionized calcium is not readily available, when investigating disorders of calcium regulation.

Sample handling errors: Animals may be falsely identified as being hypocalcaemic when blood samples for calcium measurement become contaminated with potassium EDTA. This can happen when a syringe tip is allowed to touch the anticoagulant in an EDTA collection pot. The EDTA is then introduced into a serum tube where it chelates calcium, creating artificially low calcium, low ALP and high potassium.

A second way to lower serum calcium concentrations artificially is to give a blood transfusion where the collection bag is under-filled so that there is an excess of citrate in the transfused blood. Citrate chelates calcium and will result in the transfusion recipient being transiently hypocalcaemic. This rarely occurs in practice unless small volumes of blood are taken from donors into 500 ml collection bags.

Hypoparathyroidism: Primary idiopathic hypoparathyroidism is uncommon in dogs and rare in cats but is a cause of severe hypocalcaemia (<1.5 mmol/l) with an ionized fraction <0.8 mmol/l. The diagnosis of primary hypoparathyroidism is based on the following:

- Low total calcium
- Low ionized calcium
- Concurrent low PTH concentration – either below the reference interval (20–65 pg/ml in the dog) or in the lower part of the reference interval (<30 pg/ml), which is inappropriate in the face of hypocalcaemia. In cats, where the reference interval is <25 pg/ml, a low result would be in the range 0–5 pg/ml
- High reference interval or elevated phosphate concentration
- Normal renal function.

PTH increases calcium uptake in the kidney while also reducing phosphate loss. Thus, hyperphosphataemia is a feature of hypoparathyroidism.

Iatrogenic hypoparathyroidism: This is most commonly induced in cats after thyroidectomy for hyperthyroidism although currently recommended surgical techniques are designed to avoid this problem.

Acute and chronic renal failure: Calcium dysregulation in renal failure is discussed in the section on hypercalcaemia. The eventual outcome, whether hyper-, normo- or hypocalcaemia, is variable in each individual patient and is dependent on many factors including the degree of renal compromise, degree of parathyroid hyperplasia and the acid–base balance. Symptomatic hypocalcaemia is rare in chronic renal disease but may occur in ethylene

Disease	Mechanism	Characteristics
Hypoparathyroidism	Primary hypoparathyroidism (immune-mediated destruction of parathyroid glands)	Negligible PTH levels tCa and iCa both decreased PO$_4$ normal to mildly elevated
Acute renal failure	Acutely elevated phosphate complexes with calcium with concurrent tubular loss of calcium	Azotaemia Elevated phosphate concentrations
Chronic renal failure	Reduced production of 1,25(OH)$_2$-cholecalciferol	Azotaemia, high phosphate, isosthenuria, anaemia
Protein-losing enteropathies	Poor fat absorption leads to low vitamin D levels Hypoalbuminaemia means tCa is low Hypomagnesaemia leads to low PTH secretion	tCa low iCa decreased in severe cases PO$_4$ normal Vitamin D may be measurably low
Pancreatitis	Calcium thought to be sequestered in saponified fat around pancreas and other soft tissues	Low calcium recognized as negative prognostic indicator in cats
Postpartum hypocalcaemia (eclampsia)	Massive calcium requirements for fetal skeletal development and lactation Parathyroid dysfunction and diet may play roles	Commonly seen in young, small-breed dogs, 2 weeks post-whelping Low tCa and iCa
Sepsis and acute trauma	Multifactorial, involving inhibition or inactivation of vitamin D and PTH pathways	Low tCa and iCa recognized in critical care patients Other parameters variable

8.20 The differential diagnosis of hypocalcaemia and the mechanisms leading to a decrease in calcium. iCa = ionized calcium; PO$_4$ = phosphate; PTH = parathyroid hormone; tCa = total calcium.

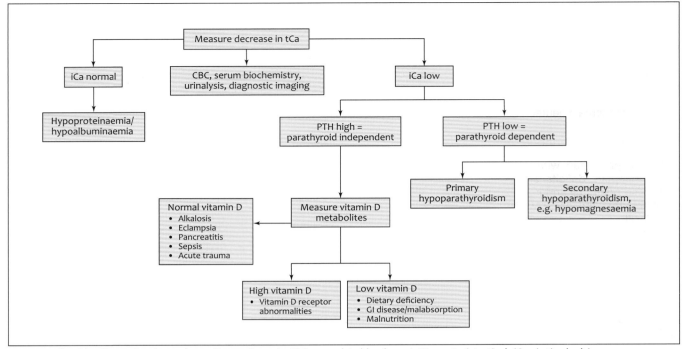

8.21 Algorithm illustrating the work-up of hypocalcaemia. CBC = complete blood count; GI = gastrointestinal; iCa = ionized calcium; PO$_4$ = phosphate; PTH = parathyroid hormone; tCa = total calcium.

glycol-induced acute renal failure where ethylene glycol is converted to oxalate, which forms complexes with calcium. Antifreeze also contains phosphate that causes hyperphosphataemia. If treatment for hypocalcaemia is required then the minimum amount of supplemental calcium should be used because supplementary calcium increases the risk of soft tissue mineralization in these patients.

Protein-losing enteropathy: In dogs or cats with protein-losing enteropathy, total calcium concentrations are expected to be low because of concurrent hypoalbuminaemia but in many cases ionized calcium is also significantly reduced (<1.0 mmol/l) because of reduced calcium uptake through the gut wall and low levels of vitamin D. Fat malabsorption is common in these patients and vitamin D is a fat-soluble vitamin, therefore vitamin D concentrations are also measurably reduced (Mellanby *et al.*, 2005). It is rare for animals to have symptomatic hypocalcaemia through this mechanism and calcium absorption can be seen to improve following improvement in the underlying disease. Vitamin D can be supplemented if there is concern that the ionized calcium is falling too much but this may not be therapeutically successful if the underlying gut disease is not addressed.

Functional hypoparathyroidism refers to a situation in which PTH synthesis and release are impaired by factors other than inherent parathyroid gland disease. It has been reported in dogs with low magnesium concentrations due to intestinal disease (Bush *et al.*, 2001). Hypoparathyroidism caused by severe hypomagnesaemia has been described in a dog that was also suffering from a protein-losing enteropathy. Magnesium is essential for parathyroid hormone synthesis and release.

Pancreatitis: Hypocalcaemia may result from pancreatitis (usually acute, severe) when calcium becomes sequestered in saponified peripancreatic fat or fat in adjacent soft tissues. Hypocalcaemia is reported equally frequently in cats with acute and chronic pancreatitis and is a negative prognostic indicator in this species (Kimmel *et al.*, 2001; Ferreri *et al.*, 2003).

Decreased calcium has also been documented in dogs with acute pancreatitis but appears to be much less common than in cats (Holowaychuk *et al.*, 2009).

Eclampsia or perparturient tetany: This syndrome is usually seen in young, small-breed dogs and is rare in cats. It occurs about 2 weeks post-whelping when lactation is at its peak and calcium requirements are at their highest in a bitch that has already suffered severe depletion of skeletal calcium stores during the ossification of the fetal skeletons.

Sepsis and critical care patients: Hypocalcaemia has been documented in veterinary patients with sepsis and following acute trauma (Holowaychuk *et al.*, 2009). Calcium concentrations are inversely correlated with the outcome and duration of hospitalization (Holowaychuk and Monteith, 2011). Many factors contribute to the development of hypocalcaemia in sepsis, including defects in the parathyroid–vitamin D axis. Similar mechanisms occur in individuals with acute severe illness and following trauma. Cats with urethral obstruction may have moderate to severe ionized hypocalcaemia although the need for calcium-specific therapy is not warranted in these patients and they respond to management directed at relieving the obstruction (Drobatz and Hughes, 1997).

Case examples

CASE 1

SIGNALMENT

13-year-old female neutered Domestic Longhair cat.

HISTORY

The cat presented with a history of hindlimb paresis, proprioceptive deficits and a plantigrade stance. She had also been dull and inappetent. Physical examination showed that the cat was depressed and weak with a grade III systolic heart murmur and significant muscle wasting.

CLINICAL PATHOLOGY DATA

Biochemistry	Result	Reference interval
Sodium (mmol/l)	**157.6**	135–155
Potassium (mmol/l)	**2.08**	3.6–4.5
Chloride (mmol/l)	111.2	104–123
Phosphate (mmol/l)	**1.57**	0.7–1.2
Creatinine (μmol/l)	131	45–150
Urea (mmol/l)	**14.6**	6.7–10.0
AST (IU/l)	**224**	0–32
CK (IU/l)	**13,979**	49–151

Abnormal results are in **bold**.

Haematology

Unremarkable.

Urinalysis	Result
Appearance	Clear, straw-coloured
Specific gravity	1.020
Dipstick	No significant findings

WHAT ABNORMALITIES ARE PRESENT?

There is a mild hypernatraemia and a severe hypokalaemia. The phosphate is mildly elevated along with urea. There are marked increases in the muscle-associated enzymes AST and CK.

WHAT ARE THE POSSIBLE CAUSES?

Chronic renal insufficiency is a common cause of hypokalaemia in the cat and this could also cause a mild hypernatraemia through mild dehydration caused by polyuria. However, although the urea is elevated, creatinine is within the reference range and this degree of hypokalaemia in the face of apparently normal renal

function or mild renal insufficiency would be unusual. Hypokalaemia can also be seen when animals are anorexic, and this cat had a reduced appetite but, again, the magnitude of the hypokalaemia is unexpected. The kidneys are responsible for potassium excretion so this clinical pathology picture could fit with enhanced renal potassium loss, perhaps mediated by an excess of aldosterone.

The elevated muscle enzymes are not unexpected given the history of muscle wastage and weakness.

WHAT FURTHER TESTS WOULD YOU PERFORM?

- Fractional excretion of potassium: in this cat the fractional excretion of potassium was 40%, where >6% in hypokalaemic animals indicates excessive renal loss.
- Fractional excretion of sodium: in this cat the functional excretion of sodium was 0.59% (<1% consistent with a prerenal azotaemia).
- Aldosterone assay: aldosterone >3300.0 pmol/l (0.0–960.0 pmol/l).

Imaging

Thoracic and abdominal radiographs, an abdominal ultrasound examination and an echocardiogram were carried out. A left adrenal mass was identified. The heart murmur was attributed to mild tricuspid regurgitation with no signs of cardiomyopathy.

Blood pressure measurement

Systolic blood pressure was normal at 160 mmHg.

DIAGNOSIS

Hyperaldosteronism (Conn's syndrome).

DISCUSSION

This cat is displaying criteria consistent with the diagnosis of hyperaldosteronism or Conn's syndrome in that she is hypokalaemic with high aldosterone levels and an adrenal mass. Unfortunately, renin was not measured in this case; this would have provided proof that aldosterone secretion was autonomous and not a result of volume depletion and subsequent renin release. This cat was not hypertensive at the time of the examination, nor did she have any signs of a hypertensive retinopathy but this would also have supported the diagnosis if found.

A left-sided, friable adrenal mass was removed. The mass was identified as an adrenal carcinoma. The cat's owners declined any further treatment although the possibility of tumour recurrence is quite high in this case. The cat remained stable without medication for several months after surgery until she was lost to follow-up.

CASE 2

SIGNALMENT

12-year-old female neutered Domestic Shorthair cat.

HISTORY

This cat was reported to have always been obsessed with water and had a history of polydipsia/polyuria (PD/PU) ever since she was first acquired as a kitten. This had been investigated through routine bloodwork but no specific reason was identified and she had lived relatively problem-free until she began to vomit and became dehydrated and depressed. Physical examination showed that the cat was dull and quiet. She was underweight with a large urinary bladder palpable. A thyroid goitre was palpable. No other significant abnormalities were found.

WHAT ARE YOUR DIFFERENTIAL DIAGNOSES?

Hyperthyroidism seemed likely in this cat given her age, weight and lack of other clinical findings. However, this does not explain why the cat was reported to have been obsessed with water throughout her life, so potentially this cat had more than one problem. Polydipsia can be caused by chronic renal insufficiency, endocrinopathy, e.g. diabetes mellitus, hypercalcaemia, liver disease, psychogenic polydipsia and central diabetes insipidus amongst other causes, but many of these diseases would not be compatible with the cat having lived for 12 years with almost no health problems. Routine blood tests were initially performed to rule in or out some of these major differentials.

CLINICAL PATHOLOGY DATA

Biochemistry	Result	Reference interval
Sodium (mmol/l)	**165**	135–155
Potassium (mmol/l)	3.9	3.8–5.6
Chloride (mmol/l)	**130**	110–127
Calcium (mmol/l)	2.33	2.0–2.7
Phosphate (mmol/l)	1.61	0.90–2.10
Creatinine (μmol/l)	107	56–153
Glucose (mmol/l)	4.5	3.9–5.8
Urea (mmol/l)	9.3	5.4–10.7
ALT (IU/l)	**80**	17–62

Abnormal results are in **bold**.

Haematology

Unremarkable.

Urinalysis	Result
Colour	Pale yellow
Specific gravity	**1.005**
pH	5.0
Protein	Trace
Glucose	Negative

Abnormal results are in **bold**.

Urinalysis *continued*	Result
Ketones	Negative
Blood	Negative
WBC	<5
RBC	<5
Sediment	Amorphous debris and occasional epithelial cell
Culture	No growth

Abnormal results are in **bold**.

Total thyroxine (T4): >90 nmol/l (19–65 nmol/l).

WHAT ABNORMALITIES ARE PRESENT?

The cat was moderately hypernatraemic and hyperchloraemic and also had mildly elevated alanine aminotransferase (ALT). The specific gravity of the urine was hyposthenuric, which is unusual in a cat; their urine is usually well into the hypersthenuric range.

WHAT ARE YOUR REVISED DIFFERENTIALS AND WHAT FURTHER INVESTIGATIONS WOULD YOU PERFORM?

Hyperthyroidism has been confirmed by the elevated T4 measurement. Renal failure has been ruled out but there is no obvious explanation for the hypernatraemia and hyperchloraemia with hyposthenuria. Hypernatraemia may develop as a result of pure water or hypotonic fluid loss, inadequate water intake (hypodipsia) or because of solute gain. The cat had no access to any salt-containing substances so salt poisoning was unlikely. Hypodipsia is ruled out owing to the marked polydipsia present. It seemed more likely, given the dilute urine, that water or hypotonic fluid losses were responsible and that these losses were renal rather than extrarenal. This left central or nephrogenic diabetes insipidus as the most likely diagnosis.

TREATMENT

The cat was sent home with treatment for hyperthyroidism with a view to reviewing the severity of the polydipsia once the hyperthyroidism had been brought under some degree of control. Hyperthyroidism is also a cause of polydipsia in the cat, so it would be difficult to look for another cause while the cat was hyperthyroid. The cat returned after 2 weeks. At this time there was still marked PD/PU and the hypernatraemia persisted.

FURTHER INVESTIGATIONS

* Repeat T4 measurement: 45 nmol/l (19–65 nmol/l).
* Imaging: no significant abnormalities.
* Systolic blood pressure: 130 mmHg.

Since the hyperthyroidism had now been controlled, and in the absence of renal and liver disease, hypercalcaemia or any other obvious cause of PD/PU, a modified water deprivation test was performed.

The urine specific gravity was monitored over 24 hours while restricting water access. It was not thought to be safe to do a full water deprivation test because the

→ CASE 2 CONTINUED

cat's water consumption exceeded 200 ml/kg/day. Urine output was also difficult to monitor as the cat urinated in its cage and not just in the litter tray. The aim was to reduce water intake to 200 ml/kg/day while monitoring specific gravity. This revealed that the cat was unable to concentrate her urine above a specific gravity of 1.005. During this time she lost weight, presumably due to dehydration. She could therefore not tolerate any degree of water deprivation, however mild. Treatment with desmopressin (DDAVP; given into the conjunctival sac) failed to raise the urine specific gravity above the hyposthenuric range even after continuing treatment for several days to allow for a degree of medullary washout inhibiting the response.

DIAGNOSIS

A diagnosis of concurrent hyperthyroidism and diabetes insipidus was made.

DISCUSSION

Diabetes insipidus in this cat could be central or nephrogenic and was apparently present from when the cat was first acquired at 9 weeks of age. The lack of response to desmopressin suggests that the diabetes insipidus is nephrogenic, though it could not be characterized further. Primary nephrogenic diabetes insipidus is extremely rare in domestic animals and in humans, though secondary nephrogenic diabetes insipidus can be caused by hypercalcaemia, hypokalaemia, endocrine diseases such as hyperadrenocorticism and some forms of renal disease. This cat did not have an obvious cause for ADH antagonism, nor did she seem to have inherent renal disease, although this was not investigated through renal biopsy. This is an unusual case that illustrates how loss of free water can lead to hypernatraemia in certain circumstances.

The cat went on to be treated with a thiazide diuretic along with treatment for hyperthyroidism but was eventually euthanased as she suffered more problems with dehydration and depression after showing gastrointestinal signs.

CASE 3

SIGNALMENT

3-year-old male neutered Jack Russell Terrier.

HISTORY

Presented with a history of chronic weight loss and being slightly less active than normal. The owner suffered from psoriasis and used a vitamin D-based cream (calcipotriol). The dog was known to enjoy licking the cream from the owner's legs. Physical examination was unremarkable. The anal sacs were normal on palpation and there was no lymphadenomegaly.

CLINICAL PATHOLOGY DATA

Biochemistry	Result	Reference interval
iCa (mmol/l)	**1.73**	1.18–1.40
tCa (mmol/l)	**3.94**	2.20–2.90
Phosphate (mmol/l)	**2.13**	0.80–1.73
Urea (mmol/l)	**43.7**	2.5–7.4
Creatinine (μmol/l)	**262**	34–136

Abnormal results are in **bold**.

Urinalysis	Result
Colour	Clear, straw-coloured
Specific gravity	1.020
Dipstick	No significant findings
Sediment examination	Calcium phosphate crystals

WHAT ARE THE ABNORMALITIES SHOWN BY THIS DOG?

The dog was severely hypercalcaemic (both total and ionized calcium were elevated) and was mildly hyperphosphataemic. He was azotaemic with a more pronounced elevation of urea than creatinine, suggesting a component of prerenal azotaemia.

WHAT ARE THE DIFFERENTIAL DIAGNOSES AND WHAT FURTHER INVESTIGATIONS WOULD YOU PERFORM?

Given the history of calcipotriol ingestion the most likely cause of the hypercalcaemia was vitamin D toxicosis. However, the amount of cream ingested was not known and it was also possible that the dog had primary hyperparathyroidism with secondary renal insufficiency or neoplasia. Hypoadrenocorticism (Addison's disease) was also a possibility, as was granulomatous disease of some sort although the site of this was not apparent.

FURTHER INVESTIGATIONS

Assessment of PTH/PTHrP

Parameter	Result	Reference interval
PTH (pg/ml)	**<16.2**	18–130
PTHrP (pmol/l)	<0.1	0.0–0.5

Abnormal results are in **bold**.

ACTH stimulation test

Parameter	Result	Reference interval
Basal cortisol (nmol/l)	102	<250
Cortisol post-ACTH (nmol/l)	150	<400–600

→ CASE 3 CONTINUED

Vitamin D

Parameter	Result	Reference interval
25(OH)-cholecalciferol (ng/ml)	20.4	8.0–60.0
1,25(OH)₂-cholecalciferol (pg/ml)	29	16–60

Survey radiographs and abdominal ultrasound examination

No abnormalities detected.

WHAT IS YOUR DIAGNOSIS?

Vitamin D intoxication with psoriasis cream (calcipotriol), with renal failure.

DISCUSSION

Calcipotriol is a synthetic vitamin D substance and is not detected using the routine assays for the two forms of vitamin D. This dog was severely hypercalcaemic but was also significantly azotaemic. Low PTHrP did not support a neoplastic cause of hypercalcaemia. The PTH result helped exclude primary hyperparathyroidism. Although a prerenal component seemed likely it was also possible that the kidneys had been damaged. The urine specific gravity showed that the dog was only able to concentrate its urine slightly above isothenuria, and some degree of renal damage was suspected; however, the extent of this was unclear at the point of diagnosis because both renal failure and hypercalcaemia affect concentrating ability.

TREATMENT

The dog was prevented from licking the owner's skin cream and was treated with aggressive fluid therapy. However, the urea and creatinine proved difficult to control, probably owing to the ongoing fluid loss through the kidney caused by hypercalcaemia antagonizing antidiuretic hormone (ADH). In addition he received:

- Gastroprotectants to help improve appetite in the face of azotaemia
- Clodronate capsules 200 mg orally
- Phosphate binder.

OUTCOME

The dog remained stable for 3 months although he suffered fluctuations in the degree of control of his hypercalcaemia. Appetite progressively became a problem as his azotaemia worsened and eventually he was euthanased owing to chronic renal failure.

CASE 4

SIGNALMENT

1-year-old male entire Miniature Poodle.

HISTORY

The dog was presented as an emergency with seizures, collapse, muscle twitching and skin bruising. The dog was collapsed, hyperaesthetic and had muscle twitching. He had petechial and ecchymotic haemorrhages in the oral cavity, on the tongue and hard palate. The rectal temperature was elevated.

CLINICAL PATHOLOGY DATA

Biochemistry	Result	Reference interval
iCa (mmol/l)	**0.75**	1.18–1.40
tCa (mmol/l)	**1.39**	2.20–2.90
Phosphate (mmol/l)	**2.15**	0.80–1.73
Urea (mmol/l)	**15.3**	2.5–7.4
Creatinine (µmol/l)	127	34–136

Abnormal results are in **bold**.

Haematology	Result	Reference interval
WBC (x 10⁹/l)	15.3	6.0–17.0
Neutrophils (x 10⁹/l)	**13.3**	3.0–11.5
Monocytes (x 10⁹/l)	0.3	0.2–1.5

Abnormal results are in **bold**.

Haematology *continued*	Result	Reference interval
Eosinophils (x 10⁹/l)	0.1	0.1–1.3
Basophils (x 10⁹/l)	0.0	0.0–0.5
RBC (x 10¹²/l)	6.3	5.5–8.5
Platelets (x 10⁹/l)	**7.0ᵃ**	175–500
Haematocrit (l/l)	0.44	0.35–0.50

ᵃ Examination of the blood smear confirmed the low platelet numbers with no clumping seen. Abnormal results are in **bold**.

Urinalysis	Result
Appearance	Clear, straw-coloured
Specific gravity	**1.013**
Dipstick	No significant findings
Microscopy	Unremarkable

Abnormal results are in **bold**.

WHAT ABNORMALITIES WERE PRESENT?

The dog had low total and ionized calcium. Calcium concentrations this low would be expected to lead to clinical signs. There was a mild hyperphosphataemia and mild elevation in urea, possibly reflecting a pre-renal azotaemia, but the urea could also reflect the fact that there was haemorrhage into the gastrointestinal tract. Low calcium alongside elevated phosphate in the face of normal renal function (creatinine was

→ **CASE 4 CONTINUED**

normal although urea was elevated) implies hypoparathyroidism. Many of the other differentials for hypocalcaemia (see Figure 8.20) were highly unlikely. Hypoparathyroidism may be caused by transient damage to the parathyroid glands during thyroid surgery, for example, or may be due to immune-mediated destruction of the glands. This latter cause would be expected to be permanent. Platelets were severely decreased in number but the haematocrit and all other haematological parameters were normal.

WHAT FURTHER TESTS WOULD BE INDICATED?

PTH should be measured to investigate possible hypoparathyroidism.

A coagulation panel should be performed to investigate the thrombocytopenia and haemorrhage, although thrombocytopenia rather than coagulopathies are most likely to cause the clinical signs seen in this case.

In addition, imaging of both body cavities should be carried out to rule out neoplasia, infectious or inflammatory diseases that may trigger an immune-mediated disease such as immune-mediated thrombocytopenia.

Assessment of PTH

Parameter	Result	Reference interval
PTH (pg/ml)	**<10.0**	10–60

Abnormal results are in **bold**.

Coagulation panel

Parameter	Result	Reference interval
Platelets (x 10⁹/l)	**7.0**[a]	175–500
OSPT (sec)	9.1	7.6–11.6
aPTT (sec)	14.3	12.5–25.0
D-dimer (ng/ml)	**500–1000**	<250–500

[a] The platelet count appeared low on the blood film. Sample checked for clots and film checked for clumps. Abnormal results are in **bold**.

Survey radiographs

No abnormalities detected.

WHAT WAS YOUR DIAGNOSIS?

Primary hypoparathyroidism with probable immune-mediated platelet destruction.

DISCUSSION

This dog presented with severe hypocalcaemia and hyperphosphataemia, which are compatible with hypoparathyroidism. Initially, ethylene glycol toxicity was considered as a possible differential but there was no supportive history and no monohydrate calcium oxalate crystals were found in the urine. Ethylene glycol toxicity typically leads to azotaemia alongside hypocalcaemia, but hypocalcaemia can be observed in the pre-azotaemic animal. The moderate increase in urea concentration with normal creatinine is likely to indicate a degree of dehydration (prerenal) as well as GI bleeding. The marked thrombocytopenia with normal coagulation times was thought to reflect immune-mediated thrombocytopenia. No other cell lines apart from platelets were affected so bone marrow aspiration or biopsy to investigate a lack of platelet production was not carried out.

This case is interesting in that the patient appeared to present with two immune-mediated diseases concurrently. Primary hypoparathyroidism is thought to be most commonly due to immune-mediated destruction of the parathyroid glands, although in most clinical cases this is not confirmed by biopsy and histological evaluation of the glands. Immune-mediated thrombocytopenia is a much more common manifestation of immune-mediated disease.

TREATMENT

Treatment was initiated using immunosuppressive doses of prednisolone and ciclosporin, vitamin D and intravenous, followed by oral, calcium supplementation.

PROBLEMS

The major problem in this case was trying to balance calcium supplementation with the calciuretic effects of steroid therapy. This was anticipated and was the reason for using ciclosporin as an additional immunosuppressive agent from the outset. This dog's steroid dose was tapered quickly (over 2 weeks) and thereafter immunosuppression was achieved through use of ciclosporin only. The dog recovered well and is currently stable on vitamin D alone.

References and further reading

Adrogue HJ and Madias NE (2000) Hypernatraemia. *New England Journal of Medicine* **324**, 1493–1499

Baylis PH (2003) The syndrome of inappropriate antidiuretic hormone secretion. *International Journal of Biochemistry and Cell Biology* **35**, 1495–1499

Boag AK, Murphy KF and Connolly DJ (2005) Hypercalcaemia associated with *Angiostrongylus vasorum* in three dogs. *Journal of Small Animal Practice* **46**, 79–84

Brofman PJ, Knostman KA and DiBartola SP (2003) Granulomatous amebic meningoencephalitis causing the syndrome of inappropriate secretion of antidiuretic hormone in a dog. *Journal of Veterinary Internal Medicine* **17**, 230–234

Brown EA, Markandu ND, Roulston JE, Jones BE, Squires M and Macgregor GA (1982) Is the renin-angiotensin-aldosterone system involved in the sodium retention in the nephrotic syndrome? *Nephron* **32**, 102–107

Bush WW, Kimmel SE, Wosar MA and Jackson MW (2001) Secondary hypoparathyroidism attributed to hypomagnesemia in a dog with protein-losing enteropathy. *Journal of the American Veterinary Medical Association* **15**, 1732–1734

Chew DJ and Schenck PA (2009) Idiopathic feline hypercalcaemia. In: *Kirk's Current Veterinary Therapy XIV*, ed. JD Bonagura and JD Twedt, pp. 236–241. Saunders Elsevier, St. Louis, Missouri

Dhupa N and Proulx J (1998) Hypocalcaemia and hypomagnesaemia. *Veterinary Clinics of North America: Small Animal Practice* **28**, 587–608

DiBartola SP (2000) *Fluid Therapy in Small Animal Practice*, 2nd edn. WB Saunders, Philadelphia

DiBartola SP, Buffington C, Chew D, Mcloughlin MA and Sparks RA (1993) Development of chronic renal disease in cats fed a commercial diet. *Journal of the American Veterinary Medical Association* **202**, 744–751

DiBartola SP, Johnson SE, Davenport DJ, Prueter JC, Chew DJ and Sherding RG (1985) Clinicopathologic findings resembling hypoadrenocorticism in dogs with primary gastrointestinal disease. *Journal of the American Veterinary Medical Association* **187**, 60–63

Djajadiningrat-Laanan S, Galac S and Kooistra H (2011) Primary hyperaldosteronism: expanding the diagnostic net. *Journal of Feline Medicine and Surgery* **13**, 641-650

Drobatz KJ and Hughes D (1997) Concentration of ionized calcium in plasma from cats with urethral obstruction. *Journal of the American Veterinary Medical Association* **211**, 1392–1395

Ferreri JA, Hardam E, Kimmel SE *et al.* (2003) Clinical differentiation of acute necrotizing from chronic nonsuppurative pancreatitis in cats: 63 cases (1996–2001). *Journal of the American Veterinary Medical Association* **223**, 469–474

Fradkin JM, Braniecki AM, Craig TM, Ramiro-Ibanez F, Rogers KS and Zoran DL (2001) Elevated parathyroid hormone-related protein and hypercalcaemia in two dogs with schistosomiasis. *Journal of the American Animal Hospital Association* **37**, 349–355

Goldkamp C and Schaer M (2007) Hypernatremia in dogs. *Compendium on Continuing Education for the Practicing Veterinarian* **29**, 148–161

Goldstein RE, Atwater DZ, Cazolli DM, Goldstein O, Wade CM and Lindblad-Toh K (2007) Inheritance, mode of inheritance, and candidate genes for primary hyperparathyroidism in Keeshonden. *Journal of Veterinary Internal Medicine* **21**, 199–203

Gow AG, Gow DJ, Bell R *et al.* (2009) Calcium metabolism in eight dogs with hypoadrenocorticism. *Journal of Small Animal Practice* **50**, 426–430

Graves TK, Schall WD, Refsal K and Nachreiner RF (1994) Basal and ACTH-stimulated plasma aldosterone concentrations are normal or increased in dogs with *Trichuris*-associated pseudohypoadrenocorticism. *Journal of Veterinary Internal Medicine* **8**, 287–289

Hodson S (1998) Feline hypokalaemia. *In Practice* **20**, 135–144

Holowaychuk MK, Hansen BD, Defrancesco TC and Marks SL (2009) Ionized hypocalcemia in critically ill dogs. *Journal of Veterinary Internal Medicine* **23**, 509–513

Holowaychuk MK and Monteith G (2011) Ionized hypocalcemia as a prognostic indicator in dogs following trauma. *Journal of Veterinary Emergency and Critical Care* **21**, 521–530

Jeffery ND, Watson PJ, Abramson C and Notenboom A (2003) Brain malformations associated with primary adipsia identified using magnetic resonance imaging. *Veterinary Record* **152**, 436–438

Jones BR (2000) Hypokalaemic myopathy in cats. In: *Kirk's Current Veterinary Therapy XIII*, ed. J Bonagura, pp. 985–987. WB Saunders, Philadelphia

Kasai CM and King R (2009) Hypernatremia. *Compendium on Continuing Education for the Practicing Veterinarian* **31**, E1-6

Khanna C, Boermans HJ and Wilcock B (1997) Fatal hypernatremia in a dog from salt ingestion. Journal of American Animal Hospital Association, **33(2)**, 113–122

Kimmel SE, Washabau RJ and Drobatz KJ (2001) Incidence and prognostic value of low plasma ionized calcium concentration in cats with acute pancreatitis: 46 cases (1996–1998). *Journal of the American Veterinary Medical Association* **219**, 1105–1109

Kreissler JJ and Langston CE (2011) A case of hyporeninemic hypoaldosteronism in the dog. *Journal of Veterinary Internal Medicine* **25**, 944–948

LeBlanc CJ, Echandi RL, Moore RR, Souza C and Grooters AM (2008) Hypercalcaemia associated with gastric pythiosis in a dog. *Veterinary Clinical Pathology* **37**, 115–120

Lobetti RG (1998) Hyperreninaemic hypoaldosteronism in a dog. *Journal of the South African Veterinary Associ*ation **69**, 33–35

Luzius H, Jans DA, Grunbaum EG, Moritz A, Rascher W and Fahrenholz F (1992) A low affinity vasopressin V2-receptor in inherited nephrogenic diabetes insipidus. *Journal of Receptor Research* **12**, 351–368

Mackay BM and Curtis N (1999) Adipsia and hypernatraemia in a dog with focal hypothalamic granulomatous meningoencephalitis. *Australian Veterinary Journal* **77**, 14–17

Martin L (1998) Hypercalcaemia and hypermagnesaemia. *Veterinary Clinics of North America: Small Animal Practice* **28**, 565–585

Mellanby RJ, Mellor PJ, Roulois A *et al.* (2005) Hypocalcaemia associated with low serum vitamin D metabolite concentrations in two dogs with protein-losing enteropathies. *Journal of Small Animal Practice* **46**, 345–351

Mellanby RJ, Mellor P, Villiers EJ *et al.* (2006) Hypercalcaemia associated with granulomatous lymphadenitis and elevated 1,25 dihydroxyvitamin D concentration in a dog. *Journal of Small Animal Practice* **47**, 207–212

Midkiff AM, Chew DJ, Randolph JF, Center SA and DiBartola SP (2000) Idiopathic hypercalcaemia in cats. *Journal of Veterinary Internal Medicine* **14**, 619–626

Peterson ME, Kintzer PP and Kass PH (1996) Pretreatment clinical and laboratory findings in dogs with hypoadrenocorticism: 225 cases (1979–1993). *Journal of the American Veterinary Medical Association* **208**, 85–91

Pouzot C, Descone-Junot C and Loup J (2007) Successful treatment of severe salt intoxication in a dog. *Journal of Veterinary Emergency and Critical Care* **17**, 294–298

Ramsey IK, Tebb A, Harris E, Evans H and Herrtage ME (2005) Hyperparathyroidism in dogs with hyperadrenocorticism. *Journal of Small Animal Practice* **46**, 531–536

Ross LA (1990) Disorders of serum sodium concentration: diagnosis and therapy. *Compendium on Continuing Education for the Practicing Veterinarian* **12**, 1277–1289

Rubin SI (1995) Management of fluid and electrolyte disorders in uraemia. In: *Kirk's Current Veterinary Therapy XII*, ed. J Bonagura, pp. 951–955. WB Saunders, Philadelphia

Sadek D and Schaer M (1996) Atypical Addison's disease in the dog: a retrospective survey of 14 cases. *Journal of the American Animal Hospital Association* **32**, 159–163

Schaefer C and Goldstein RE (2009) Canine primary hyperparathyroidism. *Compendium on Continuing Education for the Practicing Veterinarian* **31**, 382–389

Schaer M, Halling KB, Collins KE and Grant DC (2001) Combined hyponatraemia and hyperkalaemia mimicking acute hypoadrenocorticism in three pregnant dogs. *Journal of the American Veterinary Medical Association* **15**, 897–899

Schenck PA and Chew DJ (2005) Prediction of serum ionised calcium concentration by serum total calcium measurement in dogs. *American Journal of Veterinary Research* **66**, 1330–1336

Schenck PA, Chew DJ, Refsal K, Nachreiner R and Rick M (2004) Calcium metabolic hormones in feline idiopathic hypercalcaemia. *Journal of Veterinary Internal Medicine* **18**, 442

Shiel RE, Pinilla M and Mooney CT (2009) Syndrome of inappropriate antidiuretic hormone secretion associated with congenital hydrocephalus in a dog. *Journal of the American Animal Hospital Association* **45(5)**, 249–252

Skelly BJ and Franklin RJM (2007) Mutations in genes causing human familial isolated hyperparathyroidism do not account for hyperparathyroidism in Keeshond dogs. *The Veterinary Journal* **174**, 652–654

Willard MD, Fossum TW, Torrance A and Lippert A (1991) Hyponatraemia and hyperkalaemia associated with idiopathic or experimentally induced chylothorax in four dogs. *Journal of the American Veterinary Medical Association* **199**, 353–358

Wysolmerski JJ and Broadus AE (1994) Hypercalcemia of malignancy: the central role of parathyroid hormone-related protein. *Annual Review of Medicine* **45**, 189–200

Chapter 9

Blood gas analysis and acid–base disorders

Derek Flaherty and Laura Blackwood

Acid–base disturbances are common, and can have a significant impact on patient morbidity and mortality if unrecognized or if treated inappropriately. Blood gas analysis can be used to assess a patient's acid–base status and also the oxygenation of the blood. While blood gas analysis can identify the presence of these disturbances, a reasonable understanding of the underlying pathophysiology is required to manage the case adequately. Unfortunately, much of the published work on blood gas analysis is based on human sampling. The differences between normal values in small animals and humans also mean that some of the definitions used in human medicine fit awkwardly when applied to animals. For example, acidaemia is often defined as a blood pH <7.35, but many reference intervals for cats extend into this range. However, the principles applied in human medicine have been applied to small animals for decades now and, while it is likely that some of the detailed data reported in the literature are unsuitable for direct transfer to animal patients, the principles of interpretation provide useful guidelines. As for any other analyte, the reference interval should be established for each system.

This chapter will give an overview and basic guidance on blood gas analysis, but it is only with regular assessment of blood gas samples that the clinician is likely to become competent in their interpretation. Complex acid–base disorders will not be covered in detail in this chapter; the interested reader is referred to the References and further reading section. The abbreviations and terminology used in the chapter are summarized in Figure 9.1.

Term (units)	Definition
A	Alveolar
a	Arterial
A^- (mmol/l)	Anion (of a weak acid buffer pair)
AG (mmol/l)	Anion gap
BE	Base excess. Amount of acid, in mmol/l, required to return 1 litre of blood to a pH of 7.4 at a P_aCO_2 of 40 mmHg (5.3 kPa)
F_iO_2 (% or decimal of 1)	Fraction of inspired oxygen; e.g. room air has an F_iO_2 of 21% or 0.21
H^+	Hydrogen ion
$[H^+]$ (nmol/l)	Hydrogen ion concentration
HA	Weak acid

9.1 Abbreviations and terminology used in blood gas analysis. (continues) ▶

Term (units)	Definition
HCO_3^-	Bicarbonate ion
H_2CO_3	Carbonic acid
kPa	kilopascal: SI unit of pressure: 1 kPa = 7.52 mmHg (strictly speaking, it is the Pascal (Pa) that is the SI unit)
mEq/l	Milliequivalents per litre
mmHg	Millimetres of mercury; commonly used unit of pressure
P or p	Pressure (or partial pressure: the term partial pressure refers to the fact that the total pressure is due to a combination of gases)
$P_{(A-a)}O_2$ (mmHg or kPa)	Alveolar–arterial oxygen gradient, i.e. difference between calculated alveolar P_AO_2 and measured arterial P_aO_2
P_aCO_2 (mmHg or kPa)	Partial pressure of carbon dioxide in arterial blood
P_aO_2 (mmHg or kPa)	Partial pressure of oxygen in arterial blood
P_B (mmHg or kPa)	Barometric pressure
P_{H_2O} (mmHg or kPa)	Saturated vapour pressure of water
pK	Negative log of the dissociation constant; pH at which the concentrations of the ionized $[A^-]$ and unionized forms $[HA]$ are the same
P_vCO_2 (mmHg or kPa)	Partial pressure of carbon dioxide in venous blood
P_vO_2 (mmHg or kPa)	Partial pressure of oxygen in venous blood
RQ	Respiratory quotient (ratio of CO_2 exhaled to O_2 uptake). Nominal value = 0.8
S_aO_2 (%)	Saturation of haemoglobin with oxygen in arterial blood
S_pO_2 (%)	Saturation of haemoglobin with oxygen in arterial blood measured by pulse oximetry
V/Q	Ventilation–perfusion

9.1 (continued) Abbreviations and terminology used in blood gas analysis.

pH scale

The concentration of hydrogen ions ($[H^+]$) in the body is tightly controlled within a relatively narrow range of approximately 35–45 nmol/l. These tiny concentrations are awkward to work with clinically and it is more common to discuss the negative logarithm (base 10) of the H^+ concentration, i.e. the pH. However, in human medicine there has been some movement away from considering the pH and reverting back to considering the [H⁺], although at the moment most veterinary surgeons (veterinarians) tend to evaluate pH as opposed to [H⁺] *per se*.

- $pH = -\log_{10}[H^+]$.
- pH changes in the opposite direction to [H⁺]: reductions in [H⁺] lead to an increase in pH and *vice versa*.
- Because of the logarithmic scale, the changes in [H⁺] required to produce any given numerical change in pH vary at different pH values. For example, twice as many H⁺ ions are needed to change the pH from 7.5 to 7.4 as are needed to change it from 7.8 to 7.7. This means that changes in pH in acidaemic (usually defined as blood pH <7.35) animals can reflect large deviations from normal [H⁺]. Around the normal range a change of 1 nmol/l of H⁺ equates to 0.01 pH unit.

Buffering

Chemical reactions within the body produce hydrogen ions that would rapidly lead to alterations in pH incompatible with life if they were allowed to accumulate. The rate of production of H⁺ is too rapid for elimination from the body to keep pace, and *buffering* must come in to play. *Buffers* are combinations of weak acids with their 'conjugate bases'. If [H⁺] in the body starts to rise, the conjugate base can 'mop up' this excess, limiting the effect on pH. Similarly, if [H⁺] starts to drop, more weak acid can dissociate to raise the [H⁺] back towards normal.

Many different buffers exist within the body, in the intracellular fluid (ICF) and extracellular fluid (ECF) and in bone. Acutely, buffering in the ECF is most important, because it takes hours for the H⁺ load to be distributed throughout the body and for intracellular buffers to be activated. The most important buffering system is the carbonic acid (H_2CO_3)–bicarbonate (HCO_3^-) system in the ECF:

$$CO_2 + H_2O \rightleftharpoons H_2CO_3 \rightleftharpoons H^+ + HCO_3^-$$

The significance of this particular system lies in the fact that, unlike most other buffers, saturation does not occur because the end products (CO_2, water, H⁺ and HCO_3^-) are dissipated by pulmonary (CO_2) or renal routes. The pulmonary capacity to excrete CO_2 is enormous. In addition, virtually total resorption or massive excretion of HCO_3^- can occur in the kidney in response to alterations in plasma HCO_3^-. For both these reasons, the buffering potential is huge compared with that of other weak acids found in the ECF and ICF.

The H_2CO_3–HCO_3^- system links the respiratory and renal responses to changes in H⁺, which are vital for buffering purposes:

- Respiratory response: increased free H⁺ ions, reduced ECF pH, hypercapnia (an increase in PCO_2, also called hypercarbia) and hypoxaemia all stimulate ventilation. Healthy patients can excrete a great deal of CO_2. In normal lungs, the limit to CO_2 excretion is the availability of HCO_3^-
- Renal response: the kidney excretes H⁺, and also effectively regenerates the HCO_3^- supply, thus allowing buffering to continue. Renal control of plasma HCO_3^- is mediated by control of HCO_3^- resorption, and titratable acid and ammonium excretion.

The respiratory and renal responses are effectively yoked together in a continuum. If CO_2 levels within the body increase, the equation above will push to the right and the excess H⁺ (and HCO_3^-) produced can then be eliminated by the kidneys. If H⁺ concentrations rise, the equation will move to the left, generating extra CO_2, which can be eliminated via the lungs. This reaction is not limited by HCO_3^- because of the large quantities of HCO_3^- in the ECF, and also the tremendous capacity of the kidney to reabsorb and regenerate HCO_3^- as required. This is an oversimplification of what occurs *in vivo*, but gives some idea of the importance of the H_2CO_3–HCO_3^- system.

The Henderson–Hasselbalch equation relates pH, H_2CO_3 and HCO_3^- for the H_2CO_3–HCO_3^- system. The derivation of this equation (Figure 9.2) illustrates one of the most important points in acid–base physiology: provided the *ratio* of HCO_3^- to CO_2 remains at its usual value of approximately 20:1, the pH will be normal regardless of any deviation from normal in the *individual* HCO_3^- and CO_2 values. This concept is important when trying to calculate the appropriate compensatory responses for an acid–base disturbance (see below).

Derivation of the Henderson–Hasselbalch equation
$pH = -\log_{10}[H^+]$
For any weak acid, the ionization equilibrium can be expressed as: $HA \rightleftharpoons H^+ + A^-$
K is the equilibrium constant (or ionization constant) for this reaction and is defined as: $K = [H^+][A^-]/[HA]$
Rearranging this equation gives: $[H^+] = K[HA]/[A^-]$
If we express this in log form: $-\log_{10}[H^+] = -\log_{10}K + \log_{10}([A^-]/[HA])$
$-\log_{10}K = pK_a$ (the pH at which the concentrations of the ionized [A⁻] and unionized forms [HA] are the same, i.e. when the reaction is evenly balanced)
Thus: $pH = pK_a + \log_{10}([A^-]/[HA])$.
This is the Henderson–Hasselbalch equation

For carbonic acid in the bicarbonate buffering system:	
$pH = pK_a + \log_{10}([HCO_3^-]/[H_2CO_3])$ $pH = 6.1 + \log_{10}([HCO_3^-]/(0.225 \times P_aCO_2))$	(pK_a of carbonic acid = 6.1) The concentration of H_2CO_3 depends upon the dissolved CO_2, which depends upon the PCO_2. Most carbonic acid in the body exists as dissolved CO_2 and 0.225 is the solubility coefficient of CO_2 in blood in ml/kPa
$pH = 6.1 + \log_{10}(24/(0.225 \times 5.3))$	Mean [HCO_3^-] in arterial blood is 24 mmol/l, while mean P_aCO_2 is 5.3 kPa (human values)
$pH = 6.1 + \log_{10}(24/1.1925)$ $pH = 6.1 + 1.3$ $pH = 7.4$	7.4 is the midpoint of the normal pH range of body fluids

9.2 Derivation of the Henderson–Hasselbalch equation.

Blood gas analysis

A blood gas analyser will directly measure pH, PCO_2 (partial pressure of CO_2) and PO_2 (partial pressure of oxygen) in the sample, and will derive values for HCO_3^- and base excess, based on standard nomograms. In addition, most of the current analysers will also provide values for electrolytes, while some also report ionized calcium and lactate.

A variety of different analysers are now available and widely used in veterinary practice, but it is important to note that not all of them have had their accuracy confirmed for companion animal use. Much of the choice in selecting an analyser (in addition to confirming that appropriate validation has been performed for the species in which it is to be used) is based on personal preference of the clinician, but they can be generally split into larger bench-top analysers (Figure 9.3) and hand-held analysers (Figure 9.4ab). Both types of analyser have advantages and disadvantages. Hand-held analysers are truly 'point-of-care' because they can be used 'kennel side'; however, this ease of transport also makes them potentially more liable to damage during movement. Conversely, benchtop analysers are of sufficient size that they are generally relatively immobile where they are positioned, which necessitates the clinician having to take samples to the machine for analysis. However, their greater size means they are generally 'sturdier' than some hand-held analysers and this, combined with the lower likelihood of them being moved from place to place, suggests that they are potentially less likely to sustain damage.

Arterial samples are essential for assessment of respiratory function, but either venous or arterial samples can provide useful information on the animal's metabolic status. When collecting arterial blood samples:

- In dogs, arterial samples may be drawn from the dorsal pedal artery (Figure 9.5) or the femoral artery in conscious dogs, or from the central auricular, lingual or coccygeal arteries in anaesthetized dogs

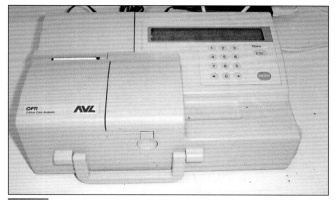

9.3 Benchtop blood gas analyser.

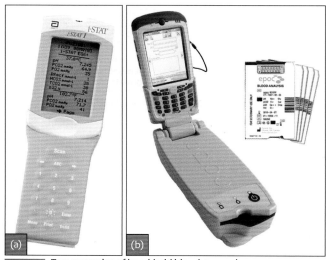

9.4 Two examples of hand-held blood gas analysers.
(Courtesy of Woodley Equipment Company Limited)

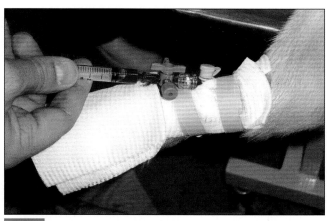

9.5 Sampling for blood gas analysis from the dorsal pedal artery.

- In cats, the femoral artery is generally the most suitable in conscious patients, but the dorsal pedal and coccygeal arteries may also be accessible in anaesthetized cats
- After sampling, pressure must be applied for an adequate period of time (5 minutes) to prevent haematoma formation
- Heparin is the standard anticoagulant for blood gas analysis
- Heparin sodium (1000 IU/ml) can be aspirated by syringe from a vial in a sterile manner, using a 23 or 25 G needle, until the syringe barrel is filled, and then the excess is expelled; this preloaded 1 or 2 ml syringe is used to collect the sample. The syringe should be 50–100% full after sampling. Too much heparin can cause a drop in P_aCO_2 (and in calculated HCO_3^-)
- Alternatively, pre-heparinized blood-gas syringes can be purchased, which ensures there is no anticoagulant excess
- Samples for blood gas analysis must be stored anaerobically, with no air/vacuum space adjacent to the blood sample into which CO_2 or O_2 could evaporate
- Commonly, samples are obtained in an anticoagulant-treated syringe and, after sampling, the syringe is capped with a rubber bung or plastic cap
- Alternatively, the needle may be bent over to form a seal, but this is less effective and more dangerous.

The sample is introduced to the blood gas analyser directly from the syringe. Transferring blood to a tube will alter gas pressures, and exchange will occur between the blood and air trapped in the tube with it. In order to minimize changes in blood gas concentrations as a result of continued cell metabolism, samples should ideally be processed immediately, but there are likely to be minimal changes in the values obtained provided analysis occurs within 10 minutes; if analysis is likely to be delayed beyond this point, the sample should be placed on ice and analysis performed within a maximum of 1 hour. Less than 200 μl of fresh whole blood or heparinized whole blood is required for hand-held analysers, and traditional (benchtop) analysers also require only small volumes of blood.

Blood gas analysers routinely analyse samples at 37°C, but some units have facilities for entry of the actual patient temperature and correction of output to allow for alterations from 37°C if the animal is either hypo- or hyperthermic, because temperature deviations affect blood solubility of both O_2 and CO_2. There is controversy over whether to 'correct' blood gases for patient temperature (i.e. input the actual patient temperature into the analyser and allow it to modify the results to account for the deviation in temperature away from 37°C), or to ignore the effect of the patient's body temperature and allow the machine to produce results for 37°C, regardless of the animal's actual temperature. Currently, the preference in humans is to ignore the effects of body temperature and use 'uncorrected results'.

Reported normal values for arterial and venous blood gases are summarized in Figure 9.6.

pH

The normal pH value of blood is approximately 7.35–7.45, although reference intervals for small animals sometimes include values slightly outside this range (Figure 9.6).

- **Acidaemia** refers to a pH value <7.35 (7.36 in some texts).
- **Alkalaemia** refers to a pH >7.45 (7.44 in some texts).
- The terms **acidosis** and **alkalosis** refer to the processes that occur at a cellular level, which may give rise to an acidaemia or alkalaemia if left uncompensated.

As a general rule, pH values of ≤7.0 and ≥7.65 are immediately life-threatening. Specific treatment of the acid–base disorder may be required if the pH is <7.2 or >7.6, but treatment of the underlying disease is most important for correction of acid–base disturbances.

Units for blood gas measurements

Two different units are in common use in relation to blood gases (O_2 and CO_2): mmHg and kPa. Although the SI unit for pressure measurement is the Pascal (Pa), many clinicians (particularly in North America, but also, not uncommonly, in the UK) continue to use the older unit mmHg. It is therefore common to see either unit used in relation to blood gas values. The relationship between the two is that 1 kPa = 7.52 mmHg.

P_aCO_2

P_aCO_2 values (the subscript 'a' signifies an arterial sample; 'v' signifies venous) indicate the ability of alveolar ventilation to remove the CO_2 produced by the body. P_aCO_2 is directly proportional to the rate of CO_2 production and inversely proportional to alveolar ventilation; i.e. if alveolar minute ventilation were to decrease by 50% without any change in CO_2 production, the P_aCO_2 would double. Measurement of P_aCO_2 is considered the 'gold standard' for assessing adequacy of ventilation in any patient. Many

clinicians use a working range of 35–45 mmHg in dogs (the reference range in humans) and, based on this, P_aCO_2 values <35 mmHg (<4.65 kPa) indicate *hyperventilation*, while values >45 mmHg (>5.98 kPa) indicate *hypoventilation*. However, the reported canine normal range is actually lower than this (30.8–42.8 mmHg, 4.10–5.69 kPa), and cats tend to have lower values again (25.2–36.8 mmHg, 3.35–4.89 kPa) (see Figure 9.6).

Normal P_vCO_2 is higher than P_aCO_2, with reported reference values of approximately 33–41 mmHg (4.47–5.48 kPa) in dogs and 33–45 mmHg (4.35–5.94 kPa) in cats. As a rough guide for an individual animal, P_vCO_2 is normally approximately 6 mmHg (~0.8 kPa) higher than P_aCO_2, although this can be affected by a number of factors.

P_aO_2

P_aO_2 values indicate the ability of the lungs to oxygenate blood. However, the P_aO_2 can only be interpreted in light of the P_AO_2 (alveolar partial pressure of oxygen), which, in turn, is based on the fraction of oxygen in the inspired air, according to the alveolar gas equation:

$$P_AO_2 = F_iO_2 (P_B - P_{H_2O}) - \frac{P_aCO_2}{0.8}$$

where:

- F_iO_2 is the fractional inspired oxygen concentration (e.g. F_iO_2 is 0.21 for room air (21% O_2) or 1.0 for 100% O_2)
- P_B is barometric pressure
- P_{H_2O} is the saturated vapour pressure of water (47 mmHg (~6.25 kPa) at normal body temperature)
- 0.8 is the respiratory quotient (RQ). The RQ is the ratio of CO_2 exhaled to O_2 uptake and is assumed to be 0.8. (Some variation in RQ occurs depending on diet, as a consequence of nitrogen excretion, but this is generally not clinically significant.)

Once the P_AO_2 has been calculated from the above equation, it can then be compared with the P_aO_2 value from the arterial blood sample. The arithmetic difference between the two is known as the alveolar–arterial oxygen difference or gradient, and is signified by $P_{(A-a)}O_2$. In normal patients breathing room air, the upper limit of normality for $P_{(A-a)}O_2$ is approximately 25 mmHg (3.3 kPa), although this can rise to around 120 mmHg (16.0 kPa) in patients breathing 100% oxygen. Calculation of the alveolar–arterial oxygen difference can be used to help assess the contribution of hypoventilation to hypoxaemia: the $P_{(A-a)}O_2$ will be normal if the low O_2 is solely due to increased P_aCO_2 (i.e. hypoventilation), but will increase with other causes of impaired oxygenation.

Parameter	Dogs		Cats	
	Arterial blood	*Venous blood*	*Arterial blood*	*Venous blood*
pH	7.35–7.46	7.35–7.44	7.31–7.46	7.28–7.41
PCO_2	30.8–42.8 mmHg 4.10–5.69 kPa	33.6–41.2 mmHg 4.47–5.48 kPa	25.2–36.8 mmHg 3.35–4.89 kPa	32.7–44.7 mmHg 4.35–5.94 kPa
PO_2 (room air)	80.9–103.3 mmHg 10.76–13.74 kPa	47.9–56.3 mmHg 6.37–7.49 kPa	95.4–118.2 mmHg 12.69–15.72 kPa	27–50 mmHg 3.59–6.65 kPa
HCO_3^-	18.8–25.6 mmol/l	20.8–24.2 mmol/l	14.4–21.6 mmol/l	18.0–23.2 mmol/l
Base excess	0 ± 4	0 ± 4	0 ± 4	0 ± 4

9.6 Approximate normal arterial and venous blood gas values for dogs and cats. The accepted SI unit for gas pressure is the Pascal, but many clinicians still use the older unit of mmHg. 1 kPa = 7.52 mmHg.
(Data from Zweens *et al.*, 1977; Rodkey *et al.*, 1978; Haskins, 1983; Senior, 1995)

P_aO_2 for dogs breathing room air is approximately 80–104 mmHg (10.76–13.74 kPa), and for cats is 95–118 mmHg (12.69–15.72 kPa). P_vO_2 is lower than P_aO_2, and venous samples should not be used to assess adequacy of oxygenation. Normal P_vO_2 values (breathing room air) are approximately 48–56 mmHg (6.37–7.49 kPa) in dogs and as varied as 27–50 mmHg (3.59–6.65 kPa) in cats.

Bicarbonate

HCO_3^- may be measured directly by the blood gas analyser but, more commonly, it is a derived value based on the PCO_2 and pH values. Some analysers give a result for only one form of HCO_3^- (usually 'actual' bicarbonate), while others provide information on two forms: 'actual' and 'standard' bicarbonate. If the analyser just gives a single bicarbonate value without specifying which of these two it is reporting, it is most likely to be actual bicarbonate, though this should be confirmed with the manufacturer. For example, the i-STAT® analyser (see Figure 9.4a) provides a calculated actual bicarbonate value.

Actual bicarbonate

Actual bicarbonate ($HCO_3^-{}_a$) is the HCO_3^- concentration in the blood that results from both metabolic and respiratory effects. The H_2CO_3–HCO_3^- equation is as follows:

$$CO_2 + H_2O \rightleftharpoons H_2CO_3 \rightleftharpoons H^+ + HCO_3^-$$

Thus, although HCO_3^- concentration can change directly as a result of a metabolic disorder (loss or gain of HCO_3^-), from the equation it can also be seen that alterations in CO_2 levels in the blood will influence the HCO_3^- levels. An increase in CO_2 causes a shift of the equation to the right, increasing HCO_3^- production, and vice versa. Consequently, $HCO_3^-{}_a$ values as reported by blood gas analysers will be abnormal with either a respiratory or a metabolic disturbance.

Standard bicarbonate

Many analysers can titrate the CO_2 back to a value of 40 mmHg (5.3 kPa), and can then calculate what the HCO_3^- value would be at this CO_2 concentration. This is reported as the standard bicarbonate ($HCO_3^-{}_s$) value, which estimates the HCO_3^- concentration in the blood that arises solely as a result of metabolic factors, but ignores the change in HCO_3^- which is brought about by altered CO_2 concentrations; i.e. standard $HCO_3^-{}_s$ only deviates from normal when there is a primary metabolic disorder or where there is metabolic compensation for a respiratory disorder.

Total CO₂

Total CO_2 (TCO_2) represents the total amount of CO_2 that can be recovered from the sample under anaerobic conditions, and encompasses CO_2 from HCO_3^-, dissolved CO_2 and H_2CO_3. As the HCO_3^- is responsible for around 95% of the total CO_2, TCO_2 gives a good index of total HCO_3^- activity. TCO_2 will be about 5% higher than plasma HCO_3^- concentration, and a difference between TCO_2 and HCO_3^- of more than 5% suggests that the patient probably has an acidosis. However, by itself, TCO_2 offers little information and, as a general rule, TCO_2 is typically ignored when HCO_3^- results are concomitantly presented. The plasma HCO_3^-, P_aCO_2 and pH are more useful in evaluating acid–base status. TCO_2 gives no direct information about respiratory function.

Base excess/base deficit

The base excess (BE) value is a parameter derived by the blood gas analyser. Like the HCO_3^- measurement, it provides an indication of the degree of metabolic dysfunction, but with slightly greater accuracy, because it takes into account all the buffering systems within the body, not just the contribution from the H_2CO_3–HCO_3^- buffer. It is defined as the amount of acid, in mmol/l, required to return 1 litre of blood to a pH of 7.4 at a P_aCO_2 of 40 mmHg (5.3 kPa). Like the HCO_3^- value, BE only deviates from normal when there is a primary metabolic disturbance, or metabolic compensation for a respiratory disorder. While some analysers report a BE result, others report a base deficit (BD) result, one simply being the negative of the other, i.e. a base excess of 6 mmol/l is the same as a base deficit of –6 mmol/l. The situation is confused by the fact that either can have a positive or negative value: normal base excess is approximately 0 ± 4 mmol/l, and negative BE values are often reported. To avoid confusion, it is recommended that BE is used.

Simple acid–base disorders

There are four primary (or simple) acid–base disturbances:

- Metabolic acidosis
- Metabolic alkalosis
- Respiratory acidosis
- Respiratory alkalosis.

Metabolic acidosis is the most common clinically encountered acid–base disturbance in conscious animals, while respiratory acidosis is the most common in anaesthetized animals.

- Metabolic disturbances primarily affect HCO_3^- concentration, and there is usually a compensatory change in P_aCO_2 (Figure 9.7).
- Respiratory disturbances primarily affect CO_2 partial pressure, and there is usually a compensatory change in HCO_3^- (Figure 9.7).

The pH is determined by the ratio of HCO_3^- to CO_2 (Henderson–Hasselbalch equation), which is normally maintained at approximately 20:1 (see Figure 9.2). Remembering this allows one always to determine the appropriate bodily response to a primary acid–base disturbance.

Metabolic acidosis

Metabolic acidosis implies a primary reduction in HCO_3^- concentration. This may arise owing to:

- Loss of HCO_3^-, e.g. as a result of severe diarrhoea
- Failure to excrete H^+, e.g. in renal failure or renal tubular acidosis
- Accumulation of acid, which is 'mopped up' by the HCO_3^-. For example, in shock the acid that accumulates is lactic acid, and in diabetic ketoacidosis ketoacids accumulate. Lactic acidosis is a common pathway in many disease processes, and lactate levels may correlate with prognosis (high and, in particular, persistently high levels being associated with a poor prognosis).

Disorder	Uncompensated			Compensated			
	pH	*HCO₃⁻*	*PCO₂*	*pH*	*HCO₃⁻*	*PCO₂*	*Compensatory response*
Metabolic acidosis	↓↓	↓	Normal	↓	↓	↓	Hyperventilation to ↓ P_aCO_2
Metabolic alkalosis	↑↑	↑	Normal	↑	↑	↑	Hypoventilation to ↑ P_aCO_2
Respiratory acidosis	↓↓	Normal	↑	↓	↑	↑	HCO₃⁻ retention by kidneys
Respiratory alkalosis	↑↑	Normal	↓	↑	↓	↓	Increased HCO₃⁻ elimination by kidneys

9.7 Simple acid–base disorders and their compensatory responses. Note that it is unusual not to have *some* respiratory compensation for a primary metabolic disturbance by the time an animal presents to the clinician (see text).

In metabolic acidosis, the body attempts to compensate for the disturbance by lowering CO_2 levels through hyperventilation to maintain the HCO_3^- : CO_2 ratio.

Anion gap

The anion gap (AG) is a useful measurement when attempting to determine the cause of a metabolic acidosis. It represents the difference between the commonly measured cations (positive ions) in plasma and commonly measured anions (negative ions). To maintain electroneutrality, the number of cations and anions in the plasma must actually be equal:

$$(Na^+ + K^+ + UC^+) - (Cl^- + HCO_3^- + UA^-) = 0$$

where:
UC = unmeasured cations
UA = unmeasured anions

However, a proportion of circulating anions and cations are not measured routinely by laboratory tests. The unmeasured anions (e.g. negatively charged proteins, phosphate, lactate) are present in larger quantities than unmeasured cations (e.g. calcium, magnesium, globulins) so there are fewer measured anions. This means that when the measured anions are subtracted from the measured cations the answer is not zero, and this is the calculated AG.

$$AG = (Na^+ + K^+) - (Cl^- + HCO_3^-)$$

(K^+ is omitted by some authors from the equation because it contributes little to the overall charge difference.)

From the first equation above, to maintain electroneutrality, a decrease in HCO_3^- (metabolic acidosis) has to be balanced by an increase in either chloride or unmeasured anions. If the chloride replaces the HCO_3^- (as usually occurs with direct HCO_3^- loss from the body), it can be seen from the second (AG) equation above that the AG will be normal, a so-called hyperchloraemic metabolic acidosis. However, if the reduction in HCO_3^- is due to accumulation of unmeasured anions (such as lactate, beta-hydroxybutyrate or acetoacetate) and the chloride concentration remains normal (normochloraemic metabolic acidosis), it can be seen from the AG equation that the AG will be high. Thus, the AG is used to determine whether metabolic acidosis is due to primary HCO_3^- loss (normal AG), or to accumulation of acids within the body (high AG).

Normal AG values have been reported to be in the range of 12–25 mmol/l in dogs and 13–27 mmol/l in cats.

Causes of metabolic acidosis and the associated AG are summarized in Figure 9.8. Changes in AG do not necessarily imply metabolic acidosis, though an increased AG is most often associated with acidosis; rather, AG is generally used to categorize an already diagnosed metabolic acidosis.

High anion gap acidosis: This occurs due to accumulation of acids in the ECF. If the ion that accumulates is readily excreted (by the kidney), then the concentration of the acid is limited and a high AG does not develop. High AG acidosis is seen most commonly in impaired tissue perfusion (e.g. hypovolaemic shock) due to accumulation of lactic acid secondary to tissue anaerobic metabolism, advanced renal failure (see below), toxicosis (ethylene glycol and salicylate) and diabetic ketoacidosis. In ethylene glycol toxicity, the high AG is due to accumulations of metabolites (organic acids) of the compound, exacerbated by lactic acidosis and acute renal failure. Further examples are given in Figure 9.8.

Normal anion gap (hyperchloraemic) metabolic acidosis: This occurs in any clinical situation in which the kidney is able to excrete the accumulating acid, and reduced HCO_3^- is balanced by increased chloride, or where there is HCO_3^- loss with subsequent chloride retention. Classic examples are shown in Figure 9.8. In the early stages of ketoacidosis, or early or mild lactic acidosis, this type of acidosis will also develop but will become a high AG acidosis as the acids accumulate.

Low anion gap: This arises less commonly, and is poorly characterized in small animals. A low AG is most often seen in the presence of hypoalbuminaemia, because albumin constitutes the majority of the unmeasured anions, and its loss leads to an increase in Cl^- and HCO_3^- to maintain electroneutrality; this, therefore, results in a decrease in the calculated AG. Less common causes of decreased AG are where there are increased unmeasured cations (globulins, calcium and magnesium), as ECF sodium is reduced to maintain electroneutrality, so measured cations fall. The calculated AG is therefore low. Low AG often occurs in the absence of acidosis.

Diabetes mellitus

Metabolic acidosis in ketoacidotic diabetics may be characterized by a normal or high AG, depending on the balance between production, metabolism and excretion of ketone anions. Ketones are filtered and resorbed by the kidneys.

In high AG ketosis, ketones produced by the liver exceed renal excretion. This is the common clinical situation, as volume contraction associated with polyuria drives renal sodium resorption, and enhanced tubular resorption of sodium is associated with enhanced resorption of accompanying anions, including the ketoacids. In addition, lactic acidosis (due to poor perfusion in volume-contracted patients) can contribute to the high AG, and result in a much more severe metabolic acidosis than diabetic ketoacidosis alone.

Cause of altered anion gap	Disease state	Mechanism
High anion gap acidosis		
Azotaemia or uraemia	Advanced renal failure	Accumulation of organic acids due to failure of renal excretion (elevation in AG may not be very marked)
Lactic acidosis	Shock, hypovolaemia, poor tissue perfusion	Lactate accumulation
Ketoacidosis	Diabetic ketoacidosis	Increased hepatic production of ketoacids (acetoacetate and beta-hydroxybutyrate) Volume contraction and acidaemia causes lactic acidosis
Hyperosmolar non-ketotic diabetes mellitus	Diabetes mellitus	Accumulation of measured cations, especially sodium NB: Will only be acidotic if volume contraction causes lactic acidosis
Toxicity	Ethylene glycol, aspirin, methanol or paraldehyde toxicosis	Accumulation of metabolic products (acids)
Normal anion gap (hyperchloraemic) acidosis		
Diarrhoea	Many gastrointestinal diseases: diarrhoea must be severe	Loss of HCO_3^-
Early renal failure	Early renal failure	Reduced excretion of ammonia with subsequent retention of H^+ and failure to regenerate HCO_3^-
Renal tubular acidosis	Proximal (Fanconi syndrome) or distal renal tubular defects	Defective renal acid processing, with failure to excrete normal quantities of metabolically produced acid
Carbonic anhydrase inhibitors		Inhibition of carbonic anhydrase conversion of H_2CO_3 to HCO_3^-
Acidifying agents		Exogenous acid load
Hyperalimentation (in parenteral nutrition)		Acid load as a consequence of metabolism of nutrients (especially amino acids)
Very rapid intravenous rehydration		Rapid dilution of plasma bicarbonate
Ketoacidosis with renal ketone loss	Diabetes mellitus	Renal excretion of ketoacids sufficient to prevent a high anion gap developing
Low anion gap (often occurs in absence of metabolic acidosis)		
Retained non-sodium cations • Paraneoplastic hyperproteinaemia (increased cations) • Hypercalcaemia • Hypermagnesaemia • Lithium toxicity		Where there are increased cations, extracellular fluid sodium is reduced to maintain electroneutrality, so measured cations fall. The calculated anion gap is therefore low
Hypoalbuminaemia, dilution		Reduced concentration of unmeasured anions (by dilution), with compensatory increase in measured anions to maintain electroneutrality. Sodium and potassium, which are physiologically maintained in a narrow range, are not greatly altered

9.8 Types of metabolic acidosis and causes of altered anion gap (AG). (Low anion gap conditions are not well characterized in small animals and some of the causes are extrapolated from human data.)

In animals with less severe hypovolaemia, renal excretion of ketoacids may be sufficient to prevent a high AG developing. These animals are acidotic, but with normal AG.

Rarely, patients develop hyperosmolar non-ketotic diabetes mellitus (HNDM), which is characterized by severe hyperglycaemia (>35 mmol/l), hyperosmolality (>350 mOsm/kg) and dehydration without ketosis or acidosis (unless there is lactic acidosis). HNDM may result in high AG due to increases in both sodium and potassium, which are measured cations, as part of the hyperosmolar state (see Chapter 8). Not all cases of HNDM are initially acidotic (though all have high AG), but most cases rapidly develop severe hypovolaemia and lactic acidosis, further increasing the AG.

Renal failure

In early renal failure, AG is normal and there is a hyperchloraemic metabolic acidosis. This is thought to be due to reduced excretion of ammonium ions (NH_4^+) (formed by ammonia (NH_3) binding H^+ in the tubule lumen), with subsequent retention of H^+ and failure to regenerate HCO_3^-. In normal animals, renal ammonium production is one method by which the kidney excretes H^+.

In advanced renal failure, reduced glomerular filtration rate and associated retention of anions (phosphate, sulphate and, sometimes, lactate) results in a high AG acidosis.

Metabolic alkalosis

Metabolic alkalosis implies a primary increase in HCO_3^- levels. This may occur iatrogenically (e.g. over-treatment of a metabolic acidosis with $NaHCO_3$ in the intravenous fluids) or, more commonly, as a result of loss of acid from the body, which leaves a relative excess of HCO_3^-. The classical clinical situation is severe protracted true gastric vomiting, for example due to pyloric outflow obstruction. Compensation is by a reduction in ventilation to allow CO_2 levels to rise to maintain the all-important HCO_3^- : CO_2 ratio. However, there is a limit to respiratory compensation for metabolic alkalosis, as the reduced ventilation may induce hypoxaemia, which will then stimulate ventilation through hypoxic drive. (Most patients with chronic vomiting due to causes other than true pyloric obstruction are acidotic, because bilious vomiting tends to lead to acidosis due to loss of HCO_3^-.) The causes of metabolic alkalosis are summarized in Figure 9.9.

Respiratory acidosis

Respiratory acidosis implies a primary rise in P_aCO_2 (hypercapnia), which the body will attempt to correct by retention of HCO_3^- and increased excretion of H^+ by the kidney (thus restoring the $HCO_3^- : CO_2$ ratio). However, metabolic compensation is slow to develop and peak in response to primary respiratory disturbances. Respiratory acidosis is seen most commonly with alveolar hypoventilation; causes are summarized in Figure 9.10.

Respiratory alkalosis

Respiratory alkalosis implies a primary reduction in P_aCO_2 levels (hyperventilation). Compensation is by increased elimination of HCO_3^- by the kidney. The causes of respiratory alkalosis are summarized in Figure 9.10.

Cause of alkalosis	Disease state	Mechanism
HCO_3^- overload	Iatrogenic (most common)	Excess supplementation
Severe and protracted gastric vomiting	Pyloric outflow obstruction	Loss of H^+ (in vomit) leads to 'relative' excess of HCO_3^-, loss of Cl^- (in vomit) leads to enhanced renal HCO_3^- retention to maintain electroneutrality; volume depletion and enhanced renal H^+ secretion in exchange for Na^+ retention maintains alkalosis
Loop or thiazide diuretics	Cardiac patients	Loss of Cl^- in amounts greater than HCO_3^- loss, and relative extracellular fluid depletion with HCO_3^- retention. Na^+ retention due to hypovolaemia maintains alkalosis (as above)

9.9   Causes of metabolic alkalosis.

Respiratory acidosis
Upper airway obstruction Pleural cavity disease: • Pleural effusion • Pneumothorax Pulmonary disease: • Severe pneumonia • Severe pulmonary oedema • Diffuse metastatic disease • Massive pulmonary thromboembolism Depression of central control of respiration: • Drugs • Toxins • Brainstem disease Depression of neuromuscular respiratory function: • Neurological/neuromuscular disease • Toxins Cardiopulmonary arrest
Respiratory alkalosis
Pulmonary disease: • Pneumonia • Interstitial lung disease Central stimulation of respiration: • Anxiety, fear • Excitement • Pain • Pyrexia • (Drug therapy)

9.10   Causes of respiratory acidosis and alkalosis.

Responses to acid–base disturbances

Whenever an acid–base disorder occurs, the body will attempt to restore pH to the normal range. Intra- and extracellular buffering systems will begin working as soon as an alteration in acid–base status is detected, thus providing rapid protection against changes in pH. Over the next few minutes, the respiratory system will start to attempt to compensate for the disturbance (provided the primary disorder is metabolic and not respiratory), either by retaining or excreting extra carbon dioxide. Although respiratory compensation begins to work fairly rapidly, it takes several hours to achieve maximum effect. Finally, metabolic compensation will come into play. This usually takes several hours to begin having a significant effect, and 2–5 days for these effects to become maximal. Although metabolic compensation will occur for a primary respiratory disorder, it is also possible to have metabolic compensation for a primary metabolic disorder. This will only occur if the kidney is not the underlying cause of the problem. Because of the rapidity with which respiratory compensation develops in response to a primary metabolic disturbance, by the time of presentation, animals with metabolic acidosis or alkalosis should already show an appropriate alteration in PCO_2 on blood gas analysis (decreased PCO_2 with metabolic acidosis, increased PCO_2 with metabolic alkalosis). If the PCO_2 is *normal* in a patient with a primary metabolic disturbance, this tends to suggest that there is actually a *mixed* disturbance occurring. On the other hand, because metabolic compensation is relatively slow to develop and reach maximum effect in animals with primary respiratory disturbances, it is not uncommon to see HCO_3^- concentrations within the normal range in these patients upon presentation. In fact, many primary respiratory disturbances do not persist long enough for full metabolic compensation to develop.

Although metabolic and respiratory compensation for simple acid–base disorders can help reduce the effect of the disorder on pH, there is a limit to the body's ability to compensate. In simple disorders, the expected responses can be quantified (Figure 9.11) but the compensatory responses listed are based on *mean* values, and some patients may lie outside the calculated compensation value. If there is marked discrepancy between the patient's blood value and expected compensatory response, however, it tends to suggest that there may be a *mixed*

Disturbance	Primary change	Expected compensation
Acute respiratory acidosis	Each 10 mmHg (1.33 kPa) ↑ P_aCO_2	HCO_3^- ↑ by 1.5 mmol/l
Chronic respiratory acidosis	Each 10 mmHg (1.33 kPa) ↑ P_aCO_2	HCO_3^- ↑ by 3.5 mmol/l
Acute respiratory alkalosis	Each 10 mmHg (1.33 kPa) ↓ P_aCO_2	HCO_3^- ↓ by 2.5 mmol/l
Chronic respiratory alkalosis	Each 10 mmHg (1.33 kPa) ↓ P_aCO_2	HCO_3^- ↓ by 5.5 mmol/l
Metabolic acidosis	Each 1 mmol/l ↓ HCO_3^-	P_aCO_2 ↓ by 0.7 mmHg (~0.1 kPa)
Metabolic alkalosis	Each 1 mmol/l ↑ HCO_3^-	P_aCO_2 ↑ by 0.7 mmHg (~0.1 kPa)

9.11   Expected compensatory responses for primary acid–base disturbances.
(Data from DiBartola, 2012)

acid–base disorder, i.e. two or more disorders occurring simultaneously. Another way to identify mixed disorders in animals with high AG metabolic acidosis is to compare the change in AG to the change in HCO_3^-. In simple acid–base disturbances, these changes will be of similar magnitude (i.e. each 1 mmol/l increase in AG should be mirrored by a fall of $[HCO_3^-]$ by 1 mmol/l).

'Complete' compensation with reference to acid–base disturbances is defined simply as a compensatory response that returns the pH to within the normal reference range; it does not imply that the primary disorder has actually been corrected.

Evaluation of samples

A systematic approach should be adopted when evaluating blood gas data.

1. Examine the pH

If pH is in the normal range, this may imply:

- There is no acid–base disturbance
- There is an acid–base disturbance which has been completely compensated
- There are two opposing acid–base disturbances (a mixed disorder), which are cancelling each other out in terms of their effect on pH.

If there is an acidaemia (pH <7.35), there must be an underlying metabolic or respiratory acidosis, or both. If there is an alkalaemia (pH >7.45), there must be an underlying metabolic or respiratory alkalosis, or both.

Even with maximal compensation for any disorder, the pH will tend not to return to the midpoint of the normal range (although it may lie just within the normal range), and the body does not usually overcompensate for an acid–base disturbance. If there were a primary metabolic or respiratory acidosis, even with respiratory or metabolic compensation respectively, the pH would still be <7.4; it would lie towards the acidaemic side of the midpoint of the pH range. Similarly, if there were a primary metabolic or respiratory alkalosis, even with appropriate compensation, the pH would still be >7.4.

2. Look at the PCO_2

- If PCO_2 is elevated, there is either a primary respiratory acidosis or a compensatory response to a metabolic alkalosis.
- If PCO_2 is low, there is either a primary respiratory alkalosis or a compensatory response to a metabolic acidosis.

3. Look at the actual and standard bicarbonate values and the base excess

In general, BE and HCO_3^- will change in a similar direction, because they are variants on the same theme (see earlier).

- If there is purely a respiratory disturbance, $HCO_3^-{}_a$ will be altered but $HCO_3^-{}_s$ and BE will be normal.
- If there is a metabolic disorder, or a metabolic compensatory response, $HCO_3^-{}_s$ and $HCO_3^-{}_a$ and BE will change.

4. Distinguish the primary disturbance from the compensatory response

In a patient with a low PCO_2 and a low HCO_3^-, for example, does the patient have:

- A primary respiratory alkalosis with metabolic compensation, *or*
- A primary metabolic acidosis with respiratory compensation?

Evaluation of the patient's history and clinical signs should help to identify the primary disturbance. It should be remembered that the pH will move in the same direction as for the primary disorder, and the body does not usually overcompensate (see above). Even with maximal compensation, if the pH returns to the normal range it usually lies at its extremes. Thus, in this case, if the pH of the sample were <7.4 (i.e. to the acidaemic side of the pH range), it would suggest that the primary problem was an acidosis, and would fit best with the second explanation above. If the pH were >7.4 (i.e. to the alkalaemic side of the pH range), the first explanation would be most appropriate. Interpretation becomes more complex if the pH is at, or close to, 7.4 as it becomes difficult to determine which is the primary problem. Because overcompensation does not usually occur, it is uncommon for even 'complete' compensation (see above) to restore the pH back to around 7.4 – it will usually lie towards the outer limits of the reference range. Therefore, a pH at, or close to, the midpoint of the normal range suggests that two opposing disorders are occurring (i.e. there is a mixed disturbance). Concurrent respiratory alkalosis and metabolic acidosis, for example, could result in a pH that is at, or close to, 7.4.

5. Assess whether the compensatory response is as expected

Refer to Figure 9.11. If the compensatory response is not as expected, this may suggest the presence of a mixed acid–base disorder.

6. Assess the patient's oxygenation

The patient's oxygenation is assessed on an arterial sample, using the alveolar gas equation, and calculating the alveolar–arterial oxygen difference. Unless the patient is exhibiting respiratory signs, this is seldom carried out and, as an alternative, a rough guide to the expected P_aO_2 is obtained by multiplying the inspired O_2 concentration by a factor of five; i.e. if the patient is breathing room air (21% O_2), the P_aO_2 should be around 100 mmHg (13.3 kPa). If it is breathing 100% O_2, the expected P_aO_2 would be around 500 mmHg (66.5 kPa).

Blood gas analysis in respiratory patients

Arterial samples must be used to assess respiratory patients, and P_aO_2 and P_aCO_2 are the most important parameters, because it is the animal's gas exchange capacity that is of interest. Arterial blood gas tensions are affected by a number of factors including hypoventilation, ventilation–perfusion (V/Q) mismatch and, rarely, diffusion abnormalities. Blood gas analysis may, however, be normal in mild respiratory conditions and in the early stages of more severe disease.

Normal arterial oxygen tension (P_aO_2) is approximately 80–100 mmHg (10.6–13.3 kPa) on room air and, at these values, haemoglobin saturation will be around 97–98%. At values less than about 60 mmHg (8 kPa) there is significant hypoxaemia, and below 40–50 mmHg (5.3–6.6 kPa) cyanosis may become evident.

Many clinicians use a value for normal P_aCO_2 of 35–45 mmHg (4.65–5.98 kPa) in the dog; however, this is based on human data and will result in overdiagnosis of hyperventilation. Normal P_aCO_2 in dogs is 30.8–42.8 mmHg (4.10–5.69 kPa), and cats tend to have lower values of 25.2–36.8 mmHg (3.35–4.89 kPa) (see Figure 9.6). Normal P_vCO_2 is higher than P_aCO_2, and values are approximately 33–41 mmHg (4.47–5.48 kPa) in dogs and 33–45 mmHg (4.35–5.94 kPa) in cats.

Hypoventilation (alveolar hypoventilation) results in hypercapnia (increased P_aCO_2, respiratory acidosis; see Figure 9.10) and may also lead to hypoxaemia, although this depends upon both the degree of hypercapnia and the F_iO_2. For example, an animal under general anaesthesia breathing 100% O_2 is unlikely to exhibit hypoxaemia, even in the face of severe hypercapnia. Hypoventilation is most often caused by upper airway obstruction, pleural effusion and drugs or disorders affecting central control of respiration (e.g. general anaesthesia), or diseases affecting the neuromuscular components of the respiratory system.

Ventilation–perfusion (V/Q) mismatch (or imbalance) occurs when there is either normal ventilation but inadequate perfusion (so there is insufficient blood passing the alveoli for oxygen to be taken up into the pulmonary capillaries, for example with a pulmonary embolus), or inadequate ventilation but adequate perfusion (where pulmonary capillary blood reaches the alveoli in adequate quantities, but ventilation to those alveoli has been insufficient to allow optimal oxygenation, for example with alveolar oedema or pulmonary fibrosis). The end result of V/Q mismatch is that oxygen transfer is inefficient and, if impairment is severe enough, it may produce hypoxaemia. However, although blood oxygenation is usually impaired in this situation, patients with V/Q mismatch are usually normocapnic, because CO_2 diffuses easily and exchange is not limited. Indeed, patients with V/Q mismatch severe enough to induce hypoxaemia may actually be hypocapnic because the hypoxaemia may stimulate ventilatory drive. Increasing the F_iO_2 will usually improve the hypoxaemia in patients with V/Q mismatch. V/Q mismatch is most often associated with significant lower airway and pulmonary parenchymal disease, where there is diffusion impairment, especially interstitial and alveolar diseases such as pneumonia and pulmonary oedema, although it can also be seen in severe hypostatic congestion (e.g. the critically ill animal that is not being turned regularly). Severe chronic bronchitis, asthma or obstructive pulmonary disease can also cause mismatch. Lastly, it is commonly seen in pulmonary thromboembolism.

In clinical practice, a simplified version of the alveolar–arterial oxygen gradient equation is often used to differentiate hypoxaemia caused by alveolar hypoventilation from that caused by V/Q mismatch:

$$P_{(A–a)}O_2 = [150 – (P_aCO_2/0.8) – P_aO_2]$$

This equation assumes values for F_iO_2 (based on room air), barometric pressure, saturated vapour pressure of water and respiratory quotient (RQ; see Figure 9.1). It will be greatly affected by the patient receiving supplemental oxygen (in which case the full alveolar gas equation should

be used) and to a lesser extent the natural variations in barometric pressure, alterations in vapour pressure with body temperature and variations in RQ (which do occur, but are never measured). However, although it is imprecise, the alveolar–arterial oxygen difference calculated in this way does provide useful information. In normal animals, it is <25 mmHg (3.32 kPa), and usually <10 mmHg (1.33 kPa). If hypoxaemia is solely due to hypoventilation, the alveolar–arterial O_2 difference should be within the normal range, whereas other causes, such as V/Q mismatch, will lead to an elevation. Calculation of the $P_{(A–a)}O_2$ is particularly useful when monitoring progression of impaired oxygenation in critically ill patients over time, because the value obtained is independent of any effect on the P_aO_2 of alterations in P_aCO_2. Simply assessing P_aO_2 in isolation would be ineffective for monitoring progression of respiratory disease, because P_aO_2 will be influenced by alterations in ventilation (P_aCO_2).

The relationship between S_aO_2 and PO_2 is illustrated in Figure 9.12, in a haemoglobin oxygenation curve. Some blood gas analysers will estimate the S_aO_2, the saturation of haemoglobin with oxygen in arterial blood. This value is calculated on the basis of the P_aO_2 but does not make any allowance for other factors that affect the haemoglobin oxygenation curve, e.g. concentrations of 2,3-diphosphoglycerate in red blood cells (see Chapter 4). The S_pO_2 (haemoglobin saturation measured by pulse oximetry) is usually similar to S_aO_2 and can be used to give an indication of P_aO_2. Owing to the almost linear relationship between S_aO_2 or S_pO_2 and P_aO_2 at P_aO_2 values <60 mmHg (7.98 kPa) (Figure 9.12), some key values are worthy of note: P_aO_2 values of 40, 50 and 60 mmHg (5.32, 6.65 and 7.98 kPa) correspond approximately to S_aO_2 or S_pO_2 values of 70, 80 and 90%, respectively. S_pO_2 values <90% are of immediate concern.

When considering oxygenation, it should be remembered that the oxygen-carrying capacity of haemoglobin is also affected by the pH. At any given P_aO_2, haemoglobin has less affinity for oxygen if the pH drops, because the oxygenation curve moves to the right. This means that oxygen is given up more readily at tissue level. However, where there is poor oxygenation, this reduced affinity also means that poorer haemoglobin saturation may be achieved and, in hypoxaemic animals, this may actually limit the delivery of oxygen to the tissues.

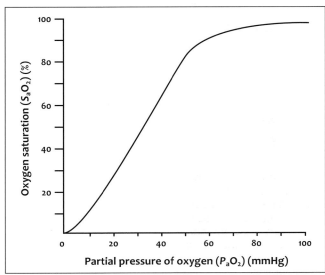

9.12 Oxygen–haemoglobin dissociation curve. Note the almost linear relationship between S_aO_2 and P_aO_2 at P_aO_2 values <60 mmHg.

Effects of blood gas disturbances on other analytes

Animals with acid–base disorders may have secondary abnormalities in other biochemical parameters, among which potassium is probably the most important. Chloride levels are often altered in metabolic acidosis, as described above, where there is compensatory hyperchloraemia in normal anion gap metabolic acidosis to maintain electrical neutrality. Less commonly, hypochloraemia may be seen with a high anion gap metabolic acidosis, most frequently with diabetic ketoacidosis or ethylene glycol toxicity.

Potassium distribution is affected by acid–base disturbances, and potassium disorders themselves can exacerbate acid–base disorders. In metabolic acidosis (and, to a much lesser extent, respiratory acidosis), potassium is translocated from the ICF to the ECF in exchange for H^+; chloride cannot follow H^+ into cells, so exchange must occur. This may result in hyperkalaemia, though measured serum or plasma potassium concentration is often normal because these patients often have an overall depletion of total body potassium. Where the acid can follow the H^+ into the cell (e.g. lactate) this effect may be less profound.

In metabolic alkalosis, the opposite can occur, and potassium shifts into cells, but this rarely causes a significant hypokalaemia. However, in potassium depletion (e.g. due to vomiting), alkalosis may be exacerbated. If there is ECF volume depletion, this may limit the normal renal response to metabolic alkalosis (rapid HCO_3^- excretion) and prevent correction. The kidney prioritizes volume expansion above acid–base balance, and sodium retention occurs to expand plasma volume. Sodium is reabsorbed in the distal tubule in exchange for H^+ or potassium, and if potassium is depleted more H^+ is exchanged. Secretion of H^+ into the tubule lumen is associated with HCO_3^- entry into the ECF, which maintains the alkalosis. Thus, the alkalosis is not corrected, and there is H^+ secretion in the urine. This results in a so-called 'paradoxical aciduria', where acid urine is produced in the face of alkalosis.

Mixed acid–base disturbances

Complex or mixed acid–base disturbances should be suspected if the expected compensation for the primary disturbance fails to develop (see Figures 9.7 and 9.11), if the PCO_2 and HCO_3^- changes are not in the same direction or if, in a high anion gap acidosis, the changes in AG and HCO_3^- are not of similar magnitude. If a mixed disturbance causes pH changes in the same direction (e.g. a combined respiratory and metabolic acidosis), life-threatening disturbances are likely and treatment of the immediate crises is vital. If the two conditions act disparately, the pH may be normal and treatment of one condition may unmask a second disturbance. However, mixed acid–base disturbances can be too complex to diagnose on blood gas analysis, and – in common with simple disturbances – it is important to attempt interpretation only in conjunction with the patient's history.

Case examples

CASE 1

SIGNALMENT

8-month-old entire female crossbred dog.

HISTORY

Presented 1 hour following a road traffic accident, the dog was laterally recumbent and extremely depressed, with minimal response to external stimulation. She also had severe conjunctival bruising of both eyes, and a fractured mandible. No other abnormalities were detected on clinical examination.

CLINICAL PATHOLOGY DATA

A basic biochemistry and haematology profile showed no significant abnormalities. Given the clinical signs that the dog was demonstrating, intracranial trauma was deemed the likeliest cause of the severe depression. Although there was no direct indication of abnormal ventilation, it was considered appropriate to assess an arterial (rather than a venous) blood gas sample to evaluate the adequacy of ventilation accurately, given that head trauma can lead to respiratory depression, and also that increases in P_aCO_2 can produce an elevation in intracranial pressure through cerebral vasodilation. Consequently, an arterial blood gas sample was obtained while the dog was breathing room air.

Blood gas analysis	Result	Reference interval
pH	**7.04**	7.35–7.46
P_aCO_2 (mmHg)	**66.0**	30.8–42.8
P_aO_2 (mmHg)	**64.0**	80.9–103.3
HCO_3^- (mmol/l) (actual)	**17.1**	18.8–25.6
BE (mmol/l)	**−6.9**	0 ± 4

Abnormal results are in **bold**.

WHAT ABNORMALITIES ARE PRESENT AND HOW WOULD YOU INTERPRET THE RESULTS?

The blood gas results demonstrate an acidaemia.

KEY POINT

An acidaemia implies the dog must have either a metabolic acidosis, a respiratory acidosis or both.

The P_aCO_2 is increased, which means the dog either has a respiratory acidosis or respiratory compensation for a metabolic alkalosis (the latter would be very unlikely to reach a P_aCO_2 of this magnitude).

KEY POINT

The body will attempt to maintain a normal ratio of HCO_3^- : CO_2 (approximately 20:1) to keep the pH as close to the normal range as possible; therefore, an increase in PCO_2 may be a primary problem or may be a compensatory response to an increased HCO_3^-.

→ **CASE 1 CONTINUED**

Both the HCO_3^- and BE are decreased, indicating a metabolic acidosis or metabolic compensation for a primary respiratory alkalosis.

KEY POINT

Remember that metabolic compensation is slow to develop and to peak; most respiratory disorders in animals do not persist long enough for full metabolic compensation to develop.

At this point the clinician should stop and consider the preceding two findings. Bearing in mind that with normal compensatory responses HCO_3^- and P_aCO_2 will change in the same direction to maintain their ratio and, therefore, pH close to the normal range, the fact that P_aCO_2 and HCO_3^- are moving in *opposite* directions in this dog (P_aCO_2 increasing; HCO_3^-/BE decreasing), indicates a *mixed* acid–base disorder; i.e. there are two separate problems, and it is not just a simple disturbance with a compensatory response.

Thus, this dog has a **combined respiratory and metabolic acidosis**; this is why the pH is so low, because there is no compensation 'pulling it back' towards the normal range. Electrolyte values were not available for this dog, so it was not possible to calculate an anion gap (AG) to ascertain the cause of the metabolic acidosis; however, given the acute presentation of this case, it is much more likely that the metabolic acidosis was due to acid gain (probable hypovolaemia) rather than direct HCO_3^- loss.

What is the alveolar–arterial oxygen difference?

$P_AO_2 = 150 - (P_aCO_2/0.8)$
$P_AO_2 = 150 - (66/0.8)$
$P_AO_2 = 67.5$ mmHg
P_aO_2 (from blood gas) $= 64$ mmHg
$\therefore P_{(A-a)}O_2 = 67.5 - 64 = 3.5$ mmHg

Thus, the $P_{(A-a)}O_2$ is normal, which tells us there is no evidence of impaired oxygenation; consequently, we can conclude that the low P_aO_2 in the blood gas sample is due solely to hypoventilation (elevated P_aCO_2).

WHAT IS THE LIKELY EXPLANATION FOR THESE FINDINGS?

Given the history of a road traffic accident and the obvious signs of head trauma, the probable diagnosis would be that there is hypovolaemia leading to metabolic acidosis (probably hyperlactataemia, although lactate was not actually measured in this dog), and the respiratory acidosis is most likely due to 'central depression' resulting from brain trauma. Although other causes of hypercapnia such as pneumothorax or haemothorax should be ruled by radiography, these are less likely to be the cause of the elevated P_aCO_2 in this particular dog because oxygenation is normal on the basis of the alveolar–arterial oxygen difference, and this gradient would be expected to be elevated in cases of pleural space disease.

OUTCOME

The dog was volume resuscitated (carefully!), treated with mannitol and placed on mechanical ventilation (under propofol anaesthesia). After 6 hours, the propofol was gradually reduced, the dog was weaned from the ventilator and she began to show signs of recovery of consciousness shortly thereafter. Subsequent arterial blood gas analysis showed that P_aCO_2 had returned to within the reference range, so anaesthesia was terminated and the trachea extubated approximately 20 minutes later. The dog went on to make a full recovery.

CASE 2

SIGNALMENT

11-year-old female neutered German Shepherd Dog.

HISTORY

Following an episode of collapse the previous evening, the owner had presented the dog to their primary veterinary surgeon, who suspected an abdominal mass. Upon presentation at a referral hospital, the dog was quiet but relatively alert and ambulatory. Heart rate was 130 beats/min with an irregular rhythm, peripheral pulses were of moderate quality, and mucous membranes were slightly pale. Electrocardiography revealed the presence of intermittent uniform ventricular premature complexes. No other significant abnormalities were detected on clinical examination. Subsequent abdominal ultrasonography revealed the presence of free fluid in the peritoneal cavity and a large splenic mass, and the dog was scheduled for exploratory coeliotomy.

CLINICAL PATHOLOGY DATA

Routine biochemistry was performed, revealing all parameters to be within the reference range. Haematology demonstrated anaemia (HCT 0.26 l/l; reference range 0.38–0.56) and mild thrombocytopenia (172 x 10^9/l; reference range 200–500) but no other abnormalities.

A venous blood gas sample was drawn while the dog was breathing room air.

Blood gas analysis	Result	Reference interval
pH	**7.31**	7.35–7.46
P_vCO_2 (mmHg)	**30.3**	33.6–41.2
P_vO_2 (mmHg)	**43.4**	47.9–56.3 (room air; difficult to interpret venous oxygen during oxygen supplementation)
HCO_3^- (mmol/l) (actual)	**17.2**	20.8–24.2
BE (mmol/l)	**-7.7**	0 ± 4

Abnormal results are in **bold**.

→ **CASE 2 CONTINUED**

The blood gas results demonstrate an acidaemia.

KEY POINT

An acidaemia implies the dog must have either a metabolic acidosis, a respiratory acidosis or both.

The P_vCO_2 is reduced, which means the dog either has a respiratory alkalosis or respiratory compensation for a metabolic acidosis.

KEY POINT

The body will attempt to maintain a normal ratio of HCO_3^- : CO_2 (approximately 20:1) to keep the pH as close to the normal range as possible; therefore, a reduction in PCO_2 may be a primary problem or may be a compensatory response to a reduced HCO_3^-.

Both the HCO_3^- and BE are decreased, indicating a metabolic acidosis or metabolic compensation for a primary respiratory alkalosis.

KEY POINT

Remember that metabolic compensation is slow to develop and to peak; most respiratory disorders in animals do not persist long enough for full metabolic compensation to develop.

Given that the dog has an acidaemia, the alterations in both P_vCO_2 and HCO_3^-/BE would fit best with the metabolic acidosis being the primary problem (if the reduced P_vCO_2 was the primary problem, i.e. a respiratory alkalosis, we would expect the pH to be alkalaemic).

IS THE DEGREE OF COMPENSATION APPROPRIATE?

From Figure 9.11, it can be seen that, in metabolic acidosis, the appropriate respiratory compensation is a decrease in PCO_2 of 0.7 mmHg for every 1 mmol/l decrease in HCO_3^-. If the midpoint of the normal HCO_3^- range in the dog is taken as 22 mmol/l, this means that there has been a decrease of approximately 5 mmol/l (22 − 17.2) in HCO_3^-; therefore, the expected decrease in PCO_2 would be 5 × 0.7 = 3.5 mmHg. If the midpoint of the normal canine P_aCO_2 range is taken as 36 mmHg, the PCO_2 would be expected to be approximately 32.5 mmHg if this blood gas represented a primary metabolic acidosis with respiratory compensation. This individual's P_vCO_2 is actually 30.3 mmHg so is not exactly what we would expect if the low PCO_2 were a normal compensatory response. However, it is important to emphasize that the values reported in Figure 9.11 are **mean** values and some patients, therefore, may deviate slightly from what is expected. In addition, the values in Figure 9.11 are based on arterial samples, so some variation should be expected from the reported values if venous samples are being analysed. The difference of only 2.2 mmHg between expected and actual compensation suggests that the P_vCO_2 value in this sample is consistent with what would be expected for respiratory compensation in this case. This perhaps demonstrates that some aspects of blood gas interpretation are not black and white but slightly 'grey'!

WHAT IS THE ANION GAP?

In cases where a primary metabolic acidosis has been diagnosed, it is worthwhile calculating the anion gap (AG) to determine whether the acidosis is due to direct bicarbonate loss (in which case the AG will usually be within the normal range), or to accumulation of acids (in which case the AG will usually be elevated). The measured electrolyte values from this dog were all within the reference range.

Electrolyte	Result	Reference interval
Na^+ (mmol/l)	151	136–159
Cl^- (mmol/l)	100	95–115
K^+ (mmol/l)	4.2	3.4–5.8

Calculating the AG:

$$AG = (Na^+ + K^+) - (Cl^- + HCO_3^-)$$
$$\therefore AG = (151 + 4.2) - (100 + 17.2)$$
$$AG = 38 \text{ (reference range 12–25 mmol/l)}$$

Thus, there is an increased AG, suggesting that the metabolic acidosis is due to acid accumulation. Given this dog's clinical presentation, it is likely that there is decreased tissue perfusion due to hypovolaemia, as well as impaired tissue oxygenation as a result of both the hypovolaemia and the anaemia. As such, it is probable that there is a degree of tissue anaerobic metabolism resulting in production of lactic acid – the cause of the high anion gap metabolic acidosis. Blood lactate was not specifically measured in this dog, but it is probable that it would have been elevated.

IS OXYGENATION NORMAL?

Given that this is a venous sample, the adequacy of oxygenation cannot be accurately appraised: while venous samples are suitable for assessment of metabolic function and disorders, arterial samples are required if analysis of oxygen status is to be evaluated.

FINAL DIAGNOSIS

Primary metabolic acidosis with respiratory compensation.

OUTCOME

Following intravenous fluid resuscitation with compound sodium lactate, the dog was anaesthetized and underwent routine splenectomy without complication.

CASE 3

1-year-old male entire Labrador Retriever.

HISTORY

The dog was a renowned scavenger, having previously had two gastroscopies to remove foreign objects. On this occasion, the dog presented with a history of reduced appetite and intermittent vomiting of 2 days' duration. Radiography revealed the presence of multiple radiopacities in the stomach, presumed to be stones on the basis of their radiographic appearance. Given the large number of objects seen on the radiograph, it was decided that gastrotomy would be preferable to gastroscopy, and the dog was scheduled for general anaesthesia. Clinical examination revealed no abnormalities and the dog was very bright and bouncy, so pre-anaesthetic blood sampling was omitted.

CLINICAL PATHOLOGY DATA

During the anaesthetic, it was decided to perform an arterial blood gas analysis to guide the choice of intravenous fluid therapy for the dog. (Note that it would have been equally effective to perform *venous* blood gas analysis for this dog because the concern was with metabolic (as opposed to respiratory) function. However, an arterial cannula had been placed for measurement of arterial blood pressure during anaesthesia, so it was elected to sample from that.)

Blood gas analysis	Result	Reference interval
pH	7.36	7.35–7.46
P_aCO_2 (mmHg)	**66.3**	30.8–42.8
P_aO_2 (mmHg)	**510.8**	80.9–103.3 when breathing room air; should be ~5 × inspired O_2% if O_2 is being supplemented
HCO_3^- (mmol/l) (actual)	**36.0**	18.8–25.6
BE (mmol/l)	**10.2**	0 ± 4

Abnormal results are in **bold**.

WHAT ABNORMALITIES ARE PRESENT AND HOW WOULD YOU INTERPRET THE RESULTS?

The pH is within the normal range.

KEY POINT

A normal pH implies that either no acid–base disturbance is present, there is a simple acid–base disturbance with complete compensation, or there are two opposing acid–base disturbances pulling the pH in opposite directions and essentially cancelling each other out (in terms of their effect on the pH).

The P_aCO_2 is high, which implies either a primary respiratory acidosis or respiratory compensation for a metabolic alkalosis.

KEY POINT

The body will attempt to maintain a normal ratio of HCO_3^- : CO_2 (approximately 20:1) to keep the pH as close to the normal range as possible; therefore, an increase in PCO_2 may be a primary problem or may be a compensatory response to an increased HCO_3^-. Note, however, that a P_aCO_2 of 66.3 mmHg is unlikely to be compensatory – it is simply too high; an elevation of this magnitude tends to imply that there must be a respiratory acidosis, rather than respiratory compensation for a metabolic disturbance.

Both the HCO_3^- and BE are increased, indicating a metabolic alkalosis or metabolic compensation for a primary respiratory acidosis.

KEY POINT

Remember that metabolic compensation is slow to develop and to peak; most respiratory disorders in animals do not persist long enough for full metabolic compensation to develop.

Thus, there are two abnormalities here; an increase in P_aCO_2 and an increase in HCO_3^- and BE. Normally the pH is evaluated to help determine which of these is the primary problem: if the pH were acidaemic, it would suggest that the elevated P_aCO_2 was primary (respiratory acidosis); if the pH were alkalaemic, it would suggest that the elevated HCO_3^-/BE was primary (metabolic alkalosis). However, in this case, the pH is within the normal range (7.36), which makes interpretation more difficult, although the fact that the pH is towards the acidaemic end of the range might suggest that the respiratory acidosis was the primary problem.

KEY POINT

Blood gas results should ALWAYS be interpreted in relation to the patient's history. With this particular case, there is no real reason to expect that a normal, relatively healthy dog (albeit with a gastric foreign body) should have a primary respiratory problem; in addition, even if there had been a primary respiratory acidosis, for metabolic compensation of this degree to occur (i.e. restoring pH back to within the normal range) would imply it must have been going on for some period of time. This simply does not fit with the presenting history of the dog. An alternative explanation is that there is actually a *mixed* disturbance occurring with both abnormal respiratory and metabolic components.

CONSIDERING THIS DOG'S HISTORY, IS IT POSSIBLE TO EXPLAIN A MIXED DISTURBANCE BEING PRESENT?

First, pure gastric vomiting commonly leads to metabolic alkalosis. This occurs for two main reasons:

- Direct loss of HCl (hydrochloric acid) in vomit (loss of acid leads to a 'relative' excess of base (HCO_3^-))
- Much of the Na^+ resorption in the renal tubules is accompanied by Cl^- to maintain electroneutrality. However, animals with gastric vomiting are often Cl^- depleted owing to the direct Cl^- losses in the HCl of the vomitus. This means that, rather than reabsorbing Cl^- in the renal tubules with the Na^+, there is reabsorption of HCO_3^-, i.e. the metabolic alkalosis commonly observed in gastric vomiting is partly due to the renal response as well as the direct acid loss from the stomach.

→ CASE 3 CONTINUED

Thus, a primary metabolic alkalosis (increased HCO_3^-) is quite common in dogs with pure gastric vomiting. The normal expected compensation for this would be for the dog to retain CO_2 in order to maintain the ratio between HCO_3^- and PCO_2; however, this would entail the animal actually reducing ventilation to lessen the amount of CO_2 being excreted via the lungs. The problem with this is that a reduction in ventilation in an attempt to retain CO_2 will simultaneously lead to a decrease in O_2 uptake by the lungs, potentially leading to the animal becoming hypoxaemic. If this occurs, hypoxic drive is then stimulated which leads to an increase in ventilation in order to restore oxygenation. The end result of all of this is that the respiratory compensatory response to metabolic alkalosis may be limited by decreased oxygenation.

WHAT IS THE EXPLANATION FOR THE ELEVATED P_aCO_2 IN THIS DOG?

Part of this may well be a compensatory response to metabolic alkalosis but, as stated above, a P_aCO_2 of 66.3 mmHg is too high to be purely due to compensation, i.e. there must be a primary respiratory acidosis to achieve a P_aCO_2 of this magnitude.

The appropriate respiratory compensation for a dog with metabolic alkalosis would be an increase in P_aCO_2 by approximately 0.7 mmHg for every 1 mmol/l increase in HCO_3^- (see Figure 9.11). For this particular dog, HCO_3^- has increased from 22 mmol/l (approximate midpoint of the HCO_3^- reference range in dogs) to 36 mmol/l, an increase of 14 mmol/l. If the animal was exhibiting a normal respiratory compensatory response to a metabolic alkalosis (see Figure 9.11), P_aCO_2 would be expected to increase by around 9.8 mmHg (14 × 0.7) from the midpoint of the normal P_aCO_2 reference range. It should certainly be nowhere near 66.3 mmHg, which again suggests there is a primary respiratory acidosis here and not just a respiratory compensatory response to metabolic alkalosis.

An alternative explanation for the blood gas results, however, would be that the elevated P_aCO_2 in this dog is actually the primary problem (respiratory acidosis) and the increase in HCO_3^- is merely a compensatory response for this rather than a primary metabolic alkalosis (based on the fact that the pH lies to the acidaemic end of the range, and despite the fact that this explanation of the results does not fit at all with the dog's history). Consequently, it is worth calculating what the results would actually be if this were the case. Thus, if there was a primary respiratory acidosis in this animal, the following compensatory changes would be expected in the HCO_3^- concentrations (see Figure 9.11).

- If the respiratory acidosis was acute, the HCO_3^- should increase by 1.5 mmol/l for every 10 mmHg increase in P_aCO_2. This dog's P_aCO_2 has increased from 36 mmHg (approximate midpoint of the normal P_aCO_2 range in dogs) to 66.3 mmHg, an increase of approximately 30 mmHg. Therefore, the expected compensatory rise in HCO_3^- would be (3 × 1.5 = 4.5 mmol/l). If the midpoint of the normal HCO_3^- range in dogs is taken as approximately 22 mmol/l, it would be anticipated that the HCO_3^- would increase to around 26.5 mmol/l if this case was a straightforward

acute respiratory acidosis with metabolic compensation. Given that this dog's HCO_3^- is actually 36 mmol/l, this does not fit with this proposed interpretation of the results.
- If the respiratory acidosis was chronic, the HCO_3^- should increase by 3.5 mmol/l for every 10 mmHg increase in P_aCO_2. This dog's P_aCO_2 has increased by approximately 30 mmHg (see above). Therefore, the expected compensatory rise in HCO_3^- would be (3 × 3.5 = 10.5 mmol/l). Accordingly, it would be anticipated that the HCO_3^- would increase to around 32.5 mmol/l (see above for fuller explanation) if this case was a chronic respiratory acidosis with metabolic compensation. Again, given that the dog's HCO_3^- is 36 mmol/l, the blood gas results suggest this is not the case.

Given that straightforward respiratory compensation for a primary metabolic alkalosis has been ruled out, and that metabolic compensation for either an acute or chronic respiratory acidosis has also been excluded, the conclusion is that we have a mixed disorder, i.e. a concurrent metabolic alkalosis and respiratory acidosis.

WHY MIGHT THIS DOG HAVE A RESPIRATORY ACIDOSIS?

The answer lies in the anaesthesia: all anaesthetic agents are respiratory depressants, and therefore will lead to an increase in P_aCO_2 in spontaneously breathing patients. Thus, this dog probably had a lower elevation in P_aCO_2 as a compensatory response to the metabolic alkalosis *prior* to anaesthesia, but this has been exacerbated by induction of anaesthesia which has superimposed a concurrent respiratory acidosis.

Calculation of the alveolar–arterial oxygen difference in this dog requires use of the full alveolar gas equation because the dog is breathing supplemental oxygen.
(NB The F_iO_2 value of 93% (0.93) below, was taken directly from the anaesthetic monitor.)

$$P_AO_2 = F_iO_2 \, (P_B - P_{H_2O}) - \frac{P_aCO_2}{0.8}$$

$P_AO_2 = 0.93 \, (760 - 47) - (P_aCO_2/0.8)$
$P_AO_2 = 663 - (66.3/0.8)$
$P_AO_2 = 580$ mmHg
P_aO_2 (from blood gas) = 510 mmHg
∴ $P_{(A-a)}O_2 = 580 - 510 = 70$ mmHg

Given that the alveolar–arterial difference is within the normal range for a dog breathing supplemental oxygen, there is no evidence of impairment of oxygenation in this dog (as would be expected given the animal's history). It would also not be 'routine' to calculate the $P_{(A-a)}O_2$ for an animal with such a high oxygen partial pressure in the absence of any clinical signs of respiratory disease; it would be more common (but less accurate!) to 'eyeball' the P_aO_2 and assume it was normal given that it is approximately 5 × the inspired oxygen concentration (93% in this case). It is included for this case simply to reinforce the concepts behind the calculation.

FINAL DIAGNOSIS

The dog has a mixed acid–base disturbance: metabolic alkalosis and respiratory acidosis.

→ **CASE 3 CONTINUED**

OUTCOME

The anaesthetic depth appeared appropriate, so intermittent positive pressure ventilation was undertaken to reduce the P_aCO_2 to a more acceptable level. In addition, the intravenous fluids were changed from compound sodium lactate to 0.9% NaCl, given that the higher Cl^- concentrations in the latter would increase the availability of Cl^- in the renal tubules and, therefore, reduce the 'inappropriate' HCO_3^- resorption by the kidneys.

Note that hypokalaemia is also commonly observed in animals with gastric vomiting, so ideally plasma K^+ concentrations should have been checked and the intravenous fluids supplemented as appropriate.

CASE 4

SIGNALMENT

5-year-old entire male Border Collie.

HISTORY

Presented with depression and anorexia to the first-opinion practice 2 days after the owner had pulled a stick from the dog's mouth, which he had run on to while playing. The veterinary surgeon had anaesthetized the dog and noted a penetrating wound in the dorsal pharyngeal area; the dog was maintained on intravenous compound sodium lactate at twice maintenance rates for 24 hours prior to referral, and was given a single subcutaneous injection of amoxicillin/clavulanic acid (co-amoxiclav).

On presentation at the referral hospital, the dog was pyrexic (40.2°C), extremely depressed and unwilling to stand or move around. Heart rate was 140 beats/min, respiratory rate 20 breaths/min, mucous membranes appeared slightly pale, and peripheral pulses were not palpable.

CLINICAL PATHOLOGY DATA

On admission, blood was drawn for routine biochemistry and haematology, and the results below obtained. (All other reported parameters were within the reference intervals.)

Parameter	Result	Reference interval
Albumin (g/l)	**16**	29–36
Globulin (g/l)	24	28–42
ALT (IU/l)	**110**	<90
ALP (IU/l)	**322**	<230
Triglycerides (mmol/l)	**1.1**	<0.6
Lactate (mmol/l)	**4.4**	<2.5
Na$^+$ (mmol/l)	151	136–159
Cl$^-$ (mmol/l)	**122**	95–115
K$^+$ (mmol/l)	3.8	3.4–5.8
Neutrophils (x 10^9/l)	**1.2**	3.0–11.8

Abnormal results are in **bold**.

WHAT ABNORMALITIES ARE PRESENT AND WHAT IS THEIR SIGNIFICANCE?

The neutropenia is probably secondary to infection. The mild elevations in triglycerides, alanine aminotransferase (ALT) and alkaline phosphatase (ALP) are probably relatively 'non-specific' changes, and are unlikely to be of significant clinical relevance (although, in conjunction with the hypoalbuminaemia, they could potentially be suggestive of liver failure, but this is unlikely given that the dog had been clinically normal until the incident with the stick). The significance of the elevated lactate and Cl^- is discussed below in relation to the blood gas results.

Arterial blood gas analysis was performed while the dog was breathing room air.

Blood gas analysis	Result	Reference interval
pH	**7.22**	7.35–7.46
P_aCO_2 (mmHg)	**24.0**	30.8–42.8
P_aO_2 (mmHg)	93.0	80.9–103.3
HCO_3^- (mmol/l) (actual)	**12.1**	18.8–25.6
BE (mmol/l)	**−15.4**	0 ± 4

Abnormal results are in **bold**.

WHAT ABNORMALITIES ARE PRESENT IN THE BLOOD GAS RESULTS AND HOW WOULD YOU INTERPRET THESE?

The blood gas results demonstrate an acidaemia.

KEY POINT

An acidaemia implies the dog must have a metabolic acidosis, respiratory acidosis, or both.

The P_aCO_2 is reduced, which means the dog either has a respiratory alkalosis or respiratory compensation for a metabolic acidosis.

KEY POINT

The body will attempt to maintain a normal ratio of HCO_3^- : CO_2 (approximately 20:1) to keep the pH as close to the normal range as possible; therefore, a reduction in PCO_2 may be a primary problem or may be a compensatory response to a reduced HCO_3^-.

Both the HCO_3^- and BE are decreased, indicating a metabolic acidosis or metabolic compensation for a primary respiratory alkalosis.

KEY POINT

Remember that metabolic compensation is slow to develop and to peak; most respiratory disorders in animals do not persist long enough for full metabolic compensation to develop.

Thus, there are alterations in both P_aCO_2 and HCO_3^-/BE in this dog; which of these is the primary problem? Given that the dog has an acidaemia, this would fit best with the metabolic acidosis being the primary problem (if the reduced P_aCO_2 was the primary problem, i.e. a respiratory alkalosis, we would expect the pH to be alkalaemic).

→

→ **CASE 4 CONTINUED**

IS THE DEGREE OF COMPENSATION APPROPRIATE? IS THE ANION GAP NORMAL AND IS THIS EXPECTED?

Having decided that the metabolic disturbance is the primary issue, it is important to check whether the alteration in P_aCO_2 is an appropriate compensatory response (quantitatively). If not, this may imply that we have a mixed acid–base disturbance.

For each 1 mmol/l reduction in HCO_3^-, we should expect a reduction in P_aCO_2 of 0.7 mmHg (see Figure 9.11). If we take the midpoint of the normal HCO_3^- as about 22 mmol/l (reference range 18.8–25.6 mmol/l) then the expected reduction in P_aCO_2 would be $(22 - 12.1) \times 0.7 = 6.93$ mmHg. This is then subtracted from the midpoint of the normal P_aCO_2 range (~36 mmHg; reference range 30.8–42.8 mmHg) to give an expected P_aCO_2 for this case of $(36 - 6.93) = 29.07$ mmHg. Given that this dog's P_aCO_2 is 24 mmHg, this would imply that the reduction is not just a straightforward compensatory response, because it is approximately 5 mmHg less than the calculated compensatory value, i.e. this blood gas result would tend to suggest the dog has a concurrent metabolic acidosis and respiratory alkalosis.

This explains the acid–base derangements, but what other information can be deduced? Since this dog has a metabolic acidosis, it is worth calculating the anion gap to determine whether this is due to primary bicarbonate loss (e.g. through the kidney), or to acid gain.

$$AG = (Na^+ + K^+) - (Cl^- + HCO_3^-)$$
$$\therefore AG = (151 + 3.8) - (122 + 12.1)$$
$$AG = 20.7 \text{ (reference range 12–25 mmol/l)}$$

Thus, the AG is normal, suggesting that the metabolic acidosis is due to bicarbonate loss, and this would fit with the concurrent increase in chloride (a hyperchloraemic metabolic acidosis). *However*, the lactate value in this dog is high, which suggests tissue hypoperfusion, and one would expect the associated accumulation of lactic acid to have resulted in an *elevated* AG. So, how do these two apparently disparate pieces of information fit together? Clinically, the dog was showing evidence of tissue hypoperfusion (tachycardia, weak peripheral pulses, pale mucous membranes), which would fit with the elevated lactate value. The likeliest explanation for the AG being within the normal range despite both the clinical appearance of hypovolaemia and the elevated lactate lies with the dog's low albumin levels: hypoalbuminaemia is one of the commoner causes of a *low* AG. In this particular dog, it is likely that the hypovolaemia and hyperlactataemia were tending to elevate the AG, but the hypoalbuminaemia was tending to reduce it, the final result being that the AG was within the normal reference range.

WHAT IS THE $P_{(A-a)}O_2$?

What about this dog's oxygenation: is it normal? On first glance, a P_aO_2 of 93 mmHg would appear to be completely normal; however, one needs to consider that hyperventilation (as demonstrated by the low P_aCO_2 in this dog) should result in an increase in P_aO_2. Calculating the alveolar–arterial oxygen difference in this dog (and the shortened form of the equation can be used because the dog is breathing room air), gives:

$$P_AO_2 = 150 - (P_aCO_2/0.8)$$
$$P_AO_2 = 150 - (24/0.8)$$
$$P_AO_2 = 120 \text{ mmHg}$$
$$P_aO_2 \text{ (from blood gas)} = 93 \text{ mmHg}$$
$$\therefore P_{(A-a)}O_2 = 120 - 93 = 27 \text{ mmHg}$$

This is just slightly outside the reference range for a dog breathing room air, and may either be normal for this animal (~5% of values from 'normal' patients will lie outside reference intervals), or may indicate that there is early (very mild, and – currently – clinically inconsequential) impairment of oxygenation. It would be advisable to repeat an arterial sample at a later point to determine whether the alveolar–arterial O_2 difference is widening.

FINAL DIAGNOSIS

- Primary metabolic acidosis, probably secondary to hypovolaemia (clinical signs and elevated lactate), with concurrent respiratory alkalosis, probably resulting from the pyrexia and/or pain.
- Normal anion gap (but see text for possible explanation).
- Possible mild impairment of oxygenation.

This is a fairly complex case from the point of view of result interpretation, and also highlights the fact that not all animals have 'read the textbooks' and fit neatly into one clinical scenario.

OUTCOME

The dog was treated with intravenous fluid therapy, intravenous antibiotics and opioid analgesics, with a view to stabilization prior to surgical exploration of the wound. Unfortunately, the dog suffered a cardiopulmonary arrest approximately 24 hours following presentation, and resuscitation was unsuccessful.

References and further reading

Adams LG and Polzin DJ (1989) Mixed acid–base disorders. *Veterinary Clinics of North America: Small Animal Practice* **19**, 307–326

Bach JF (2008) Hypoxemia: A quick reference. *Veterinary Clinics of North America: Small Animal Practice* **38**, 423–426

De Morais HAS (2008) Metabolic acidosis: A quick reference. *Veterinary Clinics of North America: Small Animal Practice* **38**, 439–442

DiBartola SP (2012) Introduction to acid–base disorders. In: *Fluid, Electrolyte, and Acid-Base Disorders in Small Animal Practice*, ed. SP DiBartola, pp. 231–252. Elsevier Saunders, Missouri

Driscoll P, Brown T, Gwinnutt C and Wardle T (1997) *A Simple Guide to Blood Gas Analysis*. BMJ Publishing Group, London

Foy D and De Morais HAS (2008) Metabolic alkalosis: A quick reference. *Veterinary Clinics of North America: Small Animal Practice* **38**, 435–438

Haskins SC (1983) Blood gases and acid–base balance: clinical interpretation and therapeutic implications. In: *Current Veterinary Therapy, 8th edn*, ed. RW Kirk *et al.*, pp. 201–215. WB Saunders, Philadelphia

Johnson RA and De Morais HAS (2012) Respiratory acid–base disorders. In: *Fluid, Electrolyte, and Acid-Base Disorders in Small Animal Practice*, ed. SP DiBartola, pp. 287–301. Elsevier Saunders, Missouri

Kaae J and De Morais HAS (2008) Anion gap and strong ion difference: A quick reference. *Veterinary Clinics of North America: Small Animal Practice* **38**, 443–447

Martin L (1999) *All You Really Need to Know to Interpret Arterial Blood Gases, 2nd edn*. Lippincott, Williams and Wilkins, Philadelphia

McGrotty Y and Brown A (2013) Blood gases, electrolytes and interpretation 1. Blood gases. *In Practice* **35(2)**, 59–65

Peterson M (1998) Endocrine emergencies. In: *BSAVA Manual of Endocrinology, 2nd edn*, ed. AG Torrance and CT Mooney, pp. 163–172. BSAVA Publications, Gloucester

Polzin DJ, Stevens JB and Osborne CA (1982) Clinical application of the anion gap in evaluation of acid–base disorders in dogs. *Compendium on Continuing Education for the Practicing Veterinarian* **4**, 1021–1032

Robertson SA (1989) Simple acid–base disorders. *Veterinary Clinics of North America: Small Animal Practice* **19**, 289–306

Rodkey WG, Hannon JP, Dramise JG *et al*. (1978) Arterialized capillary blood used to determine the acid–base and blood gas status of dogs. *American Journal of Veterinary Research* **39**, 459–464

Rubush JM (2001) Metabolic acid–base disorders. *Veterinary Clinics of North America: Small Animal Practice* **31**, 1323–1354

Senior DF (1995) Fluid therapy, electrolytes and acid–base control. In: *Textbook of Veterinary Internal Medicine, 4th edn*, ed. SJ Ettinger and EC Feldman, pp. 294–312. WB Saunders, Philadelphia

Verwaerde P, Malet C, Lagente M, de la Farge F and Braun JP (2002) The accuracy of the i-STAT portable analyser for measuring gases and pH in whole blood samples from dogs. *Research in Veterinary Science* **73**, 71–75

Zweens J, Grankena H, van Kampen EJ, Rispins P and Zijlstra WG (1977) Ionic composition of arterial and mixed venous plasma in the unanaesthetized dog. *American Journal of Physiology* **233**, F412–F415

Chapter 10

Urinalysis

Niki Skeldon and Jelena Ristić

Urinalysis is one of the most useful diagnostic tools available to the practitioner. The specimen is readily available, provides extensive information about the animal's health, and routine urinalysis tests are cheap to perform. The majority of these routine tests can be performed in-house; not only is this more economical, but it avoids any artefactual changes which can occur with delayed urine processing and hinder interpretation of the results. Routine urinalysis tests include macroscopic examination, specific gravity (SG), dipstick analysis, wet sediment examination and often culture. There are numerous indications for urinalysis: it is not only useful for animals with signs of urinary tract disease but can also be used as a screening test in older animals or as part of a thorough medical work-up. In many cases the most information is obtained if urinalysis is performed in combination with serum/plasma biochemistry. This chapter will work through the routine urinalysis tests in some detail, before discussing tests which are only relevant in specific circumstances. Tests that are still under investigation are included in order to familiarize the clinician with promising new assays that may become commercially available in the future.

Sampling: collection and storage

Sample collection

There are three methods of sample collection: free catch; catheterization of the bladder; and cystocentesis. Voided samples can be useful for basic tests: they are straightforward and cheap to collect, but do have their limitations because of the potential for contamination. Cystocentesis samples avoid contamination from the genital tract and are often less traumatic for the patient than catheterization, so are the ideal sample type in most cases. Morning samples tend to be more concentrated, which increases the chances of detecting any abnormalities, hence they are preferred where possible.

Free-catch sampling

The sample is collected either during normal micturition or by expressing the bladder. Expressing the bladder can be painful for the animal and there is a risk of rupture so it is not generally recommended, unless there is a neurological

problem which makes manual expression easy. For dogs, specially designed collection kits can make it easier for an owner to collect a sample; alternatively, many people find a shallow dish such as a kidney dish suitable. For cats, non-absorbent litter allows collection at home, using the cat's usual litter tray; the urine can then be removed with a syringe or pipette (Figure 10.1).

It is best not to collect the first portion of the stream of urine because it can be contaminated with cells and hairs. If, however, a lesion in the distal urinary tract is suspected the first stream of urine is collected, and if prostatic disease is suspected the end of the stream is most useful. Free-catch samples are not recommended for culture owing to the likelihood of contamination from the external genitalia and urethra.

Catheterization

Catheterization is rarely indicated. If a sample is to be collected directly from an animal, cystocentesis is usually preferable. Catheterization can be useful to collect a sample from a nearly empty bladder or in large dogs, where cystocentesis can be technically difficult. It can usually be performed conscious in male dogs and many bitches, but cats often require sedation or general anaesthesia.

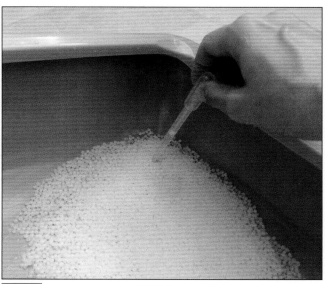

10.1 Use of non-absorbent cat litter to harvest urine.

There are disadvantages to catheterization: there is a risk of introducing infection with this technique, so care should be taken to maintain catheter sterility, and contamination from the external genitalia and urethra can complicate interpretation of bacteriology results. It is best to collect the sample directly into a sterile universal container to minimize the chances of contamination (Figure 10.2).

Cystocentesis

Provided there is sufficient urine in the bladder cystocentesis is a very useful technique and not difficult to perform, especially under ultrasound guidance. Cystocentesis provides an immediate sample and is the ideal sample type for culture. It can, however, result in microscopic haematuria which can be difficult to differentiate from *in vivo* haemorrhage. Contraindications to cystocentesis include coagulopathies such as severe thrombocytopenia or suspected bladder tumours, which can be seeded along the needle tract (Figure 10.3).

Storage

Urinalysis should be performed within 60 minutes of urine collection where possible. If a sample is left at room temperature for a number of hours the following changes can occur:

- pH can increase as bacteria break down urea to ammonia
- Cells and casts degenerate
- Crystals can dissolve or precipitate
- Levels of glucose, ketones and bilirubin can decrease
- Bacteria can multiply.

These factors should be borne in mind if a sample is posted to an external laboratory.

When storing urine in house or submitting it to a laboratory, the sample should be kept in a sterile universal container. It is best refrigerated, then warmed to room temperature and mixed before testing. Refrigeration can cause precipitation of crystals, which do not always dissolve on warming. Urine should not be frozen because this can damage the sediment. A recent study found that cystocentesis samples stored in boric acid were less likely to give a positive result on culture than those tested fresh or stored in a plain tube (Rowlands *et al.*, 2011); this may or may not apply to samples collected in other ways. If boric acid is used it is important to ensure the correct amount of powder is present because if the tube is under-filled this can affect isolation of bacteria. Some laboratories request that samples for cytology are preserved in a particular way (e.g. in ethylenediamine tetra-acetic acid (EDTA) or with the addition of formalin); it is best to check your laboratory's specific requirements before taking the sample.

General tips
• Lubricate catheter tip with sterile lubricant, to aid passage • Advance catheter until urine starts to flow, then stop to prevent knots forming in long catheters

Tom cat	Queen
• Best under general anaesthesia so the urethra is fully relaxed • 3, 3.5 or 4 Fr cat catheter with or without stylet • Fully extrude the penis • Hold penis with swab or piece of tissue to increase grip if required	• Easier under general anaesthesia or heavy sedation • 3, 3.5 or 4 Fr cat catheter or occasionally a 6 Fr dog catheter • Best performed blind • Urethral opening lies on ventral vaginal floor, in the midline, so the cat should be in ventral recumbency and kept straight

Dog	Bitch
• 6–10 Fr dog catheter unless very small dog • Usually restrained in lateral recumbency; can be performed standing • Grasp os penis in one hand and pull back prepuce with other hand, then hold penis exposed with one hand • May feel the catheter pass the start and end of the os penis • Once the catheter has passed the os penis there is no need to hold the penis extended	• Easier under sedation or general anaesthesia, especially in small patients • 6–10 Fr dog catheter; a Foley may be used if there is a reason for it to remain *in situ* • Positioning is personal preference: dorsal, ventral or lateral recumbency • Use an otoscope or vaginal speculum to identify the urethral orifice on the ventral floor of the vestibule • The vagina travels dorsocranially and then horizontally; the orifice is usually just before the change in direction • In large bitches it is possible to feel the orifice with a gloved finger • It may help if an assistant pulls the ventral vulva caudally • If catheterization is not successful, changing the dog's position may help • Once the orifice is identified insert the catheter; it should pass easily, without force

10.2 Tips for catheterization.

Cats	Dogs

• Use a fine needle – 23 G or smaller, 5/8 inch (16 mm) long – and 5 ml syringe
• Positioning is personal preference: usually the cat is standing or in lateral recumbency
• Palpate and immobilize the bladder
• Insert the needle into the ventral or lateral abdominal wall at a 45-degree angle to the bladder wall, aiming caudally
• It is best to avoid the bladder apex because as urine is aspirated and the bladder becomes smaller it can shrink off the end of the needle
	• 23 G needle, 1 inch (25 mm) long, in all but small dogs
	• Positioning is personal preference: usually the dog is in dorsal recumbency but some prefer lateral
	• Locating the site:
	  • Ideally, palpate and immobilize the bladder
	  • The procedure is easier with ultrasound guidance
	  • The site is usually halfway between the pelvic brim and the umbilicus
	  • If the dog is in dorsal recumbency some operators shave the midline, pour on surgical spirit, and use the position it pools in as the entry site
	• Aim the needle in a caudodorsal direction

10.3 Tips for cystocentesis.

Normal urine

Figure 10.4 gives details of sample preparation and examination. See Figures 10.5, 10.6, 10.9, 10.14 and 10.20 for expected physical, chemical and sediment examination findings in urine from healthy dogs and cats.

Equipment

- Conical-tip tubes
- Plastic pipette
- Centrifuge
- Specialized urine stain (e.g. Sedi-Stain) (optional)
- Glass slides and coverslips
- Microscope

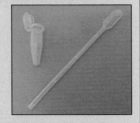

Sample preparation

- **Obtain a standard volume of urine.** Usually this is 5 ml, but in practice may be limited by the type of centrifuge available. As long as a standard volume is used each time consistent results will be seen with respect to the quantity of structures present
- **Mix gently and transfer to conical-tip tube**
- **Centrifuge at a slow speed** (e.g. 1000–2000 rpm for 5 minutes). It is important the urine is centrifuged at a slow speed so that delicate structures such as casts and cells are not damaged
- **Discard the supernatant** (or save for measurement of urine specific gravity). This can be done by pipetting, or by simply tipping it out. The chosen method should be adhered to for consistency of results
- **Flick the tube to resuspend the sediment**
- **Optional: add one drop of a suitable stain** (e.g. Sedi-Stain). With practice, many people prefer to examine unstained samples, but inexperienced microscopists can find staining useful to highlight cells and other structures
- **Pipette a drop of urine on to the slide**
- **Place a coverslip over the urine.** The size of the coverslip will affect the area over which the urine spreads and therefore the concentration of the constituent elements. This is probably of minimal clinical significance, but be consistent to gain familiarity with what is normal for the particular method of sediment preparation

Tips for examination

- Ensure the microscope's condenser is LOWERED to highlight structures
- Scan whole area using the X10 objective; most crystals are visible at this magnification
- Change to the X40 objective to search for cells, casts, small crystals and bacteria
- It is good practice to count the number of each structure in 10 fields and take an average
- Use the X100 objective to confirm the presence of bacteria if necessary and to distinguish them from stain precipitate and Brownian motion of particulate matter

10.4 Wet sediment examination: sample preparation and examination.

Parameter	Normal result	Comments
Colour	Yellow	In healthy animals, the intensity of the yellow colour is approximately proportional to urine SG (see Figure 10.6)
Clarity	Clear	Some healthy animals have slightly turbid urine due to suspended crystals and/or epithelial cells

10.5 Macroscopic examination of urine: expected findings in healthy dogs and cats. SG = specific gravity.

Macroscopic examination

The urine should be fresh and mixed thoroughly before being examined macroscopically for colour, clarity and any obvious sediment. Normal urine should be pale to deep yellow, and clear or only mildly turbid (Figure 10.6). Abnormal urine colour is described as pigmenturia. See Figure 10.7 for possible changes in the macroscopic appearance of urine and potential causes.

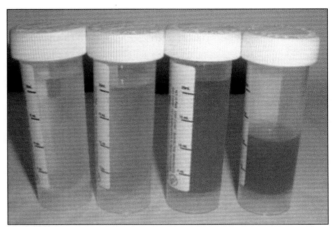

10.6 Macroscopic appearance of normal urine, demonstrating the variation in colour intensity depending on urine concentration (left to right: least to most concentrated samples).

Appearance of urine	Possible causes	Comments
Very pale, almost colourless	Low specific gravity	
Red	Erythrocytes Haemoglobin Myoglobin	
Red–brown	Erythrocytes Haemoglobin Myoglobin Methaemoglobin	Methaemoglobin forms in aged samples as haemoglobin or myoglobin is oxidized Methaemoglobinuria is also seen with severe cases of intravascular haemolytic anaemia due to erythrocyte oxidative damage
Red–pink	Consumption of beetroot or red food dyes	
Dark brown	Methaemoglobin Use of Oxyglobin™	As for methaemoglobinuria
Yellow–orange	Bilirubin	
Yellow–green or yellow–brown	Bilirubin Biliverdin (forms after *in vitro* breakdown of bilirubin)	Biliverdin is not detected by dipsticks
Turbid	Increase in any of the following: • Cells • Casts • Mucus • Bacteria • Crystals • Lipid droplets • Amorphous material	

10.7 Macroscopic examination of urine: changes in colour and clarity, and possible causes.

Specific gravity

The SG of urine is an indication of its weight compared with an equal volume of distilled water. The SG depends on the number and molecular weight of solutes dissolved in urine. Measurement of SG should always be performed on a refractometer because dipsticks are notoriously inaccurate. A refractometer measures the refractive index. As light passes through the urine sample it is refracted or bent; the degree to which it bends depends on the amount of solute or particles present, so the refractive index correlates with the SG. The scale on the refractometer gives the SG as a number compared with 1.000, which is the SG of distilled water.

Measuring SG

See Figure 10.8 for maintenance of the refractometer. Two or three drops of urine should be applied for testing. The SG can be measured on whole urine or, if the sample contains significant sediment and is turbid, it can be centrifuged and SG tested on the supernatant.

- Clean the refractometer glass with distilled water after each use
- Wipe dry, taking care to avoid scratching the glass
- 'Zero' the instrument by placing 2–3 drops of distilled water on the stage and adjusting the eyepiece until it reads 1.000. Ideally this should be performed at each use
- Check calibration with saline: a 5% solution should read 1.022

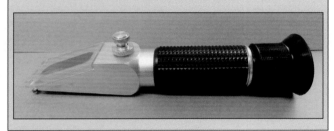

10.8   Maintenance of the refractometer.

If the SG is higher than available on the scale on the refractometer being used, concentrated samples can be diluted 1:1 with distilled or deionized water. The numbers after the decimal point are then multiplied by 2. However, this is rarely of clinical relevance.

Example

Mix 1 ml sample with 1 ml water

If the diluted sample measures 1.030
0.030 × 2 = 0.060
The SG is 1.060

The SG can increase slightly with large amounts of glucose or protein in the urine. The dogma that refractometers specially calibrated for feline urine must be used, has recently been debunked; indeed, feline-specific refractometers may underestimate SG in cats (Tvedten *et al.*, 2015).

Key point

Regularly 'zero' the refractometer with distilled water

Interpretation of SG

See Figure 10.9 for interpretation of urine SG. Note that SG can vary with time: two- to three-fold variations have been noted within hours in samples from dogs. Furthermore, the SG of urine from normal animals can be any value, and correct interpretation of this value depends on the context.

The SG is often used to distinguish prerenal and renal azotaemia. In an animal that has azotaemia and a condition affecting the kidneys' ability to concentrate urine, such as secondary diabetes insipidus (e.g. in hypercalcaemia, pyometra), or loss of medullary hypertonicity (e.g. hypoadrenocorticism) it is not possible to use SG to find the cause of the azotaemia. For example, with hypercalcaemia the azotaemia may be prerenal, reflecting hypercalcaemia and excess water loss, or the azotaemia may be renal, owing to renal damage induced by the hypercalcaemia. In both scenarios, the urine SG will be low.

It is important to note that urine SG is generally lower in very young animals than in adults. See below and Figure 10.48 for further information on urinalysis in puppies.

Key point

Urine SG cannot be used to distinguish prerenal from renal azotaemia if concurrent conditions are present that cause secondary diabetes insipidus – see text and Figure 10.10

Specific gravity (SG)	Interpretation
1.015–1.045 1.035–1.060	Normal for dogs Normal for cats
Isosthenuria: 1.008–1.012	This is the concentration of plasma, and implies the kidneys are not changing the SG. The SG can fall within this range with many conditions that cause PU/PD or in normal animals in certain circumstances. SG in this range with azotaemia supports a diagnosis of renal failure
Dilute urine (hyposthenuria): <1.008	This implies the kidneys can alter SG and make urine more dilute, and therefore excludes renal failure. Possible causes include diabetes insipidus, primary polydipsia or conditions that interfere with the action of ADH (see Figure 10.10)
Concentrated urine: >1.030 in dog >1.035 in cat	Suggests kidney disease is not present. Useful to confirm prerenal azotaemia. Approximately two-thirds of nephron function must be lost before abnormalities in renal concentrating ability occur, therefore clinically inapparent renal disease could be present with concentrated urine
Partially concentrated urine: 1.013–1.029 in dog 1.013–1.034 in cat	May be partial impairment of renal function or partial deficiency/lack of response to ADH (see Figure 10.10). If the animal is clinically dehydrated this is considered inappropriately dilute (see below)
Inappropriately dilute: <1.030 in dog <1.035 in cat With clinical evidence of dehydration or azotaemia	This can be due to renal disease, or a partial deficiency or incomplete action of ADH. Concurrent pre-renal azotaemia and a condition that causes a deficiency/reduced action of ADH is also possible
Inappropriately concentrated urine: >1.007 in an over-hydrated patient	Suggests there is renal disease because the kidneys should produce dilute urine in this situation

10.9   Interpretation of urine specific gravity. ADH = antidiuretic hormone; PU/PD = polyuria and polydipsia.
(Modified from www.iris-kidney.com)

Primary polyuria			Primary polydipsia
Osmotic diuresis	**Central diabetes insipidus** (can be complete or partial)	**Nephrogenic diabetes insipidus (NDI)** (primary or secondary) Note that many causes of PU/PD are due to a secondary NDI caused by impaired release or action of ADH	
• Diabetes mellitus • Primary renal glucosuria	• Congenital • Neoplastic • Trauma • Inflammatory • Idiopathic	• Primary congenital NDI • Renal disease • Hypercalcaemia • Hyperadrenocorticism • Pyometra • Pyelonephritis • Liver disease • Hyperthyroidism • Acromegaly • Hypoadrenocorticism • Hypokalaemia • Drugs, e.g. steroids, diuretics	• Psychogenic polydipsia

10.10 A guide to the differential diagnosis of polyuria and polydipsia (PU/PD). ADH = antidiuretic hormone.

Approach to polyuria and polydipsia

The first step is to confirm that the patient genuinely has PU/PD. It is helpful to measure thirst. A fluid intake of >100 ml/kg/24h in dogs and >45 ml/kg/24h in cats is defined as polydipsia. In households with multiple pets where it may not be possible to measure water intake accurately, urine SG can give a good guide as to whether PU/PD is genuine. If the urine SG is >1.030 in a dog or >1.035 in a cat, it is unlikely that the patient has PU/PD.

Polydipsia can result in medullary washout of solute. Normally there is a high concentration of electrolytes in the renal medulla, which draws water from the urine in the tubules. Excess water handling can decrease the concentration of electrolytes, thus affecting the kidneys' ability to draw water from the urine. This results in dilute urine and a compensatory increase in thirst. Medullary solute washout is not a diagnosis but occurs secondarily to an increase in urine flow through the kidneys in animals that are already PU/PD, for example in psychogenic polydipsia. Medullary solute washout can affect an animal's response to water deprivation testing.

See Figure 10.10 for a guide to the differential diagnoses of polyuria and polydipsia and Figure 10.11 for an approach to the investigation of PU/PD. The underlying pathophysiology has been simplified in order to help clinicians compile a logical differential list to facilitate work-up of a PU/PD case.

Parameter	Abnormality/ comment	Main differential diagnoses	Other differential diagnoses to consider
Signalment	Female entire	Pyometra	
	Breed predisposition	e.g. Burmese cat, Samoyed – DM	
History	Confirm PD	See text	
	Very severe PD	Possible DI	
	Polyphagia	DM, HAC, hyperthyroidism	
	Inappetence	Renal disease, pyometra, DKA	Pyelonephritis, hypoadrenocorticism, hypercalcaemia
	Dietary changes	Recent change to dry diet	
	Weight loss	Renal or hepatic disease, DM	Hypoadrenocorticism
	Drugs	Steroids, diuretics	
Examination	Excitable	Psychogenic polydipsia Hyperthyroidism	
	Tachycardia	Hyperthyroidism	
	Bradycardia	Hypoadrenocorticism, hyperkalaemia, hypercalcaemia	
	Lymphadenopathy	Lymphoma	
	Thyroid mass	Hyperthyroidism	
	Anal sac mass	Hypercalcaemia	
	Kidneys shrunken	CRF	
	Renomegaly	Renal neoplasia, pyelonephritis	
	Hepatomegaly	Liver disease, HAC	
	Vaginal discharge	Pyometra	
	Skin and coat changes	HAC	
	CNS signs	Hepatic encephalopathy, large pituitary mass	

10.11 Approach to the investigation of polyuria and polydipsia (PU/PD). A full history, examination, urinalysis, haematology and biochemistry are required in most cases; the results of these are used to direct further investigations. ACTH = adrenocorticotropic hormone; ADH = antidiuretic hormone; ALP = alkaline phosphatase; ALT = alanine aminotransferase; CDI = central diabetes insipidus; CKD = chronic kidney disease; CNS = central nervous system; CRF = chronic renal failure; DI = diabetes insipidus; DKA = diabetic ketoacidosis; DM = diabetes mellitus; HAC = hyperadrenocorticism; LDDST = low-dose dexamethasone suppression test; NDI = nephrogenic diabetes insipidus; SG = specific gravity; TT4 = total thyroxine; UPCR = urine protein:creatinine ratio; UTI = urinary tract infection. (continues)

▶

Parameter	Abnormality/ comment	Main differential diagnoses	Other differential diagnoses to consider
Urinalysis	Check SG	See Figure 10.9 for further details	
	SG <1.008	DI (primary or secondary), psychogenic PD. Implies the kidneys can alter SG and make urine more dilute; rules out renal failure	
	SG 1.008–1.012 'fixed range'	If azotaemic, suggests renal failure until proven otherwise. Rule out other causes; partial CDI and NDI and secondary causes of NDI (see Figure 10.10) may give SG in this range	
	SG >1.030 in dog SG >1.035 in cat	Renal failure extremely unlikely	
	SG 1.013–1.029 in dog SG 1.013–1.034 in cat	All differential diagnoses possible, except complete DI, where urine is hyposthenuric	
	Pyuria, bacteriuria, haematuria	Pyelonephritis, pyometra if free catch	Secondary to DM, HAC
	Increased UPCR	Glomerulonephritis, renal amyloidosis	HAC
	Glucosuria	DM, stress hyperglycaemia in cats	Primary renal glucosuria, Fanconi syndrome
Haematology	Neutrophilia ± left shift	Pyometra	UTI
	Non-regenerative anaemia	CKD, liver disease	Hypoadrenocorticism
	Stress leucogram	HAC, steroid therapy	
	Lymphocytosis, eosinophilia	Hypoadrenocorticism	
Biochemistry	Azotaemia	Renal failure, dehydration	
	Elevated liver enzymes	Liver disease, HAC or steroid therapy in dogs (usually ALP>ALT), hyperthyroidism	
	Hypercalcaemia	Neoplasia, e.g. lymphoma, anal sac adenocarcinoma, primary hyperparathyroidism, idiopathic hypercalcaemia in cats	Hypoadrenocorticism, renal disease, granulomatous disease, hypervitaminosis D
	Hyperglycaemia	DM (marked), stress in cats	HAC, acromegaly
	Hyperkalaemia/ hyponatraemia and hypochloraemia	Hypoadrenocorticism	
	Hypercholesterolaemia	HAC	Nephrotic syndrome
TT4	Elevated TT4	Hyperthyroidism	
ACTH stimulation test/LDDST/urine cortisol:creatinine ratio	Indicated as screening tests for hyperadrenocorticism; see Chapter 18		
Fructosamine	Elevated	DM	No or milder increase in stress-induced hyperglycaemia in cats
Water deprivation test	Adequate concentration	Psychogenic polydipsia	
	Inadequate concentration	DI	
ADH response test	Adequate concentration	CDI	
	Inadequate concentration	NDI – primary or secondary	
Osmolality	Urine osmolality low, plasma high	Suggests primary polyuria	
	Urine osmolality low, plasma low	Suggests primary polydipsia	
Imaging	Useful to evaluate kidneys, uterus, liver, adrenal glands, thyroid and parathyroid glands, brain		

10.11 (continued) Approach to the investigation of polyuria and polydipsia (PU/PD). A full history, examination, urinalysis, haematology and biochemistry are required in most cases; the results of these are used to direct further investigations. ACTH = adrenocorticotropic hormone; ADH = antidiuretic hormone; ALP = alkaline phosphatase; ALT = alanine aminotransferase; CDI = central diabetes insipidus; CKD = chronic kidney disease; CNS = central nervous system; CRF = chronic renal failure; DI = diabetes insipidus; DKA = diabetic ketoacidosis; DM = diabetes mellitus; HAC = hyperadrenocorticism; LDDST = low-dose dexamethasone suppression test; NDI = nephrogenic diabetes insipidus; SG = specific gravity; TT4 = total thyroxine; UPCR = urine protein:creatinine ratio; UTI = urinary tract infection.

Chemical analysis

Reagent strips (dipsticks) are the starting point for the chemical analysis of urine, and in most cases are all that is necessary. See Figures 10.12–10.14 for general concepts regarding the use and interpretation of dipsticks. On rare occasions it may be necessary to clarify dipstick results with a confirmatory test, especially when heavily pigmented urine interferes with reading the strip, such as when there is marked haematuria, haemoglobinuria, bilirubinuria, or Oxyglobin™ has been administered. Confirmatory tablets are available for detecting urinary glucose, ketones, bilirubin and blood, but these are rarely necessary in practice.

Key point

Read dipsticks at the stipulated time

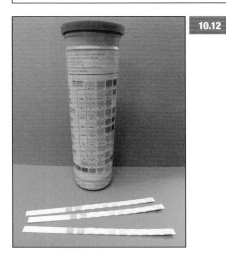

10.12	Chemical analysis of urine: dipsticks.

pH

The pH measurement is only reliable if performed on a fresh sample. It is most accurately assessed with a pH meter, but the expense of the equipment means that this is rarely performed, even in reference laboratories (one of the reasons that reference laboratories do not invest in pH meters is that samples are usually a few hours old on receipt and therefore likely to have undergone an artefactual increase in pH). In general, the accuracy of the pH as evaluated by dipsticks is sufficient for clinical needs, although it may be prudent to use a pH meter on a fresh sample for patients with urolithiasis.

Glucose

The renal tubular transport maximum for glucose is approximately 10–12 mmol/l in dogs and 12–16 mmol/l in cats. Once the glucose concentration in blood increases above this level any excess is lost in the urine. Glucosuria can result from hyperglycaemia (due to diabetes mellitus or, in cats, stress) or renal tubular dysfunction (normoglycaemic glucosuria). The latter can occur with congenital or acquired renal tubular disease such as Fanconi syndrome and primary renal glucosuria. In Fanconi syndrome, there is also loss of amino acids, phosphate and electrolytes, while in primary renal glucosuria there is loss only of glucose. Normoglycaemic glucosuria also can be due to acquired tubular pathology (e.g. ischaemic or toxic damage). Persistent glucosuria increases the risk of urinary tract infection (UTI), so sediment examination and culture are indicated.

Principle
• Urine reacts with chemicals impregnated in a pad to induce a colour change
• The colour change is compared by eye or using an automated spectrophotometer, with reference colour tones displayed on the dipstick container (see Figure 10.12)
• Reference tones relate to absolute concentrations of the various chemical constituents

Method
• Invert the sample to mix it thoroughly
• The dipstick is introduced into the urine sample, withdrawn and the excess removed by tapping lightly against the edge of the container or, in the case of a small sample, applied to the strip with a pipette
• The dipstick is allowed to 'develop' for the required length of time
• The colour on each pad is compared with the reference tones on the kit packet
• The results are recorded, usually in a semi-quantitative fashion ('negative', 'trace', '1+', '2+', '3+', etc.)

Interpretation
See text under individual parameters in 'Chemical analysis', and Figure 10.14

Important considerations
• Dipsticks are manufactured for humans; not all the available tests are appropriate for use in veterinary species (see Figure 10.14)
• Interpreting colour changes is subjective

Tips for maximizing accuracy of dipstick tests
• Store dipsticks in the manufacturer's pot, with the lid screwed on tightly. Avoid extremes of temperature, direct sunlight and moisture. Do not remove the desiccant provided
• Observe expiry dates: the chemicals in the reagent pads have a limited shelf-life (discoloration of the pads may indicate deterioration of the reagent)
• Ensure work areas and specimen containers are free from detergents and other contaminating substances
• Do not touch pads with the fingertips
• Perform testing on fresh urine at room temperature (if unable to perform on fresh urine, refrigerate but allow sample to return to room temperature before testing)
• Mix the sample well prior to testing
• Tap dipstick on removal from sample to remove excess urine. This prevents 'run-off', where chemicals from one reagent pad can affect the adjacent pad
• Wait the correct amount of time before reading the pads (this varies between tests)
• Read the pads in a good light or use an automated stick reader to improve consistency between operators

10.13	Dipstick use.

Parameter	Reported range	Normal value	Abnormal value	Possible causes	Potential sources of error	Comments
pH	5.0–8.5	6.0–7.5	>7.5	• Presence of urease-producing bacteria • Sample ageing (spontaneous urea degradation) • Transient postprandial effect • Metabolic alkalosis • Early proximal renal tubular acidosis • Distal renal tubular acidosis (see Chapter 11)	• Pigmenturia may interfere with visual assessment False decrease • 'Run-off' of buffer from protein pad	Urease-producing bacteria can be present due to UTI or sample contamination
			<6.0	• Metabolic (and some respiratory) acidosis • Hypochloraemic metabolic alkalosis ('paradoxical aciduria' – rare in dogs and cats) • Proximal renal tubular acidosis, once HCO_3^- depleted • Hypokalaemia (see Chapter 8) • Furosemide therapy • Acidifying diets		

Glucose	Negative
	Trace (5.5 mmol/l)
	1+ (14.0 mmol/l)
	2+ (28.0 mmol/l)
	3+ (55.0 mmol/l)
	4+ (>111.0 mmol/l)
		Negative	Trace or positive	• With hyperglycaemia
				  • Diabetes mellitus
				  • Transient stress hyperglycaemia (cats)
				  • Hyperadrenocorticism
				• With normoglycaemia
				  • Congenital renal tubular dysfunction (Fanconi syndrome, etc.)
				  • Acquired renal tubular dysfunction (ischaemia, toxins, etc.)
					False increase
					• H_2O_2 or sodium hypochlorite (e.g. sample contamination with cleaning products)
					• Contamination of the collection pot
					
					False decrease
					• High concentrations of ascorbic acid[a]
					• High ketone levels
					• Very concentrated urine
					• Very cold urine
					• Marked bilirubinuria
					• Presence of bacteria	

Ketones	Negative Trace (0.5 mmol/l) 1+ (1.5 mmol/l) 2+ (4.0 mmol/l) 3+ (8.0 mmol/l) 4+ (>16.0 mmol/l)	Negative	1+ or greater	• Diabetic ketosis • Severe starvation • Pregnancy ketosis • Hyperthyroidism in cats (Berent et al., 2007)	False increase • Pigmenturia • Very concentrated and acidic urine False decrease • Aged sample	Mainly detects acetoacetate; does not detect BHB
Bilirubin	Negative 1+ 2+ 3+	Dogs: negative, trace or 1+, depending on urine concentration Cats: negative	Dogs: 2+ or above Cats: trace or above	• Haemolysis • Hepatic dysfunction • Hepatic obstructive cholestasis • Post-hepatic obstructive cholestasis • Functional cholestasis (due to sepsis)	False increase • Metabolites of etodolac (NSAID) • Presence of indican (breakdown product derived from tryptophan) False decrease • Ascorbic acid[a] supplementation • Exposure to daylight (bilirubin degrades with exposure to UV light)	In dogs, interpret in context of urine concentration

Blood	Negative
	Trace (~10 RBC/µl)
	2+ (~80 RBC/µl)
		Negative	Positive	• Haemorrhage anywhere in urogenital tract
				  • Inflammation (infection, crystalluria, etc.)
				  • Neoplasia
				  • Trauma (including sampling trauma)
				  • Coagulopathy
				  • Other (see Figure 10.15)
				• Oestrus in entire bitches (voided samples)
					False increase
					• Hypochlorite (sample contamination with cleaning products)
					• Microbial peroxidase (UTI or sample contamination)
					
					False decrease
					• Sample not mixed (erythrocytes settle)
					• Very concentrated urine
					• Ascorbic acid[a]
					• Formaldehyde	

10.14 Interpretation of urine dipstick results. [a]High concentrations of ascorbic acid may be found with urinary acidifiers, vitamin therapy or drug preservatives. BHB = beta-hydroxybutyrate; NSAID = non-steroidal anti-inflammatory drug; RBC = red blood cells; UTI = urinary tract infection; UV = ultraviolet. (continues) ▶

Parameter	Reported range	Normal value	Abnormal value	Possible causes	Potential sources of error	Comments
Haemo-globin	Negative Trace (~10 RBC/µl) 1+ (~25 RBC/µl) 2+ (~80 RBC/µl) 3+ (~200 RBC/µl)	Negative	Positive	• Lysis of erythrocytes with sample aging • Intravascular haemolysis • Myoglobinuria • Methaemoglobinuria	As for blood	Methaemoglobin forms in aged haemoglobinuric samples due to spontaneous oxidization of ferrous haem

Protein	Negative
	Trace
	1+ (0.3 g/l)
	2+ (1.0 g/l)
	3+ (3.0 g/l)
	4+ (>20 g/l)
		Negative or trace	1+ or greater if urine dilute
			2+ or greater if urine concentrated
				• Prerenal
				  • Paraproteinuria (not always detected by dipstick)
				  • Intravascular haemolysis (leading to haemoglobinuria)
				  • Myoglobinuria
				• Renal
				  • Glomerular pathology: glomerulonephritis; amyloidosis
				  • Tubular pathology: toxicosis; ischaemic injury; congenital conditions
				• 'Postrenal'
				  • Includes genital tract sources, e.g. seminal fluid, prostatic disease and oestral blood
					Pigmenturia
					
					False increase
					• Very alkaline urine (pH >8)
					• Chlorhexidine
					• Quaternary ammonium salts (ammonia-based disinfectants)
						Interpret in context of urine concentration and sediment examination
						
						Detects albumin better than globulins or paraproteins
						
						Only if urine is **macroscopically bloody** will it have a clinically significant effect on protein concentration

Urobili-nogen	**Not recommended** Adds no further information to that provided by urine bilirubin and is less reliable (inconsistently positive in haemolytic states)					
Nitrite	**Not recommended** Nitrites produced by Gram-negative bacteria are only detectable if urine has been in the bladder for at least 4 hours before sampling; unreliable in dogs and cats (false negatives common)					
Leucocyte esterase	**Not recommended** Esterase produced by leucocytes is an unreliable indicator of pyuria in veterinary species owing to false negatives in dogs and false positives in cats					
Specific gravity	**Not recommended** Dipsticks estimate urine concentration by producing different colour changes depending on the ionic strength of the urine, this being related to total solute concentration. This is an unreliable way of determining urine concentration in veterinary species					

10.14 (continued) Interpretation of urine dipstick results. [a] High concentrations of ascorbic acid may be found with urinary acidifiers, vitamin therapy or drug preservatives. BHB = beta-hydroxybutyrate; NSAID = non-steroidal anti-inflammatory drug; RBC = red blood cells; UTI = urinary tract infection; UV = ultraviolet.

Ketones

Of the three types of ketone bodies which can be present in plasma, dipsticks detect acetoacetate, and – to a lesser extent – acetone. They do not detect beta-hydroxybutyrate (BHB). This is not usually of clinical significance because the detectable ketones are usually excreted in sufficient quantities concurrently with BHB; however, if in doubt, serum BHB should be tested in suspicious cases before ruling out ketosis. Ketonuria can appear to *increase* transiently upon initiation of insulin therapy for diabetic ketoacidosis, owing to increased conversion of BHB to acetoacetate. Diabetic ketoacidosis is the most common cause of ketonuria in dogs and cats, but severe starvation or hypoglycaemic disorders can also cause ketonuria. Trace ketonuria has been documented in hyperthyroid cats (Berent *et al.*, 2007).

Bilirubin

Most species (dogs especially) have a low renal threshold for bilirubin and therefore dipsticks are often positive *before* an animal has hyperbilirubinaemia or is overtly jaundiced; a positive urine dipstick may be the first warning sign of haemolysis. A small amount of bilirubin may be present in the urine of healthy dogs, particularly if the urine is concentrated. Bilirubinuria is *always* abnormal in cats. Causes of increased bilirubinuria are haemolytic anaemia and cholestatic liver disease.

> **Key point**
>
> Bilirubinuria is always abnormal in cats

Blood

Dipstick pads theoretically distinguish between haematuria and haemoglobinuria; the former produces a speckled colour change on the reagent pad (corresponding to the presence of whole erythrocytes), while the latter causes a uniform colour change. Often, however, haematuria is too marked for the speckled pattern to be appreciated, as the pad is entirely swamped with whole erythrocytes. Furthermore, a uniform colour change does not distinguish between haemoglobinuria due to haemoglobinaemia (i.e. intravascular haemolysis) and that due to lysis of erythrocytes in the urine due to sample ageing.

The significance of haematuria/haemoglobinuria depends on the sampling method, because cystocentesis and catheterization may cause iatrogenic haemorrhage. See Figures 10.15 and 10.16 for further information on the differential diagnoses and localization of haematuria, and Figure 10.17 for features distinguishing haematuria, haemoglobinuria and myoglobinuria.

Coagulopathies	Urinary tract disease	Genital tract origin	
• Thrombocytopenia • Platelet function defects • Clotting factor deficiencies • Disseminated intravascular coagulation (DIC)	• Urinary tract infection • Feline lower urinary tract disease (FLUTD) • Urolithiasis • Neoplasia of kidneys, bladder, ureters, urethra • Idiopathic renal haemorrhage • Congenital defects, e.g. urachal diverticulum • Polypoid cystitis • Drugs, e.g. cyclophosphamide • Urinary tract trauma • Granulomatous urethritis	Female • Oestrus • Infection, e.g. pyometra, vaginitis • Neoplasia of uterus or vagina • Trauma	Male • Prostatitis • Benign prostatic hyperplasia • Neoplasia of prostate gland, or penis • Trauma

10.15 A guide to the differential diagnosis of haematuria.

Parameter	Coagulopathy	Urinary tract	Genital tract
History	• Usually other sites of bleeding	• Timing may help localize • Blood at the beginning of urination may be due to urethral or genital bleeding • Bleeding at end of stream suggests pathology of the ventral bladder • Dysuria • Usually present with bladder or urethral disease • Renal or ureteral bleeding does not cause urinary tenesmus, unless there is secondary bladder disease, e.g. blood clot	• Entire or neutered? • May bleed between urinations; with prostatic disease, may bleed at end of urination • Dysuria may be present • Dyschezia may be seen with prostatic disease
Examination	• Petechiae and ecchymoses with platelet abnormalities • Haematomas and haemorrhages with clotting factor disorders	• May help to localize, e.g. renal mass, cystic calculi, empty bladder confirming pollakiuria	• May reveal prostatomegaly • May detect uterine or vaginal masses • Swollen vulva in oestrus
Localization by sample type	• Blood present in all sample types • Note that cystocentesis is not advisable when a coagulopathy is suspected	• If blood present in cystocentesis or free-catch samples may be from bladder, kidneys or ureter • Blood only present in free-catch sample suggests urethral or genital bleeding	• Blood only present in free-catch sample suggests urethral or genital bleeding
Urinalysis	• This confirms haematuria; there should be no inflammatory cells	• In idiopathic renal haemorrhage and trauma there will be increased erythrocytes, but no increase in inflammatory cells • Neoplastic cells may be found on cytology • Inflammatory conditions, infection and urolithiasis usually cause an increase in RBCs, WBCs and epithelial cells ± bacteriuria	• Features do not usually help differentiation from urinary tract disease
Fine-needle aspiration	• Not indicated	• Ideally bladder FNA/cystocentesis should be avoided in cases with bladder masses to avoid seeding of the tumour	• Prostatic fine-needle aspirates (preferred) or washes (less ideal) can be very helpful
Biopsy	• Not indicated	• Useful for specific lesions	• Useful for specific lesions
Imaging	• Not indicated	• Plain, positive-, negative- or double-contrast radiography should help to localize haematuria • Ultrasonography very useful • Advanced imaging such as CT or MRI can be helpful for renal lesions and sometimes other sites	• Radiography and ultrasonography are useful to investigate prostatic disease • Ultrasonography is useful to confirm a pyometra • Contrast radiography can be used to evaluate the vagina
Cystoscopy/ vaginoscopy	• Not indicated	• Useful for selected cases	• Useful for selected cases

10.16 Approach to the localization of haematuria. CT = computed tomography; FNA = fine-needle aspiration; MRI = magnetic resonance imaging; RBCs = red blood cells; WBCs = white blood cells.

Parameter	Haematuria	Haemoglobinuria	Myoglobinuria
Macroscopic examination	Pink to red, to frankly bloody (or brown with sample ageing)	Pink to red, to frankly bloody (or brown with sample ageing)	Pink to red (or brown with sample ageing)
Dipstick	Blood pad positive (speckled or uniform colour change)	Blood pad positive (uniform colour change)	Blood pad positive (uniform colour change)
Sediment examination	Whole erythrocytes present, unless lysis has occurred due to sample ageing	Whole erythrocytes absent/rare Haemoglobin droplets stain light green with new methylene blue	Whole erythrocytes absent/rare
Plasma colour	Normal	Red/pink (due to haemoglobinaemia) – unless the haemoglobinuria is caused by haematuria and subsequent red cell lysis	Normal
Supportive findings	Any obvious explanation for urogenital tract haemorrhage (e.g. pyuria on sediment examination, neoplasia or urolithiasis on imaging) Clinical signs of dysuria	Concurrent anaemia (usually regenerative) Blood film findings supportive of a haemolytic process (e.g. spherocytes, agglutination) Hyperbilirubinaemia Bilirubinuria	Elevated creatine kinase and AST Elevated urea and creatinine, and isosthenuria if concurrent renal failure

10.17 Distinguishing features of haematuria, haemoglobinuria and myoglobinuria. AST = aspartate aminotransferase.

Myoglobin

Distinguishing myoglobinuria from haemoglobinuria is usually possible without specific testing (Figure 10.17). Myoglobin can be precipitated using ammonium sulphate, but this is considered unreliable (Stockham and Scott, 2008). Immunological, electrophoretic and spectrophotometric methods can also be used, but are not widely available.

Protein

Proteinuria can be classified into three major types.

1. **Prerenal (or 'overflow') proteinuria:** this results from increased plasma concentration of a small protein molecule that passes through the glomerular filtration barrier. Examples include:
   - Light chain proteinuria (presence of Bence–Jones proteins, not detected by dipstick)
   - Haemoglobinuria
   - Myoglobinuria.
2. **Renal proteinuria:** in glomerular pathology, larger proteins that are not usually filtered pass through the filtration barrier, while in tubular pathology, proteins which are normally reabsorbed remain in the filtrate and are excreted. Hypoalbuminaemia is expected with glomerular pathology, but not tubular. Examples are:
   - Glomerular
     - Glomerulonephritis
     - Amyloidosis
   - Tubular
     - Toxicosis
     - Ischaemic damage
     - Congenital proximal tubular disease.

The proteinuria associated with chronic renal failure may be either glomerular or tubular in origin, or a combination of both; see Chapter 11 for further details.

3. **'Postrenal' proteinuria:** this refers to proteinuria caused by inflammation or haemorrhage within the urogenital tract or contamination with seminal fluid. It is technically a misnomer because inflammation and haemorrhage can occur anywhere within the urinary tract, including within the kidney. However, this title continues to be used because it enables a conceptually simple classification system for proteinuria. 'Postrenal' proteinuria is the most common type of proteinuria and must be ruled out before other types of proteinuria are diagnosed. It does not cause hypoalbuminaemia *per se*, but may be associated with a mild hypoalbuminaemia secondary to the inflammatory state or to chronic blood loss.

Positive dipstick results for protein should be interpreted in the context of urine concentration. A urine sample with an SG of 1.010 and urine protein 2+ on dipstick, contains twice as much protein as urine with an SG of 1.020 and the same dipstick protein result. As proteinuria can result from urinary tract inflammation, a positive dipstick result should be interpreted alongside sediment examination. Haematuria can also cause proteinuria, but only if severe enough for the urine to be macroscopically haemorrhagic (Vaden *et al.*, 2004). Dipsticks detect albumin better than globulins (though the latter do contribute to the reaction), but this is rarely an issue in practice because the only situation in which globulin would predominate is myeloma and this is uncommon. Dipsticks do not generally detect protein within epithelial cells and leucocytes.

The urine of some apparently healthy dogs contains a small amount of protein (trace or 1+ on dipstick), which is mainly albumin. False positive reactions are a problem, especially in cats. A recent study concluded that a positive dipstick result had no diagnostic value in cats (Lyon *et al.*, 2010), because when the cut-off for an abnormal result was set at ≥1+, the specificity was only 49.7% when compared with a quantitative species-specific immunoturbidimetric albumin assay (to detect microalbumin), suggesting an unacceptable number of false positive results. However, when the cut-off was raised to ≥2+, the negative predictive value was only 47.3%, consistent with an unacceptable number of false negatives. The authors of this study concluded that feline samples should be analysed with the quantitative species-specific immunoturbidimetric assay; they do not advocate the use of the urine protein:creatinine ratio (UPCR; see below) owing to its relatively poor sensitivity. However, see the section on Microalbuminuria below for a discussion of the clinical utility of the analysis of urinary microalbumin.

In summary, dipstick protein should be interpreted with caution, especially in cats, because false positive and false negative results can be seen. The UPCR can be used to quantify proteinuria but false negative results can occur. Microalbumin measurement by immunoturbidimetric assay (see below) is more sensitive for the detection of small amounts of proteinuria but has poor diagnostic specificity because levels can be increased in non-renal systemic disease.

Key point

Interpret proteinuria in the context of sediment examination

Sulphosalicylic acid turbidity

The precipitation of urinary protein in a 5% sulphosalicylic acid solution was traditionally employed to help identify false positive dipstick protein reactions, but is now rarely used because of questionable accuracy. If the veracity of a positive dipstick reaction is in doubt, the urine protein (or UPCR – see below) should be measured on a chemistry analyser.

Urine protein:creatinine ratio

The UPCR gives a quantitative measure of urinary protein. Quantification is indicated when *all of the following criteria apply*:

- Urine dipstick tests are repeatedly positive for protein
- There is no significant haematuria
- There is no evidence of inflammation on sediment examination.

If urine protein concentration is measured on a spot sample there are large variations over time due to variations in urine concentration. Creatinine is excreted constantly and is not absorbed. Therefore, protein is measured, by standard automated methods, and compared with the creatinine concentration to determine whether or not protein excretion is increased in relation to the constant excretion of creatinine. A spot sample measuring the ratio correlates with 24-hour urine protein excretion measurements.

$$UPCR = \frac{Urine\ protein\ (mg/dl)}{Urine\ creatinine\ (mg/dl)}$$

It is important that the units used are the same for both analytes. To convert SI units to conventional units:

Protein (g/l) × 100 = Protein (mg/dl)
Creatinine (mmol/l) × $\frac{1000}{88.4}$ = Creatinine (mg/dl)

The UPCR **must** be interpreted in the context of sediment examination because inflammation and gross haematuria can increase the results. If either is present, the clinician should wait until the inflammation and/or haematuria has resolved before re-testing the urine to get a meaningful UPCR.

Figure 10.18 gives the International Renal Interest Society (IRIS: http://www.iris-kidney.com/index.shtml) guidelines for interpreting UPCR. IRIS recommends that at least three samples collected over a period of at least 2 weeks are analysed when using proteinuria to stage chronic kidney disease (CKD). This will rule out spurious or transient elevations in the UPCR. The significance of proteinuria or borderline proteinuria depends on the concurrent IRIS stage of CKD.

UPCR in dogs	UPCR in cats	Significance
<0.2	<0.2	Not proteinuric
0.2–0.5	0.2–0.4	Borderline proteinuric: recheck in 2 months
>0.5	>0.4	Proteinuric: recheck in 2 weeks to determine persistence
>3.0	>3.0	Significant proteinuria. Glomerulonephropathies are frequently associated with UPCRs of this level

10.18 Interpretation of urine protein:creatinine ratio (UPCR), according to the International Renal Interest Society (IRIS).

Semi-quantitative dipsticks are now available to give an estimation of UPCR, but their accuracy has not been fully established. One study reported that the dipsticks gave fairly reliable results in dogs but not in cats (Welles *et al.*, 2006), while another reported good correlation between the dipsticks and a reference method in cats, but only fair correlation in dogs (Defontis *et al.*, 2013). These methods should probably be considered to be equivalent to interpreting the relationship between urine protein concentration and urine SG. See Chapter 11 for further details on the UPCR and IRIS staging of CKD.

Urine protein electrophoresis and immunoelectrophoresis

Urine protein electrophoresis can be used to characterize the protein fractions once proteinuria has been diagnosed. The urine is concentrated before the test is run. See Figure 10.19 for traces generated from normal and proteinuric patients.

Urine protein electrophoresis is preferred to the unreliable Bence–Jones protein heat precipitation test for the detection of immunoglobulin light chains (paraproteins), which appear as a narrow spike in the β_2 or γ-globulin fraction. Ideally, urinary light chains are definitively identified using immunoelectrophoresis, but, to the authors' knowledge, this is not available in the UK at present. Light chain proteinuria is most often associated with myeloma or, more rarely, extramedullary plasma cell tumours or chronic B-cell lymphocytic leukaemia. It has also been documented in dogs with leishmaniosis, ehrlichiosis and babesiosis (Bonfanti *et al.*, 2004).

Microalbuminuria

Microalbuminuria is defined as a concentration of urinary albumin which is increased, but is below that which is reliably identified on dipsticks. The latter is often stated to be 30 mg/dl, although in reality many dipsticks have a limit of detection considerably lower. Notwithstanding this, the conventional definition of microalbuminuria in dogs and cats is a urine albumin concentration between 1 and 30 mg/dl *in urine adjusted to a SG of 1.010.* As with other tests for proteinuria, inflammatory or haemorrhagic proteinuria must be ruled out when determining the clinical significance of a positive result.

Microalbuminuria can be detected by an immunoturbidimetric test in reference laboratories to give a quantitative result, or by commercially available point-of-care tests. These use species-specific antibody reactions to detect albumin in a semi-quantitative fashion once urine has been diluted to a SG of approximately 1.010 using distilled water. A recent study found that 29% of canine samples with measurable urine albumin by the immunoturbidimetric

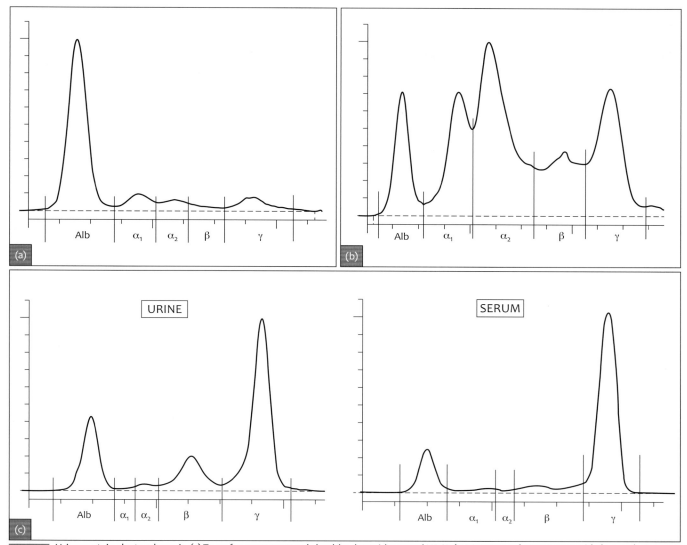

10.19 Urine protein electrophoresis. (a) Trace from an apparently healthy dog with normal UPCR (UPCR: 0.19; reference interval (RI): 0–0.5). Only albumin is present in appreciable amounts. Many apparently healthy dogs excrete a small amount of albumin in their urine. (b) Trace from a dog with suspected glomerulonephritis. The UPCR is significantly elevated (UPCR: 3.48; RI: 0–0.5), and all protein fractions are present in increased amounts in the urine, suggesting disruption of the glomerular filtration barrier. (c) Serum and urine traces from a dog with suspected myeloma. There is a monoclonal peak in the γ-globulin region in the serum and a similar monoclonal peak is present in the urine, consistent with urinary paraproteins.

assay were negative using the canine early renal disease (E.R.D.) test strips (Murgier *et al.*, 2009). Another study found that there were issues with repeatability of the test and potential false negatives when the Feline E.R.D. test strips were used (Mardell and Sparkes, 2006). Since these in-house kits have a limited shelf-life it may be preferable to send these samples to a reference laboratory for analysis.

There is also a human dipstick method for estimating the urine albumin:creatinine ratio but this has been reported to be unreliable for the detection of microalbuminuria in dogs (Pressler *et al.*, 2002).

The clinical significance of microalbuminuria remains to be fully established. Approximately 25% of the general population of dogs and cats has microalbuminuria and this percentage increases with age. Microalbuminuria has been associated with a plethora of non-renal conditions, including cardiovascular disease, dental disease, pyoderma, endocrinopathies, infectious disease and neoplasia; it may also be present in animals on glucocorticoid therapy. In one study, 56% of dogs with persistent microalbuminuria were found to have non-renal systemic

disease, while 31% were found to have renal disease (Whittemore *et al.*, 2006). Given the lack of specificity for renal pathology, it can be difficult to determine the significance of microalbuminuria. It appears to be a sensitive but non-specific indicator of early renal disease, but it has yet to be shown whether all animals with microalbuminuria will go on to develop renal failure, or whether the clinical utility of testing for microalbuminuria is superior to that of tests for overt proteinuria (i.e. protein >30 mg/dl) in the diagnosis of CKD. It is useful for detecting early renal disease in young dogs of breeds predisposed to congenital nephropathies, but may be too non-specific to be helpful in the diagnosis of CKD in older animals that are likely to have concurrent non-renal conditions. It is possible that the conventional definition of proteinuria uses an inappropriately low upper threshold for urinary protein concentration. Some authors believe that a urinary concentration of >39 mg/dl is a more clinically useful definition of proteinuria in dogs (Tvedten, 2014). If this becomes more widely accepted, then measurement of microalbumin may seem less useful.

Wet sediment examination

Wet sediment examination is a key part of routine urinalysis. It is best performed in house to avoid storage artefacts, but many practitioners refer this to an external laboratory, probably because of time constraints and lack of confidence with microscopy. The purpose of this section is to provide clinicians and technicians with the skills to perform wet sediment examination themselves. As common findings are frequently seen, practitioners will rapidly become adept at identifying them accurately. It should be necessary to send samples to a reference laboratory only for corroboration of less familiar findings.

Method

See Figure 10.4 for details of sample preparation for wet sediment examination.

> **Key point**
>
> Lower the microscope condenser when examining wet preparations

Normal findings

See Figure 10.20 for expected sediment findings in urine from healthy dogs and cats (based on a sample volume of 5 ml).

Sediment constituent	Expected quantity (from centrifugation of 5 ml urine)	Comments
Leucocytes	<5 per hpf (X400)	Some microscopes may not have a standard-sized field of view
Erythrocytes	<5 per hpf (X400)	
Epithelial cells	0–2 per lpf (X100)	Small cells from kidney and upper tract; large cells from bladder and urethra
Bacteria	None	>1 x10⁴/ml rods or >1 x 10⁵/ml cocci must be present to enable detection on sediment examination
Casts	Usually none	Low numbers of hyaline casts or rare granular casts can be seen in healthy animals
Crystals		Many types of crystal can be found in normal animals; their presence does not necessarily indicate a pathological state

10.20 Expected sediment findings in urine from healthy dogs and cats. hpf = high power field; lpf = low power field.

Interpretation

Cells

Figure 10.21 shows examples of findings on wet sediment examination.

Erythrocytes: Erythrocytes can appear as smooth round discs, or may become crenated with sample ageing (Figure 10.21e). Lysis can occur with sample storage, especially with dilute urine, so absence of erythrocytes does not rule out haematuria unless the sample is fresh. If lysis occurs, the dipstick blood pad will be positive owing to haemoglobinuria. Normal urine contains fewer than five erythrocytes per X400 high power field (hpf).

Increased numbers are seen in many situations (see Figure 10.15); the main causes are:

- Traumatic catheterization or cystocentesis
- Haemorrhage anywhere in the urogenital tract
  - Inflammation (infection, crystalluria, obstruction, etc.)
  - Neoplasia
  - Trauma
  - Coagulopathy
- Oestrus in entire females (voided samples).

> **Key point**
>
> Erythrocytes can lyse as a result of sample storage; their absence does not rule out haematuria unless the sample is fresh

Leucocytes: These are slightly larger than erythrocytes, although the difference can be subtle. Their internal contents appear more granular when unstained and they may be present individually or in clumps (Figure 10.21d–f). Inexperienced microscopists may find staining the sample useful to highlight leucocytes (Figure 10.21g). The vast majority are neutrophils, though rare macrophages, lymphocytes and eosinophils may be seen if the urine is prepared and stained for cytological examination (differentiation of leucocyte type is not reliable with wet preparations). Small epithelial cells can appear similar to leucocytes. The number of leucocytes reduces with sample storage as they rapidly deteriorate. Normal urine contains fewer than five leucocytes per X400 hpf.

Increased numbers are seen with:

- Urinary tract inflammation
- Genital tract inflammation.

Consideration of the sampling method may help to localize the inflammation: if a cystocentesis sample is pyuric, the site of inflammation must be somewhere between the kidneys and the proximal urethra. Collecting a free-catch sample midstream will minimize the chances of contamination from the genital tract because contaminants are washed away with the first part of the stream.

Some puppies, especially females, have higher numbers of white cells in their urine (see Figure 10.48). The authors of one study proposed that this may be due to the environment (e.g. bedding on litter) and a lack of grooming in puppies under 12 weeks old (Faulks and Lane, 2003).

Epithelial cells: These include renal epithelial cells, transitional epithelial cells and (in voided and catheterized samples) squamous epithelial cells originating from the distal urethra and external genitalia. Their large size generally distinguishes them from leucocytes (Figure 10.21de). Renal epithelial cells are the smallest type and have a rounded outline; these are rarely seen. Transitional epithelial cells are large, and are rounded to oval. Squamous epithelial cells are the largest cells seen and are often angular or polygonal. Figure 10.21(a–e) shows the appearance of stained and unstained epithelial cells in wet preparations.

Occasional large round (i.e. transitional) epithelial cells and (in catheterized and free-catch samples) squamous epithelial cells are seen in normal urine (0–2 per X100 low power field (lpf)).

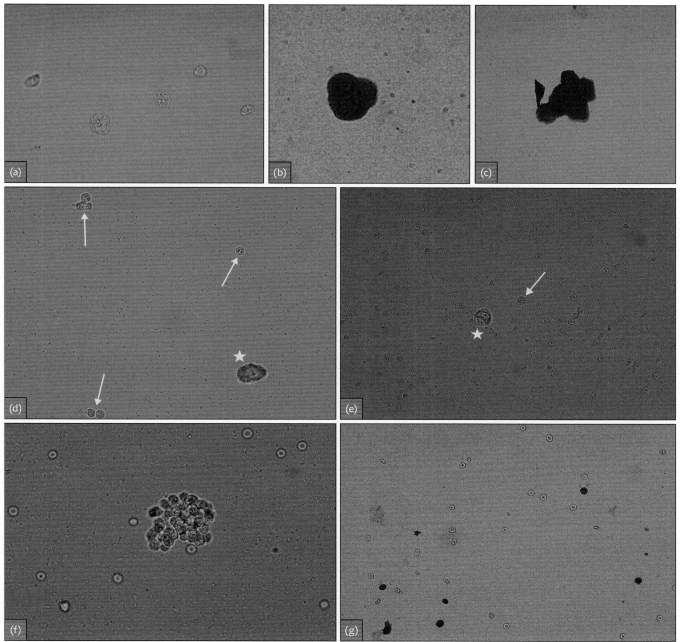

10.21 Wet sediment examination: cells. (a) Individual epithelial cells. The two smaller cells on the right could be small epithelial cells or white blood cells (WBCs). The angular object out of the plane of focus on the left is an artefact. (Original magnification X400). (b) Cluster of three epithelial cells. (Sedi-Stain; original magnification X400). (c) Sheet of squamous epithelial cells (note angular shape). (Sedi-Stain; original magnification X400). (d) Pyuria and bacteriuria. Note relative sizes of epithelial cell (asterisk) and WBCs (arrowed). (Original magnification X400). (e) Pyuria, haematuria and bacteriuria. Note relative sizes of epithelial cell (asterisk), WBC (arrowed) and erythrocytes. Some erythrocytes are crenated. Cocci and bacilli are visible in the background. (Original magnification X400). (f) Pyuria, haematuria and bacteriuria. There is a central cluster of WBCs, with individual red blood cells (RBCs) and bacteria in the background. Note the more refractile, granular quality of WBCs compared with RBCs. (Original magnificationX400). (g) Use of Sedi-Stain to highlight WBCs against the background RBCs. (Sedi-Stain; original magnification X400)

Increased numbers are seen with:

- Traumatic catheterization
- Mucosal inflammation
- Mucosal hyperplasia
- Neoplasia.

Detailed morphology is difficult to appreciate on wet sediment preparations, but if there are obvious abnormalities, numbers are significantly increased, or there is evidence of a mass on imaging that cannot be directly biopsied, then urine cytology is indicated (see below).

Crystals

Many crystals are found incidentally in healthy animals. While their presence *may* predispose to urolith formation, it is imperative to interpret their significance in the context of clinical signs, sedimentary evidence of haematuria and/ or inflammation and any evidence of uroliths on imaging. *Many animals are put on urolith prevention/treatment regimes unnecessarily.* See Figure 10.22 regarding the significance of crystalluria.

It is important to examine a fresh sample because crystals can form or dissolve on sample storage and with

Crystals are more likely to be significant if:

- They are seen in a fresh sample (less than an hour old) examined at room temperature
- There are related clinical signs (dysuria, increased frequency of urination)
- There is concurrent haematuria
- The urine is dilute
- The crystals are large
- Crystalluria is persistent on repeated sampling
- There is evidence of urolithiasis on imaging

10.22 Factors to consider when determining the clinical significance of crystalluria.

temperature change. If there is a delay until analysis, the sample should be refrigerated but then allowed to reach room temperature before examination. Crystals can vary in size depending on solute strength, urine concentration, pH, sample temperature, etc., so size guidelines will not be given. The pH of the urine affects the likelihood of formation of certain types of crystal, but this is not an absolute effect (e.g. struvites can be found in acidic urine and calcium oxalate crystals in alkaline urine). Be aware that different types of crystal can coexist. See Figure 10.23 for further information on different types of crystalluria.

Key point

Interpret crystalluria in context to determine clinical significance; it may be an incidental finding

Struvite: These are also known as magnesium ammonium phosphate crystals, are common in dogs and cats and may be an incidental finding. Alkaline and concentrated urine encourages their precipitation. They are often associated with urinary tract infection (UTI) in dogs. In cats, they are usually found in sterile samples, but can be associated with infection. Infection-induced struvite crystals are more common in older cats due to their higher incidence of UTIs. The presence of urease-producing bacteria (either as a result of UTI or as sample contaminants) leads to increased urine pH and encourages struvite formation. Classic struvites are oblong and coffin-shaped, but they can present in a variety of forms (Figure 10.24).

Calcium oxalate dihydrate: These are common in both dogs and cats and can be an incidental finding. They are generally associated with acidic urine. Rarely, they may be

Crystal	Associated urine pH	Guide to prevalence	Clinical significance
Struvite (magnesium, ammonium, phosphate)	≥7	Common	• May be incidental finding in healthy dogs and cats • Often associated with UTI, especially in dogs • *May predispose to urolithiasis*
Calcium oxalate dihydrate	≤7	Common	• May be incidental finding in healthy dogs and cats • Rarely seen in association with ethylene glycol toxicity • *May predispose to urolithiasis*
Calcium oxalate monohydrate	≤7	Rare	• Very occasionally an incidental finding in healthy dogs and cats • Associated with ethylene glycol toxicity
Calcium phosphates	All except 'brushites': ≥7 Amorphous phosphates: ≥7 'Brushites': <7	Uncommon	• May be an incidental finding in healthy dogs and cats • Associated with hypercalcaemia and other factors (see Figure 10.44) • Small numbers can be associated with UTI-induced struvite crystalluria • *May predispose to urolithiasis*
Ammonium urates and uric acid	Ammonium urate: ≥7 Uric acid: <7 Amorphous urates: ≤7	Ammonium urates: common in predisposed breeds; otherwise rare Uric acid: rare	• May be seen in healthy Dalmatians, Bulldogs and other breeds • Associated with hepatic insufficiency and PSS • Predispose to urolithiasis (it is not understood why some Dalmatians do not form uroliths)
Bilirubin	Variable, usually acidic	Common in dogs, rare in cats	• May be an incidental finding in dogs; abnormal in cats • Associated with hepatobiliary disease and intravascular haemolysis • Not associated with uroliths
Cystine	≤7	Rare	• Always abnormal • Associated with inherited tubular reabsorption defect • Bull Mastiff, mastiffs, Bulldog, Dachshund, Chihuahua, Newfoundland, Australian Cattle Dog, Scottish Deerhound, Basset Hound • *May predispose to urolithiasis*
Tyrosine	≤7	Very rare	• Always abnormal • Associated with liver disease or inherited tubular reabsorption defect
Cholesterol	Variable	Rare	• Minimal clinical significance • Not associated with uroliths
Drug-associated crystals • Sulphonamides • Ampicillin • Allopurinol • Ciprofloxacin • Tetracyclines • Primidone • Radiopaque contrast agents	Variable	Sulphonamide crystals common; others uncommon or rare	• Some drug-associated uroliths have been reported, but these are rare

10.23 Clinical significance of crystalluria. PSS = portosystemic shunt; UTI = urinary tract infection.

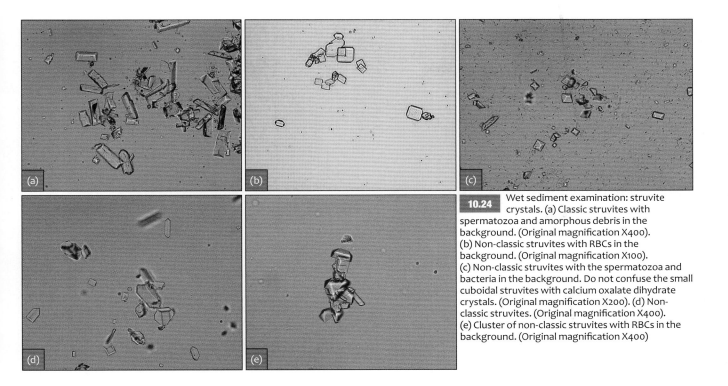

10.24 Wet sediment examination: struvite crystals. (a) Classic struvites with spermatozoa and amorphous debris in the background. (Original magnification X400). (b) Non-classic struvites with RBCs in the background. (Original magnification X100). (c) Non-classic struvites with the spermatozoa and bacteria in the background. Do not confuse the small cuboidal struvites with calcium oxalate dihydrate crystals. (Original magnification X200). (d) Non-classic struvites. (Original magnification X400). (e) Cluster of non-classic struvites with RBCs in the background. (Original magnification X400)

associated with hypercalcaemia. These are square crystals with a classic 'Maltese cross' formation (Figure 10.25). Note that (as with other crystals) they have a wide size range and are sometimes only visible at high magnification (X400).

Calcium oxalate monohydrate: These are less common than the dihydrate form. They also form in acidic urine. While they can be found in some healthy individuals, they are also associated with ethylene glycol toxicity or hypercalcaemia. The classic shape is an oblong with pointed ends ('picket fence' formation), but variations are seen (Figure 10.26).

Calcium phosphate: Relatively rare in dogs and cats, these are found in pH neutral to alkaline urine (with the exception of 'brushite' crystals). They can be found in healthy animals, or may be a consequence of hypercalcaemia; their presence is an indication to check serum calcium. There are many different forms of calcium phosphate crystals. They may be amorphous (distinguishable from amorphous urates by their presence in alkaline pH and lack of yellowish colouring), spherical (dogs only), or needle-like, sometimes aggregating into rosettes (Figure 10.27). In acidic urine, 'brushite' (calcium hydrogen phosphate dihydrate) crystals may form; these are narrow, elongated rectangular crystals often present in aggregates.

Urates and uric acid: Ammonium urates (also known as ammonium biurates) are the most common type of urate crystal, but sodium urates can also form. Uric acid crystals are much rarer than ammonium urates, but have the same clinical associations. Ammonium urates are most commonly seen in Dalmatians, which have an inborn defect in purine metabolism, leading to excretion of insoluble uric acid rather than the soluble allantoin. This genetic mutation also appears to exist in some individuals of other predisposed breeds – Bulldogs and Black Russian Terriers (Karmi *et al.*, 2010). In other breeds, urate crystals are associated with portosystemic shunts or hepatic dysfunction; if they are found it is important to evaluate the liver further by measuring hepatic enzymes and performing a bile acid stimulation test.

Ammonium urates tend to form in weakly acidic to alkaline urine, while the less common uric acid crystals tend to form in acidic urine. Ammonium urates are darkish brown/yellow spherical crystals which often appear in dense clusters. They sometimes have pointed protuberances on their surfaces ('thorn apple' formation) (Figure 10.28a), but can present in the smooth, spheroid form, especially in cats (Figure 10.28b), or they may be amorphous. Amorphous crystals can be difficult to identify; the urine pH gives a clue to their identity and their colour is usually similar to the structured crystals, e.g. amorphous urates are brown in colour and form in acidic urine, while amorphous phosphates are colourless and form in alkaline urine. Uric acid crystals are colourless crystals of a diamond or rhomboid shape.

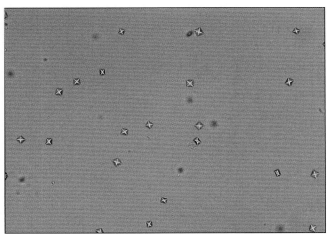

10.25 Wet sediment examination: calcium oxalate dihydrate crystals. (Original magnification X400)

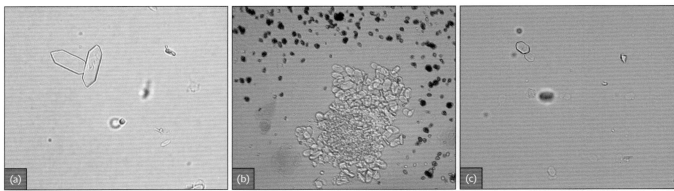

10.26 Wet sediment examination: calcium oxalate monohydrate crystals. (a) Classic 'picket fence' calcium oxalate monohydrate crystals, with spermatozoa in the background. (Original magnification X500). (b) A cluster of calcium oxalate monohydrate crystals, with erythrocytes and squamous epithelial cells also present. (Sedi-Stain; original magnification X500). (c) Non-classic calcium oxalate monohydrates from an apparently healthy cat. (Original magnification X400)

(a, First published in Ristić and Skeldon (2011), © Niki Skeldon; b, © Kathleen Tennant)

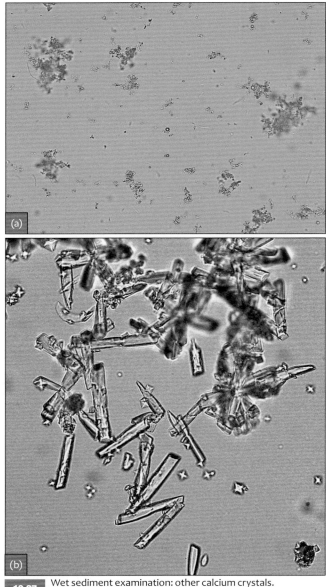

10.27 Wet sediment examination: other calcium crystals. (a) Amorphous phosphates and bacteria. (Original magnification X400). (b) Calcium phosphate crystals, with small calcium oxalate dihydrates also present. (Original magnification X400)

(Courtesy of Microbiology Dept., Axiom Veterinary Laboratories Ltd)

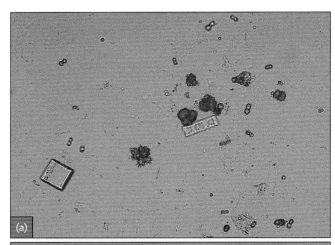

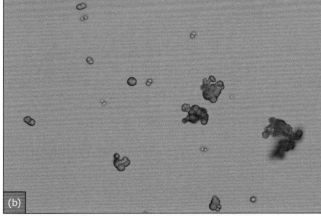

10.28 Wet sediment examination: urate crystals. (a) Classic ammonium urate crystals, with struvites and bacteria also present. (Original magnification X400). (b) Ammonium urate crystals, smooth type. (Original magnification X500)

Bilirubin: Bilirubin crystals are commonly seen in well concentrated urine from healthy dogs. They are not seen in healthy cats. In both species, bilirubin crystals can be associated with hepatobiliary disease and intravascular haemolysis. Acidic urine encourages their formation, where they are readily identified as golden needles or granules (Figure 10.29).

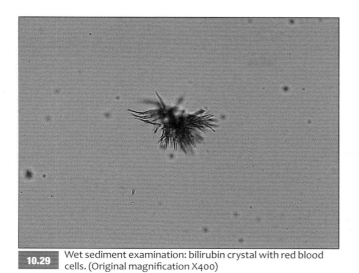

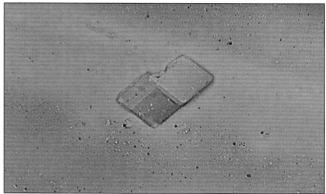

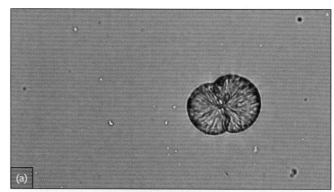

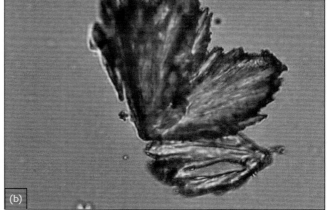

10.29 Wet sediment examination: bilirubin crystal with red blood cells. (Original magnification X400)

10.31 Wet sediment examination: cholesterol crystal. (Sedi-stain; original magnification X400)

Cystine: Cystine crystals are always abnormal and indicate a tubular transport defect. They tend to form in acidic urine. They are colourless, hexagonal crystals appearing individually or in stacks (Figure 10.30).

Tyrosine: These are always abnormal and have been associated with inherited tubular defects or liver disease. Tyrosine crystals form in acidic urine and are fine, colourless to yellow needle-like crystals which tend to aggregate into sheaves.

Cholesterol: Cholesterol crystals are rarely seen. They may indicate cell breakdown, but have been observed in the urine of apparently healthy dogs and are considered of minimal clinical significance. Their morphology is shown in Figure 10.31.

Drug crystals: It is imperative to check the drug history when faced with unexpected or unfamiliar crystals, because many drugs are excreted and can precipitate out in the urine. Sulphonamide crystals are commonly seen in animals on potentiated sulphonamides (Figure 10.32ab). Other antibiotics such as ampicillin and ciprofloxacin have also been associated with crystalluria (Escobar and Grindem, 2010). Xanthine crystals are seen in dogs medicated with allopurinol. These cannot be reliably distinguished from ammonium urate crystals or amorphous urates (Figure 10.32c).

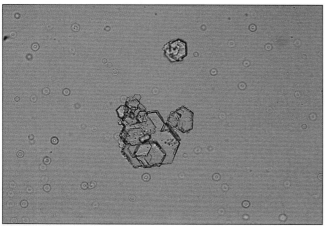

10.30 Wet sediment examination: cystine crystals with erythrocytes also present. (Original magnification X400)

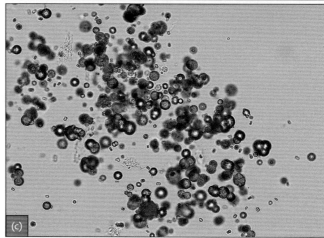

10.32 Wet sediment examination: drug crystals. (a) Sulphonamide crystal. (Original magnification X400). (b) Sulphonamide crystals. (Original magnification X1000). (c) Xanthine crystals. (Original magnification X500)

Casts

Casts are not a normal finding; they indicate renal tubular pathology. The exception is occasional hyaline or granular casts i.e. fewer than two per low power field (X10 objective), which can be found in healthy animals. Casts are thought to be formed from Tamm–Horsfall mucoprotein (secreted by renal epithelial cells), with variable incorporation of cell debris, whole cells, plasma proteins or lipid. Different types of cast can coexist, and a single cast can contain different components.

The number of casts present does not correlate with the severity of disease or give any indication of whether the pathology is permanent. They may be voided intermittently; therefore, their absence does not rule out tubular pathology (they cannot be used as a reliable indicator of nephrotoxicity when using aminoglycosides, for example). The type may give an indication of the underlying tubular pathology, but not always, and it is the presence of casts rather than the type that is most important. Suffice to say that significant numbers indicate renal tubular pathology and the type *may* provide some clue as to its nature (Osborne and Stevens, 1999).

Casts are large, cylindrical bodies with blunt, tapered or irregular ends, but perfectly parallel sides; this distinguishes them from artefacts (Figure 10.33). They may appear as short, straight fragments, or in convoluted shapes, depending on their original location and preservation. Their diameter reflects the size of the renal tubule in which they were formed. Bilirubinuria, haemoglobinuria or myoglobinuria can lead to pigmented casts. Casts are extremely fragile, especially in alkaline urine (they begin to lyse within 2 hours of sampling), so are most readily detected in fresh urine; therefore it is better to look for them in-house.

Hyaline casts: These are composed of Tamm–Horsfall mucoprotein without other inclusions and are thought to be the structural basis of all other casts. Occasional hyaline casts can be found in healthy animals, but increased numbers are seen with glomerular proteinuria or after strenuous exercise. They appear as smooth, almost transparent bodies with no internal structure (Figure 10.33a).

Granular casts: These form when cellular debris or plasma proteins are incorporated into the Tamm–Horsfall matrix, or possibly by degeneration of cellular casts. Occasional granular casts can be found in healthy animals, but increased numbers indicate tubular cell degeneration, necrosis or inflammation. They may contain fine or coarse granules, depending on their constitutive material and the time elapsed since formation (Figure 10.33b).

Cellular casts: Always pathological, these form when epithelial cells, erythrocytes or leucocytes (or a mixture of these) are incorporated into the Tamm–Horsfall matrix. Epithelial cell casts occur when there is active tubular degeneration or necrosis (e.g. toxic nephrosis; haemoglobinuria or myoglobinuria-associated nephropathy; or ischaemic damage), while leucocyte casts indicate renal tubule inflammation (i.e. tubular nephrosis and pyelonephritis). Erythrocyte casts form with glomerular or tubular haemorrhage.

Fatty casts: These form with the incorporation of lipid droplets or lipid-laden cell remnants into the Tamm–Horsfall matrix and are associated with the same pathology as epithelial cell casts (indeed, they may be aged epithelial cell casts).

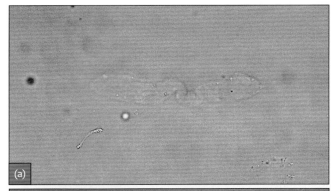
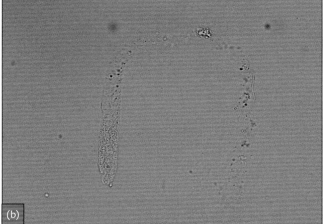
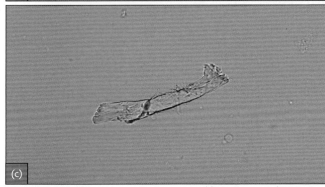

10.33 Wet sediment examination: casts. (a) Hyaline cast. (Original magnification X400). (b) Granular cast. (Original magnification X400). (c) Artefact, not to be confused with a cast, with WBCs and an epithelial cell also present. (Original magnification X400)

Waxy casts: Rarely seen, these are thought to be formed by the *in vivo* deterioration and solidification of granular or epithelial cell casts; they suggest chronic renal disease.

Organisms

Sediment examination is useful to detect bacteriuria, though absence on visual examination does not rule out the presence of bacteria: at least 1×10^4/ml rods or at least 1×10^5/ml cocci must be present to enable detection on sediment examination.

Bacteria are visible at high power magnification (X400), and in unstained specimens appear as almost colourless cocci or bacilli which may be present in clumps or chains (see Figure 10.21d–g). Their presence may be due to UTI or sample contamination, so must be interpreted in the context of sediment examination (i.e. is there evidence of pyuria?), culture results and knowledge of the sampling method (for more detail see 'Culture' section). For voided samples where there is a delay between collecting the sample and urinalysis, it can be useful to compare the quantity of bacteria in sediment obtained from a plain sample with that obtained from a boric acid sample, to help determine the proportion of bacteria present due to multiplication of potential contaminants. As the risk of contamination is minimal, the presence of bacteria in a cystocentesis sample is always considered abnormal.

Fungal hyphae (Figure 10.34a) or yeasts (Figure 10.34b) most often reflect sample contamination, but certain species such as *Candida* or *Aspergillus* species can be associated with urinary tract infection, especially if long-term antibiotic use has affected the commensal flora or if the animal is immunosuppressed.

Rarely, sediment examination may reveal the presence of adult nematodes or eggs as a result of infection with *Pearsonema* (formerly *Capillaria*) *plica* or *Dioctophyme renale* (Figure 10.35). Other parasite eggs usually reflect faecal contamination of the sample.

Findings of little or no diagnostic significance

Sometimes contaminants or artefacts may be present, which can be difficult to identify and cause confusion, such as plant material or air bubbles (Figures 10.36 and 10.37).

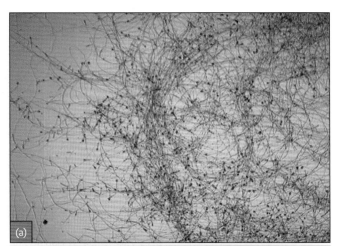

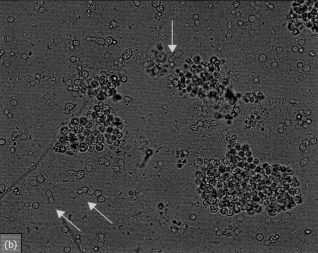

10.34 Wet sediment examination: yeasts and fungi. (a) Fungal hyphae. (Original magnification X100). (b) Yeasts (probably *Candida* spp.), demonstrating budding (arrowed). (Original magnification X400)

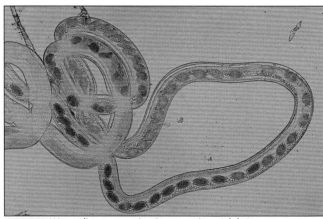

10.35 Wet sediment examination: parasites. Adult *Pearsonema* (formerly *Capillaria*) *plica* nematode containing ova. (Original magnification X100)
(Courtesy of Microbiology Dept., Axiom Veterinary Laboratories Ltd)

Structure	Origin	Comments/features
Lipid droplets	Renal tubular epithelium Lubricating gel	Especially common in cats Distinguish from erythrocytes by variable size and refractile nature
Mucus strands	Urogenital tract secretions	
Spermatozoa (Figure 10.37a)	Male gonads	Especially common in voided samples Occasionally seen in entire females after breeding
Fungal hyphae (Figure 10.34a)	Environmental contaminants of free-catch, 'off-surface' or aged samples	Usually of no diagnostic significance; rarely may indicate UTI (see text) Culture usually necessary for identification
Yeasts (Figure 10.34b)	Environmental contaminants of free-catch, 'off-surface' or aged samples	Usually of no diagnostic significance; rarely may indicate UTI (see text) Distinguish from bacteria by larger size; often oval and may be budding
Pollens	Environmental contaminants of free-catch or 'off-surface' samples	
Plant and cotton fibres (Figure 10.37b)	Environmental contaminants of free-catch or 'off-surface' samples	Distinguish from casts by coarse internal striations; sides may not be perfectly parallel
Starch granules	Glove powder	Markedly larger than bacteria Central cross may be visible
Glass shards (Figure 10.37c)	Slide or coverslip	Distinguish from crystals by very variable size and form Often located in a particular area on the slide, i.e. not throughout the sample
Air bubbles (Figure 10.37d)	Pipetting of sample	Variable size Out of plane of focus
Stain precipitate (Figure 10.37e)	Use of Sedi-Stain	Distinguish from bacteria by variable size and more amorphous appearance
Muscle fibres	Accidental FNA of skeletal muscle during cystocentesis	Distinguish from casts by internal striations

10.36 Wet sediment examination: contaminants and findings of little/no diagnostic significance (see Figure 10.37 for examples). FNA = fine-needle aspiration; UTI = urinary tract infection.

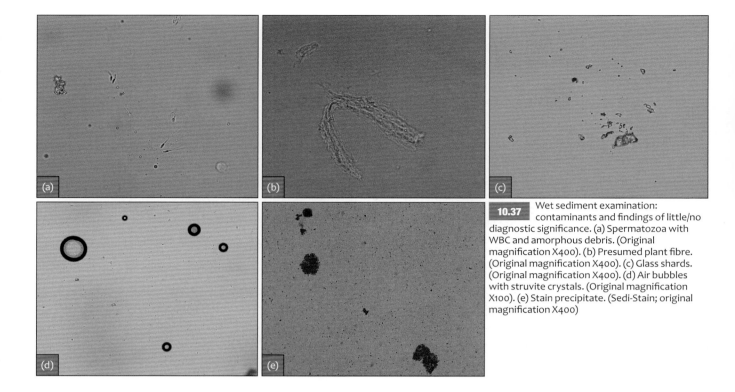

10.37 Wet sediment examination: contaminants and findings of little/no diagnostic significance. (a) Spermatozoa with WBC and amorphous debris. (Original magnification X400). (b) Presumed plant fibre. (Original magnification X400). (c) Glass shards. (Original magnification X400). (d) Air bubbles with struvite crystals. (Original magnification X100). (e) Stain precipitate. (Sedi-Stain; original magnification X400)

Urine culture

Culture is not usually considered a part of routine urinalysis, but is often indicated. It may be relevant in the work-up of animals with systemic disease, despite a lack of clinical signs indicative of UTI or evidence of inflammation on sediment examination. In one study, 42% of dogs with diabetes mellitus and/or hyperadrenocorticism had a positive urine culture, despite the fact that most did not exhibit clinical signs referable to a UTI. Of the dogs with positive culture, 19% did not have bacteriuria or pyuria on sediment examination (Forrester *et al.*, 1999). Another study reported that 58 of 344 cats with chronic kidney disease, 16 of 121 cats with diabetes mellitus and 10 of 46 cats with hyperthyroidism had positive urine cultures, despite the fact that clinical signs suggestive of lower urinary tract disease were only seen in four, six and two cats respectively (Bailiff *et al.*, 2008).

Urine can be cultured in-house using commercially available Petri dishes and antibiotic discs to determine sensitivity; this does not, however, allow identification of the bacteria involved, and interpretation of the antibiotic sensitivity results can be difficult for inexperienced operators. Mini culture trays are available to identify (to genus level) bacteria and yeasts and to give a guide to antibiotic sensitivity (Figure 10.38). In general, however, culture at a reference laboratory is infinitely preferable to in-house culture: it will yield more accurate and detailed results, and specialist microbiologists can be consulted for advice if required. In cases of refractory UTIs involving organisms resistant to multiple antibiotics, this can be invaluable (see Chapter 27).

Sample requirements vary, so it is important to check whether the reference laboratory prefers urine samples submitted in plain or boric acid containers. A recent study advocated using plain tubes rather than boric acid

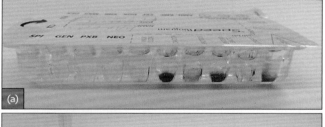

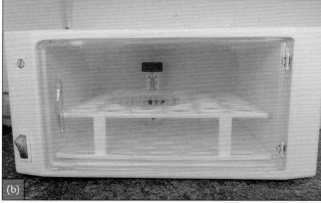

10.38 (a) A mini culture tray designed for use in general practice. It can be used to culture samples from skin, ears and urine. (b) A table-top incubator.

tubes, because false negatives were more common with boric acid tubes (Rowlands *et al.*, 2011). This study was performed on cystocentesis samples, which are less liable to contamination and so do not require the bacteriostatic effects of boric acid as much as other sample types; therefore, the conclusions may not be applicable to catheterized or free-catch samples. If using boric acid, it is important to fill the container to the line because if the boric acid is too concentrated it can kill any bacteria present (consider removing some of the boric acid powder if only a small amount of urine is obtained). It is preferable to submit a urine sample rather than just a swab for culture.

Many potential urinary tract pathogens are commensals of the urogenital or gastrointestinal tracts; therefore, cultures should be interpreted in the context of the clinical signs, sampling method and sediment examination (i.e. evidence of pyuria) to determine their clinical significance. Bacterial isolates are more likely to be significant if:

- They are cultured from a cystocentesis sample
- There is concurrent pyuria (but note that immunosuppressed animals can have a UTI without pyuria, e.g. patients with hyperadrenocorticism or those receiving exogenous steroids)
- There is a pure culture (mixed cultures are common with contamination).

Quantitative or semi-quantitative urine culture is performed by many laboratories to help determine the clinical significance of an isolate. The number of bacteria is expressed usually as colony forming units per millilitre; the higher the result, the more likely infection is to be present, rather than contamination. However, the result must still be interpreted with the sediment findings and also the identification of the organism isolated. Readers are referred to standard veterinary medical textbooks for further information (e.g. Pressler and Bartges, 2010). Occasionally a urine culture will be sterile, despite bacteria having been seen microscopically. Figure 10.39 lists possible reasons for this.

- The bacteria were not viable
  - Successful host defences
  - Previous antimicrobials
  - Exposure of sample to extremes of temperature
  - Excessive boric acid added
- The bacteria were viable but not successfully cultured
  - Fastidious isolate not cultured using routine methods
  - Too few were present to be detected (unlikely if sufficiently numerous for microscopic visualization)
  - Laboratory error
- The 'bacteria' were actually particulate debris in the urine demonstrating Brownian motion

10.39 Possible explanations for sterile culture following visualization of bacteria on microscopy.

Isolation of multidrug-resistant species of bacteria such as Extended-spectrum beta-Lactamase (ESBL) producers (most commonly *Escherichia coli* and *Klebsiella* species) is becoming increasingly common. In this situation it is important to make sure the bacteria identified are significant, and not commensals or contaminants, prior to treatment. See Chapter 27 for further information on bacterial culture.

Key point

Interpret culture results in the context of the clinical signs, sediment examination and sample collection method

Recently, a catalase based test was evaluated as an in-clinic method for the rapid detection of UTIs, for which it was shown to be more sensitive but less specific than sediment examination (Kvitko-White *et al.*, 2013). False negatives are possible so culture remains the gold standard.

Urine cytology

See Chapter 21 for general principles of cytological examination.

Key point

Urine cytology is only indicated in certain circumstances

Urine cytology is often unrewarding because the hostile urine environment leads to rapid cell deterioration and poor morphology; this can be a problem even when cytology is performed on very fresh samples if the urine has been in the bladder for a few hours before collection. Urine cytology is rarely useful when included in urinalysis as part of a routine medical work-up. It can, however, be a valuable tool in the following situations:

- Markedly increased numbers or obviously abnormal morphology of epithelial cells noted on sediment examination
- Equivocal evidence of bacteria on sediment examination
- Evidence of a urinary tract mass on imaging where direct fine-needle aspiration (FNA) or biopsy is not appropriate owing to logistical or financial considerations, or concerns regarding tumour cell seeding.

In reference laboratories, the cells are concentrated by centrifuging the urine using a dedicated cytocentrifuge which spins at a low speed to minimize cell damage. When this is not available samples are prepared in the same way as for wet sediment examination (see Figure 10.4). A drop of sediment is placed on either a plain slide or one coated with serum to encourage cell attachment (in practice, serum is rarely used; if cells are present in high enough numbers to warrant cytological examination, sufficient cells should remain on a plain slide after washing). The slide is tilted to ensure the cells spread in a monolayer, and then air-dried (urine samples can take a long time to dry). As an alternative, there are commercially available cytocentrifuge filters (e.g. Cytopro cytocentrifuge filter) for use in practice. These work by wicking away moisture to speed up the drying process. However, a recent study found that the resulting samples had such poor cell morphology that cell identification was impossible (O'Neil *et al.*, 2013). Staining is performed with a Romanowsky-type stain (i.e. a modified Wright's stain or rapid stain such as Diff-Quik®).

If the sample is to be submitted to an external laboratory, attention should be paid to that laboratory's submission protocol (most require urine to be submitted in a plain tube). If cytocentrifugation is an option in practice, a slide should be submitted in tandem with the fluid sample to avoid the problems associated with cell degeneration that occur with delayed processing.

Normal findings

Normal urine is acellular, or contains occasional transitional epithelial cells (also known as urothelial cells) and (with the exception of cystocentesis samples) squamous epithelial cells. Samples collected by catheter tend to be more cellular than other sample types, owing to the traumatic harvesting method. The epithelial cells are usually present singly (small clumps/rafts of cells are more often associated with inflammation, urolithiasis or neoplasia). Transitional epithelial cells are round cells which vary in size depending on their site of origin (cells from the renal pelvis and ureters are the smallest, with cell size increasing as the tract descends). See Figure 10.40 for

Feature	Transitional epithelial cell	Squamous epithelial cell
Size	Small to large, depending on site of origin	Large
Shape	Round	Polygonal, often angular
Cytoplasm	Moderate to abundant Palely basophilic or slightly eosinophilic	Abundant Palely basophilic cytoplasm or bright blue if keratinized (contaminating skin cells)
Nucleus	Round central nucleus N:C ratio generally higher than in squamous epithelial cells Stippled to coarse chromatin	Round central nucleus; may be pyknotic, or not visible N:C ratio generally lower than in transitional epithelial cells
	(a)	(b)

10.40 Comparative features of normal transitional and squamous epithelial cells in cytological samples. (a) Two normal transitional epithelial cells with small artefact between them. (b) Three squamous epithelial cells against a background of granular debris. (Original magnification of both photographs X500). N:C = nuclear to cytoplasmic.

comparative features of transitional and squamous epithelial cells; however, note that it is not always possible to distinguish large transitional cells from squamous epithelial cells. Rare erythrocytes and neutrophils may be present.

Inflammation

Neutrophilic inflammation is a common finding and usually reflects infection. As with other cells, neutrophils deteriorate rapidly in urine; they often appear shrunken, with loss of the characteristic lobed structure of the nucleus (sometimes it even appears smoothly round or oval), and the cytoplasm may not be intact. Macrophages, lymphocytes, eosinophils and rare plasma cells may accompany the neutrophilic inflammation.

Bacteria may be numerous in such preparations and are more readily recognizable than on wet sediment examination (Swenson *et al.*, 2004): compare Figures 10.41 and 10.21d. The presence of bacteria within neutrophils is strong circumstantial evidence of UTI, but sometimes this cannot be confirmed even in fulminant infection, owing to poor cellular preservation. Furthermore, bacterial phagocytosis by neutrophils can occur *in vitro*, and therefore it does not completely distinguish between bacterial infection and sample contamination. Even if bacteria are not visualized, neutrophilic inflammation is an indication for urine culture. Haematuria often accompanies inflammation.

Hyperplasia, dysplasia and metaplasia

Hyperplasia of transitional cell epithelium can occur with chronic inflammation due to infection, urolithiasis or exposure to toxins (notably chemotherapeutic agents). Hyperplastic cells are indistinguishable from normal cells. If the inflammation is long-standing, dysplasia and squamous metaplasia may occur. Dysplastic cells display mild anisocytosis, increased cytoplasmic basophilia or vacuolation, and the chromatin may appear coarser, although these changes are often difficult to distinguish from those associated with poor cell preservation. With squamous metaplasia, transitional cells take on the appearance of

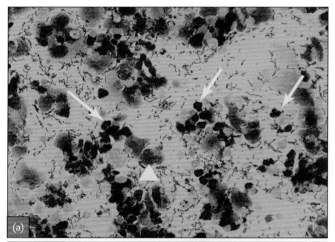

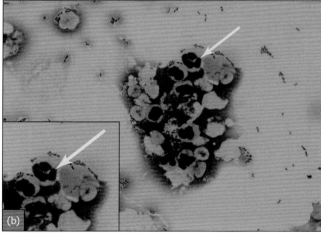

10.41 Cytology: urinary tract infection. (a) Note very poorly preserved neutrophils (arrowed), moderate numbers of erythrocytes, abundant extracellular bacteria (monomorphic population) and frequent lysed cells (arrowhead). (Modified Wright's stain; original magnification X500). (b) Same case as in (a); intracellular bacteria are just visible (arrowed). (Modified Wright's stain; original magnification X1000). Inset: higher magnification showing intracellular bacteria.

squamous epithelial cells (described under 'Normal findings'). The discovery of squamous cells in cystocentesis samples is always an abnormal finding, because squamous epithelial cells originate from the terminal urethra of males and the vagina and vulva of females; it warrants a search for metaplastic or neoplastic disease. Similarly, the presence of suspected metaplastic or dysplastic cells without accompanying inflammation should trigger a search for neoplastic disease.

Neoplasia

Neoplasia of the urinary tract is usually malignant, but it can be difficult or impossible to distinguish malignant masses from polyps and hyperplastic lesions on urine cytology alone. Urine samples containing cells with equivocal features of malignancy require assessment of cells obtained by direct FNA of the lesion, which yields cells better preserved than those exfoliated into urine (compare Figure 10.42). Although a very rare complication, there have been reports of seeding of transitional cell carcinomas (TCCs) along needle tracts or incision sites after fine-needle aspirates or surgical biopsy samples have been obtained from bladder tumours (Anderson *et al.*, 1989; Vignoli *et al.*, 2007; Higuchi *et al.*, 2013;). An alternative is to smear cells obtained by catheter suction biopsy on to a slide for cytological assessment.

The most common neoplasm diagnosed by urine cytology is TCC of the bladder (or, rarely, the urethra). Samples from animals with TCC usually have markedly increased cellularity, with cells present in clusters and rafts, although occasionally only low numbers of epithelial cells are shed. Given the variation in size of normal transitional epithelial cells, it can be difficult to identify abnormal anisocytosis; marked anisocytosis and anisokaryosis within cells within the same raft are indicators of pathological change. There may also be anisokaryosis, coarse or reticulated nuclear chromatin, multinucleation, prominent and/or abnormally shaped nucleoli, increased cytoplasmic vacuolation and/or cytoplasmic 'ballooning' ('signet ring' cells). (See Chapter 21 for more detail on cytological features of malignancy.) A characteristic feature of neoplastic transitional cells is the

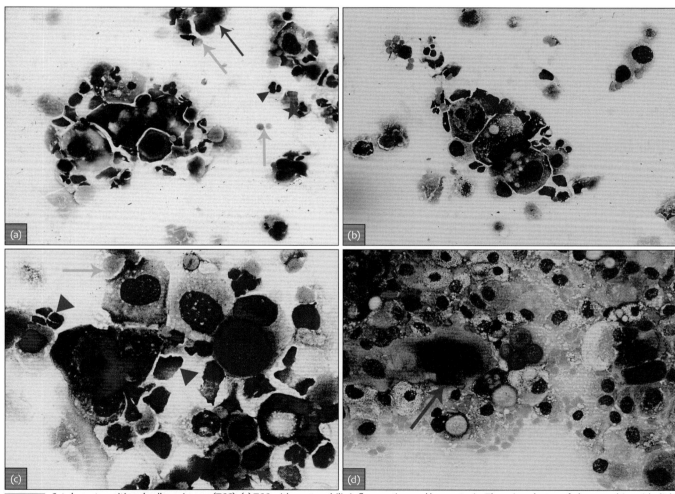

10.42 Cytology: transitional cell carcinoma (TCC). (a) TCC with neutrophilic inflammation and haematuria. There is a cluster of pleomorphic epithelial cells with deeply basophilic and variably vacuolated cytoplasm, variably shaped nuclei with coarse chromatin and multinucleation. Also present are more normal-appearing poorly preserved epithelial cells (red arrow), many poorly preserved neutrophils (arrowhead), erythrocytes (green arrows) and lysed cells (asterisk). (Modified Wright's stain; original magnification X500). (b) Same case as in (a); there is a central cluster of neoplastic epithelial cells demonstrating anisocytosis, anisokaryosis and bizarre nuclear morphology (nuclear fragmentation). Neutrophils, erythrocytes and lysed cells are also present. (Modified Wright's stain; original magnification X500). (c) Same case as in (a) showing pleomorphic epithelial cells, including small cells with a high nuclear to cytoplasmic (N:C) ratio (red arrow). One cell contains a single large pink cytoplasmic globule characteristic of TCC. Frequent poorly preserved neutrophils (arrowheads) and erythrocytes (green arrow) are also present. (Modified Wright's stain; original magnification X1000). (d) TCC, catheter biopsy sample. The sample is highly cellular with good preservation. There is a markedly pleomorphic population of epithelial cells which demonstrate multiple features of malignancy, including multinucleation with incomplete nuclear separation and prominent nucleoli of variable size (arrowed). Many cells contain the pink cytoplasmic globules characteristic of TCC. (Modified Wright's stain; original magnification X500)

presence of bright pink cytoplasmic material, often present as one or more large globules which distort the cell, giving it a 'signet ring' appearance (see Figure 10.42). Mitotic figures are variably present.

Other urogenital tract neoplasms which may shed cells into the urine include papillomas, prostatic carcinomas and adenocarcinomas, urothelial adenocarcinomas and squamous cell carcinomas. Cells shed from papillomas are indistinguishable from normal transitional cells, so diagnosis relies on clinical features, imaging and histology rather than cytology. Prostatic epithelial cell tumours include those of urothelial origin (i.e. they are TCCs) and those of glandular origin (i.e. prostatic adenocarcinomas). Cytology cannot distinguish reliably between these; both can display features as described above for TCCs, including the pink cytoplasmic globules (LeBlanc *et al.*, 2004). Squamous cell carcinomas yield particularly large cells; these display cytoplasmic keratinization and vacuolation (often perinuclear), as well as other features typical of malignant epithelial cells (see Chapter 21). Note that there is considerable overlap between the cytological features of squamous cell carcinomas and those of TCCs displaying squamous metaplasia; histology is usually necessary for definitive diagnosis in these cases.

Renal or bladder lymphomas occasionally shed large numbers of lymphoid cells into the urine; this is always an abnormal finding, even if cell morphology is unremarkable. Other tumours of the urinary tract include primary renal carcinomas, rhabdomyosarcomas, leiomyomas, leiomyosarcomas and giant cell sarcomas (Rigas *et al.*, 2012); these do not or only rarely exfoliate into the urine.

Other findings

Any of the other structures described under 'Wet sediment examination' may also be seen in cytological preparations.

Urolith analysis

Uroliths (also known as urinary calculi or stones) form within the urinary tract from aggregated crystals and organic matrix. They are believed to form when the urine is supersaturated with their constituent cations and anions, with other factors such as urinary pH and flow rate affecting the rate of formation. Urolith formation is more likely if there is a surface on which crystallization can occur, such as casts, bacterial aggregates, mucin plugs, cell debris or crystals that have already formed. Natural inhibitors exist to prevent crystallization and urolith formation: these include Tamm–Horsfall protein and citrate. Reduced levels of these inhibitors and increased amounts of the non-crystalline matrix predispose to urolith formation.

In general, predisposing factors for urolith formation are the same as those for crystalluria, but uroliths can be found in the absence of crystalluria, and can coexist with crystals of another type. Uroliths can be of mixed type, with concentric layers made of different minerals. This may reflect the dynamic environment and variable urine composition of different parts of the urinary tract, or that a urolith of any type can cause inflammation and predispose to infection, thus raising urinary pH and encouraging incorporation of struvite crystals into the outer layers.

Urolith analysis is a specialized procedure performed at particular reference laboratories. Semi-quantitative chemical methods have inherent inaccuracies, so where possible other methods are preferred. Reference laboratories analyse the physical properties of uroliths using optical crystallography, X-ray diffraction, infrared spectroscopy, electron microprobes or scanning electron microscopy. These methods can also be employed to confirm the crystal composition in a case with clinically significant crystalluria but without detectable urolithiasis: a pellet of crystals can be made by centrifuging a large volume of urine and then submitted for physical analysis. Uroliths should always be analysed so that a treatment plan can be designed to prevent recurrence. It is important not to rely on urinalysis for identification because any crystals present may not be the same type as the uroliths and, as mentioned above, mixed stones can occur.

See Figure 10.44 for further information on individual types of urolith (illustrated in Figure 10.43), and Figure 10.45 for the relative prevalence of different types of urolith submitted to the Minnesota Urolith Centre in 2007 (Osborne *et al.*, 2009). A recent study reported the composition of uroliths in small domestic animals in the UK (Rogers *et al.*, 2011).

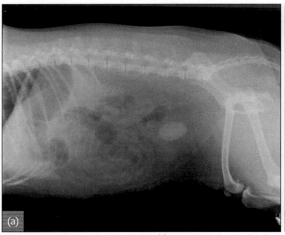 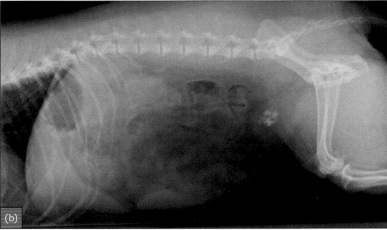

10.43 Radiographs of uroliths. (a) Lateral abdominal radiograph of a 7-year-old female entire Cavalier King Charles Spaniel. There is a single large radiopaque urolith in the bladder. This was analysed and found to be a struvite urolith. (b) Lateral abdominal radiograph of an 11-year-old male neutered Bichon Frise. There are several irregular radiopaque masses in the dependant portion of the bladder. These were removed surgically and found to be calcium oxalate uroliths.
(Courtesy of Heath and Reach Veterinary Surgery)

Type of urolith	Associated urine pH	Other predisposing factors	Radiopacity	Signalment associations (not exhaustive)	Comments
Struvite (magnesium, ammonium, phosphate)	≥7	• UTI with urease-producing bacteria • High concentrations of magnesium, phosphate and ammonium ions • High magnesium content dry diets • Reduced urine glycosaminoglycans	Radiopaque (see Figure 10.43a)	Dogs: • Bitches • Mixed breeds • Miniature Schnauzer • Lhasa Apso • Shih Tzu • Bichon Frise • Miniature Poodle Cats: • Older queens	In dogs, most often associated with UTI In cats, urine usually sterile Note: In cats, struvite calculi are rare. Most urethral obstructions are caused by plugs comprising struvite crystals and mucoid material

Calcium oxalate	≤7	• Hypercalciuria due to:
		  ∘ Hypercalcaemia
		  ∘ Increased intake of Ca^{2+}
		  ∘ Increased intake of vitamin D
		• Hyperoxaluria due to ingestion of oxalate-rich foods (e.g. chocolate, nuts and sweet potato)
		• Diet high in protein, vitamin C or sodium
		• Acidifying diets
		• Reduced urine glycosaminoglycans
		• Reduced production of compounds which inhibit calcium oxalate crystal growth (Tamm–Horsfall protein, nephrocalcin and prothrombin fragments)
			Radiopaque (see Figure 10.43b)	Dogs:
				• Older males
				• Lhasa Apso
				• Shih Tzu
				• Bichon Frise
				• Miniature Poodle
				• Miniature Schnauzer
				• Yorkshire Terrier
				
				Cats:
				• Older males
				• Burmese
				• Himalayan
				• Persian
					Urine usually sterile

Calcium phosphate; includes basic calcium phosphate, hydroxyapatite, calcium hydrogen phosphate dehydrate ('brushite')	≥7 (except brushite)	• UTI • Hypercalciuria (as for calcium oxalate uroliths) • Increased dietary phosphate • Renal tubular acidosis	Radiopaque	Dogs: • Middle-aged to older males • Cocker Spaniel • Yorkshire Terrier • Miniature Schnauzer Cats: • Middle-aged queens	Rare in cats
Ammonium urate and uric acid	Ammonium urate: variable (usually alkaline) Uric acid <7	• Inherited purine metabolic defect leads to excretion of insoluble uric acid • PSS or hepatic insufficiency	Radiolucent	Dogs: • Males • Dalmatian • Bulldog • Black Russian Terrier • Yorkshire Terrier • Miniature Schnauzer	• Dalmatians, some Bulldogs and some Black Russian Terriers are predisposed by defective purine metabolism • Yorkshire Terrier and Miniature Schnauzer are predisposed owing to their high incidence of PSS
Cystine	≤7	• Inherited renal tubular transport disorder leading to reduced renal reabsorption of cystine and some other amino acids	Relatively radiolucent	Dogs: • Young males • Bulldog • Newfoundland • Mastiffs • Bullmastiff • Dachshunds • Basset Hound • Australian Cattle Dog • Scottish Deerhound • Chihuahua	Rare in cats
Xanthine	≤7	• Allopurinol treatment (for urate urolithiasis or leishmaniosis) • Inherited xanthinuria	Radiolucent	• Cavalier King Charles Spaniel • Dachshunds	Rare in cats
Silica	≤7	• Acidifying diets containing high levels of plant gluten, soybean or maize hulls • Dogs with pica	Radiopaque	Dogs: • Middle-aged males • German Shepherd Dog • Golden Retriever • Labrador Retriever • Old English Sheepdog	Rare

10.44 Features of the different types of urolith. PSS = portosystemic shunt; UTI = urinary tract infection.

Urolith	Percentage of 40,612 samples
Struvite	40%
Calcium oxalate	41%
Compound (two or more components)	9%
Purine	5%
Other	3%
Cystine	1%
Calcium phosphate	<1%
Silica	<1%

10.45 Mineral composition of canine uroliths submitted to the Minnesota Urolith Centre in 2007.

(Data from Osborne et al., 2009)

Water deprivation testing

The water deprivation test (WDT) is used in animals with hyposthenuria to distinguish between:

- Central diabetes insipidus (CDI)
- Nephrogenic (primary) diabetes insipidus (NDI)
- Primary ('psychogenic') polydipsia (PP).

It is paramount that all other possible causes of failure to concentrate the urine have been ruled out first, because this test is potentially dangerous. Severe dehydration may lead to renal failure, and rapid rehydration at the end of the test could cause cerebral oedema. The WDT is contraindicated if an animal is azotaemic or dehydrated. See Figure 10.46 for conditions which must be ruled out prior to commencing the WDT; note that most are far more common than CDI, NDI or PP. In particular, the practitioner must be confident that hyperadrenocorticism has been ruled out because this can confound the results: some animals with hyperadrenocorticism demonstrate antidiuretic hormone (ADH) antagonism, meaning that they can concentrate their urine to >1.008, but not >1.025. When desmopressin (a synthetic ADH analogue) is administered, this over-rides the antagonism to some extent and these animals can concentrate their urine further – thus mimicking CDI. The mechanism of ADH antagonism in hyperadrenocorticism has not been fully established, but cortisol has been postulated to inhibit ADH secretion and to inhibit the responsiveness of renal tubules to ADH.

- Hyperadrenocorticism
- Diabetes mellitus
- Hypoadrenocorticism
- Renal insufficiency
- Hepatic insufficiency
- Hypercalcaemia
- Pyometra
- Pyelonephritis

10.46 Differential diagnoses that must be ruled out before performing a water deprivation test.

Principle

If a normal animal becomes dehydrated, serum osmolality increases and ADH is released from the hypothalamus to cause renal conservation of water. The idea behind the test is to determine: (i) whether ADH is released, and (ii) whether the kidneys can respond to ADH effectively. This is done by splitting the test into three consecutive parts:

1. Gradual water restriction.
2. Abrupt water deprivation.
3. Response to intravenous desmopressin (if necessary).

Because serum and urine osmolality testing is not widely available, a combination of urine SG and accurate measurement of bodyweight is used as a substitute. The same refractometer and set of weighing scales should be used throughout Stages 2 and 3.

Protocol

Various similar protocols exist. The following protocol is taken from the *BSAVA Guide to Procedures in Small Animal Practice* (Bexfield and Lee, 2010).

Stage 1. Gradual water restriction (at home)

Gradual, progressive water restriction is advisable before commencing abrupt water deprivation, to minimize the effects of medullary washout on the test. This can be done by the owner at home by gradually reducing the amount of water provided to the animal for the 3 days preceding the abrupt WDT, as follows:

1. During the initial 24 hours, allow the dog or cat twice its calculated normal daily water requirement (120–150 ml/kg), divided into six to eight small portions.
2. During the next 24 hours, give 80–100 ml/kg.
3. Over the last 24 hours, provide normal maintenance requirements (60–80 ml/kg).

During this period the owner should:

- Feed dry food and monitor the animal's bodyweight on a daily basis
- Observe for any significant change in the animal's mentation. Should this occur, the test should be stopped and veterinary attention sought immediately.

Stage 2. Abrupt water deprivation (in clinic)

The aim of this stage is to achieve maximal ADH secretion and urine concentration, which should occur once dehydration has caused a 3–5% loss of bodyweight. This stage must be carried out in a veterinary clinic (indeed, some clinicians advocate that this is only appropriate in referral facilities because of the close monitoring required), and it is advisable to commence early in the day because the duration of the procedure cannot be accurately predicted.

> **WARNING**
>
> **Throughout Stage 2, the animal must be monitored for signs of central nervous system (CNS) depression and the test immediately ceased if these are seen**

1. Completely empty the animal's bladder (consider an indwelling catheter, especially in females) and collect the urine.
2. Record the urine SG, obtain an exact bodyweight and remove all food and water.
3. At 1–2-hourly intervals, empty the bladder completely, measure the urine SG and reweigh the animal (to monitor for dehydration). Serum urea and creatinine can also be measured (optional).

4. Continue until there is a 5% loss in bodyweight *or* the urine SG is >1.030 in dogs or >1.035 in cats *or* the animal becomes azotaemic or depressed.
5. Some animals will fail to reach the 5% dehydration endpoint by the end of the working day. If it is not possible to continue the test, overnight access to water in maintenance amounts (2.5–3.0 ml/kg/h) can be provided. On the following morning, water is once again withdrawn and monitoring continued until a 5% loss of bodyweight or concentrated urine SG is reached.

Stage 3. Response to intravenous desmopressin (in clinic)

This is performed if the animal has lost 5% or more of its bodyweight, but the urine SG remains <1.015.

1. Provide water in maintenance amounts (2.5–3.0 ml/kg/h) for the duration of this stage.
2. Inject synthetic desmopressin intravenously:
   - 2.0 µg for dogs <15 kg and cats
   - 4.0 µg for dogs >15 kg.
3. Completely empty the animal's bladder (consider an indwelling catheter, especially in females) and collect the urine.
4. Record the urine SG every 30–60 minutes.
5. Stop the test when the urine SG has risen above 1.015 *or the animal shows signs of CNS depression.*
6. Continue this stage for a maximum of 8 hours.
7. Upon completion of the test, water should be offered in maintenance amounts (2.5–3.0 ml/kg/h) for 2–3 hours then provided *ad libitum.*

Interpretation of results

See Figure 10.47.

Disorder	Urine SG prior to test	Urine SG after Stage 2	Urine SG after Stage 3
Central diabetes insipidus	1.001–1.007	<1.008	Increase to >1.015
Nephrogenic diabetes insipidus	1.001–1.007	<1.008	No change (remains <1.008)
Primary polydipsia	1.001–1.020	>1.030	Stage 3 not indicated

10.47 Interpretation of results of the water deprivation test. SG = specific gravity.
(Reproduced from the *BSAVA Guide to Procedures in Small Animal Practice*)

Equivocal results

After Stage 3, if the urine SG is between 1.008 and 1.015, this is considered equivocal and may be due to medullary washout, which can be a consequence of any primary PU or PD disorder (see above). Stage 1, gradual water deprivation, is designed to minimize this problem.

Sometimes there may be partial concentration of the urine by the end of Stage 2 (i.e. the animal has lost more than 5% of its bodyweight, but the urine SG is in the range 1.016–1.029 (in a dog). This could imply partial diabetes insipidus (nephrogenic or central). In these circumstances, or if the WDT is non-diagnostic, a closely monitored therapeutic trial of synthetic desmopressin (DDAVP) can be performed over 5–7 days. In CDI, desmopressin administration will cause water intake to halve at least, whereas in NDI there will be no response.

An alternative is to measure endogenous plasma ADH levels, but this test is not widely available and is expensive.

The Hickey–Hare test, which involves intravenous injection of hypertonic saline to measure renal and pituitary responses to hyperosmolality, is not recommended owing to the risk of inducing marked hypertonicity.

Tests for glomerular pathology

See under the Protein section, above, for details of the urine protein to creatinine ratio, urine microalbumin and urine protein electrophoresis. Renal biopsy and histopathology may be necessary in the investigation of glomerular pathology.

Tests for tubular pathology

Osmolality

The gold standard for measuring urine solute concentration (i.e. osmolality), and thus renal concentrating ability, is freezing-point osmometry. This is rarely available and, because urine SG correlates well with urine osmolality, is rarely necessary. Occasionally, concurrent measurement of urine and plasma osmolality is performed to try to differentiate primary polydipsia from primary polyuria. In both cases the urine will have a low osmolality, but in primary PD the plasma also has slightly low osmolality whereas in primary polyuria the plasma osmolality is high normal to slightly increased.

Fractional excretion tests

The fractional excretion (FE) of a plasma constituent by the kidney is the proportion filtered by the glomerulus that is excreted in the urine. FE measurements are most commonly performed on electrolytes, which are reabsorbed and secreted by the renal tubules and thus give an indication of tubular function. Measurement requires either the collection of urine over 24 hours or the spot sample approach, in which urine and blood are sampled at the same time and the concentrations of the electrolyte in both are compared with those of creatinine, which provides an approximation of glomerular filtration rate (GFR). See Chapter 11 for equations and further details.

The FE values of electrolytes are subject to large inter- and intra-individual variation, depending on species, age, diet and absorption of the analyte from the gastrointestinal tract; establishment of meaningful reference values is therefore problematic. This, combined with the logistical problems of 24-hour urine sample collection and the inaccuracy of the spot sample approach, limits the clinical relevance of FE tests in veterinary medicine. The authors of a review concluded that their use should be confined to the diagnosis of canine Fanconi syndrome, nutritional investigations and nephrology research (Lefebvre *et al.*, 2008).

Urine gamma-glutamyl transferase:creatinine ratio

Renal tubular epithelial cells synthesize the enzyme gamma-glutamyl transferase (GGT; also known as γ-glutamyl transpeptidase). In acute renal tubular damage, injured epithelial cells release GGT into the urine. GGT can be measured in the urine and is expressed as a ratio with urinary creatinine to take into consideration the influence of urine concentration. An elevated GGT:creatinine ratio (GGT:Crt) suggests active renal tubular damage. One of the main indications for this test is in dogs on aminoglycoside therapy (see also Chapter 11), because the GGT:Crt is elevated prior to detectable changes in serum creatinine, urine SG or UPCR in cases of nephrotoxicosis (Grauer *et al.*, 1995).

It is important to note that the urine GGT:Crt can be increased by decreased GFR because creatinine excretion is decreased with decreased GFR whereas GGT excretion is not; therefore interpretation should be cautious when there is significant azotaemia. The aim is to use urine GGT:Crt to detect acute renal damage *before* renal function is affected. Urine GGT:Crt also may increase with severe glomerular damage owing to passage of plasma GGT into the filtrate.

Urine NAG:creatinine ratio

N-acetyl-β-D-glucosaminidase (NAG) is a lysosomal enzyme present in proximal tubule cells which leaks into the urine if the cells are damaged. It is a useful predictor of the progression of renal disease in humans. As with GGT, an increased NAG:creatinine ratio (NAG:Crt) is postulated to be a marker of active disease that is damaging the renal cells.

Two different enzymatic colorimetric assays have recently been validated for use in dogs; in both cases, the between-run coefficient of variation for urinary NAG concentration was relatively high for diagnostic purposes. The first study found a significant difference between the NAG:Crt in dogs with CKD and that in healthy dogs, but there was a large overlap between the two groups (Smets *et al.*, 2010), while the second study showed that the NAG:Crt successfully distinguished dogs with X-linked hereditary nephropathy from unaffected dogs *early in the disease process* (Nabity *et al.*, 2012). The clinical utility of the NAG:Crt ratio remains to be fully established. This test is currently available commercially.

Promising new tests for tubular pathology

Various biomarkers for detecting early tubular pathology are currently under investigation and may become more widely available in the future, including:

* **Urine cystatin C:creatinine ratio (UCysC):** this shows promise as a test for renal tubular function. A human assay was recently validated in dogs and is commercially available. The UCysC was able to distinguish dogs with renal disease, from those without (Monti *et al.*, 2012)
* **Urine retinol-binding protein (RBP) to creatinine ratio:** this may be useful for detecting early tubular damage before an obvious increase in creatinine is seen, but further work is necessary to establish its clinical utility (Nabity *et al.*, 2011, 2012). To this authors' knowledge, this test is not currently offered by commercial reference laboratories in the UK
* **Urine neutrophil gelatinase-associated lipocalin (NGAL) to creatinine ratio:** this shows promise as a biomarker for the detection of acute kidney injury (Segev *et al.*, 2013). It can be detected in both blood and urine using a commercially available canine-specific enzyme-linked immunosorbent assay (ELISA). It may be elevated in UTIs, so care must be taken when interpreting results (Daure *et al.*, 2013).

Detection of amino acid tubular transport disorders

See under 'Miscellaneous tests'.

Urinary tests for adrenal disease

Urine corticoid:creatinine ratio

The urine corticoid:creatinine ratio (UCCR) is used to determine whether there is increased urinary excretion of cortisol and its metabolites due to hypercortisolaemia; comparing it to the creatinine concentration corrects for variation in urine concentration. The UCCR is elevated in hyperadrenocorticism (HAC), but is non-specific for this disease: it can also be elevated as a result of the stress of other chronic disease or external factors. Its high sensitivity but low specificity renders it more useful for *ruling out* hyperadrenocorticism than for diagnosis. In order to minimize false positives it is important that samples for this test are collected in a non-stressful environment (i.e. at home rather than at the surgery, and also not within a few days of visiting the surgery). If possible, three separate samples should be collected; equal aliquots of each are mixed and submitted for analysis. Since the original reports of this test various reference intervals (RIs) have been used. Laboratories use different methods to assay cortisol and this can influence the result. Furthermore, a recent publication found that some assays detect various cortisol metabolites in addition to cortisol, the so-called corticoids, and this can lead to very different results (Zeugswetter *et al.*, 2013); the reader is referred to Chapter 18 (Figure 18.6) for further information. In essence, it is important to check the RI with the laboratory assaying the sample.

Using the most common methodology (chemiluminescence), dogs with UCCR $<26.5 \times 10^{-6}$ are highly unlikely to have hyperadrenocorticism. UCCR values over 161.2×10^6 are highly suggestive of HAC, but there is a large grey area between these two ratios where the increase may be due to HAC or non-adrenal illness (Zeugswetter *et al.*, 2010). See Chapter 18 for calculation and further details.

Urinary catecholamines and metadrenalines

These may be used in the diagnosis of phaeochromocytoma, although their use is hindered by the limited availability of testing and the lability of vasoactive amines and their metabolites. The urine must be collected into a plain tube, acidified, protected from light and shipped on ice to the reference laboratory, where it is analysed by high-pressure liquid chromatography with electrochemical detection. The concentrations of the catecholamines and their metabolites are expressed as a ratio to the urinary creatinine concentration, to take into account the spot nature of the sample. A recent study demonstrated that urine normetadrenaline:creatinine ratios were significantly higher in seven dogs with phaeochromocytoma than in controls, and that the performance characteristics of this metabolite were superior to those of adrenaline (epinephrine), noradrenaline (norepinephrine), dopamine and metadrenaline to creatinine ratios in distinguishing the affected dogs from healthy controls (Kook *et al.*, 2010).

Detection of systemic infectious diseases

In certain systemic infectious diseases, evidence of the organism involved can be found in urine. In leptospirosis, polymerase chain reaction (PCR) can be used to detect leptospiral DNA, or the direct immunofluorescent assay (dIFA) can be used to visualize leptospires in smears of urine sediment. These methods are more sensitive than traditional dark-field microscopy for detecting spirochaetes. However, these tests do not distinguish among serovars or between live or dead organisms, and they rely on active shedding of spirochaetes at the time of sampling.

In acute distemper, the dIFA can be used to detect canine distemper virus (CDV) antigen in urine, while in chronic cases, reverse transcriptase-PCR to detect CDV RNA in urine has been shown to be more sensitive than serum samples and of equal sensitivity to CSF analysis (Saito *et al.*, 2006). See Chapters 27–29 for further information on clinical pathology of infectious disease.

Detection of toxic substances

Ethylene glycol

In cases of suspected antifreeze ingestion, a commercially available point-of-care enzymatic kit can be used to detect ethylene glycol in plasma. Although not marketed for such use, it will also detect ethylene glycol in urine; this may be useful to diagnose toxicity once the plasma levels of ethylene glycol have declined below detectable levels as a result of rapid metabolism. False positives can be caused by the presence of propylene glycol (found in some pharmaceuticals and semi-moist diets). Ethylene glycol can also be detected by gas chromatography–mass spectrometry and enzymatic assays in reference laboratories; these are more sensitive, but turnaround time may be prohibitive (see also Figure 11.11).

Lead

Blood levels of lead do not correlate well with clinical signs: low blood lead concentrations do not rule out lead poisoning. Urinary levels of lead, before and after chelation therapy, can be used to confirm the diagnosis, because chelated lead is excreted in the urine. A urine sample is taken at baseline and then 24 hours after chelation therapy is instigated. A 10-fold (or greater) increase in urinary lead concentrations after chelation therapy is indicative of lead toxicosis. Analysis of urinary lead concentrations requires a specialized reference laboratory.

Illicit drugs

Human point-of-care kits for the detection of recreational drugs in urine are widely available. To the authors' knowledge, these have not been validated for use in veterinary species. There was a recent report of the successful diagnosis and treatment of barbiturate toxicity in a dog using a positive urine drugs screening test (Campbell *et al.*, 2009).

Extensive toxicology screening

Extensive screening for over 30,000 drugs and toxins is commercially available in the UK. The technique uses gas chromatography–mass spectrometry to detect substances in various sample types, including urine (http://ctdslab.co.uk/toxicology-and-poison-testing/).

Miscellaneous tests

Urine bile acid:creatinine ratio

When plasma bile acids are elevated, urinary excretion of bile acids is increased. The bile acid concentration in a spot urine sample relates to the plasma concentration of bile acids during the time the sampled urine was formed. Relating this to urine creatinine corrects for variation in urine concentration. The information gained from the urine bile acid:creatinine ratio (BA:Crt) is similar to that gained from measuring serum bile acids, and has the advantage of convenience compared with pre- and post-prandial blood sampling. There is limited published information regarding the diagnostic utility of the urinary BA:Crt compared with established methods of evaluating liver disease. One study found that diagnostic performance was comparable to that of serum bile acids for the identification of dogs with hepatic disorders (Balkman *et al.*, 2003).

Bladder tumour antigen test

This is used to screen for TCC in dogs. The principle behind the test is that urinary tract epithelial neoplasms degrade the basement membrane, releasing fragments of type IV collagen, fibronectin, laminin and proteoglycans into the urine. These can be detected by a commercially available rapid latex agglutination test. While it may be useful as a screening test in older dogs, or in conjunction with other diagnostic techniques in dogs suspected of having TCC, the test is poorly specific: frequent false positives are found in dogs with other lower urinary tract diseases. Therefore, the test is not recommended if there is haematuria, significant proteinuria or significant glucosuria (Billet *et al.*, 2002; Henry *et al.*, 2003).

Detection of amino acids

Taurine deficiencies in cats and dogs have been associated with dilated cardiomyopathy (DCM), retinal degeneration, reproductive failure and growth retardation. Carnitine deficiency in dogs has been associated with DCM, lipid storage myopathies and other conditions; carnitine deficiency has not been reported in cats. Urinary concentrations of taurine and carnitine can be used as indicators of total body levels; 24-hour urine taurine concentration, fractional excretion, or the taurine:creatinine ratio can be measured to assess taurine levels (Sanderson, 2009a). Only 24-hour urine carnitine concentrations (i.e. *not* spot samples) are thought to be useful in dogs (Sanderson, 2009b). Currently, blood samples are more commonly used than urine to measure these molecules owing to the ease of sampling, wider availability of testing and more readily available reference limits (see Chapter 20). On occasion, urine testing of amino acids is performed to aid the diagnosis of Fanconi syndrome or cystinuria.

Detection of organic acids

Rare, usually inherited, metabolic diseases can result in the accumulation of abnormal metabolites, resulting in organic acidaemia and neurological abnormalities. These compounds are concentrated in the urine and may be detected by gas chromatography–mass spectrometry in specialist laboratories.

Urinalysis in animals less than 6 months old

There is a paucity of information on urinalysis in young animals, but they do present with urinary tract signs, so urinalysis is sometimes necessary. It is generally accepted that urine SG is lower in the very young, though there is variation in precise values and ages quoted. Puppies less than 8 weeks old may have urine SG up to 1.018, though one study found that values reached adult levels (over 1.030) by 4 weeks of age as the kidneys matured (Faulks and Lane, 2003). Figure 10.48 details the expected findings.

Urinalysis	Percentage of puppies affected (Faulks and Lane, 2003)	Comments
Red blood cells	5% (>10/hpf)	
Blood/ haemoglobin on dipstick	17% (trace)	Note fewer puppies affected on sediment examination
White blood cells	44% (>10/hpf)	>40–70/hpf in 22% of puppies
Epithelial cells	83%	Squamous and transitional epithelial cells
Crystals	37%	Mainly struvite
pH	5–8.5	
Protein	98% (trace to 3+)	
Glucose	Negative	May be positive up to 3 weeks of age (Kruger et al., 2001)
Specific gravity (SG)	Puppies 0–3 weeks old, SG range 1.003–1.038, mean 1.018 Over 4 weeks old >1.030 (1.003–1.055)	Up to 8 weeks old may be lower, up to 1.018

10.48 Expected findings on sediment and dipstick examination of urine from puppies under 6 months old. hpf = high power field.

Case examples

CASE 1

SIGNALMENT

10-year-old entire male crossbreed dog.

HISTORY

The dog presented for difficulty with urination. Clinical examination revealed pain on palpation of the lumbar spine and mild prostatomegaly.

CLINICAL PATHOLOGY DATA

Urinalysis	Result	Reference interval
Sample type	Unknown	
Urine protein (mg/l)	1319.0	
Urine creatinine (mmol/l)	11.91	
UPCR	**0.98**	0.0–0.5
Chemistry		
pH	7.0	
Specific gravity	1.030	
Protein	++	
Glucose	Negative	
Ketones	Negative	
Urobilinogen	Negative	
Bilirubin	Negative	
Haemoglobin	Negative	▶

Abnormal results are in **bold**.

Microscopy	Result	Reference interval
WBC (per hpf)	**20–100**	<5
RBC (per hpf)	**5–20**	<5
Epithelial cells	+++	
Bacteria	+++	
Crystals	Not seen	
Casts	Not seen	
Culture		
Organism	*Escherichia coli* +++	
Amoxicillin/clavulanate (co-amoxiclav)	Sensitive	
Marbofloxacin	Sensitive	
Cefovecin	Sensitive	
Nitrofurantoin	Sensitive	
Clindamycin	Resistant	
Enrofloxacin	Sensitive	
Sulphonamide/trimethoprim	Sensitive	
Cephalexin	Sensitive	

Abnormal results are in **bold**.

HOW WOULD YOU INTERPRET THESE RESULTS?

Pyuria, an increase in epithelial cells, bacteriuria and mild haematuria all provide evidence of infection of the urinary tract or prostate gland. The pure heavy growth of *E. coli* and presence of inflammatory sediment suggests this is a clinically significant organism rather than contamination of the urine with bacteria. When the urine is contaminated a mixed growth is often identified.

→ CASE 1 CONTINUED

The UPCR cannot be interpreted in the presence of inflammation.

The dog was treated with antibiotics and a further sample collected.

FOLLOW-UP CLINICAL PATHOLOGY DATA

Urinalysis	Result	Reference interval
Sample type	Free catch	
Urine protein (mg/l)	147.1	
Urine creatinine (mmol/l)	9.14	
UPCR	0.14	0.0–0.5
Chemistry		
pH	7.0	
Specific gravity	1.025	
Protein	Negative	
Glucose	Negative	
Ketones	Negative	
Urobilinogen	Negative	
Bilirubin	Negative	
Haemoglobin	Negative	
Microscopy		
WBC (per hpf)	Not seen	<5
RBC (per hpf)	Not seen	<5

Microscopy *continued*	Result	Reference interval
Epithelial cells	++	
Bacteria	Not seen	
Yeasts	+++	
Crystals	+ Struvite	
Casts	Not seen	
Amorphous debris	++	
Sperm	++	
Fungal hyphae	+++	
Culture		
Organism	No growth	

WHAT IS YOUR INTERPRETATION OF THE FOLLOW-UP SAMPLE?

There is no longer evidence of inflammation or infection (there are no inflammatory cells, no haematuria, and bacteria are not visible on microscopy or present on culture).

The UPCR has reduced into the reference interval, suggesting the original increase was due to the haematuria and pyuria present in the first sample.

There are yeasts and fungal hyphae present in the absence of inflammatory sediment, suggesting the sample has been contaminated.

A small number of struvite crystals are noted this time; these have probably precipitated during storage. The lack of haematuria means they are less likely to be significant.

CASE 2

SIGNALMENT

13-year-old neutered female West Highland White Terrier.

HISTORY

The dog was diabetic and already on insulin therapy. She presented with increased frequency of urination and had developed urinary incontinence, which had not been present previously.

CLINICAL PATHOLOGY DATA

Urinalysis	Result	Reference interval
Sample type	Cystocentesis	
Urine protein (mg/l)	319.5	
Urine creatinine (mmol/l)	0.36	
UPCR	**7.85**	0.0–0.5
Chemistry		
pH	7.0	
Specific gravity	1.020	
Protein	+	
Glucose	+++	

Abnormal results are in **bold**.

Chemistry *continued*	Result	Reference interval
Ketones	Negative	
Urobilinogen	Negative	
Bilirubin	Negative	
Haemoglobin	Negative	
Microscopy		
WBC (per hpf)	Not seen	<5
RBC (per hpf)	<5	<5
Epithelial cells	Rare	
Bacteria	Not seen	
Crystals	Not seen	
Casts	Not seen	
Amorphous debris	+	
Culture	No growth	

Abnormal results are in **bold**.

HOW WOULD YOU INTERPRET THESE RESULTS?

Marked glucosuria is present, consistent with the diabetes mellitus. There is a marked increase in UPCR. There is no evidence of haematuria or pyuria which could lead to an artefactual increase in urine protein (so-called 'postrenal' proteinuria). Therefore genuine renal

→ CASE 2 CONTINUED

proteinuria is likely to be the cause of the increased UPCR and, with this history, may suggest a diabetic nephropathy or an unrelated nephropathy. Interestingly, diabetic dogs do not commonly develop diabetic nephropathy.

There is no evidence of urinary tract infection or inflammation, so it seems likely that the incontinence and increased frequency of urination are due to PU/PD as a result of either the diabetes mellitus or protein-losing nephropathy.

The SG is difficult to interpret here. The presence of proteinuria means there could be glomerular disease but urine SG is likely to be reduced as a result of diabetes mellitus and the associated PU/PD. Glucosuria can cause a small increase in SG too. Therefore there are potentially two conditions which could lower SG and one that could increase it, so it is very hard to decide whether renal concentrating ability is adequate.

WHAT FURTHER TESTS WOULD YOU PERFORM?

It would be useful to check serum biochemistry to search for evidence of renal failure, to evaluate serum albumin and also to exclude prerenal proteinuria. The International Renal Interest Society (IRIS) recommends checking the UPCR on at least three urine samples collected over 2 weeks when staging CRF, to check whether it is persistent, although levels this high are unlikely to occur as a transient finding. Measurement of fructosamine and blood glucose would be helpful to evaluate the stability of the diabetes mellitus.

A pre-insulin glucose concentration was 23 mmol/l and nadir blood glucose 13 mmol/l, suggesting that an increase in insulin was required. The dog was suspected of having concurrent hyperadrenocorticism, which could contribute to the raised UPCR, as well as contributing to the polyuria via secondary NDI. Unfortunately the dog was not responding well to treatment and the owners opted for euthanasia soon after these tests were performed.

CASE 3

SIGNALMENT

17-year-old neutered female Domestic Shorthair cat.

HISTORY

The cat had hyperthyroidism. Urine was being tested as part of a work-up prior to referral for radioactive iodine therapy.

CLINICAL PATHOLOGY DATA

Microscopy	Cystocentesis sample	Expressed sample	Reference interval
WBC (per hpf)	<5	<5	<5
RBC (per hpf)	<5	20–100	<5
Epithelial cells	Rare	Rare	▶

Microscopy *continued*	Cystocentesis sample	Expressed sample	Reference interval
Bacteria	Not seen	+++	
Crystals	Not seen	Not seen	
Casts	Not seen	Not seen	
Amorphous debris	+/–	+/–	

CAN YOU EXPLAIN THE REASONS FOR THE DIFFERENCES BETWEEN THE TWO SAMPLE TYPES?

There are more red cells in the expressed sample, presumably due to trauma during collection.

There are bacteria present in the expressed sample, which suggests contamination because the cystocentesis sample does not contain bacteria. This illustrates the fact that a cystocentesis sample is ideal for culture as it should reflect the true situation in the bladder. Furthermore, collection is likely to be less traumatic by this method than by manual expression.

QUIZ QUESTION

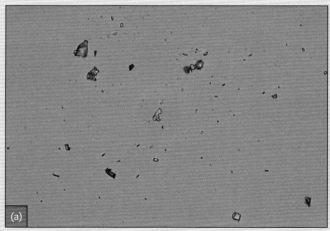

(a)

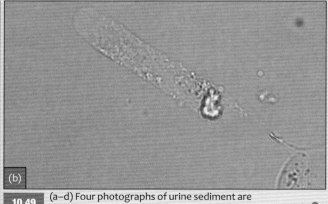

(b)

10.49 (a–d) Four photographs of urine sediment are presented. Can you identify the structures present?

(continues)

→ **QUIZ CONTINUED**

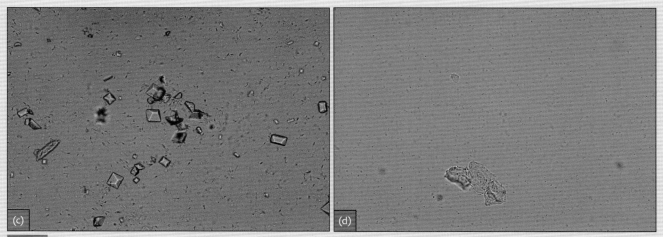

10.49 (continued) (a–d) Four photographs of urine sediment are presented. Can you identify the structures present?

Answers: (a) Glass shards. These are occasionally seen as an artefact and should not be confused with crystals. **(b)** A granular cast. Note the parallel sides. The cast is clear but with a granular internal appearance. **(c)** Struvite crystals with spermatozoa in the background. These crystals have a cuboid shape. Do not confuse them with the 'Maltese cross' feature of calcium oxalate dihydrate crystals (pH can be measured to help determine the likelihood of different crystal types). **(d)** Three clustered squamous epithelial cells. They are slightly granular structures with an angular shape and no nuclei. The smaller structure present towards the top of the picture is probably a WBC.

References and further reading

Anderson WI, Dunham BM, King JM *et al.* (1989) Presumptive subcutaneous surgical transplantation of a urinary bladder transitional cell carcinoma in a dog. *Cornell Veterinarian* **79**, 263–266

Bailiff NL, Westropp JL, Nelson RW *et al.* (2008) Evaluation of urine specific gravity and urine sediment as risk factors for urinary tract infections in cats. *Veterinary Clinical Pathology* **37**, 317–322

Balkman CE, Center SA, Randolph JF *et al.* (2003) Evaluation of urine sulfated and nonsulfated bile acids as a diagnostic test for liver disease in dogs. *Journal of the American Veterinary Medical Association* **222**, 1368–1375

Berent AC, Drobatz KJ, Ziemer L *et al.* (2007) Liver function in cats with hyperthyroidism before and after ^{131}I therapy. *Journal of Veterinary Internal Medicine* **21**, 1217–1223

Bexfield N and Lee C (2010) Water deprivation test. In: *BSAVA Guide to Procedures in Small Animal Practice*, ed. N Bexfield and C Lee, pp. 234–236. BSAVA Publications, Gloucester

Billet JPH, Moore AH and Holt PE (2002) Evaluation of a bladder tumour antigen test for the diagnosis of lower urinary tract malignancies in dogs. *American Journal of Veterinary Research* **62**, 370–373

Bonfanti U, Zini E, Minetti E *et al.* (2004) Free light-chain proteinuria and normal renal histopathology and function in 11 dogs exposed to *Leishmania infantum*, *Ehrlichia canis*, and *Babesia canis*. *Journal of Veterinary Internal Medicine* **18**, 618–624

Campbell VL, Butler AL and Lunn KF (2009) Use of a point-of-care urine drug test in a dog to assist in diagnosing barbiturate toxicosis secondary to ingestion of a euthanized carcass. *Journal of Veterinary Emergency and Critical Care* **19**, 286–291

Daure E, Belanger M, Beauchamp G *et al.* (2013) *Research in Veterinary Science* **95**, 1181–1185

Defontis M, Bauer N, Failing K *et al.* (2013) Automated and visual analysis of commercial urinary dipsticks in dogs, cats and cattle. *Research in Veterinary Science* **94**, 440–445

Escobar C and Grindem C (2010) What is your diagnosis? Urine crystals in a dog. *Veterinary Clinical Pathology* **39**, 513–514

Faulks RD and Lane IF (2003) Qualitative urinalyses in puppies 0 to 24 weeks of age. *Journal of the American Animal Hospital Association* **39**, 369–378

Forrester SD, Troy GC, Dalton MN *et al.* (1999) Retrospective evaluation of urinary tract infection in 42 dogs with hyperadrenocorticism or diabetes mellitus or both. *Journal of Veterinary Internal Medicine* **13**, 557–560

Grauer GF, Greco DS, Behrend EN *et al.* (1995) Estimation of quantitative enzymuria in dogs with gentamicin-induced nephrotoxicosis using enzyme/creatininine ratios from spot urine samples. *Journal of Veterinary Internal Medicine* **9**, 324–327

Gunn-Moore DA (2008) How to choose a cat urinary catheter. *Companion* **April**, 13–15

Henry CJ, Tyler JW, McEntee MC *et al.* (2003) Evaluation of a bladder tumour antigen test as a screening test for transitional cell carcinoma of the lower urinary tract in dogs. *American Journal of Veterinary Research* **64**, 1017–1020

Higuchi T, Burcham GN, Childess MO *et al.* (2013) Characterization and treatment of transitional cell carcinoma of the abdominal wall in dogs: 24 cases (1985–2010). *Journal of the American Veterinary Medical Association* **242**, 499–506

Karmi N, Safra N, Young A *et al.* (2010) Validation of a urine test and characterization of the putative genetic mutation for hyperuricosuria in Bulldogs and Black Russian Terriers. *American Journal of Veterinary Research* **71**, 909–914

Kook PH, Grest P, Quante S *et al.* (2010) Urinary catecholamine and metadrenaline to creatinine ratios in dogs with a phaeochromocytoma. *Veterinary Record* **166**, 169–174

Kruger JM, Osborne CA, Lulich JP *et al.* (2001). The urinary system. In: *Veterinary Pediatrics*, 3rd edn, ed. JD Hoskins, pp. 371–401. WB Saunders, Philadelphia

Kvitko-White HL, Cook AK, Nabity MB *et al*, (2013) Evaluation of a catalase-based urine test for the detection of urinary tract infection in dogs and cats. *Journal of Veterinary Internal Medicine* **27**, 1379–1384

LeBlanc CJ, Roberts CS and Bauer RW (2004) Firm rib mass aspirate from a dog. *Veterinary Clinical Pathology* **33**, 253–256

Lefebvre HP, Dossin O, Trumel C *et al.* (2008) Fractional excretion tests: a critical review of methods and applications in domestic animals. *Veterinary Clinical Pathology* **37**, 4–20

Lyon SD, Sanderson MW, Vaden SL *et al.* (2010) Comparison of urine dipstick, sulfosalicylic acid, urine protein-to-creatinine ratio, and species-specific ELISA methods for detection of albumin in urine samples of cats and dogs. *Journal of the American Veterinary Medical Association* **236**, 874–879

Mardell EJ and Sparkes AH (2006) Evaluation of a commercial in-house test kit for the semi-quantitative assessment of microalbuminuria in cats. *Journal of Feline Medicine and Surgery* **8**, 269–278

Monti P, Benchekroun G, Berlato D *et al.* (2012) Initial evaluation of canine urinary cystatin C as a marker of renal tubular function. *Journal of Small Animal Practice* **53**, 254–259

Murgier P, Jakins A, Bexfield N *et al.* (2009) Comparison of semi-quantitative test strips, urine protein electrophoresis, and an immunoturbidimetric assay for measuring microalbuminuria in dogs. *Veterinary Clinical Pathology* **38**, 485–492

Nabity MB, Lees GE, Cianciolo R *et al.* (2012) Urinary biomarkers of renal disease in dogs with X-linked hereditary nephropathy. *Journal of Veterinary Internal Medicine* **26**, 282–293

Nabity MB, Lees GE, Dangott LJ *et al.* (2011) Proteomic analysis of urine from male dogs during early stages of tubulointerstitial injury in a canine model of progressive glomerular disease. *Veterinary Clinical Pathology* **40**, 222–236

O'Neil E, Burton S, Horney B *et al.* (2013) Comparison of white and red blood cell estimates in urine sediment with hemocytometer and automated counts in dogs and cats. *Veterinary Clinical Pathology* **42**, 78–84

Osborne CA, Lulich JP, Kruger JM *et al.* (2009) Analysis of 451,891 canine uroliths, feline uroliths and feline urethral plugs from 1981 to 2007: perspectives from the Minnesota Urolith Centre. *Veterinary Clinics of North America: Small Animal Practice* **39**, 183–197

Osborne CA and Stevens JB (1999) *Urinalysis: A Clinical Guide to Compassionate Patient Care*. Bayer, Veterinary Learning Systems, Leverkusen, Germany

Pressler BM and Bartges JW (2010) Urinary tract infections. In: *Textbook of Veterinary Internal Medicine, 7th edn*, ed. SJ Ettinger and EC Feldman, pp. 2036–2047. Saunders Elsevier, St. Louis, Missouri, USA

Pressler BM, Vaden SL, Jensen WA *et al.* (2002) Detection of canine microalbuminuria using semiquantitative test strips designed for use with human urine. *Veterinary Clinical Pathology* **31**, 56–60

Rigas JD, Smith TJ, Elena Gorman M *et al.* (2012) Primary ureteral giant cell sarcoma in a Pomeranian. *Veterinary Clinical Pathology* **41**, 141–146

Ristić J and Skeldon N (2011) Urinalysis in practice – an update. *In Practice* **33**, 12–19

Rogers KD, Jones B, Roberts L *et al.* (2011) Composition of uroliths in small domestic animals in the UK. *The Veterinary Journal* **188**, 228–230

Rowlands M, Blackwood L, Mas A *et al.* (2011) The effect of boric acid on bacterial culture of canine and feline urine. *Journal of Small Animal Practice* **52**, 510–514

Saito TB, Alfieri AA, Wosiacki SR *et al.* (2006) Detection of canine distemper virus by reverse transcriptase-polymerase chain reaction in the urine of dogs with clinical signs of distemper encephalitis. *Research in Veterinary Science* **80**, 116–119

Sanderson SL (2009a) Taurine. In: *Blackwell's Five Minute Veterinary Consult: Laboratory Tests and Diagnostic Procedures, Canine and Feline, 1st edn*, ed. SL Vaden, JS Knoll, FWK Smith and LP Tilley, pp. 584–587. Blackwell, Ames, Iowa

Sanderson SL (2009b) Carnitine. In: *Blackwell's Five Minute Veterinary Consult: Laboratory Tests and Diagnostic Procedures, Canine and Feline, 1st edn*, ed. SL Vaden, JS Knoll, FWK Smith and LP Tilley, pp. 160–163. Blackwell, Ames, Iowa

Segev G, Palm C, LeRoy B *et al.*, (2013) Evaluation of neutrophil gelatinase-associated lipocalin as a marker of kidney injury in dogs. *Journal of Veterinary Internal Medicine* **27**, 1362–1367

Smets PM, Meyer E, Maddens BEJ *et al.* (2010) Urinary markers in healthy young and aged dogs and dogs with chronic kidney disease. *Journal of Veterinary Internal Medicine* **24**, 65–72

Stockham SL and Scott MA (2008) Urinary system. In: *Fundamentals of Veterinary Clinical Pathology, 2nd edn*, ed. SL Stockham and MA Scott, p. 465. Blackwell, Ames, Iowa

Swenson CL, Boisvert AM, Kruger JM *et al.* (2004) Evaluation of modified-Wright staining of urine sediment as a method for accurate detection of bacteriuria in dogs. *Journal of the American Veterinary Medical Association* **224**, 1282–1289

Tvedten H, Ouchterlony H and Lilliehöök I (2015) Comparison of specific gravity analysis of feline and canine urine, using five refractometers, to pycnometric analysis and total solids by drying. *NZ Veterinary Journal*, Jan 27: 1–6

Vaden SL, Barrak MP, Lappin MR *et al.* (2004) Effects of urinary tract inflammation and sample blood contamination on urine albumin and total protein concentrations in canine urine samples. *Veterinary Clinical Pathology* **33**, 14–19

Vignoli M, Rossi F, Chierici C *et al.* (2007) Needle tract implantation after fine needle aspiration biopsy (FNAB) of transitional cell carcinoma of the urinary bladder and adenocarcinoma of the lung. *Schweizer Archiv für Tierheilkunde Gesellschaft Schweizerischer Tierärzte* **149**, 314–318

Welles EG, Whatley EM, Hall AS *et al.* (2006) Comparison of Multistix PRO dipsticks with other biochemical assays for determining urine protein (UP), urine creatinine (UC) and UP:UC ratio in dogs and cats. *Veterinary Clinical Pathology* **35**, 31–36

Whittemore JC, Gill VL, Jensen WA *et al.* (2006) Evaluation of the association between microalbuminuria and the urine albumin–creatinine ratio and systemic disease in dogs. *Journal of the American Veterinary Medical Association* **229**, 958–963

Yam P (1994) Cystocentesis in the dog and cat. *In Practice* **16**, 319–320

Zeugswetter F, Bydzovsky N, Kampner D *et al.* (2010) Tailored reference limits for urine corticoid:creatinine ratio in dogs to answer distinct clinical questions. *Veterinary Record* **167**, 997–1001

Zeugswetter F, Neffe F, Schwendenwein I *et al.* (2013) Configuration of antibodies for assay of urinary cortisol in dogs influences analytic specificity. *Domestic Animal Endocrinology* **45**, 98–104

Useful websites

American College of Veterinary Pathologists
www.acvp.org/meeting/2014/appFiles/87_Tvedten.docx

Carmichael Torrance Veterinary Diagnostic Laboratory
http://ctdslab.co.uk/toxicology-and-poison-testing/

International Renal Interest Society
http://www.iris-kidney.com/index.shtml

Chapter 11

Laboratory evaluation of renal disorders

Harriet M. Syme

The function of the kidneys is to regulate the volume and composition of extracellular fluid. This is achieved by the initial formation of an ultrafiltrate of plasma by the passage of solutes, small proteins and other non-cellular constituents of the blood across the glomerular filtration barrier. The volume of ultrafiltrate formed is primarily determined by the hydrostatic pressure within the glomerular capillary tuft (the difference between afferent and efferent arteriolar pressures) and the number of functioning nephrons. Following filtration the fluid is further 'conditioned' accord-

ing to the physiological needs of the animal (i.e. its composition is altered by the secretion and reabsorption of solutes and water as it passes along the nephron). In a healthy animal, under normal physiological conditions, less than 1% of the fluid that is filtered by the glomerulus will eventually be excreted as urine.

Renal disease can influence these processes in a number of different ways, as outlined in Figure 11.1. Reduction in glomerular filtration rate (GFR) (acute and chronic kidney disease), defects of the glomerular filtration barrier (primary

Function	Assessment	Examples of deranged function in patients with kidney disease
Glomerular filtration	Indirect: • Creatinine • Urea • Others Direct: • Urinary clearance • Plasma clearance • Renal scintigraphy	Chronic kidney disease; CKD (many causes) Acute kidney injury; AKI (many causes)
Glomerular barrier (retention of medium–large proteins and other macromolecules)	Quantification of proteinuria (various methods; see Chapter 10) Evaluation for clinicopathological sequelae of protein-losing nephropathy (PLN; e.g. hypoalbuminaemia, hypercholesterolaemia) Specific tests for underlying causes of glomerular disease	Immune complex glomerulonephritis Amyloidosis Non-immune complex glomerulonephropathy: • Glomerulosclerosis • Primary GBM defects • Congenital or developmental glomerulonephropathies • Other
Tubular function (reabsorption and secretion)	Urinalysis Stone analysis Blood gas analysis Urine protein:creatinine ratio Fractional excretion of electrolytes	Stone formation: • Cystine • Urate • Others Renal tubular acidosis Fanconi syndrome Primary renal glucosuria Tubular proteinuria
Fluid balance	Urine specific gravity Urine/plasma osmolality	Polyuria due to osmotic diuresis and reduced medullary concentrating gradient in many renal (and non-renal) diseases Oligo- or anuria may occur in patients with AKI
Endocrine: • Erythropoietin • Calcitriol Others (renin, bradykinin, prostaglandins, nitric oxide, etc.)	PCV, haematology Calcium and phosphate (calcitriol, PTH and FGF-23 can be quantified but primarily as a research tool)	Anaemia of CKD Polycythaemia due to renal tumours Renal secondary hyperparathyroidism (CKD–MBD)
Control of blood pressure	Blood pressure measurement Fundic examination	Systemic hypertension

11.1 Renal functions, clinicopathological assessment and examples of associated diseases. CKD–MBD = chronic kidney disease–mineral bone disorder; FGF = fibroblast growth factor; GBM = glomerular basement membrane; PCV = packed cell volume; PTH = parathyroid hormone.

glomerular disease) and abnormal tubular function will be considered in turn in this chapter. Normal renal function is integral to the formation of concentrated urine in situations where this is necessary, for example when the patient is hypovolaemic or dehydrated. However, polyuria and polydipsia also have a large number of non-renal causes; these are discussed further in Chapter 10. The kidney is an endocrine organ, responsible for the secretion of a number of autocrine, paracrine and endocrine factors. These are considered as they pertain to the manifestations of acute and chronic kidney disease in this chapter but also in the sections on calcium and phosphate homeostasis in Chapter 8.

Glomerular filtration

Assessment of glomerular filtration rate

The GFR is generally considered to be the best global indicator of renal function. However, it is important to recognize that the kidney has a multitude of different functions (see Figure 11.1) and it is perfectly possible for renal disease to be present in an animal with normal GFR. Consider, for example, a Dalmatian with excessive excretion of uric acid due to defective proximal tubular transport mechanisms, or a young cat with polycystic kidney disease. In the former example, GFR is not expected to reduce as a consequence of the dog's renal disease unless urethral obstruction occurs; in the latter, GFR is expected to decline progressively, but is likely to be normal when the condition is first diagnosed.

Measurement of GFR is considered to be the most relevant assessment of overall renal function because it is correlated, albeit weakly, with the number and functionality of nephrons present within the kidneys. However, many nephrons can be lost before GFR declines significantly, particularly if the patient has time to compensate. When an animal undergoes uninephrectomy, the GFR is near normal within a few weeks of the surgery being performed owing to compensatory hypertrophy of the nephrons in the contralateral kidney. This underlines the fact that even with direct measurements of GFR early or mild renal disease may be difficult to detect (Figure 11.2).

The laboratory tests that are usually employed as indirect indicators of GFR are urea and creatinine. Some other markers (cystatin C, symmetrical dimethyl arginine (SDMA)) have recently been studied in dogs and/or cats and may become more widely available to veterinary practitioners in the near future. The general principle for the clinical use of all of these markers is that in renal failure (either acute or chronic), filtration of the marker is reduced and it accumulates in plasma. A limitation of indirect markers is that when GFR changes it takes time for a new steady state to be achieved; thus, if a patient suffers an abrupt renal insult with consequent reduction in GFR, the concentration of the marker will continue to rise for some time (potentially days) until a new equilibrium is achieved. Once this has occurred, presuming that the production of the marker remains constant, its daily excretion will be the same as it was prior to the decrement in GFR, since if this were not the case the concentration of the marker would continue to increase indefinitely. The reduction in GFR is effectively offset by the increased concentration of the marker being presented to the glomerular barrier. For all of these markers their reliability as an estimate of GFR will depend on them having a constant rate of production that is scaled to body size in the same manner that GFR is, and that the marker is eliminated solely by renal filtration and is not secreted, reabsorbed, metabolized or eliminated by non-renal routes. No marker perfectly meets all of these criteria.

Urea

Urea generation and excretion: Urea is synthesized in the liver from ammonia generated by the deamination of amino acids which are ingested in excess of nutritional requirements. Urea is a small molecule that diffuses readily throughout all body fluid compartments. It is freely filtered at the glomerulus but much of it is subsequently reabsorbed in the renal tubules and collecting ducts. Reabsorption is increased when tubular flow rates are low and is enhanced by the actions of antidiuretic hormone (ADH). Thus, urea is suggested to be a sensitive indicator of prerenal azotaemia, although it does not perform very well as a diagnostic test for this (Finco and Duncan, 1976). In fact, urea measurements are influenced by a large number of non-renal variables such as fasting, dietary protein content, gastrointestinal haemorrhage, liver function, diuresis and hyperthyroidism; these, together with its high rate of tubular reabsorption, limit its usefulness as a marker of GFR. In a recent study of nearly 5000 unselected canine serum/plasma samples submitted to a diagnostic laboratory, urea was found to exceed the laboratory reference range in 27.5% of dogs in which creatinine measurements were normal (Medaille et al., 2004). Urea remains on most biochemistry panels because, in spite of the fact that the urea molecule itself is relatively non-toxic, it is reasonably well correlated with the clinical signs of uraemia that develop with advanced renal failure.

Laboratory aspects of urea measurement: Most laboratory methods for the quantification of urea rely upon the enzyme urease to hydrolyse urea to ammonia and carbon dioxide, with the ammonia generated being detected, directly or indirectly, by a colorimetric reaction. The use of

Remaining nephrons	100%	50%	25%	10%
GFR (value compared with baseline)	Normal (100%)	Undetectably reduced unless baseline measurements available for comparison (90%)	Subnormal if using a breed-specific reference range[a] or compared to baseline measurements (50%)	Subnormal (20%)
Creatinine	Within laboratory reference range	Within laboratory reference range, not detectably different from baseline	Increased if compared with baseline but within laboratory reference range or borderline elevation	Increased, above laboratory reference range
USG	Variable, but concentrated if fluid depleted	Variable, but concentrated if fluid depleted	Usually minimally concentrated or isosthenuric[b]	Usually isosthenuric[b]

11.2 Expected alteration in glomerular filtration rate (GFR), creatinine and urine specific gravity with differing severity of renal insult. [a]This has not been directly shown in any clinical studies but can be inferred from available data. [b]Concentrating ability may be maintained in patients with primary glomerular disease, and is generally better preserved in cats than dogs with chronic kidney disease. USG = urine specific gravity.

the term blood urea nitrogen (BUN) is commonplace in the USA and some other countries and can result in confusion when converting values into SI units. This is because BUN is, as the name suggests, the mass of nitrogen in the urea molecule (historically this was how urea was measured), and so when converting BUN in mg/dl to urea in mmol/l two steps have to occur: first the BUN is converted to urea in mg/dl (by multiplying by 2.14) and then urea is converted into SI units (by multiplying by 0.167). Alternatively, this can be done in a single step by multiplying BUN (mg/dl) by 0.357 to yield urea (mmol/l). Errors occur when the terms urea and BUN are used interchangeably and the wrong conversion factors applied as a result.

Creatinine

Creatinine generation and excretion: Creatinine is a small molecule (molecular weight (MW) 113) produced by the breakdown of phosphocreatine (also known as creatine phosphate), an energy-storing molecule that is mainly present in skeletal muscle, and its precursor creatine. The formation of creatinine from these molecules is spontaneous (non-enzymatic) and irreversible. The turnover of the muscle store of phosphocreatine is relatively constant in each individual (about 2% daily). A small amount of creatine and phosphocreatine can be derived from dietary intake, although this is negligible if the patient is eating a commercial diet. A very small increase in creatinine may occur in animals consuming either raw or cooked meat. Endogenous production of creatinine is reduced (by about 25%) in dogs with renal dysfunction; this partially offsets the reduced excretion and may contribute to its limited sensitivity for detection of mild renal impairment (Watson *et al.*, 2002). Creatinine is distributed throughout the total body water compartment with very little protein binding and has a half-life in plasma of approximately 3 hours.

The relationship between plasma/serum creatinine concentration and GFR is described as hyperbolic or curvilinear, as illustrated in Figure 11.3. The shape of the curve means that when GFR is normal or high, large changes in GFR have to occur before this is reflected by a detectable change in the creatinine concentration. Conversely, when renal function is poor any further reduction in GFR will result in a large change in creatinine concentration. In practice this means that when creatinine is elevated there is little value in performing direct GFR measurements.

Laboratory aspects of creatinine measurement: Creatinine has for many years been measured in the laboratory by the Jaffé reaction, which is now being replaced progressively by specific enzymatic techniques. The Jaffé reaction relies on the formation of a yellow–orange chromogen when picrate and creatinine react at alkaline pH. Unfortunately, many other substances in plasma (so-called non-creatinine chromogens) also react with picrate, resulting in significant overestimation of creatinine measurements. The amount of non-creatinine chromogen present varies between individuals, so that a uniform correction formula cannot be applied to convert Jaffé measurements to the 'true' creatinine concentration. The amount of non-creatinine chromogens present in the sample becomes progressively less important as the 'true' creatinine concentration in plasma increases, and their concentration is insignificant in urine. This can be an issue when creatinine concentrations in plasma and urine are compared, such as in calculations of fractional excretion or creatinine clearance, because plasma concentrations will be elevated by the non-creatinine chromogens while urine concentrations will not.

The critical difference (between values that can be considered to reflect a real change and those due to combined analytical and biological variability) for creatinine measurements has been estimated as 35 µmol/l when within or close to the laboratory reference range (Jensen and Aaes, 1993). When creatinine concentrations are significantly increased the critical difference will be correspondingly larger. Studies have shown that while, as expected, analytical differences in creatinine measurements do exist between diagnostic laboratories, these are not related to the differences in quoted reference ranges. As a result patients will often be classified as having apparently 'normal' renal function by one laboratory and 'subnormal' by another, in spite of having similar measured values for creatinine (Ulleberg *et al.*, 2011). In many

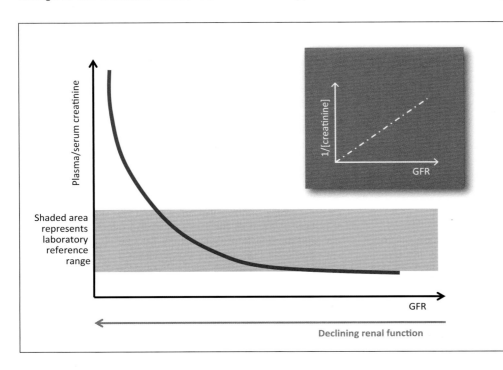

11.3 Relationship between creatinine concentration and glomerular filtration rate (GFR).

instances the number of animals from which samples were collected to derive the laboratory reference range was very small.

In dogs, creatinine concentrations tend to increase with bodyweight (Figure 11.4) and so the derived reference range may vary quite markedly depending on breed composition. Ideally, in the future, reference laboratories will report different reference ranges according to the size of the patient being tested. Part of the reason that larger dogs have higher creatinine concentrations is presumably because they have greater muscle mass than small dogs. Muscular dogs, such as greyhounds, have increased creatinine concentrations, often exceeding the standard laboratory reference ranges. However, the increased muscle mass in larger dogs would not be expected to result in higher plasma creatinine concentration if there were a corresponding mass-related increase in GFR. When GFR measurements have been compared in dogs of different sizes it is apparent that if reported as an index related to bodyweight, GFR values are lower in larger patients (Bexfield et al., 2008). Although phenotypic differences between breeds of cats are much less extreme than in dogs, breed differences in creatinine concentrations have also been observed. In particular, in one study apparently healthy Birman cats were shown to have higher creatinine concentrations than the other breeds of cat that were tested (Reynolds et al., 2010).

Weight (kg)	Number in sample	Creatinine (μmol/l)[a]	GFR (ml/min/kg)[b]
<10	36	62 ± 11 (42–90)	>2.7
11–25	130	75 ± 14 (49–110)	> 2.0
26–45	127	89 ± 23 (53–178)	>1.7
>45	24	105 ± 21 (78–161)	>1.3

11.4 Relationship between body size, creatinine concentration and glomerular filtration rate (GFR) in dogs. Creatinine values are reported as ± standard deviation (range).
([a] Data from Craig et al. (2006). [b] Data from Lefebvre (2010))

Estimating GFR from creatinine measurements: Direct measurement of GFR is infrequently performed in human medicine outside of research studies. Although GFR values are quoted in many scientific papers and in the management of clinical patients, these values have usually only been estimated from the patient's creatinine concentration with knowledge of certain other clinical details such as the patient's sex, age, race and bodyweight. It should be a goal of the veterinary community either to derive formulae for estimation of GFR or to develop narrower breed- and/or size-dependent reference ranges for creatinine concentration in dogs to compensate for differences in muscle mass. In the meantime, it is important to recognize that a Chihuahua with a high-normal creatinine value may well have kidney disease and a Saint Bernard with elevated creatinine may well have normal renal function.

Other indirect markers of GFR

Other indirect markers of GFR exist and some are offered, or are likely to be offered in the near future, by the larger commercial laboratories. Evaluation of these markers has shown that they correlate well with direct GFR measurements; however, they have not generally been demonstrated to be superior to creatinine in this regard. In some instances these tests may appear to be more sensitive than creatinine in the detection of renal dysfunction but this is usually achieved at the expense of specificity, and

similar results can be achieved for creatinine simply by reducing the upper limit of the reference range.

Cystatin C: Cystatin C is a cysteine protease inhibitor produced by all nucleated cells. It is freely filtered by the glomerulus and partially reabsorbed by the tubular epithelial cells, where it is catabolized. In dogs, plasma/serum cystatin C measurements have been evaluated as markers of GFR in several small studies, with advantages over creatinine measurement demonstrated in some studies (Wehner et al., 2008) but not in all (Almy et al., 2002). Cystatin C is increased in hyperthyroidism, probably owing to an increased rate of cellular metabolism. This is likely to confound any attempts to use cystatin C as a marker of GFR in cats.

Symmetrical dimethyl arginine: SDMA is derived from the intranuclear methylation of L-arginine and released into the circulation after proteolysis. Thereafter it is excreted renally. The concentration of SDMA in serum/plasma has been shown to correlate well with GFR measured by iohexol clearance but it does not appear to perform better than creatinine in this regard (Nabity et al., 2013).

Direct estimation of GFR

Measurement of GFR may be useful in small animal practice in the work-up of clinical patients under the following circumstances:

- In patients with suspected (non-azotaemic) kidney disease
- To determine renal function prior to the use of nephrotoxic drugs
- For assessing the response to therapeutic interventions aimed at improving renal function.

However, it has yet to be proven that direct measurement of GFR is superior to measurement of creatinine for these purposes in dogs and cats. Although it is assumed that direct measurement of GFR will be a superior (more sensitive) test, it should be recognized that the derived reference ranges for GFR are themselves very wide and vary according to bodyweight, and so this will not necessarily be the case (Figure 11.4).

Urinary clearance methods for the estimation of GFR are impractical in client-owned animals because they require the placement of urinary catheters for the collection of timed urine samples over protracted periods. Therefore, in clinical practice, GFR is usually estimated by measuring the plasma clearance of an injected substance. This in turn can be achieved in one of two ways: either repeated blood samples can be taken to monitor the disappearance of the injected analyte from the blood or, if the substance injected is radioactive, its rate of accumulation within the renal parenchyma (which relates to its rate of filtration) can be monitored using a gamma camera. This latter method confers the advantage that the relative contribution of each of the kidneys to the overall GFR can be calculated; this information may be useful, for example if nephrectomy is being contemplated. Since gamma cameras are not widely available outside of equine referral practices and universities these methods will not be considered in detail here.

To measure GFR by plasma clearance, all that is required is the ability to perform an intravenous injection of a very accurately determined quantity of the filtration marker and the ability to collect timed blood samples afterwards. Thus, the technical capability to measure GFR is well within the realms of what can be achieved in general practice. To determine the quantity of the filtration marker that is injected, accurate scales are ideally used to measure the weight of the syringe before and after injection. Although a dose of the filtration marker is recommended this is not as important as the accurate quantification of the amount that is given to the patient. Similarly, although recommendations are made for the times of sample collection post-injection, if these deviate from the timetable by a few minutes this is not all that important, provided that the actual time of sampling is accurately recorded.

Choice of marker

The fructose polymer inulin is considered the gold standard filtration marker for measurement of GFR using urinary clearance methods. However, studies suggest that inulin is cleared by non-renal (hepatic) routes, which makes it unsuitable for measurement of plasma clearance. It is also expensive and there are periodic difficulties with its availability. Thus, the filtration markers that are most often used for estimation of GFR by plasma clearance methods are exogenous creatinine and iohexol, each of which has advantages and disadvantages (Figure 11.5).

Creatinine	Iohexol
Routinely measured by laboratories	Only measured by specialist laboratories
No medical-grade injectable available	Medical-grade injectable readily available (radiographic contrast material)
Samples must be collected over a longer period	Shorter test duration

11.5 Comparison of the advantages and disadvantages of exogenous creatinine and iohexol for estimation of glomerular filtration rate.

Accurate plasma clearance methods rely on the collection of blood samples at multiple time points to create a graph of plasma concentration *versus* time. The clearance is then calculated as:

Clearance = Dose/AUC

Where AUC is the area under the plasma concentration *versus* time curve.

A two-compartment model is regarded as the most appropriate pharmacokinetic model for most filtration markers. This model is based on the concept that, following injection of the marker, equilibration occurs between the plasma (central compartment) and the peripheral compartment (extracellular water or total body water (TBW) depending on the marker). The marker is eliminated by renal clearance, which allows slow redistribution of the marker back into the plasma from the peripheral compartment from which it is cleared. Therefore, there is an initial redistribution phase of the marker within the body followed by a slower elimination phase. At least four samples (and usually many more) are required to generate the biexponential curve. Techniques which require the collection of only a limited number of samples have become an important goal for clinicians when measuring clearance in clinical practice to minimize patient stress. This can be achieved by the use of correction formulae which enable the calculation of GFR using only the second elimination phase of the curve, because the initial redistribution phase is both independent of GFR and relatively constant from subject to subject. Specific correction formulae have been developed for use in both the dog and the cat (Heiene and Moe, 1999; Finch *et al.*, 2011).

If a general practitioner wants to perform GFR measurement it is not necessary for them to be able to calculate GFR themselves from the raw data because there are laboratories that provide a protocol for evaluation of iohexol clearance and will perform all measurements and calculations (Figure 11.6).

Specialist test	Sample requirements	Laboratory availability[a]
Antithrombin	Citrate blood	Animal Health Trust (AHT) (http://www.aht.org.uk/cms-display/diag_clinpath.html) Cornell University (https://ahdc.vet.cornell.edu/sects/Coag/)
Cystinuria (SLC31A and SLC7A9 mutations)	EDTA whole blood or cheek swab from Labrador Retrievers, Newfoundlands and Australian Cattle Dogs	PennGen Laboratories (http://research.vet.upenn.edu/penngen/PennGenHome/tabid/91/Default.aspx)
Cystinuria (urine nitroprusside and/or amino acid quantification)	Urine from any breed of dog (or cat)	PennGen Laboratories (as above) Some NHS (human) laboratories
Fanconi syndrome	Urine from any breed of dog (or cat)	PennGen Laboratories (as above) NHS or specialist laboratories
Glomerular filtration rate (GFR; iohexol clearance)	Multiple timed blood (usually serum) samples	University of Michigan www.animalhealth.msu.edu/Submittal_Forms Some NHS and other specialist laboratories will measure iohexol but will not perform GFR calculations for dogs or cats
Hereditary nephritis in Cocker Spaniels	EDTA blood or cheek swab	Antagene, La tour de Salvagny, France (http://www.antagene.com/en)
Leptospirosis serology	Serum	Animal Health and Veterinary Laboratories Agency (http://www.defra.gov.uk/ahvla-en/)
N-acetyl-β-D-glucosaminidase (NAG)	Urine	Axiom Veterinary Laboratories (http://www.axiomvetlab.com/)
Neutrophil gelatinase-associated lipocalin (NGal)	Urine or serum	Not yet commercially available Validated canine ELISA kit is available (BioPorto Diagnostics; http://www.bioporto.com/)

11.6 Specialist renal testing only performed by selected laboratories. [a]Where possible, UK-based laboratories are listed. Similar services are also likely to be available in other countries. [b]Although this is the causative mutation in Dalmatians, genetic testing is unnecessary in purebred dogs because all are homozygous for the SLC2A9 mutation. EDTA = ethylenediamine tetra-acetic acid; ELISA = enzyme-linked imunoabsorbent assay. (continues)

Specialist test	Sample requirements	Laboratory availability[a]
Polycystic kidney disease	EDTA blood or cheek swab	AHT (http://www.aht.org.uk/cms-display/genetics_polycystic.html) Bristol University (http://www.langfordvets.co.uk/diagnostic-laboratories)
Protein-losing nephropathy in Soft Coated Wheaten Terriers	EDTA whole blood or cheek swab	Soft Coated Wheaten Terrier Club of America/University of Pennsylvania (http://www.scwtca.org/health/dnatest.htm)
Specialist renal histopathology	Renal biopsy samples in fixatives provided by the specialist pathology service	International Veterinary Renal Pathology Service – formerly at Texas A&M, now at Ohio State University: contact Dr. Rachel Cianciolo (rachel.cianciolo@cvm.osu.edu) Utrecht Veterinary Nephropathology Service: contact Dr Astrid M. van Dongen (a.m.vandongen@uu.nl)
Canine hyperuricosuria (SLC2A9 mutation leading to urate stones)	EDTA whole blood from Russian Black Terriers, Bulldogs and other breeds[b]	Animal Health Trust (http://www.aht.org.uk/cms-display/genetics_US.html)

11.6 (continued) Specialist renal testing only performed by selected laboratories. [a]Where possible, UK-based laboratories are listed. Similar services are also likely to be available in other countries. [b]Although this is the causative mutation in Dalmatians, genetic testing is unnecessary in purebred dogs because all are homozygous for the SLC2A9 mutation. EDTA = ethylenediamine tetra-acetic acid; ELISA = enzyme-linked imunoabsorbent assay.

Clinicopathological assessment of patients with reduced GFR

Reduced GFR is usually demonstrated in clinical practice by documenting that the plasma/serum creatinine concentration exceeds the given laboratory reference range. Such patients are said to be azotaemic (defined as an increase in the concentration of nitrogenous waste products in the blood). Although urea is also a nitrogenous waste product, it is affected by numerous non-renal variables (as discussed above) and so assessment of creatinine is preferred. Once azotaemia is documented in a patient it needs to be established first whether it is prerenal, renal or postrenal in origin, and then whether it is acute or chronic in onset.

Localization of azotaemia

- High production of nitrogenous waste substances (prerenal).
- Low GFR:
  - Reduced renal perfusion (prerenal)
  - Intrinsic or functional renal disease (renal)
  - Urinary obstruction (postrenal).
- Reabsorption of urine escaped from urinary tract (postrenal).

Differentiation of prerenal and renal azotaemia

The distinction between prerenal and renal causes of azotaemia is most often made on the basis of measurement of urine specific gravity (USG). If the USG is greater than 1.030 in a dog, or 1.035 in a cat, then the azotaemia is considered to be prerenal in origin. However, certain caveats to these rules should be noted. Cats with chronic kidney disease (CKD) will sometimes retain significant urine concentrating ability with USG >1.035 or even 1.040. Concentrated urine has been documented in cats following subtotal nephrectomy even when as much as seven-eighths of the renal tissue has been ablated. Dogs and cats with primary glomerular disease sometimes retain concentrating ability, even once they have developed azotaemia. Conversely, it is important to consider that the patient will only be able to concentrate urine in the face of prerenal azotaemia if the tubular/collecting duct mechanisms for doing so are intact. If there is a lack of medullary hypertonicity (for example in a patient with hypoadrenocorticism, or one eating a very protein-restricted diet) or interference with tubular function (patients receiving diuretics) or collecting duct function (patients with primary

or secondary causes of diabetes insipidus), then creation of concentrated urine will not be possible even when azotaemia is prerenal. In these patients the prerenal nature of the azotaemia is usually confirmed by administering intravenous fluids (or reducing the dose of diuretics) and documenting its resolution.

Postrenal azotaemia

This is usually suspected on the basis of the patient's history and physical examination, or on the basis of diagnostic imaging, rather than the results of clinicopathological testing, although there are situations in which this can be informative. In particular, if fluid is present in either the retroperitoneal or peritoneal cavity then a sample should be collected for analysis (see Chapter 22). A creatinine concentration in the fluid greater than twice that in the circulation is consistent with urinary tract rupture. The fluid may be otherwise characterized as a transudate, protein-poor; transudate, protein-rich; or exudate, due to the presence of haemorrhage or inflammatory cells. Urine is a chemical irritant so non-septic, neutrophilic inflammation is common.

Differentiation of acute from chronic azotaemia

Chronic kidney disease (CKD) is sometimes defined as a problem that has been present for a prescribed period of time (typically 3 months); however, it may be more useful to consider CKD as a condition characterized by a permanent reduction in the number of functioning nephrons. This means that, regardless of how long the problem has been present, it is irreversible without any possibility of true recovery (although the remaining nephrons may hypertrophy and the single-nephron GFR increase). In contrast, in patients with acute kidney injury (AKI) recovery is possible, although depending on the severity these patients may be critically ill and many will die or be euthanased as a result of this disease syndrome. It is also relatively common for patients to suffer from an episode of AKI that is superimposed on a pre-existing state of CKD, described as acute-on-chronic kidney disease.

Differentiation of acute and chronic disease is predominantly based on the patient's history and physical examination findings. Weight loss may be seen if the disease is chronic. Non-regenerative anaemia may be present in patients with CKD. The causes are multifactorial but relative erythropoietin deficiency is thought to be the most important. Anaemia may also occur in patients with AKI for a number of reasons; for example, patients with over-hydration, leptospirosis or hypoadreno-corticism may be anaemic. Additionally, haemorrhage or haemolysis resulting in hypoxia/hypotension may serve as an inciting cause for AKI. Documentation of anaemia should not, therefore, be considered to indicate invariably that azotaemia is chronic in nature, and particularly if the anaemia is regenerative, then alternative causes for anaemia and possible AKI should be sought.

Hyperkalaemia is most often associated with AKI and particularly with postrenal causes of AKI. Hyperkalaemia may, however, occasionally develop in dogs with CKD that are eating renal diets, especially if they are concurrently treated with angiotensin converting enzyme (ACE) inhibitors or angiotensin receptor blockers.

Complete urinalysis is mandatory in the investigation of azotaemia and may provide valuable clues to its underlying cause; for example, pyuria, bacteriuria and white cell casts would be consistent with pyelonephritis, calcium oxalate monohydrate crystals suggest ethylene glycol poisoning, and glucosuria indicates proximal tubular dysfunction. However, pyelonephritis and proximal tubular dysfunction can be either acute or chronic in nature. Large numbers of granular casts, and renal epithelial tubular cell casts, are indicative of acute tubular necrosis.

Renal size and shape may provide valuable clues to whether the azotaemia is acute (normal or enlarged size, normal shape, occasionally abnormally turgid feeling) or chronic (small and/or irregular in shape). Renal palpation is usually much more informative in cats than it is in dogs. Diagnostic imaging can be used to provide further information. This allows a more objective assessment of renal size and contour, together with evaluation for mineralization and loss of internal architecture, changes consistent with chronicity.

Laboratory abnormalities in patients with kidney disease

Phosphate

When GFR is reduced, the amount of phosphate that is filtered will decline and the plasma/serum phosphate concentration will tend to increase. This occurs with both acute and chronic kidney disease. However, downstream consequences of long-standing hyperphosphataemia, such as enlargement of the parathyroid glands and bone demineralization, take time to develop and so can be used to evaluate disease chronicity. In the normal animal, a large proportion of the filtered phosphate is reabsorbed in the proximal tubules, a process that is inhibited by the actions of parathyroid hormone (PTH) and fibroblast growth factor-23 (FGF-23). Thus, in the earliest stages of kidney disease plasma phosphate concentrations are normalized by the actions of these hormones.

However, once renal disease is moderately advanced, rates of renal phosphate excretion are reduced in parallel with GFR. Hyperphosphataemia will usually occur unless prevented by dietary phosphate restriction. Hyperphosphataemia in CKD is associated with patient morbidity and decreased survival (Boyd et al., 2008), and amelioration of hyperphosphataemia by the feeding of phosphate-restricted ('renal care') diets and use of intestinal phosphate binders prolongs survival in both dogs and cats. This has led to the recommendation of targets for plasma/serum phosphate concentrations in dogs and cats being treated for CKD. The targets shown in Figure 11.7

IRIS stage (see text)	Target plasma/serum phosphorus[a] (mmol/l)
1	Not applicable
2	0.81–1.45
3	0.81–1.61
4	0.81–1.94

11.7 Proposed targets for plasma/serum phosphate concentration stratified according to severity of azotaemia. [a]Laboratory reference ranges vary but a typical range would be 0.81–2.2 mmol/l. IRIS = International Renal Interest Society.

differ according to the International Renal Interest Society (IRIS) staging scheme (detailed below), to reflect the fact that a low normal phosphate concentration is very difficult to achieve in patients with severe renal disease. When targeting phosphate concentrations with therapy it is important to pay attention to sample quality; phosphate concentrations will be increased in samples that are haemolysed or where there is delayed separation of the serum/plasma from cells.

Calcium

Plasma/serum concentrations of ionized calcium are typically normal or low in patients with CKD. Decreases in ionized calcium are a stimulus for PTH secretion. Limited data exist for patients with AKI, other than cats with urethral obstruction, but ionized calcium is also expected to be low or low normal. This is thought to occur, at least in part, as a result of abrupt increases in plasma phosphate concentration due to decreased renal excretion; this complexes calcium, reducing the amount that is in the ionized form. In spite of the tendency for ionized calcium to be low in patients with CKD, total calcium concentration is often high or high-normal. This is because total calcium is the sum of ionized calcium, protein-bound calcium and complexed calcium.

Complexed calcium, and as a result total calcium, concentrations increase in patients with renal failure owing to retention of organic and inorganic anions such as citrate, phosphate and sulphate (Schenck and Chew, 2003). When total calcium concentrations are increased it is important to differentiate patients in which hypercalcaemia is the primary problem from those with intrinsic renal disease and (total) hypercalcaemia as a consequence. These conditions can be discriminated by measurement of ionized calcium (see Chapter 8). If the ionized calcium is normal or low then azotaemia is the primary problem. If ionized calcium concentration is high in an azotaemic patient then this is the primary problem and the azotaemia is likely to be secondary. Prerenal azotaemia can develop in hypercalcaemic patients as a consequence of intrarenal vasoconstriction or volume depletion (due to vomiting and/or inadequate fluid intake in a polyuric animal), in which case it may be corrected by fluid administration. Although the azotaemia is prerenal, the USG may still be inappropriately low because calcium interferes with the actions of ADH in the distal nephron. However, if hypercalcaemia is long-standing then irreversible injury may occur owing to deposition of calcium phosphate within the renal parenchyma (hypercalcaemic nephropathy).

PTH, FGF-23 and vitamin D

The excessive secretion of PTH in patients with CKD is referred to as renal secondary hyperparathyroidism. Traditionally this has been a focus for monitoring and treatment of patients with CKD because it is correlated with patient morbidity and mortality in humans and, it is presumed, in animals. Diets with low phosphate content have been shown to decrease the severity of hyperparathyroidism and improve survival. However, in human medicine attention has widened in the last decade to encompass changes in the concentrations of other hormones as well as PTH. The preferred term is now CKD–mineral and bone disorder (MBD); this is defined as a systemic disorder of mineral and bone metabolism manifested by either one or a combination of the following:

- Abnormalities of calcium, phosphorus, PTH or vitamin D metabolism
- Abnormalities in bone turnover, mineralization, volume, linear growth or strength
- Vascular or other soft tissue calcification.

The relative importance of the various humoral factors that are responsible for CKD–MBD varies according to the stage of the disease. In the earliest stages of CKD, even when the patient is non-azotaemic, FGF-23 secretion by osteoblasts and osteocytes is increased in response to decreased renal clearance of phosphate. FGF-23 reversibly inhibits the activity of the enzyme 1-alpha hydroxylase, so reducing the formation of active 1,25-dihydroxyvitamin D ($1,25(OH)_2$-vitamin D, also known as calcitriol). The reduction in $1,25(OH)_2$-vitamin D, in turn, allows secretion of PTH to increase in the later stages of disease. Both FGF-23 and PTH act to increase phosphate excretion by the kidney. PTH also increases mobilization of calcium and phosphate from bone. In early CKD the actions of FGF-23 and PTH are sufficient to normalize plasma phosphate concentration. As the disease progresses, however, reabsorption of phosphate by the nephron is at a minimum, and further increases in PTH and FGF-23 concentrations cannot decrease this any further. Phosphate excretion becomes entirely dependent on GFR, and as this falls further hyperphosphataemia results. In advanced CKD, -vitamin hydroxylase activity is irreversibly reduced owing to the paucity of nephrons, and hyperphosphataemia and ionized hypocalcaemia also directly stimulate the secretion of PTH (Figure 11.8).

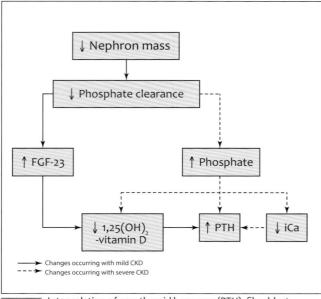

Inter-relation of parathyroid hormone (PTH), fibroblast growth factor (FGF)-23 and $1,25(OH)_2$-vitamin D in CKD. iCa = ionized calcium.

Although changes in PTH, $1,25(OH)_2$-vitamin D and FGF-23 have all been associated with a worse prognosis in human patients with CKD, their inter-related regulatory mechanisms make the contribution of individual factors difficult to dissect. It is also unclear whether interventions to normalize their concentrations will improve patient outcomes. It is not, therefore, routinely recommended that the concentrations of these hormones be measured when managing canine and feline patients with CKD, although they are an area of active clinical research and the situation may change in the future.

Potassium

Hypokalaemia is relatively common in cats with azotaemic CKD. The reasons for this are unclear but likely to be multifactorial. Proposed mechanisms include inadequate dietary intake, increased renal losses and relative hyperaldosteronism. Hypokalaemia is uncommon in dogs with CKD unless they are receiving intravenous fluids without potassium supplementation. Hyperkalaemia is common in patients with AKI, particularly if they are anuric.

Acid–base status

Patients with AKI usually have metabolic acidosis, the severity of which is proportional to that of the azotaemia. The exception to this is ethylene glycol toxicity, where the acidosis is particularly severe owing to the presence of its metabolite, glycolic acid, in the circulation. Metabolic acidosis may also occur in patients with CKD but usually only when the condition is advanced (usually IRIS stage 4) (Elliott et al., 2003). This occurs as a result of reduced renal ammoniagenesis, and thus an inability to excrete hydrogen ions, caused by the reduced number of functional nephrons. Retention of phosphate and organic acids (uric, hippuric and lactic acids) may also result in an increased anion gap (see Chapter 9).

Cholesterol

Hypercholesterolaemia is common in canine and feline patients with CKD, even those with predominantly tubulointerstitial rather than glomerular disease. The mechanisms for this have not been investigated. Concentrations of other lipids are probably also altered, although this has not been well characterized in animals.

Urinalysis

Urinalysis is critical for the differentiation of prerenal and renal azotaemia when diagnosing renal disease, as discussed above. However, the value of urinalysis in monitoring patients with established CKD is often underestimated. Urinary tract infections (UTIs) are common in patients with CKD and often do not result in lower urinary tract signs. If untreated, patients may develop pyelonephritis and this may lead to progression of their azotaemia. Thus, whenever a patient with CKD is having bloodwork performed to monitor the severity of their azotaemia, it is always indicated to perform a urinalysis at the same time. Quantification of proteinuria by measurement of the urine protein:creatinine ratio (UPCR) is also indicated in staging of kidney disease (see below) and in the differentiation of tubulointerstitial (with relatively mild proteinuria), and glomerular (moderate–severe proteinuria) diseases. Measurement of UPCR should only be performed once postrenal causes for proteinuria (such as UTIs) have been ruled out.

Staging chronic kidney disease

In the last few years the International Renal Interest Society (IRIS) has proposed a staging scheme for CKD (http://www.iris-kidney.com) and this has been adopted by both American and European nephrology/urology special-ity groups. The idea underlying the scheme is to stratify disease severity (Figure 11.9) by measurement of plasma or serum creatinine, UPCR and blood pressure, so that when examining the results of clinical trials it is apparent which groups of patients were studied. It can also be used when making general recommendations regarding the diagnostic work-up and the different treatments that are appropriate according to disease severity.

It should be noted that patients with stage 1 (and some with stage 2) CKD are actually non-azotaemic. This reflects the fact that kidney disease can be present with-out there being any appreciable decline in GFR; in fact, hyperfiltration may occur in the earliest stages of some renal diseases. In these patients the presence of non-azotaemic CKD is established by means other than the direct or indirect estimation of GFR. For example, a Persian cat with polycystic kidney disease or a dog with glomerulonephritis might have stage 1 disease when first diagnosed.

This staging scheme should only be applied to patients with stable renal function, ideally corroborated by repeated measurement of creatinine concentration, after correction of any prerenal component to the azotaemia. Complete staging of CKD using this scheme should also include assessment of proteinuria (see Chapter 10) and measure-ment of blood pressure. Proteinuria is a significant finding in patients with CKD because it is associated with a worse prognosis and is a potential target for therapy. The origin of the protein in patients with CKD may be either glomerular, tubular or a combination of both. Glomerular proteinuria may occur owing to structural changes to the glomerulus, but may also result from increased hydrostatic pressure within the glomerular capillaries. This, in turn, is a result of adaptive hyperfiltration (i.e. increased single-nephron GFR) of the remaining functional nephrons and may be worsened if systemic hypertension is also present. Tubular proteinuria occurs when the reabsorptive capacity of the tubular epi-thelial cells is overwhelmed, either because the cells are poorly functional or due to the very high tubular flow rates.

Discussion of the management of CKD is beyond the scope of this manual, and readers are directed to the *BSAVA Manual of Canine and Feline Nephrology and Urology* for detailed consideration of how to manage patients with CKD. In broad terms, patients with stage 1 and 2 disease are not expected to have clinical signs related to a decrease in GFR. They will either be asymp-tomatic or they could have signs referable to their under-lying disease. Management of these patients is therefore primarily directed at identifying and treating their underly-ing disease if at all possible. In patients with stage 2 and 3 disease where GFR is reduced, even if they remain non-azotaemic, treatments (for example 'renal-care' diets) that are directed at attempting to slow intrinsic progression of CKD may be appropriate. Patients with stage 4 disease are likely to require symptomatic treatment to ameliorate urae-mic signs. This illustrates how staging of the disease may be useful in devising a diagnostic and/or therapeutic plan for patients. In time it is envisaged that the staging scheme will be used to devise evidence-based guidelines.

Acute kidney injury

Acute renal failure (ARF) is characterized by excretory fail-ure that is abrupt in onset, resulting in rapid development of azotaemia. Clinical signs in the patient with ARF relate to accumulation of metabolic (uraemic) toxins within the body and derangements of fluid, electrolyte and acid–base balance. Since the term ARF is usually only applied to patients that have developed azotaemia and/or oligo-anuria, this term does not encompass mild renal insults or the early stages of disease. For this reason the term acute kidney injury (AKI) has been adopted in preference; this term encompasses the entire spectrum of disease sever-ity and includes patients with either intrinsic or functional (including prerenal and postrenal) problems.

AKI is recognized by an increase in plasma/serum creatinine concentration, decrease in GFR or reduction in urine output. There are several schemes that have been employed to classify the severity of AKI in humans; the first of these to be put into widespread clinical use was the RIFLE scheme (an acronym relating risk, injury and failure for AKI of increasing severity, loss and end-stage renal failure for eventual clinical outcome). The RIFLE scheme has been superseded by other schemes with even greater sensitivity for detecting minor changes in renal function that can be observed when serial monitoring is performed on the same patient. Attempts have been made to utilize or adapt such schemes for veterinary patients. In

CKD stage	Plasma/serum creatinine (μmol/l)		Comments
	Dogs	Cats	
1	<125	<140	Non-azotaemic Some other renal abnormality present, such as persistent proteinuria or morphological abnormalities detected by imaging
2	125–180	140–250	Non-azotaemic to mildly azotaemic Clinical signs usually mild or absent
3	181–440	250–440	Mild to moderately azotaemic With or without clinical signs of uraemia
4	>440	>440	Severe azotaemia With or without clinical signs of uraemia
Sub-stage proteinuria	UPCR		
	Dogs	Cats	
Non-proteinuric (NP)	<0.2	<0.2	
Borderline proteinuric (BP)	0.2–0.5	0.2–0.4	
Proteinuric (P)	>0.5	>0.4	
Sub-stage blood pressure[a]			
Risk of end-organ damage	Systolic (mmHg)	Diastolic (mmHg)	
None (N)	<150	<95	
Low (L)	150–159	95–99	
Moderate (M)	160–179	100–119	
High (H)	>180	>120	

11.9 IRIS staging of chronic kidney disease (CKD). [a]Cut-offs are the same for dogs and cats. UPCR = urine protein:creatinine ratio.

one study, RIFLE-like categorization (according to serum creatinine concentration) of dogs with AKI showed that this approach could be prognostically useful (Lee *et al.*, 2011). Another study evaluated data from dogs that had been managed within a critical care facility, with creatinine concentrations compared with baseline values from the same individual (Thoen and Kerl, 2011). Nearly 15% of dogs included in the study developed AKI, and even if this was very mild (increase of creatinine to 150–200% of baseline or absolute increase of ≥28.5 μmol/l) it had prognostic significance.

An IRIS grading scheme for AKI has been proposed and is outlined in Figure 11.10. In addition to staging according to creatinine concentration, AKI is further sub-graded according to current urine production as oligoanuric (O; <1 ml/kg/h) or non-oliguric (NO), and on the requirement for renal replacement therapy (RRT; dialysis or transplantation). Just as IRIS staging for CKD has facilitated the development of standardized management recommendations and provision of prognostic information, it is hoped that IRIS staging will allow earlier recognition, therapeutic stratification and outcome assessment for AKI in dogs and cats.

If possible, it is helpful to establish the cause of AKI, because this will determine whether any specific treatment will be helpful and it also informs prognosis. For example, once azotaemia has developed in patients with ethylene glycol toxicosis the prognosis is hopeless, even in situations where dialysis is available. In a recent study of 182 dogs being treated with haemodialysis, the cause of the AKI was determined to be leptospirosis (31%), ethylene glycol (27%), haemodynamic (10%), other toxins including non-steroidal anti-inflammatory drugs (6%) or miscellaneous (4%); the cause was unidentified in 22% of cases (Segev *et al.*, 2008). In a study of 132 cats treated at the same centre, the cause of AKI was unidentified in 40% of cases. Identified causes of AKI were ureteral obstruction (35%), ethylene glycol (9%), pyelonephritis (5%), lily poisoning (4%) and lymphoma (3%) (Segev *et al.*, 2013a). Of course, the aetiology of AKI in patients receiving dialysis is likely to be somewhat different from that in patients seen in general practice because the kidney injury in dialysis cases will have been severe and the clinical status of the patients prior to development of AKI is likely to have been relatively good or the owners would not consider such an expensive and involved therapy. However, comparable data for patients presenting to general practice are not available. Some of these causes of AKI are established on the basis of history (for example, known exposure to toxins) but for others clinical pathology can play an important role in diagnosis (for details see Figure 11.11).

Early diagnosis of acute kidney injury

Most veterinary patients diagnosed with AKI have developed the problem at home and are presented to the veterinary surgeon for evaluation once clinical signs have developed. However, AKI can also develop in patients that are hospitalized. It is probable that with an increase in the complexity of medical and surgical care that is provided for veterinary patients in the future, the incidence of hospital-acquired AKI will increase. In these patients, additional diagnostic strategies may be helpful, because if AKI can be detected early in its clinical course therapeutic interventions may be more effective and outcomes more positive.

N-acetyl-beta-D-glucosaminidase and gamma-glutamyl transferase

Detection of enzymuria (enzyme activity within the urine) can be utilized as a more sensitive indicator of renal damage than changes in creatinine concentration. Several different enzymes can be used for this purpose but those that have been most studied in dogs and cats are *N*-acetyl-β-D-glucosaminidase (NAG) and gamma-glutamyl transferase (GGT; also known as γ-glutamyl transpeptidase). These enzymes are large proteins that originate from proximal tubular cells: GGT from the brush border of the proximal tubule and NAG from tubular lysosomes. Enzymuria increases with tubular injury. In clinical practice, measurement of enzymuria can be useful when repeatedly administering a drug that is known to be nephrotoxic (e.g. aminoglycocides, amphotericin B). Before initiating therapy a urine sample is collected for baseline measurement of NAG or GGT and this is indexed to the creatinine concentration in the urine. Measurement is repeated after 3 days, and then every other day, until the NAG or GGT:creatinine ratio increases significantly (usually considered to be a doubling of the ratio), at which point the nephrotoxic drug is discontinued. This method has been shown to be more sensitive than serial evaluation of serum creatinine concentration in the early detection of renal damage (Rivers *et al.*, 1996).

Neutrophil gelatinase-associated lipocalin

Neutrophil gelatinase-associated lipocalin (NGal) is a promising biomarker for the detection of AKI. It is normally expressed at low concentrations within renal and other tissues, but this is markedly increased when tubular injury occurs. Measurement of NGal within blood or urine can be useful as a sensitive marker of renal damage; in laboratory animal studies values rise with either ischaemic or toxic causes of renal damage. A specific enzyme-linked immunosorbent assay (ELISA) for detection of NGal in blood or urine has been validated for use in dogs but unfortunately does not detect NGal in feline samples. Using this assay, the urine NGal:creatinine ratio has been shown to increase in AKI in dogs; it also increases to a lesser extent in CKD and with urinary tract infections (Segev *et al.*, 2013b). NGal has also been shown to increase in a model of gentamicin-induced renal injury in

Stage	Serum/plasma creatinine (μmol/l)	Clinical description
I	<140	Non-azotaemic or volume-responsive AKI Historical, clinical, laboratory or imaging evidence of renal injury Progressive non-azotaemic increase in creatinine ≥26 μmol/l (0.3 mg/dl) in 48 hours Measured oliguria (<1 ml/kg/h) or anuria over 6 hours
II	141–220	Mild AKI: historical, clinical, laboratory or imaging evidence of AKI and mild static or progressive azotaemia Progressive non-azotaemic increase in creatinine ≥26 μmol/l (0.3 mg/dl) in 48 hours Measured oliguria (<1 ml/kg/h) or anuria over 6 hours
III	221–439	Moderate to severe AKI: documented AKI and increasing severity of azotaemia and functional renal failure
IV	440–880	
V	>880	

11.10 IRIS staging scheme for acute kidney injury (AKI) in dogs and cats. Each stage is further sub-staged depending on whether the patient is oligoanuric (O) or non-oliguric (NO) and on the requirement for renal replacement therapy (RRT).

Cause of AKI	Test methodology	Findings
Leptospirosis	Routine testing (haematology, biochemistry and urinalysis)	No findings are specific for leptospirosis but clinical suspicion should increase in the presence of thrombocytopenia, anaemia, increased liver enzyme activities (particularly ALP), hyperbilirubinaemia, hyperbilirubinuria or glucosuria
	Serology (microagglutination test)	Titres may be negative/low initially (low sensitivity) necessitating a convalescent titre
		Initial titre of ≥1/800 for a non-vaccinal serovar or doubling of a convalescent titre considered confirmatory
	PCR (blood and/or urine)	Performs well in experimental infections but in clinical practice rarely positive, possibly because patients have often received antibiotics before testing occurs
Ethylene glycol	Routine testing (haematology, biochemistry and urinalysis)	Hypocalcaemia, high anion gap, acidosis, calcium oxalate monohydrate crystalluria
	Kacey test strips	False positive and false negative results reported
	Catachem ethylene glycol test kit	Evaluation of the test *in vitro* using spiked canine blood samples appears promising; not yet tested in clinical practice but recommended by the ASPCA toxicology service
	Urine fluorescence under ultraviolet light	Only positive (green) in the first 6 hours after ingestion, false positives can occur with certain drugs and not all sources of antifreeze contain fluorescein
	Gas chromatography–mass spectroscopy	Reference method – results not available fast enough for ante-mortem diagnosis
Pyelonephritis	Urinalysis	Diagnosis of infection in the lower urinary tract (pyuria, bacteriuria, positive urine culture) should increase suspicion of pyelonephritis as the cause of AKI
		White cell casts indicate tubular inflammation
		Collection of urine directly from the renal pelvis using ultrasound guidance is possible when this is dilated
	Haematology	An inflammatory leucogram ± left shift can support a diagnosis of pyelonephritis but is infrequently documented
Lymphoma	FeLV test	Most cats with renal lymphoma are FeLV negative
	Cytology	Renal aspirates can be useful in confirming the diagnosis. Where a subcapsular 'halo' of anechoic material is present this should be aspirated in addition to the parenchymal tissue

11.11 Clinical pathology findings for specific causes of acute kidney injury (AKI). ALP = alkaline phosphatase; ASPCA = American Society for the Prevention of Cruelty to Animals; FeLV = feline leukaemia virus; PCR = polymerase chain reaction.

dogs, so it may prove useful in the serial evaluation of patients receiving nephrotoxic drugs. Widespread clinical use of urinary biomarkers is only likely to occur if cage-side assays are developed.

Glomerular barrier function

Assessment of the glomerular barrier

An important renal function is to maintain an intact glomerular barrier so that macromolecules (primarily proteins) are retained within plasma and not lost into the urine. The size of the molecules that are retained is not absolute because it is partly dependent on charge, with negatively charged molecules being repelled by the glomerular barrier. Albumin, with a mass of approximately 69 kDa and negative charge, is almost completely retained by the barrier, but proteins smaller than albumin will also be partially impeded. The filtration barrier is composed of three layers: fenestrated endothelium, which lines the glomerular capillaries; the glomerular basement membrane; and the slit diaphragm, which is formed by the interdigitating foot processes of the podocytes. Damage to any one of these three layers, but particularly the basement membrane or the podocytes, will result in loss of barrier function, leading to glomerular proteinuria. Glomerular barrier function can also be compromised if there is increased hydrostatic pressure within the glomerular capillaries, resulting in a small net increase in protein passage into the primary filtrate. Increases in hydrostatic pressure may occur as a consequence of systemic hypertension or the adaptive hyperfiltration that occurs when the number of functioning nephrons is significantly reduced.

Broadly speaking, causes of primary glomerular disease include congenital abnormalities of the glomerular barrier (e.g. hereditary nephritis due to a mutation in type IV collagen), immune-complex glomerulonephritis (e.g. membranous nephropathy and membranoproliferative glomerulonephritis), acquired non-immunological glomerular disease (e.g. glomerulosclerosis) and amyloidosis. Primary glomerular disease is less common in the cat than in the dog. Immune-complex glomerulonephritis can occur in apparent isolation or be secondary to infection, inflammation or neoplasia elsewhere in the body.

Laboratory abnormalities associated with glomerular disease

Proteinuria is the main laboratory abnormality seen. There is no absolute cut-off point for the magnitude of proteinuria that signifies that primary glomerular disease is present, but UPCR values are typically greater than 2 or 3. Quantification of proteinuria is discussed in Chapter 10.

When proteinuria is marked, hypoalbuminaemia and/or hypercholesterolaemia may develop. Hypoglobulinaemia does not generally occur because the large size of the globulin molecule prevents its passage through the glomerular barrier even when the barrier is damaged. Hypercholesterolaemia is caused by an increase in hepatic biosynthesis, defective lipolysis of lipoproteins and defective conversion of cholesterol to bile acids. Although it is not well documented in dogs and cats, hypertriglyceridaemia is also likely to occur, as it does in humans. Only a small proportion of patients with primary glomerular disease will develop nephrotic syndrome. Nephrotic syndrome is the concurrent presence of proteinuria, hypoalbuminaemia, hypercholesterolaemia and interstitial or third-space fluid accumulation, recognized most often as ascites or peripheral oedema. Fluid collected from the body cavities of patients with nephrotic syndrome is expected to have low protein (<25 g/l) and cell counts (<1500 cells/μl), characteristic of a pure transudate (or transudate; protein-poor).

The severity of proteinuria cannot, in general, be used to predict the type of glomerular disease that is present. Ultimately, in most instances the diagnosis can only be made by collection of renal biopsy samples. Although evaluation of formalin-fixed tissue is adequate for identification of amyloidosis, renal dysplasia and renal lymphoma, differentiation of other types of primary glomerular disease usually requires immunofluorescence testing and electron microscopy to be performed (Cianciolo et al., 2013). Thus, it is important to check the appropriate fixatives with specialist veterinary nephropathology centres (see Figure 11.6) before biopsies are obtained.

In some breeds, specific types of glomerular disease are well characterized and a diagnosis can be made by genetic testing without the need to resort to a renal biopsy. For example, Cocker Spaniels suffering from hereditary nephropathy have a mutation resulting in a defect in type IV collagen in the glomerular basement membrane. Genetic associations have also been characterized in Soft Coated Wheaten Terriers with protein-losing nephropathy, although the pattern of inheritance is unclear. It is possible that not all dogs with the identified risk alleles (which encode the slit diaphragm proteins nephrin and Neph3/filtrin) will develop disease, although it appears that the risk is high in animals that are homozygous (Littman et al., 2013).

Complications of glomerular disease

Patients with primary glomerular disease are at increased risk of thromboembolism. The reason for this is multifactorial but due in part to loss of antithrombin (a protein of similar size to albumin) through the glomerular barrier. Many patients with glomerular disease also have elevated fibrinogen, which may increase platelet aggregation. It has previously been recommended that therapy to inhibit platelet aggregation be instituted in patients with hypoalbuminaemia or decreased antithrombin activity. In a recent study the majority of dogs with protein-losing nephropathy (PLN), had changes consistent with hypercoagulation when assessed by thromboelastography (Lennon et al. 2013). However, albumin concentration and antithrombin activity were only weakly correlated and did not relate to changes on the thromboelastogram. The authors of the study recommended the routine evaluation of patients using thromboelastography, but this is not a test that can be easily performed from general practice, since samples must be tested a set time after collection (see Chapter 6 for further information).

Investigation of glomerular disease

The initial work-up of a patient with PLN should be directed at trying, if possible, to identify an underlying cause for the glomerular disease. A proposed schematic approach for this is outlined in Figure 11.12. Immune-mediated glomerulonephritis may be triggered by a variety of infectious, inflammatory, immune-mediated or neoplastic conditions, so an extensive diagnostic work-up can be justified, although this can ultimately be frustrating because in the majority of cases no underlying cause can be identified. Amyloidosis may also be triggered by chronic inflammatory/neoplastic conditions.

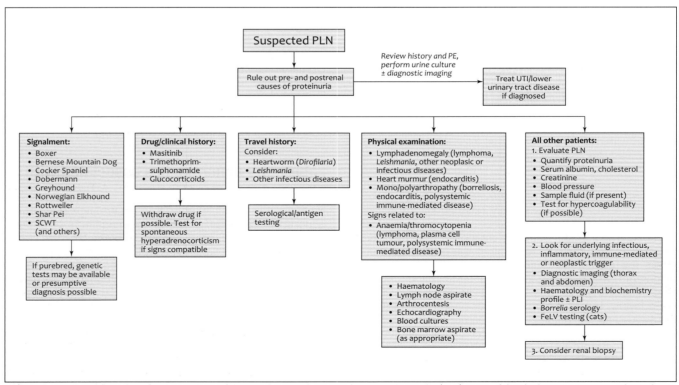

11.12 Suggested flow chart for the work-up of dogs and cats with protein-losing nephropathy (PLN). FeLV = feline leukaemia virus; PE = physical examination; PLI = pancreatic lipase immunoreactivity; SCWT = Soft Coated Wheaten Terrier; UTI = urinary tract infection.

Many of the specific infectious agents and parasites that have been associated with immune-mediated glomerulonephritis in the dog are not endemic in the United Kingdom. The one exception is *Borrelia burgdorferi* (and other closely related organisms from the genus). Infection with *Borrelia* has been associated with the development of 'Lyme nephritis', an acute progressive proteinuric renal disease of dogs. Anecdotally, however, very few, if any, dogs with PLN in the UK have been diagnosed with borreliosis. If testing for this disease, serology is preferred over Polymerase chain reaction (PCR) testing (Littman *et al.* 2006; see Chapter 29). One non-endemic cause of glomerular disease in dogs that warrants particular mention is leishmaniosis. This disease is highly prevalent in southern Europe and is commonly associated with glomerular proteinuria (see Chapter 29).

Although amyloidosis may cause proteinuria it does not invariably do so. Many Shar Pei dogs and Abyssinian cats with amyloidosis have deposits that are predominantly in the renal medulla, and these patients may develop azotaemia without PLN. Indeed some animals will present with signs referable to hepatic deposition of amyloid, including acute haemorrhage as a result of hepatic rupture, without any evidence of renal involvement.

Monitoring the response to treatment in patients with protein-losing nephropathy

It is recommended that before instituting therapy for PLN that three baseline UPCR measurements are obtained (Lees *et al.*, 2005). This is because of a very high degree of day-to-day variability in proteinuria. This can lead to owner frustration and increase costs, although it has been shown that pooling samples (combining several 1 ml aliquots of refrigerated urine collected over a 48-hour period) also provides a valid estimate (LeVine *et al.*, 2010). It is also important to recognize that the severity of proteinuria may actually decline with disease progression as the number of functional nephrons decreases. Dogs with PLN may be non-azotaemic, especially when first diagnosed.

Tubular function

Assessment of tubular function

Fractional excretion

Measurement of the fractional excretion (FE) of solutes, usually electrolytes, is sometimes advocated as an indicator of the tubular handling of the solute being measured. Before contemplating measurement of FE it is important to understand that many non-tubular influences severely limit its usefulness as a test in individual clinical patients, particularly when based on spot measurements (reviewed by Lefebvre *et al.*, 2008). FE can be useful when repeated measurements are made in the same individual, or groups, under controlled conditions, such as in the conduct of nutritional research, but the results are very difficult to interpret in individuals where dietary intake of electrolytes is not strictly controlled and in patients with reduced renal function, as will be explained below.

The FE of a solute is defined as the fraction of a filtered solute which is excreted into the urine. If reabsorption of the solute occurs in the tubules then FE will be less than 100% (as occurs for most electrolytes), but if the substance is actively secreted by the tubules FE could, in theory, exceed 100%. The amount of solute that is filtered is determined

by its plasma concentration and GFR, resulting in the following equation:

Equation 1:

$$FE = \frac{\text{Solute (electrolyte) excreted}}{\text{Solute (electrolyte) filtered}} = \frac{U_e \times V}{P_e \times GFR}$$

Where U_e = urine concentration of electrolyte (e)
P_e = plasma concentration of electrolyte (e)
V = urine volume

GFR is usually estimated from the endogenous creatinine clearance ($U_{creat} \times V/P_{creat}$); substitution into Equation 1 results in the following formula:

Equation 2:

$$FE = \frac{U_e \times P_{creat}}{P_e \times U_{creat}}$$

Use of Equation 2 allows estimation of the FE from spot urine samples. However, this requires that the eventual urine concentration of electrolyte and creatinine when the sample was collected is reflective of the concentration presented to the glomerulus at the time of filtration. For this to be even approximately true the patient should have been fasted for at least 12 hours, then allowed to urinate so that the bladder is emptied, and sufficient time allowed for fresh urine to collect in the bladder prior to simultaneous collection of the spot urine and blood samples. FE should not be calculated for patients that are receiving intravenous fluids or diuretics. Ideally, patients would be eating a standardized diet prior to collection of samples for measurement of FE, and this would be identical in composition to that eaten by the population of animals that were used to derive the reference intervals. In reality, published reference intervals are generally used, and these were often obtained from small numbers of animals eating a non-standardized diet.

The use of FE in patients with reduced renal function is particularly problematic, with measures of FE generally increasing as renal function deteriorates. To understand this it can be helpful to consider the example of sodium excretion in a dog that develops mild CKD; the dog is not systemically unwell, retains a good appetite and the diet has not been changed. The plasma concentration of sodium is the same as before the renal disease developed. Given that the patient is in a state of equilibrium, with the amount of the sodium that is ingested each day balanced by the amount that is excreted, Equation 1 above, shows that the numerator (i.e. daily excretion of sodium) is unchanged but since the denominator (i.e. GFR) is reduced, the FE of sodium must be increased. This presents a particular problem because calculation of FE is most often considered for patients with altered renal function, but laboratory reference intervals are usually obtained using data from healthy individuals, which does not provide a valid comparison.

Other tests of tubular function

Routine urinalysis can be considered in some instances to serve as a marker of tubular function. Tubular dysfunction may result in glucosuria or changes in urine pH detected by routine laboratory evaluation. Crystalluria may also signify a specific tubular function defect. In addition, blood gas analysis may be useful in patients suspected to have renal tubular acidosis (RTA), as discussed below.

The early markers of AKI discussed above (for example NAG and NGal) are essentially tests of proximal tubular function/injury. They may also increase in more chronic disease states, representing ongoing tubular injury or increased cellular workload (such as the processing of filtered protein).

Cystatin C is usually measured in serum/plasma as a marker of GFR. Following filtration, cystatin C is taken up and catabolized by proximal tubular cells, so the concentration in the urine is very low. In patients with renal disease, cystatin C concentrations in the urine increase and this may prove to be a useful additional marker of tubular dysfunction (Monti et al., 2012).

Syndromes associated with tubular dysfunction

Fanconi syndrome

Fanconi syndrome is a term that describes a generalized defect in the function of proximal tubular cells, resulting in a failure of reabsorption of solutes from the tubular lumen. This results in excessive urinary losses of glucose, phosphate, amino acids, bicarbonate, calcium and potassium along with low molecular weight proteins. Affected animals may have metabolic acidosis due to renal bicarbonate loss (see below) and obligatory polyuria due to the osmotic effect of the glucose in the urine. Glucosuria may also predispose to urinary tract infections. Other non-specific signs may include weight loss, poor hair coat and muscular weakness. Azotaemia may occur in patients with Fanconi syndrome but is not always present, particularly when the condition is first diagnosed.

It should be noted that both acute and chronic kidney disease may result in defective proximal tubular function, and such patients may present with renal glucosuria and potentially other components of the Fanconi syndrome. This is most often evident in patients that are severely azotaemic. However, the term Fanconi syndrome is usually reserved for patients where the signs of proximal tubular dysfunction, rather than azotaemia, predominate.

Fanconi syndrome may be familial or acquired (Figure 11.13). The familial syndrome is most commonly encountered in Basenjis although there have been occasional reports in other dog breeds. Although familial, the abnormalities are not evident at birth and the condition is most often diagnosed in middle age. If pre-emptive screening for the condition is performed, euglycaemic glucosuria may be detected before any clinical signs or other biochemical abnormalities are evident. Affected Basenjis are reported to have a fairly normal lifespan, although the eventual cause of death is renal failure in about half of the dogs (Yearley et al., 2004). Dogs with acquired forms of Fanconi syndrome, such as those associated with the consumption of 'jerky' treats, may have azotaemia at the time of first presentation. However, if further exposure to the treats is prevented, and with appropriate supportive care, recovery of renal function may occur.

The diagnostic approach to a patient suspected to have Fanconi syndrome should include the simultaneous measurement of blood and urine glucose. In Basenjis the blood glucose concentration is typically normal but hypoglycaemia may occur with some of the acquired forms of Fanconi

syndrome if the patient is anorexic (Thompson et al., 2013). Ketonuria may also develop in patients with acquired Fanconi syndrome as a result of increased fat metabolism and possibly reduced proximal tubular reuptake of filtered ketones. Other biochemical changes that may be evident in patients with Fanconi syndrome, regardless of its cause, include hypophosphataemia and hypokalaemia. Even where the concentrations of these electrolytes in plasma remain normal the FE may be increased, helping to confirm a diagnosis of Fanconi syndrome, although, as discussed above, interpretation of FE is problematic in patients with azotaemia because their values would be expected to increase even in the absence of a specific tubular absorptive defect.

It is important to evaluate for UTIs in patients with Fanconi syndrome because the glucosuria may make patients vulnerable, but also because pyelonephritis has been reported as a potential cause of Fanconi syndrome. It is also possible, but not absolutely necessary, to test the urine for excessive excretion of amino acids, which is most often generalized but may be limited to cystine, methionine, glycine and some dibasic amino acids (see Figure 11.6). The reporting of amino acid excretion varies between laboratories, with some reporting FE values and others providing amino acid:creatinine ratios. Proteinuria, resulting from reduced tubular uptake of predominantly low molecular weight proteins, is usually mild.

In patients other than Basenjis, serum biochemistry may also provide potential clues as to the underlying cause for the Fanconi syndrome (Figure 11.13). Particular attention should be paid to liver enzyme activities and bilirubin; these may be elevated in dogs with copper storage hepatopathy (see Chapter 12) or patients with leptospirosis, while hypocalcaemia is present in hypoparathyroidism and vitamin D deficiency.

Isolated (familial) renal glucosuria

Isolated (familial) renal glucosuria is a term that is applied to patients that have euglycaemic glucosuria and no other signs of proximal tubular dysfunction. Some of these patients may have progressive disease and eventually manifest other components of Fanconi syndrome. Others may only ever have glucosuria, a condition that is considered benign, and it can be speculated that they may have mutations in the sodium–glucose co-transporters present in the cell membrane of the proximal tubule, as described in humans. Norwegian Elkhounds are reported to have a high prevalence of renal glucosuria (Heiene et al., 2010), but they are also known to develop a hereditary nephropathy characterized by marked periglomerular fibrosis and progressive azotaemia. It is unclear whether these conditions are related or represent two different renal diseases occurring in the same breed and occasionally in the same individuals.

Renal tubular acidosis

RTAs are a rare group of disorders resulting in hyperchloraemic (normal anion gap) metabolic acidosis (see Chapter 9). Clinical signs are typically mild and nonspecific. Occasionally symptomatic hypokalaemia may occur. RTAs are usually only considered once other more common causes of metabolic acidosis (diarrhoea, lactic or ketoacidosis, renal failure and intravenous fluid therapy with 0.9% NaCl) have been excluded. RTAs can be divided into type I (distal) and type II (proximal) forms. Hypoaldosteronism has been referred to as type IV RTA but really represents a subtype of distal (type I) RTA. In distal RTA, urine cannot be maximally acidified because of impaired H^+ secretion (and thus bicarbonate generation)

- Dried meat 'jerky' treats
- Drug therapy
  - Tetracycline (out-of-date product)
  - Aminoglycosides
  - Streptozotocin
  - Cisplatin
- Copper-associated hepatopathy
- Pyelonephritis
- Hypoparathyroidism/vitamin D deficiency

11.13 Causes of acquired Fanconi syndrome.

in the collecting duct. Urine pH is usually >6.0 despite moderate to marked decreases in plasma bicarbonate concentration. Nephrolithiasis, bone demineralization and potassium wasting may occur. The diagnosis of distal RTA can be confirmed by performing an ammonium chloride challenge test (see specialist texts for details).

Proximal RTA occurs due to failure by the proximal tubule to reclaim filtered bicarbonate. Proximal RTA is most often accompanied by other signs of proximal tubular dysfunction and, as such, is just one component of Fanconi syndrome. In patients with metabolic acidosis as a result of proximal RTA the urine pH is usually appropriately low (<6.0). This is because distal acidification mechanisms are intact and also because, when the plasma concentration of bicarbonate falls, less is filtered at the glomerulus. The small amount of bicarbonate that is filtered can be reabsorbed by the distal tubules; thus, proximal RTA can be considered to be a 'self-limiting' disorder. If plasma pH is returned to normal by the administration of bicarbonate then the urine pH becomes alkaline owing to failure to reclaim this, and the patient may develop hypokalaemia.

Urolithiasis

Tubular defects underlie the formation of several different types of stone in dogs and cats, notably those composed of uric acid and cystine. In both of these conditions there is a failure of tubular reabsorption of filtered solute, causing a high urine concentration and subsequent stone formation in some individuals. Xanthinuria may occur as a primary tubular defect or, more commonly, when dogs are treated with allopurinol. The crystals that may be evident in the urinalysis of affected animals are shown in Chapter 10. Genetic tests for these disorders are available for some breeds (see Figure 11.6).

Case examples

CASE 1

SIGNALMENT

14-year-old male neutered Domestic Shorthair cat.

HISTORY

The cat was presented for weight loss and polyphagia. On questioning, the owner also reported that the cat had an increase in thirst. On physical examination the cat was in poor body condition (score 3/9) with moderate dental disease, tachycardia (heart rate 220 bpm) and bilateral goitre. The kidneys palpated as small, smooth and bilaterally symmetrical.

CLINICAL PATHOLOGY DATA

Haematology

Unremarkable.

Biochemistry

Biochemistry	Initial result	3 months post I-131	Reference interval
Glucose (mmol/l)	**7.8**	6.2	3.5–6.5
Total protein (g/l)	62	63	61–80
Albumin (g/l)	31	33	28–42
Globulin (g/l)	31	30	25–46
Urea (mmol/l)	**22**	**18**	4–15
Creatinine (µmol/l)	145	**214**	70–177
Sodium (mmol/l)	146	152	145–158
Potassium (mmol/l)	4.1	5.4	3.8–5.5
Chloride (mmol/l)	122	118	111–123
Calcium (mmol/l)	2.1	2.3	2.1–2.8
Phosphate (mmol/l)	1.9	1.6	0.7–1.9
ALT (IU/l)	**340**	**101**	20–100
ALP (IU/l)	**78**	42	10–60
Total bilirubin (µmol/l)	0	1	0–3

Abnormal results are in **bold**.

Biochemistry continued	Initial result	3 months post I-131	Reference interval
GGT (IU/l)	2	2	0–2
Creatinine kinase (IU/l)	193	476	52–506
Cholesterol (mmol/l)	5.9	**9.5**	2.2–6.7
Total T4 (nmol/l)	**>300**	**<5.1**	10–55

Abnormal results are in **bold**.

Urinalysis	Initial result	Post I-131
Specific gravity	**1.022**	**1.024**
pH	6.5	6.0
Protein	1+	1+
Glucose	Negative	Negative
Ketone	Negative	Negative
Bilirubin	Negative	Negative
Blood/Hb	1+	trace
Sediment	5–10 RBCs per hpf, 1–2 WBCs per hpf, many fat droplets	1–2 RBCs per hpf
UPCR	0.45	0.18

Abnormal results are in **bold**.

WHAT ABNORMALITIES ARE PRESENT INITIALLY AND HOW SHOULD THEY BE INTERPRETED?

The elevated total thyroxine (T4) result initially, in combination with the clinical signs the cat is exhibiting, secure a diagnosis of hyperthyroidism. Diabetes mellitus is an important differential diagnosis for weight loss in the face of a good appetite, especially with the reported polydipsia, but the hyperglycaemia is very mild and not accompanied by glucosuria so the cat is unlikely to be diabetic. Concern could be raised for intrinsic liver disease in view of the increased liver enzyme activity; however, this is most likely to be attributable to the hyperthyroidism.

An additional concern could be raised for this cat's renal function. It is very difficult to predict whether cats will develop azotaemia following treatment for hyperthyroidism. Polydipsia can be noted in cats with hyperthyroidism that remain non-azotaemic following

→ CASE 1 CONTINUED

treatment; it does not necessarily indicate that renal function is compromised. The occurrence of polydipsia seems to be quite unpredictable, although it is most often associated with marked elevation of total T4 (as in this case). It has been ascribed to a psychogenic mechanism. The USG is consistent with the history of polydipsia. The elevation in urea is common in cats with hyperthyroidism (even when fasted) and does not indicate that the cat is at increased risk for development of azotaemia; the urea:creatinine ratio decreases with treatment of hyperthyroidism regardless of the patient's eventual renal status. Similarly, UPCR is often elevated in hyperthyroid cats, and although it has been associated (weakly) with survival, it does not predict the development of azotaemia.

Ultimately, the usual manner of determining whether a cat will develop azotaemia is to treat it and monitor to see what happens. This pragmatic approach is sensible because survival times are actually not notably different in cats with and without azotaemia following treatment for hyperthyroidism, provided they are euthyroid. The owner of this cat was unable to medicate him so he was treated instead with radioactive iodine. Following treatment the owner felt that he was clinically much improved, he had a normal appetite and had gained a significant amount of weight. His drinking was unchanged.

HOW WOULD YOU INTERPRET THE DATA OBTAINED FOLLOWING RADIOACTIVE IODINE THERAPY?

The cat has developed azotaemia and the USG of 1.024 is consistent with the azotaemia being renal in origin.

The total T4 value is undetectable, the cat may now be hypothyroid and this may be contributing to the azotaemia. In addition, in hypothyroidism the rate of creatinine generation is reduced, so this cat's GFR may actually be less than would otherwise be thought by considering the plasma creatinine concentration in isolation. The cat is also hypercholesterolaemic; this is common in hypothyroidism but also in cats with azotaemia, even if they are not proteinuric.

WHAT FURTHER TESTS WOULD YOU RECOMMEND?

Cats often have low total T4 measurements immediately after radioactive iodine treatment because all the hyperfunctioning tissue is destroyed. It takes a few months for the hypothalamus–pituitary axis to resume secretion of thyroid-stimulating hormone (TSH) and then for any remaining thyroid cells to recover and produce thyroid hormone. Three months is probably adequate time for thyroid function to recover but one way to establish whether the cat is hypothyroid would be to measure the endogenous TSH concentration. If this is elevated it is consistent with a diagnosis of hypothyroidism and supplementation with oral thyroid hormone would be recommended. With this treatment it would be anticipated that the creatinine concentration will fall, although it is difficult to predict whether it would be within the laboratory reference interval. An alternative explanation for the low total T4 would be depression of the hormone due to non-thyroidal illness. This is possible (in which case the TSH would be expected to be low normal) but does not seem as likely in view of the lack of clinical signs.

The cat's blood pressure should be measured if this has not been performed.

CASE 2

SIGNALMENT

7-year, 6-month old female neutered Labrador Retriever.

HISTORY

The dog was presented for inappetence and weight loss over a 3-month period. There was a more recent history of polyuria and polydipsia. Physical examination was unremarkable except for mild icterus.

CLINICAL PATHOLOGY DATA

Haematology	Result	Reference interval
WBC (x 10⁹/l)	12.9	6.0–17.1
Neutrophils (x 10⁹/l)	9.93	3.0–11.5
Lymphocytes (x 10⁹/l)	1.42	1.0–4.8
Monocytes (x 10⁹/l)	1.16	0.15–1.5
Eosinophils (x 10⁹/l)	0.39	0–1.3
Basophils (x 10⁹/l)	0	
RBC (x 10¹²/l)	6.01	5.5–8.5
Haemoglobin (g/dl)	15.3	12.0–18.0
Haematocrit (%)	46.1	37–55 ▶

Haematology *continued*	Result	Reference interval
MCV (fl)	76.8	60–77
MCHC (g/dl)	33.1	31–37
Platelet (x 10⁹/l)	294	150–500
Plasma colour	Moderate icterus	
Comment	Mild anisocytosis, no polychromasia	

Biochemistry	Result	Reference interval
Total protein (g/l)	66	49–71
Albumin (g/l)	32	28–39
Globulin (g/l)	34	21–41
Sodium (mmol/l)	147	142–153
Potassium (mmol/l)	4.3	3.9–5.5
Chloride (mmol/l)	113	105–118
Calcium (mmol/l)	2.51	2.13–2.70
Phosphorus (mmol/l)	0.8	0.8–2.0
Urea (mmol/l)	4.8	3.0–9.1
Creatinine (μmol/l)	129	59–138
Cholesterol (mmol/l)	5.3	3.3–8.9 ▶

Abnormal results are in **bold**.

→ **CASE 2 CONTINUED**

Biochemistry *continued*	Result	Reference interval
Bilirubin (μmol/l)	**74.9**	0–2.4
Amylase (IU/l)	1017	176–1245
Lipase (IU/l)	171	72–1115
ALT (IU/l)	**968**	13–88
ALP (IU/l)	**497**	19–285
Creatinine kinase (IU/l)	206	61–394
Glucose (mmol/l)	6.0	3.4–6.2

Abnormal results are in **bold**.

Urinalysis	Result
Specific gravity	1.015
pH	7
Protein	1+
Glucose	**3+**
Ketone	Negative
Bilirubin	**2+**
Blood/Hb	**2+**
Sediment	RBCs 6–10/hpf, WBCs 6–8/hpf, some stained organic debris

Abnormal results are in **bold**.

WHAT ABNORMALITIES ARE PRESENT AND HOW SHOULD THEY BE INTERPRETED?

The haematology is unremarkable, effectively ruling out a prehepatic cause for the icterus. The clinical finding of icterus is confirmed by documentation of moderate hyperbilirubinaemia and associated bilirubinuria. There is moderate–marked elevation of liver enzyme activities but no biochemical changes indicative of hepatic synthetic failure. Glucosuria is present despite euglycaemia, which could indicate proximal tubular dysfunction. Alternative explanations include certain drugs, out-of-date urine dipsticks or transient hyperglycaemia. The urine sediment is mildly inflammatory; this could indicate that a urinary tract infection is present, which in turn could either be a cause of Fanconi-like syndrome or have been made more likely by the glucosuria. The finding of 1+ protein in a relatively dilute urine sample could be significant but would have to be further quantified by measurement of UPCR to determine whether it is abnormal. If proteinuria is confirmed, it could be postrenal (if a UTI is present) or tubular in origin.

WHAT FURTHER TESTS WOULD YOU RECOMMEND?

This dog appears to have a hepatic (or posthepatic) disease causing icterus and a proximal tubular disorder causing euglycaemic glucosuria. These could be related but do not have to be. There is no evidence for pancreatitis (a common cause of posthepatic icterus) on the basis of history, physical examination or initial diagnostic tests since the mildly elevated lipase is non-specific. This could be further investigated by measurement of pancreatic lipase immunoreactivity (PLI), although with such a chronic problem it might not be elevated even if pancreatitis had been present initially. This was not performed in this case because a posthepatic cause of icterus was ruled out by diagnostic imaging: the biliary tract appeared normal ultrasonographically. In preparation for potential liver biopsies, coagulation times (and potentially blood typing) are advisable.

To further characterize the proximal tubular dysfunction, numerous tests can be performed. It is possible to quantify amino acid excretion, and this may be abnormal in patients with Fanconi syndrome. This was not performed in this case because the results can take some time and it tends not to have a direct impact on management of the case. Blood gas analysis (if available) is more helpful because the results are immediate. Urine culture should also be performed.

Two conditions that are associated with both hepatic and renal tubular dysfunction should be given particular consideration in this case. The first is leptospirosis. Although the history is rather long for a diagnosis of this, it is an important consideration owing to its zoonotic potential. It can be tested for by serology and/or PCR. The second is copper-associated hepatitis, which has been documented quite frequently in Labrador Retrievers. This diagnosis can only be confirmed by taking hepatic and/or renal biopsy samples.

SUBSEQUENT DIAGNOSTIC TEST RESULTS

Blood type: DEA 1.1 positive.

Coagulation times (prothrombin time (PT) and activated partial thromboplastin time (aPTT): normal.

Urine culture: negative.

Venous blood gas: pH **7.28** (reference interval 7.36–7.44), bicarbonate **8.0 mmol/l** (reference interval 16–24 mmol/l).

Leptospirosis MAT titres

L. ballum	negative: 1/100.
L. canicola	positive: 1/200.
L. copenhageni	positive: 1/200.
L. icterohaemorrhagiae	negative: 1/100.

Hepatic biopsy specimens

Widespread moderate mixed inflammation (lymphocytic and neutrophilic) with bridging fibrosis. Rhodanine staining identified excess copper accumulation.

Hepatic copper quantification: **2239 ppm** (<400 ppm is considered normal).

INTERPRETATION

The venous blood gas results are consistent with a metabolic acidosis and, with the rest of the clinical picture, point to this patient having Fanconi syndrome. Leptospirosis seems unlikely in view of the low titres and the fact that the highest titre is to a vaccinal serovar. In an acute presentation serology could be repeated to check for a rising titre but that is unnecessary in this case because copper-associated hepatopathy was confirmed on the liver biopsy.

References and further reading

Almy FS, Christopher MM, King DP and Brown SA (2002) Evaluation of cystatin C as an endogenous marker of glomerular filtration rate in dogs. *Journal of Veterinary Internal Medicine* **16**, 45–51

Bexfield NH, Heiene R, Gerritsen RJ *et al.* (2008) Glomerular filtration rate estimated by 3-sample plasma clearance of iohexol in 118 healthy dogs. *Journal of Veterinary Internal Medicine* **22**, 66–73

Boyd LM, Langston C, Thompson K, Zivin K and Imanishi M (2008) Survival in cats with naturally occurring chronic kidney disease (2000–2002). *Journal of Veterinary Internal Medicine* **22**, 1111–1117

Cianciolo RE, Brown CA, Mohr FC *et al.* (2013) Pathologic evaluation of canine renal biopsies: methods for identifying features that differentiate immune-mediated glomerulonephritides from other categories of glomerular diseases. *Journal of Veterinary Internal Medicine* **27**, S10–S18

Craig AJ, Seguela J, Queau Y *et al.* (2006) Redefining the reference interval for plasma creatinine in dogs: Effect of age, gender, body weight, and breed. *Journal of Veterinary Internal Medicine* **20**, 740

Elliott J, Syme HM, Reubens E and Markwell PJ (2003) Assessment of acid–base status of cats with naturally occurring chronic renal failure. *Journal of Small Animal Practice* **44**, 65–70

Finch NC, Syme HM, Elliott J *et al.* (2011) Glomerular filtration rate estimation by use of a correction formula for slope-intercept plasma iohexol clearance in cats. *American Journal of Veterinary Research* **72**, 1652–1659

Finco DR and Duncan JR (1976) Evaluation of blood urea nitrogen and serum creatinine concentrations as indicators of renal dysfunction: a study of 111 cases and a review of related literature. *Journal of the American Veterinary Medical Association* **168**, 593–601

Heiene R, Bjørndal H and Indrebø A (2010) Glucosuria in Norwegian elkhounds and other breeds during dog shows. *Veterinary Record* **166**, 459–462

Heiene R and Moe L (1999) The relationship between some plasma clearance methods for estimation of glomerular filtration rate in dogs with pyometra. *Journal of Veterinary Internal Medicine* **13**, 587–596

Jensen AL and Aaes H (1993) Critical differences of clinical chemical parameters in blood from dogs. *Research in Veterinary Science* **54**, 10–14

Lee Y-J, Chang C-C, Chan JP-W, Hsu W-L, Lin K-W and Wong M-L (2011) Prognosis of acute kidney injury in dogs using RIFLE (risk, injury, failure, loss and end-stage renal failure)-like criteria. *Veterinary Record* **168**, 264

Lees GE, Brown SA, Elliott J, Grauer GE and Vaden SL (2005) Assessment and management of proteinuria in dogs and cats: 2004 ACVIM Forum Consensus Statement (small animal). *Journal of Veterinary Internal Medicine* **19**, 377–385

Lefebvre HP (2010) Normal kidney function: from small to extra-large. *Proceedings of the World Small Animal Veterinary Association World Congress*, Geneva

Lefebvre HP, Dossin O, Trumel C and Braun J-P (2008) Fractional excretion tests: a critical review of methods and applications in domestic animals. *Veterinary Clinical Pathology* **37**, 4–20

Lennon EM, Hanel RM, Walker JM and Vaden SL (2013) Hypercoagulability in dogs with protein-losing nephropathy as assessed by thromboelastography. *Journal of Veterinary Internal Medicine* **27**, 462–468

LeVine DN, Zhang D, Harris T and Vaden SL (2010) The use of pooled vs serial urine samples to measure urine protein:creatinine ratios. *Veterinary Clinical Pathology* **39**, 53–56

Littman M, Wiley C, Raducha M and Henthorn P (2013) Glomerulopathy and mutations in NPHS1 and KIRREL2 in Soft Coated Wheaten Terrier dogs. *Mammalian Genome* **24**, 119–126

Littman MP, Goldstein RE, Labato MA, Lappin MR and Moore GE (2006) ACVIM small animal consensus statement on Lyme disease in dogs: diagnosis, treatment, and prevention. *Journal of Veterinary Internal Medicine* **20**, 422–434

Medaille C, Trumel C, Concordet D, Vergez F and Braun JP (2004) Comparison of plasma/serum urea and creatinine concentrations in the dog: a 5-year retrospective study in a commercial veterinary clinical pathology laboratory. *Journal of Veterinary Medicine A, Physiology Pathology Clinical Medicine* **51**, 119–123

Monti P, Benchekroun G, Berlato D and Archer J (2012) Initial evaluation of canine urinary cystatin C as a marker of renal tubular function. *Journal of Small Animal Practice* **53**, 254–259

Nabity MB, Lees GE, Boggess M *et al.* (2013) Correlation of symmetric dimethylarginine with glomerular filtration rate in dogs with chronic progressive renal disease. *Journal of Veterinary Internal Medicine* **27**, 733 (abstract)

Reynolds BS, Concordet D, Germain CA, Daste T, Boudet KG and Lefebvre HP (2010) Breed dependency of reference intervals for plasma biochemical values in cats. *Journal of Veterinary Internal Medicine* **24**, 809–818

Rivers BJ, Walter PA, O'Brien TD, King VL and Polzin DJ (1996) Evaluation of urine gamma-glutamyl transpeptidase-to-creatinine ratio as a diagnostic tool in an experimental model of aminoglycoside-induced acute renal failure in the dog. *Journal of the American Animal Hospital Association* **32**, 323–336

Ross LA and Finco DR (1981) Relationship of selected clinical renal function tests to glomerular filtration rate and renal blood flow in cats. *American Journal of Veterinary Research* **42**, 1704–1710

Schenck PA and Chew DJ (2003) Determination of calcium fractionation in dogs with chronic renal failure. *American Journal of Veterinary Research* **64**, 1181–1184

Segev G, Kass PH, Francey T and Cowgill LD (2008) A novel clinical scoring system for outcome prediction in dogs with acute kidney injury managed by hemodialysis. *Journal of Veterinary Internal Medicine* **22**, 301–308

Segev G, Nivy R, Kass PH and Cowgill LD (2013a) A retrospective study of acute kidney injury in cats and development of a novel clinical scoring system for predicting outcome for cats managed by hemodialysis. *Journal of Veterinary Internal Medicine* **27**, 830–839

Segev G, Palm C, LeRoy B, Cowgill LD and Westropp JL (2013b) Evaluation of neutrophil gelatinase-associated lipocalin as a marker of kidney injury in dogs. *Journal of Veterinary Internal Medicine* **27**, 1362–1367

Thoen ME and Kerl ME (2011) Characterization of acute kidney injury in hospitalized dogs and evaluation of a veterinary acute kidney injury staging system. *Journal of Veterinary Emergency and Critical Care* **21**, 648–657

Thompson MF, Fleeman LM, Kessell AE, Steenhard LA and Foster SF (2013) Acquired proximal renal tubulopathy in dogs exposed to a common dried chicken treat: retrospective study of 108 cases (2007–2009). *Australian Veterinary Journal* **91**, 368–373

Ulleberg T, Robben J, Nordahl KM and Heiene R (2011) Plasma creatinine in dogs: intra- and inter-laboratory variation in 10 European veterinary laboratories. *Acta Veterinaria Scandinavica* **53**, 25

Watson ADJ, Lefebvre HP, Concordet D *et al.* (2002) Plasma exogenous creatinine clearance test in dogs: comparison with other methods and proposed limited sampling strategy. *Journal of Veterinary Internal Medicine* **16**, 22–33

Wehner A, Hartmann K and Hirschberger J (2008) Utility of serum cystatin C as a clinical measure of renal function in Dogs. *Journal of the American Animal Hospital Association* **44**, 131–138

Yearley JH, Hancock DD and Mealey KL (2004) Survival time, lifespan, and quality of life in dogs with idiopathic Fanconi syndrome. *Journal of the American Veterinary Medical Association* **225(3)**, 377–383

Chapter 12

Laboratory evaluation of hepatic disease

Edward J. Hall and Alexander J. German

The recognition and diagnosis of hepatobiliary diseases can be challenging. The associated clinical signs are varied and often quite vague and non-specific (Figure 12.1), and while there is a wide range of laboratory tests of both hepatic damage and function, there is rarely a single test that definitively identifies the disease. It is the synthesis of the clinicopathological results with information gathered from the history, physical examination and imaging that usually leads to a potential diagnosis, although ultimately, in many cases, the definitive diagnosis depends on histological examination of liver tissue.

In some instances, specific laboratory abnormalities, such as hyperammonaemia in an encephalopathic animal, may directly indicate hepatobiliary disease (Figure 12.2). However, many laboratory findings are not a direct reflection of liver disease and, indeed, other systemic diseases can cause abnormal hepatic test results. Awareness that underlying diseases can cause so-called secondary or reactive hepatopathies is necessary when interpreting clinicopathological results. To compound the difficulties associated with the lack of specificity of clinical signs, the liver has great functional reserve capacity, and no clinical signs may be apparent until advanced liver disease is present. Consequently, laboratory analyses may allow early detection of subclinical liver disease and hopefully, through earlier intervention, lead to a better outcome.

The aims of the clinicopathological evaluation of hepatic disease are to:

- Identify and characterize hepatic damage and dysfunction
- Identify primary causes of secondary hepatopathies
- Differentiate causes of icterus
- Evaluate potential anaesthetic risks
- Assess the effect of xenobiotics, i.e. drugs and toxins
- Monitor response to therapy
- Assess prognosis.

• Depression, decreased appetite and lethargy	
• Ascites	
• Icterus	
• Altered liver size	
• Encephalopathy	
• Stunting and/or weight loss	
• Vomiting and/or diarrhoea	
• Grey, acholic faeces (rare)	
• Polydipsia and polyuria	
• Bleeding tendency	
• Abdominal pain (rare)	

12.1 The range of clinical signs seen, in various combinations, in hepatobiliary disease.

Function	Abnormal laboratory test associated with hepatobiliary dysfunction
Carbohydrate metabolism: • Glucose homeostasis	Hyper- or hypoglycaemia
Lipid metabolism: • Cholesterol • Fatty acids • Lipoproteins • Bile acids	Hypo- or hypercholesterolaemia Hypertriglyceridaemia Lipaemia Elevated bile acids
Protein metabolism: • Albumin • Globulins • Coagulation proteins	Hypoalbuminaemia Increased acute phase proteins, immunoglobulins Coagulopathies
Vitamin metabolism	?Decreased folate, cobalamin, vitamin E, vitamin K
Immunological functions	Hyperglobulinaemia Increased acute phase proteins
Detoxification	Hyperammonaemia Decreased urea Hyperbilirubinaemia
Portosystemic shunt	Elevated bile acids Hyperammonaemia

12.2 Clinicopathological abnormalities associated with the disturbance of specific hepatobiliary functions.

Diagnostic approach to liver disease

The diagnostic approach to liver disease includes:

- Clinical history
- Physical examination
- Laboratory tests
- Analysis of any ascitic fluid (see Chapter 22)
- Imaging
- Liver and/or bile cytology and culture
- Liver biopsy.

During the early stages, a list of possible differential diagnoses is developed, and knowledge of the age, sex and breed of the patient helps to refine this list. For example, chronic hepatitis is prevalent in middle-aged female Dobermanns. The speed of onset may also offer clues. Acute diseases have a sudden onset; however, chronic diseases may also appear to develop acutely, as signs may only manifest once the functional reserve capacity of the liver is exhausted. Despite an apparent sudden onset, careful questioning of owners may elicit a history of previous (recurrent) low-grade illness. A history of weight loss and/or ascites also suggests that the disease is chronic.

Physical examination may identify signs of liver disease such as jaundice or hepatomegaly, but it is equally important in identifying underlying disorders causing secondary hepatopathies. For example, in hyperadrenocorticism, cutaneous changes (e.g. thin skin, comedones and calcinosis cutis) may be seen in conjunction with hepatomegaly and increased serum alkaline phosphatase (ALP) activity. Indeed, the importance of history and physical examination cannot be overemphasized, and any test results must always be interpreted in the light of these findings.

Laboratory testing is a key part of the investigation and diagnosis of hepatobiliary disease, but it does not necessarily differentiate primary liver diseases from secondary hepatopathies. Part of the art of interpreting laboratory abnormalities is the awareness that any changes may not be indicators of primary liver disease and the liver may not actually need to be investigated further. Serum biochemistry, haematology and urinalysis are performed routinely, when investigating animals with suspected hepatic disease, before performing more specific tests. Biochemical findings are often the most useful in the identification and characterization of liver disease.

Serum biochemistry

Serum markers of liver damage

Increased activities in serum of liver-specific enzymes are generally considered to be sensitive markers of liver disease because they reflect 'liver damage'. However, it can be difficult to decide, first, whether the magnitude of liver enzyme elevations is significant and, second, whether the increases represent primary or secondary liver disease or enzyme induction. Increased liver enzyme activities are common but are not necessarily associated with clinically significant *primary* liver disease. Systemic diseases and various drugs can cause misleading increases in serum enzyme activities, which are potentially reversible without any specific therapy for liver disease (i.e. *secondary* or *reactive* hepatopathies).

It is important to interpret increases in serum enzyme activities in light of the results from other diagnostic investigations, in particular the history and physical examination. For example, feline hyperthyroidism causes secondary increases in liver enzyme activity, and therefore assessment of thyroid function is indicated before obtaining liver biopsy samples in older cats with increased enzyme activities, particularly if they have typical signs such as polyphagia, weight loss and/or goitre (see Chapter 17).

Even when increased serum activities are associated with primary liver disease, it is a popular misconception that these are 'liver *function* tests'. Serum enzyme activities do not reflect the liver's ability to function. They actually depend not only on the extent and/or severity of the hepatic damage but also on the enzymes':

- Total hepatic activity
- Intracellular location (and thus their propensity to leak from hepatocytes)
- Potential for induction by drugs and xenobiotics
- Serum half-life.

In summary, serum enzyme activities give little indication of the type of disease present, the overall functional state of the liver, or the reversibility of the disease. For example, in severe chronic hepatopathies such as cirrhosis, and also in congenital portosystemic shunts (PSS), there may be marked hepatic dysfunction with no or minimal marker enzyme release. This occurs because there is either insufficient functional hepatic mass to synthesize and release the enzymes (e.g. cirrhosis, PSS) or no active hepatic damage (e.g. PSS).

The magnitude of the increase in serum activity is not necessarily important. Less than 2-fold increases in liver enzymes in dogs are generally considered to be insignificant. Only in acute disease might the magnitude of the increase in enzyme activity correlate with severity of the damage although, again, it gives no indication of the potential reversibility of the damage or the prognosis. For example, an increase in liver enzymes of a similar magnitude may be seen if the liver is contused in a road traffic accident (RTA) or if the patient is poisoned with carbon tetrachloride, but the outcome may be completely different: the bruised liver will recover, but carbon tetrachloride poisoning inevitably leads to liver failure.

Persistently increased liver enzymes at any level usually indicate chronic disease but, occasionally, persistent increases occur without abnormal hepatic function and histopathological changes. This situation may reflect the presence of macroenzymes, which are large antibody-bound complexes of enzymes cleared from the circulation more slowly than normal and which have no clinical significance. So, paradoxically, mild increases in serum liver enzyme activities may either be of no consequence or reflect loss of almost all hepatocytes in end-stage disease.

Liver enzyme activities that can be measured in serum can be classified into two major types:

- Hepatocellular enzymes that are released by cell damage (leakage/damage markers)
- Biliary enzymes whose synthesis is induced by drugs and retained bile (cholestatic markers).

A number of enzymes are available for measurement but, within either class, one enzyme rarely offers greater diagnostic advantage over the others. Therefore, the routine biochemical profile usually only offers one or two enzymes within each class, and with which the clinician becomes familiar.

Enzyme activities are measurable in serum or heparinized plasma and are stable over several days, as long as the sample is not exposed to excessive heat. The effects of haemolysis, icterus and lipaemia are variable depending on the analyser and method being used. Reference ranges vary among laboratories depending on the assay methodology, and comparison of results from different laboratories is better achieved by comparing the magnitude of any increase with respect to the relevant upper reference range than by comparing absolute numbers. For example, an alanine aminotransferase (ALT) concentration of 300 IU/l represents a 5-fold increase if the upper limit of the reference range is 60 IU/l, but only a 3-fold increase if the limit is 100 IU/l.

Hepatocellular/leakage enzymes

Alanine aminotransferase: ALT is a cytosolic enzyme found in hepatocytes at concentrations ~10,000-fold greater than in normal serum. Measurement of ALT activity following release into serum is considered to be the test of choice for hepatocellular damage in dogs and cats because of its reported high sensitivity. It is routinely measured in clinical practice as a screening test for hepatic damage because the likelihood of false negative results, i.e. ALT within the reference range despite significant active liver damage, is considered to be very low. However, Fieten *et al.* (2012) suggested that the sensitivity of ALT for subclinical damage is relatively poor: in a group of Labrador Retrievers with subclinical hepatitis, the sensitivity of increased ALT for predicting histological abnormalities was only 64%.

The serum half-life of ALT in dogs is variously reported to be between 3 hours and 4 days but, whichever value is used, the half-life is significantly shorter in cats. Therefore, in cats, the normal reference range is lower and smaller increases are considered more significant because it is cleared more rapidly from serum.

ALT is considered to be liver-specific in dogs and cats, although there are some other tissue sources (e.g. heart, kidney and muscle). However, these other isoenzymes are either present in low concentrations or their serum half-life is very short and they rarely contribute to increased serum activity. ALT may increase in very severe muscle diseases, e.g. muscular dystrophy in dogs, severe muscle trauma and muscle necrosis following an aortic saddle thrombus in cats. In addition, increases in ALT are not specific for *primary* liver damage; increases of equal magnitude may be seen in *secondary* hepatopathies.

Primary hepatocellular damage: Immediate increases in serum ALT activity are found following release, due to either hepatocyte necrosis or 'leakage' resulting from altered cell membrane permeability and/or altered cell metabolism (Figure 12.3a). Acute hepatopathies, such as infectious canine hepatitis or caused by liver toxins, may cause a rapid 100-fold increase in activity (Figure 12.4). The magnitude of the rise in ALT in acute liver disease is roughly proportional to the number of hepatocytes affected, but a common mistake in the interpretation of ALT is to place too much significance on the magnitude of the rise in chronic disease. As stated previously, at least a 2-fold increase is needed before any significance is attached, but the magnitude of the rise in ALT beyond this does not directly reflect the severity of the disease, its reversibility or the prognosis, and it is not an indicator of liver function or dysfunction.

Increases may not be marked in chronic hepatopathies and may fluctuate; they will be persistent but in end-stage liver disease, when there is little active damage occurring, ALT activities may be almost within the reference range (Figure 12.5), suggesting that only a few hepatocytes are left to leak enzyme. Yet, recovery from acute hepatitis is more likely than with chronic disease, and it is the duration of enzyme elevation that is often of more diagnostic and, particularly, prognostic importance.

While decreased serum ALT activity can be a bad prognostic sign if it reflects loss of hepatocytes, a gradual but steady decline in ALT following an acute insult usually indicates a good prognosis. Serum ALT activity declines more slowly than would be predicted from the enzyme's half-life, because it is derived both from leaky damaged cells and from regenerating hepatocytes. Therefore, in dogs, activities should fall by 50% every 3–4 days, and should have returned to the reference range in 2–3 weeks (Figure 12.4).

Cholestasis: As expected, ALT rises immediately following acute hepatocyte injury, but it increases more slowly in

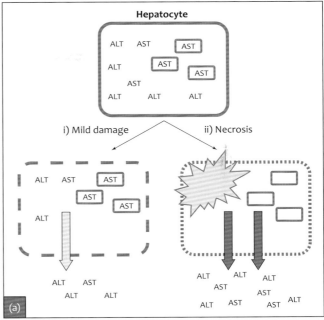

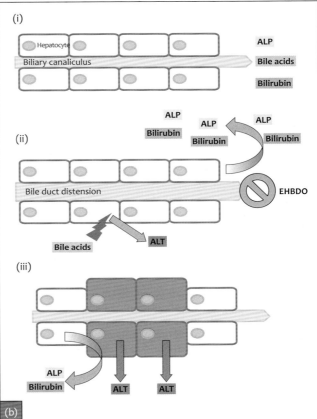

12.3 Mechanism of hepatic enzyme release. (a) Hepatocellular damage: (i) Mild damage causes release of cytosolic ALT and a small amount of aspartate aminotransferase (AST) through increased cell membrane permeability; (ii) Hepatocyte necrosis causes liberation of more ALT and mitochondrial AST is also released. (b) Intra- and extrahepatic cholestasis: (i) ALP is normally secreted in bile with excreted bilirubin; (ii) Common bile duct obstruction causes extrahepatic cholestasis (EHBDO), leading to increased serum ALP because ALP is both regurgitated into the blood and its synthesis is induced. Bilirubin cannot be excreted and the patient becomes icteric. Accumulation of bile acids damages the hepatocyte membrane, leading to the release of ALT; (iii) Hepatocyte damage causes release of ALT, but swelling of the hepatocytes occludes the narrow biliary canaliculi that run between hepatocytes. This causes intrahepatic cholestasis. Jaundice sometimes occurs if there is significant hepatocyte dysfunction.

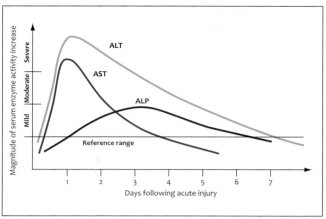

12.4 Pattern of changes in serum liver enzymes after an acute hepatic injury and during resolution. Note that there is a parallel increase in ALT and AST but a longer persistence of ALT because of its longer serum half-life and continued synthesis and release during hepatic repair. The increase in ALP lags behind the hepatocellular marker enzymes, as hepatocyte swelling causes intrahepatic cholestasis.

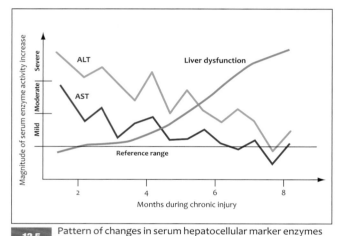

12.5 Pattern of changes in serum hepatocellular marker enzymes (ALT, AST) with chronic injury and progressive hepatic dysfunction. Note that ALT and AST fluctuate but remain persistently elevated, although there is an overall decrease as liver function (assessed by serum bile acids) declines, and terminally, serum enzyme activity may be within the reference range.

cholestatic liver disease (Figure 12.6). Extrahepatic bile duct obstruction and consequent bile stasis leads to intrahepatic accumulation of toxic bile salts, which eventually cause hepatocyte damage and enzyme leakage (see Figure 12.3b), although the rises in serum ALT activity (e.g. 2- to 10-fold) often do not reach the magnitude of the increase in cholestatic marker enzymes (e.g. 10- to 100-fold). Similarly, cholangitis only causes a moderate (5- to 10-fold) increase in serum ALT activity in comparison to cholestatic marker enzyme activity.

Neoplasia: Rises in ALT activity are also seen in some cases of primary and metastatic hepatic neoplasia, if there is enzyme leakage from tumour cells of hepatic origin or from tumour-associated necrosis. However, significant hepatic infiltration with lymphoma or mast cell tumours may be associated with minimal increases in ALT because there is minimal hepatocyte destruction.

Drug induced: Small increases in ALT can also be caused by microsomal enzyme induction after administration of hepatotoxic drugs (Figure 12.7), and the rise in activity tends to be dose-dependent:

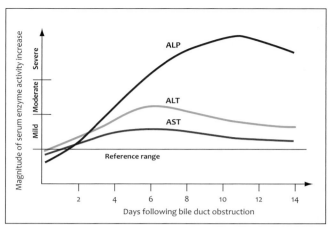

12.6 Pattern of changes in serum liver enzymes following extrahepatic bile duct obstruction. Note the rise and plateau of ALP, which will parallel the rise in bilirubin. Lesser increases in ALT and AST follow the accumulation of toxic bile acids that increase hepatocyte cell membrane permeability.

- Azathioprine
- Barbiturates (including phenobarbital, primidone)
- Doxycycline (cats)
- Glucocorticoids (dogs)
- Griseofulvin
- Halothane
- Ketoconazole
- Mebendazole
- Methimazole (cats)
- Paracetamol (acetaminophen)
- Sulphonamides

12.7 Important hepatotoxic drugs known or suspected to cause increases in ALT.

- Therapeutic doses of anticonvulsants such as phenobarbital usually produce a mild increase, whereas toxic doses can cause a 50-fold rise. Idiosyncratic reactions with the development of significant liver dysfunction are likely to be associated with greater rises in ALT activity
- Doxycycline and methimazole/carbimazole are occasionally associated with large increases in ALT activity in cats. Glucocorticoids can also induce ALT activity (doses of prednisolone >4 mg/kg can cause a 10-fold rise in ALT), but the increase is usually disproportionately less than the induced rise in ALP (see below). Increased activity may persist for several weeks following a single dose of steroids owing to enzyme induction and steroid hepatopathy.

Reactive hepatopathies: Another major problem in the interpretation of ALT activities is that changes are also sensitive markers of secondary and clinically insignificant hepatopathies. For example, it is not unusual to see up to 5-fold increases in ALT in dogs with primary inflammatory gastrointestinal (GI) disease, due to the portal delivery of bacteria and/or toxins and/or cytokines from the inflamed gut. Liver biopsy is not indicated in most of these cases, especially as liver function tests (see below) are typically normal. If histological analysis is performed, changes are absent or mild, and are often reported as a 'vacuolar hepatopathy'. It is believed that the release of cytokines by activated Kupffer cells results in mild reversible hepatocyte damage.

Increased ALT activity can occur secondary to fatty infiltration in diabetes mellitus. ALT activity can also be increased secondary to hypoxic liver damage, and consequent increases in haemolytic anaemia may mislead clinicians into thinking that a primary hepatopathy is present. Given the large number of Kupffer cells in, and large blood supply to, the liver, increased ALT activity may be seen in response to haemolysis or sepsis and endotoxaemia from any site; even severe periodontal disease can cause mildly elevated serum ALT activities. Thus, the careful clinician usually checks at least one other liver enzyme and if necessary performs a liver function test and/or imaging before embarking on liver biopsy. However, persistent elevation of ALT activity over 1–2 months is indication for further investigations such as liver biopsy, even if clinical signs are not yet apparent and liver function tests are normal, and provided no primary underlying disorder can be found.

When a clinician is faced with a patient with apparently non-specific increases in ALT, found either on a routine biochemical screen or during illness, a logical approach to be taken is shown in Figure 12.8.

Aspartate aminotransferase: AST is another hepatocellular enzyme that is released by cell damage, but unlike ALT it is also found in significant quantities in cardiac and skeletal muscle. Muscle inflammation is relatively uncommon in the dog and cat but muscle trauma is common, e.g. following an RTA, and can be identified by simultaneous measurement of a muscle-specific enzyme activity, e.g. creatine kinase (see Chapter 24). In liver disease, rises in AST activity usually parallel ALT. Thus, an increase in AST and creatine kinase, but not ALT, probably indicates muscle damage. AST may also be increased by haemolysis and release from red blood cells (RBCs).

Since AST appears to have no advantage over ALT as a marker of hepatocyte damage in terms of sensitivity, its measurement is of limited value. However, because some of the hepatocellular AST is mitochondrial-bound rather than all free in the cytosol, some clinicians argue that release requires more severe injury, i.e. cell necrosis rather than increased cell membrane permeability. Therefore, release

of AST often lags slightly behind ALT (see Figure 12.4) and, because its half-life is shorter, its presence probably suggests more profound or persistent injury than an increase in ALT alone (see Figure 12.3). Consequently, increased serum AST may be a more specific marker of *significant* liver damage than ALT as it is less likely to be increased in secondary hepatopathies e.g. glucocorticoid hepatopathy. In humans, differentiation of the cytosolic and mitochondrial isoforms of AST has prognostic implications, but this test is not currently available in veterinary medicine.

Increases in AST in acute hepatitis parallel increases in ALT (see Figure 12.4) although they are rarely more than 50-fold. Although they decline over several weeks, they usually normalize before ALT; persistently elevated AST is a poor prognostic sign. Smaller increases in AST are seen in chronic hepatitis (see Figure 12.5) and cholestatic disease (see Figure 12.6). Once again, the plasma half-life of 1 hour in cats is less than in dogs (5 hours), and therefore smaller increases are as significant; indeed, it has been suggested that AST is a more sensitive marker of *significant* liver disease in cats.

Other serum enzymes: In most cases ALT and AST are the only hepatocellular marker enzymes that need to be measured. However, there are a number of other candidate markers, developed primarily for ruminants, which have been proposed for use in dogs and cats. These include arginase, glutamate dehydrogenase (GLDH), lactate dehydrogenase (LDH), succinate dehydrogenase (SDH) and ornithine carbamoyltransferase (OCT). None has been shown to have any significant advantages and some, such as LDH, are so ubiquitous as to be unhelpful. Arginase and SDH are perhaps potentially useful (although SDH is not liver specific), because their release tends to be less in secondary hepatopathies as they are localized in mitochondria and, unlike ALT and AST, their leakage ceases during recovery. Therefore, persistent increases carry a poorer prognosis.

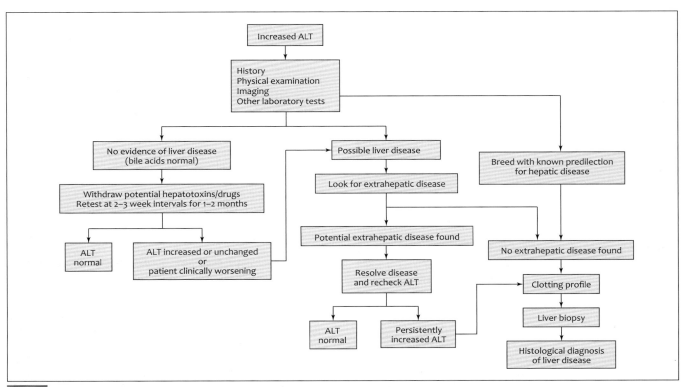

12.8 Logical approach to a patient with an unexplained increase in serum ALT activity.

Biliary/cholestatic marker enzymes

Enzymes bound to the membranes of the biliary canaliculi and bile duct cells, and that are normally secreted or shed into bile, can be released into the circulation in response to cholestasis. They are usually measured in a serum biochemistry profile in conjunction with ALT. However, their specificity for cholestatic disease is limited; increases are frequently seen in other diseases, and in the dog a corticosteroid-induced isoenzyme is a frequent complication.

Alkaline phosphatase: In the liver, alkaline phosphatase (ALP; also known as AP or serum AP (SAP)) is anchored in the microsomal and biliary canalicular membranes of hepatocytes and cholangiocytes, and is normally secreted into bile. Hepatic ALP is released into the blood in response to cholestasis (extra- or intrahepatic, see Figure 12.3b) and drug induction. The level of ALP activity cannot be used to distinguish between intra- and extrahepatic cholestasis, and the value of ALP even as a test of cholestasis is limited by the presence of a number of isoenzymes, particularly in dogs, which have a steroid induced isoenzyme (Figure 12.9).

ALP has higher specificity for cholestasis in cats than in dogs because there are no steroid-induced isoenzymes (see below). In addition, the half-life of liver ALP in cat serum is only 6 hours, compared with 3 days in dogs; there is also a smaller total ALP activity in feline liver and therefore lesser rises are more significant in cats than in

Primary liver disease

• Cholestasis:
  • Intrahepatic
• Hepatic inflammation:
  • Parenchymatous
  • Cholangitis
• Nodular hyperplasia
• Neoplasia

Extrahepatic conditions

• Bile duct obstruction
• Bone metabolism:
  • Growth
  • Osteomyelitis
  • Fracture repair
  • Osteosarcoma
  • Secondary renal hyperparathyroidism
• Gastrointestinal disease:
  • Gastroenteritis
  • Pancreatitis
• Hyperthyroidism
• Pregnancy
• Right-sided heart failure
• Sepsis:
  • Systemic infections
  • Pyometra
• Urological disease:
  • Nephritis
  • Cystic calculi

Drug-induced

• Corticosteroids (dogs):
  • Iatrogenic
  • Hyperadrenocorticism
  • Endogenous (stress)?
• Anticonvulsants:
  • Phenobarbital
  • Primidone
  • Phenytoin
• Azathioprine

12.9 Causes of increased ALP in dogs. Cats do not produce a steroid-induced ALP isoenzyme, and increased activities are less notable in extrahepatic disease in cats.

dogs. However, ALP is not as sensitive in cats as in dogs and can even be normal in jaundiced cats.

ALP isoenzymes of non-hepatic origin: ALP isoenzymes are present in the liver, bone, intestine, kidney and placenta. However, renal and intestinal sources rarely contribute to increased serum levels and placental ALP is obviously only detectable in pregnancy. The ALP content of intestine is actually higher than that of liver but, because the plasma half-life of the intestinal isoenzyme (~6 minutes) is much shorter than the liver isoenzyme (~3 days), and because it is a brush border enzyme that is largely lost into the intestinal lumen, increased serum activities of the alimentary isoenzyme are rarely seen, even in severe intestinal disease. Indeed, any increase in serum ALP in primary intestinal disease is more likely to be the result of secondary hepatic damage than intestinal isoenzyme release. Similarly, renal ALP is excreted in urine and urinary ALP may be a useful marker of renal damage, but it is of no significance when measuring serum ALP. Thus, the key causes of increased serum ALP are cholestasis, drug/hormone induction and increased osteoblastic activity.

Bone ALP is released in response to osteoblastic activity. In young growing dogs and cats the normal total serum ALP range is approximately twice the adult level because of the presence of this isoenzyme. Increases in ALP are seen in adult dogs with active bone lesions (e.g. fractures, osteomyelitis and bone tumours) and in secondary renal hyperparathyroidism, but are rarely more than 5-fold. With osteosarcoma, there is some correlation between the magnitude of ALP increase and the volume of tumour tissue. If there is any confusion, assay of another cholestatic marker (e.g. gamma-glutamyl transferase; GGT), which has no bone isoenzyme (see below), will be helpful. Increases in ALP activity are even lower in cats with bone lesions, although the bone isoenzyme is reported to be induced by hyperthyroidism.

ALP in cholestasis: As stated above, hepatic ALP is released into the blood as a result of cholestasis (extra- or intrahepatic) and drug induction. In cholestasis, the increases in serum hepatic ALP do not simply reflect regurgitation from within hepatocytes, but also both solubilization of ALP from membranes by accumulated bile salts and induction of *de novo* synthesis. Thus, after an acute hepatic insult, ALP increases are delayed compared with ALT rises, because of the slower induction of synthesis. In dogs, ALP begins to rise 8 hours after biliary obstruction, and increases up to 15-fold in 2–4 days. Peak activity, ~100-fold above normal, is reached in 1–2 weeks, and then activity plateaus (see Figure 12.6). ALP is also usually the last enzyme to return to the reference range after an acute insult because impairment of bile flow is usually the last functional disturbance to resolve and increased synthesis may persist beyond resolution of the injury.

A wide range of intra- or extrahepatic lesions may cause cholestasis. There is a tendency for periportal injury to cause greater increases in ALP than centrilobular damage. However, intrahepatic cholestasis is associated with increased ALP and can be caused not only by biliary disease (e.g. cholangitis) but also by hepatitis because consequent hepatocyte swelling occludes small biliary canaliculi. Extrahepatic (posthepatic) bile duct obstruction (e.g. by pancreatitis, pancreatic neoplasia or choleliths) causes a rise in ALP and hyperbilirubinaemia in both cats and dogs (see Figure 12.9).

Other hepatic causes of increased ALP: Primary hepatic neoplasia (hepatocellular and biliary carcinomas) has also been associated with increased ALP, and this is presumed to be the result of aberrant synthesis, although intrahepatic cholestasis is also likely to be present. Similarly, metabolic diseases such as canine diabetes mellitus and idiopathic feline hepatic lipidosis can cause a rise in ALP, because of fatty infiltration of the liver and hepatocyte swelling.

Increased serum ALP activity has been recorded in older Scottish Terriers in association with a vacuolar hepatopathy and hepatic fibrosis (Chevallier *et al.*, 2012). An association with hepatocellular carcinoma has also been noted (Bento *et al.*, 2013), and may reflect abnormal adrenal hormone hyperactivity causing atypical hyperadrenocorticism, through increased synthesis of progesterone and androstenedione.

Steroid-induced ALP: In dogs, interpretation of serum ALP activity is complicated by the presence of a so-called (cortico)steroid-induced ALP isoenzyme (CIALP or SIALP). It is found particularly in canine hyperadrenocorticism, or after exogenous steroid administration (oral, parenteral or topical), but synthesis can also be induced by barbiturate anticonvulsants. SIALP comprises <15% of the total serum ALP activity in normal dogs, but after glucocorticoid administration this may rise to 85%, with a resultant rise in total ALP.

The proportion of the SIALP isoenzyme in the total ALP activity can be quantified by electrophoretic separation methods, but chemical manipulations have also been described, and the levamisole inhibition assay appears the most reliable. SIALP does not appear to occur in cats but, in dogs, the response to exogenous corticosteroids varies with the type of steroid, dosage, frequency and route of administration, and also between individuals, resulting in unexpectedly large increases in some patients. Thus, SIALP complicates the interpretation of increases in total ALP, as endogenous and exogenous steroids may induce it. Furthermore, any increase may persist for 6 weeks after the steroid administration has ceased.

Most dogs with hyperadrenocorticism have increased SIALP and therefore the absence of SIALP makes a diagnosis of hyperadrenocorticism less likely. However, induction of SIALP by steroids is unpredictable, and excessive steroid concentrations may also cause intrahepatic cholestasis and increases in the hepatic ALP isoenzyme. Furthermore, SIALP may be expressed in diabetes mellitus, hypothyroidism and pancreatitis as well as with anticonvulsant therapy.

Hyperbilirubinaemia is not a feature seen concurrently with steroid-induced increases in ALP and its presence can help to indicate primary cholestatic disease, although sometimes bilirubinuria and a mild increase in serum bile acid concentrations (see below) are actually found. Most confusingly, varying proportions of SIALP may also be produced in primary liver disease, perhaps due to stress-induced increases in concentrations of endogenous steroids that are sufficient to induce SIALP synthesis. Thus, specific measurement of the SIALP isoenzyme has fallen from favour and is not generally used in the UK. However, increases in ALP are not specific for biliary disease, and the magnitude of any increase in ALP does not correlate with the severity of the disease process. Indeed, the finding of increased total ALP in isolation (i.e. with no or minimal increase in ALT) is suggestive of hyperadrenocorticism, but increased ALP may also be seen in benign nodular hyperplasia of the liver. Isolated increases in serum ALP activities are seen in nodular hyperplasia, a benign condition seen in virtually all dogs over 9 years of age. A review of the clinical signs and/or evaluation of adrenal function (see Chapter 18) should be performed to distinguish the two conditions.

Gamma-glutamyl transferase: GGT, or γ-glutamyl trans-peptidase (γ-GT), is another microsomal membrane-bound glycoprotein associated with the biliary tree whose activity increases in serum in response to cholestasis. It generally parallels rises in ALP activity, but is perhaps less influenced by hepatocyte necrosis. There are GGT isoenzymes in other tissues, notably the kidney, pancreas, intestine, heart, lungs, muscle and RBCs, but most circulating GGT is presumed to be of hepatic origin. There is no bone isoenzyme and, therefore, increased GGT is not seen in growth or bone disease. However, colostrum and milk do contain GGT and may cause an increase in nursing animals up to 10 days of age. As with ALP, a steroid-induced isoenzyme is also present, but its synthesis is apparently less likely to be induced by barbiturate anticonvulsants.

Differences in the zonal distribution of GGT within the liver and biliary tree compared with ALP may influence the sensitivity of GGT in various diseases. GGT is also found in the lower biliary tree but, like ALP, GGT lacks complete specificity in differentiating cholestatic from hepatocellular disease. It has been suggested that measurement of ALP and GGT together increases their diagnostic value. In dogs, GGT is probably more specific and less sensitive than ALP but, in cats, the converse appears true. In cats, most cholestatic disease causes greater increases in GGT than ALP. The exception is idiopathic hepatic lipidosis, where increases in ALP may occur in the absence of a significant rise in GGT. It has been postulated that this discordance reflects either delayed clearance of ALP or excess production, or differences in the localization of the two enzymes.

In summary, measurement of ALP as a cholestatic marker in dogs is generally preferred to GGT, with the converse in cats, but in some situations measurement of both enzymes may provide additional information.

MicroRNAs

MicroRNAs (miRNAs) are small conserved tissue-specific regulatory non-coding RNAs that modulate a variety of biological processes and play a fundamental role in the pathogenesis of some liver diseases. The concentrations of circulating liver-specific miRNAs in experimental animals and humans correlate with the degree of hepatic damage, and measurement of their plasma levels may be used as a highly sensitive biomarker (Tryndyak *et al.*, 2012). However, veterinary assays are not yet commercially available.

Other routinely assessed biochemical parameters commonly altered in liver disease

Abnormalities occur in many biochemical tests in liver disease but are not specific. However, they can offer a crude assessment of liver status, or aid recognition of diseases that either mimic the clinical signs of liver disease or actually cause secondary liver disease.

Cholesterol

Cholesterol is derived from both the diet and hepatic synthesis, and undergoes enterohepatic recycling. However, the usefulness of serum cholesterol concentration as a marker of liver disease is limited because its concentration may be decreased, normal or increased depending on the type of liver disease and the dietary intake.

Hypercholesterolaemia is common with extrahepatic bile duct occlusion in dogs and cats, but may also be seen in diseases that secondarily affect the liver, e.g. diabetes mellitus, hyperadrenocorticism, hypothyroidism, hyperlipidaemia, pancreatitis and nephrotic syndrome. While hypocholesterolaemia can be found in cases of PSS, cirrhosis and liver failure, it can also be a consequence of malabsorption or anorexia.

Triglycerides

Abnormalities of lipid metabolism in hepatic disease are not well characterized. Hypertriglyceridaemia may be seen in biliary obstruction, and reduced concentrations may be seen in chronic hepatitis. Lipaemia is seen in a number of metabolic diseases, e.g. diabetes mellitus, hyperadrenocorticism, hypothyroidism, and in pancreatitis, all of which can secondarily affect the liver (see Chapter 15).

Glucose

Glucohomeostatic mechanisms are so effective that significant fasting hypoglycaemia is only seen occasionally in dogs and cats with primary liver diseases when there is severe hepatic compromise e.g. massive hepatic necrosis, PSS or end-stage liver disease. Congenital hepatic enzyme deficiencies, termed glycogen storage diseases, are very rare but may cause hypoglycaemia and hepatic engorgement with stored glycogen. Juvenile hypoglycaemia is recognized in young toy breed dogs; this appears to be a metabolic abnormality because ketonaemia also develops. Sepsis and large or diffuse tumours, such as hepatic lymphoma, may also cause hypoglycaemia through excessive glucose utilization or release of insulin-like factors (see Chapter 16).

Urea and creatinine

Decreased serum urea concentration, or a decrease relative to serum creatinine, is sometimes seen in animals with PSS or severe liver dysfunction because of failure to convert ammonia to urea (see below).

Azotaemia (increased serum urea and creatinine concentrations) indicates decreased glomerular filtration, which can be a consequence of primary hepatic disease among *many* other causes. In a fasting sample, a disproportionate increase in urea compared with creatinine can be seen with gastrointestinal (GI) haemorrhage. A combination of coagulopathy and portal hypertension in liver disease can lead to occult GI haemorrhage that may be detected by changes in the urea:creatinine ratio before haematemesis or melaena is noticeable.

Serum proteins

Given that the liver is the source of all albumin and most globulins (except γ-globulins), serum total protein and, especially, albumin concentrations are crude markers of liver function. The differential diagnosis for hypoproteinaemia includes liver disease, protein-losing nephropathies (PLN), protein-losing enteropathies (PLE) and blood loss. These diseases can often be distinguished by their clinical signs, their relative changes in albumin and globulin concentrations, and simple confirmatory laboratory tests (see Chapter 7).

Albumin: Mild decreases (typically <20%) in albumin concentration are seen in anorexia, as an acute phase response in inflammatory diseases (with the down-regulation of synthesis inversely related to the increases in serum globulin), and in ascitic animals because of the increased volume of distribution (third-space effect). PLE or PLN are more common causes of severe hypoalbuminaemia leading to ascites.

Given that the half-life of albumin is reported to be between 1 and 3 weeks in dogs, significant decreases in albumin concentration develop slowly in liver disease, and indicate the existence of chronic disease. Dogs and cats also have a large reserve capacity for albumin synthesis through muscle catabolism, and profound hypoalbuminaemia in liver disease is usually only seen with PSS and severe hepatocellular dysfunction. In end-stage liver disease there is both decreased albumin synthesis and dilution of serum by sodium and water retention. Thus, serum albumin measurements have some prognostic value, as well as the presence of ascites indicating a poorer prognosis.

Globulins: Hyperglobulinaemia is common in acquired liver disease, not just because there may be an inflammatory aetiology, but also because of acute phase responses and decreased clearance of antigen by Kupffer cells resulting in a systemic immune response. Therefore, most globulins are increased in inflammatory liver diseases: α- and β-globulins include acute phase proteins and increase in inflammation in parallel with γ-globulins. Hyperglobulinaemia is particularly seen in cats with feline infectious peritonitis (FIP) and lymphocytic cholangitis, two conditions that can cause jaundice and ascites. The hyperglobulinaemia may be sufficient to mask hypoalbuminaemia if only total protein concentration is measured.

Routine haematology

Red cell series

Mild to moderate anaemia (haematocrit ranging from 0.20 to 0.35 l/l in dogs, and 0.18 to 0.24 l/l in cats) is common in liver disease, and usually results from chronic illness and/or GI bleeding and/or haemostatic disorders (see Chapter 4). Profound anaemia most typically results from profuse bleeding or from primary haemolytic disease, which may be associated with icterus and secondary increases in liver enzyme activities.

Chronic or intermittent internal bleeding from hepatic tumours, such as haemangiosarcoma, more typically results in moderate regenerative anaemia, and schistocytes may be present; cases with more severe haemorrhage are likely to present with hypovolaemic shock and haemoabdomen, rather than anaemia. Other hepatic diseases can result in profuse haemorrhage, e.g. hepatic trauma, peliosis and hepatic amyloidosis (i.e. conditions that can result in spontaneous hepatic rupture) or GI bleeding secondary to portal hypertension.

Microangiopathic haemolytic anaemia with the presence of RBC fragments (schistocytes) can be associated with inflammatory and benign or malignant neoplastic hepatic (and splenic) diseases (see Chapter 4).

Microcytosis (Figure 12.10a) is relatively common in dogs with congenital PSS, and is seen occasionally in acquired liver disease; it is believed to reflect abnormal

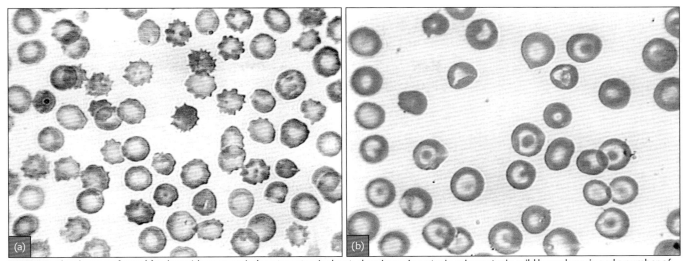

12.10 Blood smears from: (a) a dog with a congenital portosystemic shunt, showing anisocytosis, microcytosis, mild hypochromia and a number of acanthocytes (spur cells); (b) a Cocker Spaniel with chronic hepatitis showing slight anisocytosis, hypochromia and target cells. (Wright–Giesma stain; original magnification X1000)

iron metabolism. Chronic occult GI blood loss, with iron deficiency anaemia, is the major differential diagnosis.

Variable red cell shapes (poikilocytosis) with irregularly spiculated erythrocytes (acanthocytes or spur cells) are seen in chronic liver disease (Figure 12.10b) and are probably the result of changes in phospholipid metabolism.

White cell series

There are no white blood cell (WBC) changes pathognomonic for hepatic disease. The total WBC count may be increased and an inflammatory leucogram seen in acute infectious disease (e.g. leptospirosis) and sometimes in severe chronic inflammatory hepatopathies and neoplastic liver diseases with necrosis of tumour nodules (see Chapter 5).

Platelets

Moderate decreases in platelet numbers and abnormal platelet function are non-specific changes sometimes seen in severe liver disease.

Urinalysis

Discoloured (i.e. orange) urine may be the first indication to owners that their pet is jaundiced, but further biochemical and microscopic examination of urine may provide the clinician with additional information about liver dysfunction.

Specific gravity

If polyuria is suspected from the history, this can be confirmed by documenting a consistently low urine specific gravity (<1.020).

Bilirubin

The normal degradation and metabolism of bilirubin are shown in Figure 12.11 and discussed below. In healthy dogs, small quantities of bilirubin may be found in the urine because renal tubular cells, especially in male dogs, can metabolize some haemoglobin to bilirubin; if there is proteinuria any urinary albumin will have bilirubin bound to it. Thus, only a large total amount of urinary bilirubin is significant and semi-quantitative dipstick results should be interpreted in light of the overall urine concentration and protein content. For example, 2+ bilirubin on a dipstick test of an isosthenuric urine sample is probably significant, but this same result is likely to be normal in a very concentrated urine sample. In addition, in dogs, the glomerular threshold for conjugated bilirubin is low and, as a consequence, bilirubinuria may be an early indicator of liver disease, i.e. prior to the onset of icterus. In contrast, cats have a higher renal threshold and feline bilirubinuria is always significant, and usually associated with overt jaundice.

Urobilinogen

Urobilinogen is synthesized from bile pigments by intestinal bacteria. Some is reabsorbed, most of which undergoes enterohepatic recycling and re-excretion in bile. However, about 20% passes the glomerulus. Thus, the presence of urobilinogen in urine is normal (although it is not always present) and a marker of enterohepatic recycling of bile (Figure 12.11). Increased amounts in the urine are associated with hyperbilirubinaemia, unless complete biliary obstruction is present, when urobilinogen will be absent. Although the test is found on most 'multi-test' urine dipsticks, its usefulness in any icteric patient is minimal because severe bilirubinuria frequently obscures any colour change on the dipstick test.

Urate crystalluria

Abnormal uric acid metabolism and hyperammonaemia in liver disease can result in precipitation of ammonium biurate crystals in the urine. Occasionally, massive crystalluria causes obvious brown turbidity (Figure 12.12a) but, most often, characteristic crystals are found by microscopic examination of urine sediment. The crystals resemble mites or thorn-apples (Figure 12.12b). Ammonium biurate crystals can be found on serial urinalyses in approximately two-thirds of dogs with congenital PSS. Amorphous urate and uric acid can also be found on sediment examination.

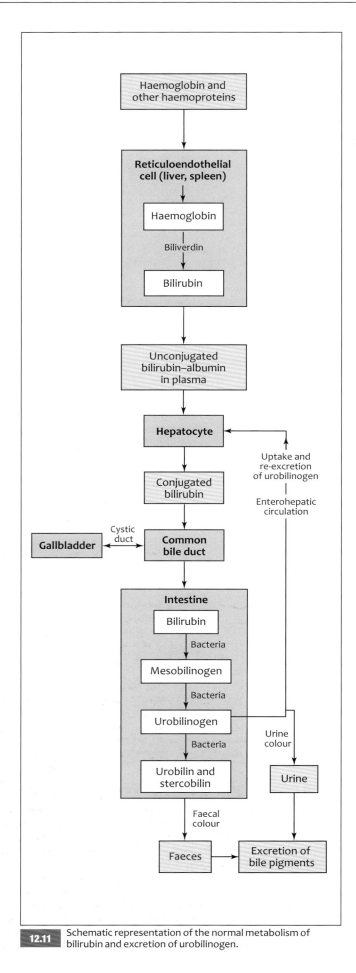

Haemoglobin and other haemoproteins

Reticuloendothelial cell (liver, spleen)

Haemoglobin

Biliverdin

Bilirubin

Unconjugated bilirubin–albumin in plasma

Hepatocyte

Conjugated bilirubin

Uptake and re-excretion of urobilinogen

Enterohepatic circulation

Gallbladder

Cystic duct

Common bile duct

Intestine

Bilirubin

Bacteria

Mesobilinogen

Bacteria

Urobilinogen

Bacteria

Urine colour

Urine

Urobilin and stercobilin

Faecal colour

Faeces

Excretion of bile pigments

12.11 Schematic representation of the normal metabolism of bilirubin and excretion of urobilinogen.

12.12 (a) Gross appearance of massive amounts of ammonium biurate crystals in urine from a dog with chronic hepatitis. (b) Microscopic appearance of urate crystals in urine sediment from a dog with a congenital portosystemic shunt. (Original magnification X400)

Liver function tests

Increases in liver marker enzymes do not necessarily correlate with the degree of liver damage and do not distinguish localized from diffuse disease. Therefore, they do not offer any information on overall liver function, and in cases of congenital PSS may actually be normal. In these situations specific tests are available to measure liver function.

Liver function tests may be crude markers of overall liver function, e.g. albumin synthesis and bilirubin excretion, or they may dynamically assess certain functional pathways in the liver, e.g. enterohepatic recycling of bile acids. The former are often adequate when hepatic dysfunction is severe, while the latter are useful in confirming the requirement for further investigation when clinical signs are equivocal. In the presence of jaundice, many dynamic liver function tests (e.g. bile acid assay) will invariably be abnormal, do not assist in identifying the disease process and do not need to be performed. Therefore, once haemolytic (prehepatic) jaundice has been ruled out, evidence of hyperbilirubinaemia is a specific marker of hepatobiliary dysfunction and no other function test is required.

Markers of liver function

Bilirubin

Hyperbilirubinaemia results in jaundice (icterus), which is the yellow discoloration of tissues by accumulated bile pigments. Jaundice may be indicative of liver disease, but can be caused by other conditions (Figure 12.13) and does not occur in all hepatic disorders. For example, it is *not* seen in congenital PSS or steroid hepatopathy and is only rarely seen in metastatic liver disease.

Clinically, jaundice is first and most readily detected in the white of the sclera when bilirubin concentrations exceed 25 μmol/l, because the human eye can only detect the yellow colour against pink mucous membranes at about 45 μmol/l. Similarly, hyperbilirubinaemia can be identified in separated serum at approximately 15 μmol/l, before clinical jaundice can be observed. Thus, chemical measurements of serum bilirubin are most sensitive, and should be carried out to detect incipient jaundice or to quantify the magnitude of overt hyperbilirubinaemia. Given its low renal threshold, bilirubinuria usually precedes

Dogs	Cats
Prehepatic	
Haemolytic anaemia: • Immune-mediated haemolytic anaemia • *Babesia* • Oxidant damage, e.g. onion poisoning and zinc toxicity	Haemolytic anaemia: • *Haemoplasma* • Immune-mediated haemolytic anaemia
Primary liver disease	
Acute hepatitis: • Drugs • Leptospirosis • Infectious canine hepatitis	Acute hepatitis
Chronic hepatitis and cirrhosis	Idiopathic hepatic lipidosis
Cholangitis: • Neutrophilic (suppurative)	Cholangitis: • Neutrophilic (suppurative) • Lymphocytic
Neoplasia: • Carcinoma • Lymphosarcoma	Neoplasia: • Lymphosarcoma • Mast cell tumour
Secondary liver disease	
Septicaemia and endotoxaemia	Feline infectious peritonitis Diabetes mellitus ± pancreatitis Toxoplasmosis Paracetamol (acetaminophen) Hyperthyroidism (rarely)
Posthepatic disease	
Extrahepatic biliary disease: • Common bile duct or gallbladder rupture • Obstruction by gallstones • Pancreatitis • Pancreatic carcinoma • Biliary carcinoma	Extrahepatic biliary disease Pancreatitis

12.13 Potential causes of jaundice in dogs and cats.

jaundice in dogs and can be the first sign of impending jaundice; the renal threshold is higher in cats and bilirubinuria is usually associated with obvious jaundice.

In order to understand jaundice, it is necessary to understand bilirubin metabolism (see Figure 12.11). Bilirubin is the major bile pigment and is a product of the degradation of haemoprotein from haemoglobin, myoglobin and haem-containing enzymes (e.g. cytochromes). The phagocytic cells of the mononuclear phagocyte system (MPS), particularly in the liver, spleen and bone marrow, engulf senescent and abnormal RBCs, and convert haemoglobin to bilirubin via biliverdin. Free bilirubin is insoluble in water and is carried in the plasma to hepatocytes, reversibly bound to albumin. Here it is taken up and, along with bilirubin produced within the hepatocytes, from intracellular haemoproteins, conjugated to bilirubin diglucuronide. Conjugation of bilirubin aids aqueous solubilization and excretion via the biliary canaliculi.

After biliary excretion and gallbladder storage, bile is passed to the intestine via the common bile duct. Bile pigment is converted by intestinal bacteria to a number of faecal pigments, including stercobilin, which produce the normal brown faecal colour (see Figure 12.11). The pigment urobilinogen is also produced (see above).

Hyperbilirubinaemia can be caused by three basic mechanisms (see Figure 12.13):

• Prehepatic causes: increased production of bilirubin exceeding the capacity for hepatic excretion
• Hepatic causes: abnormal uptake, conjugation or excretion by hepatocytes

• Posthepatic causes: obstruction of either intra- or extrahepatic biliary excretion or biliary tract rupture.

These three types of hyperbilirubinaemia can often be distinguished by a combination of other laboratory tests such as haematocrit, cholesterol, and hepatocellular and cholestatic marker enzymes, and other findings such as the ultrasonographic appearance of the extrahepatic biliary system.

Historically, the van den Bergh test, measuring the relative proportions of unconjugated (insoluble) and conjugated (soluble) bilirubin, was advocated for the differentiation of the types of jaundice. However, the results are unreliable and the test is *not* recommended. Even in haemolysis, which theoretically should lead to a rise in unconjugated bilirubin, there is consequent hepatocyte dysfunction, and the accumulation of conjugated bilirubin as well. The van den Bergh test is also unreliable, in part, because of the variable presence of bilirubin bound irreversibly to serum proteins.

This δ-bilirubin (biliprotein) is covalently bound to serum proteins and cannot be taken up by hepatocytes, so adding to the hyperbilirubinaemia. It is found in variable amounts, between 2 and 96% of circulating bilirubin. Its clearance is as slow as the turnover of albumin (i.e. half-life up to 3 weeks), and jaundice and hyperbilirubinaemia can occasionally persist well beyond the time of resolution of the disease that initially caused the jaundice. Such persistent jaundice, after clinical recovery, occurs most frequently in dogs with biliary obstruction caused by acute pancreatitis. Therefore, prolonged jaundice does not necessarily indicate persistent disease, and persistent hyperbilirubinaemia should be interpreted in the light of other clinical features.

Prehepatic jaundice: Increased production of bilirubin and consequent jaundice is almost invariably associated with severe haemolysis, and typically a low haematocrit is present. Mild hyperbilirubinaemia (often without clinically overt jaundice) may occur in some hyperthyroid cats, probably secondary to accelerated haemoprotein turnover in the cat's hypermetabolic state.

Increased bilirubin production may also occur during resorption of large haematomas, but is rarely sufficient to produce jaundice. Intracavitary haemorrhage (e.g. haemoperitoneum) does not produce jaundice because many RBCs (approximately 40%) are resorbed intact. Similarly, GI haemorrhage does not cause jaundice because the haemoglobin is metabolized by bacteria to non-absorbable porphyrins.

Immune-mediated haemolytic anaemia is the most common cause of prehepatic jaundice, although other non-immune causes of haemolysis occur (see Chapter 4). Given that the capacity of the liver for hepatic bilirubin processing is normally large, development of jaundice depends not only on haemolysis of a large number of RBCs, but also on the presence of concurrent hypoxic liver damage associated with the anaemia.

Initially, during haemolytic jaundice, the accumulated bilirubin is predominantly unconjugated, but conjugated bilirubin accumulates gradually. Spherocytosis and a positive Coombs' test support a diagnosis of immune-mediated haemolytic anaemia (see Chapter 4). The faeces may be orange-coloured (due to excess bilirubin excretion), significant bilirubinuria will be present and urinary urobilinogen in the urine will be increased. Hypoxia may cause some increase in liver-specific enzymes (ALT, AST) that may be misleading but, if the haematocrit is normal or there is only mild anaemia, any jaundice and liver enzyme elevations are **not** of haemolytic origin.

Hepatic jaundice: In primary liver disease, hepatocyte abnormalities affecting bilirubin uptake and conjugation usually coexist with intrahepatic cholestasis. Thus, increases in both hepatocellular and cholestatic enzymes associated with jaundice are highly suggestive of primary hepatic disease, although it should be remembered that enzymes may be increased in haemolytic anaemia and may not be increased in terminal cirrhosis.

Altered RBC integrity in liver diseases, and consequent increased destruction, may also contribute to the jaundice and, thus, both unconjugated and conjugated bilirubin may appear in the blood. Bilirubinuria and urobilinogen are expected on urinalysis.

Extrahepatobiliary disease can also cause cholestatic jaundice, but the exact mechanisms are poorly defined. Sepsis outside the hepatobiliary system can cause intrahepatic cholestasis and jaundice in dogs, probably through an effect of inflammatory cytokines and/or bacterial endotoxin. However, it is not clear how FIP causes jaundice.

Posthepatic jaundice: Posthepatic jaundice occurs with bile duct obstruction, often associated with pancreaticoduodenal disease. Extrahepatic bile duct obstruction is characterized by hyperbilirubinaemia in association with hypercholesterolaemia and increases in cholestatic enzymes of a magnitude greater than increases in hepatocellular enzymes. Lack of hypertriglyceridaemia in posthepatic jaundice helps narrow the differential diagnoses.

Although an increase in conjugated bilirubin alone might be expected because the defect in bilirubin excretion occurs after hepatocellular conjugation, this is rarely found because, by the time clinical signs occur, there is also bile salt-induced damage and significant dysfunction of hepatocyte conjugation mechanisms. Increased cholestatic markers (ALP, GGT) and hypercholesterolaemia are found. Urine urobilinogen is absent if obstruction is complete but it can be absent normally. Ultrasonographic examination of the biliary tree can be helpful in confirming the obstruction and identifying its cause.

Passage of acholic faeces, from which bile pigments are absent (Figure 12.14), is usually the result of persistent mechanical extrahepatic bile duct obstruction. In cats with severe cholangitis, obstruction is most commonly due to the accumulation of biliary sludge, but occasionally a clear viscous bile which lacks pigment is produced, resulting in acholic faeces even in the absence of obstruction.

Rupture of the biliary tract results in another form of posthepatic jaundice. It is either a result of trauma or

of spontaneous pathology (e.g. necrotizing cholecystitis, ruptured mucocoele or obstruction and perforation during passage of a gallstone), and leads to accumulation of bile in the peritoneal cavity (Figure 12.15). The severity of jaundice gradually increases as bile accumulates. Identification of bile peritonitis is discussed in Chapter 22.

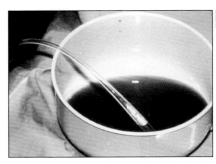

12.15 Abdominal fluid drained from a dog with bile peritonitis.

Serum proteins

Total concentrations of albumin and globulin offer crude indices of liver function, and hypoalbuminaemia is indicative of chronic disease. Serum protein electrophoresis offers some prognostic information, and may demonstrate increased acute phase protein synthesis associated with inflammatory hepatopathies, or may identify production of abnormal proteins in certain liver diseases.

Serum hyaluronic acid has been proposed as a marker of hepatic fibrosis but was not helpful in the diagnosis of PSS (Seki *et al.*, 2010). Liver autoantibodies (anti-nuclear antibody, anti-mitochondrial antibody) develop in human liver disease, and have been noted in canine chronic hepatitis. Their significance is not clear, and they are not routinely measured.

Coagulation times

The liver plays a central role in the coagulation and fibrinolytic systems, and subtle abnormalities may be detected by assay of individual factor activities. However, overall coagulation ability assessed by one-stage prothrombin time (OSPT or PT) and activated partial thromboplastin time (aPTT) (see Chapter 6) is usually only significantly prolonged in severe disease. While a bleeding diathesis should be expected if there is a history of GI bleeding, an occult bleeding tendency should always be suspected, and evaluation of coagulation is mandatory before a liver biopsy is performed. If coagulation times are prolonged, administration of vitamin K is indicated before retesting and biopsy.

As well as deficiencies of clotting factors and failure of vitamin K-dependent activation, bleeding tendencies in liver disease may also reflect increased fibrinolysis, demonstrable as increased fibrin degradation products (FDPs) and D-dimers, and platelet dysfunction, which is most easily assessed by determining the buccal mucosal bleeding time (BMBT; see Chapter 6). It is recommended that a BMBT is obtained prior to hepatic biopsy, because some studies have suggested that complications arise more commonly as a result of platelet dysfunction, rather than secondary (coagulation factor) haemostatic abnormalities. Thromboelastography may detect subtle changes in coagulation and fibrinolysis, although currently the clinical significance of a variety of detectable changes is not clear.

Bleeding can also occur because of acquired vitamin K deficiency in complete bile duct obstruction; absence

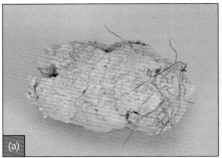
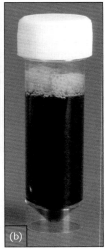

12.14 Extrahepatic bile duct obstruction. (a) Acholic faeces. Pale faeces lacking bile pigments from a dog with complete bile duct obstruction. (b) Massive bilirubinuria. Urine collected from the dog with complete bile duct obstruction that passed the acholic faeces in (a). Urinary urobilinogen is absent but the bilirubinuria obscures all dipstick test results.

of bile salts and intestinal malabsorption preclude uptake of this fat-soluble vitamin, particularly following antibiotic therapy when bacterial synthesis of vitamin K is impaired. Consequently, both PT and aPTT are abnormal. This problem has been reported in feline biliary disease and in feline exocrine pancreatic insufficiency. It appears to be a rarer feature of canine biliary disease, and in fact a hypercoagulable state has been demonstrated (Mayhew *et al.*, 2013).

Urea

Decreased serum concentrations of urea are sometimes seen in animals with PSS or severe liver dysfunction, as a consequence of failure to convert ammonia to urea. However, this marker is unreliable because the normal lower limit for serum urea concentration is close to the limit of sensitivity of the assay, and prolonged anorexia can produce very low urea concentrations.

Uric acid

Uric acid is an excretory metabolite of hepatic purine degradation, but increased serum uric acid concentration is rarely used as a marker of hepatic dysfunction. It has a sensitivity and specificity of 65 and 59%, respectively (Hill *et al.*, 2011). In contrast, the identification of urate crystalluria can suggest the presence of hepatic dysfunction (see Figure 12.12). However, uric acid also accumulates in dogs such as Dalmatians with inherited abnormalities of purine metabolism.

Ascites

The accumulation of free fluid in the peritoneal cavity can be indicative of liver disease. Mechanisms of fluid accumulation can be identified by diagnostic abdominocentesis and measurement of the protein and cellular content. Classification of the fluid as: transudate, protein-poor (transudate); transudate, protein-rich (modified transudate); or exudate can be helpful (see Chapter 22). Assessment of the serum–ascites albumin gradient can help in classification of the effusion (Pembleton-Corbett *et al.*, 2000), but this is not often calculated in veterinary species.

A pure transudate will accumulate if there is marked hypoalbuminaemia (i.e. albumin ≤15 g/l). However, liver disease in dogs and cats very rarely causes ascites by this mechanism alone, and consequently hydrothorax or subcutaneous oedema is rarely seen in liver disease. Ascites in liver disease usually arises through a combination of hypoalbuminaemia and portal hypertension, resulting in accumulation of a protein-rich (modified) transudate, although this is variable and sometimes the transudate may be low in protein, especially if the cause of the portal hypertension is presinusoidal.

The term *modified* transudate is a misnomer in liver disease, because the fluid is not necessarily 'modified' after formation. While modification of ascitic fluid by infection and inflammation can occur in liver disease, the fluid is more commonly a transudate that has developed secondary to increased hydrostatic pressure (i.e. portal hypertension). As hepatic sinusoids are highly permeable, the fluid entering the extracellular hepatic tissue spaces contains approximately 80% of serum proteins. Therefore, hepatic lymph is protein-rich and, when vessels are obstructed by intrahepatic causes or due to obstruction of blood flow between the liver and the heart, (posthepatic portal hypertension), it tends to accumulate as a protein-rich transudate. However, increased resistance in the extrahepatic portal vein, which is termed prehepatic portal hypertension (e.g. due to portal vein thrombosis, over-zealous PSS ligation) or simple hypoalbuminaemia will cause a typical low-protein transudate, although this can also be seen in some animals with chronic liver disease, including cirrhosis. A protein-rich transudate may indicate either primary hepatic disease or a 'posthepatic' problem, such as cardiac tamponade or right-sided heart failure, causing hepatic venous congestion and portal hypertension. The presence of a protein-rich cellular exudate is more suggestive of bacterial peritonitis. Protein-rich exudates are also seen in cats with lymphocytic cholangitis and FIP infection, which can be associated with jaundice, although these may not have high cell counts.

The presence of significant amounts of blood, chyle or urine in an abdominal effusion suggests extrahepatic disease. The presence of a bile-like fluid is consistent with bile peritonitis associated with rupture of the extrahepatic biliary tree. Although the patient is jaundiced as a result of bile peritonitis, the bilirubin concentration, if measured, is much greater in the peritoneal fluid than in the serum. However, the gross appearance of the abdominal effusion is generally sufficient to make a diagnosis of bile peritonitis (see Figure 12.15).

Dynamic liver function tests

Dynamic function tests rely on analysis of paired blood samples to assess the capacity of the liver to clear substances (e.g. bile acids, ammonia) from the circulation. Impaired clearance is suggestive of hepatocellular dysfunction and/or PSS, but does not differentiate the cause. Therefore, additional tests including portovenography, ultrasonography and biopsy are required. Dynamic tests are not useful if the patient is already icteric, as hyperbilirubinaemia is indicative of hepatic dysfunction. Scintigraphy is also a dynamic test that can be used to assess both hepatic MPS function and vascular shunting, but the need for radioisotopes and expensive equipment precludes its use in general practice.

Function tests often only interrogate one of the many functions of the liver; they may not identify focal disease, and do not necessarily give a global picture of all liver functions. For example, liver function is clearly abnormal in patients with congenital PSS, according to invariably abnormal serum bile acids (SBA), and yet the patient is rarely jaundiced. This suggests that bile acids are actually a better marker of hepatic blood flow, while bilirubin is a better indicator of hepatocyte function and biliary excretion.

Although an abnormal function test may provide an indication to perform a liver biopsy, biopsy may still be indicated despite a normal function test. For example, there may be hepatic neoplasia that must be sampled to obtain a definitive diagnosis, and yet there is still sufficient hepatic function that these tests are normal.

Endogenous metabolism tests

These tests assess the metabolic capacity of the liver to process endogenous metabolites, and are feasible for veterinary surgeons (veterinarians) in general practice.

Serum bile acids: Bile acids (bile salts) are a major constituent of bile, but are *not* the same as bile pigments (e.g. bilirubin). Fasting serum total bile acid concentration (FSBA) is a reflection of the enterohepatic circulation of bile acids (Figure 12.16). Bile acids are synthesized in the

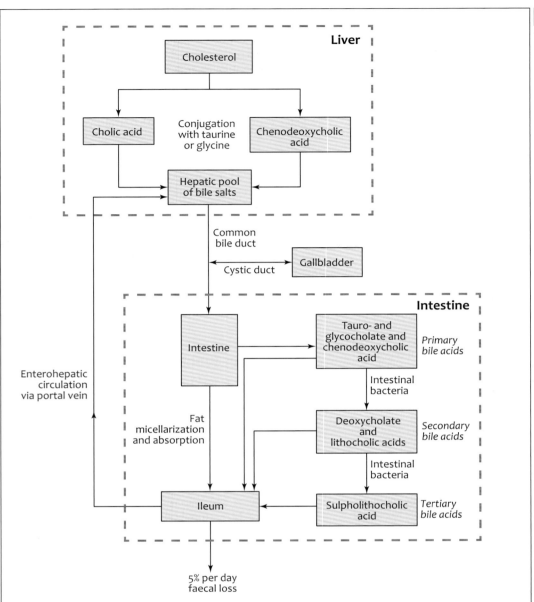

12.16 Schematic representation of the normal enterohepatic recycling of bile salts.

liver at a rate to compensate for small faecal losses, while the enterohepatic circulation maintains a larger pool of bile acids that is recycled several times per meal. Hepatic dysfunction and/or PSS permits increased amounts of bile acids to reach the systemic circulation, where such increases can be measured. Measurement of urinary bile acids has also been proposed as a test of liver function (see below).

Bile acids (cholic and chenodeoxycholic acids) are synthesized in the liver from cholesterol, and are conjugated, predominantly with taurine, before biliary secretion as salts. Conjugated bile acids are ionized at the pH of the intestinal lumen and are lipid insoluble, preventing their absorption through the intestinal mucosa. Only when fat absorption, facilitated through micellarization, has been completed are bile acids reabsorbed via specific receptors in the ileum. Some of the primary bile acids (cholic and chenodeoxycholic acids) are metabolized by intestinal bacteria to secondary bile acids (deoxycholic and lithocholic acids) and even tertiary bile acids (sulpholithocholic acid) before

reabsorption, and about 5% escape recycling and are lost in the faeces, to be replaced by *de novo* synthesis. On return to the liver, bile acids are efficiently removed from the portal blood by hepatocytes and are re-excreted.

Commercial bile acid assays measure total concentrations and do not distinguish among primary, secondary and tertiary bile acids. In the future, fractionation of SBA into specific acids may have diagnostic utility in the identification of specific hepatopathies. Measurement of unconjugated bile acids has been suggested as a test of intestinal bacterial metabolism (see Chapter 13), but results have not been helpful.

The rate of synthesis and the size and distribution of the bile acid pool can be abnormal in liver disease if there is:

- A reduction in hepatocellular mass
- Impaired hepatocyte function
- Disturbed enterohepatic circulation, including:
  - Impairment of bile flow from the liver
  - Disruption of the flow of portal blood to the liver.

Thus, SBA can be abnormal if hepatic function is sub-optimal, if there is a PSS or if biliary obstruction occurs, and increases in SBA are *not* specific for certain disease types. Increases will be present in extrahepatic bile duct obstruction as well as primary liver disease and congenital PSS. SBA are most valuable for the detection of PSS and chronic hepatitis/cirrhosis before the development of jaundice.

The bile acid test is simple and sensitive and is readily available to veterinary practitioners. However, given that secondary hepatopathies can increase SBA (often up to ~50 μmol/l, and very occasionally up to 100 μmol/l), the specificity for detecting primary hepatic diseases is not good. Using the upper limit of their laboratory reference intervals (20 μmol/l), Ruland *et al.* (2010) showed a sensitivity and specificity for the diagnosis of PSS of 93% and 67% in dogs, and 100% and 71% in cats, respectively, compared with healthy animals; specificity is inevitably poorer if patients with other hepatopathies are tested.

The sensitivity of the test is improved by measurement of a 2-hour postprandial SBA concentration (PPSBA). Ingestion of food causes release of bile through stimulation of gallbladder contraction, and increases the amount of bile acids available for enterohepatic recycling. Thus, dynamic bile acids (i.e. the bile acid stimulation test) provides a safe endogenous test of hepatic function.

The value of the PPSBA measurement is debated. In cholestasis, FSBA concentrations can be high and often do not increase much postprandially, whereas some patients with PSS have normal FSBA and massively abnormal PPSBA concentrations. Owing to the repeated enterohepatic recycling of bile acids, the exact timing of the PPSBA sample is not absolutely critical, but confusing decreases in the postprandial sample are sometimes found. Possible explanations include inherent variability, failure to store all new bile in the gallbladder, random gallbladder contraction, incomplete gallbladder contraction on feeding, and intestinal bacterial metabolism. The general recommendation is to assign significance to the higher of the two results.

Bile acids can be most accurately measured by radio-immunoassay but, in most veterinary laboratories, enzymatic fluorimetric or spectrophotometric methods are used, and these may not be as accurate. Poor laboratory technique as well as haemolysis and lipaemia can produce spurious results. Reference ranges for bile acids are somewhat controversial, not only because of methodological problems in some laboratories, but because of the effect of secondary hepatopathies. The initial criteria of <5 μmol FSBA and <10 μmol PPSBA when this test was validated may be too stringent and, in clinical practice, normal individuals can sometimes have bile acid concentrations that are double these concentrations. Furthermore, the presence of microvascular dysplasia cannot be excluded in clinically healthy dogs without liver biopsy. Specificity is improved by increasing the upper limit of the reference range, but at the expense of sensitivity. Concentrations above 25 μmol/l, for both FSBA and PPSBA, correlate with the presence of histological lesions although, in some cases, these may still be secondary hepatopathies.

A FSBA concentration of >50 μmol/l is usually taken as good evidence of primary hepatic dysfunction and a need to perform further tests, such as a biopsy, unless an underlying disease can be identified. The magnitude of the FSBA once it exceeds ~100 μmol/l apparently has little predictive value for the severity of any particular hepatopathy, and some cases of PSS have normal FSBA and massively raised (>1000 μmol/l) PPSBA.

The interpretation of FSBA concentrations between 20 and 50 μmol/l is a grey area, and recommendations for these patients are to:

- Look for extrahepatic disease
- Repeat FSBA with a PPSBA and look for at least a 2-fold increase
- Repeat FSBA in 2–4 weeks

or

- If clinical signs and other results suggest primary liver disease, carry out other investigations.

Urinary bile acids: Measurement of urinary bile acids has also been proposed as a test of liver function in dogs and cats because, in theory, it provides an assessment of the cumulative production and excretion of bile acids. Results are normalized as the bile acid:creatinine ratio to correct for the effects of urine dilution. However, the test is not in common usage.

Plasma ammonia and ammonia tolerance test: Ammonia, produced by intestinal bacteria, is normally cleared from the portal blood by the liver: normal portal blood contains up to 350 μmol/l ammonia, but <50 μmol/l enters the systemic circulation from the liver. Increased resting plasma ammonia concentration is evidence of hepatic dysfunction and/or PSS (Figure 12.17). Very rarely, hyperammonaemia is caused by an abnormality in the urea cycle. This may be either due to a genetic defect or secondary to cobalamin deficiency, which can impair enzyme activity in the urea cycle (Battersby *et al.*, 2005). In these circumstances, SBA will be normal.

Sample storage increases the ammonia content of blood and, to produce meaningful results, plasma must be harvested on ice and ammonia concentration assayed within 30 minutes. Although dry chemistry ammonia tests are available in veterinary practice, the results are frequently unreliable. Therefore, measurement of plasma ammonia should be limited to institutions and practices with immediate access to a wet chemistry analyser.

The severity of hepatic encephalopathy correlates crudely with the degree of hyperammonaemia, and so it is a reasonable marker for the condition, although the clinical signs of encephalopathy can develop secondary to the accumulation of other toxic metabolites. Fasting blood ammonia concentration only provides a relatively insensitive measure of hepatic function, because resting concentrations are frequently normal in patients with liver disease, including some with PSS. Using the upper limit of their laboratory reference intervals (59 μmol/l), Ruland *et al.* (2010) showed the sensitivity and specificity for the diagnosis of PSS to be 85% and 86% in dogs, and 83% and 76% in cats, respectively.

The sensitivity of the test can be improved by performing an ammonia tolerance test (ATT), administering exogenous ammonia, either orally or *per rectum*, to determine whether ammonia intolerance exists. Ammonium chloride is usually administered (100 mg/kg; maximum 3 g) by either stomach tube or enema, and a blood sample is taken 30 minutes later. Plasma ammonia concentration does not increase significantly in normal patients; marked increases are seen in PSS. The oral ATT is quite sensitive and will detect PSS, but is not able to detect subtle hepatic dysfunction. It can cause vomiting and can be potentially dangerous in patients, especially cats, that are already encephalopathic.

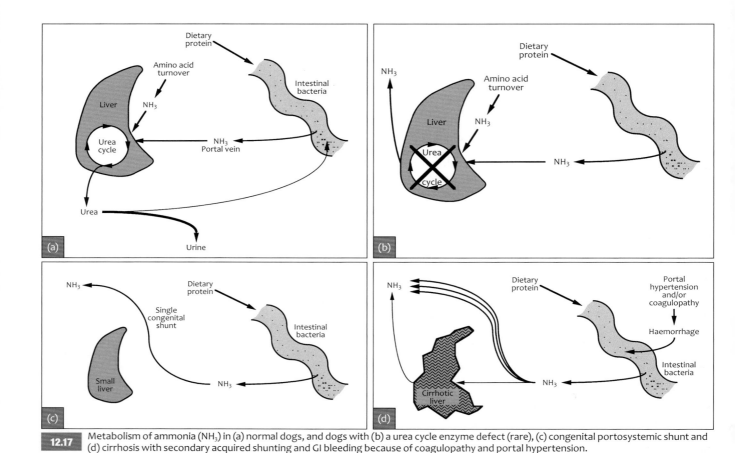

12.17 Metabolism of ammonia (NH$_3$) in (a) normal dogs, and dogs with (b) a urea cycle enzyme defect (rare), (c) congenital portosystemic shunt and (d) cirrhosis with secondary acquired shunting and GI bleeding because of coagulopathy and portal hypertension.

The rectal ATT has the advantage over the oral ATT of not provoking immediate vomiting, but the absorption of ammonia is more variable and plasma samples must be collected at 20 and 40 minutes. Further, the colon must first be prepared by enema and, since the results are less sensitive, this method is rarely used. Measurement of postprandial ammonia (6 hours after a meal) has been advocated as a safer test of ammonia tolerance (Walker et al., 2001). It is sensitive for detecting congenital PSS but not for hepatocellular disease.

Exogenous metabolism tests

These tests use exogenously administered substances (e.g. aminopyrine, caffeine, lidocaine) to detect dysfunction of specific metabolic pathways, either by using labelled tracer compounds or by the measurement of novel products. However, none is used in general practice.

Exogenous excretion tests

The bromosulphthalein (BSP) and indocyanine green (ICG) retention tests measure the excretion of exogenous dyes administered intravenously, but are of historical interest having been superseded by dynamic bile acid measurements.

Genetic testing

Canine chronic hepatitis and feline lymphocytic cholangitis show significant breed associations, e.g. with Dobermanns, Cocker Spaniels and Labrador Retrievers, and Persian cats, respectively. In the future, specific genetic tests may be available. For copper hepatotoxicosis of Bedlington Terriers, there is a commercial test for a mutation in the COMMD-1 (formerly MURR-1) gene, although suspicion remains that there may be a second gene involved (see Chapter 30).

Liver biopsy

Indications and techniques

While a tentative diagnosis of liver disease can often be deduced from the results of laboratory tests, in conjunction with a variety of imaging techniques, a definitive diagnosis of specific primary liver diseases usually depends on histological examination of biopsy specimens. Hopefully, extrahepatic causes of secondary liver disease will have been identified before biopsy is considered, but the finding of a 'vacuolar hepatopathy' is an indication that an underlying disease may have been missed. Indications for liver biopsy include:

- Persistent elevations of liver enzymes with no apparent underlying disease
- Increased FSBA or PPSBA without imaging evidence of a single PSS
- Altered liver size or ultrasonographic architecture without imaging evidence of a single PSS
- Progressive signs of liver disease, e.g. continuing poor appetite and weight loss, or the development of ascites or jaundice.

Cytology

It is possible to perform cytological examination of liver cells either by fine-needle aspiration (FNA) or by a touch preparation of a liver biopsy specimen (see Chapter 21). However, the accuracy of cytology, even when ultrasound-guided, is limited (Wang *et al.*, 2004; Bahr *et al.*, 2013). There is only 30% and 50% agreement between the cytological and histopathological diagnoses in canine and feline liver diseases, respectively. Ultrasound-guided cytology, in particular, is relatively accurate for the diagnosis of primary and metastatic neoplastic disease and for the recognition of vacuolar hepatopathies, although it will not often identify the cause of the vacuolation. However, the absence of the architectural structure of the liver in cytological specimens prevents an accurate diagnosis of chronic inflammatory diseases. Thus, cytology is best reserved for suspected cases of neoplasia and hepatic lipidosis, or if there is likely to be a delay in obtaining a histopathological diagnosis. The value of checking a coagulation profile before performing cytology is debated, as significant bleeding is rare after FNA and results correlate poorly with any tendency to bleed.

There are many causes of vacuolar hepatopathies (Figure 12.18) and, therefore, the cytological finding of enlarged cells with vacuolated cytoplasm may not be of diagnostic value in dogs. Small foamy vacuoles may indicate glycogen accumulation, e.g. in steroid hepatopathy. Numerous larger discrete vacuoles in enlarged hepatocytes are highly suggestive of hepatic lipidosis in cats (Figure 12.19a), although this may be secondary to underlying primary disease in the liver such as inflammation and metabolic abnormalities or disease elsewhere such as pancreatitis.

The presence of intranuclear inclusion bodies is considered to be diagnostic of infectious canine hepatitis (Figure 12.20), but this cytological examination is usually only performed post-mortem. Copper hepatotoxicosis (in Bedlington Terriers and other dog breeds) can be identified by staining FNA for copper granules with rubeanic acid, but histopathological staining and biochemical quantitation of copper content are necessary to avoid false negatives.

Canine inflammatory liver disease cannot be diagnosed reliably by cytology: differentiation of chronic hepatitis and cirrhosis cannot be made because observation of the tissue architecture is needed. Similarly, it is not usually possible to diagnose cholangitis in cats without solid biopsy.

Infiltration with malignant cells may be detected by FNA in primary and metastatic liver disease: malignant hepatic neoplasia, haemopoietic neoplasia (lymphoma, mast cell tumour) and disseminated metastatic neoplasia may all be diagnosed cytologically.

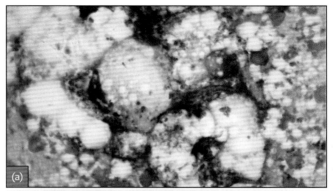
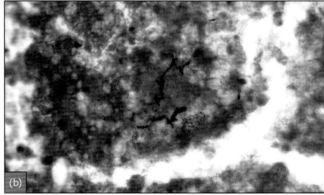
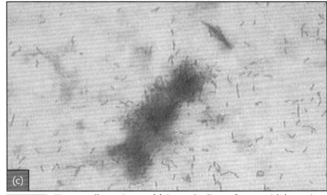

12.19 Fine-needle aspirates. (a) From the liver of a cat with hepatic lipidosis, showing foamy vacuolated hepatocytes. (Original magnification X1000). (b) From the liver of a dog with intrahepatic cholestasis, showing hepatocyte vacuolation and darkly staining bile plugs. (Original magnification X500). (c) From the gallbladder of a dog with cholecystitis showing bacterbilia. (Original magnification X1000)
(a, Courtesy of Marta Costa, Langford Veterinary Services; b, Courtesy of Kathleen Tennant, Langford Veterinary Services; c, Courtesy of Emma O'Neil, University College Dublin)

- Chronic infections and systemic inflammation:
  - Abscesses
  - Pyelonephritis
  - Severe dental disease
- Diabetes mellitus
- Haemolytic anaemia
- Hepatic lipidosis (cats)
- Hyperadrenocorticism (dogs)
- Hyperlipidaemia
- Hyperthyroidism (cats)
- Intestinal inflammation including idiopathic inflammatory bowel disease
- Neoplasia
- Pancreatitis
- Right-sided heart failure
- Shock
- Treatment with glucocorticoids (dogs)

12.18 Some causes of vacuolar hepatopathy in dogs and cats.

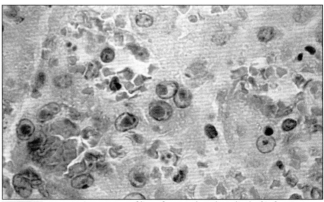

12.20 Impression smear of liver from a dog that died of infectious canine hepatitis, showing characteristic intranuclear inclusions. (Haematoxylin and eosin stain; original magnification X400)

Histopathology

Liver biopsy specimens for histopathological examination can be collected by a number of methods, but a coagulation profile and BMBT are recommended before biopsy because of the dangers of potential haemorrhage. In practice, liver biopsy is often limited to wedge biopsy at exploratory coeliotomy. The techniques used are described in detail in the *BSAVA Manual of Canine and Feline Gastroenterology*.

Percutaneous biopsy techniques provide a core of tissue, and are safest if performed under ultrasonographic guidance. The main limitation of percutaneous biopsy is the size of the specimen collected, which can be inadequate for making an accurate histopathological diagnosis. Indeed, the diagnostic accuracy of two needle biopsies has been shown to be less than 50% when compared with surgical biopsy, and therefore multiple needle biopsies are required. Laparoscopic biopsy is now considered best practice because focal lesions can be examined directly, larger biopsy samples obtained and excessive bleeding identified. The main limitations of laparoscopy include the cost, as well as a lack of availability of equipment and expertise.

In addition to histological examination, tissue specimens should be submitted for culture. However, both Gram staining of tissue and routine culture are insensitive. Bile, obtained by cholecystocentesis (at surgery or under ultrasound guidance), can be used for cytology and culture to try to identify cholecystitis (see Figure 12.19c). Percutaneous cholecystocentesis is relatively safe but should not be performed in cases of biliary obstruction because persistent leakage and bile peritonitis may occur. Bacterial culture of bile is more often positive than culture of a paired tissue sample. Furthermore, fluorescent *in situ* hybridization (FISH) of the samples is more sensitive and is now available commercially, enabling previously unidentified organisms to be demonstrated: leptospires can be identified in liver tissue even when they are not detectable using Gram staining.

A number of stains, in addition to routine haematoxylin and eosin, are available to facilitate characterization of hepatic pathology (Figure 12.21). However, the clinician needs to work with the pathologist, providing all the relevant historical, clinical and clinicopathological information, so that appropriate stains are used and a relevant diagnosis reached. Pieces of hepatic tissue about the size of 1 cm cubes are required for accurate determination of hepatic copper content by atomic absorption spectrophotometry; formalin-fixed tissue can be used.

Pattern recognition in liver disease

Apart from liver biopsy and identification of PSS (i.e. by portovenography or ultrasonography), there is rarely any one test that provides a definitive diagnosis in liver disease. Laboratory tests are only capable of identifying suspected liver disease, but particular patterns of clinicopathological abnormalities, when interpreted in light of the clinical findings, can often provide a high index of suspicion of specific diseases. The characteristic clinicopathological features of certain conditions are described below and summarized in Figure 12.22. However, while pattern recognition can assist the diagnostic approach, all results must be interpreted in light of the clinical picture. In this regard, laboratory artefacts may produce abnormal results, and laboratory errors may occur. The bile acid assay can be problematic, and some dry chemistry analysers are inaccurate, especially when measuring ammonia. Further, if poor quality or unsuitable samples are presented to the laboratory, the results may be inaccurate and misleading. Some of the common artefacts are summarized in Figure 12.23.

Primary hepatopathies

Benign nodular hyperplasia

A common incidental finding in old dogs, nodular hyperplasia is usually considered to have no significant effect on overall liver function. However, there can be a marked rise in serum ALP with minimal changes in ALT. In this situation the major differential diagnosis would be hyperadrenocorticism because there may be hepatomegaly but no

Feature	Special stain
Amyloid	Congo red
Bacteria	Gram, Ziehl–Neelsen Fluorescent *in situ* hybridization (FISH)
Bile	Fouchet's, van Gieson
Collagen	Masson's trichrome, van Gieson
Copper	Rhodanine, rubeanic acid
Copper-associated protein	Orcein
Elastin	Elastic van Gieson, Weigert's
Fibrin, fibrinoid	Martius scarlet blue (MSB)
Glycogen	Periodic acid–Schiff (PAS) diastase positive Best's carmine, Bauer–Feulgen (frozen tissue)
Iron (ferric)	Perl's Prussian blue
Lipid	Oil-red-O (frozen tissue)
Lipofuscin	Schmorl, Ziehl–Neelsen
Reticulin	Reticulin stain

12.21 Some of the special stains available for the characterization of hepatic histopathological changes.

Condition	ALT	ALP	Bilirubin	FSBA	PPSBA	Ammonia
Acute hepatitis	++ to +++	+ to ++	N to +++	N to ++	N to ++	N to ++
Chronic hepatitis	+ to +++	+ to ++	N to ++	N to ++	N to ++	N to ++
Cirrhosis	N to ++	N to ++	N to +++	+ to +++	+ to +++	N to ++
Congenital PSS	N to +	N to +	N	N to ++	++ to +++	+ to +++
Non-obstructive biliary disease	N to ++	+ to +++	N	N	N	N
EHBDO	N to ++	+++	++ to +++	++ to +++	++ to +++	N
Hepatic neoplasia	N to ++	N to ++	N to +	N to +	N to +	N to +

12.22 Typical patterns of clinicopathological results in liver disease. + = mild increase; ++ = moderate increase; +++ = marked increase; ALP = alkaline phosphatase; ALT = alanine aminotransferase; EHBDO = extrahepatic bile duct obstruction; FSBA = fasting serum total bile acid concentration; N = normal; PPSBA = postprandial serum bile acid concentration, PSS = congenital portosystemic shunt.

Analyte	False increase	False decrease
Bilirubin[a]	Severe haemolysis Lipaemia	Ultraviolet light Viscous serum (dry chemistry)
Bile acids	Hypertriglyceridaemia Increased serum dehydrogenases	Severe chylomicronaemia Haemolysis
Ammonia	Delayed assay Strenuous exercise Dry chemistry analyser	
ALT	Severe haemolysis Lipaemia	
AST	Severe haemolysis Lipaemia Ketosis	
ALP	Jaundice Lipaemia Storage (haemolysis)	Fluoride–oxalate Citrate EDTA
GGT	Lipaemia Fluoride–oxalate	

12.23 Potential laboratory artefacts affecting liver test results. The effects are variable with different analysers and different biochemical methods. [a] Severe hyperbilirubinaemia precludes measurement of serum creatinine by colorimetric assays, and obscures colour changes on urine dipsticks. ALP = alkaline phosphatase; ALT = alanine aminotransferase; AST = aspartate aminotransferase; EDTA = ethylenediamine tetra-acetic acid; GGT = γ-glutamyl transferase.

other signs consistent with liver disease. Nodular hyperplasia may, therefore, explain occasional cases where hyperadrenocorticism is suspected because of increased ALP and hepatomegaly, but the endocrine status is normal on dynamic hormone testing.

Feline idiopathic hepatic lipidosis

Massive fatty infiltration of the liver in cats is associated with marked hepatic dysfunction with increased FSBA and jaundice. In theory, cholestatic markers should be increased, but interestingly there is often an increase in ALP but no significant rise in GGT. The reason for this unique discrepancy between ALP and GGT is not understood. Nonetheless, differential increases in these two enzymes can provide useful diagnostic information, and it is worth running both tests whenever a hepatopathy is suspected in cats. The diagnosis of hepatic lipidosis can be confirmed by hepatic biopsy, although biopsy is potentially dangerous when cats are presented in a critical situation and FNA cytology may be sufficient for a diagnosis (see Figure 12.19).

Congenital portosystemic shunts

Given the absence of hepatic inflammation and cholestasis in most cases of congenital PSS, liver enzyme concentrations are often only mildly increased or can even be normal. Haematology quite frequently shows microcytic anaemia and poikilocytosis (see Figure 12.10a); urate crystalluria (see Figure 12.12) may be found.

Shunting and hepatic bypass is characterized by increased FSBA and/or PPSBA; a typical 'shunt pattern', with normal FSBA and markedly increased PPSBA, has been described. Hyperammonaemia and/or ammonia in-tolerance may also be seen. Serum urea, albumin, cholesterol and occasionally glucose may all be decreased. A decline in albumin may indicate a poorer prognosis, but can also be caused by severe dietary protein restriction used in an attempt to control hepatoencephalopathy.

Portal vein hypoplasia/microvascular dysplasia

Microvascular anomalies within the canine liver, in the absence of a single congenital PSS, are considered to be a consequence of portal vein hypoplasia. However, this may be a spectrum of conditions, with complete aplasia of the portal vein being the most extreme and lethal example.

At the mild end of the spectrum there may be no or just subtle clinical signs. This condition has also been termed microvascular dysplasia, and is most commonly reported in terrier breeds. Its only real significance is that dynamic bile acid testing is abnormal and may lead to a suspicion of a PSS, yet none can be found on imaging.

More severe portal vein hypoplasia is believed to lead to progressive hepatic fibrosis without overt inflammation, and is seen in young dogs of certain breeds, e.g. Standard Poodles, German Shepherd Dogs, Rottweilers. It has been termed juvenile hepatic fibrosis and non-cirrhotic portal hypertension. It can lead to the classic signs of end-stage liver disease with jaundice, ascites and hepatoencephalopathy. Liver function tests are abnormal, particularly when secondary acquired shunts develop because of portal hypertension, and there are increases in liver enzymes and decreases in urea.

Acute hepatitis and hepatic necrosis

Acute inflammatory conditions (whether due to toxic or infectious causes) usually cause rapid, moderate to marked increases in ALT (see Figures 12.3 and 12.4). Other hepatocellular enzymes are likely to be increased, but rises in AST and arginase activity may be indicative of more severe damage. Intrahepatic cholestasis, caused by hepatocyte swelling, induces a rise in ALP and GGT, but more slowly. Depending on the severity of the hepatic damage, there will be variable impairment of bile acid circulation, and in severe cases hyperbilirubinaemia will follow. Marked hypoalbuminaemia is not a feature because of the acute nature of the condition, but a mild negative acute phase response may be seen.

Chronic hepatitis

Histopathological assessment of liver tissue is usually required to differentiate specific types of chronic hepatitis; clinicopathological testing merely provides evidence of persistent damage and dysfunction, identifying the need for biopsy. In most disorders, moderate to severe and persistent increases in ALT (or AST) and ALP (or GGT) are characteristic (see Figure 12.5). The absolute activities can fluctuate spontaneously, and the clinician should not assume that a decrease in enzyme activity at a single timepoint is necessarily indicative of clinical improvement. Similarly, the magnitude of any change in bile acids is not indicative in a change in the severity of the disease; for example, a decrease from 500 to 400 μmol/l is not necessarily a sign that the liver is recovering.

Liver biopsy is indicated if there are persistent increases in enzyme activity and/or bile acids. Jaundice suggests significant hepatic impairment and may herald the development of cirrhosis. Late in the disease, serum albumin is likely to be decreased and this may be a poor prognostic indicator.

Cirrhosis

Hepatic fibrosis and nodular regeneration in cirrhosis, the end result of various forms of chronic hepatitis, are associated with significant hepatic dysfunction as demonstrated by increased SBA and eventually jaundice. Hypoalbuminaemia, low blood urea and, ultimately, coagulopathies and ascites may develop, and animals often develop multiple secondary (acquired) PSS.

Hypoglycaemia is a marker for end-stage cirrhosis, and is a poor prognostic indicator. Serum protein electrophoresis may demonstrate hypoalbuminaemia and decreases in acute phase proteins. Serum enzyme activities may be increased, but can be normal if there is no active inflammation or very little hepatocellular tissue remains (see Figure 12.5).

Primary hepatic neoplasia

Primary hepatocellular tumours may be associated with increases in ALT and/or ALP, depending on the presence of associated inflammation/necrosis and/or intrahepatic cholestasis. Biliary carcinomas may cause increases in ALP and obstructive jaundice, and occasionally increased serum albumin; other tumours cause jaundice infrequently. Hypoglycaemia has been noted with large hepatomas, but many are clinicopathologically 'silent'.

Metastatic liver disease

In primary hepatic or metastatic haemangiosarcoma there may be minimal increases in enzyme activity despite extensive tumour infiltration. Presentation with haemoperitoneum, and haematological abnormalities such as mild anaemia (which may be regenerative) and an inflammatory leucogram are more commonly seen; schistocytes are sometimes observed. None of these findings is specific for primary hepatic or metastatic disease. Focal metastatic disease is best detected ultrasonographically and confirmed by FNA or biopsy because many, particularly older, animals will have areas of increased or decreased echogenicity due to pathology other than neoplasia, such as nodular hyperplasia.

Hepatic lymphoma

Enzyme elevation is an unreliable indicator of hepatic involvement in lymphoma, but hepatomegaly, other clinical signs of lymphoma, increases in bile acids and, sometimes, hypercalcaemia are usually enough to indicate the need for FNA or, if required, biopsy.

Cholangitis

In dogs, cholangitis and associated cholecystitis appear to be most commonly associated with ascending infection, and an inflammatory leucogram may be seen. Increases in ALT as well as ALP suggest extension of the inflammation into the hepatic parenchyma, in addition to intrahepatic cholestasis. The presence of gallbladder sludge, detected ultrasonographically, in cats is associated with increased liver enzymes and hyperbilirubinaemia (Harran et al., 2011).

Cholecystitis may be suspected from ultrasonographic changes in the gallbladder wall and cytological and microbiological examination of bile. A diagnosis of cholangitis may be suspected if cholecystitis is present, but it is confirmed by histological examination of liver biopsy tissue, supported by bacteriological culture of bile and/or liver tissue.

Lymphocytic cholangitis is the other major form of cholangitis and is not uncommon in cats. Increases in liver enzymes and liver dysfunction are expected; occasionally lymphocytosis is seen. Sometimes protein-rich ascitic fluid is present, and the major differential diagnosis would be FIP.

Gallbladder mucocoele

A diagnosis of a gallbladder mucocoele is made on its ultrasonographic appearance, and histology after cholecystectomy. It is typically associated with marked increases (100-fold) in the serum activity of cholestatic enzymes, although it is not always clear whether this is primary or occurs because there is concurrent cholangitis or another hepatopathy present (Malek et al., 2013). There may also be an association with hyperadrenocorticism.

Extra-hepatic bile duct obstruction

Bile duct obstruction is classically associated with jaundice, hypercholesterolaemia and increased ALP; increases in hepatocellular marker enzymes are often smaller in magnitude. Initially, obstruction is associated with increases in ALP and GGT but, if persistent, bilirubinuria and then hyperbilirubinaemia develop. The onset of obstruction is gradual if caused by biliary and pancreatic tumours or by chronic inflammatory lesions. Acute pancreatitis can also cause temporary, acute bile duct obstruction with elevated bile acids; any onset of jaundice is often sudden and may be preceded by the more typical signs of pancreatitis. Abnormalities in hepatic parameters will reflect not only the bile duct obstruction but also toxic hepatic changes secondary to pancreatic inflammation (see Chapter 14). In cases of biliary obstruction, ultrasonographic examination can be very helpful in determining a cause before exploratory surgery.

Secondary hepatopathies
Reactive hepatopathies

The circulation of cytokines and toxins produced by diseases elsewhere in the body can produce a range of clinicopathological changes that are easily misinterpreted by the unwary as markers of primary liver disease. The most extreme example is cholestasis and jaundice in sepsis, but **any** infectious or inflammatory disease (see Figure 12.18) can produce increases in both hepatocellular and cholestatic marker enzymes. Something as apparently innocuous as marked periodontal disease is sufficient to cause 2–3-fold increases in ALT and ALP. In these situations, overall liver function is rarely impaired, and dynamic function tests (e.g. bile acids) are either within the reference range or only very slightly elevated. Similarly, there is no permanent histological change, and biopsy samples typically show only vacuolar changes.

Metabolic/hormonal diseases

Various hormonal and metabolic diseases cause secondary hepatopathies. Vacuolar hepatopathies with accumulation of lipid (e.g. diabetes mellitus, feline idiopathic hepatic lipidosis) or glycogen (e.g. hyperadrenocortism) can cause increases in liver enzymes, but usually overall hepatic function is minimally impaired. Feline hyperthyroidism is often associated with increased serum liver enzyme activities. Identification of the primary disorder usually precludes the need to investigate the liver even if mild increases in SBA are found.

Drugs

Toxic hepatopathies may be associated with increases in hepatocellular or cholestatic enzyme markers, if hepatocellular damage or cholestasis, respectively, is present. Drugs such as barbiturate anticonvulsants induce production of 2–5-fold increases in ALP/GGT and, to a lesser extent, can induce synthesis of ALT. Figure 12.7 lists some of the more important known or suspected hepatotoxic drugs that can cause increases in ALT in dogs and cats. Dogs with epilepsy on chronic primidone or phenobarbital therapy sometimes develop chronic hepatitis and cirrhosis. However, as barbiturates regularly induce liver enzymes, increased serum enzyme activities cannot be considered an indication of active liver damage. Such dogs should have liver function monitored by dynamic bile acid testing every 6 months.

Glucocorticoids

In dogs, both endogenous and exogenous glucocorticoids induce an increase in ALP/GGT, with minimal increases in ALT/AST. However, cats appear to be resistant to these changes. The response in individual dogs is quite variable (ranging from none to 30-fold), but can persist for at least 6 weeks after the administration of even a single dose of steroid in some individuals. When severe steroid hepatopathy is present, moderate increases in ALT may develop but the increase is generally disproportionate to the magnitude of the increase in ALP. There may be mild hepatic impairment and mild to moderate increases in SBA (50–70 µmol/l, very occasionally reaching as high as 100 µmol/l), but jaundice is exceptionally rare. There may also be hyperglycaemia and hypercholesterolaemia. If there is no history of exogenous steroid administration (and topical steroids should not be discounted), dynamic hormone tests for hyperadrenocorticism (see Chapter 18) should be considered if the clinical signs are compatible with the diagnosis.

Summary

In summary, there are a variety of markers of hepatic pathology with variable sensitivity and specificity. At a minimum, measurement of ALT, ALP and FSBA should be performed in suspected liver disease, and these will identify most conditions. However, imaging and, ultimately, liver biopsy (after a coagulation profile) will be needed to reach a definitive diagnosis.

Prognostic indices

As well as identifying and helping to characterize hepatopathies, laboratory testing can provide some prognostic information.

Good prognostic signs

- Decreasing hyperbilirubinaemia.
- Decreasing liver enzymes. With resolution of an acute hepatic insult, ALT should fall by approximately 50% every 3–4 days in the dog, and even more quickly in cats. Initially increasing ALT may indicate regeneration rather than continued hepatocyte damage. ALP may continue to rise after the injury as a result of enzyme induction and can take several weeks to normalize (see Figure 12.4).
- Normoglycaemia.
- Normal coagulation times and BMBT.
- Increases in serum albumin not due to dehydration. In inflammatory disease, albumin is frequently subnormal as a negative acute phase response, but serum protein electrophoresis at that time will show normal to elevated haptoglobin and alpha-1 antitrypsin. This is a good prognostic sign.
- Increasing cholesterol concentration (if previously low).

Poor prognostic signs

- Increases in AST as well as ALT, suggesting more severe hepatocellular damage.
- Persistent elevation of ALT and AST, indicative of continuing damage.
- Hypoglycaemia and prolonged PT in chronic hepatitis. In Dobermanns with copper-associated chronic hepatitis, these abnormalities were shown to be indicators for imminent death.
- Hypoalbuminaemia due to failure of synthesis. A decrease in albumin and other acute phase proteins on serum protein electrophoresis is suggestive of end-stage disease and carries a poor prognosis.

Case examples

CASE 1

SIGNALMENT

7-year-old neutered female Cocker Spaniel.

HISTORY

Acute onset of anorexia and vomiting with haemorrhagic diarrhoea. Dehydration with discomfort on abdominal palpation.

CLINICAL PATHOLOGY DATA

Haematology	Result	Reference interval
RBC (x 10^{12}/l)	8.8	5.50–8.50
Haematocrit (l/l)	0.57	0.39–0.55
Haemoglobin (g/dl)	18.5	12.00–18.00
MCV (fl)	65.0	60.0–77.0
WBC (x 10^9/l)	29.1	6.0–15.0
Neutrophils (segmented) (x 10^9/l)	25.9	3.60–12.00
Band neutrophils (x 10^9/l)	1.3	0.0–0.3
Lymphocytes (x 10^9/l)	0.3	0.70–4.80
Monocytes (x 10^9/l)	1.6	0.0–1.50
Eosinophils (x 10^9/l)	0.0	0.0–1.0
Basophils (x 10^9/l)	0.0	0.0–0.2
Platelets (x 10^9/l)	235	200–500

Abnormal results are in **bold**.

Biochemistry	Result	Reference interval
Total protein (g/l)	75	58–73
Albumin (g/l)	37	26–35
Globulin (g/l)	38	18–37
ALT (IU/l)	195	15–60
AST (IU/l)	35	7–50
ALP (IU/l)	775	20–60
GGT (IU/l)	12	0–8
Bilirubin (µmol/l)	8	0–10
Fasting bile acids (µmol/l)	25	0–30
Creatinine (µmol/l)	131	30–90
Urea (mmol/l)	12.5	1.7–7.4
Glucose (mmol/l)	6.1	3.0–5.0
Calcium (mmol/l)	2.41	2.30–3.00
Phosphate (mmol/l)	1.2	0.90–1.20
Sodium (mmol/l)	153	139–154
Potassium (mmol/l)	3.6	3.60–5.60

Abnormal results are in **bold**.

> **Urine specific gravity:** 1.065.
> **Urine dipstick and sediment:** unremarkable.

WHAT ABNORMALITIES ARE PRESENT?

- Haemoconcentration and increased serum proteins.
- Leucocytosis with a neutrophilia and left shift, mild monocytosis, lymphopenia.
- 3-fold increase in ALT but normal AST.
- 10-fold increase in ALP and mild increase in GGT.
- Mild hyperglycaemia.
- Serum potassium concentration bordering on hypokalaemia.
- Mild azotaemia with a maximally concentrated urine.

HOW WOULD YOU INTERPRET THESE RESULTS AND WHAT ARE THE LIKELY DIFFERENTIAL DIAGNOSES?

There is evidence of:

- Dehydration: the azotaemia is likely to be prerenal as the urine is appropriately concentrated
- An inflammatory leucogram
- A hepatopathy.

The problem appears predominantly cholestatic (markedly increased cholestatic enzymes and lack of increase in AST). If it is a primary hepatopathy, cholangitis is more likely on the basis of the history and laboratory results. However, it is more likely to be a secondary, reactive hepatopathy as the major clinical signs are gastrointestinal and there is no evidence of hepatic dysfunction (normal bilirubin and FSBA, with increased albumin).

Differential diagnoses

- Acute gastroenteritis.
- Acute pancreatitis.
- Acute (or acute exacerbation of chronic) hepatitis/cholangitis.

Hypoadrenocorticism is virtually ruled out by normal serum electrolytes.

WHAT FURTHER TESTS WOULD YOU RECOMMEND?

- If there were any doubt, liver function could be assessed by measuring postprandial serum bile acids, but only once the vomiting and anorexia have been addressed.
- Abdominal ultrasonography is likely to be helpful in evaluating the biliary tree, pancreas and GI tract.
- Canine pancreatic lipase (Spec cPL®) is indicated as it is the most sensitive test for pancreatitis, especially when combined with abnormal ultrasonographic findings. The dehydration, mild hyperglycaemia and inflammatory leucogram could all be consistent with acute pancreatitis.
- Ascending biliary infection could be identified by cholecystocentesis and/or liver biopsy for cytology and/or histology with culture, but it would be reasonable to wait to see the outcome of symptomatic treatment for the GI signs and possible pancreatitis first.

OUTCOME

Abdominal ultrasound examination findings were consistent with pancreatitis. The dog was managed symptomatically (intravenous fluids, analgesia and antiemetics) and made a full recovery with normalization of liver enzymes, which suggests that this dog had a secondary (reactive) hepatopathy.

CASE 2

SIGNALMENT

6-year-old neutered male Labrador Retriever.

HISTORY

3-month history of reduced appetite and weight loss.

CLINICAL PATHOLOGY DATA

Haematology	Result	Reference interval
RBC (x 10¹²/l)	**4.8**	5.50–8.00
Haematocrit (l/l)	**0.31**	0.39–0.55
Haemoglobin (g/dl)	**9.8**	12.0–18.0
MCV (fl)	65.0	60.0–77.0
Reticulocytes (x 10⁹/l)	10	<60
WBC (x 10⁹/l)	13.5	6.00–15.00
Neutrophils (segmented) (x 10⁹/l)	11.0	3.60–12.00
Lymphocytes (x 10⁹/l)	1.0	0.70–4.80
Monocytes (x 10⁹/l)	1.4	0.0–1.50
Eosinophils (x 10⁹/l)	0.1	0.0–1.0
Basophils (x 10⁹/l)	0.0	0.0–0.2
Platelets (x 10⁹/l)	325	200–500

Abnormal results are in **bold**.

Biochemistry	Result	Reference interval
Total protein (g/l)	62	58–73
Albumin (g/l)	**19**	26–35
Globulin (g/l)	**43**	18–37
ALT (IU/l)	**621**	15–60
AST (IU/l)	**63**	7–50
ALP (IU/l)	**435**	20–60
GGT (IU/l)	**17**	0–8
Bilrubin (μmol/l)	**15**	0–10
Fasting bile acids (μmol/l)	**75**	0–30
Creatinine (μmol/l)	56	30–90
Urea (mmol/l)	**1.1**	1.7–7.4
Glucose (mmol/l)	4.6	3.0–5.0
Calcium (mmol/l)	**2.1**	2.30–3.00
Cholesterol (mmol/l)	**2.3**	3.5–9.0
Phosphate (mmol/l)	1.1	0.90–1.20
Sodium (mmol/l)	151	139–154
Potassium (mmol/l)	4.7	3.60–5.60

Abnormal results are in **bold**.

WHAT ABNORMALITIES ARE PRESENT?

There is:
* Mild normocytic, normochromic, non-regenerative anaemia
* Mild hyperbilirubinaemia, but insufficient to cause overt jaundice
* Abnormal FSBA
* Moderate to marked increase in both hepatocellular and cholestatic marker enzymes
* Hypoalbuminaemia and hyperglobulinaemia
* Low urea concentration
* Hypocholesterolaemia.

HOW WOULD YOU INTERPRET THESE RESULTS AND WHAT ARE THE LIKELY DIFFERENTIAL DIAGNOSES?

* The anaemia is mild and likely to be an anaemia of chronic inflammatory disease.
* The low urea concentration may reflect poor appetite, diuresis or hepatic dysfunction.
* Changes in serum proteins in the context of the other results are consistent with an inflammatory hepatopathy or necrosis of a liver tumour.
* Hypocholesterolaemia is consistent with a hepatopathy or anorexia.
* The hyperbilirubinaemia is unlikely to be prehepatic in origin because the anaemia appears non-regenerative and not severe, plus elevated FSBA suggest hepatic dysfunction. Pre-regenerative anaemia is unlikely considering the chronic history. Posthepatic disease is unlikely because of the similar magnitude of the increases in both hepatocellular and cholestatic marker enzymes and the hypocholesterolaemia.

A chronic hepatopathy is likely, owing to:

* Prolonged history
* Evidence of hepatic dysfunction (hyperbilirubinaemia, increased FSBA)
* Hypoalbuminaemia suggests chronic disease
* Evidence of hepatic damage.

The most likely differentials are:

* Chronic hepatitis
  * Lobular dissecting hepatitis
  * Chronic hepatitis
  * Copper hepatotoxicosis
* Extensive primary hepatic tumour (hepatocellular or biliary carcinoma)
* Hepatic lymphoma.

WHAT FURTHER TESTS WOULD YOU RECOMMEND?

* Postprandial bile acid measurement is superfluous because the FSBA already confirms hepatic dysfunction.
* Ultrasonographic imaging of the liver will indicate whether there are architectural changes in the liver that need to be sampled.
* Assessment of coagulation profile (platelet count, PT, aPTT) and buccal mucosal bleeding time to check for safety of liver biopsy.
* Fine-needle aspirates may detect hepatic neoplasia but are unreliable in the diagnosis of chronic hepatitis, unless staining for copper identifies copper-containing hepatocytes.
* Liver biopsy, with samples for culture and copper analysis (staining with rhodanine or rubeanic acid, and atomic absorption spectrophotometry), will provide a definitive diagnosis.

OUTCOME

Percutaneous liver biopsy confirmed chronic hepatitis in association with copper accumulation. The dog was treated with D-penicillamine and S-adenosyl methionine and fed a low copper/high zinc diet.

CASE 3

SIGNALMENT

6-month-old entire female Maltese.

HISTORY

Poor appetite and slightly underweight but normal stature.

CLINICAL PATHOLOGY DATA

Haematology	Result	Reference interval
RBC (x 10^{12}/l)	7.13	5.50–8.00
Haematocrit (l/l)	0.41	0.39–0.55
Haemoglobin (g/dl)	13.1	12.0–18.0
MCV (fl)	**57**	60.0–77.0
MCHC (g/dl)	32.0	32.0 – 36.0
WBC (x 10^9/l)	9.8	6.00–15.00
Neutrophils (segmented) (x 10^9/l)	8.1	3.60–12.00
Lymphocytes (x 10^9/l)	1.3	0.70–4.80
Monocytes (x 10^9/l)	0.3	0.0–1.50
Eosinophils (x 10^9/l)	0.1	0.0–1.0
Basophils (x 10^9/l)	0.0	0.0–0.2
Platelets (x 10^9/l)	398	200–500

Abnormal results are in **bold**.

Biochemistry	Result	Reference interval
Total protein (g/l)	59	58–73
Albumin (g/l)	31	26–35
Globulin (g/l)	28	18–37
ALT (IU/l)	**75**	15–60
ALP (IU/l)	**151**	20–60
Bilirubin (μmol/l)	1.2	0–10
Fasting bile acids (μmol/l)	**45**	0–30
Creatinine (μmol/l)	35	30–90
Urea (mmol/l)	2.1	1.7–7.4
Glucose (mmol/l)	4.5	3.0–5.0
Calcium (mmol/l)	**3.1**	2.30–3.00
Cholesterol (mmol/l)	3.8	3.5 – 9.0
Phosphate (mmol/l)	**1.4**	0.90–1.20
Sodium (mmol/l)	145	139–154
Potassium (mmol/l)	4.2	3.60–5.60

Abnormal results are in **bold**.

Urine specific gravity: 1.018.

WHAT ABNORMALITIES ARE PRESENT?

- Microcytosis; no anaemia.
- Mild increase in FSBA.
- Mild increases in ALT and ALP.
- Mild increases in calcium and phosphate.

HOW WOULD YOU INTERPRET THESE RESULTS AND WHAT ARE THE LIKELY DIFFERENTIAL DIAGNOSES?

- Microcytosis is associated with iron-deficiency anaemia and hepatic disease, especially portosystemic shunting. There is no anaemia and no history of blood loss; hypochromia (reduced mean corpuscular haemoglobin concentration (MCHC)) and thrombocytosis, characteristic of blood loss anaemia, are not present.
- Increase in ALT less than 2-fold and not considered significant.
- Mild increase in ALP is consistent with ongoing bone growth in a young dog.
- Raised calcium and phosphate are also consistent with growth.

The history and laboratory results are suggestive of:

- Congenital portosystemic shunt
- Microvascular dysplasia due to portal vein hypoplasia
- Acquired juvenile hepatopathy
  - Lobular dissecting hepatitis
  - Portal vein hypoplasia leading to idiopathic juvenile hepatic fibrosis.

WHAT FURTHER TESTS WOULD YOU RECOMMEND?

- FSBA are suspicious of a primary hepatopathy, but measurement of PPSBA may be more sensitive in a non-icteric dog.
- Radiographs to assess liver and kidney sizes: microhepatica and renomegaly are typical of congenital PSS.
- Ultrasonography to assess liver size and vasculature.
- Portovenography or computed tomography (CT) with contrast to detect congenital vascular anomaly.

The lack of signs of encephalopathy and poor growth make a congenital shunt less likely, and the lack of an increase in liver enzymes is not consistent with lobular dissecting hepatitis. Microvascular dysplasia is a mild form of portal vein hypoplasia, typically seen in terrier breeds. Intrahepatic microvascular shunting leads to abnormal bile acid tests, but no single congenital shunt can be identified by imaging. The liver is of normal size and clinical signs are mild or even absent. More severe portal vein hypoplasia may lead to progressive fibrosis and clinicopathological changes consistent with a chronic, progressive hepatopathy.

OUTCOME

Doppler ultrasonography and contrast-enhanced CT failed to demonstrate a macroscopic portosystemic shunt. Liver biopsy showed a vascular anomaly, with no significant fibrosis. A diagnosis of microvascular dysplasia due to portal vein hypoplasia was made. There is no specific treatment for portal vein hypoplasia; symptomatic treatment of any hepatoencephalopathy may improve clinical signs.

References and further reading

Bahr KL, Sharkey LC, Murakami T *et al.* (2013) Accuracy of US-guided FNA of focal liver lesions in dogs: 140 cases (2005–2008). *Journal of the American Animal Hospital Association* **49**, 190–196

Balkman CE, Center SA, Randolph JF *et al.* (2003) Evaluation of urine sulfated and nonsulfated bile acids as a diagnostic test for liver disease in dogs. *Journal of the American Veterinary Medical Association* **222**, 1368–1375

Battersby IA, Giger U and Hall EJ (2005) Hyperammonaemic encephalopathy secondary to selective cobalamin deficiency in a juvenile Border collie. *Journal of Small Animal Practice* **46**, 339–344

Bento PAL, Center SA, Randolph JF *et al.* (2013) Hepatocellular carcinoma/adenoma in 94 dogs: association with vacuolar hepatopathy and adrenal hyperactivity. *Journal of Veterinary Internal Medicine* **27**, 716–716 (abstract)

Center SA (2007) Interpretation of liver enzymes. *Veterinary Clinics of North America: Small Animal Practice* **37**, 297–333

Chevallier M, Guerret S, Pagnon A, Lecoindre P and Peyron C (2012) Liver histological lesions in 43 Scottish terriers with hyperactivity of alkaline phosphatases. *Journal of Veterinary Internal Medicine* **26**, 780–781 (abstract)

Cole TL, Center SA, Flood SN *et al.* (2002) Diagnostic comparison of needle and wedge biopsy specimens of the liver in dogs and cats. *Journal of the American Veterinary Medical Association* **220**, 1483–1490

Day MJ and Williams JM (2005) Biopsy collection, processing and interpretation. In: *BSAVA Manual of Canine and Feline Gastroenterology, 2nd edn,* ed. EJ Hall, JW Simpson and DA Williams. BSAVA Publications, Gloucester

Favier RP, Spee B, Schotanus BA *et al.* (2012) COMMD1-deficient dogs accumulate copper in hepatocytes and provide a good model for chronic hepatitis and fibrosis. *PLOS One* **7**, e42158

Fieten H, Leegwater PAJ, Watson AL and Rothuizen J (2012) Hepatic copper concentration and blood parameters in subclinical Labrador Retrievers and association with diet. *Proceedings of the 22nd ECVIM Congress*, Maastricht

Harran N, d'Anjou M-A, Dunn M *et al.* (2011) Gallbladder sludge on ultrasound is predictive of increased liver enzymes and total bilirubin in cats. *Canadian Veterinary Journal* **52**, 999–1003

Hill JM, Leisewitz AL and Goddard A (2011) The utility of uric acid assay in dogs as an indicator of functional hepatic mass. *Journal of the South African Veterinary Association* **82**, 86–93

Lidbury JA and Steiner JM (2013) Liver: diagnostic evaluation. In *Canine and Feline Gastroenterology*, ed. RW Washabau and MJ Day, pp. 863–869. Elsevier, St Louis

Malek S, Sinclair E, Hosgood G *et al.* (2013) Clinical findings and prognostic factors for dogs undergoing cholecystectomy for gall bladder mucocele. *Veterinary Surgery* **42**, 418–426

Mayhew PD, Savigny MR, Otto CM *et al.* (2013) Evaluation of coagulation in dogs with partial or complete extrahepatic biliary tract obstruction by means of thrombo-elastography. *Journal of the American Veterinary Medical Association* **242**, 778–785

Pembleton-Corbett JR, Center SA, Schermerhorn T *et al.* (2000) Serum-effusion albumin gradient in dogs with transudative abdominal effusion. *Journal of Veterinary Internal Medicine* **14**, 613–618

Rothuizen J and Twedt DC. (2009) Liver biopsy techniques. *Veterinary Clinics of North America: Small Animal Practice* **39**, 469-480

Ruland K, Fischer A and Hartmann K (2010) Sensitivity and specificity of fasting ammonia and serum bile acids in the diagnosis of portosystemic shunts in dogs and cats. *Veterinary Clinical Pathology* **39**, 57–64

Seki M, Asano K, Sakai M *et al.* (2010) Serum hyaluronic acid in dogs with congenital portosystemic shunts. *Journal of Small Animal Practice* **51**, 260–263

Trainor D, Center SA, Randolph JF *et al.* (2003) Urine sulfated and nonsulfated bile acids as a diagnostic test for liver disease in cats. *Journal of Veterinary Internal Medicine* **17**, 145–153

Tryndyak VP, Latendresse JR, Montgomery B *et al.* (2012) Plasma microRNAs are sensitive indicators of inter-strain differences in the severity of liver injury induced in mice by a choline- and folate-deficient diet. *Toxicology and Applied Pharmacology* **262**, 52–59

Walker MC, Hill RC, Guilford WG *et al.* (2001) Postprandial venous ammonia concentrations in the diagnosis of hepatobiliary disease in dogs. *Journal of Veterinary Internal Medicine* **15**, 463–466

Wang KW, Panciera DL, Al-Rukibat RK and Radi ZA (2004) Accuracy of ultrasound-guided fine-needle aspiration of the liver and cytological findings in dogs and cats: 97 cases (1990–2000). *Journal of the American Veterinary Medical Association* **224**, 75–78

Chapter 13

Laboratory evaluation of gastrointestinal disease

Edward J. Hall and Alexander J. German

The gastrointestinal (GI) tract is relatively inaccessible, and laboratory investigations are an important component of the diagnostic approach to GI diseases. Although alone they often do not provide a definitive diagnosis, they are helpful in ruling out non-GI causes of GI signs, narrowing the list of differential diagnoses and directing further more specialized and potentially more invasive diagnostic procedures (Figure 13.1).

The major clinical signs associated with GI disease are:

- Vomiting
- Diarrhoea
- Weight loss
- GI bleeding: haematemesis and/or melaena or haematochezia
- Abdominal pain.

Each problem may dictate which specific laboratory investigations are performed. However, most cases of GI disease are acute, non-fatal and self-limiting, and only require symptomatic support without laboratory investigation. Therefore, the extent of the diagnostic investigations required varies, and often no or minimal laboratory assessment is needed; even the simple assessment of dehydration, by the measurement of the packed cell volume (PCV) and total solids by refractometry, may not be necessary if signs are acute and the patient is bright and alert. More detailed investigations are appropriate if systemic signs accompany vomiting and diarrhoea, or signs are chronic and/or unresponsive to symptomatic treatment.

A diagnostic approach to gastrointestinal problems

There is a battery of tests available for the investigation of GI diseases, although many lack sensitivity and/or specificity. Thus, the usual diagnostic approach is first to eliminate diseases not involving the GI tract. It is important to take a history and to perform a physical examination. See the *BSAVA Manual of Canine and Feline Gastoenterology* for further information.

For emergency and critical care cases, an emergency database should be collected at admission (Figure 13.2) to enable selection of appropriate intravenous fluid therapy and initial treatment. In more chronic cases, it is usually necessary to submit concurrent blood and urine samples,

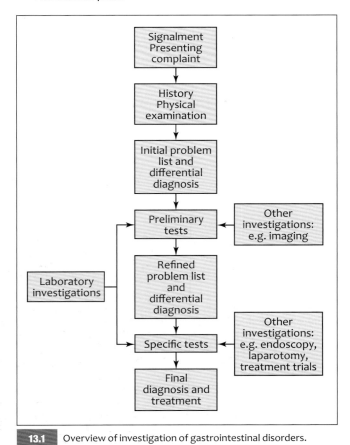

13.1 Overview of investigation of gastrointestinal disorders.

Haematology
• Packed cell volume (PCV)
• Total solids (refractometer)
• Blood smear examination
Biochemistry
• Urea
• Glucose
• Electrolytes
Urinalysis
• Dipstick tests
• Specific gravity by refractometer
Additional (if available)
• Blood gas analysis (acid–base): PCO_2, P_aO_2, HCO_3^-

13.2 Emergency database.

for haematological and serum biochemical analyses and full urinalysis, respectively; routine faecal analyses include bacteriological and parasitological examination and are clearly indicated if the patient has diarrhoea. From this point, further investigations may be necessary, including diagnostic imaging (radiography and ultrasonography), exclusion of exocrine pancreatic insufficiency (EPI), indirect tests of intestinal function and damage and, ultimately, direct examination by endoscopy or surgery with histological examination of GI biopsy samples (Figures 13.3 and 13.4).

Vomiting

Vomiting is a reflex act that originates from the central nervous system (CNS) and can result from numerous causes. It is an active process and, when investigating the patient, the first aim is to differentiate this sign from retching due to expectoration and from regurgitation.

A detailed history is essential to classify the nature of vomiting. The vomitus may contain food, fluids, saliva, mucus, bile or blood (fresh red blood, or digested blood resembling 'coffee grounds' in appearance). Direct examination of the vomitus may assist in diagnosis. In this regard, the presence of bile, digested blood or acidic

---

Preliminary tests (all cases)

- Haematology
- Serum biochemistry
- Urinalysis
- Faecal parasitology
- Folate and cobalamin (for suspected small intestinal disease)

Additional tests to eliminate non-gastrointestinal diseases

- Exocrine pancreatic insufficiency (all cases):
  - Trypsin-like immunoreactivity
- Tests for pancreatitis (occasional indication):
  - Canine or feline pancreatic lipase immunoreactivity (PLI)
  - Serum lipase
    - DGGR lipase
- Endocrinopathies (occasional indication):
  - Basal cortisol or ACTH stimulation test
  - Total T4 (cats)
  - Gastrin measurement (for gastrinoma)

Tests specific for gastrointestinal disease

- Histopathological assessment of stomach and small intestine (all cases)
- Cytological assessment (occasional cases)

Additional tests with limited indication

- Tests for gastric spiral organisms
- Cytological examination

Suggested approach

- Preliminary tests should be performed in all cases
- If abdominal pain is present and/or there is supportive evidence of pancreatitis on diagnostic imaging, tests for pancreatitis should be performed
- Older cats should be tested for hyperthyroidism
- An ACTH stimulation test should be considered (in both species), especially if supportive electrolyte changes are present
- Gastrin measurement should be considered if a pancreatic mass is detected and/or hypertrophic gastropathy is detected on gastric biopsy specimens
- Assuming non-gastrointestinal diseases have been eliminated, biopsy specimens should be procured for histopathological assessment
- Exploratory laparotomy should be considered subsequent to endoscopic biopsy, if results do not fit or response to chosen therapy is poor
- Additional tests listed have rare indications and further advice should be sought prior to their consideration

13.3 Approach to laboratory testing for chronic vomiting.

Preliminary tests (all cases)

- Haematology
- Serum biochemistry
- Urinalysis
- Faecal bacteriology
- Faecal parasitology
- Folate and cobalamin

Additional tests to eliminate non-gastrointestinal diseases

- Exocrine pancreatic insufficiency (all cases):
  - Trypsin-like immunoreactivity
- Tests for pancreatitis (occasional indication):
  - Canine or feline pancreatic lipase immunoreactivity (PLI)
  - Feline trypsin-like immunoreactivity (fTLI)
  - Serum lipase
    - DGGR lipase
- Endocrinopathies (occasional indication):
  - ACTH stimulation test
  - Total T4/free T4 (cats)

Tests specific for gastrointestinal disease

- Histopathological assessment of stomach and small intestine (all cases)
- Cytological assessment (occasional cases)

Additional tests with limited indication

- Tests of intestinal function
- Protein loss: faecal alpha-1 protease inhibitor
- Malabsorption: sugar probe tests, breath hydrogen testing
- Permeability: sugar probe tests
- Immune function: serum IgA concentrations

Suggested approach

- Preliminary tests should be performed in all cases
- TLI should always be performed to eliminate the possibility of EPI
- If abdominal pain is present and/or there is supportive evidence of pancreatitis on diagnostic imaging, tests for pancreatitis should be performed
- Older cats should be tested for hyperthyroidism
- An ACTH stimulation test should be considered (in both species), especially if supportive electrolyte changes are present
- Assuming non-gastrointestinal diseases have been eliminated, biopsy specimens should be procured for histopathological assessment
- Exploratory laparotomy should be considered subsequent to endoscopic biopsy, if results do not fit or response to chosen therapy is poor
- Additional tests listed have rare indications and further advice should be sought prior to their consideration

13.4 Approach to laboratory testing for chronic diarrhoea.

---

contents (i.e. pH <5, measured by litmus paper) confirms the material to be vomitus. Urine dipsticks can be used to detect blood but are not suitable to detect gastric acid as they do not distinguish a pH below 5. However, the absence of these findings does not exclude the presence of vomiting. For example, if vomiting occurs shortly after eating, the contents will not be acidified; if intestinal contents are present, the contents may have a pH greater than 6; and bile will be present if intestinal contents are vomited in addition to gastric contents, and not if there is a pyloric obstruction.

Once vomiting has been confirmed, non-GI causes should be investigated next, and an integrated approach is required to achieve a diagnosis. Physical examination findings may assist in making a diagnosis although, in many cases, findings are unremarkable. Subsequently, a combination of laboratory investigations and diagnostic imaging (radiography and transabdominal ultrasonography) is most often employed. It is sensible to perform investigations of other organ systems before focusing on the GI tract, for example haematological and serum biochemical analysis, dynamic bile acid measurement, adrenocorticotropic hormone (ACTH) stimulation test, and tests for pancreatic disease. The most pertinent initial laboratory investigations for primary GI disease include haematological and serum biochemical analysis, electrolyte measurement, faecal analyses and, in some cases, acid–base measurement.

Diarrhoea

There are also numerous causes of diarrhoea in dogs and cats. Again, a history which includes information on the frequency, nature, severity and timing of clinical signs is necessary. A full dietary history should also be recorded. The aim is to determine whether the diarrhoea is secondary to disease in other organ systems or, if primary, whether the diarrhoea originates in the small or large intestine (Figure 13.5). While such an approach may be useful in narrowing the list of differential diagnoses and targeting further investigations, there are limitations. First, diseases of the small intestine (SI) can provoke secondary large intestinal diarrhoea. Second, in some cases there are signs consistent with both small and large intestinal diarrhoea and it is not possible to localize the condition further. Also of importance in the history is detailed information on environment, past medical history and the health status of in-contact animals.

Clinical sign	Small intestine	Large intestine
Tenesmus	Rare	Common
Frequency	2–3 x normal/day	>3 x normal/day
Urgency	Uncommon	Common
Stool volume	Increased	Multiple small volumes
Mucus	Rare	Common
Fresh blood	Uncommon (melaena typical)	Common
Vomiting	Occasionally	Uncommon
Weight loss	Common	Rare

13.5 Differentiation of small from large intestinal signs.

Again, physical examination findings can be helpful but, for most cases of chronic diarrhoea, further diagnostic tests are required. In dogs with chronic diarrhoea a trypsin-like immunoreactivity (TLI) test for EPI should be performed first, as clinical signs of malabsorption are not specific (see Chapter 14). Cats >5 years of age with diarrhoea should have serum thyroxine (basal T4) measured.

The integration of history, physical examination, laboratory analyses and diagnostic imaging should allow non-GI disorders to be eliminated, and many infectious causes of diarrhoea to be identified. If a diagnosis has not been reached, GI biopsy may be indicated, and a decision must be made on whether endoscopy or exploratory laparotomy is appropriate.

Weight loss

There are numerous differential diagnoses for weight loss in dogs and cats, and a complete discussion is outside the scope of this chapter. However, GI diseases are common causes: in some cases, intestinal disease can present with weight loss and no other localizing signs (i.e. no vomiting or diarrhoea). In the diagnostic approach to weight loss, it is first essential to record the exact amount and type of food fed, to exclude the possibility of inadequate feeding, and to rule out dysphagia. The subsequent diagnostic approach is similar to that for other GI signs although a

wider battery of tests for systemic disease may be required (e.g. echocardio-graphy and electrocardiography for suspected cardiac disease). In dogs with weight loss, a TLI test should be performed early in the investigation to rule out EPI, before more involved investigations of the intestine are attempted. Similarly, in older cats, thyroxine (T4) should be measured to exclude hyperthyroidism before commencing GI investigations.

Haematemesis and melaena

Haematemesis refers to vomiting with blood; the blood may be either fresh or altered by digestion/acidification (usually grossly resembling 'coffee grounds'). Information derived from the history generally enables haematemesis to be identified but, if there is any doubt, the vomitus should be examined. The presence of microscopic amounts of blood can be simply identified by testing the vomitus with a urine dipstick, unless the patient vomits meat, which contains haemoglobin or myoglobin and would give a positive result on the dipstick. Melaena refers to passage of faeces containing digested blood; the colour of the stool usually becomes black, resembling tar. However, significant quantities of blood can be present without altering the nature of the faeces; this is termed occult bleeding.

History and physical examination findings may reveal abnormalities that help to explain the presence of haematemesis and/or melaena, e.g. a history of non-steroidal anti-inflammatory drug (NSAID) use or identification of a cutaneous mast cell tumour as causes of gastric ulceration. Haematological parameters may confirm the presence of chronic blood loss, sometimes with features typical of iron deficiency (i.e. microcytosis, hypochromia and thrombocytosis); they may also enable the severity of blood loss to be determined. Serum biochemical parameters provide information on underlying causes of GI blood loss such as renal disease, hepatic disease and endocrinopathies. If GI haemorrhage is suspected, but melaena has not been noted, faecal occult blood can be tested. Associated iron deficiency can be confirmed by measurement of serum iron and total iron-binding capacity with calculation of the percentage saturation, or measurement of ferritin (where available) or, in dogs, assessment of iron stores by Prussian blue staining of bone marrow biopsy material (see Chapter 4). However, while both faecal occult blood and assessment of iron status may confirm blood loss, they provide no information on the underlying cause. Other laboratory testing may be necessary in some circumstances, including dynamic bile acid measurement, ACTH stimulation testing, and measurement of plasma gastrin concentrations. Diagnostic imaging may also provide supportive information on the likely cause, but endoscopy and exploratory laparotomy are usually necessary to establish a definitive diagnosis.

Abdominal pain

Abdominal discomfort/pain is typically caused by over-distention of the GI tract secondary to obstruction (e.g. foreign body, neoplasia), GI inflammation (e.g. gastric ulceration, inflammatory bowel disease) or intraperitoneal inflammation (e.g. pancreatitis, peritonitis). Laboratory tests directly relevant to a primary GI disease are likely to be unhelpful, and abdominal imaging is likely to be more fruitful. Haematology may demonstrate an inflammatory leucogram, and there may be a degenerative left shift with toxic neutrophils if there is bacterial peritonitis. Serum pancreatic lipase immunoreactivity can be measured as a marker for pancreatitis (see Chapter 14).

Lead poisoning is rare, but can cause abdominal pain, and is characterized by the presence of inappropriate numbers of nucleated red blood cells (RBCs) in the face of a normal haematocrit. Apparent abdominal pain is sometimes seen in hypoadrenocorticism (perhaps related to GI ischaemia), and an ACTH stimulation test should be undertaken before embarking on any invasive investigations.

Routine diagnostic procedures

Routine laboratory testing is an essential early step in the investigation of most GI diseases and usually includes routine haematological and serum biochemical analyses and urinalysis in the first instance. However, such investigations may not provide a definitive diagnosis and indeed are often unremarkable in primary GI disease; their value lies more in being able to rule out non-GI causes of secondary GI signs. This is an important concept to convey to owners, especially if using a stepwise approach in general practice. Thus, they should be used in conjunction with other clinical interventions in an integrated diagnostic approach (see Figures 13.1–13.4). Other general tests include routine faecal analyses such as parasitology and bacteriology.

Routine haematological analysis

Red cell parameters

An increase in haematocrit, especially in conjunction with increased serum total protein, is often a marker of dehydration and is typically associated with acute GI diseases. Depending on the severity, it may indicate the need for parenteral fluid therapy. The most marked haemoconcentration is typically seen in canine acute haemorrhagic gastroenteritis (HGE). The increase in haematocrit is marked (usually >0.60 l/l) because of rapid fluid and protein shifts between the intravascular compartment and intestinal tract. In HGE, total protein is usually normal or slightly increased, but proportionately lower than would be expected from the corresponding increase in haematocrit.

Anaemia might accompany non-GI disorders that cause secondary GI signs, such as chronic kidney disease and endocrinopathies (e.g. hypoadrenocorticism and hypothyroidism), but can also be associated with GI disorders, reflecting either chronic inflammation or intestinal blood loss. Anaemia secondary to chronic inflammation in GI disease is typically mild, normocytic, normochromic and non-regenerative. In contrast, the anaemia associated with acute blood loss is usually markedly regenerative, assuming there has been sufficient time for a bone marrow response to occur (see Chapter 4).

Characteristics that suggest chronic iron-deficient blood-loss anaemia include microcytosis, hypochromia (with decreased red cell haemoglobin) and thrombocytosis. Iron-deficiency anaemia is seen more often with chronic low-level occult GI bleeding associated with ulcers or GI tumours. Given that microcytic anaemia can accompany some hepatic disorders that can also produce GI signs (e.g. portosystemic shunting), it is important that such abnormalities are interpreted in light of the entire clinical picture.

White cell parameters

In GI disorders with an inflammatory aetiology (e.g. inflammatory bowel disease, IBD), neutrophilia with or without a left shift may be seen. However, such changes are usually mild and are not invariably present, and do not assist in differentiating GI inflammation from inflammation in other organ systems. The most marked abnormalities are likely to be associated with severe inflammation, for example in acute pancreatitis or haemorrhagic gastroenteritis and in diseases associated with bacteraemia/septicaemia. Typically the latter occurs when the mucosal barrier is severely compromised, i.e. mucosal ulceration is present, such that there is transmural inflammation or even perforation leading to peritonitis. Neutrophilia is also a common finding in feline infectious peritonitis (FIP), and may be associated with anaemia and lymphopenia.

Eosinophilia may be associated with parasitism, dietary sensitivity and eosinophilic gastroenteritis (EGE); it has also been reported in feline hyperthyroidism but it is not clear whether this might actually be due to concurrent disease. However, an eosinophil count slightly above the reference range established for healthy dogs of most breeds can be normal in German Shepherd Dogs (which are prone to GI disease) and Rottweilers. If eosinophilia is genuine, non-GI causes need to be excluded, e.g. ectoparasitism and hypoadrenocorticism, before considering intestinal parasites, food allergy or EGE. Furthermore, EGE can be seen with no, or just a non-specific, white blood cell (WBC) response. Eosinophilia can occasionally be seen as a paraneoplastic effect of lymphoma in the GI tract or elsewhere, and as part of hypereosinophilic syndrome.

If leucopenia is seen in cases of acute gastroenteritis in dogs or cats, parvovirus infection (canine parvovirus and feline panleucopenia respectively) should be suspected, as these enteric viruses attack the rapidly dividing cells of the bone marrow as well as the intestinal crypts. Cytotoxic drugs may also cause GI signs and leucopenia. Lymphopenia can be seen in lymphangiectasia but other laboratory abnormalities would be expected, i.e. panhypoproteinaemia and hypocholesterolaemia. Circulating atypical lymphocytes are uncommon but may be associated with lymphoproliferative disorders affecting the GI tract.

Routine serum biochemistry

A full panel of routine biochemical tests is recommended in all cases with chronic or severe acute GI signs although, in most instances, the main purpose of performing such tests is to exclude dysfunction of other body systems including renal, hepatic and endocrine disorders.

Albumin and globulin

Increased protein concentrations usually indicate dehydration if the accompanying clinical picture fits and especially if the haematocrit is increased. However, decreases in protein concentrations may be noted in GI disease, particularly chronic intestinal diseases (e.g. protein-losing enteropathy, PLE). In rare cases, protein-losing gastropathies are recorded. Causes of PLE are listed in Figure 13.6. In most cases of PLE, panhypoproteinaemia is noted, and this is in contrast to hepatic dysfunction or protein-losing nephropathy (PLN), where hypoalbuminaemia alone is typical (Figure 13.7).

Historical and physical examination findings and the results of other laboratory analyses (e.g. haematology, urinalysis) assist in differentiating causes of hypoalbuminaemia, so that PLN, liver dysfunction and other causes, (e.g. blood loss, vasculitis, burns) can be ruled out relatively easily. Serum protein concentrations are an insensitive indicator of GI protein loss, and more sensitive tests (e.g. measurement of alpha-₁ proteinase inhibitor

Lymphangiectasia

• Primary:
  ○ Intestinal
  ○ Generalized
• Secondary:
  ○ Venous hypertension, e.g. right-sided cardiac failure, hepatic cirrhosis

Infectious
• Parvovirus • Salmonellosis
Structural
• Intussusception
Neoplasia
• Lymphoma
Inflammation
• Inflammatory bowel disease: lymphoplasmacytic enteritis; eosinophilic enteritis; granulomatous enteritis
Endoparasitism
• *Giardia* • *Ancylostoma* (not in UK)
Gastrointestinal haemorrhage
• Haemorrhagic enteritis • Neoplasia • Ulceration

13.6 Causes of protein-losing enteropathies.

Cause[a]	Albumin	Globulin	Clinical signs	Confirmatory test
Liver disease	↓	Normal or ↑	Varied (includes diarrhoea and weight loss)	Liver function test e.g. serum bile acids
Protein-losing enteropathy	↓	↓	Diarrhoea and weight loss	None readily available in UK, e.g. faecal α_1-PI
Protein-losing nephropathy	↓	Normal	Nephrotic syndrome and weight loss	Proteinuria (dipstick urine, UPCR)

13.7 Differentiation of the main underlying causes of hypoproteinaemia. [a]Third-space effect and haemorrhage can also cause hypoalbuminaemia. α_1-PI = alpha-1 proteinase inhibitor; UPCR = urine protein:creatinine ratio.

(α_1-PI) in faeces) are available, though rarely used because they do not alter the diagnostic approach. Hyperglobulinaemia can be seen in some GI disorders, including those associated with intense inflammation (e.g. Basenji enteropathy), some infections (e.g. FIP) and lymphoproliferative diseases (e.g. lymphoma, myeloma).

Sodium and potassium

Electrolyte abnormalities can be a feature of persistent vomiting, intestinal obstruction and secretory diarrhoea. Thus, electrolyte measurements, ideally in association with blood gas analysis, are important in determining the most appropriate type of fluid for initial replacement. Hypokalaemia is a common finding in GI disease as a result of anorexia and/or GI losses.

Hyponatraemia and hyperkalaemia are suggestive of hypoadrenocorticism, which itself can cause GI signs. However, similar electrolyte changes (i.e. hyponatraemia and hyperkalaemia) can be associated with primary GI disease especially with whipworm infection and salmonellosis (see Chapter 8). Other potential laboratory abnormalities in hypoadrenocorticism include azotaemia, hypercalcaemia, non-regenerative anaemia, lymphocytosis and eosinophilia but, ideally, an ACTH stimulation test should be performed to confirm hypoadrenocorticism. If ACTH is not available, a basal cortisol concentration ≥50 µmol/l helps rule out hypoadrenocortisolism, assuming that exogenous steroids have not been administered. See Chapter 18 for further information on the diagnosis of hypoadrenocorticism.

Liver enzymes

The activities of liver enzymes that can be measured in serum samples from small animals are broadly characterized as hepatocellular/leakage enzymes and biliary/cholestatic markers (see Chapter 12). Alanine aminotransferase (ALT) and alkaline phosphatase (ALP), respectively, act as such markers and are the enzymes most commonly measured in routine serum biochemical screening panels. Mild to moderate increases in the serum activities of these enzymes may be seen in primary GI disease. Such changes are likely to represent a reactive hepatopathy caused by delivery of lumen-derived antigens, endotoxins and bacteria from the GI tract to the liver via the portal circulation. This is probably associated with the alterations of the permeability of the mucosal barrier that accompany many GI diseases. Therefore, it can be difficult to differentiate primary GI disease with a secondary hepatopathy from primary hepatopathies causing vomiting and diarrhoea. Measurement of serum bile acid concentrations can be helpful in making the distinction, although some types of GI disease can be associated with mild increases in bile acid concentrations. In cats with IBD, moderate to marked increases in liver enzyme activities may suggest significant concurrent biliary pathology as well as GI disease, since simultaneous inflammatory changes in related organs (small intestine (SI), liver and pancreas in so-called triaditis) are recognized.

Cholesterol

Increased serum cholesterol concentrations are rarely associated with primary GI disease, but may be seen in diseases of other body systems that cause secondary GI signs (e.g. endocrinopathies, renal disease, hepatic disease, pancreatic disease). Hypercholesterolaemia can be associated with PLN, which is also an important differential diagnosis for hypoalbuminaemia (see above). As cholesterol is synthesized in the liver, low serum cholesterol concentrations are typically associated with diseases involving hepatocellular dysfunction, but hypocholesterolaemia may also be a feature of primary pancreatic and intestinal diseases, most notably diseases that cause fat malabsorption. Marked hypocholesterolaemia is quite often seen in lymphangiectasia.

Urea and creatinine

Increased urea and creatinine concentrations can be associated with prerenal (e.g. dehydration), intrinsic renal, or postrenal azotaemia. Numerous diseases that cause vomiting and diarrhoea cause dehydration and, therefore, are associated with increased urea and creatinine concentrations.

Low serum concentrations of urea, relative to serum creatinine, are sometimes seen in animals with GI signs secondary to either portosystemic shunting (PSS) or severe liver dysfunction because of failure to convert ammonia to urea. Given that digestion and assimilation of protein lead to increased urea synthesis in the liver, increased urea relative to serum creatinine can also be associated with recent dietary protein intake or gastric or upper intestinal haemorrhage. Subnormal creatinine concentrations may be seen if there has been significant weight loss and loss of muscle mass due to GI disease.

Calcium and magnesium

Decreased total calcium and magnesium concentrations can be seen in patients with a PLE. The reduction in total serum calcium can, in part, be explained by the concurrent hypoalbuminaemia (see Chapter 8). However, ionized hypocalcaemia and ionized hypomagnesaemia have been reported in some cases of PLE and other mechanisms are likely to be involved, e.g. vitamin D, calcium and magnesium malabsorption, and the GI loss of vitamin D-binding protein.

Serum bile acids

Serum total bile acid concentration is a reflection of the enterohepatic circulation of bile acids, and increased concentrations are associated with hepatic dysfunction and/or PSS (see Chapter 12). The bile acid concentrations are increased as a result of primary hepatopathies but hepatopathies secondary to a number of diseases, including those affecting the GI tract, can cause milder increases. Potential malabsorption of bile acids by the ileum cannot result in subnormal serum bile acids because the reference range is 0–15 μmol/l.

Urinalysis

Routine urinalysis, involving biochemical assessment (dipstick analysis), assessment of specific gravity by refractometer and sediment analysis (Chapter 10), rarely provides any definitive information on GI disorders. However, it is an important component of the preliminary diagnostic database and, as part of an emergency database, urinalysis can assist in the choice of initial therapy (including fluid therapy). Urine specific gravity, measured before the administration of any intravenous fluids, enables assessment of renal tubular concentrating ability and identification of prerenal azotaemia. Abnormalities can also sometimes be identified on sediment analysis, and these may assist in differentiating causes of vomiting and diarrhoea. Most notably, the presence of ammonium biurate crystals (see Figure 12.12) is suggestive of a PSS, or hepatocellular dysfunction. Finally, identification of proteinuria, confirmed by a raised urine protein:creatinine ratio (UPCR), indicates the presence of PLN in cases of hypoalbuminaemia, although concurrent PLE and PLN can occur in Soft Coated Wheaten Terriers.

Serum folate and cobalamin

Folate is predominantly absorbed in the proximal small intestine, while cobalamin, bound to intrinsic factor, is absorbed by a specific carrier mechanism in the distal small intestine (Figure 13.8). Therefore, a subnormal concentration of folate suggests proximal small intestinal disease, a low cobalamin concentration can occur in diseases involving the distal small intestine as well as in EPI, and both low folate and low cobalamin may be seen if diffuse disease is present.

These water-soluble vitamins can be measured in both canine and feline serum, but the assays must be validated for the relevant species because non-specific binders in feline serum can interfere. Serum folate shows limited stability at room temperature. Therefore, serum samples for folate analysis should be frozen if they cannot be measured within 48 hours. Historically, folate and cobalamin were considered light sensitive and it was recommended that samples were stored in the dark or wrapped in foil to avoid spurious decreases in measured concentrations; this has now been refuted (Clement and Kendal, 2009).

Many factors other than GI disease can affect serum concentrations of both folate and cobalamin (Figure 13.9), and concentrations can be within the reference range despite severe GI disease. Currently, the main value of these tests is in documenting the presence of malabsorption and, by inference, identifying small intestinal disease and in indicating when supplementation is necessary.

Small intestinal bacterial overgrowth/antibiotic-responsive diarrhoea

Small intestinal bacterial overgrowth (SIBO), an absolute increase in the number of small intestinal bacteria, is a controversial diagnosis. There is little doubt that true overgrowth can occur secondary to a number of underlying disorders such as partial intestinal obstruction and EPI. However, the existence of a primary (idiopathic) SIBO is doubted. Diagnosis is hampered by the lack of clear definitions of both normal bacterial numbers and the disease phenotype and, as a result, the term antibiotic-responsive diarrhoea (ARD) is normally used in preference to SIBO for the primary idiopathic condition (Figure 13.10). A positive response to antibiotics can be measured objectively but whether this response reflects an effect on bacterial numbers or an effect on bacteria–host interactions is not known.

Serum folate and cobalamin assays have been used historically as indicators of SIBO. Given that many bacterial species synthesize folate, while others can bind cobalamin, increased numbers of small intestinal bacteria could increase serum folate concentrations, decrease serum cobalamin concentrations, or do both. However, the results do not correlate with a diagnosis of ARD. Furthermore, measurement of serum folate and cobalamin concentrations has poor sensitivity and specificity for canine SIBO, and the results do not correlate with quantitative duodenal juice culture. Moreover, changes in folate or cobalamin (or both) cannot reliably discriminate dogs with idiopathic ARD from those with other aetiologies (German et al., 2003a). Thus, measurement of folate and cobalamin concentrations is of very limited value in the diagnosis of idiopathic SIBO/ARD. In theory, these tests should be helpful in documenting secondary SIBO although, in practice, it is preferable to diagnose the underlying cause instead (e.g. EPI, intestinal obstruction).

Malabsorption

Although folate and cobalamin concentrations are of no use in the diagnosis of SIBO, they can identify the presence of GI diseases associated with malabsorption. Decreased serum concentrations are likely to reflect malabsorption because dietary deficiency is extremely unlikely if the patient has been eating a normal diet. However, these tests are limited by their lack of specificity for particular primary diseases and the fact that both folate and cobalamin can be affected by other factors (see Figure

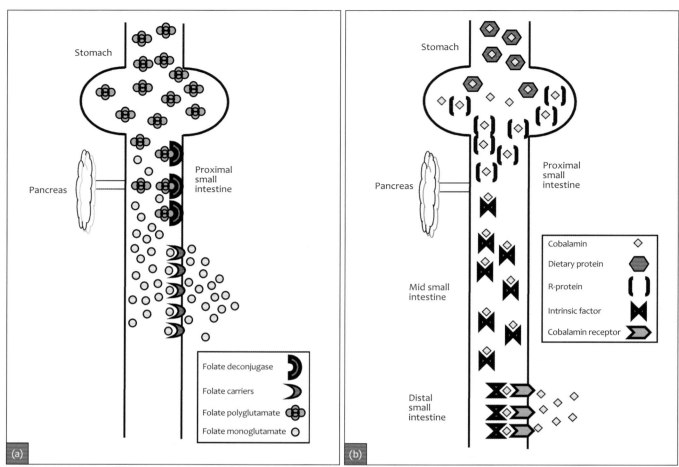

13.8 Assimilation of folate and cobalamin. (a) Dietary folate is present in food as a conjugated form, folate polyglutamate. This conjugate is digested by folate deconjugase, an enzyme on the microvillar membrane, which removes all but one residue. The resultant folate monoglutamate is taken up by specific carriers in the mid small intestine. (b) Following ingestion, cobalamin is released from dietary protein in the stomach. It then binds to non-specific binding proteins (e.g. 'R-proteins'). In the small intestine, cobalamin transfers on to intrinsic factor (IF), which is synthesized by the stomach (dog) and pancreas (dog and cat). Cobalamin–IF complexes pass along the intestine until the distal small intestine, where cobalamin is transported across the mucosa and into the portal circulation.

Vitamin	Increased	Decreased
Cobalamin	High dietary intake Parenteral supplementation Liver disease Solid neoplasm	Dietary deficiency Exocrine pancreatic insufficiency (EPI) Ileal disease[a] Ileal resection Intestinal bacterial metabolism
Folate	EPI Haemolysis High dietary intake Intestinal bacterial metabolism Low intestinal pH Parenteral supplementation	Dietary deficiency Drugs, e.g. sulfasalazine Proximal small intestinal disease[a] Sample aging

13.9 Factors influencing serum folate and cobalamin concentrations. [a]See Figure 13.10.

13.9). Nevertheless, the presence of malabsorption can be confirmed and the need for vitamin supplementation assessed. However, not all intestinal diseases causing malabsorption are sufficiently severe or long-standing to deplete body stores of either vitamin. Therefore, not all dogs and cats with GI diseases have abnormal test results.

Cobalamin deficiency is documented more commonly as a sequel to small intestinal disease, particularly in cats, and systemic metabolic consequences and loss of appetite have been recognized (Worhunsky et al., 2013). Elevated concentrations of serum and urinary methylmalonic acid (MMA), a consequence of cobalamin deficiency, correlate with the severity of the deficiency, and increased serum MMA concentrations are at least partly responsible for clinical signs such as anorexia and worsening diarrhoea. However, the MMA assay is not readily available, and measurement of serum cobalamin concentration is adequate and readily available in the UK.

Although many GI diseases (and some pancreatic diseases) can potentially cause a decreased serum cobalamin concentration in cats, the most severe decreases have been documented in association with IBD and lymphoma; there is a weak correlation between the histological severity of canine IBD and serum cobalamin concentration. Deficiency can develop within 6 weeks in cats because they lack the transport protein necessary for hepatic storage of cobalamin, which also undergoes rapid enterohepatic recycling. In dogs, the genetic cause of a specific intrinsic factor–cobalamin receptor deficiency was first identified in Giant Schnauzers (Fyfe et al., 2013); it is associated with severe cobalamin deficiency. Selective cobalamin deficiency has also been identified in Australian Shepherd Dogs, Beagles (http://research.vet.upenn.edu/Default.aspx?TabId=7620), Border Collies (http://www.mmg.msu.edu/fyfe.html) and Shar Peis, and specific genetic tests are now available for all of these breeds except the Shar Pei.

Parameter	Small intestinal bacterial overgrowth	Antibiotic-responsive diarrhoea
Causes	Always occurs secondary to underlying disease: • Exocrine pancreatic insufficiency • Other causes of malabsorption? • Partial obstruction • Decreased gastric acid production (e.g. drug therapy, gastric surgery)	Idiopathic
Signalment	Cats and dogs Any age or gender Any breed	Dogs only Young dogs of either sex German Shepherd Dogs predisposed
History	Predominantly small intestinal diarrhoea, although other signs possible Signs of underlying disease? If partial obstruction, could be cyclical pattern	Predominantly small intestinal diarrhoea and weight loss/failure to gain weight
Physical examination	Signs of underlying disease If partial obstruction, may have abnormalities on abdominal palpation	Varies from no signs to poor body condition
Preliminary laboratory tests	Signs of underlying disease? No specific findings	No specific findings
Faecal analysis	Negative	Negative
Folate/cobalamin	Variable results	Variable results
Diagnostic imaging	Findings specific to underlying disease Evidence of partial obstruction	No specific findings
Intestinal biopsy	Not required	Normal or mild inflammatory change only
Recommended method of diagnosis	Diagnose underlying disease: e.g. TLI for EPI; ultrasonography for partial obstruction	Rule out all other GI diseases (see Figure 13.4) Response to antibacterial trial Relapses often requiring repeated antibacterials

13.10 Comparison of small intestinal bacterial overgrowth (SIBO) and antibiotic-responsive diarrhoea (ARD). EPI = exocrine pancreatic insufficiency; GI = gastrointestinal; TLI = trypsin-like immunoreactivity.

If cobalamin deficiency is documented, parenteral supplementation with cobalamin is recommended, or the response to treatment of the underlying GI disease may remain suboptimal. Cobalamin is injected weekly until intracellular stores are restored and serum concentrations at least are at the top of the reference range, and ideally are supranormal. Thereafter, rechecking serum concentrations will indicate whether further weekly supplementation is required, or whether less frequent supplements (every 3–6 months) will help maintain the replete status. Decreased folate concentrations can be caused by malabsorption. If documented, supplementation with oral folic acid can be considered.

Serology

In cats with GI signs, serological tests for feline leukaemia virus (FeLV) and feline immunodeficiency virus (FIV) should always be performed, while coronavirus serology may be useful in some cases (see Chapter 28). Serology for infectious diseases such as parvovirus can sometimes be useful, although it is often complicated by titres derived from vaccination and the need to document either increased immunoglobulin (Ig)M or rising IgG titres to prove current infection.

Tests of endocrine disease

Routine haematological, serum biochemical and urinalysis findings can often increase the index of suspicion for an endocrinopathy as the cause of GI signs. For example, the presence of electrolyte abnormalities and azotaemia would suggest hypoadrenocorticism, hypercholesterolaemia may suggest hypothyroidism, and increased liver enzyme activity can be seen in cats with hyperthyroidism. However, more specific diagnostic tests are required for a definitive diagnosis, e.g. assessment of adrenal and thyroid function (see Chapters 17 and 18). Measurement of serum T4 is mandatory in older cats with GI signs.

Faecal analysis

Information on faecal character can be derived from the history and/or by direct examination of a stool sample which, if necessary, can be collected at the time of digital rectal examination. The presence of diarrhoea can be confirmed, and the likely site of pathology can be deduced. In this regard, if fresh blood or mucus is present, a large intestinal disorder is most likely, while changes in colour or volume suggest small intestinal disease, with or without malabsorption (see Figure 13.5).

Laboratory-based faecal examinations are an important part of the investigation of GI disease. However, many tests, such as quantification of faecal fat excretion and measurement of proteolytic activity, are unhelpful or unsuitable for practice; but bacteriological culture and identification of parasites are performed routinely. Newer faecal markers of intestinal disease have been developed (e.g. alpha-1 protease inhibitor, calprotectin) but currently have limited availability, although they may yet prove useful once they become more widely available.

Microscopic examination of stool specimens is the cornerstone of the detection of intestinal parasites (Dryden et al., 2005). Generally, fresh non-preserved stool specimens are used but because intestinal parasites are shed intermittently, multiple stool samples may need to be examined. Three-day pooled samples may increase sensitivity, but the limitation of this approach is that detection of the vegetative stages of protozoa may be missed because of delays in processing and/or low compliance with submitting multiple samples.

Bacterial, viral and protozoal causes of GI signs are typically sought in cases with acute disease, but bacteria and viruses are rarely responsible for chronic GI disease. Indeed, isolation of acute bacterial pathogens in chronic cases is often confusing because organisms can also sometimes be isolated from asymptomatic animals (Marks *et al.*, 2011). Helminths are more likely to be associated with chronic signs, and investigations in chronic GI disease are perhaps better restricted to searching for protozoal and helminth infections. The dog and cat can be the definitive hosts of various cestodes, but clinical signs are rarely associated with their infection. In acute diarrhoea, testing for bacterial pathogens such as *Salmonella*, *Campylobacter* and *Clostridium* spp. can be performed although its value is debated because these organisms can be found in the stool of clinically healthy animals.

Direct faecal examination

Faecal smears: Although it is possible to stain faeces for undigested starch granules (Lugol's iodine), fat globules (Sudan stain) and muscle fibres (Wright's or Diff-Quik® stains), this is generally not helpful because these are insensitive markers of malabsorption and are very non-specific. However, on occasion, a microscopic examination of a direct smear of fresh faeces can demonstrate an enteropathogen (e.g. the 'seagull' shape of *Campylobacter*), although the sensitivity is poor.

Given that *Clostridium perfringens* is a potential cause of diarrhoea, Diff-Quik® stained faecal smears can be examined for the characteristic subterminal clostridial endospores. If large numbers of spores (>5 per oil field) are detected, *C. perfringens* enterotoxicosis is possible but not necessarily confirmed: the correlation between sporulation and toxin elaboration is unreliable because endospores and endotoxin can be found in stool samples from normal dogs, and toxin can be found in the absence of endospores and *vice versa*. Overall tests for the detection of *C. perfringens* enterotoxin (see below) are now preferred. For *Campylobacter*, examination of a stained faecal smear for slender, seagull-shaped bacteria can yield a presumptive diagnosis, although *Campylobacter* and a number of other spiral organisms are found in normal stool.

Examination of a direct smear of faeces can also be used to detect fungal elements, such as *Histoplasma* and *Pythium*, and is important if fungal/oomycete diseases are endemic in the area, although rectal cytology may be more appropriate (see below). *Cryptosporidium* spores can be detected if a direct smear is stained with an acid-fast stain, or by immunofluorescence. However, this organism is more commonly assessed using special faecal flotation techniques (see below).

Wet faecal preparations: Unstained wet mounts can be used to identify motile protozoal trophozoites, such as *Giardia* spp., while identification of *Trichomonas*, *Tritrichomonas*, *Pentatrichomonas*, *Balantidium* and *Entamoeba* spp. may be significant in cases of large intestinal (LI) diarrhoea. The sample must be fresh (warm) because the trophozoites rapidly encyst as they cool. Cysts are better identified by faecal concentration methods (see below).

Differentiation of the most significant protozoal pathogens in cats, i.e. *Giardia* and *Tritrichomonas* spp., can be made by their characteristic motion in a faecal wet mount. Although both organisms are flagellated, *Giardia* trophozoites tumble like a falling leaf while *Tritrichomonas* are highly motile cells and progress rapidly across the field of view. Traditionally, *Tritrichomonas* has been considered a feline (and bovine genital) infection, but it has also been identified using polymerase chain reaction (PCR) in faecal samples collected from dog breeding kennels. Rapid fixation and staining allows more accurate identification from the characteristic morphology of the various protozoa that can be present in faeces, but the pathogenicity of most enteric protozoa (e.g. *Pentatrichomonas*, *Balantidium*) is still debated, with the exception of *Giardia* and *Tritrichomonas*.

Faecal concentration methods

Although direct examination of faecal samples can identify metazoan endoparasites, faecal concentration methods are more sensitive. Faeces can be 'concentrated' either with flotation (using a sugar or salt solution) or sedimentation techniques. Formalin is often added to preserve organisms, and because of the relatively high fat content of canine and feline faeces, methods using ether or ethyl acetate are generally preferred.

The methodologies are described in Figure 13.11 and their relative advantages and disadvantages listed in Figure 13.12. However, in most cases samples are submitted for analysis at commercial laboratories where, because these concentrating techniques are laborious, semi-automated separation techniques are often employed.

Wet preparation
1. The sample must be fresh (warm).
2. A tiny drop of faecal material is put on a slide with a similar volume of warm saline.
3. A cover slip is immediately placed over the sample.
4. The slide is examined immediately at dry high power (X400) magnification.

Faecal flotation
1. Place 2–3 g of faeces in 15 ml of saturated sugar or salt solution:
   - Sugar solution = 454 g sugar + 355 ml water (specific gravity = 1.27) (+ 6 ml formaldehyde in Modified Sheather's solution)
   - Salt solutions (specific gravity = 1.18–1.20):
     - Sodium chloride = 350 g/l water
     - Sodium nitrate = 338 g/l water
     - Zinc sulphate = 330 g/l water.
2. Mix thoroughly, then strain through tea strainer or cheesecloth.
3. If there is excess fat after filtration, mix with 2–3 ml of ethyl acetate or ether, centrifuge and discard the supernatant.
4. Place in 15 ml polypropylene tube.
5. Centrifuge at 1500 rpm for 5 minutes.
6. Place coverslip on top, touching the meniscus, for 3–4 minutes (alternatively use bacteriology loop).
7. Place coverslip on microscope slide and examine.
   - Stain with Lugol's iodine for zinc sulphate flotation, if desired.

Faecal sedimentation

Water
1. Mix sample of fresh faeces with water and strain to remove debris.
2. Allow sample to settle for between 30 minutes and 2 hours.
3. Place the sediment on a microscope slide, place a coverslip over the sediment and examine.

Formalin ether
1. Mix sample of fresh faeces with water and strain to remove debris.
2. Centrifuge strained faeces and resuspend in 9 ml of 5% formalin solution.
3. Add 3 ml of ethyl acetate and shake vigorously.
4. Re-centrifuge and discard the debris at the formalin–ethyl acetate interface.
5. Examine the sediment as above.

13.11 Methodologies for performing faecal examination for parasites (Dryden *et al.*, 2005). (Note that the Parasep® faecal filtration system method simplifies the technique).

Technique	Advantages	Disadvantages
Direct smear	• Fast • No distortion of parasites if isotonic saline is used as diluent • Only way to see live trophozoites	• Insensitive especially if concentration is too low or if too much debris or fat is present

Saturated sucrose or salt flotation	• Inexpensive
	• Suitable for most common helminth ova and coccidian oocysts
		• Ideally requires centrifugation
		• Unsuitable for:
		  • Fatty stool samples
		  • Tapeworm ova
		  • *Giardia* cysts

Zinc sulphate (ZnSO₄) flotation	• Recommended for most faecal examinations
	  • Floats most helminth eggs
	  • Best for protozoan cysts, especially *Giardia*
		• Procedure will not float some trematode ova and some tapeworm ova
		• Unsuitable for fatty stool samples
		• ZnSO₄ is relatively expensive

Formalin ether sedimentation	• Procedure recovers *all* types of helminth ova, larvae and most protozoan cysts • Best technique for formalin-fixed samples and for stools with high fat content	• More difficult to perform than other techniques • Ether and ethyl acetate are flammable and subject to various handling precautions • More debris remains

13.12 Relative advantages and disadvantages of different techniques for performing faecal examination for intestinal parasites.

The Parasep® faecal filtration system is available for veterinary practice laboratories (Saez *et al.*, 2011). The basis of the Parasep® system is that the faecal sample is placed in a mixing tube with plastic granules to break up the sample, and a filtrate is collected while gross debris is collected by a filter. The filtrate is then examined using a modified McMaster technique. Further details can be found on the distributor's website. Similarly the Flotac® system is convenient, mess-free and potentially more sensitive than routine flotation methods (Cringoli, 2006; Becker *et al.*, 2011).

Flotation with sugar or salt solutions generally detects the majority of parasites (Figures 13.12–13.19) including coccidia and *Cryptosporidium* spp., but the fat content of

canine and feline faeces makes the formalin ether sedimentation technique more suitable for metazoan ova (roundworms, hookworms and whipworms). Zinc sulphate flotation is recommended for detecting *Giardia* oocysts.

A direct smear, sedimentation or the Baermann technique can identify larvae of *Strongyloides* spp., although the last technique is most commonly used to detect lungworm (*Angiostrongylus vasorum* and *Oslerus osleri*) larvae. Lungworm larvae are also detected using the Parasep® tube technique.

As with any diagnostic test, reliable interpretation is as important as methodology. In this regard, identification of a parasite may not necessarily prove causation, particularly in cases presenting with chronic GI signs. Indeed,

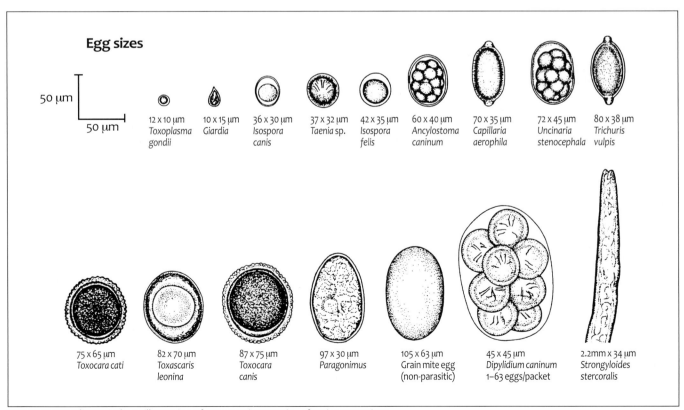

13.13 Faecal parasitology: illustration of comparative egg size of various parasites.
(Courtesy of Hoechst–Roussel-AGri Vet Company, USA; permission requested)

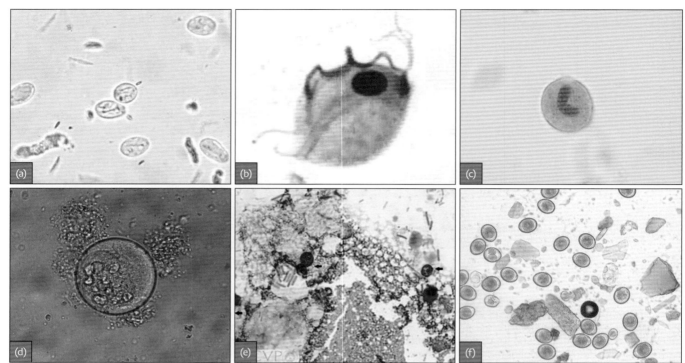

13.14 Faecal parasitology: protozoal parasites. (a) Zinc suphate flotation showing *Giardia* cysts. (b) Stained faecal smear showing characteristic appearance of *Tritrichomonas foetus* with its long undulating membrane. (c) *Balantidium coli* cyst (stained). Note the large kidney bean-shaped macronucleus. (d) *Balantidium coli* cyst (not stained). Note that the large kidney bean-shaped macronucleus is not easily observed. (e) Modified Kinyoun's acid-fast stain of *Cryptosporidium* sp. oocysts. *Cryptosporidium* spp. are now considered gregarines. (f) Oocysts of *Cystoisospora* spp. in a canine faecal float. Note the two different sizes and that several are sporulated.

(a–b, Reproduced from the *BSAVA Manual of Canine and Feline Gastroenterology, 2nd edition*; c–f, © The National Center for Veterinary Parasitology at Oklahoma State University, www.ncvetp.org/)

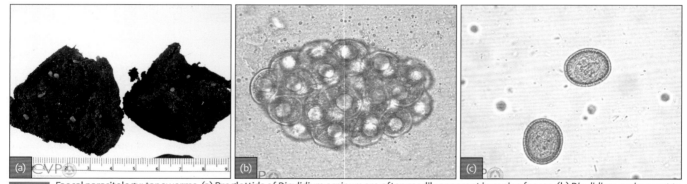

13.15 Faecal parasitology: tapeworms. (a) Proglottids of *Dipylidium caninum* are often readily apparent in canine faeces. (b) *Dipylidium caninum* eggs are found in clusters 120–200 μm in size. Individual eggs measure 35–60 μm in diameter and contain an embryo bearing hooks. (c) Taeniid eggs of *Taenia* spp. and *Echinococcus* spp. are morphologically indistinguishable, measure 25–40 μm, and consist of a thick, striated wall surrounding a hexacanth embryo.

(© The National Center for Veterinary Parasitology at Oklahoma State University, www.ncvetp.org/)

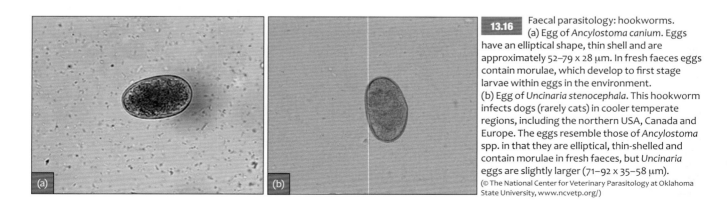

13.16 Faecal parasitology: hookworms.
(a) Egg of *Ancylostoma canium*. Eggs have an elliptical shape, thin shell and are approximately 52–79 x 28 μm. In fresh faeces eggs contain morulae, which develop to first stage larvae within eggs in the environment.
(b) Egg of *Uncinaria stenocephala*. This hookworm infects dogs (rarely cats) in cooler temperate regions, including the northern USA, Canada and Europe. The eggs resemble those of *Ancylostoma* spp. in that they are elliptical, thin-shelled and contain morulae in fresh faeces, but *Uncinaria* eggs are slightly larger (71–92 x 35–58 μm).
(© The National Center for Veterinary Parasitology at Oklahoma State University, www.ncvetp.org/)

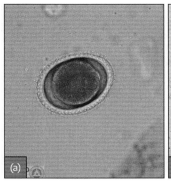

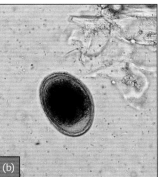

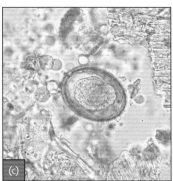

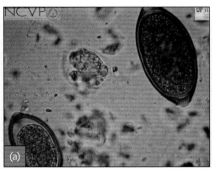

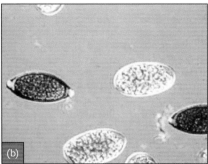

13.17 Faecal parasitology: ascarids. (a) Egg of *Toxocara canis*. The eggs are 85–90 x 75 μm, subspherical and have a thick and pitted shell. (b) Egg of *Toxocara cati*. The eggs are similar to those of *Toxocara canis*, but are 65 x 75 μm and tend to be more elliptical. (c) Egg of *Toxascaris leonina*. The eggs are approximately 70–80 μm and resemble those of *Toxocara* spp., but have a smooth shell and the embryo takes up less space within the egg.
(© The National Center for Veterinary Parasitology at Oklahoma State University, www.ncvetp.org/)

13.18 Faecal parasitology. (a) Comparative image of *Eucoleus aerophilus* (left) and *Trichuris vulpis* (right) eggs found in a faecal flotation from a dog. Though similar in appearance, *Eucoleus* is asymmetrical and smaller in size. (b) Faecal flotation showing *Trichuris vulpis* ova (darker appearing biperculate ova) and *Ancylostoma caninum* ova.
(a, © The National Center for Veterinary Parasitology at Oklahoma State University, www.ncvetp.org/; b, Reproduced from the *BSAVA Manual of Canine and Feline Gastroenterology, 2nd edition*)

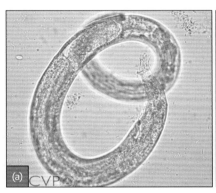

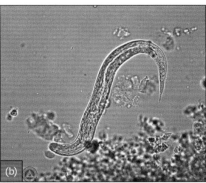

13.19 Faecal parasitology. (a) Larva of *Ollulanus tricuspis*. Third-stage larvae are approximately 500 μm and have a tricuspid tail similar to that of the adult female (2nd- and 4th-stage larvae also have this type of tail). Adults and larvae are found in the stomachs of domestic cats and other felids. Diagnosis is based on the identification of larvae or small adults (1 mm) in vomitus using the Baermann test. (b) In fresh faeces, *Strongyloides* spp. larvae rapidly develop to the infective filariform stage, which enters the host via skin or mucosal penetration. Filariform refers to the elongated shape of the oesophagus. In dogs and cats, *Strongyloides* eggs frequently hatch before leaving the body, thus free larvae are most often found in fresh faeces.
(© The National Center for Veterinary Parasitology at Oklahoma State University, www.ncvetp.org/)

most cestodes and roundworms do not cause clinical signs in adult dogs; ascarid roundworms can cause clinical signs in immature animals but rarely, if ever, cause significant clinical disease in adults. Further, coccidia species and many other protozoans are usually incidental findings on faecal examination in adults.

In contrast, parasites such as hookworms, whipworms, *Giardia*, *Tritrichomonas* and *Cryptosporidium* are more often associated with clinical disease which starts acutely but which might then become chronic. Nevertheless, the presence of an underlying disease may actually be allowing such parasites to colonize the GI tract and therefore all positive findings should be interpreted in the light of the clinical presentation. If any doubt exists as to whether a particular agent is causal, a treatment trial is indicated.

Tests for bacterial pathogens

Bacterial culture of faeces is generally performed for animals with acute GI signs, with either small or large intestinal or mixed diarrhoea. It can also be argued that culture is important because a number of the organisms that can be isolated from dog and cat faeces are potentially zoonotic. However, the zoonotic risk is small compared with the risk of eating contaminated food, assuming basic hygiene is practised.

Bacterial culture is most important if cases present with haemorrhagic diarrhoea, and/or pyrexia, and/or an inflammatory leucogram, and/or if neutrophils are identified on rectal cytology (see below). Yet bacterial culture is also often performed in practice as a preliminary diagnostic screen for cases with chronic diarrhoea, although the interpretation of a positive culture is problematic because it may not equate with causation (Marks *et al.*, 2011).

Use of inappropriate techniques is a common reason for false negative cultures, and samples of fresh faecal material, rather than rectal swabs, should be submitted promptly to laboratories that are equipped to culture the major pathogenic bacteria. In particular, *Campylobacter* is quite labile and may die before postal samples reach the laboratory. If shipment to a laboratory is required, placing a swab in Amies transport medium (containing charcoal) is recommended in addition to sending in faecal material.

Some laboratories recommend routine aerobic culture of faecal samples on the basis that changes in predominant populations of bacteria correlate with disease. However, there are currently no published studies to support such an approach, and the effects of postal delay on the relative growth rates of different organisms cannot be quantified. Given that many of the bacteria classed as pathogens can be found not only in the faeces of normal individuals but often at the same isolation rates, all results must be interpreted in light of the clinical presentation (Marks *et al.*, 2011).

The faecal bacterial flora may be representative of colonic bacterial populations but stool culture correlates poorly with the small intestinal flora, and so is *not* suitable for the diagnosis of so-called small intestinal bacterial overgrowth (SIBO). Evaluation of the whole microbiome, by high-throughput molecular sequencing of bacterial ribosomal 16S RNA, gives a global assessment of the intestinal microbial population but is a technique most applicable to assessing perturbations at the population level. For example, a shift towards predominance of Enterobacteriaceae has been demonstrated in feline IBD. Indeed, this technique is arguably not applicable to individual patients and is not available to practitioners. Therefore, targeted evaluation for potential pathogens, e.g. *Salmonella* spp., *Campylobacter* spp., *Escherichia coli*, *Clostridium perfringens* and *Clostridium difficile*, by culture on selective media can be performed. However, *E. coli* can be cultured from almost all faecal samples yet only certain strains are pathogenic, and it is more appropriate to use molecular probes to detect pathogenicity markers. Similarly the presence of clostridia may be more reliably detected by assays of their toxins in faeces. Molecular tests and toxin assays are probably more sensitive, may be positive even when there is a negative stool culture, and potentially are more clinically relevant.

Given that all of these organisms can be isolated from the faeces of both healthy animals and those with diarrhoea, determining the clinical significance of positive cultures can be difficult; however, because it is a potential zoonosis, the isolation of *Salmonella* is invariably important. The decision to treat a particular animal shedding *Salmonella* depends upon its individual circumstances because the carrier state develops during not after therapy.

Salmonella *spp.*: This organism is a potential pathogen in dogs and cats, although not all species appear equally pathogenic, and isolation from the faeces of healthy animals occurs. It is a fairly rare isolate from dogs and cats, with most reports suggesting a prevalence of <2%, but isolation rates up to 30% are reported. However, these are typically from dogs fed raw meat diets or untreated rawhide chews, and faecal isolation may represent passage of the organism through the GI tract rather than true infection.

Diagnosis is typically made by culture of faeces on selective media to allow the rapid identification of *Salmonella* spp. in faeces: they are facultative anaerobes that grow readily at 37°C. Most laboratories use a combination of selective enrichment broth followed by subculture to selective agar plates and will then identify presumptive salmonella colonies using biochemical techniques. Isolates identified as salmonella can be further discriminated by serotyping, and this is usually performed at reference laboratories. Although PCR assays are available, they are not used routinely despite a single routine culture being less sensitive. If the sensitivity of any culture method is ≥45%, three consecutive negative cultures are needed to be ~90% confident that the sample is truly negative, and six cultures would be required to be ~99% confident (Marks *et al.*, 2011).

Campylobacter *spp.*: Isolation of *Campylobacter* spp. by culture is more likely to be successful if attempted from fresh faeces; the organism is fastidious and grows best on selective media at 42°C. However, campylobacter isolates are usually only identified to genus rather than species level as standard microbiological culture and biochemical techniques cannot distinguish the species reliably, and it is then often assumed that most isolates are the potential pathogen *C. jejuni*.

Molecular techniques to aid accurate speciation are now commercially available; such an approach will be important in the future because recent research shows that many current isolates are actually different species for which pathogenicity is not established. *Campylobacter jejuni* has been shown to be potentially pathogenic in dogs and *C. coli* may be associated with diarrhoea in cats. However the most common isolate from dogs is *C. upsaliensis*, and its pathogenicity in dogs is unproven. Indeed a variety of campylobacter species can be found in the stool of clinically healthy animals, and inappropriate treatment in these circumstances may allow the development of antimicrobial resistance.

As stated, *C. upsaliensis* is actually the most common isolate from faeces from UK dogs whether or not they have diarrhoea. *Campylobacter* spp. are typically found in the faeces of approximately 30% of dogs in the UK, and more than 90% of the isolates are *C. upsaliensis* (Parsons *et al.*, 2010); *C. coli* can also be found in the faeces of healthy and diarrhoeic cats (Cogan T, personal communication).

In a longitudinal study of a small cohort of dogs ($n = 25$) in Denmark, which sampled faeces every month from weaning to 2 years of age, all dogs excreted campylobacter at least once during the study. Three-quarters of the isolates were *C. upsaliensis* and, interestingly, molecular techniques showed that repeat isolations from the same dog were clonal, suggesting persistent infection and intermittent shedding. In contrast, any repeated isolates of *C. jejuni* were genetically dissimilar, suggesting repeated new infections (Hald *et al.*, 2004).

Clostridia *spp.*: Clostridia are ubiquitous isolates from the faeces of healthy cats and dogs, and disease is thought to be more associated with their periodic production of enterotoxin.

Clostridium difficile: This is a Gram-positive anaerobic, spore-forming rod responsible for antibiotic-associated pseudomembranous colitis in humans; it has been incriminated as a rare cause of acute and chronic diarrhoea in dogs and cats and a potential nosocomial infection. Tests for *C. difficile* include:

- Culture
- Common antigen enzyme-linked immunosorbent assay (ELISA)
- PCR for toxigenic strains
- ELISA for toxins A and B.

Often considered fastidious to grow, the organism has been isolated by culture from the faeces of healthy dogs at isolation rates varying from 0 to 58%, depending on the study. The organism can also be identified by the presence of the common clostridial antigen (GLDH enzyme), although this test is insensitive for *C. difficile*. A negative culture or common antigen test does not necessarily rule out the presence of the organism. An ELISA can be used to detect toxins A and B. Alternatively, PCR for toxigenic strains can be performed either on faeces or cultured organisms.

However, the presence of the organism, and indeed the presence of toxigenic strains, does not necessarily correlate with the presence of disease. It is the secretion of an enterotoxin (toxin A) and a cytotoxin (toxin B) that is associated with virulence, and it is the presence of toxins in faeces that is probably most significant clinically. Indeed only about 50% of isolates have the genes for toxins A and/or B. Therefore, ELISAs that identify both the A and B toxins simultaneously are preferred to identification of potentially pathogenic organism. Even then, the presence of either toxin does not necessarily correlate with disease, because they can both be found in the stool of some clinically healthy animals.

Clostridium perfringens: *C. perfringens* has been associated with acute and chronic large bowel diarrhoea in dogs, which may or may not be accompanied by the presence of mucus, blood and tenesmus. The disease can range from mild and self-limiting to severe, but systemic signs are unusual. Unfortunately bacterial culture for the isolation of *C. perfringens* has little clinical value, as it appears to be a commensal organism that can be detected in the faeces of most dogs and cats. However *C. perfringens* is considered to be a cause of nosocomial diarrhoea, often occurring a few days after hospitalization.

The main virulence factor of this organism is *C. perfringens* enterotoxin (CPE), which is encoded by the *cpe* gene. CPE is produced during sporulation and released after bacterial cell lysis, and can induce mucosal damage, increase intestinal permeability and reduce water absorption, mechanisms which are all likely to lead to diarrhoea. As sporulation has been assumed to coincide with enterotoxin elaboration, examination of a Diff-Quik® stained faecal smear for 'safety-pin' shaped sporulating *C. perfringens* (>5 per oil field) has been suggested as a simple screening test but has subsequently been shown to be unreliable and is no longer recommended. Endospores can be seen in the faeces of healthy dogs as well as those with clinical signs, not all sporulating organisms produce CPE, and toxin can be found in the faeces of both healthy and diarrhoeic dogs in the absence of spores. Thus neither the presence of endospores nor CPE invariably confirms the diagnosis.

PCR can be used to identify organisms carrying the *cpe* gene but 20% of healthy cats, 37% of healthy dogs and 37% of diarrhoeic dogs and cats have been shown to carry organisms with the gene, and so the test has no discriminatory value. The detection of CPE is more likely to be indicative of disease. CPE can be detected in faeces by reverse passive latex agglutination or by ELISA, but the ELISA gives fewer false positive and false negative results. However, again, CPE can be found in the faeces of clinically healthy animals.

Virological examination

Viral diarrhoea is usually acute and self-limiting and there is rarely a need to make a positive diagnosis. Serological confirmation of viral enteritis is theoretically possible, but antibody conversion resulting from vaccination can obscure the significance of a positive titre.

Electron microscopy can be used directly to identify characteristic viral particles of rotavirus, coronavirus, astrovirus, norovirus and parvovirus, but is not readily available in the UK. Of these viruses, parvovirus is the most significant pathogen, and a rapid faecal ELISA for parvovirus is available (see below). Canine coronavirus identification is perhaps less important except in situations of high stocking density (e.g. kennels) where vaccination may be indicated, although a recent study suggested it may be a significant pathogen in dogs (Stavisky *et al.*, 2011).

Viruses in faeces can also be identified by PCR, and species such as coronaviruses are now included in screening panels offered by some commercial laboratories. However, as many of these viruses are only mildly pathogenic, a positive isolation does not confirm causation, and in some cases a mixed infection is present. It must also be noted that identification of feline coronavirus in faeces is not proof of FIP.

Parvovirus: A variety of tests are available for the identification of parvovirus: immunochromatography; haemagglutination; virus isolation; and conventional and real-time PCR. Using these techniques it was possible to detect canine parvovirus (CPV-2) antigen or nucleic acid in 46%, 56%, 61%, 76% and 82%, respectively, of samples in one study (Desario *et al.*, 2005). PCR has been shown overall to be most sensitive for the identification of parvovirus in faeces, but may actually be too sensitive because virus can also be found in the stool of dogs with chronic diarrhoea and healthy dogs (Schmitz *et al.*, 2009), when it presumably has no clinical significance. Although more sensitive than antibody-based tests, immune-electron microscopy (IEM) is not as sensitive as PCR and is also not available in the UK.

Antibody-based tests tend to be poorly sensitive (15.8–26.3%) compared with PCR and IEM (Schmitz *et al.*, 2009). Nevertheless, the faecal immunochromatographic (SNAP®) test is still the most applicable test to detect parvovirus antigen in the practice setting (Figure 13.20). The test has a reported sensitivity of 98% and a specificity of 100% for samples collected between days 4 and 7 post infection, when the shedding rate is highest and a positive test result is most likely to be clinically relevant.

Signalment and history
• Young animal • Unvaccinated animal • Exposure or potential exposure to parvovirus (e.g. affected in-contact animal or contaminated environment)
Clinical signs

• Acute/peracute gastrointestinal signs with or without:
  • Haematemesis, melaena or severe haematochezia
  • Pyrexia
  • Leucopenia or neutropenia

13.20 Indications for performing faecal parvovirus antigen ELISA.

For the faecal immunochromatographic (SNAP®) test, fresh faecal samples should be tested and, ideally, should be taken 24–36 hours after the onset of clinical signs. Given that false negatives can arise if samples are taken too early in the course of the disease, the test should be repeated after 36–48 hours if it is negative and the clinical signs are still consistent with parvovirus. False negative results can also occur if samples are taken too late in the disease process because shedding decreases after the first week, although the patient is still contagious. Theoretically, false negatives can also occur owing to interference from coproantibody, while weak false positives occur transiently between 5 and 15 days after vaccination with a modified live vaccine. PCR may be able to distinguish native from vaccinal virus shedding depending on the PCR primers used and the vaccine strain and, potentially, quantitative PCR may differentiate low copy numbers associated with live vaccination from true infections.

A diagnosis of parvovirus can also be made on the basis of a positive IgM titre against CPV-2. Alternatively the diagnosis can be confirmed retrospectively by documenting rising serum IgG titres in paired samples at a 2–3-week interval. Thus serology is of most use in assessing immune status and determining whether booster vaccination is necessary.

Protozoal infections

Giardia intestinalis (syn. G. lamblia, G. duodenalis): Motile, pear-shaped *Giardia* trophozoites (9–21 × 5–12 μm) (see Figures 13.13 and 13.14) can sometimes be identified in very fresh stained or unstained faecal smears. *Motile* trophozoites can also be detected in duodenal fluid, collected endoscopically, but this has not been shown to be superior to faecal methods.

Ovoid cysts, measuring 8–15 × 7–10 μm, can be detected in direct wet mounts of faeces or by faecal flotation/centrifugation. Because of fluctuating excretion, three samples collected over 3–5 days are recommended. Oocysts are best found by zinc sulphate flotation or using Parasep® centrifugation because cysts become deformed if salt flotation is attempted. Performing zinc sulphate flotation on three consecutive unpooled samples has a reported sensitivity of over 90%.

Immunofluorescent antibody (IFA) staining is used in diagnostic laboratories and is considered the gold standard, but ELISA detection of antigen in faeces is also used. A rapid immunochromatographic (SNAP®) method can be used to detect *Giardia* in faeces and is suited to in-house use; furthermore, only a small volume of diarrhoea is required (Figure 13.21). However, while convenient to perform, it does not necessarily have greater accuracy than zinc sulphate (ZNSO₄) flotation performed by an experienced technician, and does not correlate well with IFA (Rishniw *et al.*, 2010). Assuming 100% prevalence in samples, Rishniw *et al.* (2010) demonstrated that the *Giardia* SNAP® test had a sensitivity of 70%, compaired with 45% for an ELISA (*Giardia* II test Direct ELISA), 45% for a single ZnSO₄ flotation and 72% for pooled samples undergoing ZnSO₄ flotation, in comparison to 90% for the gold standard IFA. At lower prevalences (e.g. 10%), the antigen tests performed better than ZnSO₄ flotation. All had low positive predictive values (58%, 51%, 48% and 19% respectively), but negative predictive values greater than 90%.

There are seven (A–G) recognized genotypes/strains of *Giardia*. Typing assays are not readily available, but assemblages C and D are most commonly found in dogs, while F has been isolated from cats. Humans are usually infected with assemblages A and B; assemblage A has been found in both dogs and cats but assemblage B very rarely.

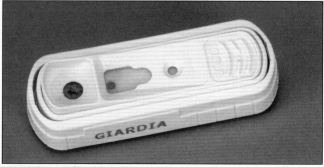

13.21 SNAP® immunochromatographic test for in-house testing for *Giardia* infection.

Tritrichomonas foetus: Recent studies suggest the organism may actually be *Tritrichomonas blagnurni* n.sp. (Walden *et al.*, 2013), but this protozoal organism is a cause of diarrhoea of emerging importance in cats. It primarily colonizes the large intestine and causes chronic large bowel diarrhoea; anal irritation and faecal incontinence can be features of infection.

Its prevalence in samples submitted from symptomatic UK cats has been estimated to be 20% (Gunn–Moore *et al.*, 2007). Cats of any age, breed or sex can be infected, but young cats and pedigree cats from densely housed catteries, rehoming centres, or multi-cat households are most at risk. Persistent infection is most common and, although signs may spontaneously resolve, infection is latent and cats will often suffer recrudescence when stressed. It is, therefore, most appropriate to look for the organism in kittens and younger cats, especially those from appropriate environments, and also in older cats with recurrent colitis-like signs. However, infection of any cat is possible and it should not be considered to be restricted to pedigree cats; there is also some limited evidence of canine infection. Furthermore, cats that are unresponsive to treatment for *Giardia* infection should be tested in case of misdiagnosis.

The organism may be recognized on colonic biopsy samples, but it is preferable to make a diagnosis of a *T. foetus* infection by examination of faeces. There are a number of methods available, but none is 100% sensitive, and repeat testing should be considered where there is a negative result and a high index of suspicion. Test sensitivities can be improved by only examining diarrhoeic samples. High colonic washing provides the best sample and is a relatively easy technique to perform. The saline washings are centrifuged or allowed to settle and the sediment submitted for examination. A loop can also be used to collect liquid faeces. The results are usually negative if formed faeces are examined, even though the cat may be carrying the infection, and antibiotic usage in the previous 7 days may also cause a false negative result.

Methods of diagnosis include:

- **Identification of motile organisms on a direct wet faecal mount:** for this, very fresh samples must be used, ideally kept warm before examination, and even then there is a very low sensitivity (reported as 14%). Specificity can also be low if the organism is misdiagnosed as *Giardia* spp. or *Pentatrichomonas hominis*. *T. foetus* organisms have a characteristic forward progressive motion with an undulating membrane
- **Faecal culture:** the organism can be cultured using a commercially available culture system Feline InPouch™TF originally developed for the diagnosis of bovine venereal *T. foetus* infection. Pouches containing medium are inoculated with approximately 0.05 g of freshly voided faeces and incubated at 25°C. The pouches are then examined under a microscope every couple of days until motile organisms are seen; this can take from 1 to 12 days from initial inoculation. Although more sensitive than direct smear examination, the method is laborious and the diagnosis potentially delayed because the results can only be considered negative after 12 days
- **PCR analysis of faeces:** this is relatively quick and is the most sensitive method of detecting *T. foetus* because as few as 10 organisms per gram of faeces can be detected. Ideally fresh faeces should be tested, but if there is a delay between collection and

submission, the faeces can be kept refrigerated for up to a week although sensitivity declines with time. Quantitative PCR allows measurement of the number of organisms present, and can be used to monitor the response to treatment. Again sensitivity is improved by providing liquid faeces or colonic washings, and samples should not include cat litter, which can contain inhibitors of the PCR; reliable laboratories include an internal amplification control to check for inhibition of the reaction.

Cystoisospora *(syn.* Isospora*) spp.*: Identification of the presence of *Cystoisospora* coccidia in the faeces of dogs and cats is by microscopic examination using centrifugal flotation. However, their presence is not, in itself, adequate proof that coccidiosis is the cause of any accompanying clinical signs. Indeed *Cystoisospora* are generally considered to be of little clinical significance except in puppies and kittens, or perhaps as a marker of another underlying problem.

Several genera of *Cystoisospora*-like organisms may be present in canine and feline faeces. *Cystoisospora* is host specific: *Cystoisospora canis*, *C. ohioensis* and *C. burrowsi* are the common species that infect dogs, while *C. felis* and *C. rivolta* infect cats. They can be differentiated on the basis of size, state of sporulation, and the presence/absence of oocysts or sporocysts (http://www.esccap.org). However, *C. ohioensis* and *C. burrowsi* are often grouped as the *C. ohioensis* complex because they are not readily separated morphologically. Oocysts of *Eimeria* spp. are also sometimes observed in canine and feline stool samples, but dogs and cats are not hosts to this organism.

Cryptosporidium parvum: *Cryptosporidium* is a genus with low host specificity that can occasionally parasitize cats and (rarely) dogs, causing diarrhoea particularly in kittens and puppies. The classification of this genus and the naming of species is rapidly changing owing to emerging molecular information, and *Cryptosporidium parvum*, a significant pathogen in humans and calves, may not be a single species. Twenty-one *C. parvum* genotypes are currently recognized and include cat and dog 'species', sometimes termed *C. felis* and *C. canis* respectively, which are only likely to be zoonotic in immunocompromised humans.

The diagnostic method of choice is faecal smear and staining (Ziehl–Neelsen, Heine or safranin stains) or direct immunofluorescence. Identification by faecal flotation or centrifugation requires oil immersion microscopy but is difficult without staining. Oocysts are extremely small, round, red or orange bodies when stained, and approximately one-tenth the size of *Isospora* oocysts. Organisms may also be recognized in intestinal biopsy samples.

As with *Giardia*, coproantigen tests are commercially available and can detect infections even if the number of excreted oocysts is low. Molecular detection is both sensitive and specific but PCR tests are not commercially available.

Occult blood

This test is used to search for GI bleeding that is not grossly visible as melaena or haematochezia, particularly when iron-deficiency anaemia is detected. Haemorrhage can potentially occur at any level of the GI tract and the test is sensitive enough to detect 2 ml blood per 30 kg bodyweight. Given that the test merely detects haemoglobin, false positive results often arise from the ingestion of diets containing meat (and blood). Fresh, uncooked vegetables can also give a false positive result due to the presence of interfering peroxidases, although any negative result rules out the presence of blood whatever the diet. For a positive test to be meaningful the patient must be fed a meat-free diet for at least 72 hours before samples are obtained; a vegetarian or hydrolysed diet is recommended.

Rectal cytology

Samples can be taken for cytological analysis by mildly abrading the rectal wall with a gloved finger after digital rectal examination. The material is then rolled on to a microscope slide and the smear stained. The test is easy to perform and non-invasive, but the results are most often negative. Such examinations are of limited use for small intestinal disease, and are instead most appropriate for diseases involving the large intestine, and particularly the rectum.

Rectal lymphoma can occasionally be identified, and increased numbers of neutrophils may be suggestive of a bacterial infection and indicate the need for faecal culture. Clostridial endospores and fungal/oomycete elements (*Aspergillus*, *Candida*, *Histoplasma*, *Pythium*) may also be identified. *Aspergillus* is ubiquitous in the environment and is most likely to have been ingested accidentally; it is likely only to be of any significance in severely immunocompromised patients, and histological evidence of infection is required for diagnosis. *Candida* infection may follow antibacterial usage but yeast-like organisms are frequently seen in faeces and seem to be of little significance. *Histoplasma* and *Pythium* are pathogenic but infections are not seen in Europe. Perhaps the most specific and useful result to come from rectal cytology is when a palpable mass is present within the rectum.

Analysis of cells and tissue specimens
Histopathology

Histopathological assessment of gastric and intestinal biopsy samples remains the gold standard for the diagnosis of GI disease (Figure 13.22), although it has many limitations. Biopsy specimens can be normal by light microscopy in almost half of cats and dogs with chronic GI disease, and this suggests either that many diseases have a functional rather than morphological abnormality or that sampling problems have occurred. For example, the findings in duodenal and ileal biopsy specimens from the same patient show poor correlation. Another major problem with reliance on histopathological diagnoses is poor agreement between histopathologists. Standardized reporting criteria have been established as a means of improving agreement (Day *et al.*, 2008) but, despite this, substantial inconsistency remains among pathologists, at least partly because of differences in slide processing (Willard *et al.*, 2010). Thus, the primary clinician should always interpret results cautiously in light of the clinical presentation, and results should be questioned if the histopathological diagnosis does not fit the clinical picture or the response to apparently appropriate therapy is poor.

Cytology

Cytological examination of endoscopic biopsy squash preparations or mucosal brushings (Figure 13.23) can occasionally be a useful adjunct to diagnosis of GI disease.

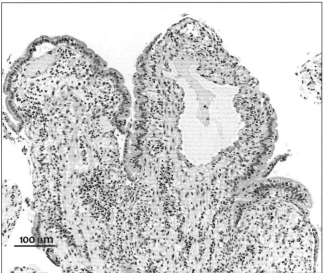

13.22 Photomicrograph of a biopsy specimen from the duodenum of an 8-year-old neutered male crossbred dog with diarrhoea, ascites and severe panhypoproteinaemia (albumin 10 g/l, reference interval: 25–31 g/l; globulins 20 g/l, reference interval: 27–40 g/l). There is evidence of villous atrophy, epithelial erosions and mild lacteal dilatation. There is a variable, mixed inflammatory cell infiltrate within the mucosa. These findings are consistent with mixed intestinal inflammation. (Haematoxylin and eosin stain; original magnification X10)
(Courtesy of R Fox, University of Liverpool)

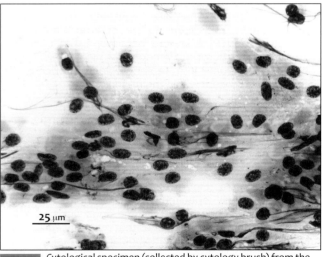

13.23 Cytological specimen (collected by cytology brush) from the duodenum of a 6-year-old neutered male Staffordshire Bull Terrier with chronic vomiting and diarrhoea. The preparation demonstrates clumps of normal epithelial cells. Streaks of nuclear material are due to rupture during smearing. The histopathological specimens from this case were unremarkable and the dog responded to dietary management, suggesting an adverse reaction to food. (Rapid Romanowsky stain; original magnification X40)

Brush cytology provides superior cytological information, and complements (rather than replaces) histopathological analysis because it does not provide architectural information. Its greatest benefit is likely to be in the differentiation of severe lymphocytic–plasmacytic enteritis from alimentary lymphoma, because the cellular and nuclear characteristics of malignancy can be better assessed. Brush cytology or touch preparations of gastric biopsy samples allow identification of *Helicobacter* spp. in the stomach (see below).

Specialized diagnostic tests

Numerous tests have been developed in an attempt to investigate GI diseases non-invasively. However, many of these specialized tests are not available commercially, many have not been properly validated and many are only applicable to referral and/or research institutions, rather than general practice. What follows is a summary of the main tests developed, and their indications. These tests are *not* recommended for routine use.

Further tests for gastric disease

Gastric enzyme assays (gastric lipase, pepsinogen)

Measurement of serum gastric lipase does not aid in the diagnosis and differentiation of gastric diseases. Assays for canine and feline pepsinogen-like immunoreactivity are not yet available.

Tests for gastric spiral organisms

A number of tests assess the presence of gastric spiral organisms (GSOs), usually presumed to be *Helicobacter* spp. Infection in dogs and cats appears to be almost ubiquitous, seroconversion is common and, because the pathogenic potential of the organisms remains unclear, specifically looking for organisms is largely an academic exercise.

Most of the detection methods have been modified from techniques used for the detection of *Helicobacter pylori* in humans. However, the species of GSOs seen in companion animals differ from humans, and their true significance as pathogens remains to be established; indeed they may be commensal organisms in the majority of healthy dogs and cats and the presence of organisms does not necessarily correlate with the presence of clinical disease. Thus, the significance of any positive test for GSO should be interpreted in light of the clinical presentation.

Histopathology: While GSOs can be detected by brush cytology of the gastric mucosa, histopathology permits their microscopic identification within biopsy material, especially if special staining procedures, e.g. Warthin–Starry silver staining, are performed. Sensitivity is also improved if multiple biopsy samples are submitted from different gastric regions, and especially from the fundus and corpus. Some histopathologists comment on the presence of GSO within gastric glands, but there is no evidence to suggest that this correlates with pathogenicity. The presence of an inflammatory (lymphocytic–plasmacytic) infiltrate within the mucosa and lymphoid nodular hyperplasia may suggest an associated gastritis. Although similar findings have been documented in studies involving experimental infection of dogs and cats with *Helicobacter* organisms, the histopathological changes did not correlate with the presence of clinical signs.

Other techniques for identifying GSOs: Given that the morphology of all GSOs is similar under light microscopy, techniques such as electron microscopy and PCR are required to identify the exact species of GSO that is present. However, such tests are not widely available.

Urease test: Helicobacter spp. produce urease, which can split urea, leading to ammonia production. Inoculation of a mucosal biopsy sample into a special medium which changes colour when ammonia is produced can be used to detect helicobacters.

Urea breath test: This is a non-invasive means of confirming the presence of urease-producing organisms but is rarely used in veterinary medicine.

Gastrin

Gastrin is normally secreted by G-cells in the gastric and duodenal mucosa, and stimulates the secretion of gastric acid by parietal cells. On occasion, it is necessary to measure gastrin in vomiting dogs, for example when gastrinoma, a neuroendocrine tumour usually located in the pancreas, is a possible differential diagnosis. This can be done either by radioimmunoassay or ELISA (using antibodies that cross-react with human gastrin). Special sample handling is required to prevent gastrin degradation. The reference range for serum gastrin concentration in dogs in one assay (http://vetmed.tamu.edu/gilab/service/assays/gastrin) was established as <27.8 ng/l, but most healthy dogs have undetectable serum gastrin concentrations.

Serum gastrin concentrations vary inversely with the concentration of hydrogen ions in the gastric lumen, and many gastric diseases can elevate serum gastrin concentrations if there is acid hyposecretion. These conditions include chronic gastritis (atrophic and ulcerative types), gastric outflow obstruction including pyloric stenosis, and gastric dilatation–volvulus. Increased serum gastrin concentrations may also occur in chronic kidney disease, after small intestinal resection and secondary to drug administration (e.g. glucocorticoids). Given that high gastrin concentrations also arise if hyposecretion of gastric acid occurs when H_2 antagonists or proton pump inhibitors are in use, it is usually sensible to measure gastric luminal pH concurrently and to withdraw acid blockers for at least 1 week before measurement.

Serum concentrations of gastrin 10 times above the upper limit of the reference range are considered abnormal. This cut-off is extrapolated from humans; it is probably rather conservative in dogs and reflects a high prevalence in humans of atrophic gastritis related to *Helicobacter pylori* infection, which frequently causes severely elevated serum gastrin concentrations. Therefore, a <10-fold elevation of serum gastrin concentration may still be sufficient to diagnose a canine gastrinoma if other differential diagnoses have been carefully ruled out. Endoscopy and biopsy may provide supportive evidence for a gastrinoma by demonstrating gastric mucosal hypertrophy and ulceration. If gastrinoma is suspected, but only moderate increases in serum gastrin concentration are documented, a provocative test could be considered.

Further tests for chronic diarrhoea

Tests of pancreatic function

Exocrine pancreatic insufficiency (EPI) should be excluded in all cases presenting with chronic diarrhoea by testing serum trypsin-like immunoreactivity (TLI). This test and diagnostic tests for pancreatitis, which can cause vomiting and diarrhoea, are discussed in Chapter 14.

Alternative tests for SIBO/ARD

The current diagnostic gold standard for SIBO is quantitative bacterial culture of duodenal juice, although a number of other 'indirect' tests have been reported including measurement of serum parameters (cobalamin, folate, unconjugated bile acids) and performing breath hydrogen studies.

Quantitative bacterial culture of duodenal juice: Duodenal juice can be cultured quantitatively and, if both aerobic and strict anaerobic conditions are used, values can be obtained for total bacterial numbers and for numbers of aerobes and anaerobes. However, there is no clear definition of normal bacterial numbers, and molecular analysis of the intestinal microbiome shows that many organisms are never actually cultured. Consequently, this test has fallen out of favour in veterinary medicine, not least because it does not aid decision-making in cases of GI disease (German *et al.*, 2003a). Similarly, indirect chemical tests of SIBO are not recommended.

Tests of gastrointestinal function

A number of indirect tests are available to assess for malabsorption, protein loss, altered permeability and GI dysfunction. Such tests confirm the presence of GI disease and any associated complications (e.g. PLE). However, a definitive diagnosis is rarely obtained and most cases of primary GI disease require biopsy for histopathological assessment.

Tests of malabsorption

Before detailed assessment of GI function is performed, EPI should be ruled out by a TLI test, because signs of malabsorption are non-specific (see Chapter 14). Historical tests that have been used to document malabsorption, including the fat absorption test, the oral glucose absorption test, the starch digestion test and the D-xylose absorption test, are unreliable and not recommended. Indeed, all such methods required multiple blood samples or urine collection, were insensitive and were not capable of differentiating among different types of GI disease. Protocols for diagnosing malabsorption using breath hydrogen analysis have also been described but are no longer used. Therefore, the only widely available tests are measurement of serum folate and cobalamin (see above).

Faecal elastase measurement

Tests to measure faecal proteolytic activity are of no value when investigating intestinal disease. They are also unreliable for diagnosing EPI (see Chapter 14). Measurement of faecal elastase concentrations has been validated for dogs, and is a reasonably sensitive and specific test of EPI although still poorer than serum TLI measurement. Therefore, it is not commonly used in clinical practice.

Tests of gastrointestinal protein loss

Historically, intestinal protein loss has been detected by measuring the faecal loss of [51]chromium-labelled albumin. Since this compound is radioactive, this procedure is rarely used clinically, but remains the standard by which other tests have been judged. In reality, the laboratory parameter most widely used for documentation of GI protein loss is a reduction in serum proteins, although faecal markers such as faecal α_1-PI may detect protein loss before serum albumin concentrations fall.

Serum protein concentrations: Measurement of serum protein concentrations is currently the only practicable test outside North America for detecting GI protein loss. Decreased albumin concentrations are reasonably specific for intestinal protein loss, once other causes of hypoalbuminaemia (i.e. renal loss, blood loss and lack of hepatic production) have been excluded (see Figure 13.7). Further, the index of suspicion for intestinal protein loss is increased when hypoglobulinaemia accompanies hypoalbuminaemia. However, albumin concentrations are insensitive and cannot detect early or mild disease because concentrations only decline once the capacity for hepatic production is exceeded.

Faecal alpha-1 proteinase inhibitor concentrations: In human gastroenterology, faecal α_1-PI is a reliable marker of GI protein loss. An assay for this marker in dogs and cats has been developed at Texas A&M University, initially as a radioimmunoassay, and now as an ELISA. α_1-PI is a serum protein with a molecular weight similar to albumin and intestinal protein loss will, therefore, lead to loss of both proteins at a similar rate. However, in contrast to albumin, α_1-PI is relatively resistant to proteolysis and thus can be measured in the faeces. The reference range for dogs is 2.2–18.7 µg/g faecal material with a mean 3-day faecal α_1-PI of ≥13.9 µg/g or an α_1-PI of one individual sample of ≥21.0 µg/g faeces being considered abnormal. The reference range for cats is 0.04–1.6 µg/g faecal material, but PLEs are rarer in this species.

Early work suggested that this test is of value for the diagnosis of PLE, and a more sensitive marker than serum albumin concentrations for the detection of early disease. However, the assay is invalidated by the presence of any blood in the faecal sample, and digital rectal evacuation of faeces can cause enough mucosal abrasion and bleeding to increase faecal α_1-PI concentrations and invalidate the result. Further, α_1-PI measurement is unreliable in puppies and kittens, which have greater concentrations normally. To improve diagnostic accuracy, three fresh faecal samples should be collected within a 48-hour period, and then shipped on ice to the laboratory. Given that no other laboratory currently offers the test, its use is currently limited, although it may become more widely available in the future.

Tests of GI inflammation

Faecal calprotectin: Calprotectin (syn. neutrophil elastase) is a cytosolic protein complex that is contained in neutrophils and released at sites of inflammation; it is a sensitive non-invasive marker for the diagnosis of GI inflammation in humans. A canine immunoassay for the measurement of faecal canine calprotectin has been developed and validated (Heilmann et al., 2008), but is currently only available in the USA from the GI Laboratory, Texas. Its value in detecting GI inflammation, and for monitoring the response to treatment in dogs, is as yet unproven.

Other faecal markers: The development of potential markers of GI inflammation is ongoing: increased nitric oxide has been demonstrated in colitis, and lactoferrin is a potential future marker.

Tests of intestinal permeability

Intestinal permeability is an index of mucosal integrity and is assessed by measuring unmediated uptake of non-digestible probe markers that after permeation are not metabolized, and are fully excreted in the urine. The permeability probe ^{51}Cr-ethylenediamine tetra-acetic acid (EDTA) was used in the original studies, but its radioactivity as a γ-emitter limited its use.

Errors related to non-mucosal factors (including gastric emptying rate, intestinal transit and completeness of urine collection) can be eliminated by concurrently measuring the absorption of two probes with different pathways of absorption. Calculation of their excretion ratio eliminates variability from extramucosal factors, because both probes should be affected equally. The ratio will be altered by villous atrophy or epithelial damage or both, but not affected by non-mucosal factors, and potentially offers a simple and sensitive diagnostic test. Recent studies show that single probe markers such as iohexol are equally sensitive (Frias et al., 2012).

Lactulose/rhamnose test: Sequential blood sampling or a 5-hour urine collection is performed after oral administration of the permeability probe(s). There are a number of candidates for the probe molecules and a mixture of one large (e.g. lactulose, cellobiose, raffinose) and one small (e.g. rhamnose, arabinose, mannitol) simple sugar is usually chosen. After advances in the high-performance liquid chromatography (HPLC) assay of these sugars, the lactulose/rhamnose test has become the standard test of SI permeability, but iohexol may offer greater utility because it is easier to measure (Frias et al., 2012). Inclusion of a sugar probe such as sucrose, which is rapidly digested in the upper SI, provides a potential marker for assessing gastroduodenal permeability.

Laboratory tests of gastric emptying time and orocaecal transit time

A ^{13}C-octanoic acid breath test has been developed and standardized for dogs, and may detect delayed gastric emptying. Breath hydrogen analysis protocols have been used to estimate orocaecal transit time, although the protocols have not yet been properly established.

Analysis of cells and tissue specimens

Diagnostic investigations other than histopathology: Other examinations of biopsy specimens are largely research tools, but can provide significant information. Possibilities include: electron microscopy; biochemical assay of brush border enzymes by subcellular fractionation; immunohistochemistry; cytokine expression; assessment of T-cell clonality (German et al., 2003b). Only a few of these tests are available to practitioners, and they are only indicated where the histological diagnosis is not clear-cut.

PCR for antigen receptor rearrangement (PARR): The PARR test can be used to look for lymphocyte clonality to try to distinguish alimentary lymphoma from IBD (see Chapter 5).

Immunohistochemistry: This can be used for the immunocytochemical characterization of B cells, T cells and their subsets (CD4, CD8, etc.) and major histocompatibility complex (MHC) expression, but is most useful for differentiating B- and T-cell lymphomas.

Fluorescent* in situ *hybridization (FISH): FISH is a sensitive way of demonstrating bacteria adherent to and within the GI mucosa (Recordati et al., 2008). A shift to adherent Enterobacteriaceae has been demonstrated in feline IBD (Janeczko et al., 2008), and the demonstration of attaching and invading E. coli (AIEC) in the colonic mucosa of Boxer dogs with granulomatous (histiocytic ulcerative) colitis has shed new light on this condition (Mansfield et al., 2009). Depending on the fluorescent molecular probes used, FISH analysis of intestinal biopsy samples can show attaching and invading organisms (Figure 13.24); the technique is now available from commercial laboratories.

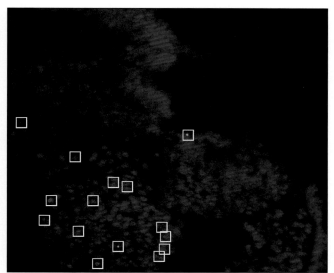

13.24 Fluorescent *in situ* hybridization (FISH) in a sample of small intestine from a dog with diarrhoea, fed a raw meat diet. The positions of bacteria are highlighted by the surrounding white boxes. A eubacterial probe shows green fluorescence and *Campylobacter* appears red.

Tests of GI immune function and inflammation

Humoral immunity: Given that IgA deficiency may predispose to GI disease, measurement of immunoglobulins has been advocated to assess mucosal immunity. However, serum immunoglobulin concentrations do not reflect those at mucosal surfaces and, while measurement of faecal immunoglobulins may be more useful, concentrations again correlate poorly with intestinal production. Therefore, routine measurement of serum or faecal immunoglobulins is not recommended currently.

Food-specific antibodies: Antigen-specific serum antibodies to food components can be measured *in vitro* (by a radioallergosorbent test (RAST) or ELISA), and a number of laboratories now offer this commercially. In most situations, IgG and/or IgE responses to different food components are assessed. Subjectively, clinicians who use such tests believe them to be of value, but critical appraisal suggests they are unhelpful (Foster *et al.*, 2003).

There are many reasons why the use of such tests is flawed. First, antibodies to food components can be found in normal individuals and, therefore, the presence of antibody in an affected individual may be incidental. Second, because vaccines may contain bovine serum albumin, individuals may develop antibodies to beef antigens. Third, because these tests only measure antibodies, they do not assess cell-mediated responses. Fourth, since the affinity of antibodies formed to a particular antigen in different individuals may vary, not all may be detected in the immunoassay, and some may not react at all (if the *in vitro* antigen is not relevant). Fifth, the presence of antibodies does not necessarily prove primary food hypersensitivity; they may have arisen secondary to another underlying disease process, e.g. IBD.

It has been shown that dogs with chronic GI disease due to a variety of causes had greater levels of food-specific IgG than healthy and atopic dogs (Foster *et al.*, 2003). However, the results did not correlate with their response to exclusion diet trials, and any perceived benefit of dietary modification may be coincidental. Thus, these tests cannot be recommended.

Immune cell populations: Flow cytometry and immunohistochemistry have been used to quantify and map the distribution of immune cell populations within the inflamed GI mucosa but are not yet practical for routine diagnostic use.

Humoral factors:
Cytokines: Semi-quantitative and quantitative real-time reverse transcriptase (RT)-PCR techniques can determine the expression of mRNA encoding various cytokines and any differences between control tissues and diseased samples. However, the results so far have often been contradictory, and the method is not suitable for clinical diagnosis in individual patients.

Acute phase proteins: In other recent studies, serum acute phase proteins (APP) have been measured, and increases in some markers (e.g. C-reactive protein) have been documented in samples from dogs with IBD. Given that APP are non-specific markers of inflammation, these tests alone are not diagnostic for IBD. However, assessment of APP may provide a non-invasive means of assessing disease severity (in conjunction with a canine IBD activity index), and for monitoring response to treatment.

Case examples

CASE 1

SIGNALMENT

6-year, 7-month old entire female Airedale Terrier.

HISTORY

3-week history of anorexia, vomiting and occasional diarrhoea, then rapid deterioration prior to presentation. On physical examination the dog was 8% dehydrated, with a normal body temperature and a pulse rate of 160 beats/min. The abdomen was tense, which made palpation difficult.

WHAT DIFFERENTIAL DIAGNOSES WOULD YOU CONSIDER AND WHAT IN-HOUSE TESTS MIGHT YOU USE TO TRY AND RULE THEM IN OR OUT?

Differential diagnosis	Discriminatory tests
Acute bacterial gastroenteritis	• Unlikely because of chronic history • Stool culture of debatable value • Haematology, serum biochemistry and imaging are only helpful in ruling out other causes and assessing degree of dehydration
Parvovirus	• Unlikely because of chronic history • SNAP® faecal antigen test, but may be negative if more than 10 days post infection • Serology
Acute (on chronic) pancreatitis	• Canine pancreatic lipase immunoreactivity (SNAP® cPL™ initially, followed by Spec cPL®) • Abdominal ultrasonography
Acute hepatitis	• Serum biochemistry: ALT, ALP, bile acids • Abdominal ultrasonography
Intestinal obstruction	• Plain radiography and ultrasonography
Hypoadrenocorticism with Addisonian crisis	• Sodium:potassium ratio • Basal cortisol or ACTH stimulation test
Acute (on chronic) renal failure	• Serum biochemistry: urea, creatinine, phosphate • Urine specific gravity

CLINICAL PATHOLOGY DATA

Haematology	Result	Reference interval
RBC (x 10¹²/l)	6.21	5.50–8.50
Haematocrit (l/l)	0.42	0.37–0.55
Haemoglobin (g/dl)	13.9	12.0–18.0
MCV (fl)	68.0	60.0–77.0
WBC (x 10⁹/l)	**18.5**	5.5–16.9
Neutrophils (segmented) (x 10⁹/l)	**14.2**	3.00–12.00
Lymphocytes (x 10⁹/l)	1.89	0.50–4.90
Monocytes (x 10⁹/l)	**2.23**	0.30–2.00 ▶

Abnormal results are in **bold**.

Haematology *continued*	Result	Reference interval
Eosinophils (x 10⁹/l)	**0.07**	0.10–1.40
Basophils (x 10⁹/l)	0.00	0.00–0.10
Platelets (x 10⁹/l)	215	175–500

Abnormal results are in **bold**.

Biochemistry	Result	Reference interval
Total protein (g/l)	**50**	58–78
Albumin (g/l)	**21**	23–31
Globulin (g/l)	29	18–37
ALT (IU/l)	24	7–50
ALP (IU/l)	**116**	0–100
Bilirubin (μmol/l)	8	0–10
Creatinine (μmol/l)	**131**	20–110
Urea (mmol/l)	**12.3**	3.5–6.0
Calcium (mmol/l)	2.41	2.20–2.70
Phosphate (mmol/l)	1.2	0.80–2.00
Sodium (mmol/l)	151	140–153
Potassium (mmol/l)	4.40	3.80–5.30
Semi-quantitative pancreas-specific lipase test (SNAP® cPL™)	Darkly positive	>400

Abnormal results are in **bold**.

Urine specific gravity: 1.045.
Urine dipstick and sediment: unremarkable.

WHAT ABNORMALITIES ARE PRESENT?

- Mild leucocytosis with a mature neutrophilia, monocytosis and eosinopenia.
- Hypoproteinaemia resulting from mild hypoalbuminaemia.
- Azotaemia as shown by the mild–moderate increase in serum urea concentration, and mild increase in creatinine.
- Mild increase in ALP.
- Positive pancreas-specific lipase result on the cage-side test.

HOW WOULD YOU INTERPRET THESE RESULTS AND WHICH OF YOUR DIFFERENTIAL DIAGNOSES REMAIN?

- The mature neutrophilia, monocytosis and eosinopenia would be consistent with a stress leucogram.
- The azotaemia is more likely to be the result of dehydration, given the hypersthenuric urine. Increased urea concentration secondary to gastrointestinal haemorrhage would be an alternative possibility, but would not explain the mild increase in creatinine concentration.
- Possible causes for hypoalbuminaemia include hepatocellular dysfunction, renal protein loss, gastrointestinal protein loss and albumin loss secondary to haemorrhage. There is no other evidence for hepatocellular dysfunction or renal

→ **CASE 1 CONTINUED**

protein loss (given the absence of proteinuria on urinalysis) and, although there is a mild decrease in red cell mass, this is unlikely to be significant enough to account for the degree of hypoalbuminaemia. Therefore, the most likely reason for the hypoalbuminaemia is gastrointestinal protein loss.

- The mild increase in ALP is not likely to be of clinical significance, and may reflect a reactive hepatopathy. More marked increases in liver enzyme activity are often seen in acute pancreatitis.
- Serum sodium and potassium are within reference ranges, making hypoadrenocorticism very unlikely. A basal cortisol or an ACTH stimulation test could be considered because atypical hypoadrenocorticism is still possible.
- The positive cage-side pancreas-specific lipase test is consistent with acute pancreatitis. However, confirming the result with a quantitative assay (i.e. Spec cPL®) is recommended.
- Other investigations including abdominal imaging should be considered.

Remaining differential diagnoses

- Acute pancreatitis.
- Acute gastrointestinal diseases, including:
  - Acute gastroenteritis
  - Canine parvovirus infection
  - Intestinal foreign body.

WHAT FURTHER TESTS WOULD YOU RECOMMEND?

- A quantitative pancreas-specific lipase assay (i.e. Spec cPL®) is indicated to confirm the positive cage-side test results.
- Abdominal radiography and ultrasonography are also recommended to examine the pancreas and GI tract because pancreatitis cannot be confirmed on the basis of laboratory findings alone.

FURTHER RESULTS

Canine pancreas-specific lipase (Spec cPL®) was 519 µg/l (reference interval <200; suggestive of pancreatitis >400). A lateral abdominal radiograph was also taken (Figure 13.25).

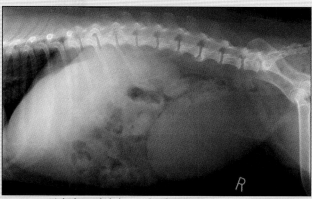

13.25 Right lateral abdominal radiograph of the Airedale Terrier with anorexia, vomiting and occasional diarrhoea.

HOW WOULD YOU INTERPRET THESE FURTHER TESTS AND THE RADIOGRAPH, AND WHAT IS THE DIAGNOSIS?

- Canine pancreas-specific lipase was again suggestive of pancreatic inflammation.
- The abdominal radiograph demonstrated poor abdominal contrast with multiple 'tear-drop' (comma-shaped) gas patterns in the cranial abdomen, suggesting possible bunching of the small intestine secondary to a linear foreign body.

OUTCOME

Abdominal ultrasonography demonstrated normal pancreatic architecture and plication of the small intestine, again consistent with a linear foreign body.

Exploratory coeliotomy was performed and a small intestinal obstruction caused by a 6 cm foreign body was identified. An enterotomy was performed and the foreign body removed; this was subsequently identified as a soft toy. The dog made a complete recovery.

CONCLUSIONS

Although serum pancreas-specific lipase tests are the most sensitive and specific clinicopathological tests for pancreatitis in dogs (see Chapter 14), the results should be interpreted in light of the clinical findings and in conjunction with other tests, most notably diagnostic imaging.

CASE 2

SIGNALMENT

10-year-old male neutered Shetland Sheepdog.

HISTORY

4-month history of watery diarrhoea passed twice daily. No report of melaena or haematochezia. Marked weight loss (12.5 kg to 9.1 kg) with a poor appetite. Not wormed since puppyhood. Body condition score 3/9. Rectal examination revealed a small, smooth, bilaterally symmetrical prostate gland, full anal sacs and a small polypoid mass on the dorsal wall of the rectum; fresh blood was found on the glove.

CLINICAL PATHOLOGY DATA

Haematology	Result	Reference interval
RBC (x 10^{12}/l)	5.71	5.50–8.50
Haematocrit (l/l)	**0.32**	0.37–0.55
Haemoglobin (g/dl)	**7.9**	12.00–18.00
MCV (fl)	**56.0**	60.0–77.0
MCH (pg)	**13.8**	22–25
MCHC (g/dl)	**24.7**	34–37
WBC (x 10^9/l)	**22.8**	5.50–16.90
Neutrophils (segmented) (x 10^9/l)	**21.1**	3.00–11.5
Band neutrophils	0.0	0.0–0.3
Lymphocytes (x 10^9/l)	**0.7**	0.8–3.80
Monocytes (x 10^9/l)	0.9	0.30–1.8
Eosinophils (x 10^9/l)	0.1	0.10–1.40
Basophils (x 10^9/l)	0.00	0.00–0.10
Platelets (x 10^9/l)	**748**	175–500
Smear comment	Microcytosis ++ Hypochromasia ++ Polychromasia + Anisocytosis +	

Abnormal results are in **bold**.

Biochemistry	Result	Reference interval
Total protein (g/l)	**32.9**	58.0–73.0
Albumin (g/l)	**15.1**	26.0–35.0
Globulin (g/l)	**17.8**	18.0–37.0
ALT (IU/l)	77	15–60
ALP (IU/l)	83	20–60
Bilirubin (μmol/l)	2.9	0–10
Fasting bile acids (μmol/l)	7.5	<25.0
Creatinine (μmol/l)	52	30–90
Urea (mmol/l)	5.1	1.7–7.4
Glucose (mmol/l)	5.0	3.0–5.0
Calcium (mmol/l)	**2.11**	2.30–3.00
Phosphate (mmol/l)	1.17	0.90–1.20
Sodium (mmol/l)	147	139–154
Potassium (mmol/l)	3.7	3.60–5.60
Cholesterol (mmol/l)	**2.9**	3.5–7.0

Abnormal results are in **bold**.

Urine specific gravity: 1.050.
Urine dipstick and sediment: unremarkable.
UPCR: 0.3 (reference interval <0.5).

Faecal examination

- *Toxocara*: ova seen.
- *Giardia* (ZnSO$_4$ flotation): oocysts seen.
- Faecal occult blood: positive.
- Stool culture: *Campylobacter* spp. positive.

WHAT ABNORMALITIES ARE PRESENT?

- Moderate hypochromic, microcytic anaemia.
- Thrombocytosis.
- Leucocytosis with mature neutrophilia and lymphopenia.
- Hypoproteinaemia resulting from marked hypoalbuminaemia and mild hypoglobulinaemia.
- Very mild increase in serum ALP and ALT activities, considered to be of no significance and probably secondary to GI disease.
- Mild hypocalcaemia.
- Hypocholesterolaemia.
- Positive faecal occult blood.
- Stool positive for *Toxocara*, *Giardia* and *Campylobacter* spp.

HOW WOULD YOU INTERPRET THESE RESULTS AND WHAT ARE THE LIKELY DIFFERENTIAL DIAGNOSES?

- There is evidence of a mild microcytic, hypochromic anaemia with reduced mean corpuscular haemoglobin (MCH) and mean corpuscular haemoglobin concentration (MCHC), but with some signs of regeneration. In conjunction with the thrombocytosis, the changes are consistent with iron-deficiency anaemia, probably due to chronic GI bleeding.
- The WBC response is most consistent with a stress response.
- The hypoalbuminaemia is too severe to be just due to chronic GI bleeding: a PLE is likely, and hypocholesterolaemia may indicate small intestinal malabsorption.
- Liver disease and a PLN as the cause of the hypoalbuminaemia are ruled out by normal liver function tests and normal urinalysis, respectively.
- The mild hypocalcaemia largely reflects reduction in the concentration of protein-bound calcium, although there may be a component of ionized hypocalcaemia if there is a PLE.
- The presence of faecal occult blood can suggest occult GI bleeding. However, even if the dog had been fed a meat-free diet before testing, the presence of a polyp and fresh blood on rectal examination negates the significance of the result, although a negative result might have helped rule out GI bleeding.
- *Toxocara* and *Giardia* infections are present but are unlikely to be the cause of this dog's problems. Adult dogs can harbour a few roundworms with no clinical significance and can be carriers of *Giardia*, but the infections should be treated anyway.

→ **CASE 2 CONTINUED**

- The presence of *Campylobacter* is unlikely to be a significant cause of chronic diarrhoea and hypoproteinaemia; speciation by PCR might indicate whether *C. jejuni* is present, but again the signs are not consistent with campylobacteriosis.

There is evidence of chronic GI haemorrhage. The rectal polyp may be the source of the GI bleeding, but does not explain the diarrhoea, weight loss and hypoproteinaemia; this suggests a PLE is also present.

WHAT ARE YOUR DIFFERENTIAL DIAGNOSES FOR THESE TWO PROBLEMS?

- Iron-deficiency anaemia due to GI bleeding. The presence of fresh blood on rectal examination indicates large intestinal bleeding, so specific causes of gastric and small intestinal ulceration causing occult GI bleeding are not listed, but might also be present:
  - Part of a generalized bleeding problem, although there was no evidence of bleeding elsewhere
  - Gastric ulceration
  - Small intestinal ulceration
  - Large intestinal ulceration:
    - Bleeding colorectal mass:
      - Polyp
      - Carcinoma
      - Lymphoma
    - Hookworms (*Ancylostoma caninum* not recorded in UK)
    - Whipworms (*Trichuris vulpis*)
    - Caeco-colic intussusception (caecal inversion)
    - Vascular malformation (rare).
  An adenomatous polyp is most likely considering the findings on rectal examination.
- Protein-losing enteropathy:
  - Inflammatory bowel disease
  - Lymphangiectasia
  - Alimentary lymphoma
  - Systemic mycoses (*Histoplasma*, *Pythium*) – not in UK.

WHAT FURTHER TESTS WOULD YOU RECOMMEND?

- Iron deficiency could be confirmed by measuring serum iron, total iron-binding capacity and percentage saturation.
- A serum TLI would rule out exocrine pancreatic insufficiency as a cause of the diarrhoea and weight loss, but EPI would not cause hypoalbuminaemia.
- Abnormal serum folate and cobalamin concentrations would indicate small intestinal disease, and a need to supplement.
- A repeat faecal flotation to look for hookworms and whipworms could be performed, but treatment for *Giardia* and *Toxocara* with fenbendazole would eliminate them anyway.
- Imaging to look for intestinal masses and alterations in gut wall thickness and layering.
- Duodenoscopy and ileoscopy to look for causes of a PLE, and colonoscopy to look for the source of bleeding.

RESULTS

- Abdominal imaging was unremarkable μg/l.
- Serum TLI (6.5 μg/l) was within reference range (5.0–35 μg/l).
- Serum folate (7.5 μg/l) was within reference range (2.5–13.0 μg/l), but serum cobalamin concentration (105 μg/l) was low (>225 ng/l).
- Colonoscopy revealed a small pedunculated bleeding mass in the rectum (Figure 13.26). The mass was removed at the time of endoscopy by submucosal resection after exteriorization through the anus. Histopathological examination of the tissue confirmed it was an adenomatous polyp.
- Duodenoscopy and ileoscopy revealed a markedly irregular small intestinal mucosa, and endoscopic biopsy samples confirmed moderate to marked lymphoplasmacytic enteritis, more severe in the ileum.

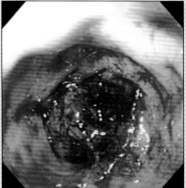

13.26 Small pedunculated bleeding rectal mass identified during colonoscopy and confirmed histologically as an adenomatous polyp.

OUTCOME

- The dog was treated with iron dextran injection and oral iron supplements after removal of the polyp. The anaemia resolved within 1 month.
- The dog was treated with fenbendazole while awaiting the results of the endoscopic biopsy but this produced no improvement in the diarrhoea. The presence of intestinal parasites was probably an incidental finding, but required treatment.
- The dog was then treated for intestinal inflammation and the consequent hypocobalaminaemia. He was given:
  - A hydrolysed diet
  - Weekly injections of vitamin B_{12}
  - Immunosuppressive doses of prednisolone.

The diarrhoea and hypoalbuminaemia had resolved 2 months later, when the steroid dosage could then be tapered.

CONCLUSIONS

- Iron-deficiency anaemia is the result of external haemorrhage and is most commonly associated with occult GI bleeding. The polyp in this case was a probable source of the blood loss anaemia but not the other signs.

> **→ CASE 2 CONTINUED**
>
> - Small intestinal inflammation explained the hypoalbuminaemia and weight loss, and was successfully treated as a case of idiopathic IBD because treatment of the *Giardia* infection did not resolve the problem.
>
> - The long-term prognosis for this dog remains guarded because anorexia, hypoalbuminaemia and hypocobalaminaemia are associated with a poorer outcome in canine chronic enteropathies.
> - The presence of *Campylobacter* spp. was of little significance. It was not the cause of the signs, and the zoonotic risk is small. Treatment might be indicated if the owner is immunocompromised.

References and further reading

Becker SL, Lohourignon LK, Speich B *et al.* (2011) Comparison of the Flotac-400 dual technique and the formalin-ether concentration technique for diagnosis of human intestinal protozoon infection. *Clinical Microbiology* **49**, 2183–2190

Clement NF and Kendall BS (2009) Effect of light on vitamin B12 and folate. *Laboratory Medicine* **40**, 657–659

Cringoli G (2006) FLOTAC, a novel apparatus for a multivalent faecal egg count technique. *Parasitologia* **48**, 381–384

Day MJ, Bilzer T, Mansell J *et al.* (2008) Histopathological standards for the diagnosis of gastrointestinal inflammation in endoscopic biopsy samples from the dog and cat: A report from the World Small Animal Veterinary Association Gastrointestinal Standardization Group. *Journal of Comparative Pathology* **138**, S1–S40

Desario C, Decaro N, Campolo M *et al.* (2005) Canine parvovirus infection: which diagnostic test for virus? *Journal of Virological Methods* **126**, 179–185

Dryden MW, Payne PA, Ridley R and Smith V (2005) Comparison of common fecal flotation techniques for the recovery of parasite eggs and oocysts. *Veterinary Therapeutics* **6**, 15–28

Foster AP, Knowles TG, Moore AH, Cousins PDG, Day MJ and Hall EJ (2003) Serum IgE responses to food antigens in normal and atopic dogs, and dogs with gastrointestinal disease. *Veterinary Immunology and Immunopathology* **92**, 113–124

Frias R, Strube K, Ternes W *et al.* (2012) Comparison of (51)Chromium-labeled ethylenediamine tetra-acetic acid and iohexol as blood markers for intestinal permeability testing in Beagle dogs. *Veterinary Journal* **192**, 123–125

Fyfe JC, Hemker SL, Venta PJ *et al.* (2013) An exon 53 frameshift mutation in CUBN abrogates cubam function and causes Imerslund–Grasbeck syndrome in dogs. *Molecular Genetics and Metabolism* **109**, 390–396

German AJ, Day MJ, Ruaux CG, Steiner JM, Williams DA and Hall EJ (2003a) Comparison of direct and indirect tests for small intestinal bacterial overgrowth and antibiotic-responsive diarrhea in dogs. *Journal of Veterinary Internal Medicine* **17**, 33–43

German AJ, Hall EJ and Day MJ (2003b) Chronic intestinal inflammation and intestinal disease in dogs. *Journal of Veterinary Internal Medicine* **17**, 8–20

Gunn-Moore DA, McCann TM, Reed N, Simpson KE and Tennant B (2007) Prevalence of *Tritrichomonas foetus* infection in cats with diarrhoea in the UK. *Journal of Feline Medicine and Surgery* **9**, 214–218

Hald B, Pedersen K, Waino M, Jorgensen JC and Madsen M (2004) Longitudinal study of the excretion patterns of thermophilic *Campylobacter* spp. in young pet dogs in Denmark. *Journal of Clinical Microbiology* **42**, 2003–2012

Hall EJ, Simpson JW and Williams DA (2005) *BSAVA Manual of Canine and Feline Gastroenterology, 2nd edn.* BSAVA Publications, Gloucester

Heilmann RM, Suchodolski JS and Steiner JM (2008) Development and analytic validation of a radioimmunoassay for the quantification of canine calprotectin in serum and feces from dogs. *American Journal of Veterinary Research* **69**, 845–853

Janeczko S, Atwater D, Bogel E *et al.* (2008) The relationship of mucosal bacteria to duodenal histopathology, cytokine mRNA, and clinical disease activity in cats with inflammatory bowel disease. *Veterinary Microbiology* **128**, 178–193

Mansfield CS, James FE, Craven M *et al.* (2009) Remission of histiocytic ulcerative colitis in Boxer dogs correlates with eradication of invasive intramucosal *Escherichia coli*. *Journal of Veterinary Internal Medicine* **23**, 964–969

Marks SL, Rankin SC, Byrne BA and Weese JS (2011) ACVIM Consensus Statement: Enteropathogenic bacteria in dogs and cats: diagnosis, epidemiology, treatment, and control. *Journal of Veterinary Internal Medicine* **25**, 1195–1208

Parsons BN, Porter CJ, Ryvar R *et al.* (2010) Prevalence of *Campylobacter* spp. in a cross-sectional study of dogs attending veterinary practice in the UK and risk indicators associated with shedding. *Veterinary Journal* **184**, 66–70

Recordati C, Radaelli E, Simpson KW and Scanziani E (2008) A simple method for the production of bacterial controls for immunohistochemistry and fluorescent in situ hybridization. *Journal of Molecular Histology* **39**, 459–462

Rishniw M, Liotta J, Bellosa M, Bowman D and Simpson KW (2010) Comparison of 4 *Giardia* diagnostic tests in diagnosis of naturally acquired canine chronic subclinical giardiasis. *Journal of Veterinary Internal Medicine* **24**, 293–297

Saez AC, Manser MM, Andrews N and Chiodini PL (2011) Comparison between the Midi Parasep and Midi Parasep Solvent Free (SF) faecal parasite concentrators. *Journal of Clinical Pathology* **64**, 901–904

Schmitz S, Coenen C, König M, Thiel HJ and Neiger R (2009) Comparison of three rapid commercial canine parvovirus antigen detection tests with electron microscopy and polymerase chain reaction. *Journal of Veterinary Diagnostic Investigation* **21**, 344–345

Stavisky J, Radford AD, Gaskell R *et al.* (2011) A case-controlled study of pathogen and lifestyle risk factors for diarrhoea in dogs. *Preventative Veterinary Medicine* **99**, 185–192

Walden HS, Dykstra C, Dillon A *et al.* (2013) A new species of Tritrichomonas (Sarcomastigophora; Trichomonida) from the domestic cat (*Felis catus*), June **112(6)**, 2227–2235. doi:10.1007/s00436–013–3381–8

Willard MD, Moore GE, Denton BD *et al.* (2010) Effect of tissue processing on assessment of endoscopic intestinal biopsies in dogs and cats. *Journal of Veterinary Internal Medicine* **24**, 84–89

Worhunsky P, Toulza O, Rishniw M *et al.* (2013) The relationship of serum cobalamin to methylmalonic acid concentrations and clinical variables in cats. *Journal of Veterinary Internal Medicine* **27**, 1056–1063

Useful websites

APACOR – Parasep® faecal filtration system
http://www.apacor.com/products/parasitology/

European Scientific Counsel Companion Animal Parasites (ESCCAP)
http://www.esccap.org

Michigan State University
http://www.mmg.msu.edu/fyfe.html

National Center for Veterinary Parasitology (NCVP) at Oklahoma State University
http://www.ncvetp.org/

Texas A&M University
http://vetmed.tamu.edu/gilab/service/assays/gastrin

University of Pennsylvania
http://research.vet.penn.edu/Default.aspx?TabId=7620

Woodley Equipment – Parasep® faecal filtration system
http://www.woodleyequipment.com

Chapter 14

Laboratory evaluation of exocrine pancreatic disease

Penny Watson

The pancreas is located in the abdomen caudal to the stomach and is composed of: a left limb or lobe, which lies caudal to the greater curvature of the stomach and adjacent to the cranial aspect of the transverse colon; a right limb or lobe, which lies just medial to the proximal duodenum; and a body between these two limbs. There are important differences between dogs and cats in pancreatic structure, function and disease associations, which are summarized in Figure 14.1.

Exocrine acinar cells comprise about 98% of the normal pancreas, and insulin-secreting endocrine islets about 2%. The acinar cells secrete enzymes involved in the initial digestion of food, including lipase (for which the pancreas is the main source), alpha-amylase, phospholipase, nucleases and the proteolytic enzymes trypsin, chymotrypsin and elastase. Proteases are stored and released as inactive zymogens, which are cleaved in the small intestine to active enzymes. Trypsin is stored as an inactive zymogen, trypsinogen, in the pancreas and is activated in the small intestine by cleavage of a peptide (the trypsin activation peptide, TAP) from the trypsinogen molecule, by the brush border enzyme enterokinase. In fact, in the small intestine, not only enterokinase but also

other activated trypsin molecules will activate trypsinogen by cleaving TAP. Recently, another pancreatic enzyme, chymotrypsin C, has also been implicated in activating trypsinogen in the small intestine, at least in humans, although its role in small animals is unknown. Activated trypsin then activates the other enzymes.

Activation of trypsin is affected by calcium concentration and pH. Calcium concentration is very low in acinar cells but high within the pancreatic duct and small intestinal lumen, favouring trypsin activation. Activation of trypsin is also pH dependent: although trypsin requires a relatively high pH to function (i.e. the alkaline pH of the small intestine), its activation appears to be exquisitely pH sensitive. The autoactivation of trypsinogen is relatively slow at the high pH within the pancreatic duct (typically 8.5 in humans and guinea pigs), whereas autoactivation is progressively stimulated when the pH is decreased from 8.5 to 7 (Pallagi et al., 2011). These interesting results suggest that pancreatic bicarbonate secretion is important not only for neutralizing gastric acid in the duodenum but also for keeping pancreatic enzymes in an inactive state in the pancreatic ducts, where the pH is higher than in the small intestine.

Feature	Dogs	Cats
Anatomy	Usually two pancreatic ducts: • Large accessory duct from right limb to minor papilla in duodenum • Small pancreatic duct from left limb to major duodenal papilla in duodenum next to (but not joining) bile duct	Usually single major pancreatic duct joins the common bile duct before entering duodenum at duodenal papilla 3 cm distal to pylorus; 20% of cats have second, accessory duct. Occasionally bile duct and major pancreatic duct remain separate
Disease associations	Pancreatitis commonly associated with endocrine disease (see text). Associated with gallbladder mucocoele in some breeds and polysystemic immune-mediated disease in Cocker Spaniels. Association with other diseases in other breeds not recognized	Common association with pancreatitis and cholangiohepatitis and/or inflammatory bowel disease Often concurrent hepatic lipidosis May also be association with nephritis, neoplasia, pyelonephritis and other diseases (Ferreri et al., 2003)
Pancreatitis: spectrum of disease	Acute disease traditionally considered most common. Chronic disease increasingly recognized	Chronic disease traditionally considered most common. Acute disease increasingly recognized
Pancreatitis: diagnosis	Histology gold standard. Variety of catalytic and immunoassays available. Ultrasonography quite sensitive. Obvious/suggestive clinical signs particularly in acute cases	Histology gold standard. Traditional catalytic assays no help. DGGR lipase and immunoassays of some value. Ultrasonography less sensitive than in dogs. More low-grade, non-specific clinical signs even in severe acute cases
Causes of exocrine pancreatic insufficiency	Often pancreatic acinar atrophy – increased incidence in certain breeds (especially German Shepherd Dogs). End-stage chronic pancreatitis does occur	Most cases end-stage chronic pancreatitis. Pancreatic acinar atrophy not reported

14.1 Comparison of pancreatic structure and disease in cats and dogs.

Diseases of the exocrine pancreas are relatively common in dogs and cats but may not be recognized because of non-specific clinical signs and a lack of sensitive and specific clinicopathological tests. Pancreatitis, acute and chronic and varying from severe to subclinical, is the most common disease of the exocrine pancreas in both species. Exocrine pancreatic insufficiency, although less common, is also often recognized. Pancreatic abscesses, cysts, pseudocysts and pancreatic neoplasia are uncommon.

Pancreatitis

Pathophysiology

The aetiopathogenesis of pancreatitis is incompletely understood, but the 'final common pathway' of pancreatitis appears to be the inappropriate early activation of trypsinogen within the pancreas, as a result of increased autoactivation and/or reduced autolysis. Activated trypsin then activates other enzymes and the result is pancreatic autodigestion, inflammation and peripancreatic fat necrosis. Mitochondrial damage and oxidant release are involved in the perpetuation of acute pancreatitis. The neighbouring gut wall becomes inflamed and there is a high risk of bacterial translocation into the blood from the gut lumen in dogs. There is a systemic inflammatory response (SIR) associated with local and systemic release of inflammatory cytokines and neutrophil activation. The circulating protease inhibitors α_1-antitrypsin (α_1-protease inhibitor) and α-macroglobulin attempt to remove trypsin and other proteases from the circulation. Damage to vascular endothelium throughout the body causes tissue oedema and hypoxia, with organs such as the lungs, kidneys and liver being particularly susceptible to damage (Talukdar and Vege, 2011). This inflammatory response is balanced with a compensatory anti-inflammatory response. However, if this is overwhelmed, multiorgan failure and disseminated intravascular coagulation (DIC) ensue. Multiorgan failure is usually the cause of death in severe acute pancreatitis (Talukdar and Vege, 2011).

The cause of pancreatitis is often known in humans, although it is increasingly recognized to be the result of a complex interaction between genes and environment (LaRusch and Whitcomb, 2011). The same is likely to be true in dogs and cats, although very little is understood about the causes of the disease in these species. Potential causes and trigger factors for pancreatitis in dogs and cats include hypertriglyceridaemia, duct obstruction, dietary indiscretion, ischaemia, trauma, and drugs and toxins. English Cocker Spaniels in the UK are believed to suffer from chronic pancreatitis as part of a polysystemic autoimmune disease which also causes keratoconjunctivitis sicca and glomerulonephritis in some dogs and may be responsive to steroids (Watson et al., 2011, 2012). However, chronic pancreatitis in other breeds appears histologically and clinically very different from the disease in Cocker Spaniels, and steroids are not indicated in these other breeds. Unlike human cases, most canine and feline cases remain idiopathic. Some of these are likely to represent hereditary disease, although genetic studies of canine pancreatitis are contradictory to date. The interested reader is referred to the author's review in JSAP (Watson, 2015) for more details on definitions and potential causes of pancreatitis in small animals.

Diagnosis

Overview

Pancreatitis may be defined as acute or chronic (Figures 14.2 and 14.3), but these terms are histopathological rather than clinical: disease severity does not differentiate acute from chronic pancreatitis. In dogs, chronic pancreatitis is often recurrent, and a long subclinical phase can culminate in a dramatic acute-on-chronic episode, which is clinically and clinicopathologically identical to a single acute bout of pancreatitis. In one study, 40% of dogs with fatal acute pancreatitis actually had underlying chronic disease (Hess et al., 1998). Differentiating acute from chronic disease is not important for short-term management. However, chronic disease may lead to more significant long-term sequelae, such as the development of exocrine pancreatic insufficiency (EPI) and/or diabetes mellitus, so it is important to recognize that some apparently acute cases already have significant tissue destruction. In general, chronic disease is more challenging to diagnose, because the clinical signs, diagnostic imaging findings and clinicopathological changes are less dramatic than in acute disease. Cats show low-grade non-specific clinical signs in both acute and chronic pancreatitis. They also have a high incidence of concurrent disease, particularly cholangiohepatitis and/or inflammatory bowel disease, making the diagnosis of pancreatitis difficult. In dogs, acute disease is believed to be commonest, but chronic disease is also frequent, particularly in certain breeds such as English Cocker Spaniels, Cavalier King Charles Spaniels, collies and Boxers in the UK and non-sporting toy breeds in the USA (Watson et al., 2007, 2010, 2011; Bostrom et al., 2013).

The gold standard for the diagnosis of pancreatitis is biopsy and histopathological examination, but this is often neither practical nor indicated because it is invasive and does not usually change the treatment plan. Even histology of a pancreatic biopsy sample is not 100% sensitive because the lesions of pancreatitis are patchy, particularly early in the disease process, so a small surgical biopsy may miss the disease. No single clinicopathological test currently available has 100% sensitivity and specificity for the diagnosis of pancreatitis in dogs and cats, and non-invasive diagnosis often remains presumptive, based on supportive results from clinical and diagnostic imaging findings, as well as the results of blood tests. The pancreas may also become inflamed secondary to other diseases, such as septic peritonitis. It is therefore very important for the clinician to remember to work-up suspected pancreatitis cases in the same way as any

Parameter	Definition
Acute pancreatitis	Histologically, pancreatic inflammation with neutrophils and varying degrees of pancreatic necrosis, oedema and peripancreatic fat necrosis. Potentially completely reversible without permanent disruption of pancreatic architecture. Clinically varies in severity from severe, necrotizing and fatal to mild interstitial subclinical disease.
Chronic pancreatitis	Histologically, inflammation with mononuclear cells with fibrosis, nodular hyperplasia and permanent disruption of pancreatic architecture. Generally clinically mild, unless acute-on-chronic ('chronic active') with neutrophils as well as mononuclear cells, which may be clinically severe and become necrotizing and fatal, and clinically indistinguishable from a single bout of acute disease.

14.2 Definitions of acute and chronic pancreatitis.

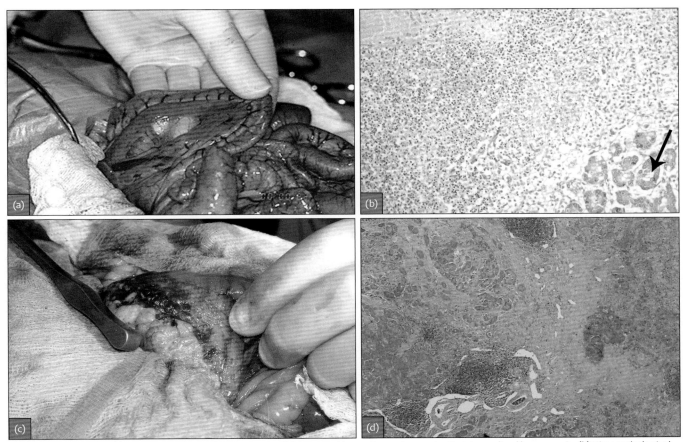

14.3 Pancreatitis. (a) Gross appearance of acute pancreatitis in a cat at laparotomy, demonstrating generalized hyperaemia. (b) Histopathological appearance of acute (fatal) pancreatitis in a dog. Note the extensive neutrophilic infiltrate and inflammatory exudate but the absence of fibrosis. A normal acinus is arrowed. (Haematoxylin and eosin stain; original magnification X100). (c) Gross appearance of chronic pancreatitis at laparotomy (right, duodenal limb). Note the nodular appearance of the pancreas and extensive adhesions to the duodenum obscuring the mesentery. (d) Histological section from a cat showing typical chronic pancreatitis. There are large bands of fibrous tissue (light pink) separating islands of remaining acinar tissue (purple) and dense patches of lymphocytes. (Haematoxylin and eosin stain; original magnification X10)

(a, Courtesy of Jane Ladlow, University of Cambridge; b, Courtesy of *In Practice* and Aude Roulois; c, Courtesy of *In Practice* and Dr Stephen Baines; d, Reproduced from Watson (2015) with permission from the *Journal of Small Animal Practice* and courtesy of Jane Ladlow, University of Cambridge)

other case, and not jump immediately to a diagnosis on the basis of a positive enzyme test. Other investigations, such as diagnostic imaging and analysis of free abdominal fluid, will often be necessary to rule out other concurrent serious disease such as intestinal perforation.

Haematology and biochemistry

Haematological and biochemical screening are important in animals with pancreatitis.

- Significant changes often occur due to the SIR associated with pancreatitis. Assessing the amount of organ compromise at presentation is important, because it affects the prognosis in animals with pancreatitis and may affect the decision to treat. Prognostic factors are detailed at the end of this section, and potential acute sequelae in Figure 14.4. In addition, it is very important to identify electrolyte and other abnormalities to facilitate early and effective treatment in severe cases. In humans, early aggressive fluid therapy improves the outcome in severe acute pancreatitis and the same may be true in small animals. This therapy should be carefully tailored to correct any measured electrolyte abnormalities and preserve renal function.
- Pancreatitis may be secondary to another disease, which may be suggested by biochemical changes, and which requires treatment or prevention to control the

Acute sequelae

- Dehydration
- Metabolic acidosis
- Prerenal azotaemia
- Electrolyte disturbances
  - Hypokalaemia: *most important*
  - Hyponatraemia
  - Hypochloraemia
  - Mild hypocalcaemia and hypomagnesaemia (not usually clinically significant)
- Hepatopathy
- Systemic inflammatory response syndrome
- Systemic hypotension
- Acute respiratory distress syndrome
- Cardiac arrhythmias
- Coagulopathies
- Diffuse intravascular coagulation
- Pancreatic abscesses and pancreatic pseudocysts (both acute and chronic)

Chronic sequelae

- Exocrine pancreatic insufficiency (90% enzyme loss)
- Diabetes mellitus (80% β-cell loss)
- Fibrosis around bile duct causing chronic or transient biliary obstruction
- Potentially neoplastic transformation
- Pancreatic abscesses and pancreatic pseudocysts (both acute and chronic)

14.4 Potential sequelae of acute and chronic pancreatitis.

pancreatitis. Concurrent disease is common, particularly in severe pancreatitis. The most important concurrent diseases in dogs are diabetes mellitus (especially ketoacidotic diabetes), hyperadrenocorticism and hypothyroidism; up to 50% of dogs with severe pancreatitis have one or more of these endocrinopathies and the prognosis is worse if they are present. There are also associations in some dogs with gastrointestinal (GI) disease and with epilepsy (which may represent the effects of treatment). English Cocker Spaniels with chronic pancreatitis often have evidence of immune-mediated disease in other organs including the kidneys and also often have concurrent liver disease, although the pathogenesis of the latter remains unclear (Watson *et al.*, 2012). The most important associated diseases in cats are diabetes mellitus, hepatic lipidosis, inflammatory bowel disease and cholangiohepatitis. Cats with pancreatitis may also have an increased incidence of interstitial nephritis.

- Pancreatitis itself may lead to secondary complications and sequelae that require recognition and treatment (see Figure 14.4).

Haematological and biochemical abnormalities seen with pancreatitis in dogs and cats are summarized in Figures 14.5 and 14.6. Overall, studies have not shown a significant difference between dogs and cats with chronic and acute pancreatitis, except that one study showed that serum alanine aminotransferase (ALT) and alkaline phosphatase (ALP) were significantly higher in cats with chronic disease than in those with acute disease (Ferreri *et al.*, 2003).

Electrolytes: Electrolyte changes seen with acute pancreatitis often include significant hypokalaemia due to loss through vomiting, reduced intake and fluid therapy increasing renal loss. Hypokalaemia must be recognized and treated, because it can cause ongoing GI atony and become life-threatening if severe. Hypocalcaemia is uncommon in dogs but common in cats and has been identified as a poor prognostic indicator in this species.

Urea and creatinine: Azotaemia is commonly prerenal, and assessment of a concurrent urine sample, before commencing fluid therapy, is important to determine whether there is also intrinsic renal compromise (see Chapter 10 for information on differentiating renal from prerenal azotaemia). English Cocker Spaniels with chronic pancreatitis often have concurrent glomerulonephritis, so it is important to check a urine sample in these dogs (see below), and they may also have azotaemia in more advanced cases.

Liver enzymes and bilirubin: Pancreatic oedema, fibrosis or neoplasia can cause partial or complete biliary obstruction, and consequent increases in liver enzymes. Typically, extrahepatic biliary obstruction like this will cause moderate to marked elevations in bilirubin and in biliary enzymes (alkaline phosphatase (ALP) and gamma-glutamyl transferase (GGT)). Hepatocellular enzymes are also often elevated significantly because of the toxic effects of refluxed bile on hepatocytes (see Chapter 12). Dogs with pancreatitis may present with jaundice; evidence from the literature suggests this is due to an 'acute-on-chronic' bout in the majority of cases, rather than a single acute episode. This is presumably because the underlying fibrosis in the pancreas makes it stiffer and more likely to obstruct the neighbouring bile duct when it is inflamed and oedematous. Most of these cases will resolve in time without surgery. In cats, pancreatitis and cholangiohepatitis often occur concurrently. There is also a high incidence of hepatic lipidosis in cats with severe acute pancreatitis. Bilirubin will be elevated in both diseases but, typically, cats with lipidosis have

Parameter	Change	Dogs (% of cases)	Cats (% of cases)	Reason
Neutrophils	Increased ± left shift	Common (55–91%)	Less common than dogs (~30%)	Systemic inflammatory response
	Decreased ± left shift and toxic change	Very uncommon	Uncommon (≤15%)	'Degenerative' response due to overwhelming inflammation – poor prognostic indicator in cats?
PCV/Hb/RBC	Increased	Moderately common (≤20%)	Moderately common (up to 13–20%)	Dehydration (may become low in some once rehydrated)
	Decreased (both regenerative and non-regenerative anaemia seen)	Moderately common (19–24%)	Common (26–55%)	Anaemia of chronic inflammatory disease ± bleeding GI ulcers ± shortened red cell lifespan (azotaemia and sepsis) ± reduced production (above + anorexia)
Fibrinogen	Increased	Common	?	Inflammatory response
	Decreased	Uncommon	?	Consumption in DIC
Fibrin degradation products (D-dimers also likely)	Increased	Uncommon (16% of severe cases)	?	Coagulation abnormalities associated with circulating proteases ± DIC
Platelets	Decreased	Common in severe cases (59%) Moderately common in chronic disease (19%)	Uncommon – usually normal or only slightly decreased	Coagulation abnormalities associated with circulating proteases ± DIC
Coagulation times	Increased	Common (prolonged prothrombin time 43%, prolonged partial thromboplastin time 61%)	Only measured in small numbers of cases but often prolonged in those – note ≤20% of cats have thrombosis	Coagulation abnormalities associated with circulating proteases ± DIC

14.5 Potential non-specific findings on haematology screens in dogs and cats with pancreatitis. These figures are from dogs and cats with both acute and chronic pancreatitis – published studies on chronic pancreatitis suggest very similar findings to acute disease in both dogs and cats. DIC = disseminated intravascular coagulation; GI = gastrointestinal; Hb = haemoglobin; PCV = packed cell volume; RBC = red blood cells.
(Data from: for dogs – Schaer, 1979; Hess *et al.*, 1998; Pápa *et al.*, 2011; Bostrum *et al.*, 2013; for cats – Hill and Van Winkle, 1993; Mansfield and Jones, 2001)

Parameter	Change	Dogs (% of cases)	Cats (% of cases)	Reason
Urea ± creatinine	Increased	Common Urea 34–65%; creatinine 21–59%	Common Urea 57%; creatinine 33%	Prerenal failure due to dehydration ± hypotension (classically urea elevated more) ± intrinsic renal failure (sepsis, immune complexes, underlying/pre-existing disease)
Potassium	Decreased	Relatively common (20%)	Very common (more than dogs) (56%)	Increased loss in vomiting, with fluid therapy, with reduced intake and with aldosterone release secondary to hypovolaemia
Sodium	Increased	Uncommon (12%)	Uncommon (4%)	Dehydration
	Decreased	Relatively common (33%)	Relatively common (23%)	Loss in GI secretions with vomiting
Chloride	Decreased	Very common (32–81%)	?Probably common	As sodium
Calcium	Increased	Uncommon (9%)	Uncommon (5%)	May be cause rather than effect?
	Decreased	Uncommon (3%); not a prognostic indicator	Very common and poor prognostic indicator (Kimmel et al., 2001). (Up to 40–45% reduced total calcium, up to 60% reduced ionized calcium)	?Saponification in peripancreatic fat (unproven), increased glucagon release, increasing calcitonin (shown in some)
Phosphate	Increased	Common (19–55%)	Quite common (27%)	Usually due to reduced renal clearance, concurrent azotaemia
	Decreased	Rare (0% in one study)	Quite common (14%)	Usually secondary to diabetes mellitus (DM)/increased insulin increasing cellular uptake. Can become clinically important in cats
Magnesium	Decreased	Reported but unknown %	Reported but unknown %	?Saponification in peripancreatic fat
Glucose	Increased	Common (30–88%)	Common (64%)	Increased glucagon, cortisol and catecholamines and reduced insulin; 40% became normal, 30% permanent DM in dogs (Hess et al., 1998)
	Decreased	Common (≤40%)	Uncommon (4%)	Sepsis/systemic inflammatory response, anorexia and malnutrition (especially small breeds), concurrent liver disease
Albumin	Increased	Common (39–50%)	Quite common (8–30%)	Dehydration
	Decreased	Quite common (17%)	Quite common (24%)	Gut loss, anorexia/malnutrition, concurrent liver disease ± renal loss
Total protein	Increased	Common (27%)	Common (24%)	Dehydration and inflammation increasing globulins
	Decreased	Common (45%)	Uncommon (14%)	As albumin
ALT and AST	Increased	Common (47%–61%)	Common (68%)	Hepatic necrosis and lipidosis due to sepsis, pancreatic enzymes ± concurrent disease (most important in cats) + reactive hepatopathy
ALP and GGT	Increased	Very common (79–88%)	Common (50%) (ALP high but GGT normal if lipidosis)	Concurrent biliary stasis (common in cats and dogs) ± primary disease (cholangitis in cats) ± hepatic lipidosis in cats (typically ALP only) ± steroid-induced ALP isoenzyme in dogs only + reactive hepatopathy
Bilirubin	Increased	Common (53%)	Very common (64%)	As ALP
Cholesterol	Increased	Common (48–80%)	Common (64%)	Commonly elevated – see discussion in text on cause versus effect. May also increase with secondary cholestasis
Triglycerides	Increased	Common – lipaemic serum	Uncommon (10%?) (but rarely measured)	Commonly elevated – see discussion in text on cause versus effect

14.6 Potential non-specific changes on biochemical analysis in dogs and cats with pancreatitis. ALP = alkaline phosphatase; ALT = alanine aminotransferase; AST = aspartate aminotransferase; GGT = gamma glutamyl transferase; GI = gastrointestinal.
(Data from: for dogs – Schaer, 1979; Hess et al., 1998; Pápa et al., 2011; Bostrum et al., 2013; for cats – Hill and Van Winkle, 1993; Mansfield and Jones, 2001)

marked elevations in ALP but normal GGT, whereas cats with cholangitis have moderate to marked elevations in both biliary enzymes. However, the clinician should not rely on liver enzyme patterns to make a diagnosis because the presence of concurrent cholangitis and lipidosis or other diseases can confuse enzyme patterns. Therefore, cytology and ideally histology of the liver are required for a definitive diagnosis of associated liver disease in cats (see Chapter 12).

Cholesterol and triglycerides: Increased cholesterol and triglycerides are common and may represent either a cause or an effect of the disease. Experimental pancreatitis does not cause elevations in cholesterol and triglycerides in dogs, even though it alters the patterns of lipoproteins (Whitney et al., 1987). However, familial hypertriglyceridaemia is a recognized cause of acute pancreatitis in humans and it is probable that the same is true in dogs. A recent study in Miniature Schnauzers showed that those with a history of pancreatitis were 5 times more likely to have hypertriglyceridaemia, which persisted after clinical resolution of pancreatitis, and almost 15 times more likely to have moderate to severe hypertriglyceridaemia than healthy Miniature Schnauzer controls (Xenoulis et al., 2010). Finding elevated triglycerides and/or cholesterol in a dog with pancreatitis should also trigger a search for an underlying endocrinopathy, particularly hypothyroidism or hyperadrenocorticism, which can elevate serum lipids and are also risk factors for fatal acute pancreatitis (see Chapters 17 and 18 for more details on diagnosis of these endocrinopathies). The risk of gallbladder mucocoele is also increased in dogs with hyperlipidaemia with or without pancreatitis and endocrinopathies, giving another possible reason for elevated liver enzymes in dogs with pancreatitis. Ultrasonography is indicated to rule this out in high-risk cases.

Other clinicopathological tests

Urinalysis: A high urine specific gravity (SG) with azotaemia suggests acute prerenal failure due to dehydration and shock. However, dogs with severe pancreatitis often have isosthenuric urine, suggesting concurrent intrinsic renal damage. Proteinuria is seen in up to 78% of dogs with acute pancreatitis (Hess *et al.*, 1998), probably due to a combination of SIR and tubular damage. In English Cocker Spaniels with chronic and acute-on-chronic pancreatitis, glomerulonephritis is often also recognized as part of a polysystemic immune-mediated disease targeting ducts. These dogs should be screened for proteinuria and treated long term for glomerulonephritis if it is found. Glucosuria may be seen in both dogs and cats with pancreatitis and may be temporary due to increased insulin resistance and a 'prediabetic' response, although this is unusual. More commonly, it represents the development of diabetes mellitus. Blood and urine glucose should therefore be monitored carefully during and after resolution of the pancreatitis to assess whether the animal is truly an insulin-dependent diabetic. The presence of ketones, in addition to glucosuria, in the urine in both dogs and cats with pancreatitis usually indicates diabetic ketoacidosis, which requires immediate and urgent treatment. Ketonuria is occasionally seen in dogs and cats with negative calorie balance, once they have depleted their hepatic glycogen reserves and are relying on fat breakdown for calories. In these circumstances, it would be very unusual to see concurrent glucosuria because affected animals are usually hypoglycaemic. Concurrent pancreatitis in a diabetic animal increases the risk of ketoacidosis and mortality.

Coagulation screens: Coagulation abnormalities are common, particularly in severe acute disease, in both dogs and cats, and are attributable to DIC (see Chapter 6). In addition, proteolytic enzymes (proteases) released from the pancreas catabolize complement and von Willebrand factor, contributing to the haemostatic abnormalities. Pancreatitis was a common diagnosis in dogs with a low blood antithrombin activity in one study, suggesting that dogs with pancreatitis are at increased risk of hypercoagulability and thrombosis, but there was no significant difference in antithrombin activity between survivors and non-survivors with pancreatitis in the same study (Kuzi *et al.*, 2010).

C-reactive protein: C-reactive protein (CRP) is often elevated in dogs with pancreatitis but the degree of elevation does not appear to be prognostic. In one study, the concentration of CRP measured 2 days after onset of clinical signs was significantly higher in dogs that died than in dogs that survived, but the numbers were small and there was no real correlation between CRP and outcome (Mansfield *et al.*, 2008).

Analysis of effusions: Body cavity effusions are common in pancreatitis and may be pleural as well as peritoneal.

They are usually serosanguineous exudates, although transudates and chylous effusions have been reported in cats. Effusions form as a consequence of focal peritonitis and fat necrosis in the abdomen, and more generalized vasculitis, inflammation and fat necrosis in the pleural space. Amylase and lipase levels in the fluid may be elevated, as may pancreatic lipase immunoreactivity (Guija de Arespacochaga and Hittmair, 2006; Chartier *et al.*, 2013). Lipase and amylase concentrations may be much higher in the abdominal fluid than in the serum, helping diagnosis in some cases. Equally importantly, measuring pancreatic enzymes in the fluid helps to diagnose the cause of a sterile exudate and differentiate it from the other possible causes of sterile exudate: urine peritonitis or bile peritonitis.

Blood gas analysis: Blood gas analysis in animals with pancreatitis shows metabolic acidosis in most cases, and one study found metabolic acidosis to be a negative prognostic indicator in dogs with acute pancreatitis. There may also be concurrent respiratory acidosis and hypoxia if acute respiratory distress syndrome is associated with the pancreatitis.

Specific enzyme assays

Non-invasive diagnosis of pancreatitis in dogs and cats requires the use of specific pancreatic enzyme assays, which are interpreted together with findings on clinical examination and diagnostic imaging. The pancreatic enzyme assays vary greatly in sensitivity and specificity among species and individuals, and no single assay is totally sensitive and specific. It is also very important to remember that a diagnosis of pancreatitis, even with a highly specific assay such as the pancreatic lipase immunoreactivity (PLI) test, does NOT indicate that pancreatitis is the animal's most serious problem and does not replace a full clinical work-up. In one study, the primary cause of death in 9 out of 11 dogs with histologically confirmed pancreatitis was another serious disease such as a small intestinal foreign body or intestinal neoplasia (Mansfield *et al.*, 2012).

In dogs and cats, the time of onset of the episode of pancreatitis is rarely known. Pancreatic enzymes have distinct half-lives: in dogs the half-life of pancreatic amylase is approximately 5 hours and that of lipase is approximately 2 hours. Many animals are examined an unknown period, often days, after the onset of the disease, by which time the enzymes may have returned to normal. In addition, the pancreas can respond to inflammation by shutting off production of enzymes and, in ongoing chronic disease, there is progressive loss of pancreatic mass with an associated overall reduction in enzyme production. All these factors contribute to the variable, often poor, sensitivity of enzyme assays. Finally, assays are often affected by renal clearance and by drug therapy, particularly steroids. Each assay has advantages and disadvantages which are summarized, together with published data on sensitivity and specificity, in Figure 14.7.

Pancreatic enzyme assays currently available for use in dogs and cats are divided into catalytic assays and immunoassays. Immunoassays are considered the most specific.

Catalytic assays: These measure plasma levels of the pancreatic acinar enzymes, amylase and lipase, by measuring the enzyme's ability to catalyse a specific reaction. Catalytic assays do not measure inactive precursors, such as zymogens, so are not used for proteases (e.g. trypsin).

Assay	Advantages	Disadvantages	Sensitivity and specificity
Immunoassays			
Canine PLI/Spec cPL®/SNAP® (see text for details)	Most sensitive and specific test currently available. Organ specific so no interference from extra-pancreatic sources. Patient-side SNAP® test available. Appears not to be increased by exogenous steroids and remains stable in serum for 21 days at room temperature (Steiner et al., 2009)	SNAP® does not give a value and is not as accurate as the Spec cPL® in the borderline range between normal and elevated (see text). Most studies show lower sensitivity with chronic and mild disease than severe acute disease. May be inappropriately low in severe ± chronic cases due to pancreatic depletion ± loss of tissue mass	Reported sensitivity varies from as low as 21% (Spec cPL®) in mild disease (Trivedi et al., 2011) to as high as 71% in moderate to severe disease histologically confirmed, or 94% in one study (McCord et al., 2012). Sensitivity in chronic disease varies from 26% to 67% depending on cut-off (Watson et al., 2010; Bostrom et al., 2013). Specificity of Spec cPL® and SNAP® varies from 66% to 88% depending on test used, study protocol and cut-off (Mansfield et al., 2012; McCord et al., 2012)
Feline PLI/Spec fPL®/SNAP®	As dogs. Feline SNAP® also available	As dogs	Fewer published studies than for dogs. Overall sensitivity in one study 67% (100% in cats with moderate to severe pancreatitis and 54% in cats with mild pancreatitis). Specificity 91% (Forman et al., 2004)
Canine TLI	Elevations are highly specific but sensitivity lower than lipase and lipase immunoreactivity	Said to rise and fall more quickly than amylase and lipase during an episode. Renal excretion also elevated 2–3 times in renal disease. May be inappropriately low in severe ± chronic cases owing to pancreatic depletion ± loss of tissue mass. Does not appear to be affected by steroids	Sensitivity varies from as low as 17% in chronic disease (Watson et al., 2010) to as high as 30% in mild to moderate pancreatitis (Trivedi et al., 2011)
Feline TLI	As dogs except less specific	As dogs but less specific and false positives reported in thin cats	Sensitivity varies from 33% to 62% depending on assay and cut-off. Specificity reported to be 56% (Gerhardt et al., 2001; Swift et al., 2000)
Catalytic assays	**NB DOGS ONLY**	**NO USE IN CATS**	
Amylase	Widely used and available on in-house analysers. Steroids do NOT elevate it (may reduce it)	High background level so low sensitivity and specificity. Much from other sources including small intestine. Renal excretion – elevated 2–3 times in azotaemia	Sensitivity in acute and chronic disease ranges from 7% to 69% in most studies (Hess et al., 1998; Watson et al., 2010; Trivedi et al., 2011). Specificity reported to be between 43% and 100% depending on study and severity of disease
Traditional lipase	Widely used and available on in-house analysers. Most specific catalytic assay (also new DGGR lipase assay, which appears more sensitive and specific; see text for details)	Extra-pancreatic sources, so high background level. Renal excretion – elevated 2–3 times in azotaemia. Falsely elevated by steroids up to 5x	Sensitivity varies from 28 to 71% depending on cut-off and severity of disease. Specificity varies from 3 to 92% depending on study (same references as amylase)

14.7 Advantages, disadvantages, sensitivities and specificities of enzyme assays in the diagnosis of pancreatitis in dogs and cats. PLI = pancreatic lipase immunoreactivity; TLI = trypsin-like immunoreactivity.

They are neither species nor organ specific: a catalytic lipase assay will potentially detect any lipase reaching the circulation, including gastric lipase, intestinal acidic lipase, lipoprotein lipase and other extra-pancreatic lipases. There is a high background non-pancreatic activity for both amylase and lipase: plasma levels of amylase and lipase are normal in dogs after total pancreatectomy. Plasma lipase is also often normal in dogs with EPI, which equates to loss of 90% of exocrine enzyme output (Steiner et al., 2006). In addition, both amylase and lipase are excreted via the kidney, so circulating levels can be increased in animals with renal disease or prerenal azotaemia. Lipase can be increased greater than 5-fold in renal disease, and mean concentrations of both amylase and lipase were greater in dogs with renal disease than in dogs with pancreatitis in one study (Mansfield and Jones, 2000). Thus these assays are neither 100% sensitive nor specific. However, as detailed in Figure 14.7, the sensitivity and specificity of lipase in particular are often similar to those of pancreatic lipase immunoreactivity, so lipase remains a useful test for the diagnosis of canine pancreatitis.

Small elevations in amylase or lipase are unlikely to be significant because of the high background level; generally only elevations of ≥3–5 times normal are considered suggestive of pancreatitis (provided none of the secondary causes of elevation outlined in Figure 14.7 is present). In the cat, plasma amylase and lipase, although measurable, are of no use at all in the diagnosis of pancreatitis because they may be elevated in normal cats and normal in cases of pancreatitis. However, work on newer substrates for enzymatic lipase is ongoing and these may prove to be more specific in cats than the current catalytic assay.

Recently, studies have been published that used a new type of lipase assay which appears to be more sensitive and specific than the traditional lipase assay. This is the 1,2-o-dilauryl-rac-glycero glutaric acid-(6'-methyl-resorufin) ester (DGGR) lipase assay. The enzyme and substrate interactions in this assay are more selective than with the traditional multistep colorimetric lipase assay which uses 1,2-diglyceride as the substrate. It is proposed that, with the new assay, hydrolysis with other lipases and esterases is less likely to occur (Graca et al., 2005). A recent study in dogs suggested good agreement between the DGGR lipase assay and pancreatic lipase immunoreactivity (PLI) in dogs (Kook et al., 2014), and another study suggests that it may also be useful in cats, unlike the older lipase assay (Oppliger et al., 2013).

Immunoassays: These are organ specific, and may be species specific, and they can measure precursors in addition to active enzymes. They use an antibody directed against part of the enzyme molecule (usually distinct from the active site) which is detected by either radioimmunoassay (RIA) or an enzyme-linked immunosorbent assay (ELISA).

Pancreatic lipase immunoreactivity (PLI): This measures lipase of pancreatic origin only. Therefore, it is pancreas specific and, unlike lipase, PLI is not only high in pancreatitis but also very low in EPI. Median serum PLI concentration is significantly lower in dogs with EPI (0.1 μg/l) than in healthy dogs (16.3 μg/l). It is species specific, and both canine and feline PLI assays are available. There is accumulating evidence that canine PLI is the most sensitive and specific test for canine pancreatitis, although its sensitivity varies depending on the severity and chronicity of disease (see Figure 14.7). The first canine PLI assay developed was an RIA. This was followed by an ELISA using two purified polyclonal antibodies and a streptavidin detection system – known as canine pancreatic lipase immunoreactivity (cPLI). This was not easily applicable to commercial use, so an ELISA using dual monoclonal antibodies and a direct enzyme-labelled detection reagent was developed, the Spec cPL® (Huth *et al.*, 2010). This ELISA has been found to be comparable in accuracy to the older ELISA.

More recently still, a dog-side SNAP® test has been developed for canine PLI which has a reported accuracy of 96% when compared with the Spec cPL® (95% confidence interval 94–97%; Beall *et al.*, 2011). Most disagreements between the SNAP® and the Spec cPL® occur in the mid-range, in deciding the cut-off between normal and abnormal, and it is recommended that these results are confirmed by sending blood to the laboratory for Spec cPL® testing, which gives a quantitative (numerical) result. Strongly positive or negative SNAP® results are generally accurate.

Current evidence suggests that the sensitivity and specificity of the cPLI, Spec cPL® and SNAP® tests are very similar and these are summarized in Figure 14.7. All three assays have a 'grey area' or indeterminate zone in the diagnostic range, which maximizes sensitivity but is not as specific as the higher cut-off. For example, for the Spec cPL®: values <200 μg/ml are classed as negative; values between 200 and 400 μg/ml are indeterminate; and values >400 μg/ml are positive for pancreatitis. There is a wide variety of sensitivities reported in the literature. Generally, the more severe and acute the disease, the higher the sensitivity in both cats and dogs, and the milder and more chronic the disease, the lower the sensitivity. The important clinical point to note is that none of these tests is 100% sensitive or specific so it is possible to have a normal result in a dog or cat with pancreatitis and, conversely, although the specificity is high, it is also possible to have a high value in a dog or cat without pancreatitis. Discordant results are also not uncommon. For example, trypsin-like immunoreactivity (TLI) could be elevated in a dog with pancreatitis with a normal cPLI and *vice versa*. This is probably due to the different half-lives of the enzymes in the plasma after the onset of pancreatitis: TLI has been shown to increase within 24 hours of the onset of pancreatitis in dogs, and to peak and decrease more quickly than lipase (Simpson *et al.*, 1989), returning to the reference interval within 5 days. There are no published studies on the half-life of cPLI although one conference abstract suggested a half-life of 2 hours in dogs, which implies that it will have returned to normal within 24 hours of an acute insult.

Early work on the clinical use of feline PLI suggested it may be more sensitive and specific than fTLI and may remain elevated for longer than fTLI in experimental feline pancreatitis (Williams *et al.*, 2003). This has been supported by more recent studies, although there is less published work on the sensitivity and specificity of the feline test (Forman *et al.*, 2004). As in dogs, the early feline PLI has been replaced by a Spec fPL® and SNAP® test.

Trypsin-like immunoreactivity (TLI): This test measures trypsin and trypsinogen and is species specific. Canine and feline (and human) TLI assays are available in the UK but there is no dog- or cat-side SNAP® test. The TLI test was originally developed in cats and dogs for the diagnosis of EPI, where the concentration is very low (see later). However, it can be used as an additional test in pancreatitis, although its sensitivity appears to be low in both species, probably due to rapid clearance from the circulation in acute cases (see Figure 14.7). In dogs, TLI does appear to be highly specific, and in early studies, before the development of the cPLI assay, TLI was considered the most specific test for pancreatitis in dogs (Simpson *et al.*, 1989). A cut-off of 35 ng/ml is generally used and any value above this is highly suggestive of pancreatitis in dogs. Because of the observation of discordant results in some dogs, an elevated TLI in dogs should not be ignored but should be considered highly likely to show pancreatitis. However, in cats, TLI has a lower sensitivity and specificity for the diagnosis of pancreatitis than in dogs. Most importantly, false positives have been reported in cats with hepatic or GI disease, which are the conditions most likely to be confused clinically with pancreatitis in cats; therefore, unlike in dogs, a high TLI in cats does not confirm pancreatitis.

Swift *et al.* (2000) found a sensitivity of 55% and a specificity of 56% for the diagnosis of pancreatitis in cats using fTLI. However, they used a lower cut-off than currently recommended (>82 ng/l) and used the RIA rather than the ELISA. Gerhardt *et al.* (2001) used the ELISA and found a sensitivity of 62% if the cut-off was 82 ng/l, a sensitivity of 33% with a cut-off of 100 ng/l (the currently accepted cut-off for diagnosis of feline pancreatitis) and a sensitivity of 86% if the cut-off was 49 ng/l (top of the normal range).

Alternative diagnostic tests: Clearly none of the enzyme tests currently used, among either immunoassays or catalytic assays, is perfect, and they have particularly low sensitivities in mild and chronic disease in dogs and cats. Therefore, new tests continue to be developed.

Trypsin activation peptide (TAP): An assay for TAP was developed as a possible alternative diagnostic test but is not currently commercially available. TAP is the peptide cleaved from trypsinogen by enterokinase in the small intestine, resulting in active trypsin. It is highly conserved among species, so the human ELISA can be used for both dogs and cats. Theoretically, there should be no TAP in the plasma in healthy animals if all the trypsinogen is activated within the small intestine. However, the finding of low but significant levels of TAP in the plasma of healthy dogs (Mansfield and Jones, 2000) suggests that a small amount of normal trypsinogen autoactivation occurs in the pancreas. Elevations in plasma TAP levels should be diagnostic of pancreatitis, but elevated plasma TAP has a specificity of only 76% and sensitivity of 53% for pancreatitis in dogs, and renal disease elevates mean plasma TAP as much as pancreatitis. The urine TAP:creatinine ratio has a higher specificity but lower sensitivity than plasma TAP. There is a much wider range of urinary TAP concentrations in healthy dogs than in humans, and urinary TAP is also increased in renal disease (Mansfield and Jones, 2000).

Serum canine pancreatic elastase-1 (cPE-1): An ELISA for serum cPE-1 has been developed for dogs, and was demonstrated in one study to have a sensitivity of 61.4% and specificity of 91.7% for diagnosis of all types of pancreatic disease. The sensitivity rose to 78.26% for the diagnosis of severe acute pancreatitis (Mansfield *et al.*, 2011). However, this test is not currently commercially available for dogs.

Summary

The non-invasive diagnosis of pancreatitis is problematical. In both dogs and cats, a combination of the history, clinical findings, diagnostic imaging findings (radiography to rule out intestinal obstruction as a cause of acute vomiting and other pathology, and ultrasonography of the pancreas) and the results of appropriately chosen pancreatic enzyme assays should be used to reach a presumptive diagnosis of pancreatitis. Ultrasonography has a high specificity but relatively low sensitivity for diagnosis of pancreatitis in dogs and even lower sensitivity in cats. The sensitivity is highest for acute disease, where the typical appearance is of a diffusely hypoechoic pancreas (due to oedema), surrounded by a hyperechoic mesentery (due to fat necrosis). In chronic disease, the appearance can be similar or the pancreas can have a mixed echogenicity corresponding to fibrosis and oedema. However, many chronic cases in dogs and cats have a normal pancreas on ultrasonography. Definitive diagnosis is only obtained by histological examination of the pancreas, which is not appropriate in many acute cases.

Prognostic indicators

The degree of elevation of pancreatic enzymes does not appear to be an accurate prognostic indicator in dogs with acute pancreatitis. Attempts to define the best prognostic indicator have led to the development of an organ score system (Ruaux and Atwell, 1998) and a clinical severity scoring system (Mansfield *et al.*, 2008), neither of which is perfect. The organ scoring system described by Ruaux and Atwell (1998) uses the results of haematology and biochemistry screens at presentation to define the number of organs compromised in addition to the pancreas. The following systems were assessed: leucogram; kidneys; liver and endocrine pancreas; and acid–base balance. The higher the score, on a scale of 0 to 4, the poorer the prognosis and the more expensive and intensive the management required.

Mansfield *et al.* (2008) did not find a correlation between this organ scoring system and outcome in their cases, but did find a correlation with a clinical severity scoring system which included clinical as well as blood test findings and measured cardiovascular and respiratory systems, vascular forces, and an assessment of intestinal integrity. 'Vascular forces' were assessed using a combination of blood pressure changes and serum albumin. The cardiovascular and respiratory systems and intestinal integrity were all assessed clinically. In this study, coagulation abnormalities, local abnormalities (such as peritonitis and pancreatic pseudocyst) and renal function were not correlated with outcome.

Overall, therefore, the ideal severity scoring system has yet to be identified in dogs. In human medicine, the most important negative prognostic indicator is persistent organ failure for more than 48 hours after presentation, although local complications such as peripancreatic fluid accumulation are also scored (Banks *et al.*, 2012). Human patients with no systemic inflammatory response syndrome (SIRS) or organ failure on presentation are defined as having mild acute pancreatitis, and have an excellent prognosis. Individuals with organ failure which resolves on treatment within 48 hours of presentation are defined as having moderately severe pancreatitis, and they also have a good prognosis when intensively managed. Humans with persistent organ failure are defined as having severe acute pancreatitis and have a mortality rate as high as 50% in spite of intensive treatment. It may be that such a dynamic system would work best prognostically in dogs and cats, where the response to treatment over the first few days may be a better indicator of prognosis than the findings on presentation, but this has yet to be investigated in small animals.

Of the individual clinicopathological tests, the urine TAP:creatinine ratio is the most useful prognostically (Mansfield *et al.*, 2003), although elevations in serum lipase, creatinine and phosphate, and low urine SG, have shown some value as negative prognostic indicators. One Hungarian study of 80 dogs with acute pancreatitis found hypothermia and metabolic acidosis to be negative prognostic indicators (Pápa *et al.*, 2011).

The degree of elevation of TLI does not appear to be prognostically useful. The prognostic relevance of the degree of elevation in cPLI in pancreatitis is unclear. In one study, dogs with inflammatory bowel disease and an elevated cPLI (although no histological or ultrasonographic confirmation of pancreatitis) were more likely to be euthanased than dogs with inflammatory bowel disease and a normal cPLI (Kathrani *et al.*, 2009).

Recognized negative prognostic indicators in cats include low ionized calcium and leucopenia (Kimmel *et al.*, 2001). Urinary or plasma concentrations of TAP do not seem to be prognostically helpful in cats.

Other tests which have been assessed as prognostic indicators but are not clinically useful include α-macroglobulin (circulating protease inhibitor) and circulating α$_1$-protease inhibitor–trypsin complexes, which have too short a half-life to be applied clinically.

Exocrine pancreatic insufficiency

Exocrine pancreatic insufficiency (EPI) is a functional lack of pancreatic enzymes resulting in clinical signs of steatorrhoea and weight loss. Unlike pancreatitis, it is readily diagnosed by clinical signs and pancreatic function tests.

Causes

Pancreatic acinar atrophy (PAA) is believed to be the predominant cause of EPI in dogs but end-stage chronic pancreatitis is also important (Watson *et al.*, 2010). PAA is particularly recognized in German Shepherd Dogs, in whom an autosomal mode of inheritance has been suggested, although more recent studies refute this. It has also been described in Rough Collies, English Setters and sporadically in other breeds. Histological studies in German Shepherd Dogs suggest an immune-mediated disease directed against the acini, although the disease shows no response to steroids or other immunosuppressive drugs. The islet cells are spared and dogs with PAA are not typically diabetic. Most dogs develop the disease in young adulthood, but a proportion of German Shepherd Dogs remain subclinical for a prolonged period, in spite of clinicopathological evidence of pancreatic enzyme insufficiency, and only develop clinical signs late in life. PAA has not been recognized in cats and end-stage pancreatitis is the commonest cause of feline EPI.

EPI can also develop as a consequence of chronic pancreatitis in dogs in whom there is extensive loss of pancreatic acini. As chronic pancreatitis may be largely subclinical or only present as occasional clinical acute-on-chronic episodes, the degree of underlying pancreatic damage may be underestimated. Many dogs with end-stage chronic pancreatitis also develop diabetes mellitus, either before or after EPI, as a result of concurrent islet cell destruction (Watson *et al.*, 2010) and the situation is likely to be similar in cats. English Cocker Spaniels and Cavalier King Charles Spaniels in the UK appear to be particularly predisposed to developing EPI as an end stage of chronic pancreatitis, as demonstrated in both clinical and clinicopathological studies (Batchelor *et al.*, 2007a; Watson *et al.*, 2010).

EPI may develop secondary to pancreatic tumours in dogs and cats, usually due to blockage of pancreatic ducts by the tumours, although destruction of acinar tissue by the mass and associated pancreatitis also play a role.

Finally, clinical EPI may develop in the presence of adequate pancreatic output as a result of hyperacidity of the duodenum inactivating lipase in the intestinal lumen. This is rare in small animals.

Diagnosis

The diagnosis of EPI relies on demonstrating reduced pancreatic enzyme output. The most sensitive and specific way of doing this is by measuring reduced circulating enzyme activity. However, there are problems interpreting these results in the presence of concurrent pancreatitis. In these cases, measurement of reduced enzyme activity in the gut, by measuring reduced faecal enzyme activity, may be useful, although is not widely used commercially.

Blood tests: immunoassays

TLI: Measurement of reduced TLI in the blood has a high sensitivity and specificity for the diagnosis of EPI in dogs and cats, and is currently the single test of choice in small animals. A fasting serum sample is required because the release of pancreatic enzymes associated with feeding can raise the levels, although in practice this is not usually a significant problem. It is **not** necessary to stop exogenous pancreatic enzyme supplementation before measuring TLI because the test is an immunoassay, which does not cross-react with the TLI of other species (and very little exogenous pancreatic enzyme is absorbed). There are some problems in interpreting the results, particularly in dogs, as outlined below.

- A low serum TLI (<2.5 ng/l in dogs) alone does not diagnose clinical EPI if there are no compatible clinical signs. Serum TLI should be measured several times, over several weeks to months, and must be persistently low to demonstrate EPI.
- Occasionally, a single TLI may be low in a dog with pancreatitis, as a result of a temporary reduction in enzyme production. A dog with persistently low TLI but no steatorrhoea or weight loss would be considered to have 'subclinical' EPI and should not be treated but be monitored for any evidence of clinical disease.

Subclinical EPI is uncommon but has been reported in a small number of German Shepherd Dogs with PAA (Wiberg *et al.*, 1999); it has not yet been reported in cats. A TLI stimulation test may give more information about the status of the animal but is rarely performed (Wiberg *et al.*, 1999). A TLI in the 'grey area' (2.5–5.0 ng/l in dogs) is not diagnostic of EPI and the test needs to be repeated a few weeks to months later. In a proportion of dogs (45% in one study: Wiberg *et al.*, 1999), the TLI will return to the normal range. In about 10% of dogs, the TLI will drop to the level diagnostic of EPI, while in the rest it remains in the grey area.

- A single normal or high TLI in a breed of dog other than a German Shepherd Dog, with suspicious clinical signs, does not rule out EPI. TLI can increase to or above the normal range in dogs with EPI secondary to chronic end-stage pancreatitis, if it is measured during a bout of disease (Watson *et al.*, 2010). This is because EPI reduces TLI, but pancreatitis elevates it. A similar situation may arise in cats, but this has not been well documented. Therefore, in any animal with suspected EPI secondary to chronic pancreatitis, TLI measurements should be repeated, preferably when the animal is showing no clinical signs of pancreatitis. Clinicians should take a proactive approach in treating such animals with enzymes as soon as clinically justified, and not wait for an abnormal TLI result. Clinical response to enzyme supplementation in such cases is very suggestive of developing EPI even in the face of a normal TLI. Alternatively, a test for enzyme activity in the gut, such as a faecal elastase test, could be used in these animals, because pancreatitis leads to enzyme release into the abdomen and bloodstream, but not into the pancreatic ducts, which drain into the gut.

cPLI: A low cPLI also has good sensitivity and specificity for the diagnosis of EPI in dogs (Steiner *et al.*, 2006), but it is not superior to TLI and the latter is more readily available. PLI is also likely to be low in cats with EPI.

Catalytic assays

Unlike in humans, amylase and lipase are **not** consistently low in dogs and cats with EPI. This is because of the high background levels of the enzymes from other organs.

Faecal tests

Faecal trypsin activity: Measurement of faecal trypsin activity has such a low sensitivity and specificity for the diagnosis of EPI that it is not worth doing.

Faecal fat: Likewise, microscopic examination of faeces for undigested fat, starch and muscle fibres is not helpful: other conditions apart from EPI can cause maldigestion/malabsorption. Observation of a subjectively 'marked' increase in faecal fat is usually associated with EPI, but this has a very low sensitivity; most dogs with EPI have only mild to moderate increases in faecal fat, overlapping with normal dogs and dogs with other diseases. In addition, animals with EPI often have intermittently normal faeces. Faecal proteolytic activity can be assessed in a number of ways, but again these tests generally have poor sensitivity and specificity. Bacteria in the gut can also produce proteolytic enzymes, and these certainly produce false negative results in tests such as the gelatine (radiographic film) digestion tests, particularly in aged samples. Normal dogs, unlike humans, show intermittent excretion of pancreatic proteases, so levels may be low on single faecal samples from normal animals. The tests can be improved by stimulation with a test food (e.g. soybean) but the tests remain difficult to perform and interpret (Westermarck and Sandholm, 1980).

Faecal elastase: This appears to have higher sensitivity and specificity than the other faecal tests for the diagnosis of EPI in dogs. Elastase is a pancreatic enzyme, and a species-specific ELISA for canine elastase has been developed (Spillmann et al., 2001). Levels are low in dogs with EPI. As with canine TLI, there is no cross-reaction with elastase from other species, so dogs can remain on enzyme supplementation while the test is performed. There is marked variation in elastase levels in normal canine faeces compared with human faeces. The sensitivity and specificity of the test are improved by taking three separate faecal samples on 3 days or using a cut-off value for the diagnosis of EPI which is below this variation in most dogs. Values of about 40 μg/g of faeces are considered normal and values below 10 μg/g of faeces are considered diagnostic of EPI. (For further information on this test, the reader is referred to the manufacturer's website). Measurement may be particularly useful in animals with end-stage pancreatitis and/or pancreatic duct blockage where TLI results might be misleading (Spillmann et al., 2000).

Faecal culture and sensitivity, and parasite examination: At least one faecal culture and sensitivity and parasite examination (see Chapter 13) should be carried out on all animals with EPI. Concurrent GI infections are not uncommon in these dogs, secondary to disruption of the GI environment and immunity. Treatment of the EPI will not be successful unless concurrent infections are also recognized and treated.

Additional tests

Cobalamin and folate: It is advisable to measure serum cobalamin (B12) concentration in animals with EPI because cobalamin is often reduced owing to a deficiency of pancreatic intrinsic factor, which is required for absorption of cobalamin, and this has been shown to be a negative prognostic indicator in these cases in dogs (Batchelor et al., 2007b). In cats with end-stage pancreatitis, cobalamin is even more likely to be reduced than in dogs, because cats only produce intrinsic factor in the pancreas, whereas dogs also produce some in the stomach. This is compounded in cats by the high incidence of concurrent inflammatory bowel disease, which often further reduces cobalamin by reducing ileal absorption. In one study of cats with EPI, all 10 cats that were tested had low serum cobalamin (Thompson et al., 2009). Cobalamin deficiency has been reported to cause villous atrophy and reduced GI function, weight loss and diarrhoea in cats. If low cobalamin is documented in dogs and cats with EPI it is important to supplement with parenteral B12 injections. In one case of marked cobalamin deficiency in a cat with EPI, hyperammonaemia developed with encephalopathy due to accumulation of methylmalonic acid (Watanabe et al., 2012).

Serum folate concentrations may also be measured in these animals, and they are elevated in about one-third of dogs and cats with EPI. This may indicate small intestinal bacterial overgrowth (SIBO) in dogs, although the sensitivity and specificity of a high serum folate for the diagnosis of SIBO are poor (see Chapter 13). Up to 75% of dogs with EPI also have SIBO, secondary to increased undigested nutrients in the gut, reduction in the antibacterial effects of pancreatic secretions, and chronic maldigestion leading to malnutrition and reduced gut immunity. The definition and diagnosis of SIBO is problematical (see Chapter 13 for more details); it is better to assume SIBO in newly diagnosed dogs with EPI and treat appropriately, rather than rely on the results of diagnostic tests. The importance of SIBO in cats with EPI is unknown.

A small number of dogs with EPI have low serum folate levels (2% in the study of Batchelor et al., 2007b). In some cases, this may be due to concurrent inflammatory bowel disease, reducing jejunal absorption of folate.

Haematology and biochemistry: Haematology and biochemistry screens are often normal in dogs with EPI. In very cachexic animals, they may show subtle changes associated with malnutrition, negative nitrogen balance and breakdown of body muscle, such as low albumin and globulin, mildly elevated liver enzymes, low cholesterol and triglycerides, and lymphopenia. Animals with EPI, particularly German Shepherd Dogs, often present with dermatological problems due to poor coat quality and may have a neutrophilia resulting from chronic pyoderma.

Cats with EPI have a high prevalence of concurrent disease – which in many cases reflects similar concurrent diseases to those accompanying chronic pancreatitis in this species. Diseases of the gut, liver and kidney are particularly common (Thompson et al., 2009). Therefore, it is also common to see concurrent changes on haematology and biochemistry screens in cats with EPI. A mild normochromic, normocytic anaemia is seen in about half of cases, and over one-third have increases in liver enzymes, bilirubin and glucose (Thompson et al., 2009).

Finding a marked hypoproteinaemia or more severe changes on haematology and biochemistry in an animal with EPI should trigger a search for another disease. Cats and dogs with end-stage pancreatitis may present with more severe secondary changes on blood screens, as outlined in the Pancreatitis section. A high percentage of these animals with end-stage pancreatitis (up to 50%) will also have concurrent diabetes mellitus and will show typical clinicopathological changes.

Pancreatic neoplasia

Neoplasia of the exocrine pancreas is uncommon in cats and dogs. However, pancreatic adenocarcinomas are generally very malignant and have usually disseminated widely by the time of diagnosis. They are often subclinical but can result in single or repeat bouts of pancreatitis and/or the development of EPI. Although the development of EPI secondary to neoplasia is rare (<10% of cases in humans), it has been reported in both dogs and cats. It occurs as a result of a combination of duct blockage and pancreatic parenchymal destruction. Occasionally, pancreatic carcinomas can cause paraneoplastic hypercalcaemia, although this is rare.

Pancreatic adenomas are rare in small animals but have been reported in cats (Bjorneby and Kari, 2002). Nodular hyperplasia of the exocrine pancreas is common in older dogs and cats. This usually presents as multiple small masses, whereas pancreatic tumours are usually single; histology is necessary to differentiate hyperplasia from neoplasia.

Pancreatic tumours are not associated with any specific clinicopathological changes and they may cause no changes in enzyme activities at all. However, some cases have been associated with very marked elevations in serum lipase concentration (Quigley *et al.*, 2001). Alternatively, they can result in recurrent bouts of pancreatitis, with typical associated blood changes, and EPI can develop. In the latter cases, TLI may be low or normal, or even elevated if the EPI is due to duct blockage and there is plenty of remaining acinar tissue to produce trypsin. In cases with suspected EPI due to pancreatic tumours, tests of enzyme function, such as the faecal elastase test, are likely to be a more sensitive means to diagnose the insufficiency. Marked elevations in liver enzymes and jaundice may be seen in some cases as a result of extrahepatic obstruction of the bile duct by the mass.

Ultrasound-guided fine-needle aspiration cytology may help to differentiate between inflammatory and neoplastic lesions of the pancreas (Bjorneby and Kari, 2002). Care must be taken, because dysplastic changes in epithelial cells in the presence of inflammation may appear very similar to neoplasia.

Pancreatic abscesses, cysts and pseudocysts

Pancreatic abscesses, cysts and pseudocysts are uncommonly reported in dogs and cats and are usually a complication of pancreatitis.

- Pancreatic cysts may be congenital (e.g. as a component of polycystic renal disease in Persian cats) or secondary to cystic neoplasia, but most commonly are secondary to pancreatitis.
- Pseudocysts have been recognized in association with pancreatitis in both cats and dogs. A pseudocyst is a collection of fluid containing pancreatic enzymes and debris in a non-epithelialized sac. Fluid analysis generally shows a modified transudate, and the levels of amylase and lipase can be measured. In humans, the enzymes are more elevated in pseudocysts associated with pancreatitis than in those associated with cystic carcinomas, but the value of this measurement in small animals is unknown. Cytologically, a pseudocyst contains amorphous debris, some neutrophils and macrophages and, rarely, small numbers of reactive fibroblasts.
- A true pancreatic abscess is a collection of septic exudate which results from secondary infection of necrotic pancreatic tissue or a pancreatic pseudocyst. Cytologically, there are many degenerative neutrophils and variable numbers of pancreatic acinar cells, which may appear atypical or dysplastic, as a result of inflammation. They are fortunately rare in dogs and cats as they are associated with a poor prognosis.

Case examples

CASE 1

SIGNALMENT

8-year, 2-month old neutered male English Cocker Spaniel.

HISTORY

The dog has a long history of intermittent mild GI upsets when he scavenges; these have not required veterinary attention. He is fed on a low-fat canned supermarket brand. Over the last 6 months, these episodes have become more severe and he presents during a bout for further investigation. The owner reports that he was anorexic and vomited bile and some food the previous day and now has diarrhoea. On clinical examination, his temperature is mildly elevated at 39.1°C. He has a dry nose and mouth and a lot of dental tartar. There is focal pain on palpation of his cranial abdomen. His anal sacs are full.

CLINICAL PATHOLOGY DATA

Haematology	Result	Reference interval
WBC (x 10⁹/l)	9.0	6.0–17.0
Neutrophils (x 10⁹/l)	6.6	3.0–11.5
Band neutrophils (x 10⁹/l)	0	<0.5
Lymphocytes (x 10⁹/l)	1.3	1.0–4.8
Monocytes (x 10⁹/l)	**1.62**	0.2–1.5
Eosinophils (x 10⁹/l)	0.3	0.1–1.3
Platelets (x 10⁹/l)	287	175–500

Abnormal results are in **bold**.

Haematology *continued*	Result	Reference interval
HCT (l/l)	0.53	0.37–0.55
RBC (x 10¹²/l)	7	5.5–8.5
Hb (g/dl)	17.4	12–18
MCV (fl)	76	61–80
MCHC (g/dl)	33	30–36

Abnormal results are in **bold**.

Biochemistry	Result	Reference interval
Sodium (mmol/l)	149	135–155
Potassium (mmol/l)	5.1	3.6–5.6
Glucose (mmol/l)	4.1	3.6–7.0
Urea (mmol/l)	6.0	3.3–6.7
Creatinine (mmol/l)	87	70–170
Calcium (mmol/l)	2.7	2.45–3.0
Phosphate (mmol/l)	1.27	0.6–1.6
Total protein (g/l)	63	55–80
Albumin (g/l)	30	25–45
Globulins (g/l)	33	20–45
Cholesterol (mmol/l)	**10**	3–6
Triglyceride (mmol/l)	**3.8**	0.3–1.2
ALT (IU/l)	**90**	5–60
ALP (IU /l)	**163**	0–130
Amylase (IU/l)	**1477**	100–1200
Lipase (IU/l)	**750**	<200
Canine Spec cPL® (μg/l)	**717**	<200

Abnormal results are in **bold**.

→ CASE 1 CONTINUED

Film comment: red cells appear normal. No abnormal white cells seen. Some platelet clumping. True count probably higher than indicated.

Urinalysis	Result	Reference interval
Specific gravity	SG 1.014	
Protein	2+ protein	
Protein:creatinine ratio	**0.9**	0–0.5
pH	9.0	
White and red cells	Negative	

Abnormal results are in **bold**.

WHAT ABNORMALITIES ARE PRESENT?

- Elevated canine Spec cPL®.
- Elevated cholesterol.
- Elevated triglycerides.
- Mild elevations in ALP and ALT.
- Mild elevation in amylase; more marked elevation in lipase.
- Poorly concentrated urine with alkaline pH and increased protein:creatinine ratio.

HOW WOULD YOU INTERPRET THESE RESULTS?

The elevated Spec cPL® suggests pancreatitis, supported by the elevated lipase. The amylase is only slightly raised and would not be diagnostic of pancreatitis alone without other evidence. The elevated cholesterol could be postprandial but, if this is a fasting sample, it may be caused by pancreatitis or a protein-losing nephropathy (PLN), although hypothyroidism should also be considered. The elevations in liver enzymes are very mild and probably secondary, although a primary hepatopathy cannot be ruled out at this stage. The urine is poorly concentrated, suggesting some renal compromise or interference with renal concentrating ability. There is a significant proteinuria in the face of an inactive sediment, which suggests glomerular disease. The urine is alkaline which could suggest urinary tract infection or may be postprandial.

WHAT FURTHER TESTS WOULD BE INDICATED?

- Blood pressure measurement because dogs with PLN can be hypertensive.
- Schirmer tear tests:
  - There is a dry nose and a suspicion of polysystemic immune-mediated disease in the breed.
- Serum B$_{12}$, folate and TLI.
- Urine culture.
- Abdominal imaging.

RESULTS OF FURTHER TESTS

- Blood pressure was normal.
- Schirmer tear tests were borderline reduced bilaterally at 10 mm (normal 12–27; borderline 5–10).
- Urine culture was negative.
- Serum B$_{12}$, folate and TLI were measured and were normal.

- An abdominal radiograph was unremarkable.
- Abdominal ultrasonography was unremarkable apart from a slightly enlarged, hypoechoic left pancreatic limb, with slightly hyperechoic surrounding mesentery suggestive of pancreatitis.

WHAT IS YOUR DIAGNOSIS?

A diagnosis of probable pancreatitis was made on the basis of the blood results and ultrasonography findings. Because of the dog's breed and history of previous bouts, this was considered most likely to be chronic and probably typical of the polysystemic Cocker Spaniel disease (chronic pancreatitis ± glomerulonephritis ± dry eye ± anal sacculitis).

TREATMENT

Analgesia was provided with buprenorphine followed by oral paracetamol and codeine, and the owners were advised to continue feeding a low-fat diet. Topical ciclosporin was dispensed for the eyes. The disease is thought to be autoimmune in Cocker Spaniels, so immunosuppression was discussed and the owner elected to try a course of corticosteroids at 1 mg/kg/day followed by gradual reduction.

FOLLOW-UP

The dog initially did well but was presented again 2 weeks later with acute-onset vomiting and anorexia followed by diarrhoea. On clinical examination, the rectal temperature was 38.6°C; mucous membranes were dry and very yellow and the abdomen was very painful on palpation. Bloods tests were repeated.

Haematology	Result	Reference interval
WBC (x 10⁹/l)	18	6.0–17.0
Neutrophils (x 10⁹/l)	8.8	3.0–11.5
Band neutrophils (x 10⁹/l)	**6.3**	<0.5
Lymphocytes (x 10⁹/l)	1.3	1.0–4.8
Monocytes (x 10⁹/l)	**1.62**	0.2–1.5
Eosinophils (x 10⁹/l)	0.6	0.1–1.3
Platelets (x 10⁹/l)	**171**	175–500
HCT (l/l)	0.39	0.37–0.55
RBC (x 10¹²/l)	6.3	5.5–8.5
Hb (g/dl)	15.4	12–18
MCV (fl)	61.9	61–80
MCHC (g/dl)	**38.8**	30–36
OSPT (seconds)	10.6	7.6–11.6
aPTT (seconds)	19.2	12.5–25
D-dimers (ng/ml)	**>2000**	<250

Abnormal results are in **bold**.

→ CASE 1 CONTINUED

Biochemistry	Result	Reference interval
Sodium (mmol/l)	143	135–155
Potassium (mmol/l)	4.1	3.6–5.6
Glucose (mmol/l)	**7.2**	3.6–7.0
Urea (mmol/l)	**9.3**	3.3–6.7
Creatinine (mmol/l)	116	70–170
Calcium (mmol/l)	2.7	2.45–3.0
Phosphate (mmol/l)	**1.7**	0.6–1.6
Total protein (g/l)	69	55–80
Albumin (g/l)	28	25–45
Cholesterol (mmol/l)	**12.8**	3.3–6.5
Triglyceride (mmol/l)	**1.3**	0.4–1.2
ALT (IU/l)	**222**	14–67
ALP (IU/l)	**4274**	26–107
Total bilirubin (μmol/l)	**156**	0–12
Amylase (IU/l)	1346	256–1609
Lipase (IU/l)	**1416**	0–200

Abnormal results are in **bold**.

Urine protein:creatinine ratio was **6.4** (reference interval 0.0–0.5) with inactive sediment.

cSpec cPL® not performed, it was considered unnecessary after ultrasonography (see below).

Film comment: marked left shift but no toxic change.

WHAT ABNORMALITIES ARE PRESENT?

- Cholesterol remains elevated although triglycerides are now almost normal.
- There is a moderate elevation in ALT, with markedly elevated ALP and bilirubin.
- Amylase is normal but lipase is markedly elevated.
- The urine protein:creatinine ratio has increased since the last visit.
- There is a leucocytosis made up predominantly of band neutrophils.
- The platelet count is slightly reduced (and much lower than on the last visit).
- D-dimers are elevated.

HOW WOULD YOU INTERPRET THESE RESULTS?

The marked elevation in ALP could be partly steroid induced. However, the concurrent marked increase in bilirubin with a normal packed cell volume (PCV) suggests biliary tract disease. In this case, extrahepatic biliary obstruction with acute-on-chronic pancreatitis

would be the top differential. The inflammatory leucogram supports an acute exacerbation of disease. The mild elevation in urea is probably due to dehydration and prerenal failure. The increased D-dimers raise the suspicion of DIC, although coagulation times are currently normal and the platelets are only borderline low.

RESULTS OF FURTHER TESTS

On ultrasonography, the pancreas appeared very different from at the previous visit. It was very painful on probing with multiple anechoic cystic areas. The surrounding mesentery was very hyperechoic. The liver was mildly hyperechoic and heterogeneous and there was distension of the biliary tract and gallbladder. Fluid was obtained by fine-needle aspiration from one of the pancreatic cysts. Cytological examination showed moderate numbers of degenerate neutrophils and occasional foamy macrophages. There were focal sheets of adipocytes with small amounts of fat necrosis. No bacteria were seen. The findings were consistent with a pancreatic abscess.

DIAGNOSIS AND TREATMENT

The dog appeared to have suffered an acute exacerbation of its pancreatitis and consequent extrahepatic biliary tract obstruction. It was impossible to know whether this had been caused by the steroids, or caused by too low a dose or too rapid a drop in the steroid therapy, or whether it was unrelated. The prognosis was considered to be poor because of the pancreatic abscesses and the suspicion of early DIC. The dog was managed with: aggressive intravenous fluid therapy; analgesia; early enteral feeding; antiemetics; ursodeoxycholic acid; potentiated amoxicillin to protect against infection of the apparently sterile pancreatic abscesses; and continued steroid therapy to prevent iatrogenic hypoadrenocorticism through sudden cessation. He recovered well and was discharged a week later on continued ursodeoxycholic acid and steroid therapy.

After 1 month, the dog was clinically well and the serum bilirubin concentration was normal but Spec cPL® was >1000 μg/l (reference interval <200 μg/l). He was gradually weaned down to a low daily dose of prednisolone. The owner reported that attempts to stop the steroids resulted in a recurrence of mild clinical signs, so he was maintained on a low dose long term.

Note that this case demonstrates well that repeated measurement of Spec cPL® in a patient with chronic pancreatitis is of no prognostic or therapeutic value. Measurement is very helpful to make a diagnosis but not to monitor treatment. Spec cPL® would be expected to be elevated long term, or to go up and down, in a dog with chronic pancreatitis, and the disease can be clinically controlled while Spec cPL® remains elevated.

CASE 2

SIGNALMENT

6-year, 6-month old neutered female Siamese cat.

HISTORY

The cat had a 6-month history of waxing and waning anorexia and lethargy. She had started vomiting during the previous week and had vomited three times. There was no diarrhoea. The cat was fed a manufactured canned cat food. Clinical examination was unremarkable – there was no evidence of abdominal pain on palpation and rectal temperature was normal.

CLINICAL PATHOLOGY DATA

The cat was negative on tests for feline leukaemia virus (FeLV) antigen and feline immunodeficiency virus (FIV) antibody.

Haematology	Result	Reference interval
WBC (x 10⁹/l)	12.5	5.5–19.5
Neutrophils (x 10⁹/l)	10.8	2.5–12.5
Lymphocytes (x 10⁹/l)	**0.7**	1.5–7.0
Monocytes (x 10⁹/l)	0.2	0.0–1.5
Eosinophils (×x 10⁹/l)	0.8	0.0–1.5
Platelets (x 10⁹/l)	365	200–800
HCT (l/l)	0.41	0.26–0.45
RBC (x 10¹²/l)	9.86	5.5–10
Hb (g/dl)	14.3	8–15
MCV (fl)	42	39–55
MCHC (g/dl)	35	30–36
PT (seconds)	**12.2**	7.0–11.0
aPTT (seconds)	12.8	10–15
D-dimers (ng/ml)	<250	<250

Abnormal results are in **bold**.

Biochemistry	Result	Reference interval
Sodium (mmol/l)	153	135–155
Potassium (mmol/l)	4	3.6–4.5
Urea (mmol/l)	7	6.7–10
Creatinine (μmol/l)	116	45–150
Calcium (mmol/l)	2.3	1.9–2.4
Phosphate (mmol/l)	0.8	0.7–1.2
Glucose (mmol/l)	**8.5**	4.0–5.3
ALP (IU/l)	**90**	16–68
ALT (IU/l)	**232**	16–44
AST (IU/l)	**90**	0–32
Creatine kinase (IU/l)	98	49–151
Total protein (g/l)	73	55–80
Albumin (g/l)	33	25–45
Bilirubin (μmol/l)	5.6	0–15
Cholesterol (mmol/l)	4.4	1–4.2
Spec fPLi® (ng/ml)	0.9	0–3.5

Abnormal results are in **bold**.

WHAT ABNORMALITIES ARE PRESENT?

- Elevated glucose.
- Elevated ALP, ALT and AST.
- Very mild elevation in prothrombin time (PT).

HOW WOULD YOU INTERPRET THESE RESULTS?

The moderate glucose elevation is consistent with stress in a cat and is still below the renal threshold. ALP, ALT and AST are all mildly to moderately elevated. A normal creatine kinase (CK) level suggests the elevated AST is of hepatic origin and not from muscle. This magnitude of elevation in liver enzymes is much more significant in a cat than in a dog because of the short half-lives of the enzymes and the lack of a steroid-induced ALP in cats (see Chapter 12).

WHAT ARE YOUR DIFFERENTIAL DIAGNOSES?

In a cat, these findings suggest primary liver disease. Hyperthyroidism might also cause this pattern, although this cat is younger than usual for hyperthyroidism. Increases in both hepatocellular (ALT and AST) and induced biliary (ALP) enzymes suggest hepatobiliary disease. Normal bilirubin reduces the suspicion of biliary tract obstruction, although bilirubin can be normal in chronic biliary tract obstruction in cats, so more investigations will be necessary to rule this out. The most common differential for primary hepatic disease in a middle-aged cat would be chronic cholangitis, although acute cholangitis and hepatic lipidosis should be considered. Feline infectious peritonitis (FIP) and neoplasia are less likely differentials. Measuring GGT might help differentiate hepatic lipidosis from cholangitis, although diagnostic imaging and biopsy will be necessary for a definitive diagnosis. Inflammatory bowel disease may also be present. Pancreatitis is less likely because of the normal fPLI, but is not ruled out because of the limited sensitivity of this test in cats with chronic disease. The very mild elevation in PT is probably not significant, generally a prolongation of 25–30% above the upper limit is considered significant, but because of the high prevalence of coagulation abnormalities in cats with liver disease, parenteral supplementation with vitamin K prior to any biopsy would be wise.

RESULTS OF FURTHER TESTS

- Total thyroxine (T4) was normal.
- On ultrasonography, the liver had a slightly increased echogenicity diffusely. The gallbladder and bile duct appeared unremarkable. The pancreas was not found. The stomach was unremarkable. The small intestines had normal wall thickness but were slightly 'uneven' in diameter. The abdominal lymph nodes were normal size but very hypoechoic.

FOLLOW-UP

The option of obtaining biopsy samples was discussed with the owners, who were very keen to have a complete diagnosis. The cat was pretreated with parenteral vitamin K for 24 hours prior to laparotomy. The liver looked unremarkable. Both pancreatic limbs appeared

→ CASE 2 CONTINUED

inflamed. Biopsy samples were taken of the liver, pancreas and small intestine. A gallbladder aspirate was taken for culture and cytology. An oesophagostomy feeding tube was placed.

Histology showed chronic lymphocytic and neutrophilic cholangitis, moderate periductular lymphoplasmacytic pancreatitis and moderate lymphoplasmacytic enteritis. Culture and cytology of bile were negative.

The cat was treated with: a single protein source hypoallergenic diet; prednisolone at a tapering dose; ursodeoxycholic acid; and S-adenosylmethionine. The feeding tube was only necessary for a few days postoperatively. She did very well, with normalization of liver enzymes and resolution of vomiting over the following 6 months.

This cat had histologically confirmed chronic pancreatitis in spite of a normal fPLI. This is not unusual, particularly with the more chronic, low-grade pancreatitis cases where fPLI has a lower sensitivity than in more severe acute cases.

CASE 3

SIGNALMENT

12-month-old neutered female German Shepherd Dog.

HISTORY

Weight loss, polyphagia, vomiting bile and intermittent diarrhoea with mucus passed 3–4 times a day for several months. Clinical examination revealed poor body condition with a dry coat, but was otherwise unremarkable.

CLINICAL PATHOLOGY DATA

Haematology	Result	Reference interval
RBC (x 10¹²/l)	**8.76**	5.5–8.5
Hb (g/dl)	**19.1**	12–18
HCT (l/l)	**0.60**	0.37–0.55
MCV (fl)	68.7	60–77
MCHC (g/dl)	**31.7**	32–37
WBC (x 10⁹/l)	13.1	6.0–17.0
Neutrophils (x 10⁹/l)	11.4	3.0–11.5
Lymphocytes (x 10⁹/l)	**0.4**	1.0–4.8
Monocytes (x 10⁹/l)	1.0	0.2–1.5
Eosinophils (x 10⁹/l)	0.2	0.1–1.3
Platelets (x 10⁹/l)	180	175–500
Fibrinogen (g/l)	**1.0**	2.0–4.0

Abnormal results are in **bold**.

Biochemistry	Result	Reference interval
Sodium (mmol/l)	149.3	135.0–155.0
Potassium (mmol/l)	5.13	3.7–5.8
Glucose (mmol/l)	**2.9**	3.4–5.3
Urea (mmol/l)	5.7	3.3–6.7
Creatinine (µmol/l)	112	70–170
Calcium (mmol/l)	2.64	2.2–2.7
Inorganic phosphate (mmol/l)	0.87	0.6–1.3
Total protein (g/l)	63	55–80
ALT (IU/l)	52	21–59
AST (IU/l)	**57**	20–32
ALP (IU/l)	42	3–142

Abnormal results are in **bold**.

Gastrointestinal panel	Result	Reference interval
TLI (ng/ml)	**<1.5**	EPI <2.5 Normal >5.0
Folate (ng/ml)	**2.6**	3–13
Cobalamin (pg/ml)	534	>200

Abnormal results are in **bold**.

Faecal culture

Campylobacter cultured. Negative parasitology and *Giardia*.

WHAT ABNORMALITIES ARE PRESENT?

Haematology
- Lymphopenia.
- Mild erythrocytosis.

Biochemistry
- Hypoglycaemia.

Gastrointestinal panel
- Subnormal TLI.
- Low folate.
- Normal cobalamin.

Faecal culture
- *Campylobacter* isolated.

HOW WOULD YOU INTERPRET THESE RESULTS?

Haematology is normal except for a lymphopenia (most likely to be stress related), and a mild erythrocytosis, possibly secondary to mild hypovolaemia. The mild reduction in glucose may be due to malnutrition, or inappropriate sample handling (wrong anticoagulant).

A low TLI in a German Shepherd Dog with this history is highly suggestive of clinical EPI due to PAA, but at least one repeat test is advisable. The low folate is unusual (it should be increased due to small intestinal bacterial overgrowth). Cobalamin is normal, although it is often reduced in EPI. The *Campylobacter* infection is probably secondary, but should be treated as it may worsen the clinical signs.

DIAGNOSIS AND TREATMENT

EPI was diagnosed, probably due to PAA, and concurrent *Campylobacter* infection. The dog was treated with a low-fat diet, pancreatic enzyme supplementation and a

→

> **→ CASE 3 CONTINUED**
>
> course of erythromycin for the *Campylobacter* infection followed by metronidazole for possible secondary small intestinal bacterial overgrowth. The faecal quality improved and she gained a little weight but the vomiting continued.
>
> | Parameter | 2 months later | 5 months later |
> |---|---|---|
> | TLI (ng/ml) | **1.8** | **1.5** |
> | Folate (ng/ml) | **1.1** | 4.1 |
> | Cobalamin (pg/ml) | 294 | **<100** |
>
> Abnormal results are in **bold**.

> **FINAL DIAGNOSIS AND OUTCOME**
>
> The persistently low TLI confirmed EPI. The persistently low folate and progressive reduction in cobalamin, inspite of enzyme supplementation, suggested infiltrative disease in the small intestine reducing absorption. The owner declined any further work-up or biopsies, so a novel protein diet and steroid therapy were commenced with a presumptive diagnosis of concurrent inflammatory bowel disease. The improvement was dramatic: the vomiting stopped and the dog gained weight.

References and further reading

Banks PA, Bollen TL, Dervenis C *et al*. Acute Pancreatitis Classification Working Group (2012) Classification of acute pancreatitis – 2012: Revision of the Atlanta Classification and definitions by international consensus. *Gut* **62(1)**, 102–111

Batchelor DJ, Noble PJM, Cripps PJ *et al*. (2007a) Breed associations for canine exocrine pancreatic insufficiency. *Journal of Veterinary Internal Medicine* **21(2)**, 207–214

Batchelor DJ, Noble PJM, Taylor RH, Cripps PJ and German AJ (2007b) Prognostic factors in canine exocrine pancreatic insufficiency: Prolonged survival is likely if clinical remission is achieved. *Journal of Veterinary Internal Medicine* **21(1)**, 54–60

Beall MJ, Cahill R, Pigeon K, Hanscom J and Huth SP (2011) Performance validation and method comparison of an in-clinic enzyme-linked immunosorbent assay for the detection of canine pancreatic lipase. *Journal of Veterinary Diagnostic Investigation* **23(1)**, 115–119

Bjorneby JM and Kari S (2002) Cytology of the pancreas. *Veterinary Clinics of North America: Small Animal Practice* **32**, 1293–1312

Bostrom BM, Xenoulis PG, Newman SJ, Pool RR, Fosgate GT and Steiner JM (2013) Chronic pancreatitis in dogs: a retrospective study of clinical, clinicopathological, and histopathological findings in 61 cases. *The Veterinary Journal* **195(1)**, 73–79

Chartier M, Hill S, Sunico S, Steiner JM, Suchodolski JS and Robertson J (2013) Evaluation of canine pancreas-specific lipase (Spec cPL®) concentration and amylase and lipase activities in peritoneal fluid as complementary diagnostic tools for acute pancreatitis in dogs. Abstract for 2013 ACVIM Congress, Seattle. *Journal of Veterinary Internal Medicine* **27**, 696; Abstract GI-3

Ferreri JA, Hardam E and Kimmel SE (2003) Clinical differentiation of acute necrotizing from chronic nonsuppurative pancreatitis in cats: 63 cases (1996–2001). *Journal of the American Veterinary Medical Association* **223**, 469–474

Forman MA, Marks SL, Cock HEV *et al*. (2004) Evaluation of serum feline pancreatic lipase immunoreactivity and helical computed tomography versus conventional testing for the diagnosis of feline pancreatitis. *Journal of Veterinary Internal Medicine* **18(6)**, 807–815

Gerhardt A, Steiner JM, Williams DA *et al*. (2001) Comparison of the sensitivity of different diagnostic tests for pancreatitis in cats. *Journal of Veterinary Internal Medicine* **15(4)**, 329–333

Graca R, Messick J, McCullough S, Barger A and Hoffmann W (2005) Validation and diagnostic efficacy of a lipase assay using the substrate 1,2-o-dilauryl-rac-glycero glutaric acid-(6' methyl resorufin)-ester for the diagnosis of acute pancreatitis in dogs. *Veterinary Clinical Pathology* **4(1)**, 39–43

Guija de Arespacochaga A and Hittmair KM (2006) Comparison of lipase activity in peritoneal fluid of dogs with different pathologies – a complementary diagnostic tool in acute pancreatitis? *Journal of Veterinary Medicine A, Physiology, Pathology and Clinical Medicine* **53**(3), 119–122

Hess RS, Saunders HM, Van Winkle TJ, Shofer FS and Washabau RJ (1998) Clinical, clinicopathologic, radiographic, and ultrasonographic abnormalities in dogs with fatal acute pancreatitis: 70 cases (1986–1995) *Journal of the American Veterinary Medical Association* **213(5)**, 665–670

Hill RC and Van Winkle TJ (1993) Acute necrotizing pancreatitis and acute suppurative pancreatitis in the cat: a retrospective study of 40 cases (1976–1989) *Journal of Veterinary Internal Medicine* **7**, 25–33

Huth SP, Relford R, Steiner JM, Strong-Townsend MI and Williams DA (2010) Analytical validation of an ELISA for measurement of canine pancreas-specific lipase. *Veterinary Clinical Pathology* **39(3)**, 346–353

Kathrani A, Steiner JM, Suchodolski J *et al*. (2009) Elevated canine pancreatic lipase immunoreactivity concentration in dogs with inflammatory bowel disease is associated with a negative outcome. *Journal of Small Animal Practice* **50(3)**, 126–132

Kimmel SE, Washabau RJ and Drobatz KJ (2001) Incidence and prognostic value of low plasma ionised calcium concentration in cats with acute pancreatitis: 46 cases (1996–1998). *Journal of the American Veterinary Medical Association* **219**, 1105–1109

Kook PH, Kohler N, Hartnack S, Riond B and Reusch CE (2014) Agreement of serum Spec cPL with the 1,2-o-dilauryl-rac-glycero glutaric acid-(6'-methylresorufin) ester (DGGR) lipase assay and with pancreatic ultrasonography in dogs with suspected pancreatitis. *Journal of Veterinary Internal Medicine* **28(3)**, 863–870

Kuzi S, Segev G, Haruvi E and Aroch I (2010) Plasma antithrombin activity as a diagnostic and prognostic indicator in dogs: a retrospective study of 149 dogs. *Journal of Veterinary Internal Medicine* **24(3)**, 587–596

LaRusch J and Whitcomb DC (2011) Genetics of pancreatitis. *Current Opinion in Gastroenterology* **27(5)**, 467–474

Mansfield CS, Anderson GA and O'Hara AJ (2012) Association between canine pancreatic-specific lipase and histologic exocrine pancreatic inflammation in dogs: assessing specificity. *Journal of Veterinary Diagnostic Investigation* **24(2)**, 312–318

Mansfield CS, James FE and Robertson ID (2008) Development of a clinical severity index for dogs with acute pancreatitis. *Journal of the American Veterinary Medical Association* **233(6)**, 936–944

Mansfield CS and Jones BR (2000) Plasma and urinary trypsinogen activation peptide in healthy dogs, dogs with pancreatitis and dogs with other systemic diseases. *Australian Veterinary Journal* **78(6)**, 416–422

Mansfield CS and Jones BR (2001) Review of feline pancreatitis part two: clinical signs, diagnosis and treatment. *Journal of Feline Medicine and Surgery* **3**, 125–132

Mansfield CS, Jones BR and Spillman T (2003) Assessing the severity of canine pancreatitis. *Research in Veterinary Science* **74**, 137–144

Mansfield CS, Watson PD and Jones BR (2011) Specificity and sensitivity of serum canine pancreatic elastase-1 concentration in the diagnosis of pancreatitis. *Journal of Veterinary Diagnostic Investigation* **23(4)**, 691–697

McCord K, Morley PS, Armstrong J *et al*. (2012) A multi-institutional study evaluating the diagnostic utility of the Spec cPL™ and SNAP® cPL™ in clinical acute pancreatitis in 84 dogs. *Journal of Veterinary Internal Medicine* **26(4)**

Oppliger S, Hartnack S, Riond B, Reusch CE and Kook PH (2013) Agreement of the serum Spec fPL™ and 1,2-O-dilauryl-rac-glycero-3-glutaric acid-(6'-methylresorufin) ester lipase assay for the determination of serum lipase in cats with suspicion of pancreatitis. *Journal of Veterinary Internal Medicine* **27**, 1077–1082

Pallagi P, Venglovecz V, Rakonczay Z Jr *et al*. (2011) Trypsin reduces pancreatic ductal bicarbonate secretion by inhibiting CFTR Cl⁻ channels and luminal anion exchangers. *Gastroenterology* **141**, 2228–2239

Pápa K, Máthé A, Abonyi-Tóth Z *et al*. (2011) Occurrence, clinical features and outcome of canine pancreatitis (80 cases). *Acta Veterinaria Hungarica* **59**, 37–52

Quigley KA, Jackson ML and Haines DM (2001) Hyperlipasemia in 6 dogs with pancreatic or hepatic neoplasia: evidence for tumor lipase production. *Veterinary Clinical Pathology* **30**, 114-120

Ruaux CG and Atwell RB (1998) A severity score for spontaneous canine acute pancreatitis. *Australian Veterinary Journal* **76(12)**, 804–808

Schaer M (1979) A clinicopathological survey of acute pancreatitis in 30 dogs and 5 cats. *Journal of the American Animal Hospital Association* **15**, 681–687

Simpson KW, Batt RM, McLean L and Morton DB (1989) Circulating concentrations of trypsin-like immunoreactivity and activities of lipase and amylase after pancreatic duct ligation in dogs. *American Journal of Veterinary Research* **50**, 629–632

Spillmann T, Wiberg ME, Teigelkamp S *et al*. (2000) Canine pancreatic elastase in dogs with clinical exocrine pancreatic insufficiency, normal dogs and dogs with chronic enteropathies. *The European Journal of Comparative Gastroenterology* **5**, 1–6

Spillmann T, Wittker S, Teigelkamp S *et al*. (2001) An immunoassay for canine pancreatic elastase 1 as an indicator of exocrine pancreatic insufficiency in dogs. *Journal of Veterinary Diagnostic Investigation* **13**, 468–474

Steiner JM, Rutz GM and Williams DA (2006) Serum lipase activities and pancreatic lipase immunoreactivity concentrations in dogs with exocrine pancreatic insufficiency. *American Journal of Veterinary Research* **67**, 84–87

Steiner JM, Teague SR, Lees GE, Willard MD, Williams DA and Ruaux CG (2009) Stability of canine pancreatic lipase immunoreactivity concentration in serum samples and effects of long-term administration of prednisone to dogs on serum canine pancreatic lipase immunoreactivity concentrations. *American Journal of Veterinary Research* **70(8)**, 1001–1005

Swift NC, Marks SL, MacLachlan NJ and Norris CR (2000) Evaluation of serum feline trypsin-like immunoreactivity for the diagnosis of pancreatitis in cats. *Journal of the American Veterinary Medical Association* **217(1)**, 37–42

Talukdar R and Vege SS (2011) Early management of severe acute pancreatitis. *Current Gastroenterology Reports* **13(2)**, 123–130

Thompson KA, Parnell NK, Hohenhaus AE, Moore GE and Rondeau MP (2009) Feline exocrine pancreatic insufficiency: 16 cases (1992–2007). *Journal of Feline Medicine and Surgery* **11(12)**, 935–940

Trivedi S, Marks SL, Kass PH *et al.* (2011) Sensitivity and specificity of canine pancreas-specific lipase (cPL) and other markers for pancreatitis in 70 dogs with and without histopathologic evidence of pancreatitis. *Journal of Veterinary Internal Medicine* **25(6)**, 1241–1247

Watanabe T, Hoshi K, Zhang C, Ishida Y and Sakata I (2012) Hyperammonaemia due to cobalamin malabsorption in a cat with exocrine pancreatic insufficiency. *Journal of Feline Medicine and Surgery* **14(12)**, 942–945

Watson PJ (2015) Pancreatitis in dogs and cats: definitions and pathophysiology. *Journal of Small Animal Practice,* **56(1)**, 3–12

Watson PJ, Archer J, Roulois AJ, Scase TJ and Herrtage ME (2010) Observational study of 14 cases of chronic pancreatitis in dogs. *Veterinary Record* **167(25)**, 968–976

Watson PJ, Constantino-Casas F, Saul CJ and Day MJ (2012) Chronic pancreatitis in the English Cocker Spaniel shows a predominance of IgG4+ plasma cells in sections of pancreas and kidney. Presented at the *American College of Veterinary Internal Medicine Forum*, New Orleans, May 30–June 2

Watson PJ, Roulois AJA, Scase T, Johnston PEJ, Thompson H and Herrtage ME (2007) Prevalence and breed distribution of chronic pancreatitis at post-mortem examination in first-opinion dogs. *Journal of Small Animal Practice* **48(11)**, 609–618

Watson PJ, Roulois A, Scase T, Holloway A and Herrtage ME (2011) Characterization of chronic pancreatitis in English cocker spaniels. *Journal of Veterinary Internal Medicine* **25(4)**, 797–804

Westermarck E and Sandholm M (1980) Faecal hydrolase activity as determined by radial enzyme diffusion: a new method for detecting pancreatic dysfunction in the dog. *Research in Veterinary Science* **28**, 341–346

Whitney MS, Boon GD, Rebar AH and Ford RB (1987) Effects of acute pancreatitis on circulating lipids in dogs. *American Journal of Veterinary Research* **48**, 1492–1497

Wiberg ME, Nurmi AK and Westermarck E (1999) Serum trypsin-like immunoreactivity measurement for the diagnosis of subclinical exocrine pancreatic insufficiency. *Journal of Veterinary Internal Medicine* **13**, 426–432

Williams DA, Steiner JM, Ruaux CG and Zavros N (2003) Increases in serum pancreatic lipase immunoreactivity (PLI) are greater and of longer duration than those of trypsin-like immunoreactivity (TLI) in cats with experimental pancreatitis. *Journal of Veterinary Internal Medicine* **17**, 445–446

Xenoulis PG, Levinski MD, Suchodolski JS and Steiner JM (2010) Serum triglyceride concentrations in miniature Schnauzers with and without a history of probable pancreatitis. *Journal of Veterinary Internal Medicine* **25(1)**, 20–25

Useful websites

ScheBo Biotech AG – faecal elastase test
www.schebo.com

Chapter 15

Laboratory evaluation of lipid disorders

Jon Wray

Increased plasma cholesterol and/or triglyceride concentration in the fasted state is a relatively common abnormality detected in dogs, and less frequently in feline patients, and is termed hyperlipidaemia. Both cholesterol and triglyceride are water insoluble in plasma and are therefore transported in a water-soluble form complexed with proteins, such lipid–protein complexes being termed lipoproteins. The term 'hyperlipoproteinaemia' is often used synonymously with hyperlipidaemia. Lipaemia describes the milky/opalescent character of serum or plasma in which an increased concentration of large triglyceride-carrying lipoproteins is present.

Abnormalities may arise, both as a result of alterations in normal lipoprotein metabolism (usually described as primary hyperlipidaemias or hyperlipoproteinaemias), and secondary to systemic disorders (secondary hyperlipidaemias or hyperlipoproteinaemias).

Triglycerides provide a source of chemical energy within the body, and cholesterol performs many roles including, but not limited to, providing a structural component of cell membranes and the myelin sheaths of nerves and acting as a precursor for steroid hormone synthesis. The majority of cholesterol is synthesized within the body by the liver, whereas triglycerides are almost equally derived from dietary sources and hepatic synthesis.

This chapter reviews normal lipid metabolism and the clinical assessment of lipid/lipoprotein disorders in dogs and cats.

Normal lipid metabolism

Lipoprotein structure and function

Normal lipoprotein metabolism in dogs and cats has been reviewed previously (Watson and Barrie, 1993; Johnson, 2005; Xenoulis and Steiner, 2010). As previously mentioned, owing to their hydrophobic nature, both cholesterol and triglycerides are transported in the form of water-soluble lipid–protein complexes called lipoproteins. A schematic cartoon of a lipoprotein molecule is shown in Figure 15.1. Most cholesterol is transported in the form of cholesteryl esters which, with triglycerides, form the core of the lipoprotein complex. This hydrophobic core is bounded by a hydrophilic 'shell' which principally comprises membrane phospholipid, in which sit 'blocks' of unesterified cholesterol and special proteins called apolipoproteins (referred to by the prefix 'apo-').

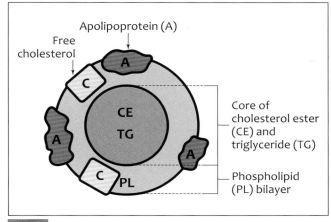

15.1 Schematic illustration of a lipoprotein molecule.

Four types of lipoprotein exist: chylomicrons; very low-density lipoproteins (VLDLs); low-density lipoproteins (LDLs); and high-density lipoproteins (HDLs). Their relative size and composition is shown in Figure 15.2. Chylomicrons represent the largest of these and are principally involved in the transport of dietary lipid from the small intestine into the circulation. The remaining lipoproteins are concerned mainly with transport of endogenously produced lipids. Three subtypes of HDL (HDL_1, HDL_2, HDL_3) are recognized. A summary of lipoprotein metabolism is shown in Figure 15.3 and explained below.

Dietary-derived lipid (chylomicrons)

Most foods fed to dogs and cats are relatively rich in dietary fats, mainly triglyceride with smaller amounts of cholesterol and phospholipid. Following ingestion, pancreatic lipase hydrolyses dietary triglyceride in the small intestine to fatty acids and mono- and diglycerides (see top part of Figure 15.3). These combine with bile acids, cholesterol and phospholipid to form mixed micelles which are transferred into adjacent enterocytes. Here the glycerides are re-esterified with fatty acids and packaged along with cholesterol, and stabilized by the apolipoprotein $apoB_{48}$ to form chylomicrons. Chylomicrons enter the intestinal lacteals and drain via the local lymphatics and thoracic duct into the bloodstream.

Within the circulation, chylomicrons acquire apoC and apoE from HDLs. These acquired apolipoproteins are responsible for the distribution of chylomicron lipid into the

Lipoprotein	Chylomicron	VLDL	LDL	HDL₁	HDL₂	HDL₃
Species	Dog, cat	Dog, cat	Dog, cat	Dog, cat	Cat	Dog, cat
Relative size and composition	75–1200 nm	26–80 nm	16–25 nm	18–35 nm	9–12 nm	5–9 nm
Composition by mass (%)	90 / 3 / 5 / 2	62 / 12 / 14 / 12	8 / 42 / 23 / 12 / 27	1 / 36 / 40 / 23	2 / 30 / 35 / 33	1 / 21 / 35 / 43

■ Triglyceride ☐ Cholesterol ▨ Phospholipid ■ Protein

15.2 Relative size and composition of canine and feline lipoproteins. HDL = high-density lipoprotein; LDL = low-density lipoprotein; VLDL = very low-density lipoprotein.

(Data from Watson and Barrie, 1993)

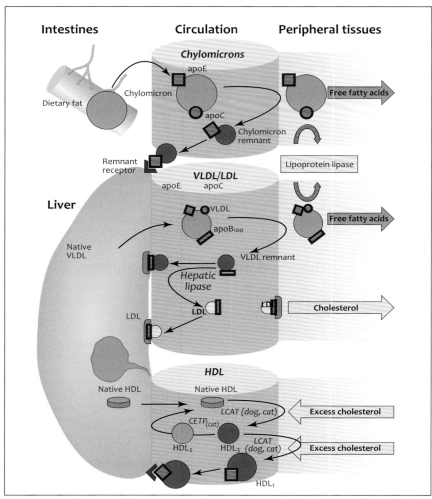

15.3 Normal lipid metabolism. apo = apolipoprotein; CETP = cholesteryl ester transfer protein (cats only); HDL = high-density lipoprotein; LCAT = lecithin:cholesterol acyl transferase; LDL = low-density lipoprotein; VLDL = very low-density lipoprotein.

tissues. In capillary beds of striated muscle and adipose tissue, the enzyme lipoprotein lipase (LPL) hydrolyses chylomicron triglyceride to fatty acid and glycerol, which is liberated from the chylomicron (to either be stored after re-esterification as triglyceride in tissue, or used immediately as an energy source in muscle). LPL activity in adipose tissue correlates positively with plasma insulin concentration and is therefore increased in the postprandial period.

A cholesterol-rich chylomicron 'remnant' is left, which is removed from the circulation by hepatocytes which recognize the remaining apoE, and which therefore ultimately receive cholesterol of dietary origin for storage, excretion or conversion to bile acids.

Endogenous lipid

The liver continually produces VLDL and HDL. LDL is essentially a remnant of VLDL after lipolysis. HDL acts as both a source and reservoir of apoC and apoE and a means of reuptake of peripheral unesterified cholesterol which is excess to metabolic requirements.

VLDL/LDL

VLDL is the main means of transport of hepatically derived triglyceride to the peripheral tissues. Triglyceride, cholesteryl esters, phospholipid and apoB$_{100}$ are packaged in the hepatocytes to form VLDL, which is then secreted continuously (middle part of Figure 15.3). ApoC and apoE are acquired from HDLs in the circulation. In adipose tissue and striated muscle, the enzyme LPL hydrolyses triglyceride to fatty acid and glycerol. Thus, VLDL becomes progressively depleted of triglyceride and apoC-II and becomes relatively more cholesterol rich. Some of the 'remnant' VLDL after triglyceride depletion is removed by the liver and the remainder is acted on by another enzyme, hepatic lipase, liberating further triglyceride and leaving a smaller molecule, LDL, which comprises mainly cholesteryl esters and apoB$_{100}$. The remaining LDL is taken up by hepatocytes, where cholesterol is received for storage, excretion or conversion to bile acids.

HDL

HDLs are the smallest lipoproteins and act both as a reservoir for apoC and apoE (transferring these to chylomicrons and VLDLs) and to transport excess peripheral cholesterol to the liver (bottom part of Figure 15.3). HDL is initially secreted from the liver as a disc-shaped bilayer of phospholipid. More cholesterol enters and transforms the disc to a spherical lipoprotein, HDL$_3$, under the action of the plasma enzyme lecithin:cholesterol acyl transferase (LCAT). In humans, cholesterol in HDL$_3$ is exchanged for triglyceride from chylomicrons, VLDLs and LDLs under the action of cholesteryl ester transfer protein (CETP). Dogs lack CETP and instead HDL$_3$ becomes further enriched with excess cholesterol from the peripheral tissues and with apoE to form a lipoprotein class called HDL$_1$, which is removed from the circulation in the liver. In cats, both HDL$_1$ and HDL$_2$ are found, suggesting that two routes of cholesterol reuptake are utilized in this species.

Hyperlipidaemia

Clinical consequences of hyperlipidaemia

Hyperlipidaemia is often recognized serendipitously on detecting lipaemic whole blood, serum or plasma after blood sampling, or detecting elevations in cholesterol and/or triglyceride on biochemical panels. However, clinical signs associated with hyperlipidaemia are listed in Figure 15.4. These effects may be broadly characterized as ophthalmic, neurological, gastrointestinal/abdominal and vascular. In the case of primary hyperlipidaemias, it has been variably suggested that hypertriglyceridaemia exceeding 5.65 mmol/l and hypercholesterolaemia exceeding 13 mmol/l should be treated in order to avoid possible complications (Whitney, 1992; Ford, 1996). However, clinical studies to stratify the risk of adverse consequences of hyperlipidaemia are lacking, though it has been reported that cholesterol values >19.5 mmol/l predispose dogs to atherosclerosis (Whitney, 1992; Bauer, 1996).

- Abdominal pain
- Vomiting and diarrhoea
- Lethargy
- Hepatomegaly
- Seizures
- Ocular manifestations of hyperlipidaemia:
  - Lipaemia retinalis
  - Arcus lipoides
  - Lipaemic aqueous
  - Lipid keratopathy[a]

15.4 Clinical signs associated with hyperlipidaemia. [a] May sometimes be associated with hyperlipidaemia but usually seen in animals without hyperlipidaemia.

The ophthalmic manifestations of hyperlipidaemia include lipaemia retinalis, crystalline stromal dystrophy (though this is only rarely associated with hyperlipidaemia, most cases having normal lipid levels), lipid keratopathy, arcus lipoides (Figure 15.5a) and lipid aqueous (Figure 15.5b). Hypertriglyceridaemia has been associated with abdominal pain but because it is also associated with pancreatitis (which also causes abdominal pain) it is often difficult to determine whether the hyperlipidaemia or the pancreatitis is the cause of the pain and whether the

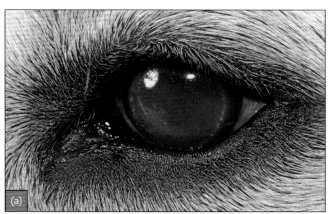

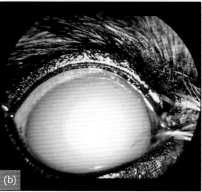

15.5 (a) Arcus lipoides in a 1-year-old Labrador Retriever. A stippled white penumbra of lipid can be seen circumferentially at the margin of the cornea. (b) Lipid aqueous in a dog with diabetes mellitus. The anterior chamber is obscured by the presence of lipid within the aqueous which is opacifying it. (Courtesy of David Gould)

hyperlipidaemia is a cause or effect of the pancreatitis. Although dogs appear naturally resistant to the development of atherosclerosis, very high levels of serum cholesterol (>19.5 mmol/l) have been associated with *in vivo* and *in vitro* accumulation of lipid by aortic medial cells (Mahley *et al.*, 1977) and dogs with atherosclerosis were found to have a 53 and 51 times increased likelihood of having diabetes mellitus or hypothyroidism respectively (Hess *et al.*, 2003). Reported neurological effects of hyperlipidaemias include development of peripheral neuropathy associated with compression by, and extension of, nerve root xanthomata (especially in cats with inherited primary hyperchylomicronaemia; Jones *et al.*, 1986) and the development of seizures. It is not clear whether seizures in these animals relate to cerebrovascular effects of hyperlipidaemia or occur as a result of some other mechanism. Cats with hyperchylomicronaemia may also sometimes present with cutaneous xanthomata.

Differential diagnosis of hyperlipidaemia

The differential diagnosis and classification of hyperlipidaemia in dogs and cats are listed in Figure 15.6. Hyperlipidaemia may be physiological (postprandial), primary (usually due to inherited defects in LPL) or secondary.

Physiological hyperlipidaemia

Absorption of dietary fats from the intestine produces a peak in chylomicrons starting approximately 2 hours after eating that usually clears by 4–6 hours postprandially (though sometimes as long as 16 hours). Cholesterol is usually minimally affected by this. Age and breed were not shown to have any significant effect on lipoprotein concentrations in one study, though intact bitches had higher concentrations of HDL than intact male dogs (Barrie *et al.*,

---

Physiological
- Postprandial hyperlipidaemia

Primary hyperlipidaemia
- Primary hypertriglyceridaemia of Miniature Schnauzers
- Primary hypertriglyceridaemia of Brittany Spaniels
- Primary hypercholesterolaemia of Rough Collies
- Primary hypercholesterolaemia of Briards
- Primary hypercholesterolaemia of Dobermanns
- Primary hypercholesterolaemia of Shetland Sheepdogs
- Primary hypercholesterolaemia of Rottweilers
- Primary mixed hypercholesterolaemia and hypertriglyceridaemia in Beagles
- Primary hypertriglyceridaemia in Domestic Shorthair, Persian, Himalayan and Siamese cats

Secondary hyperlipidaemia
- Pancreatitis (mainly hypertriglyceridaemia, less often hypercholesterolaemia)
- Protein-losing nephropathy (hypercholesterolaemia)
- Hypothyroidism (hypercholesterolaemia and hypertriglyceridaemia)
- Hyperadrenocorticism (hypercholesterolaemia and hypertriglyceridaemia)
- Diabetes mellitus (hypertriglyceridaemia, hypercholesterolaemia)
- Cholestasis (elevated cholesterol only)
- Obesity

Drug-induced hyperlipidaemia
- Corticosteroids
- Oestrogens
- Cholestyramine
- Phenytoin
- Methimazole
- Phenobarbital

15.6 Causes of hyperlipidaemia in dogs and cats.

1993b). High-fat diets have also been reported to result in hyperlipidaemia (Xenoulis and Steiner, 2010), which may persist for more than 4–6 hours.

Drug therapy

Hypertriglyceridaemia may be caused by corticosteroids, oestrogens and cholestyramine, and hypercholesterolaemia is reported to be caused by corticosteroids, phenytoin and methimazole (Burkhard and Meyer, 1995).

Primary hyperlipidaemia

Primary hyperlipidaemia has been reported in Domestic Shorthair, Persian, Himalayan and Siamese cats as an autosomal recessive trait resulting in familial lipoprotein lipase deficiency and characterized by fasting hyperchylomicronaemia and a mild elevation in VLDL (Jones *et al.*, 1983; Johnstone *et al.*, 1990; Watson *et al.*, 1992). In dogs, the most well-reported primary hyperlipidaemia is idiopathic hyperlipidaemia of Miniature Schnauzers, which is characterized by an abnormal accumulation of VLDLs, or VLDLs and chylomicrons (with or without hypercholesterolaemia). It is seemingly common in Miniature Schnauzers in the USA: in one study 32.8% of 192 apparently healthy Miniature Schnauzers investigated had fasting hypertriglyceridaemia (Xenoulis *et al.*, 2007), with both prevalence and severity increasing with age. A high prevalence has also been noted in Japan (Mori *et al.*, 2010), and experience in the UK is similar. Although a hereditary basis is strongly implicated, a genetic cause of this condition has yet to be characterized. Proposed mechanisms of the idiopathic hyperlipidaemia are either a deficiency in LPL activity, or absence or mutation in apoC-II, although studies to date have not supported either of these mechanisms (Xenoulis and Steiner, 2010).

Primary hypercholesterolaemia without hypertriglyceridaemia has been reported in Briards and Rough Collies in the UK (Watson *et al.*, 1993; Jeusette *et al.*, 2004) and hypercholesterolaemia with or without hypertriglyceridaemia has also been reported in Shetland Sheepdogs (Sato *et al.*, 2000; Mori *et al.*, 2010). Primary hypertriglyceridaemia has been reported in two related Brittany Spaniels (Hubert *et al.*, 1987), primary hypercholesterolaemia in the Dobermann and Rottweiler (Armstrong and Ford, 1989), and mixed hypercholesterolaemia and hypertriglyceridaemia in two related Beagles (Wada *et al.*, 1977).

Secondary hyperlipidaemia

Pancreatitis: An association between pancreatitis and the development of hyperlipidaemia (principally hypertriglyceridaemia and less so hypercholesterolaemia) in dogs has been suspected for many years, but it is not clear whether the pancreatitis is the cause of the hypertriglyceridaemia or whether, conversely, the presence of hypertriglyceridaemia predisposes to development of pancreatitis. In an experimental model of pancreatitis, hypertriglyceridaemia did not occur (Whitney *et al.*, 1987). Studies in Miniature Schnauzers with both laboratory evidence to support pancreatitis and a clinical history of pancreatitis show an association between hypertriglyceridaemia and elevated canine pancreatic lipase immunoreactivity (cPLI), or a history of pancreatitis, in this breed; whether the hypertriglyceridaemia is cause or effect remains unanswered (Xenoulis *et al.*, 2010, 2011) .

Protein-losing nephropathy: Proteinuric renal disease is commonly associated with development of hypercholesterolaemia and occurred in 65–89% of dogs with a familial protein-losing nephropathy (Cook and Cowgill, 1996; Littman *et al.*, 2000). The mechanism of development of hyperlipidaemia in these patients is unknown but may relate to upregulation of hepatic lipoprotein elaboration in response to systemic hypoalbuminaemia or due to impairment of LPL activity.

Endocrine diseases: Hypothyroidism and hyperadrenocorticism are commonly associated with the presence of both hypertriglyceridaemia and hypercholesterolaemia, with the latter seen most commonly. Very high serum cholesterol levels (>15 mmol/l) are often reported to occur more commonly in the presence of hypothyroidism than in any other secondary hyperlipidaemic state. Both triglyceride and cholesterol may also be elevated in patients with diabetes mellitus, although more commonly hypertriglyceridaemia is present with mildly elevated or normal serum cholesterol. Both thyroxine and insulin enhance the activity of LPL, and deficiency of either may lead to hyperlipidaemia. Increased mobilization of body fat stores in diabetes mellitus may also contribute. The mechanisms of hyperlipidaemia in hyperadrenocorticism may include downregulation of LDL receptors and development of insulin resistance. It should be noted that there is considerable overlap in both the degree and the pattern of elevation of serum cholesterol and/or triglyceride and in the lipoprotein electrophoretic patterns of dogs with endocrine disease (Rogers *et al.*, 1975b).

Cholestasis: Cholestasis may lead to mild to moderate hypercholesterolaemia and mild hypertriglyceridaemia in dogs (Whitney, 1992).

Obesity: Increases in serum triglyceride and/or cholesterol have been reported in obese dogs, and this condition worsens with the severity and duration of obesity, decreasing if weight loss is achieved (Jeusette *et al.*, 2005).

Miscellaneous causes: Hyperlipidaemia has also been reported in dogs with lymphoma, heart failure due to dilated cardiomyopathy, infection with *Leishmania infantum* and in dogs with parvoviral enteritis (Nieto *et al.*, 1992; Ogilvie *et al.*, 1994; Tidholm and Jonsson, 1997; Yilmaz and Senturk, 2007).

Hypolipidaemia

Recognition of subnormal serum triglyceride seldom occurs in canine and feline patients; this finding is generally considered of low clinical significance and investigation is therefore not pursued. Hypocholesterolaemia is most frequently recognized in patients with severely impaired hepatic function, either due to congenital disorders such as portovascular anomalies or in patients with acquired causes of hepatic failure such as cirrhosis. Hypocholesterolaemia may also be seen in patients with severe gastrointestinal disorders such as malabsorption (especially due to exocrine pancreatic insufficiency) and in the presence of protein-losing enteropathies and hypoadrenocorticism.

Investigation of hyperlipidaemia

Hyperlipidaemia is usually suspected when whole blood, serum or plasma is found to be grossly lipaemic. Lipaemia describes the turbid/opalescent appearance of blood due to increased triglyceride concentration. Increases in cholesterol concentration usually do not cause lipaemia. Lipaemia usually develops when serum triglyceride concentration exceeds 2.3 mmol/l, and the degree of lipaemia worsens with increasing concentration, the blood becoming progressively more milky (Xenoulis and Steiner, 2010). Refrigeration of a lipaemic sample for 10–12 hours may result in the formation of a creamy layer at the top of the sample (Figure 15.7). Where seen, this represents chylomicrons which, owing to their low density, will float to the surface of serum or plasma. If no chylomicron layer forms, the lipaemia is most likely due to an excess of other lipoproteins, usually VLDL (Whitney, 1992).

Routinely, total cholesterol and triglycerides are assessed by spectrophotometric or enzymatic methods, and typical values are shown in Figure 15.8, although the reference range for the specific laboratory and method used should always be referred to. Where hypercholesterolaemia >10 mmol/l or hypertriglyceridaemia >2.5 mmol/l is detected, it should first be verified that fasting has been undertaken for a period of 12–16 hours prior to sample collection and, in case of doubt, a second sample taken after the requisite fast should be assessed.

Where persistent elevations occur, systematic evaluation for causes of hyperlipidaemia (see below) should be undertaken; this might include:

* Checking whether the patient is of a breed affected by primary hyperlipidaemia
* Evaluation of tests for endocrinopathy such as serum and urine glucose, assessment of thyroid function and assessment for hyperadrenocorticism. It should be borne in mind that tests for the latter two conditions are frequently affected by non-thyroidal/non-adrenal illness and are most easily interpreted when applied to patients with compatible clinical signs and within the likely age range

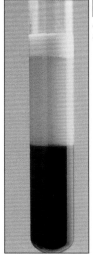

15.7 A cream-coloured layer of chylomicrons above an opalescent plasma sample containing VLDLs, obtained from a dog with concurrent diabetes mellitus and hypothyroidism.

Dogs	
Cholesterol	3.8–7.0 mmol/l
Triglyceride	0.5–1.1 mmol/l
Cats	
Cholesterol	1.9–3.9 mmol/l
Triglyceride	0.2–1.1 mmol/l

15.8 Typical reference ranges for serum lipids.

- Concomitant interpretation of analytes suggestive of cholestasis, such as hyperbilirubinaemia and elevated alkaline phosphatase (ALP)
- Assessment of urine protein:creatinine ratio (in conjunction with urine sediment examination)
- Assessment of tests for pancreatitis, bearing in mind that false negative results are seen with variable frequency with all such tests.

Evaluation of lipoprotein subclasses may be undertaken semi-quantitatively by lipoprotein electrophoresis or quantitatively by ultracentrifugation/precipitation methods (Rogers *et al.*, 1975b; Whitney, 1992; Barrie *et al.*, 1993ab). A typical lipoprotein electrophoretic pattern along with the likely composition of lipoproteins occurring at each 'peak' is shown in Figure 15.9. Although this is not commonly performed, it is available at a number of veterinary laboratories in the UK and the results are displayed as either an electrophoretic plot or a numerical breakdown of absolute cholesterol content of different lipoprotein classes. Findings in patients with idiopathic hyperlipoproteinaemia and in patients with secondary hyperlipoproteinaemias have been reported (Rogers *et al.*, 1975ab; Whitney *et al.*, 1987; Barrie *et al.*, 1993b; Jeusette *et al.*, 2004). It should be noted that electrophoretic and ultracentrifugation/precipitation patterns lack specificity for the identification of a specific aetiology for secondary hyperlipidaemias because there is considerable overlap in findings (Whitney, 1992).

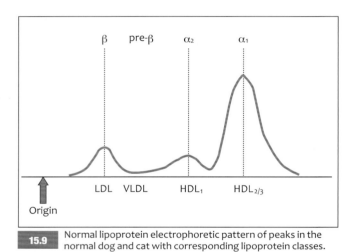

15.9 Normal lipoprotein electrophoretic pattern of peaks in the normal dog and cat with corresponding lipoprotein classes.

LPL deficiency, which is suspected of involvement in some primary hyperlipidaemias, is difficult to assess because specific canine and feline assays are not commercially available. Both LPL and hepatic lipase may be assayed by human reference laboratories and results compared with reference values obtained from control animals, though specific reference ranges in cats and dogs are not available. Intravenous heparin at 90 IU/kg bodyweight (dogs) or 10–40 IU/kg bodyweight (cats) is given to stimulate release of LPL from the capillary endothelium, and samples are collected for assay 10–15 minutes after injection. Assessment of triglyceride and cholesterol before and after heparin administration may also give indirect evidence of LPL activity or its absence. Work by Peritz *et al.* (1990) and Watson *et al.* (1992) suggests that normal feline LPL activity is similar to human reference activity and can be assayed by the same methodology. LPL activity may also be indirectly assessed by the demonstration of gross clearance of lipaemia in samples taken before and after the administration of heparin.

Laboratory effects of hyperlipidaemia

The presence of hyperlipidaemia also has important consequences for the measurement of other analytes, and some of these potential effects are summarized in Figure 15.10. The effects vary with the method used, and the effect of hyperlipidaemia on individual test performance should be verified with the equipment supplier or reference manual. Refrigeration of samples and the use of lipid clearing agents such as 'Lipoclear™' may help to reduce these effects. Separation of plasma or serum before transportation to a laboratory also helps to reduce the concurrent effects of haemolysis on sample quality.

Increased	Decreased	Variable effect	*No effect
Haemoglobin MCHC MCH Total protein (refractometer and spectrophotometer) Phosphate Calcium	Sodium (indirect ISE) Chloride (indirect ISE)	Urea GGT Cholesterol Albumin Amylase Lipase Glucose Creatinine ALT AST ALP Bile acids Bilirubin	Electrolytes when using direct ISE

15.10 Laboratory effects of hyperlipidaemia. ALP = alkaline phosphatase; ALT = alanine aminotransferase; AST = aspartate aminotransferase; GGT = gamma-glutamyl transferase; ISE = ion-specific electrode; MCH = mean corpuscular haemoglobin; MCHC = mean corpuscular haemoglobin concentration.

Case examples

CASE 1

SIGNALMENT

14-year-old female neutered Cocker Spaniel.

HISTORY

Progressive polyuria, polydipsia, nocturia and panting over a 4–6-week period.

CLINICAL PATHOLOGY DATA

Biochemistry	Result	Reference interval
Total protein (g/l)	77	54–77
Albumin (g/l)	34	25–40
Globulin (g/l)	43	23–45
Urea (mmol/l)	6.4	2.5–7.4
Creatinine (µmol/l)	128	40–145
Potassium (mmol/l)	5.0	3.4–5.6
Sodium (mmol/l)	145	139–154
Chloride (mmol/l)	108	105–122
Calcium (mmol/l)	2.9	2.3–3.0
Inorganic phosphate (mmol/l)	1.3	0.6–1.4
Glucose (mmol/l)	5.8	3.3–5.8
ALT (IU/l)	**141**	0–55
AST (IU/l)	29	0–49
ALP (IU/l)	**1376**	0–50
Bilirubin (µmol/l)	3	0–16
Bile acids (µmol/l)	3.5	0–10
Postprandial bile acids (µmol/l)	12.4	0–15
Cholesterol (mmol/l)	**18.1**	3.8–7.0
Triglyceride (mmol/l)	**4.8**	0.56–1.14
Creatine kinase (IU/l)	63	0–190

Abnormal results are in **bold**.

WHAT ABNORMALITIES ARE PRESENT?

Increased levels of hepatic enzymes are present, although the proportional rise in ALP is much higher than that of alanine aminotransferase (ALT), the latter only being modestly elevated. Marked hypercholesterolaemia is present, and less marked but still elevated hypertriglyceridaemia is notable. The bile acid stimulation test is normal.

HOW WOULD YOU INTERPRET THESE RESULTS?

A hyperlipidaemia is present, of both cholesterol and triglyceride. Assuming that this patient was fasted, this is a marked abnormality. In the presence of polyuria and polydipsia and with the markedly elevated ALP and modest ALT elevation, hyperadrenocorticism would be the principal consideration.

WHAT FURTHER TESTS WOULD YOU RECOMMEND?

The two tests most commonly employed for the diagnosis of canine hyperadrenocorticism are the adrenocorticotropic hormone (ACTH) stimulation test and the low-dose dexamethasone suppression test, which are described in more detail in Chapter 18. If hyperadrenocorticism is confirmed on the basis of a combination of compatible clinical signs and specific diagnostic testing, ultrasound examination of the adrenal glands, perhaps combined with assessment of endogenous ACTH, may help distinguish pituitary- from adrenal-dependent forms and allow therapy to be targeted appropriately.

CASE OUTCOME

In this case a low-dose dexamethasone suppression test was performed.

LDDS test results
0 hours: 125 nmol/l (27.5–125).
3 hours: <27.6 nmol/l (<27.6).
8 hours: **58** nmol/l (<27.6).

The results of this test in the presence of compatible clinical signs and clinical laboratory data, supported a diagnosis of hyperadrenocorticism. Bilaterally symmetrical mild adrenomegaly without evidence of mass lesions was identified on abdominal ultrasonography, and endogenous ACTH levels were elevated, both supporting a diagnosis of pituitary-dependent hyperadrenocorticism.

CASE 2

SIGNALMENT

3-year-old female neutered Golden Retriever.

HISTORY

There was a 6-month history of progressively worsening body condition despite an excellent appetite. No vomiting or diarrhoea has been noted. Recently more marked generalized muscle wastage has been reported and mild ascites has developed.

CLINICAL PATHOLOGY DATA

Biochemistry	Result	Reference range
Total protein (g/l)	**52**	54–77
Albumin (g/l)	**15**	25–40
Globulin (g/l)	37	23–45
Urea (mmol/l)	7.3	1.7–7.4
Creatinine (μmol/l)	92	40–145
Potassium (mmol/l)	4.7	3.4–5.6
Sodium (mmol/l)	143	139–154
Chloride (mmol/l)	109	105–122
Calcium (mmol/l)	2.3	2.3–3.0
Inorganic phosphate (mmol/l)	1.4	0.6–1.4
Glucose (mmol/l)	4.8	3.3–5.8
ALT (IU/l)	38	0–55
AST (IU/l)	43	0–49
ALP (IU/l)	44	0–50
Bilirubin (mmol/l)	1	0–16
Cholesterol (mmol/l)	**10.8**	3.8–7.0
Triglyceride (mmol/l)	0.6	0.56–1.14
Creatine kinase (IU/l)	134	0–190

Abnormal results are in **bold**.

SAMPLE QUALITY

Normal.

WHAT ABNORMALITIES ARE PRESENT?

A marked hypoalbuminaemia and a moderate rise in cholesterol are the most notable abnormalities.

HOW WOULD YOU INTERPRET THESE RESULTS?

Severe hypoalbuminaemia is most commonly associated with protein-losing nephropathies (PLNs; in which globulin is usually normal), hepatic failure and protein-losing enteropathies (PLEs). In the latter case concurrent hypoglobulinaemia is usually seen, but in early disease or when significant inflammation is present globulins may be normal. Hypoalbuminaemia may also be seen (usually less severe) in situations where a negative acute phase response is occurring and with loss into 'third-space' fluids. In this case there is concurrent hypercholesterolaemia, which would be unusual in the presence of either hepatic failure or a PLE, both of which are more normally associated with hypocholesterolaemia. This would make a PLN most likely. Note that the absence of azotaemia *never* excludes the possibility of PLN because changes in glomerular 'perm-selectivity' which characterize PLN do not necessarily imply that the glomerular filtration rate will be altered.

WHAT FURTHER TESTS WOULD YOU RECOMMEND?

Assessment of the ascitic fluid should be performed; it is expected in the presence of severe hypoalbuminaemia to be a pure transudate (transudate: protein-poor). Urine should be analysed for protein content by a urine protein:creatinine ratio (UPCR) but this result should be interpreted in light of whether any active inflammatory urine sediment is present, because this may also elevate the UPCR. Assessment of a bile acid stimulation test may help to exclude severe functional liver disease. Diagnostic imaging of the kidneys by ultrasonography (or less usefully radiography) may be helpful, particularly to evaluate for renal neoplasia or congenital renal dysplasia. If PLN is confirmed, renal biopsy may be considered, but only after very careful analysis of the balance of risk and clinical benefit inherent in this procedure.

CASE OUTCOME

In this case a very marked elevation in UPCR of 16.67 (reference range <0.5) was identified in the absence of an active urinary sediment. Bile acid stimulation was normal. A PLN was diagnosed, and ultrasound examination of the kidneys identified bilateral renomegaly with preservation of normal renal architecture. Renal cortical biopsies were performed after assessment of coagulation status and under ultrasound guidance. A final diagnosis of focal multisegmental glomerulosclerosis was made.

References and further reading

Armstrong PJ and Ford RB (1989) Hyperlipidaemia. In: *Kirk's Current Veterinary Therapy X*, ed. RW Kirk, pp. 1046–1050. WB Saunders, Philadelphia

Barrie J, Nash AS and Watson TDG (1993a) Quantitative analysis of canine plasma lipoproteins. *Journal of Small Animal Practice* **34**, 226–231

Barrie J, Watson TDG, Stear MJ *et al.* (1993b) Plasma cholesterol and lipoprotein concentrations in the dog: The effects of age, breed, gender and endocrine disease. *Journal of Small Animal Practice* **34**, 507–512

Bauer JE (1995) Evaluation and dietary considerations in idiopathic hyperlipidaemia in dogs. *Journal of the American Veterinary Medical Association* **206(11)**, 1684–1688

Bauer JE (1996) Comparative lipid and lipoprotein metabolism. *Veterinary Clinical Pathology* **25(2)**, 49–56

Burkhard MJ and Meyer DJ (1995) Causes and effects of interference with clinical laboratory measurements and examinations. In: *Kirk's Current Veterinary Therapy XII*, ed. JD Bonagura, pp. 14–20. WB Saunders, Philadelphia

Cook AK and Cowgill LD (1996) Clinical and pathological features of protein-losing glomerular disease in the dog: a review of 137 cases (1985–1992). *Journal of the American Animal Hospital Association* **32(4)**, 313–322

Crispin SM (1993) Ocular manifestations of hyperlipoproteinaemia. *Journal of Small Animal Practice* **34**, 500–506

Ford RB (1996) Clinical management of lipaemic patients. *Compendium on Continuing Education for the Practicing Veterinarian* **18**, 1053–1060

Hess RS, Kass PH and Van Winkle TJ (2003) Association between diabetes mellitus, hypothyroidism or hyperadrenocorticism, and atherosclerosis in dogs. *Journal of Veterinary Internal Medicine* **17**, 489–494

Hubert B, Braun JP, de la Farge F *et al.* (1987) Hypertriglyceridaemia in two related dogs. *Companion Animal Practice* **1**, 33–35

Jeusette I, Grauwels M, Cuvelier C *et al.* (2004) Hypercholesterolaemia in a family of rough collie dogs. *Journal of Small Animal Practice* **45**, 319–324

Jeusette IC, Lhoest ET, Istasse LP *et al.* (2005) Influence of obesity on plasma lipid and lipoprotein concentrations in dogs. *American Journal of Veterinary Research* **66**, 81–86

Johnson MC (2005) Hyperlipidaemia disorders of dogs. *Compendium on Continuing Education for the Practicing Veterinarian* **27**, 361–364

Johnstone AC, Jones BR, Thompson JC *et al.* (1990) The pathology of an inherited hyperlipoproteinaemia of cats. *Journal of Comparative Pathology* **102**, 125–137

Jones BR, Johnstone AC, Cahill JI *et al.* (1986) Peripheral neuropathy in cats with inherited primary hyperchylomicronaemia. *Veterinary Record* **119**, 268–272

Jones BR, Wallace A, Harding DR *et al.* (1983) Occurrence of idiopathic, familial hyperchylomicronaemia in a cat. *Veterinary Record* **112**, 543–547

LeBlanc CJ, Bauer JE, Hosgood G *et al.* (2005) Effect of dietary fish oil and vitamin E supplementation on hematologic and serum biochemical analytes and oxidative status in young dogs. *Veterinary Therapeutics* **6**, 325–340

Lenox CE and Bauer JE (2013) Potential adverse effects of omega-3 fatty acids in dogs and cats. *Journal of Veterinary Internal Medicine* **27(2)**, 217–226

Littman MP, Dambach DM, Vaden SL *et al.* (2000) Familial protein-losing enteropathy and protein-losing nephropathy in soft coated wheaten terriers: 222 cases (1983–1997). *Journal of Veterinary Internal Medicine* **14(1)**, 68–80

Mahley RW, Innerarity TL, Rall SC *et al.* (1977) Canine hyperlipoproteinemia and atherosclerosis. Accumulation of lipid by aortic medial cells in vivo and in vitro. *American Journal of Pathology* **87(1)**, 205–226

Mori N, Lee P, Muranaka S *et al.* (2010) Predisposition for primary hyperlipidemia in miniature schnauzers and Shetland sheepdogs as compared to other canine breeds. *Research in Veterinary Science* **88**, 394–399

Nieto CG, Barrera R, Habela MA *et al.* (1992) Changes in the plasma concentrations of lipids and lipoprotein fractions in dogs infected with *Leishmania infantum. Veterinary Parasitology* **44(3–4)**, 175–82

Ogilvie GK, Ford RB, Vail, DM *et al.* (1994). Alterations in lipoprotein profiles in dogs with lymphoma. *Journal of Veterinary Internal Medicine* **8(1)**, 62–66

Peritz LN, Brunzell JD, Harvey-Clarke C *et al.* (1990) Characterization of a lipoprotein lipase class III type defect in hypertriglyceridemic cats. *Clinical and Investigative Medicine* **13**, 259–263

Rogers WA, Donovan EF and Kociba GJ (1975a) Idiopathic hyperlipoproteinemia in dogs. *Journal of the American Veterinary Medical Association* **166**, 1087–1091

Rogers WA, Donovan EF and Kociba GJ (1975b) Lipids and lipoproteins in normal dogs and in dogs with secondary hyperlipoproteinemia. *Journal of the American Veterinary Medical Association* **166**, 1092–1100

Sato K, Agoh H, Kaneshige T *et al.* (2000) Hypercholesterolemia in Shetland sheepdogs. *Journal of Veterinary Medical Science* **62**, 1297–1301

Thompson JC, Johnstone AC, Jones BR *et al.* (1989) The ultrastructural pathology of five lipoprotein lipase-deficient cats. *Journal of Comparative Pathology* **101**, 251–262

Tidholm A and Jonsson L (1997) A retrospective study of canine dilated cardiomyopathy (189 cases). *Journal of the American Animal Hospital Association* **33(6)**, 544–550

Wada M, Minamisono T, Ehrhart LA *et al.* (1977) Familial hyperlipoproteinemia in beagles. *Life Sciences* **20**, 999–1008

Watson P, Simpson KW and Bedford PG (1993) Hypercholesterolaemia in Briards in the United Kingdom. *Research in Veterinary Science* **54**, 80–85

Watson TDG and Barrie J (1993) Lipoprotein metabolism and hyperlipidaemia in the dog and cat: A review. *Journal of Small Animal Practice* **34**, 479–487

Watson TDG, Gaffney D, Mooney CT *et al.* (1992) Inherited hyperchylomicronaemia in the cat: Lipoprotein lipase function and gene structure. *Journal of Small Animal Practice* **33**, 207–212

Whitney MS (1992) Evaluation of hyperlipidemias in dogs and cats. *Seminars in Veterinary Medicine and Surgery (Small Animal)* **7**, 292–300

Whitney MS, Boon GD, Rebar AH *et al.* (1987) Effects of acute pancreatitis on circulating lipids in dogs. *American Journal of Veterinary Research* **48**, 1492–1497

Whitney MS, Boon GD, Rebar AH *et al.* (1993) Ultracentrifugal and electrophoretic characteristics of the plasma lipoproteins of miniature schnauzer dogs with idiopathic hyperlipoproteinemia. *Journal of Veterinary Internal Medicine* **7**, 253–260

Xenoulis PG, Levinski MD, Suchodolski JS *et al.* (2011) Serum triglyceride concentrations in Miniature Schnauzers with and without a history of probable pancreatitis. *Journal of Veterinary Internal Medicine* **25**, 20–25

Xenoulis PG and Steiner JM (2010) Lipid metabolism and hyperlipidemia in dogs. *The Veterinary Journal* **183**, 12–21

Xenoulis PG, Suchodolski JS, Levinski MD *et al.* (2007) Investigation of hypertriglyceridemia in healthy Miniature Schnauzers. *Journal of Veterinary Internal Medicine* **21**, 1224–1230

Xenoulis PG, Suchodolski JS, Ruaux CG *et al* (2010) Association between serum triglyceride and canine pancreatic lipase immunoreactivity concentrations in miniature schnauzers. *Journal of the American Animal Hospital Association* **46**, 229–234

Yilmaz Z and Senturk S (2007) Characterisation of lipid profiles in dogs with parvoviral enteritis. *Journal of Small Animal Practice* **48(11)**, 643–650

Zicker SC, Ford RB, Nelson RW and Kirk CA (2000). Endocrine and lipid disorders. In: *Small Animal Clinical Nutrition*, ed. MS Hand, CD Thatcher, RL Remillard and P Roudebush, pp. 869-881. Mark Morris Institute, Walsworth Publishing, Topeka

Chapter 16

Laboratory evaluation of hypoglycaemia and hyperglycaemia

Lucy Davison

Glucose homeostasis

Glucose homeostasis refers to the processes involved in the production, storage and release of glucose from storage. Glucose is derived by the ingestion, digestion and absorption of carbohydrates, and blood glucose is maintained within tight limits by several different mechanisms. In addition, in processes particularly important in cats, gluconeogenesis and glycogenolysis allow glucose to be made within the body from other substrates. Reference ranges vary according to the laboratory and testing method but 3.0–6.5 mmol/l in dogs and 3.1–7.2 mmol/l in cats are generally acceptable glucose concentrations that are unlikely to cause clinical signs in most animals. Glucose is stored in a readily accessible form, known as glycogen, in the liver and muscles, and can be released when needed by a process called *glycogenolysis*. In addition, dogs and cats can use a pathway called *gluconeogenesis* to make glucose from amino acids and other non-carbohydrate precursors such as pyruvate in the liver.

Glucose is vitally important for many metabolic processes. Consequently, aberrations in blood glucose may have a significant clinical impact and require emergency treatment. Cells which are deficient in glucose cannot use glycolysis to make adenosine triphosphate (ATP), the main energy source of the cell, and this is particularly problematic for highly glucose-dependent cells such as neurons. When blood glucose is too high, the renal threshold of glucose absorption from the filtrate is exceeded, leading to osmotic diuresis and predisposing to urinary tract infection. While in some cases hypoglycaemia and hyperglycaemia may lead to only subtle clinical signs, in other cases, particularly where rapid changes in blood glucose concentration have occurred, permanent damage or even death may ensue.

Several hormones work together to prevent hyper- and hypoglycaemia, and Figure 16.1 illustrates the basic processes involved in balancing blood glucose. *Insulin* is released by the beta cells of the pancreas in response to hyperglycaemia and acts by several different mechanisms to reduce blood glucose. *Glucagon*, released from the alpha cells of the pancreas during times of hypoglycaemia, antagonizes insulin by promoting gluconeogenesis and glycogenolysis and reducing peripheral glucose utilization. *Cortisol*, *growth hormone* and *adrenaline* (epinephrine) also antagonize insulin, as well as the latter promoting the sympathetic 'flight or fight' response, which helps the animal cope with the hypoglycaemic state. In fact many of the clinical signs associated with hypoglycaemia are a result of the adrenergic response.

There are some differences in glucose metabolism between cats and dogs. Cats are less well prepared for

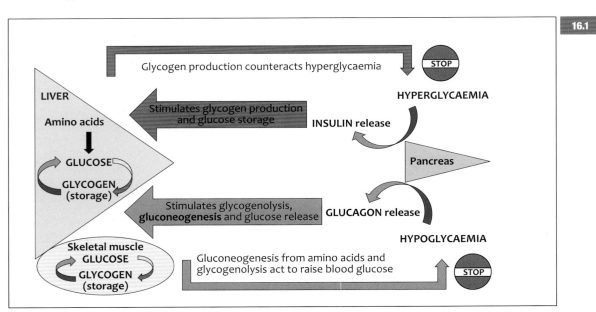

16.1 Control of blood glucose.

carbohydrate metabolism as they have lower concentrations of salivary amylase than dogs. Additionally, while glucokinase is used to metabolize glucose within cells in dogs, a slower enzyme called hexokinase is used in cats. Cats are therefore more susceptible to postprandial hyperglycaemia.

Measurement of blood glucose

Blood glucose is measured using standard spectrophotometric methods by biochemistry analysers and can also be measured using point-of-care devices and hand-held blood glucose monitors.

Storage of samples for glucose measurement

Red and white blood cells within a blood sample will carry on consuming glucose after the blood has been collected. This means that unless the sample is analysed immediately after collection, or centrifuged to remove cells, or collected into a fluoride oxalate tube to prevent further glucose utilization by cells, the measured blood glucose concentrations will be spuriously low. This effect becomes marked in animals with leucocytosis or erythrocytosis.

Use of point-of-care glucose monitors

Both human and veterinary point-of-care glucometers are available and are designed for glucose measurement in whole blood. Glucose is distributed in the water component of both plasma and cells, but there is less water per unit volume of cells compared with plasma and so glucometers may give falsely low results when compared with standard plasma measurements. There is species-specific variation in the distribution of glucose between red cells and plasma. Veterinary glucometers (e.g. AlphaTRAK™; Figure 16.2) are calibrated to correct for this variation between red cells and plasma. In humans, glucose is distributed between plasma and red cells in an approximately 60:40 ratio, while in dogs and cats most of the glucose is carried in the plasma. In animals with normal haematocrits, veterinary-specific glucometers correlate with standard serum methods. However, where the animal is anaemic or polycythaemic the haematocrit will influence the glucose measurement. Spuriously low results are obtained with all types of glucometer when the haematocrit is elevated over 50% (the sample contains less water), while in anaemic

animals (haematocrit <20%), the glucometer glucose correlates more closely with plasma glucose using human glucometers, but may be falsely high with veterinary-specific glucometers. In a recent study, glucose values were found to differ by up to 2–3 mmol/l from reference measurements in cases of altered haematocrit or when human *versus* veterinary devices were used (Paul *et al.*, 2011). The accuracy of hand-held glucometers can also be adversely affected by temperature, humidity, altitude, hyperbilirubinaemia or hypercholesterolaemia.

When taking serial blood glucose measurements, it is important to be consistent with the device that is used so that trends can be observed accurately. In addition, glucometers that draw up the correct volume of blood into a small chamber are generally more reliable than those in which a variably sized drop of blood is placed on to a measurement stick. Careful maintenance of glucometers is vital, including quality control steps such as:

- Scheduled evaluation of variation within the same sample measurement, e.g. repeated measurement of the same sample (at both the high and low end of the range) on one instrument or across all instruments in the practice
- The regular use of control calibration samples where they are available
- Frequent battery changes
- Regular cleaning of accessible parts
- Ensuring that all consumables associated with the device are stored correctly and not out of date
- The use of the correct volume of a fresh, non-haemolysed sample for each test.

Evaluation of blood glucose over a longer period

Fructosamine

If a single unexpectedly high or low blood glucose concentration is obtained, it is useful for the clinician to be able to determine whether this abnormal glycaemic level has been present for a week or more by measurement of blood fructosamine. Fructosamine is a term used to describe plasma proteins (e.g. albumin) which have undergone non-enzymatic, irreversible glycosylation in proportion to their surrounding glucose concentration (Jensen, 1992). In dogs, the serum fructosamine concentration is related to the average blood glucose concentration over the previous 1–2 weeks (Kawamoto *et al.*, 1992), and *in vitro* studies suggest that persistent hyperglycaemia is required for 4 days before an increase in fructosamine concentration is seen (Jensen, 1995). In cats, fructosamine is reported to exceed the upper limit of the reference range after 3–5 days of marked hyperglycaemia, taking around 20 days to plateau and 5 days to return to baseline when euglycaemia is restored. Conversely, hypoglycaemia will decrease fructosamine concentration.

Fructosamine concentration can also be influenced by factors other than blood glucose concentration (Reusch and Haberer, 2001). For example, fructosamine may be reduced in normoglycaemic dogs and cats with hypoproteinaemia, although the converse does not appear to be true for hyperproteinaemia. Hyperlipidaemia and azotaemia have also been reported to reduce fructosamine in dogs but not in cats (Reusch and Haberer, 2001). Additionally, fructosamine concentration can also be reduced in states of increased protein turnover such as hyperthyroidism in cats (Reusch and Tomsa, 1999) and

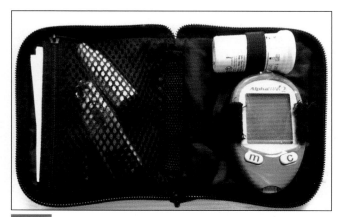

16.2 AlphaTRAK™ device.

elevated in states of decreased protein turnover such as hypothyroidism in dogs (Reusch *et al.*, 2002).

Methodology and the laboratory have a profound impact on fructosamine measurement so it is important to be consistent when comparing samples from the same patient longitudinally. Similarly, fructosamine should be interpreted in the light of clinical signs. Fructosamine should not be used in isolation to provide reassurance in a patient with clinical evidence of glycaemic instability, nor should a single measurement be the sole reason for prompting investigation if there are no associated clinical signs of instability.

Glycosylated haemoglobin

Other long-term indicators of glycaemic control such as glycosylated haemoglobin are also available and widely used in human medicine for assessing the stability of diabetic patients. The term glycosylated haemoglobin is used to describe any type of haemoglobin that has gradually and irreversibly become chemically bound to glucose, which occurs in proportion to the concentration of glucose in the surrounding medium. Although such assays have shown promise in veterinary medicine, and may provide a longer-term measurement of average blood glucose than fructosamine, they are not currently widely available to veterinary practitioners.

Home serial glucose monitoring

There are circumstances in which repeated blood glucose measurements over a longer period, such as 24 hours, are required, particularly in the care of unstable diabetic dogs and cats. The use of blood glucose curves is discussed in more detail later in this chapter, in relation to the management of diabetic patients.

In most cases, such measurements are undertaken in the veterinary practice, provided that the animal does not become too stressed during the procedure. An alternative which is gaining popularity is the home glucose curve, performed by the owner under the supervision of the veterinary practice (Casella *et al.*, 2005). The owner may be trained to take small samples of capillary blood, e.g. from the pinna or footpad, using a lancet or vacuum device. This could be considered for the management of patients who will not eat or become highly stressed in the practice, are aggressive with anyone apart from the owner, are intermittently very 'brittle' in their glycaemic control and suffer from hypoglycaemic episodes or, in the case of cats, are only intermittently diabetic and have periods of diabetic remission. Great care must be taken, however, with owner selection and training because unsupervised, poorly carried out or inappropriate testing (and/or alteration of the insulin dose) has the potential to have a significant detrimental effect on the welfare of the patient. Veterinary hand-held glucose monitoring devices such as the AlphaTRAK™ are designed for both in-clinic and at-home use, and therefore are a sensible choice for home monitoring, because many resources are available online to support training given by the practice. While some owners purchase their own devices, a recommended arrangement, which allows the practice greater control of how and when owners test blood glucose, is to have a device available which owners can borrow from the practice when a glucose curve has been scheduled or if hypoglycaemic episodes are suspected. This also ensures that regular quality control testing can be carried out on the device.

Continuous glucose monitoring

When undertaking blood glucose monitoring frequently during the course of a day, repeated blood sampling can be stressful and painful for the patient and, in addition, there is a risk that a significant blood glucose peak or nadir will fall between two sampling times and will not be recorded. Some of these issues can now be overcome by the use of continuous glucose monitoring (CGMS) devices, which are widely used in human medicine and have been successfully validated in the management of diabetic dogs and cats (Davison *et al.*, 2003; Ristic *et al.*, 2005). The MiniMed® CGMS system requires the subcutaneous implantation of a glucose sensor, using a 22 G needle attached to a spring-loaded implantation device (Figure 16.3). The subcutaneous sensor can be left in place, usually in the lateral thoracic area, for up to 72 hours. The CGMS contains a glucose oxidase-coated platinum electrode at a constant potential to a reference electrode (Figure 16.3). When glucose flows on to the membrane in the electrode in the presence of oxygen it is oxidized, producing a current that is proportional to the surrounding glucose concentration. Interstitial fluid glucose concentrations are measured every 10 seconds; an average value is recorded every 5 minutes during the time the sensor is connected, and can be downloaded on to a computer for full analysis.

It has been demonstrated in humans that the interstitial fluid glucose concentration mimics the blood glucose concentration, and in dogs the time delay between changes in

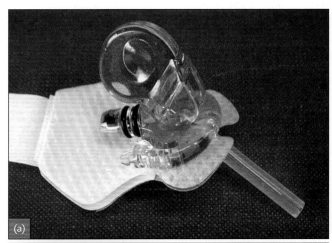

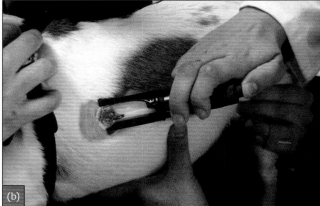

16.3 Using a continuous glucose monitoring device. (a) A subcutaneous disposable platinum electrode for use with a continuous glucose monitoring device. (b) Using the spring-loaded device to implant the electrode below the skin over the thorax of a diabetic dog, prior to initiation of continuous glucose monitoring.

the blood and in the interstitial fluid compartments is less than 10 minutes. In further clinical studies using canine and feline patients, the CGMS has been shown to correlate well with blood glucose samples taken concurrently (Surman and Fleeman, 2013).

In practical terms, CGMS technology has evolved over the past 10 years to become more user-friendly and accessible for general practitioners and owners. In early studies, the device was not wireless and the monitor (approximately the size of a pager) had to be 'worn' by the patient on a harness, as it was connected to the sensor by a short wire. In current models, however, the sensor transmits data by radiotelemetry as long as the patient and data recording device are within a few metres of each other. This is a particular advantage for cats, although they do need to stay indoors. In addition, while the working range of early devices was only 2.2–22.2 mmol/l, it is now possible to calculate values above this range, although the blood glucose must be below 22.2 mmol/l at the time the device is initiated.

One potential drawback is that the sensor must still be calibrated 2–3 times within each 24-hour period using data obtained from a blood glucose measurement with a standard glucometer, meaning that several venous or capillary blood samples are still necessary within the monitoring period. However, data are now available from the device in real time rather than having to 'dock' it in a computer terminal to check glucose measurements, allowing more informed decisions to be taken about how long to continue with monitoring. The cost of disposable platinum sensors, in addition to the device, and the limited shelf-life of the sensors, have thus far prevented many first-opinion practices from using the CGMS, but costs are gradually reducing. Each sensor can give up to 72 hours of data and can add valuable information to a standard glucose curve.

Figure 16.4 illustrates a 24-hour continuous (interstitial fluid) glucose curve, with data obtained from blood glucose samples superimposed on the graph. The CGMS system is particularly useful in the management of diabetic patients in whom periods of hypoglycaemia are suspected and when animals are difficult to blood sample. It can be used at home, within certain practical limits, if animals refuse to eat or become very stressed during hospitalization for blood glucose sampling.

Hypoglycaemia

Hypoglycaemia is a life-threatening condition generally defined by a blood glucose lower than 3 mmol/l. Clinical signs (Figure 16.5) are not always apparent at a blood glucose level of 3 mmol/l, although a rapid fall in blood glucose, for example following an accidental insulin overdose in a diabetic patient, may lead to clinical signs at a higher blood glucose concentration if there has not been sufficient time for counter-regulatory mechanisms to take effect. Similarly, a slow fall in glucose may allow an animal to appear clinically well with a blood glucose between 2 and 3 mmol/l. Hypoglycaemia can result in permanent neurological damage if not recognized and managed quickly, and is far more common in dogs than cats. Fasting in healthy dogs and cats does not normally lead to hypoglycaemia.

Clinical signs of hypoglycaemia

The severity of clinical signs of hypoglycaemia depends on many factors, not least the speed at which the animal has become hypoglycaemic and the ability of the body to

Early
• Changes in behaviour: agitation, nervousness, disorientation, aggression • Increased appetite (occasionally anorexia) • Sleepiness • Muscle fasciculation • Episodic weakness • Bradycardia or tachycardia
Late (may be influenced by catecholamine response)
• Generalized collapse • Seizure activity • Vomiting • Panting • Hypertension • Shock • Diarrhoea • Blindness or apparent blindness • Temporary neurological deficits (cerebral vasospasm, brain oedema) • Permanent neurological deficits (cortical damage, anoxia)

16.5 Clinical signs of hypoglycaemia.

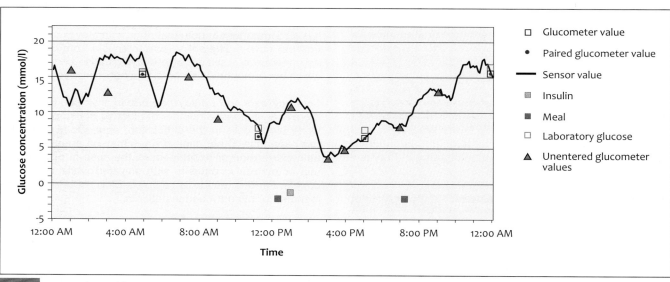

16.4 A trace obtained from a continuous glucose monitoring device implanted in a dog.

respond appropriately. Sometimes hypoglycaemia is an apparently incidental finding in an otherwise healthy animal, but investigation is warranted if there is:

- Any history of accompanying clinical signs
- Hypoglycaemia documented on more than one occasion
- Blood glucose <3 mmol/l.

Where seen, the majority of clinical signs are neurological in origin and are commonly exacerbated by the accompanying adrenergic response.

Glucose cannot be made or stored in the brain, so the central nervous system is entirely dependent on blood glucose for provision of energy and is very vulnerable to permanent damage during prolonged hypoglycaemia. Although glucose transport into the majority of neurons is not insulin dependent, a concentration gradient is still required for facilitated diffusion and hypoglycaemia leads to a serious condition called *neuroglycopenia*.

Causes of hypoglycaemia and their recognition

There are many potential causes of hypoglycaemia, which can be broadly divided into the categories of excess glucose utilization, decreased glucose production and the presence of excess insulin or hypoglycaemic agents. Causes of hypoglycaemia in these categories are listed in Figure 16.6 and discussed in more detail below.

Excess utilization of glucose

Sepsis: Sepsis is a common cause of hypoglycaemia, and is particularly associated with bacterial infection and certain parasitic infections rarely seen in the UK, such as *Babesia* spp. infections. In sepsis a state of increased glucose consumption develops which may be exacerbated by reduced food intake. Mechanisms thought to underlie septic hypoglycaemia are the production of inflammatory

Excess utilization of glucose

• **Sepsis**
• **Neoplasia**
• Pregnancy
• Seizure activity
• Exercise/working dog hypoglycaemia
• *In vitro* utilization/laboratory error
  • Sample aging with *in vitro* metabolism of glucose when sample separation is delayed
  • Leucocytosis (may only be relevant in cases of delayed sample separation)
  • Polycythemia (may only be relevant in cases of delayed sample separation)

Decrease in glucose production
• Hepatic disease, e.g. fibrosis, portosystemic shunting, **copper storage disease** • Hypoadrenocorticism • **Neonatal hypoglycaemia** • Glycogen storage diseases • Enzyme deficiencies
Presence of excess insulin or hypoglycaemic agent
• **Insulin overdose** • **Insulinoma** • Xylitol toxicity • Treatment with oral hypoglycaemic agent, e.g. sulfonylureas • Tumours producing insulin-like substances, e.g. leiomyoma

16.6 Causes of hypoglycaemia. The most common causes are in bold.

mediators, decreased blood pressure and tissue perfusion, alongside hypoxaemia-induced anaerobic metabolism. Common scenarios for hypoglycaemia associated with sepsis are pyometra and peritonitis, and clinical signs of the underlying disease usually predominate. Laboratory diagnosis involves evaluation of a complete blood count, where a neutrophilia with or without a left shift is expected.

Pregnancy: Pregnancy, dominated by progesterone, tends to cause insulin resistance, which suppresses the intracellular transport of glucose and increases blood glucose concentration. However, late in pregnancy (days 40–63), to ensure a constant supply of glucose to the growing fetuses, the normal multisystemic responses to hypoglycaemia are reduced. The metabolic demands of late pregnancy may also lead to ketosis in the presence of hypoglycaemia, but this is usually reversible with treatment (Johnson, 2008; Klein and Peterson, 2010). The presence of ketones can be detected in blood or urine. When testing urine for ketones it is important to use as fresh a sample as possible and to read the dipstick at the exact time interval indicated. In addition, the clinician must be aware that urine dipsticks test only for acetoacetate, rather than beta-hydroxybutyrate, which can be the predominant ketone in blood, so false negative results may be obtained.

Neoplasia (non-beta cell tumour): In theory, any neoplasm may cause hypoglycaemia as it consumes glucose during a phase of rapid growth. In reality, certain large tumours are more likely to have this effect, such as hepatomas, hepatocellular carcinomas, leiomyomas and leiomyosarcomas (Boari *et al.*, 1995). In addition, other types of tumour may cause hypoglycaemia either by increased consumption of glucose or an alternative mechanism such as the release of insulin-like peptides or a detrimental effect on gluconeogenesis.

Seizure activity: While seizures may be a clinical sign of hypoglycaemia, it is also important to note that a fall in blood glucose concentration may arise as a consequence of prolonged seizure activity. Hence the detection of mild hypoglycaemia in a patient after a long period of seizuring does not necessarily confirm that the primary cause of the seizure was hypoglycaemia. While the sympathetic nervous system tends to elevate blood pressure and blood glucose as a compensatory mechanism at the time of a seizure, tonic–clonic seizure activity may increase glucose consumption in muscle and in turn act to reduce blood glucose. It is also important to note that dogs with previously existing epilepsy have a different seizure threshold from other dogs and may have a seizure at a blood glucose concentration which would not be detrimental to a non-epileptic patient.

Leucocytosis and polycythaemia: In any condition where there is an increased number of glucose-consuming red or white blood cells in the circulation, spurious hypoglycaemia may arise. Other clinical signs may be apparent, such as hypertension or nosebleeds in the case of polycythaemia or pyrexia in patients with elevated white blood cell counts. For this reason, a complete blood count is recommended for hypoglycaemic patients.

Exercise-induced/working dog hypoglycaemia: Exertional hypoglycaemia is a diagnosis of exclusion and is seen in lean, healthy dogs who undertake periods of intense physical activity such as hunting. Clinical signs may range from mild weakness with muscle tremors to profound signs of hypoglycaemia resulting in seizures and coma. The exact mechanism for this condition is unclear, and many endocrinological and neurological conditions can cause similar signs. It is thought that these dogs exhaust their glycogen stores during heavy work, so they must be allowed rest periods and receive frequent meals of complex carbohydrates to maintain blood glucose concentrations during such work.

Artefactual: As previously discussed, artefactual hypoglycaemia is common, especially if samples have not been collected or stored properly, so genuine hypoglycaemia without apparent clinical signs must usually be documented more than once, including in a fresh sample, to prompt investigation.

Decrease in glucose production

Hepatic disease: Most animals with liver disease will remain euglycaemic until around 70% of liver function is lost but, nonetheless, hepatic disease is an important cause of hypoglycaemia. The liver is a major site of glycogen storage and gluconeogenesis, and therefore any type of liver disease may have an impact on blood glucose concentration. Portosystemic shunts, hepatic fibrosis, glycogen storage diseases and copper storage diseases are among the many conditions affecting the liver that may lead to hypoglycaemia. Liver disease may be accompanied by a fall in plasma albumin and urea concentrations, and in some cases liver enzymes and/or total bilirubin may also be elevated. In the non-jaundiced animal, a bile acid stimulation test will help to evaluate liver function or detect portosystemic shunting. Prolonged blood clotting times may also occur with liver disease.

Hypoadrenocorticism: Animals with hypoadrenocorticism usually lack both aldosterone and cortisol, but a proportion of 'atypical' cases are deficient in cortisol only. In the fasting dog or cat, glucocorticoids such as cortisol help to preserve normoglycaemia by increasing lipolysis and gluconeogenesis while decreasing peripheral glucose utilization. Lack of cortisol in both typical and atypical hypoadrenocorticism can lead to hypoglycaemia, which may occur in the absence of classical electrolyte abnormalities (hyperkalaemia and hyponatraemia) in atypical disease. Suggestive clinical signs accompanying hypoglycaemia in hypoadrenocorticism include vague anorexia, shivering, inability to cope with stress (e.g. cattery or kennels), gastrointestinal disturbances and lack of a stress leucogram on a complete blood count, due to hypocortisolaemia. Diagnosis is usually straightforward because patients with both atypical and typical hypoadrenocorticism fail to show a cortisol response on an adrenocorticotropic hormone (ACTH) stimulation test. The disease is much more common in dogs, but has also been reported in a number of cats.

Neonatal hypoglycaemia: Hypoglycaemia is common in young puppies and kittens secondary to a combination of an immature liver, high energy requirements and inadequate substrate availability for gluconeogenesis and glycogenolysis. Puppies and kittens are born with minimal glycogen stores and this condition is exacerbated by prematurity, prolonged feeding intervals, low body temperature, infection and increased activity. Neonatal hypoglycaemia is avoided by ensuring that all puppies or kittens are fed either by their mother or by hand every 2–3 hours and are kept in a warm environment. Puppies usually grow out of this tendency by 12–20 weeks, but some toy breeds remain susceptible to hypoglycaemia throughout their lives.

Other rarer causes of hypoglycaemia: There are several rare diseases such as glycogen storage diseases and enzyme deficiencies which can also cause hypoglycaemia. These are better documented in dogs than cats.

Presence of excess insulin or a hypoglycaemic agent

Insulin overdose: Although every care is taken to ensure that diabetic animals receive the correct dose and type of insulin by the correct route, using the correct type of syringe, accidental insulin overdose is not uncommon. In addition, signs of hypoglycaemia can be seen if a diabetic cat who is entering diabetic remission (see later in this chapter) carries on receiving the same dose of insulin, which it no longer needs. Additionally, diabetic animals who are anorexic, vomiting, suffering from exocrine pancreatic insufficiency, beginning treatment for another endocrinopathy which has been causing insulin resistance (e.g. hyperadrenocorticism) or have lost a large amount of weight (especially cats), without any insulin dose adjustment; may also become hypoglycaemic from a relative insulin overdose.

In the case of accidental or relative insulin overdose, a careful history is the key to diagnosis, although emergency management must take precedence if a known overdose has been administered (see below). It is important to check the insulin and syringes the owner is using and observe the owner drawing up insulin and injecting their pet. The seriousness of insulin overdose must not be underestimated as it can have an impact on glycaemic control for several days, may lead to permanent neurological damage or even be fatal, so it is vital to know exactly how much has been given and at what time. Counter-regulatory mechanisms provide some protection, but once they are overwhelmed, animals can seizure or become comatose very quickly. Even if no clinical signs are apparent, careful supervision and monitoring of blood glucose is necessary for at least 24 hours. Consideration should be given to pre-emptive treatment (see later), in the absence of clinical signs, if more than double the usual dose has been administered or if the animal has received its usual insulin dose without eating any food.

Insulinoma (pancreatic beta cell neoplasia): Insulinomas are tumours of the pancreatic beta cells. They are more common in dogs than cats and are found more frequently in animals of middle age and older; larger dogs are predisposed. An insulinoma is a differential diagnosis for confirmed hypoglycaemia in any older animal, particularly if accompanied by clinical signs of shivering, exercise intolerance, intermittent collapse, increased appetite, weight gain or bizarre behaviour. Typically, animals with insulinoma are 'normal' between bouts of exercise-associated episodic weakness, from which they recover after being rested and fed. In the absence of other haematological and biochemical abnormalities, patients with insulinoma often have a resting blood glucose of 1.5–3 mmol/l and a low to low normal serum fructosamine concentration. Occasionally, clinical signs of a peripheral neuropathy can also be seen. Laboratory testing involves measuring serum insulin concentration at a time when blood glucose is low and detecting an inappropriately high insulin concentration (this may still fall within the upper half of the reference range). It is imperative to measure glucose and insulin concurrently. The cut-offs for identifying insulinoma vary depending on the method being used to measure insulin, and interpretation should be guided by the laboratory.

Care should be taken when measuring serum insulin that the sample is handled correctly, according to the instructions of the laboratory being used, because insulin is labile and subject to degradation in transit, with the potential to see artefactually low values as a result. Diagnosis is not always straightforward and while insulin:glucose ratios and amended insulin:glucose ratios have been used as a diagnostic tool to try and simplify insulinoma diagnosis, these may be misleading and separate evaluation is recommended.

Confirmation of an insulinoma can be challenging, because the tumour itself may be microscopic and impossible to detect even with advanced diagnostic imaging. In addition, several other neuromuscular (e.g. myasthenia gravis) and cardiovascular (e.g. intermittent cardiac arrhythmia) conditions may mimic the clinical signs of collapse, so these must also be ruled out carefully.

In some cases, however, a pancreatic mass is detectable by ultrasonography, computed tomography (CT) or magnetic resonance imaging (MRI), and in 30–50% of insulinoma cases there is evidence of metastasis to the lungs, liver, or throughout the abdomen. Provocative testing such as 12-hour starvation, or exercise to induce collapse, is not usually needed and must only be undertaken in controlled circumstances, with an intravenous cannula in place and suitable emergency treatment for hypoglycaemia available should it be necessary.

Toxicity: In addition to insulin, several drugs and toxins can result in hypoglycaemia if ingested. Oral hypoglycaemic drugs such as sulfonylureas and glipizide, used to treat human type 2 diabetes and some cases of feline diabetes, will cause hypoglycaemia if ingested. Hypoglycaemic agents work by various mechanisms, including increasing peripheral insulin sensitivity and decreasing glucose production by gluconeogenesis. Beta-blockers such as propranolol and atenolol can also exacerbate hypoglycaemia by interfering with the adrenergic counter-regulatory responses. The artificial sweetener xylitol, commonly found in 'sugar-free' products such as chewing gum, may also cause signs of hypoglycaemia by stimulating the release of insulin from beta cells (Dunayer, 2004).

General diagnostic and emergency therapeutic approach to hypoglycaemia

Figure 16.7 is a flow chart indicating a diagnostic approach and emergency therapeutic approach to hypoglycaemia. As previously mentioned, if the patient is symptomatic or has received a known insulin overdose, emergency management must take precedence over diagnostic investigations.

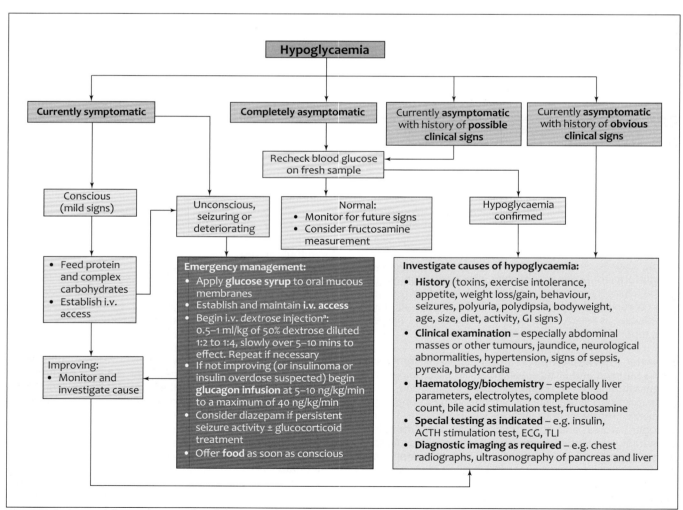

16.7 A suggested diagnostic approach and emergency therapeutic approach to hypoglycaemia. [a] Avoid dextrose bolus in insulinoma cases if possible because this may lead to further insulin release. ACTH = adrenocorticotropic hormone; ECG = electrocardiography; GI = gastrointestinal; TLI = trypsin-like immunoreactivity.

Hyperglycaemia

Hyperglycaemia is most commonly encountered in stressed animals and in patients with diabetes mellitus; common causes of this condition are listed in Figure 16.8.

• **Stress** (cortisol and adrenaline response – especially cats) • **Diabetes mellitus or a prediabetic state** • Other endocrine causes of insulin resistance: acromegaly, hyperadrenocorticism, dioestrus • Iatrogenic causes: total parenteral nutrition, exogenous glucocorticoids, glucose-containing fluid therapy, progestagens, megoestrol acetate, propranolol, ketamine, medetomidine • **Postprandial** (cats) • Pancreatitis • Neuroendocrine tumour, e.g. glucagonoma • Other causes of insulin resistance (may only be relevant in diabetes/prediabetes) e.g. infection, inflammation, hyperlipidaemia, hyperthyroidism (cat), hypothyroidism (dog)

16.8 Causes of hyperglycaemia in dogs and cats. The most common causes are in **bold**.

Clinical signs of hyperglycaemia

In dogs and cats, glucose is usually freely filtered at the glomerulus and entirely reabsorbed in the proximal tubule of the kidney, only appearing in the urine when the renal threshold is exceeded (10–12 mmol/l in dogs and 12–16 mmol/l in cats). The presence of glucose in the urine leads to an osmotic diuresis and polyuria, with a secondary polydipsia. When elevations in blood glucose concentration are severe and chronic, clinical signs can progress to altered behaviour and even coma as the osmotic effect of glucose in the blood results in the movement of water from other body compartments, causing interstitial dehydration.

Causes of hyperglycaemia

Stress hyperglycaemia

Stress hyperglycaemia in cats is an especially common phenomenon, with stress hormones such as adrenaline and cortisol potentially driving glucose higher than 16–20 mmol/l (Rand et al., 2002). Stress hyperglycaemia in cats has also been related to lactate release, associated with a cat struggling against restraint for blood sampling. 'Stress' hyperglycaemia can also be caused in critical illness by mechanisms that are not fully understood, but the potential consequences of hyperglycaemia in this situation include dehydration (via osmotic diuresis), depressed immune function, excessive inflammatory responses, oxidative stress and prothrombotic effects. Stress hyperglycaemia may also be seen in dogs, but is generally less dramatic, raising blood glucose to around 10–12 mmol/l. In both dogs and cats, stress hyperglycaemia is usually distinguished from chronic hyperglycaemia by fructosamine measurement (see earlier).

Diabetes mellitus

Diabetes mellitus is caused by a relative or absolute lack of insulin and is discussed in more detail below. Diabetic animals are at particular risk of hyperglycaemia, and although this is rarely as immediately life-threatening as hypoglycaemia, poorly controlled diabetes mellitus has a significant detrimental impact on quality of life and can progress to diabetic ketoacidosis or non-ketotic hyperosmolar syndrome, which may be fatal. The diagnosis of diabetes mellitus is discussed in more detail later in this chapter.

Obesity

There is strong evidence for obesity causing peripheral insulin resistance in cats, which can progress to diabetes mellitus (Hoenig, 2012). In dogs, there is evidence for obesity-associated insulin resistance but it is less clear whether this predisposes dogs to diabetes (Mattheeuws et al., 1984).

Hormonal antagonism

Hyperglycaemia can also arise as a result of the presence of hormones that antagonize insulin, causing peripheral insulin resistance.

Glucocorticoids: Excess glucocorticoids, such as cortisol, may elevate blood glucose in dogs or cats either iatrogenically or in the presence of a cortisol-secreting adrenal tumour (adrenal-dependent hyperadrenocorticism) or an ACTH-secreting pituitary mass (pituitary-dependent hyperadrenocorticism). Diagnosis of hyperadrenocorticism is discussed in Chapter 18.

Growth hormone: Growth hormone (GH) can also antagonize insulin and cause insulin resistance. Acromegaly in the cat, caused by excess GH from a pituitary macroadenoma, is an increasingly commonly recognized cause of hyperglycaemia and diabetes mellitus in cats (Niessen, 2010). Diagnosis is achieved by detection of an elevated serum insulin-like growth factor (IGF)-1 (which is made in the presence of GH and reflects average serum GH concentration) combined with imaging of the pituitary gland with CT or MRI. The disease is most commonly found in male cats over the age of 10 years, and in addition to insulin resistance may be characterized by a change in facial features, organomegaly, widened interdental spaces and eventually signs of hypertension and renal failure.

Acromegaly is exceptionally rare in the dog; however, during the progesterone-dominated phase of dioestrus in entire females, in a physiological phenomenon unique to this species, GH is released into the circulation from the mammary glands. Thus, bitches in dioestrus may be susceptible to hyperglycaemia and even diabetes mellitus because both progesterone and GH will contribute to peripheral insulin resistance.

Pancreatitis

Acute and chronic pancreatitis can affect beta cell function, making animals more susceptible to hyperglycaemia. In addition, hyperglycaemia itself can worsen pancreatitis, and also damage the islets further – a phenomenon sometimes referred to as 'glucose toxicity'. Signs of acute pancreatitis in dogs and cats may include inappetence, vomiting, abdominal pain, diarrhoea and depression, but it can be especially difficult to detect acute pancreatitis clinically in cats because the signs may be very vague. In addition, in both dogs and cats, chronic pancreatitis may lead to only minor clinical signs while having a significant effect on endocrine and/or exocrine pancreatic function. Usually a combination of clinical signs, testing for markers of pancreatic inflammation such as canine or feline pancreatic lipase immunoreactivity, and diagnostic imaging such as pancreatic ultrasonography is sufficient to achieve a diagnosis (Xenoulis and Steiner, 2008; Mansfield, 2012; see Chapter 14 for further information on diagnosis).

Diagnostic approach to hyperglycaemia

A diagram illustrating a suggested approach to hypergly-aemia is shown in Figure 16.9. The significance of hyper-glycaemia in isolation, in a non-starved animal with no other clinical signs or biochemical abnormalities, must be determined by the clinician. Although it may simply relate to stress, as discussed, hyperglycaemia may imply a preclinical state of reduced pancreatic endocrine reserve (e.g. from chronic pancreatitis) or peripheral insulin resist-ance (e.g. an endocrinopathy, obesity in cats) which may eventually progress to diabetes, and therefore hyper-glycaemia should not be ignored.

Diabetes mellitus

Canine diabetes

Canine diabetes is usually the result of insulin deficiency and a classification scheme has been described, illustrated in Figure 16.10 (Catchpole et al., 2005). The disease has an esti-mated prevalence in the UK of 0.32% (Davison et al., 2005). In some cases insulin deficiency may be preceded by a phase of insulin resistance, but by the time of diagnosis most dogs

are unable to synthesize and secrete adequate amounts of endogenous insulin from the pancreatic beta cells in response to hyperglycaemia. Certain breeds are predisposed to the disease, such as the Samoyed, Tibetan Terrier and Cairn Terrier, whereas others have a reduced risk such as the Boxer, German Shepherd Dog and the Golden Retriever.

A small number of cases of canine diabetes mellitus (DM) are diagnosed when young animals (<6 months of age) become hyperglycaemic, and these are considered to be congenital in origin. As already discussed, the insulin resistance that precedes diagnosis in an estimated 20–40% of canine diabetic patients may be caused by exogenous corticosteroid or progestagen treatment, or endocrinopathies such as hyperadrenocorticism. Chronic hyperglycaemia in dogs has been shown to result in permanent beta cell damage and obesity may also con-tribute to insulin resistance in dogs. In addition, diabetes associated with pancreatitis may account for 28–40% of cases of canine DM, and is especially prevalent in DM cases with accompanying diabetic ketoacidosis (see later).

The remaining cases of canine DM are thought to be associated with pancreatic autoimmunity, similar to type 1 diabetes in humans, with serological evidence of reactiv-ity to pancreatic autoantigens being reported in a number of cases.

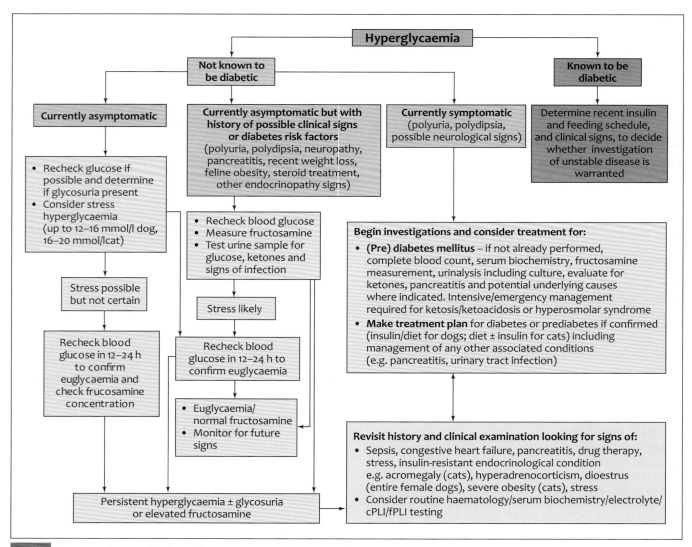

16.9 A suggested approach to hyperglycaemia. cPLI = canine pancreatic lipase immunoreactivity; fPLI = feline pancreatic lipase immunoreactivity.

Insulin deficiency diabetes (IDD)
Primary IDD in dogs is characterized by a progressive loss of pancreatic beta cells. The aetiology of beta cell deficiency/destruction in diabetic dogs is currently unknown but a number of disease processes are thought to be involved:
- Congenital beta cell hypoplasia/abiotrophy
- Beta cell loss associated with exocrine pancreatic disease
- Immune-mediated beta cell destruction
- Idiopathic

Insulin resistance diabetes (IRD)
Primary IRD usually results from antagonism of insulin function by other hormones:
- Dioestrous/gestational diabetes
- Secondary to other endocrine disorders:
  - Hyperadrenocorticism
  - Acromegaly
- Iatrogenic:
  - Synthetic glucocorticoids
  - Synthetic progestagens
- Glucose intolerance associated with obesity may contribute to insulin resistance but is not a primary cause of diabetes in dogs

16.10 Classification of canine diabetes mellitus.
(Data from Catchpole et al., 2005)

Feline diabetes

Feline DM has an estimated UK prevalence of 1 in 230 cats, and in contrast to canine DM is usually characterized by insulin resistance (Rand *et al.*, 2004). Feline DM appears to be more common with increasing age, and in certain breeds such as the Burmese (McCann *et al.*, 2007; Lederer *et al.*, 2009). The disease has a multifactorial aetiology which includes genetic factors and environmental influences such as obesity and physical inactivity, but the exact underlying cause is unclear because not all obese cats become diabetic. Other diseases can lead to diabetes in non-obese cats either directly via beta cell damage (e.g. pancreatic neoplasia or pancreatitis) or via insulin resistance (e.g. acromegaly or hyperadrenocorticism), as already discussed. In addition, just as in dogs, overt diabetes may be triggered by drug therapy with pharmacological agents which antagonize insulin, e.g. corticosteroids or progestagens.

Overt DM in cats usually results from a combination of impaired insulin secretion from the pancreatic beta cells in addition to peripheral insulin resistance. Most cats are thought to undergo a *prediabetic glucose-intolerant phase* before the islets are unable to keep up with the extra demand for insulin created by insulin resistance in the tissues. Diabetic cats may also present with 'dropped hocks' caused by a hyperglycaemia-associated peripheral neuropathy, which is often, gradually, reversible with treatment of the diabetes.

The phenomenon of a *remission* or 'honeymoon' phase once a diabetic cat is treated with insulin occurs because, in contrast to dogs, who are unlikely to have any islets left at the time of diagnosis, feline diabetic patients usually have impaired islet function rather than absolute loss of beta cells at diagnosis. Hence diabetic remission, when it occurs, is the result of beta cell recovery as the blood glucose is controlled by exogenous insulin. Recent studies suggest that achievement of remission may be facilitated by a restricted carbohydrate diet and intensive insulin therapy to maintain blood glucose within tight limits.

Confirmation of a diagnosis of diabetes

In both dogs and cats, the diagnosis of diabetes mellitus is confirmed by the presence of appropriate clinical signs, persistent hyperglycaemia, glycosuria and an elevated serum fructosamine concentration. It can be challenging to differentiate chronic stress from prediabetes or diabetes mellitus in cats because both cause hyperglycaemia and can lead to glycosuria. Persistent hyperglycaemia in a cat aged 7 years or older, in combination with obesity, a history of exocrine pancreatic disease, recent weight loss, polyphagia or polydipsia should raise suspicion of diabetes mellitus and prompt measurement of serum fructosamine concentration. If fructosamine is elevated this confirms diabetes mellitus; however, mild elevations can occur early in the course of diabetes or with chronic stress in cats, so sometimes fructosamine measurement may have to be repeated after 1–2 weeks. Evaluation of glucose in a urine sample collected in a stress-free manner at home may also help to distinguish genuine insulin resistance from diabetes or prediabetes, because a lack of glycosuria implies a non-stressed blood glucose concentration below 12–14 mmol/l. Urinalysis in diabetic patients usually reveals glycosuria in addition to possible ketonuria. Urine sediment analysis may demonstrate evidence of urinary tract infection, although infection may be asymptomatic. Therefore, urine culture is recommended in all diabetic patients at diagnosis, because glycosuria predisposes to bacterial infection. Urine specific gravity may be higher than expected in a polyuric diabetic patient because of the presence of a high concentration of glucose.

Compatible serum biochemical abnormalities in untreated diabetic dogs and cats often include mild prerenal azotaemia, as a result of dehydration, and moderate to marked elevations in liver enzymes, cholesterol and triglycerides associated with secondary lipidosis. In dogs, marked elevations in alkaline phosphatase (ALP) can be seen as a result of diabetes alone; this is not always the result of concurrent hyperadrenocorticism. Further investigation for the cause of liver enzyme elevation may be required if liver enzyme concentrations do not reduce once diabetes mellitus is stabilized. In particular, it is recommended that diagnostic testing for hyperadrenocorticism is not undertaken concurrently with diabetes stabilization unless convincing clinical signs are present, because stress may lead to a false positive diagnosis. Further investigation for pancreatitis by measurement of canine or feline pancreatic lipase immunoreactivity (PLI) is indicated at the time of diagnosis of diabetes and is especially important if there are compatible clinical signs such as abdominal discomfort, vomiting or inappetence.

In untreated diabetic patients, further changes may also be apparent on measurement of serum electrolytes, particularly in patients who are developing ketosis or ketoacidosis. In addition to metabolic acidosis, most animals with diabetic ketoacidosis have total body sodium depletion, but serum sodium levels may be high (reflecting dehydration), normal or low (as a result of hyperosmolality causing water to shift into the vascular space, leading to dilutional hyponatraemia). Insulin deficiency and acidosis can also cause movement of potassium from the intracellular to the extracellular fluid so diabetic animals, especially those with ketoacidosis, may be hyperkalaemic prior to treatment, despite whole-body depletion of potassium. Many untreated diabetic patients are also hypochloraemic due to renal loss of chloride alongside hydrogen ions.

Monitoring of diabetes mellitus

For optimal clinical management, all canine and feline diabetic patients should be examined regularly. It is particularly important to monitor cats very carefully and frequently after the instigation of insulin treatment because there is a risk of hypoglycaemia as the beta cells recover from glucose toxicity. Once stabilized, diabetic patients should be examined at least every 3 months.

Clinical signs

It is helpful if owners are able to keep records of appetite, demeanour and water intake, and regular appointments are important to monitor the health of the diabetic patient once stabilized, so that any problems with instability can be detected early. Specific issues which may arise during treatment and affect glucose control include poor dental health, urinary tract infection and formation of fatty or fibrotic lumps at injection sites.

Water intake over 24 hours

Measurement of water intake at home over 24 hours, performed on a regular basis, provides an excellent and cheap method of monitoring in single-animal households.

Urine testing

If owners are able to collect urine easily from their dog or cat, urine glucose measurement offers a further method of assessing glycaemic control, because semi-quantitative dipsticks allow assessment of glycosuria and ketonuria. It is, however, important that urine glucose is assessed at the same time of day on each occasion, preferably in the morning, and that values are interpreted alongside other clinical data. A small amount of urine glucose in a morning sample is acceptable, but if the amount rises in a consistent pattern or ketones are also present, the owner should be instructed to seek veterinary advice. Conversely, if no glucose is detected in a morning urine sample, then it is possible that the dog or cat is at risk of hypoglycaemia and the insulin dose should be reviewed. Urinary glucose measurements, however, must be interpreted in the light of other clinical findings and not used as the sole means of adjusting insulin dose because glycosuria may reflect inadequate duration of insulin activity rather than inadequate dose.

Glucose measurement

Ideally, in treated diabetic dogs, blood glucose should be maintained between 5 and 10–12 mmol/l, and in treated cats between 5 and 14–16 mmol/l, for the majority of the day.

Fructosamine measurement

Regular fructosamine measurements are useful to show trends in glycaemic control within an individual patient. Reference ranges and guidelines vary among laboratories so it is important to be consistent when comparing samples longitudinally. High fructosamine concentration implies poor glycaemic control over the preceding 1–2 weeks, and low or normal fructosamine concentration may be consistent with periods of hypoglycaemia.

Investigation of unstable diabetes mellitus

The aims of therapy in canine and feline diabetes mellitus include:

- Resolution of clinical signs (e.g. polyuria and polydipsia)
- Maintenance of a good appetite and stable bodyweight
- Owner perception that the patient has a good quality of life and is able to undertake a reasonable amount of daily exercise
- Minimal complications, such as ketosis, neuropathy hypoglycaemia, infections and cataracts.

It is important to note that most of these aims are subjective and can be achieved in some animals despite small elevations in fructosamine and intermittent mild glycosuria. However, where patients are losing weight, remain polyuric or polydipsic, have frequent periods of inappetence or have hypoglycaemic episodes, then investigation of diabetic instability is warranted. This must be undertaken in a methodical fashion and a suggested approach to the management of unstable diabetes is outlined in Figure 16.11.

Stage 1. History: factors relating to treatment and management
• Insulin type, dose, storage, handling, injection technique, feeding, diet, exercise, monitoring • Check bitches have been spayed • Look for evidence of concurrent disease, e.g. vomiting, urinary signs, abdominal pain, and check whether any other treatment is being given which may antagonize insulin, e.g. topical steroids • In cats, determine whether periods of remission have previously occurred and how long they lasted
Stage 2. Clinical examination
• Full physical examination including lymph node palpation, rectal examination (prostate gland, anal sacs), dental, ophthalmological and neurological examinations, measure blood pressure
Stage 3. Problem list and differential diagnoses
• Include all abnormalities discovered during history and clinical examination • Consider and investigate any differential diagnoses that might not be related to diabetes mellitus (e.g. renal disease, malignancy)
Stage 4. Evaluation of potential underlying causes of poor glycaemic control
• Baseline information: Blood glucose curve in practice, at home or using continuous monitoring (is the patient responding to insulin? How long is the insulin lasting? Is the nadir dangerous?), urinalysis (including culture), routine haematology, serum biochemistry
Stage 5. Categorization of possible mechanism of instability with special testing only if appropriate clinical signs
• Rule out management factors, e.g. insulin storage, injection technique, feeding (history) **If patient is receiving a high insulin dose (usually >1.5 IU/kg per injection):** • Rule out Somogyi overswing (history ± blood glucose curve) • Rule out infection or inflammation – particularly pancreatitis, urinary tract infection, dental disease (history, clinical examination, blood glucose curve, urine culture, cPLI, TLI, diagnostic imaging – radiography and ultrasonography) • Rule out hormonal antagonism, e.g. progesterone, hypo- or hyperadrenocorticism, hypo- or hyperthyroidism, acromegaly (reproductive and clinical history, ACTH simulation test, T4/TSH ratio, IGF-1 measurement), exogenous steroids or progestagens **If patient is showing erratic response to insulin:** • Investigate the possibility of poor insulin activity – test response to intramuscular dose of soluble insulin **If poor response:** • Recheck for infection, inflammation, hormonal antagonism. If good, consider change of insulin preparation or route of delivery **If good response:** • Consider a change of insulin preparation or route of delivery

16.11 A suggested approach to the management of unstable diabetes mellitus. ACTH = adrenocorticotropic hormone; cPLI = canine pancreatic lipase immunoreactivity; IGF = insulin-like growth factor; T4 = thyroxine; TLI = trypsin-like immunoreactivity; TSH = thyroid-stimulating hormone.

History and clinical examination

The importance of an accurate and thorough history and clinical examination in the unstable diabetic patient cannot be overemphasized, in addition to a problem-orientated approach. No amount of laboratory testing or diagnostic imaging will substitute for a long and detailed conversation with the owner about the patient, the timing and reasoning behind dose adjustments, the clinical signs and the practicalities of insulin administration, insulin storage, feeding, exercise, administration of other drug treatments and potential clinical signs of other diseases.

Laboratory testing

Routine haematology and serum biochemistry, as well as urinalysis (including urine culture, since urinary tract infection may be a cause or consequence of poor glycaemic control) are useful in ruling out other causes of weight loss, polyuria or polydipsia and highlighting abnormalities which may be present as a result of other diseases, e.g. hypercalcaemia, neutrophilia and azotaemia.

Blood glucose curves

Blood glucose curves (Figure 16.12) may also be important in understanding how well a patient is responding to treatment, but must be interpreted with caution. However, research has shown that blood glucose curves show considerable day-to-day variability, even in stable diabetic patients. In addition, following an event such as a hypoglycaemic episode, the blood glucose curve may be significantly affected by other factors such as the adrenergic response, discussed

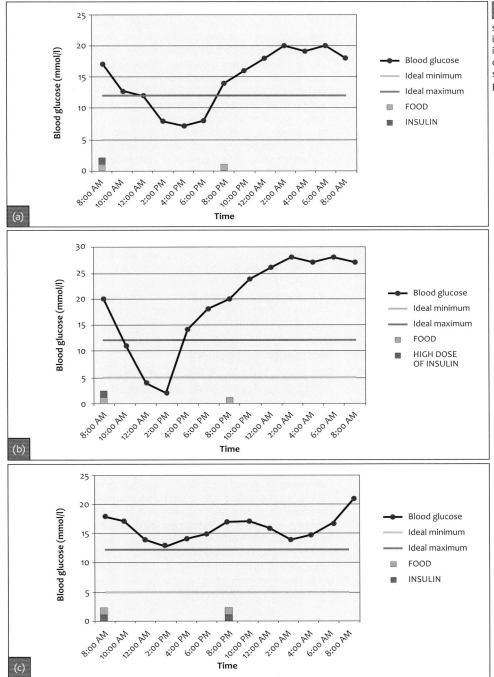

16.12 Blood glucose curves in the dog. (a) Blood glucose curve showing inadequate duration of action of insulin. (b) Blood glucose curve showing insulin-induced hyperglycaemia (Somogyi overswing). (c) Blood glucose curve showing inadequate insulin response in a patient with a urinary tract infection.

earlier in this chapter (Alt *et al.*, 2007; Sieber-Ruckstuhl *et al.*, 2008). Nonetheless, blood glucose curves can give important information in certain patients, provided the animals do not become too stressed or fail to eat during the process.

The main questions to be addressed by obtaining a curve include:

- Whether the insulin is working consistently
- How long the insulin is lasting
- Whether the nadir concentration of glucose is dangerously low.

Although the schematic figures on the previous page illustrate glucose curves with lines in between each point, in clinical practice, it is important to avoid 'joining up' the various points on an hourly or 2-hourly curve with lines, because this makes an assumption that no peaks or troughs are occurring in between samples, and can be misleading. It is also important to wait for several days for a patient to 'equilibrate' to a new insulin dose before obtaining a curve, for example by sending them home for a few days in between repeated curves, if it is safe and practical to do so.

Causes of diabetic instability
Management factors

Problems with injection technique, insulin storage, diet or exercise can only be discovered by discussion with the owner and are an important cause of poor glycaemic control.

Short duration of insulin action

A glucose curve illustrating inadequate duration of action of insulin and ideal glycaemic control is illustrated in Figure 16.12a. An inadequate duration of action will be avoided by switching once-daily treated patients to twice-daily insulin if they appear to be unstable. Patients that would benefit from such a change can be usually be identified by their history of instability on once-daily insulin, frequent morning hyperglycaemia and glycosuria, and history of overnight polyuria and polydipsia. In rare cases, insulin may last less than 8 hours and a long-acting PZI preparation may be required if treatment three times a day is not practical, although at present there is no PZI insulin licensed for veterinary use in the UK.

Insulin-induced hyperglycaemia (Somogyi overswing)

A glucose curve illustrating a Somogyi overswing is illustrated in Figure 16.12b, although owing to day-to-day variability in blood glucose curves, and the effects of hormones which counteract hypoglycaemia as discussed below, this phenomenon is not always apparent with serial blood samples.

The administration of a high dose of insulin (usually >1.5 IU/kg) once daily can lead to the phenomenon of a paradoxical insulin-induced hyperglycaemia. This occurs because of the rapid drop in blood glucose caused by the high insulin dose. As discussed earlier in this chapter, the body's natural response to a low blood glucose (usually below 3.5 mmol/l), particularly if it has occurred rapidly, is to counteract this with the secretion of a combination of hormones and activate the sympathetic nervous system to antagonize the hypoglycaemic effect of insulin, often raising blood glucose to very high levels (>20 mmol/l) for several hours to days afterwards.

As this 'overswing' effect is not always apparent on blood glucose curves, other factors such as the history must also be used to determine whether this is the cause of instability in a patient. If a Somogyi overswing is detected or suspected, then switching to 0.5 IU/kg insulin twice daily and making small adjustments every 3–5 days from that point is recommended.

Infection or inflammation

A glucose curve illustrating glycaemic control in a patient with a urinary tract infection is illustrated in Figure 16.12c. It is important to note that this type of pattern may also be seen early in the course of treatment, before the optimal insulin dose is reached, and does not necessarily require intense investigation if the insulin dose is still in the 0.5–1.0 IU/kg per injection range.

Infection and inflammation are very common causes of poor glycaemic control in diabetic dogs and cats. Any focus of infection or inflammation can result in insulin resistance in a diabetic patient and signs may be very obvious, e.g. a cat-bite abscess, or very subtle, e.g. a low-grade urinary tract infection. Bacterial or fungal infection can result in a vicious circle because it causes insulin resistance and worsens hyperglycaemia, which in turn can exacerbate infection. Screening for infection or inflammation can include routine haematology, urinalysis (ideally collected by cystocentesis) and diagnostic imaging (e.g. thoracic radiography, abdominal ultrasonography), as well as other more specific tests if indicated by the history and clinical signs (e.g. blood culture, joint aspirates, pancreatic enzyme measurement, echocardiography, rhinoscopy). Pancreatitis is another common potential complication of canine and feline diabetes, and can cause 'brittle' glycaemic control. During the history taking, should there be any suggestion that the patient has 'off days' or has experienced any signs of abdominal pain, consideration should be given to assessment for pancreatitis (see Chapter 14), as previously discussed. In diabetic patients with pancreatitis, there is also a risk of the development of exocrine pancreatic insufficiency over time, which may also affect glycaemic control.

Hormonal antagonism

As already discussed, many hormones can antagonize the effect of insulin, including corticosteroids, growth hormone and progestagens, and hypothyroid dogs can also suffer from insulin resistance. Excess hormone may be endogenously produced or administered exogenously – even topical treatment can destabilize an otherwise well controlled patient. Hormonal antagonism usually leads to insulin resistance (defined as poorly controlled signs in a patient receiving an insulin dose of >2.2 IU/kg/injection where a Somogyi overswing has been ruled out (see above)). If insulin resistance is present along with signs of any endocrinopathy, as already discussed, appropriate further testing should be carried out such as an adrenocorticotropic hormone (ACTH) stimulation test for hyperadrenocorticism, thyroxine (T4)/thyroid-stimulating hormone (TSH) measurement for hypothyroidism or insulin-like growth factor (IGF)-1 measurement for acromegaly.

Inadequate insulin activity

If other causes of insulin resistance (infection, inflammation, hormonal antagonism) and management factors have been ruled out as discussed above, it is possible that the insulin is being antagonized by some other mechanism in the periphery or that the insulin is being poorly absorbed, although very few practical tests exist to confirm this. Insulin may be poorly absorbed subcutaneously, and assessment of the glycaemic response (every 30 minutes for 2–3 hours) to a test dose of 0.2 IU/kg neutral (soluble) insulin given by the intramuscular route may be useful. This is especially useful if the skin has become thickened at the site of insulin injection.

Anti-insulin antibodies, induced by the injected insulin being from a 'foreign' species, are often quoted as a cause of insulin resistance. In practice, however, recent research has shown that, although anti-insulin antibodies are present in the majority of dogs who have received heterologous bovine insulin therapy, they do not appear to be generally associated with instability or deleterious side effects (Davison et al., 2008), and such antibodies are rare in cats (Hoenig et al., 2000). In addition, the prevalence of anti-insulin antibodies in the canine diabetic population is likely to be reducing as there is no longer a bovine insulin preparation licensed for dogs.

Diabetic ketosis, ketoacidosis and non-ketotic hyperosmolar syndrome

Diagnosis of diabetic ketoacidosis

Diabetic ketoacidosis (DKA) is a serious and life-threatening complication of chronic hyperglycaemia due to diabetes. Insulin deficiency, cellular glucose starvation and an excess of diabetogenic hormones such as glucagon result in hyperglycaemia, mobilization of free fatty acids and formation of ketones (acetoacetate and beta-hydroxybutyrate) as an alternative energy source for tissues (Sieber-Ruckstuhl et al., 2008; Usher-Smith et al., 2011). This results in ketosis and eventually progresses to acidosis. Ketones cause vomiting by direct stimulation of the chemoreceptor trigger zone and ketonuria worsens osmotic diuresis, as well as promoting urinary loss of sodium and potassium. A ketotic episode in an otherwise stable patient is usually precipitated by either a treatment failure (e.g. missed insulin injections) or concurrent disease (e.g. pancreatitis, infection, renal disease), although DKA may be present at the time of initial diagnosis. Dogs and cats are susceptible to DKA, but the condition appears more common in dogs, most likely because cats often have some islet tissue remaining, which is able to secrete a small amount of 'protective' endogenous insulin.

Clinical signs of ketoacidosis include acute depression, weakness, dehydration, vomiting, tachypnoea (due to respiratory compensation for metabolic acidosis) and a smell of acetone. Confirmation of the diagnosis can be achieved by detection of the ketone acetoacetate with a urine dipstick or, alternatively, more sensitive assessment can be achieved by measurement of the ketone beta-hydroxybutyrate in serum or plasma at an external laboratory. It is also important to evaluate the patient for possible precipitating causes of DKA such as urinary tract infection or pancreatitis.

In addition to severe hyperglycaemia, laboratory findings in DKA include:

* Ketonaemia
* Ketonuria (be aware, as previously mentioned, that urine test strips will detect acetoacetate but will not detect beta-hydroxybutyrate)
* Marked metabolic acidosis, with increased anion gap (blood pH of less than 7.10–7.15, and bicarbonate (HCO_3^-) values in the range 8–12 mmol/l)
* Non-regenerative anaemia, left shift neutrophilia, or thrombocytosis in 50% of cases (Bruskiewicz et al., 1997; Hume et al., 2006)
* Occasionally marked red blood cell Heinz body formation (cats)
* Prerenal azotaemia (more common in cats than dogs)
* Initial hyperkalaemia (due to decreased renal excretion and acidosis), which may then develop into hypokalaemia as insulin treatment is instigated and potassium is driven into cells along with glucose (Bruskiewicz et al., 1997; Hume et al., 2006)
* Hypophosphataemia may also develop with treatment, when phosphate shifts from the intracellular space to the extracellular space, and this increases the risk of haemolytic anaemia or seizures (Willard et al., 1987).

Measurement of beta-hydroxybutyrate (blood) and acetoacetate (urine) can be used to monitor the progress of the patient with DKA. In the early phase of treatment, an apparent increase in urinary dipstick ketones may actually be indicative of successful therapy as the most prevalent ketone, beta-hydroxybutyrate, is broken down to acetoacetate.

An important differential diagnosis for DKA is *non-ketotic hyperosmolar syndrome* (NKHS), which appears very similar clinically and biochemically to DKA but there is an absence of ketones. NKHS is a complication of diabetes defined by extreme hyperglycaemia (>30 mmol/l), hyperosmolality (>350 mOsm/l), severe dehydration, central nervous system (CNS) depression, no ketone body formation and absent or mild metabolic acidosis (Macintire, 1995). Plasma sodium can be low, normal or high and the clinical signs are the consequence of an elevation in plasma solutes such as glucose, chloride and urea. Clinical management is broadly similar to that for DKA but it can be more challenging to monitor progress in the absence of detectable ketones to measure.

Case examples

CASE 1

SIGNALMENT

14-year-old male neutered Domestic Shorthair cat in overweight body condition.

HISTORY

The cat was presented for a dental scale and polish. Pre-anaesthetic blood tests were performed as the owner was also concerned that the cat might be drinking slightly more than usual. Clinical examination was unremarkable apart from dental disease.

CLINICAL PATHOLOGY DATA

Haematology	Result	Reference interval
RBC (x 10¹²/l)	7.8	6.7–11.0
Hb (g/dl)	13	11–17
HCT (l/l)	0.40	0.31–0.46
MCV (fl)	41	39–53
MCH (pg)	22.0	19.5–24.5
MCHC (g/dl)	22	20–25
WBC (x 10⁹/l)	**20.0**	5.5–19.5
Neutrophils (segmented) (x 10⁹/l)	**19.4**	3.0–11.5
Neutrophils (band) (x 10⁹/l)	0	0–0.3
Lymphocytes (x 10⁹/l)	**0.1**	1.0–4.8
Monocytes (x 10⁹/l)	0.4	0.2–1.5
Eosinophils (x 10⁹/l)	0.1	0.1–1.3
Basophils (x 10⁹/l)	0	0
Platelets (x 10⁹/l)	180	175–500

Abnormal results are in **bold**.

Biochemistry	Result	Reference interval
Sodium (mmol/l)	136	135–155
Potassium (mmol/l)	3.9	3.6–5.8
Chloride (mmol/l)	119	117–123
Glucose (mmol/l)	**18.9**	3.8–8.3
Urea (mmol/l)	3.8	2.5–7.0
Creatinine (µmol/l)	121	40–130
Calcium (mmol/l)	2.3	2.0–3.0
Inorganic phosphate (mmol/l)	1.3	0.8–1.6
Total protein (g/l)	56	55–77
Albumin (g/l)	23	23–40
Globulin (g/l)	32	24–45
ALT (IU/l)	**28**	10–25
ALP (IU/l)	**49**	0–40
GGT (IU/l)	5	0–5
Cholesterol (mmol/l)	**4.6**	2.0–3.9

Abnormal results are in **bold**.

WHAT ABNORMALITIES ARE PRESENT?

Haematology

- Neutrophilia.
- Lymphopenia.

Biochemistry

- Hyperglycaemia.
- Mildly increased alkaline phosphatase (ALP) and alanine aminotransferase (ALT).
- Increased cholesterol.

HOW WOULD YOU INTERPRET THESE RESULTS AND WHAT ARE THE LIKELY DIFFERENTIAL DIAGNOSES?

The haematology profile is consistent with a stress leucogram, but neutrophilia may also be caused by infection or inflammation (e.g. dental disease).

The hyperglycaemia is a concern, especially in view of the fact that the owner reports a possibility of polydipsia, as it may reflect undiagnosed diabetes mellitus. However, if the cat was stressed at the time of blood sampling, it is possible that this simply reflects stress hyperglycaemia. The mild increase in liver enzymes is most likely secondary either to the dental disease as a result of a reactive hepatopathy or due to diabetes mellitus if present. Increased cholesterol may be postprandial or due to endocrine disease.

WHAT FURTHER TESTS WOULD YOU RECOMMEND?

In the first instance, if practical, it would be advisable to perform urinalysis to confirm glycosuria and check for ketones. Measurement of serum fructosamine is recommended as the most important test, to determine whether there has been consistent hyperglycaemia over the preceding 2–3 weeks.

Urinalysis	Result
Specific gravity	1.040
Dipstick analysis	No blood, protein or ketones Glucose +++

Additional measurement	Result
Fructosamine	**493** µmol/l (<350 µmol/l in normoglycaemic cats)

HOW WOULD YOU INTERPRET THESE RESULTS AND WHAT ARE THE LIKELY DIFFERENTIAL DIAGNOSES?

The urinalysis confirms the presence of glucose in the urine and is supportive of a diagnosis of diabetes mellitus, but fructosamine is required for confirmation of persistent hyperglycaemia. Importantly there are no ketones. Although chronic stress can lead to mild elevations in fructosamine, the clearly elevated fructosamine measurement here, combined with clinical signs of polydipsia and raised blood glucose, confirms a diagnosis of diabetes mellitus. The raised liver enzymes and cholesterol are likely to be secondary to hepatic changes associated with the diabetes.

→ CASE 1 CONTINUED

WHAT ADVICE WOULD YOU GIVE THE OWNER?

It would be advisable to delay the dental procedure after the initial blood tests until the diagnosis is established. It is likely that the fact that this cat is obese has contributed to the development of diabetes, although consideration should be given to other potential underlying causes such as pancreatitis and acromegaly. Control of diabetes mellitus can be achieved in cats with a combination of dietary and insulin therapy, and it will be important to reschedule the dental procedure once therapy has been initiated, because poor dental hygiene can compromise glycaemic control.

CASE 2

SIGNALMENT

5-year-old (estimated) female neutered Jack Russell Terrier in poor body condition.

HISTORY

The dog was presented after several days boarding in a rescue centre. During that time, she had been inappetent and had developed haemorrhagic diarrhoea. She had become progressively weaker and was now collapsed.

On clinical examination the dog was dehydrated but her temperature, pulse and respiratory rate were within normal limits. She was markedly depressed and had mild abdominal discomfort on palpation. Her mucous membranes were pink, with a capillary refill time of <2 seconds. The remainder of the clinical examination was within normal limits.

CLINICAL PATHOLOGY DATA

Haematology	Result	Reference interval
RBC (x 10¹²/l)	6.3	5.5–8.5
Hb (g/dl)	14.0	12.0–18.0
HCT (l/l)	0.44	0.37–0.55
MCV (fl)	66	60–77
MCH (pg)	22.1	19.5–24.5
MCHC (g/dl)	36	32–37
WBC (x 10⁹/l)	9.0	6–17
Neutrophils (segmented) (x 10⁹/l)	**2.9**	3.0–11.5
Neutrophils (band) (x 10⁹/l)	0	0–0.3
Lymphocytes (x 10⁹/l)	**5.0**	1.0–4.8
Monocytes (x 10⁹/l)	0.6	0.2–1.5
Eosinophils (x 10⁹/l)	1.1	0.1–1.3
Basophils (x 10⁹/l)	0	0
Platelets (x 10⁹/l)	278	175–500

Abnormal results are in **bold**.

Film comment: occasional toxic neutrophil. No left shift.

Biochemistry	Result	Reference interval
Sodium (mmol/l)	145	135–155
Potassium (mmol/l)	4.2	3.5–5.8
Chloride (mmol/l)	99	95–115
Glucose (mmol/l)	**2.3**	3.3–5.5
Urea (mmol/l)	**9.0**	2.5–8.5
Creatinine (μmol/l)	124	45–155
Calcium (mmol/l)	2.8	2.3–3.0
Inorganic phosphate (mmol/l)	1.6	1.3–1.9
Total protein (g/l)	66	50–78
Albumin (g/l)	26	25–35
Globulin (g/l)	39	25–40
ALT (IU/l)	67	0–90
ALP (IU/l)	224	0–230
GGT (IU/l)	12	0–20
Cholesterol (mmol/l)	6.9	2.0–7.0

Abnormal results are in **bold**.

WHAT ABNORMALITIES ARE PRESENT?

Haematology
- Neutropenia (mild).
- Lymphocytosis (mild).

Biochemistry
- Hypoglycaemia.
- Elevation in urea (mild).

HOW WOULD YOU INTERPRET THESE RESULTS AND WHAT ARE THE LIKELY DIFFERENTIAL DIAGNOSES?

Unusually, for a collapsed dog with haemorrhagic diarrhoea, the haematology profile is not consistent with a stress leucogram. This finding would be consistent with cortisol deficiency, but classical hypoadrenocorticism (deficiency of cortisol and aldosterone) is unlikely because the electrolytes are within normal limits. Neutropenia can also be associated with bone marrow disease and increased consumption/sequestration of neutrophils in bacterial infections.

The hypoglycaemia is a concern, especially in a stressed animal, and may be contributing to the depressed presentation. The mild urea elevation could be consistent with dehydration or gastrointestinal bleeding.

→ CASE 2 CONTINUED

At this stage, if hypoglycaemia is confirmed on a fresh (non-stored) sample, the main differential diagnoses for this patient include bacterial infection, insulinoma, atypical hypoadrenocorticism (cortisol deficiency), neoplasia, gastrointestinal disease/malabsorption, toxin exposure or glycogen storage disease. In the presence of normal urea, liver enzymes and albumin concentrations, liver disease is an unlikely cause of the hypoglycaemia.

The haemorrhagic diarrhoea may be a consequence of one of the diseases listed above (e.g. bacterial infection, atypical hypoadrenocorticism, neoplasia or toxin exposure) but may also be unrelated to the hypoglycaemia. Although there are no clinical signs of pyrexia the case should be handled as a potential infectious disease and nursed in isolation, if possible, because vaccination status, travel history and in-contact dogs are all unknown.

WHAT FURTHER TESTS WOULD YOU RECOMMEND?

The age of the dog is uncertain, and although insulinomas usually occur in older dogs, it would be useful to rule out a beta cell tumour here, especially because this might affect the capacity of the shelter to rehome the dog. This can be evaluated by measuring blood glucose and insulin in the same blood sample. If insulin is raised, or at the upper end of normal, in the presence of hypoglycaemia this is inappropriate and strongly suggestive of an insulinoma.

In addition, an ACTH stimulation test is recommended, because patients with *atypical* hypoadrenocorticism may show signs only of cortisol deficiency (including hypoglycaemia) in the absence of electrolyte changes.

There are several other potential courses of action here, as well as symptomatic management and supportive care of the patient. Faecal analysis for bacteria and parasites is indicated and diagnostic imaging may help to determine other underlying causes of the gastrointestinal signs. In addition, fructosamine measurement could be used to determine whether the hypoglycaemia has been chronic.

Insulin and glucose measurement:

Glucose	**2.2** mmol/l	(3.3–5.5 mmol/l)
Insulin	**<8.3** IU/ml	(8.3–29 IU/ml)

ACTH stimulation test:

Cortisol pre-ACTH	**<20** nmol/l	(50–250 nmol/l)
Cortisol post-ACTH	**<20** nmol/l	(50–400 nmol/l)

HOW WOULD YOU INTERPRET THESE RESULTS AND WHAT ARE THE LIKELY DIFFERENTIAL DIAGNOSES?

The insulin and glucose measurements are not supportive of a diagnosis of insulinoma. The ACTH stimulation test confirms lack of cortisol as the cause of the hypoglycaemia, giving a diagnosis of atypical hypoadrenocorticism.

WHAT ADVICE WOULD YOU GIVE?

The clinical signs are all likely to be related to cortisol deficiency, precipitated by the stressful experience of being in kennels. Supportive care to correct the dehydration and a daily replacement dose of corticosteroid (prednisolone) should result in complete control of the clinical signs, but the prednisolone will need to be continued indefinitely.

CASE 3

SIGNALMENT

10-year-old Cavalier King Charles Spaniel (weight 10 kg, average body condition).

HISTORY

The dog had been receiving 10 IU Caninsulin twice daily for treatment of diabetes mellitus for approximately 18 months. The dog also had a history of intermittent episodes of acute pancreatitis, resulting in abdominal pain and inappetence, although the most recent episode had been more than 12 months previously. The dog was presented because there had been a recent increase in thirst (2–3 weeks) and weight loss, as well as increased frequency of urination over the past 7 days. Clinical examination was unremarkable apart from the development of early diabetes-related cataracts bilaterally. Routine haematology and serum biochemistry were performed on a blood sample taken 5 hours after insulin and feeding.

CLINICAL PATHOLOGY DATA

Haematology	Result	Reference interval
RBC (x 10^{12}/l)	7.1	5.5–8.5
Hb (g/dl)	14	12–18
HCT (l/l)	0.47	0.37–0.55
MCV (fl)	65	60–77
MCH (pg)	22.2	19.5–24.5
MCHC (g/dl)	35	32–37
WBC (x 10^9/l)	**22**	6–17
Neutrophils (segmented) (x 10^9/l)	**18**	3.0–11.5
Neutrophils (band) (x 10^9/l)	0	0–0.3
Lymphocytes (x 10^9/l)	1	1–4.8
Monocytes (x 10^9/l)	0.7	0.2–1.5
Eosinophils (x 10^9/l)	0.1	0.1–1.3
Basophils (x 10^9/l)	0	0
Platelets (x 10^9/l)	179	175–500

Abnormal results are in **bold**.

→ CASE 3 CONTINUED

Biochemistry	Result	Reference interval
Sodium (mmol/l)	139	135–155
Potassium (mmol/l)	4.9	3.5–5.8
Chloride (mmol/l)	103	95–115
Glucose (mmol/l)	**22.9**	3.3–5.5
Urea (mmol/l)	8.0	2.5–8.5
Creatinine (μmol/l)	124	45–155
Calcium (mmol/l)	2.4	2.3–3.0
Inorganic phosphate (mmol/l)	1.3	1.3–1.9
Total protein (g/l)	69	50–78
Albumin (g/l)	33	25–35
Globulin (g/l)	36	25–40
ALT (IU/l)	**170**	0–90
ALP (IU/l)	**309**	0–230
GGT (IU/l)	19	0–20
Cholesterol (mmol/l)	**8.0**	2.0–7.0

Abnormal results are in **bold**.

WHAT ABNORMALITIES ARE PRESENT?

Haematology
- Neutrophilia.

Biochemistry
- Hyperglycaemia.
- Elevated ALP, ALT and cholesterol.

HOW WOULD YOU INTERPRET THESE RESULTS AND WHAT ARE THE LIKELY DIFFERENTIAL DIAGNOSES?

The haematology profile is consistent with a stress leucogram, although it could be associated with infectious or inflammatory disease.

The hyperglycaemia is a concern as it is above the level expected in a well-controlled diabetic dog and would lead to clinical signs of polyuria and compensatory polydipsia. There are no other laboratory abnormalities which would explain the polyuria and polydipsia (e.g. hypercalcaemia, renal disease). The mild elevations in liver enzymes and cholesterol are likely to be secondary to diabetic hepatopathy.

The haematology and biochemistry suggest that the diabetes has become unstable but do not give a clear indication of why this is. The most likely causes of poor glycaemic control are practical issues associated with insulin injections, infection, inflammation, hormonal antagonism (although there are no signs of other endocrinopathies in this case), poor insulin absorption (although there are no reports of lumps or fibrosis at injection sites here) or Somogyi overswing (which is unlikely because insulin is being given twice daily at 1 IU/kg and the dose has not been changed recently).

WHAT FURTHER TESTS WOULD YOU RECOMMEND?

It would be useful to measure fructosamine concentration and compare this to the fructosamine concentration the last time the dog's diabetes was considered to be well controlled symptomatically. A thorough review of the history and evaluation of whether there are any practical factors associated with the current level of poor glycaemic control (e.g. incorrect injection technique, change in routine) is indicated in this case.

Complete urinalysis is essential to check for urinary tract infection as a cause or consequence of poor glycaemic control. It would also be useful to evaluate pancreatic inflammatory markers in this dog, in case a pancreatitis flare-up is contributing to the apparent poor control of blood glucose.

If no clear cause for the apparent poor response to insulin can be found, a blood glucose curve and diagnostic imaging should be considered.

Fructosamine:
> Fructosamine at presentation
> **521** μmol/l　　　(<400 μmol/l for good control)
> Fructosamine 2 months earlier
> **420** μmol/l　　　(<400 μmol/l for good control)

Urinalysis performed on a sample collected by cystocentesis:
> Specific gravity　1.032
> Dipstick analysis　No protein or ketones
> 　　　　　　　　　　Glucose +++, Blood ++
> Sediment　　　　　Struvite crystalluria
> Culture　　　　　　White cells and bacteria seen
> 　　　　　　　　　　Moderate growth of *Escherichia coli* sensitive to multiple antibiotics

Pancreatic inflammatory marker:
> Canine pancreatic lipase immunoreactivity
> **512** μg/l (201–399 μg/l possible pancreatitis, >400 μg/l consistent with pancreatitis)

HOW WOULD YOU INTERPRET THESE RESULTS AND WHAT ARE THE LIKELY DIFFERENTIAL DIAGNOSES?

The fructosamine confirms a trend of worsening glycaemic control and the urinalysis confirms urinary tract infection which will be contributing to the clinical signs.

The cPLI also provides valuable information about ongoing pancreatic inflammation, and would be consistent with pancreatitis, another potential cause of the worsening response to insulin.

It is impossible to determine whether the urinary tract infection is the primary cause of the insulin resistance or whether this arose secondarily. Secondary urinary tract infection can arise as a consequence of glycosuria, which itself may arise from any number of infectious or inflammatory conditions leading to insulin resistance. Whether it is primary or secondary, the presence of a urinary tract infection in a diabetic patient will exacerbate any problems with glycaemic control.

WHAT ADVICE WOULD YOU GIVE?

The urinary tract infection will need a suitable course of antibiotics and confirmation by culture and sediment analysis after 2–3 weeks that the infection and crystalluria have resolved. There is no need to change the insulin dose at this stage if a convincing underlying cause of the clinical signs and hyperglycaemia has been identified. Since struvite crystals are present, diagnostic imaging to check for struvite uroliths should also be considered because these could act as a nidus for future infections. Chronic pancreatitis can be managed symptomatically and with a low-fat diet. In addition, the possibility of recurrent episodes of pancreatitis causing insulin resistance and the potential for progression to exocrine pancreatic insufficiency should be noted. A fructosamine measurement in 2–3 weeks' time could be used to confirm improved glycaemic control.

References and further reading

Alt N, Kley S, Haessig M and Reusch CE (2007) Day-to-day variability of blood glucose concentration curves generated at home in cats with diabetes mellitus. *Journal of the American Veterinary Medical Association* **230**, 1011–1017

Boari A, Barreca A, Bestetti GE, Minuto F and Venturoli M (1995) Hypoglycemia in a dog with a leiomyoma of the gastric wall producing an insulin-like growth factor II-like peptide. *European Journal of Endocrinology* **132**, 744–750

Bruskiewicz KA, Nelson RW, Feldman EC and Griffey SM (1997) Diabetic ketosis and ketoacidosis in cats: 42 cases (1980–1995). *Journal of the American Veterinary Medical Association* **211**, 188–192

Casella M, Hassig M and Reusch CE (2005) Home-monitoring of blood glucose in cats with diabetes mellitus: evaluation over a 4-month period. *Journal of Feline Medicine and Surgery* **7**, 163–171

Catchpole B, Ristic JM, Fleeman LM and Davison LJ (2005) Canine diabetes mellitus: can old dogs teach us new tricks? *Diabetologia* **48**, 1948–1956

Davison LJ, Herrtage ME and Catchpole B (2005) Study of 253 dogs in the United Kingdom with diabetes mellitus. *Veterinary Record* **156**, 467–471

Davison LJ, Slater LA, Herrtage ME *et al.* (2003) Evaluation of a continuous glucose monitoring system in diabetic dogs. *Journal of Small Animal Practice* **44**, 435–442

Davison LJ, Walding B, Herrtage ME and Catchpole B (2008) Anti-insulin antibodies in diabetic dogs before and after treatment with different insulin preparations. *Journal of Veterinary Internal Medicine* **22**, 1317–1325

Dunayer EK (2004) Hypoglycemia following canine ingestion of xylitol-containing gum. *Veterinary and Human Toxicology* **46**, 87–88

Hoenig M (2012) The cat as a model for human obesity and diabetes. *Journal of Diabetes Science and Technology* **6**, 525–533

Hoenig M, Reusch C and Peterson ME (2000) Beta cell and insulin antibodies in treated and untreated diabetic cats. *Veterinary Immunology and Immunopathology* **77**, 93–102

Hume DZ, Drobatz KJ and Hess RS (2006) Outcome of dogs with diabetic ketoacidosis: 127 dogs (1993–2003). *Journal of Veterinary Internal Medicine* **20**, 547–555

Jensen AL (1992) Serum fructosamine in canine diabetes mellitus. An initial study. *Veterinary Research Communications* **16**, 1–9

Jensen AL (1995) Glycated blood proteins in canine diabetes mellitus. *Veterinary Record* **137**, 401–405

Johnson CA (2008) Glucose homeostasis during canine pregnancy: Insulin resistance, ketosis, and hypoglycemia. *Theriogenology* **70**, 1418–1423

Kawamoto M, Kaneko JJ, Heusner AA, Feldman EC and Koizumi I (1992) Relation of fructosamine to serum protein, albumin, and glucose concentrations in healthy and diabetic dogs. *American Journal of Veterinary Research* **53**, 851–855

Klein SC and Peterson ME (2010) Canine hypoadrenocorticism: part I. *Canadian Veterinary Journal* **51**, 63–69

Lederer R, Rand JS, Jonsson NN, Hughes IP and Morton JM (2009) Frequency of feline diabetes mellitus and breed predisposition in domestic cats in Australia. *Veterinary Journal* **179**, 254–258

Macintire DK (1995) Emergency therapy of diabetic crises: insulin overdose, diabetic ketoacidosis, and hyperosmolar coma. *Veterinary Clinics of North America: Small Animal Practice* **25**, 639–650

Mansfield C (2012) Acute pancreatitis in dogs: advances in understanding, diagnostics, and treatment. *Topics in Companion Animal Medicine* **27**, 123–132

Mattheeuws D, Rottiers R, Kaneko JJ and Vermeulen A (1984) Diabetes mellitus in dogs: relationship of obesity to glucose tolerance and insulin response. *American Journal of Veterinary Research* **45**, 98–103

McCann TM, Simpson KE, Shaw DJ, Butt JA and Gunn-Moore DA (2007) Feline diabetes mellitus in the UK: the prevalence within an insured cat population and a questionnaire-based putative risk factor analysis. *Journal of Feline Medicine and Surgery* **9**, 289–299

Niessen SJ (2010) Feline acromegaly: an essential differential diagnosis for the difficult diabetic. *Journal of Feline Medicine and Surgery* **12**, 15–23

Paul AE, Shiel RE, Juvet F, Mooney CT and Mansfield CS (2011) Effect of hematocrit on accuracy of two point-of-care glucometers for use in dogs. *American Journal of Veterinary Research* **72**, 1204–1208

Rand JS, Fleeman LM, Farrow HA, Appleton DJ and Lederer R (2004) Canine and feline diabetes mellitus: nature or nurture? *Journal of Nutrition* **134**, 2072S–2080S

Rand JS, Kinnaird E, Baglioni A, Blackshaw J and Priest J (2002) Acute stress hyperglycemia in cats is associated with struggling and increased concentrations of lactate and norepinephrine. *Journal of Veterinary Internal Medicine* **16**, 123–132

Reusch CE, Gerber B and Boretti FS (2002) Serum fructosamine concentrations in dogs with hypothyroidism. *Veterinary Research Communications* **26**, 531–536

Reusch CE and Haberer B (2001) Evaluation of fructosamine in dogs and cats with hypo- or hyperproteinaemia, azotaemia, hyperlipidaemia and hyperbilirubinaemia. *Veterinary Record* **148**, 370–376

Reusch CE and Tomsa K (1999) Serum fructosamine concentration in cats with overt hyperthyroidism. *Journal of the American Veterinary Medical Association* **215**, 1297–1300

Ristic JM, Herrtage ME, Walti-Lauger SM *et al.* (2005) Evaluation of a continuous glucose monitoring system in cats with diabetes mellitus. *Journal of Feline Medicine and Surgery* **7**, 153–162

Sieber-Ruckstuhl NS, Kley S, Tschuor F *et al.* (2008) Remission of diabetes mellitus in cats with diabetic ketoacidosis. *Journal of Veterinary Internal Medicine* **22**, 1326–1332

Surman S and Fleeman L (2013) Continuous glucose monitoring in small animals. *Veterinary Clinics of North America: Small Animal Practice* **43**, 381–406

Usher-Smith JA, Thompson MJ, Sharp SJ and Walter FM (2011) Factors associated with the presence of diabetic ketoacidosis at diagnosis of diabetes in children and young adults: a systematic review. *British Medical Journal* **343**, d4092.

Willard MD, Zerbe CA, Schall WD, Johnson C, Crow SE and Jones R (1987) Severe hypophosphatemia associated with diabetes mellitus in six dogs and one cat. *Journal of the American Veterinary Medical Association* **190**, 1007–1010

Xenoulis PG and Steiner JM (2008) Current concepts in feline pancreatitis. *Topics in Companion Animal Medicine* **23**, 185–192

Chapter 17

Laboratory evaluation of hypothyroidism and hyperthyroidism

Peter A. Graham and Carmel T. Mooney

Hypothyroidism and hyperthyroidism are the most common endocrine disorders of dogs and cats, respectively, and testing for these diseases is frequently carried out in practice. Interpretation relies on a good understanding of thyroid physiology and the myriad factors, other than thyroid disease and including assay methodology, that can affect tests of thyroid function.

Physiology of the thyroid gland

The thyroid gland of dogs and cats exists as two separate lobes located on either side of the trachea, extending downwards over the first five or six tracheal rings. Each thyroid lobe is composed of microscopic spherical follicles lined by a single layer of thyroid epithelium, the lumen of which contains colloid, a gelatinous storage substance for thyroglobulin secreted by the follicular cells (Figure 17.1). Thyroglobulin is a large glycoprotein containing iodotyrosines that serve as precursors for thyroid hormone synthesis. Most of the steps involved in thyroid hormone synthesis are catalysed by the enzyme thyroid peroxidase (TPO).

The metabolically active thyroid hormones are the iodothyronines: 3,5,3',5'-L-tetraiodothyronine (thyroxine (T4)) and 3,5,3'-L-triiodothyronine (triiodothyronine (T3)). T4 is the main secretory product of the thyroid gland. Only small amounts of T3, the more metabolically active hormone, and 3,3',5'-L-triodothyronine (reverse T3 (rT3)), an inactive product, are produced by the thyroid gland. The majority of circulating T3 and rT3 is produced by peripheral monodeiodination of T4, which occurs mainly in the liver and kidney, so T4 is often considered to be a pro-hormone. Its activation to T3 is potentially autoregulated in the periphery.

The thyroid hormones circulate bound to plasma proteins. The exact proteins and their binding affinities vary between species. In dogs, circulating T4 is bound to thyroxine-binding globulin (TBG) and to a lesser extent transthyretin (TTR), albumin, a high-density lipoprotein (HDL$_2$) and a very low-density lipoprotein (VLDL). Cats depend primarily on albumin and TTR. Approximately 99.9% of T4 is protein bound in both species, and the remaining fraction is metabolically active free T4. T3 is slightly less protein bound, with a free fraction of approximately 1%. For both hormones, the bound fraction acts as a reservoir to buffer hormone delivery to target tissues.

Control of thyroid hormone production is mediated via negative feedback (Figure 17.2). The hypothalamus secretes thyrotropin-releasing hormone (TRH) into the hypophyseal portal system, and this acts on the anterior pituitary to promote the synthesis and secretion of thyrotropin (thyroid-stimulating hormone (TSH)). TSH acts on the thyroid cells, promoting trapping of iodide and the synthesis and release of the thyroid hormones. The presence of excess circulating free T4 and T3 produces a negative feedback effect on the hypothalamus and anterior pituitary, which serves to decrease synthesis and release of TRH and TSH and, subsequently, thyroid hormone production. Peripherally, protein binding, cytosolic buffers, and the activities of the deiodinase enzymes offer additional areas for control of thyroid hormone action.

Thyroid hormones have numerous functions but their major influence is on metabolic rate, growth and tissue turnover. They also interact with the nervous system by increasing overall sympathetic drive. The clinical presentations in animals with a deficiency of thyroid hormone, therefore, can include stunting in growing animals, skin and hair abnormalities, lethargy and increased bodyweight. Conversely, in hyperthyroid individuals, there is weight loss, hyperactivity, intermittent vomiting/diarrhoea, tachycardia and development of hypertrophic cardiomyopathy. The effect of thyroid hormone on tissues is relatively slow and therefore clinical signs can take some time (weeks to months) to develop after loss of thyroid function or as hyperfunction commences. Similarly, it takes time for clinical signs to disappear after appropriate treatment has been initiated. The spectrum and severity of clinical signs in any individual will vary, depending on the duration of the condition, its severity, the ability of the animal to cope and/or the existence of concurrent disorders.

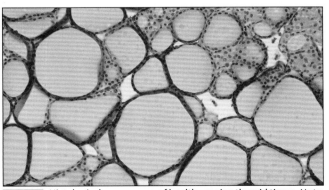

17.1 Histological appearance of healthy canine thyroid tissue. Note the follicular architecture. (Haematoxylin and eosin stain)

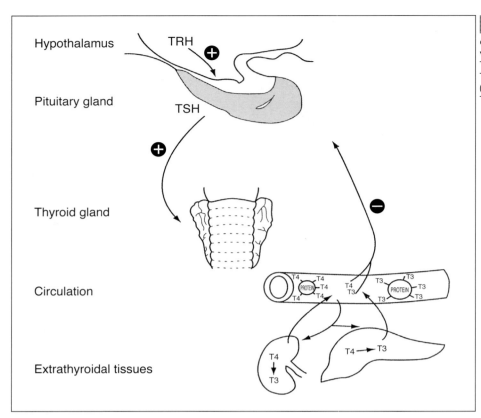

Hypothalamus

Pituitary gland

Thyroid gland

Circulation

Extrathyroidal tissues

17.2 The hypothalamic–pituitary–thyroid–extrathyroid axis, demonstrating the interactions among the various factors controlling thyroid function. TRH = thyrotropin-releasing hormone; TSH = thyroid-stimulating hormone (thyrotropin); T3 = triiodothyronine; T4 = thyroxine; + = stimulation; – = inhibition.

Laboratory methods for assessment of thyroid function

A variety of tests and methodologies are available for measurement of total and free thyroid hormone concentrations, thyroid autoantibodies and pituitary hormones that may play a role in assessment of thyroid function. In addition, the hypothalamic–thyroid–pituitary axis can be manipulated through the administration of various stimulatory and suppressive agents. A more detailed description of the methodologies available for the most commonly used tests is provided elsewhere (see the *BSAVA Manual of Canine and Feline Endocrinology*).

In general, thyroid hormones are robust and stable, with some notable exceptions (Figure 17.3). There is no effect of time of day for diagnostic sampling, but time post medication is important for certain therapeutic monitoring. Haemolysis and lipaemia rarely affect the results of radioimmunoassays (RIAs) but this is not always the case for non-isotopic methods.

Total thyroid hormone measurement

Total (free and protein-bound) concentrations of T4 and T3 circulate at nanomolar concentrations and can be readily measured in serum (or plasma) samples from dogs and cats. Methodologies have evolved from RIAs through non-isotopic assays to liquid chromatography–tandem mass spectrometry (LC-MS), although the latter is generally confined to human research laboratories. Total T4, in particular, remains largely constant across different methodologies. RIAs are relatively cheap, require extremely small sample volumes and are considered by many to be a superior technology, but because of the restrictions surrounding radioisotope use are usually only used by large commercial or research laboratories. The development of non-isotopic immunoassays has transformed the availability of thyroid hormone measurement. Such methods can be performed on fully or semi-automated platforms that use enzymes (e.g. SNAP T4™ (semi-quantitative), Vetscan™, DRI-EMIT™), fluorescence (e.g. AIA 360™) or chemiluminescence (e.g. Immulite™) as signals. They offer several advantages over RIAs, including use of hormone kits with a longer shelf-life, reduced exposure to radioactive material, easier disposal and potential application in the practice laboratory. For obvious reasons, for both diagnosing thyroid diseases and monitoring the effect of therapy, quantitative assays are preferred over semi-quantitative. Generally, studies evaluating various different assays have shown reasonable correlation between the values obtained. However, as there are differences in methodologies, and a possibility of consistent under- or overestimation of concentrations, it is usually recommended that individual reference intervals are derived for each individual laboratory and test. Anecdotally at least, erroneous values that can affect clinical decision-making appear to be more common with assays that use enzymes and fluorescence as signals, and inconsistencies with some of these cannot be rectified with method-specific reference intervals.

Several of the kits now available for measurement of total thyroid hormone concentrations have been designed specifically for use with dog or cat serum. However, human kits are still frequently used. In dogs and cats, the binding affinities and overall concentrations of the major binding proteins are lower than in humans. Consequently, kits designed for human use must be modified to allow for the measurement of the lower circulating total thyroid hormone concentrations in dogs and cats, and validated to account for differences in plasma protein binding.

Analyte	Sample type	Sampling and handling considerations	Indications
Total T4	Serum/heparin plasma	4–6 hours post thyroxine administration (Check data sheet for any specific recommendations)	Diagnosing hyperthyroidism Diagnosing hypothyroidism (with TSH) Therapeutic monitoring TRH/TSH response tests T3 suppression test
Total T3	Serum/heparin plasma	None	No advantage over total T4 for diagnostic purposes Assessment of absorption for T3 suppression test
Free T4	Serum/heparin plasma	Severe hyperlipaemia Avoid delayed transport/analysis	Diagnosing hypo- and hyperthyroidism
cTSH	Serum/heparin plasma	None	Diagnosing canine (± feline) hypothyroidism (with T4) ?Diagnosing feline hyperthyroidism Therapeutic monitoring TRH response test
Thyroglobulin autoantibody	Serum	None	Assessment of autoimmune thyroid pathology
T4 and T3 autoantibodies	Serum/heparin plasma	None	Assessment of thyroid autoimmune pathology Assessment of immunoassay interference Detect interference in T3 and T4 measurements

17.3 Sampling, special handling considerations and uses of the analytes for assessment of thyroid disease. T3 = triiodothyronine; T4 = thyroxine; TRH = thyrotropin-releasing hormone; (c)TSH = (canine) thyroid-stimulating hormone (thyrotropin).

Free thyroxine measurement

Despite the differences in circulating concentrations of total T4 between dogs, cats and humans, absolute free T4 concentrations are similar. Free T4 is responsible for the biological activity of T4 at the cellular level and its measurement is thought to better reflect thyroid physiological status. Free T4 measurement is difficult, not least because of its circulation in minute picomolar concentrations (rather than nmol/l). Several methods of measurement are available, including those that do and do not employ a physical separation (e.g. by equilibrium dialysis or ultrafiltration) of the free from the protein-bound hormone.

In dogs and cats, measurement of circulating free T4 concentration has largely been performed using equilibrium dialysis. In this method, the patient sample undergoes a dialysis step to separate the free hormone from the protein-bound fraction. Subsequently, the dialysate containing free T4 is subjected to an ultrasensitive RIA. An all-inclusive kit method is available (manufactured previously by Nichols Institute Diagnostics and now by Antech Manufacturing) and, although designed for human free T4, it is applicable to dogs, cats and other species. It is often considered as the gold standard because it is largely unaffected by altered protein binding and cross-reacting substances such as T4 autoantibodies. However, care should be taken to avoid prolonged transport times (>5 days) as measured free T4 concentrations can increase with time. Where high environmental temperatures occur, this effect can be seen in as little as 2 days. This presumably results from degradation or loss of affinity of the binding proteins, allowing the free fraction to become greater. High serum concentrations of non-esterified fatty acids have a similar effect and can exacerbate the effect of transport.

Other methodologies available for human clinical use include two-step, labelled hormone/back-titration, one-step labelled hormone-analogue or analogue-based labelled antibody assays. While the former is reportedly in use by some commercial veterinary laboratories, published studies are not yet available. Most assays thus far used are analogue based. These assays employ a T4 analogue that purportedly does not react with serum binding proteins but is able to compete with the free hormone present within the sample. While newer analogue-based

assays (e.g. Immulite Veterinary Free T4™) have not yet been fully studied in dogs and cats, it is clear from previous studies that results from analogue methods offer no further information over total T4 measurement alone. The ability of such assays to measure free T4 concentrations accurately in humans remains controversial, and they are often considered only to estimate such concentrations. They are known to be affected by autoantibodies that cross-react with T4, and an additional major concern relates to their inability to provide accurate results in the face of non-thyroidal illness.

Thyrotropin measurement

Species-specific chemiluminescent assays are widely available for measurement of canine TSH (cTSH). However, a species-specific feline assay is not yet available. It has been shown that, while not identical, feline TSH is more similar to cTSH than to human TSH (Rayalam et al., 2006b). Thus, there has been growing interest in using the canine assays for assessment of feline TSH, despite other studies suggesting that the canine assay detects less than 40% of recombinant feline TSH (Rayalam et al., 2006a).

Thyroid autoantibody measurement

A variety of antibodies can be produced during immune-mediated thyroid disease. A species-specific method for measurement of canine thyroglobulin autoantibodies (TgAA) is readily available commercially (Canine TgAA™). In recent years the assay has been modified to decrease non-specific IgG binding, thereby reducing the rate of false positive and equivocal results. Results are expressed as a percentage of a standardized positive control.

In a proportion of TgAA-positive cases, T3 and T4 autoantibodies (T3AA and T4AA) are produced when a subset of TgAA is formed against an epitope containing an iodothyronine site. These antibodies have limited impact on the availability of thyroid hormones in vivo. However, they can have a dramatic impact on laboratory test procedures because of their ability to bind labelled hormone which can result in spuriously high or low total thyroid hormone concentrations, depending on the particular assay and separation system used. A commonly used total T4 assay employs a coated tube system in which the test sample and labelled T4 are added to a tube coated with anti-T4 antibodies. The test sample T4 competes with labelled T4 for these binding sites, hence a low sample T4 concentration leads to relatively more labelled T4 binding, which reads as a low result (the measured T4 is inversely proportional to the amount of bound labelled T4). If autoantibodies are present in the test sample, these bind to the labelled T4 and so less of this is available for binding to the tube antibodies, giving falsely high test sample total T4 results. Occasionally, assays separate unbound labelled hormone only, and the presence of autoantibody-bound labelled T4 will therefore falsely decrease the test sample results.

Dynamic thyroid function tests

Dynamic thyroid function tests are often recommended to confirm or refute a diagnosis of thyroid dysfunction, particularly when baseline test results are equivocal. They can also be used to determine the site of the lesion.

In most cases, the total T4 response to exogenous TRH, TSH or synthetic T3 is assessed, and cTSH can also be measured after administration of TRH. Both exogenous TRH and T3 are readily available. Bovine TSH, previously used for the TSH response test, is no longer available as a pharmaceutical preparation. Recombinant human TSH (rhTSH) is now available and, although expensive, appears to work well in healthy dogs and cats (Campos et al., 2012). The most commonly used protocols for these tests are outlined in Figure 17.4.

Hypothyroidism

Investigating hypothyroidism is primarily a concern in dogs because it represents a relatively common disorder in this species. Naturally occurring hypothyroidism is rare in cats. However, there has been emergent interest in the potential development of hypothyroidism in cats after treatment for hyperthyroidism, and as such its investigation is more common now than previously.

Canine hypothyroidism

A range of possible causes of canine hypothyroidism exists. Primary hypothyroidism refers to disease arising as a consequence of pathology within the thyroid gland itself. Hypothyroidism may also arise because of a deficiency of TSH or TRH, so-called secondary and tertiary hypothyroidism. Although the former has been recognized in dogs and cats, the latter has only once been convincingly reported (Shiel et al., 2007a). Given similar underlying neoplastic causes and limited impact on eventual thyroid hormone supplementation, a distinction between the two is not strictly necessary and many simply refer to either type of hypothyroidism as central. The overwhelming majority of hypothyroid cases arise from irreversible acquired thyroid gland disease. Only a small percentage of hypothyroidism results from nutritional, congenital, central or other conditions.

Adult-onset hypothyroidism

Primary, irreversible, destruction of the thyroid gland accounts for almost all of the naturally occurring cases of hypothyroidism in adult dogs. The histopathological description is either lymphocytic thyroiditis or idiopathic thyroid degeneration (atrophy), each of which is observed with approximately equal frequency.

Lymphocytic thyroiditis, also referred to as autoimmune thyroiditis, is characterized by lymphocytic infiltration of the thyroid glands with progressive destruction of thyroid follicles. There is a variation in the rate of progression of this process but extensive pathological changes must have occurred prior to the appearance of clinical signs of hypothyroidism (Graham et al., 2007). This condition is recognized as a heritable trait.

Idiopathic thyroid degeneration is characterized by a loss of thyroid parenchyma with replacement by adipose or fibrous tissue. The cause is not yet defined, but there is some compelling evidence that these lesions may be an end stage of lymphocytic thyroiditis and hypothyroidism a slowly progressive disease of different stages.

A positive TgAA test is an indirect marker of lymphocytic thyroiditis. Dogs that are TgAA positive but euthyroid are younger than TgAA-positive dogs with hypothyroidism, and both these groups are younger than dogs with TgAA-negative hypothyroidism (Graham et al., 2007). In theory, the complete destruction of all thyroid tissue leads to a reduction in immune stimulation, absence of any histological thyroiditis and conversion to autoantibody negativity. As such, the disorder can be described in different stages, as outlined in Figure 17.5. The rate of progression through the different stages is variable both from stage to stage and in their respective durations. The presence of

Parameter	T3 suppression	TSH stimulation	TRH stimulation
Use	Confirming hyperthyroidism in cats	Confirming hypothyroidism in dogs and hyperthyroidism in cats	Confirming hypothyroidism in dogs and hyperthyroidism in cats
Drug	Liothyronine	TSH	TRH
Dose	20 μg 8-hourly for seven doses (cats only)	75–150 μg/dog[a] 25 μg/cat	100–600 μg (dogs) 0.1 mg/kg (cats)
Route	Oral	Intravenous	Intravenous
Sampling times	0 and 2–4 hours after last dose	0 and 6 hours (dogs and cats)	0 and 4 hours
Assay	Total T4	Total T4	Total T4
Reference interval	<20 nmol/l with >50% suppression	50% increase exceeding approximately 25–30 nmol/l (dogs) >100% increase (cats)	At least 20% increase or increment >6 nmol/l (dogs) >60% increase (cats)

17.4 Commonly used protocols for dynamic thyroid function tests in dogs and cats. Values quoted for interpretation are guidelines only. Each individual laboratory should furnish its own reference range. [a] This higher dose is particularly recommended for dogs with known non-thyroidal illness or for those receiving thyroid-suppressive medications. ND = not determined; T3 = triiodothyronine; T4 = thyroxine; TRH = thyrotropin-releasing hormone; TSH = thyroid-stimulating hormone (thyrotropin).

Stage	Thyroid tissue histopathology	TgAA	Thyroid hormone concentrations	
			TSH	T4/T3
Silent	Majority normal, mild infiltration	Positive	Normal	Normal
Subclinical/ compensating	More marked infiltration	Positive	Increased	Normal
Clinical	>75% replaced	Positive	Increased	Decreased
	Minimal thyroid tissue, limited inflammation	Negative	Increased/ decreased	Decreased

17.5 The progressive stages of canine lymphocytic thyroiditis. Such a classification system is largely based on studies indirectly assessing lymphocytic thyroiditis by measurement of circulating thyroglobulin autoantibody status. T3 = triiodothyronine; T4 = thyroxine; TgAA = thyroglobulin autoantibody; TSH = thyroid-stimulating hormone (thyrotropin).

(Reproduced and modified from Mooney (2011) with permission from the *New Zealand Veterinary Journal*)

lymphocytic thyroiditis does not always imply the development of biochemical or clinical hypothyroidism in all cases. Preliminary data suggest that approximately 20% of antibody-positive euthyroid dogs develop thyroid hormone abnormalities suggestive of declining thyroid function (usually increased circulating TSH values with or without low free T4) and one in 20 (5%) become overtly hypothyroid within 1 year. A small proportion (approximately 15%) become antibody negative without the development of thyroid dysfunction and the majority maintain evidence of lymphocytic thyroiditis. Assuming a similar proportion would progress in each subsequent year, the majority could be hypothyroid within 4 years or so. However, longer-term studies are currently lacking. There appears to be a difference in the rate of progression among breeds, given the variable proportion of TgAA-positive hypothyroidism across breeds. Alternatively, lymphocytic thyroiditis and thyroid atrophy may be two distinct entities with different breed prevalences.

Congenital hypothyroidism

Dogs that are hypothyroid at birth fail to grow and develop normally and are usually described as having disproportionate dwarfism. If goitre is present a defect in one of the steps of hormonogenesis or, less commonly, iodine deficiency is the likely cause. Defects in thyroid peroxidase have been described in toy Fox, Rat and more recently Tenterfield Terriers with congenital hypothyroidism and goitre. These disorders are inherited as simple autosomal recessive traits for which DNA-based tests are available for affected and carrier individuals. However, goitre is absent in most reports of congenital hypothyroidism. A lack of production of TSH is the suspected cause of juvenile hypothyroidism in Giant Schnauzer and Boxers. However, most reports were published prior to the availability of the cTSH assay, which remains insufficiently sensitive to low concentrations, so this is largely unproven. There are isolated case reports of thyroid dysgenesis causing congenital hypothyroidism.

Laboratory diagnosis of canine hypothyroidism

Canine hypothyroidism is difficult to diagnose because of the long preclinical phase, the variety of presenting complaints and the poor specificity of several of the diagnostic tests commonly used. It is probably one of the most over-diagnosed conditions in veterinary medicine, but certain circumstances can lead to underdiagnosis.

Both breed and age can have significant effects on thyroid hormone concentrations (especially Greyhounds – see below). Additionally, a common physiological response to any illness and many drug therapies is a lowering of circulating thyroid hormone concentrations. It is, therefore, often difficult to distinguish between pathological and physiological thyroid-deficient states, and the diagnostic specificity of certain thyroid hormone measurements is consequently less than ideal. Early in the course of the disease, animals may be overtly hypothyroid on laboratory testing but may not display classical or well-defined clinical features for many months thereafter. Finally, albeit only occasionally, hypothyroid dogs may have serum thyroid hormone concentrations within/above the reference interval because of analytical interference by cross-reacting antithyroid hormone antibodies.

Routine clinicopathological features

A variety of clinicopathological abnormalities can be seen in hypothyroid dogs although none is truly specific (Figure 17.6; Panciera, 1994; Dixon *et al.*, 1999). However, the larger the increase in cholesterol, the more likely hypothyroidism is over other possible differentials.

Abnormality	Percentage of hypothyroid dogs
Haematology	
Mild non-regenerative anaemia	18–40
Serum biochemistry	
Hypercholesterolaemia	73–78
Hypertriglyceridaemia	88
Increased creatine kinase	18–35
Increased alkaline phosphatase	30

17.6 Common routine clinicopathological abnormalities in hypothyroid dogs.

(Data from Panciera, 1994 and Dixon *et al.*, 1999)

The anaemia associated with hypothyroidism is usually mild; it is a consequence of reduced peripheral metabolic activity and a reduction in tissue oxygen demand, leading to reduced erythropoietin production. In non-anaemic hypothyroid animals, red blood cell indices are typically at the lower end of their respective laboratory reference intervals. Regenerative anaemia should prompt consideration of another underlying cause.

Hypercholesterolaemia and hypertriglyceridaemia develop primarily because of a reduction in the rate of lipid degradation. Although it is often a feature of other endocrine disorders, notably diabetes mellitus and hyperadrenocorticism, the magnitude of the cholesterol increase in hypothyroidism is typically greater, and circulating cholesterol concentrations in excess of 20 mmol/l are not uncommon. Extreme elevations in cholesterol concentrations should always prompt investigation for hypothyroidism.

Increased creatine kinase (CK) activity develops because of reduced clearance, and is typically mild. Similar mild increases in liver enzyme activities, particularly alkaline phosphatase (ALP), occur presumably because of mild hepatic lipid deposition.

Circulating fructosamine concentration may increase in hypothyroidism as a result of a reduction in protein turnover rather than any change in glycaemic control. However, values rarely reach those expected in diabetes mellitus but more typically hover at the upper end of the reference interval. In diabetic dogs with concurrent hypothyroidism, fructosamine should be interpreted cautiously as an indicator of glycaemic control.

Assessment of thyroid function/pathology

Laboratory tests for investigating thyroid disease directly can be divided into those that assess thyroid function and those that provide indirect evidence of thyroid pathology (thyroiditis).

Thyroid hormones: Low concentrations of thyroid hormones are relatively sensitive but poorly specific for hypothyroidism. Concentrations can be decreased in response to general non-thyroidal illness or administration of many drugs, or may simply reflect age and breed differences. Exogenous thyroid hormone supplementation therapy can also interfere with diagnostic testing, and a greater than 4-week withdrawal period is required before re-testing (Panciera *et al.*, 1990).

Total thyroxine: Total T4 is a reasonably sensitive test (up to 100% in some studies) but it is poorly specific (as low as 70%) (Figure 17.7). (For discussions of sensitivity and specificity, see Chapter 2.) Unfortunately, total T4 concentrations can be low in a variety of situations other than hypothyroidism. If it is used as the sole diagnostic test for hypothyroidism, many false positive results will ensue.

Total T4 is lowered in non-thyroidal illness as a normal physiological response to that illness. Although several mechanisms are responsible, not all are clearly defined in the dog. Possible explanations include:

- Reduced serum protein binding
- Altered peripheral hormone metabolism
- Glucocorticoid-mediated TSH suppression.

The suppressive effect of non-thyroidal illness can be profound and has been demonstrated in both acute and chronic illnesses (Mooney, 2011). It has been suggested that an initial response to illness is a decline in total T3 concentration, followed by a simultaneous decline in total T4 concentration (Mooney *et al.*, 2008). In general thereafter, the more severe the illness, the greater the suppression of total T4 concentrations (Figure 17.8). Values below the reference interval and the limit of detection of the assay are not uncommonly observed. Once dubbed the 'euthyroid sick syndrome' or 'low-T4 state of medical illness', the preferred terminology for these effects is the

Severity of illness	Hormone			
	Total T3	**Total T4**	**Free T4**	**TSH**
Mild	↓	↔	↔	↔
Moderate	↓↓	↓	↔/↓↑	↔/↓
Severe	↓↓↓	↓↓	↔/↓	↓↓
Recovery	↔/↓	↔/↓	↔/↓	↑

17.8 The potential effect of non-thyroidal illness on thyroid hormone concentrations in dogs. These effects are largely known for T3 and T4. In the case of TSH, data are extrapolated from humans. Most research concerning dogs has not implicated any effect of illness on TSH but this is complicated because of the poor sensitivity of the currently used canine TSH assays. T3 = triiodothyronine; T4 = thyroxine; TSH = thyroid-stimulating hormone (thyrotropin); ↓ = concentrations decrease; ↔ = concentrations remain the same; ↑ = concentrations increase (the number of arrows indicates increasing severity).
(Reproduced and modified from Mooney (2011) with permission from the *New Zealand Veterinary Journal*)

'non-thyroidal illness syndrome'. In some chronic conditions such as osteoarthritis there appears to be little effect on total T4 (Paradis *et al.*, 2003).

A similar phenomenon occurs with a variety of drugs, including but not confined to glucocorticoids, long-term phenobarbital, aspirin, ketoprofen, carprofen, clomipramine and sulphonamide-containing antibiotics (Daminet and Ferguson, 2003; Daminet *et al.*, 2003; Gulikers and Panciera, 2003; Panciera *et al.*, 2006; Figure 17.9). It has been suggested that an additional 15% decrease in total T4 concentration is expected in sick dogs that are also treated with thyroid-suppressive medications (Mooney *et al.*, 2008). As with non-thyroidal illness, values below the reference interval and the lower limit of detection of the assay are possible.

Sulphonamide therapy warrants specific mention because it potentially causes a true but reversible hypothyroidism, presumably mediated through inhibition of TPO, an enzyme essential for thyroid hormone production. As a result, circulating total T4 concentrations can be severely depressed. The effect of sulphonamide therapy is relatively long-lived after withdrawal, with full recovery in a few weeks. A withdrawal period of at least 3 weeks is recommended prior to assessing thyroid function.

While total T4 concentrations should be interpreted cautiously in dogs being treated with the drugs listed above, other studies have shown that some drugs have no or minimal effects on thyroid function, including potassium bromide, propranolol, meloxicam, deracoxib and chondroitin sulphate/glucosamine (Daminet and Ferguson,

Published work	Total T4		FT4d		TSH		Total T4/TSH		FT4d/TSH		TgAA	
	Sen	**Spec**	**Sen**	**Spec**	**Sen**	**Spec**	**Sen**	**Spec**	**Sen**	**Spec**	**Sen**	**Spec**
Iversen *et al.*, 1998											91	97
Nachreiner *et al.*, 1998											100	100
Beale and Torres, 1991											86	94
Nelson *et al.*, 1991	98	73	97	78								
Peterson *et al.*, 1997	89	82	98	93	76	93	67	98	74	98		
Scott-Moncrieff *et al.*, 1998	100	78			63	88	63	100				
Dixon and Mooney, 1999	100	75	80	94	87	82	87	92	80	97		
Boretti and Reusch, 2004					57.7	100						

17.7 Published diagnostic performance of tests used in the diagnosis of canine hypothyroidism. Values involving TgAA relate to the diagnosis of lymphocytic thyroiditis. All values expressed as percentages. FT4d = free thyroxine by equilibrium dialysis; Sen = sensitivity; Spec = specificity; T4 = thyroxine; TSH = thyroid-stimulating hormone (thyrotropin); TgAA = thyroglobulin autoantibodies.

Drug	Hormone		
	Total T4	Free T4	TSH
Prednisone/ prednisolone	↓↔	↓↔	↔↓
Phenobarbital	↓↔	↓↔	↔↓ *
Potassium bromide	↔	↔	↔
Potentiated sulphonamides	↓	↓	↑
Propranolol	↔	↔	↔
Clomipramine	↓	↓	↔
Aspirin	↓	↓↔	↔
Ketoprofen	↓	↔	↔
Carprofen	↓↔	↓↔	↔↓
Deracoxib	↔	↔	↔

*Although concentrations may increase, they rarely exceed the upper limit of the reference interval

17.9 The potential effect of drug therapy on thyroid hormone concentrations in dogs. T4 = thyroxine; TSH = thyroid-stimulating hormone (thyrotropin); ↓ = concentrations decrease; ↔ = concentrations remain the same; ↑ = concentrations increase.

(Data from Daminet and Ferguson, 2003; Daminet et al., 2003; Gulikers and Panciera, 2003; Sauve et al., 2003; Panciera et al., 2006). (Reproduced and modified from Mooney (2011) with permission from the New Zealand Veterinary Journal)

2003; Daminet et al., 2003; Sauve et al., 2003; Panciera et al., 2006). Thyroid function can be reasonably reliably assessed in animals receiving these particular medications. Where specific studies have not yet been carried out using other drugs, a potential effect should always be presumed until proven otherwise.

Several physiological mechanisms are also responsible for low circulating total T4 concentrations in dogs. Of the potential factors, time of year, age, dioestrus, exercise and nutritional status do not affect total T4 concentrations enough to misdiagnose eu- or hypothyroidism, although extreme diet alteration may (Castillo et al., 2001). Total T4 concentrations decline with age, and values may be below the reference interval in old age. Breed appears to be very important. Greyhounds, other sighthounds and sled dogs usually have values at the low end or below the general reference interval (Shiel et al., 2007b). Values may even be undetectable in healthy individuals of these breeds, creating difficulties in defining a breed-specific reference interval. Unfortunately, hypothyroidism continues to be mistakenly diagnosed in a large proportion of sighthounds purely on the basis of low serum thyroid hormone concentrations alone (Shiel et al., 2010).

Relying on a reference interval total T4 concentration alone to rule out a diagnosis of hypothyroidism also has its drawbacks. Such a value may make hypothyroidism less likely but does not rule it out completely, particularly if T4AAs are present (see below). Thus, neither a reference interval nor a low total T4 concentration result can be relied upon accurately to confirm or refute hypothyroidism. The use of a serial testing protocol, only progressing to additional thyroid tests if an initial 'screening' total T4 is abnormal, is therefore a flawed approach.

Assessment of total T4 concentrations has several advantages, including its relative cheapness and ready availability.

Free thyroxine by equilibrium dialysis: Measurement of free T4 concentrations is a more specific diagnostic test for hypothyroidism than measurement of total T4 alone (see Figure 17.7). It is most helpful when:

- There is significant non-thyroidal illness present, suppressing total T4 concentrations
- The animal is receiving medications that can influence protein binding and ultimately total T4 concentrations
- T4AA are present, resulting in falsely elevated total T4 concentrations.

In these cases, serum free T4 concentrations are expected to remain within the reference interval. However, although they are less affected by non-thyroidal illness and drug therapies, free T4 concentrations may be suppressed by severe illness and certain drugs, including glucocorticoids, aspirin, long-term phenobarbital therapy and clomipramine (see Figures 17.8 and 17.9). Free T4 concentrations may also be affected by breed. Certainly, Greyhounds and Salukis can have free T4 concentrations below the lower limit of the reference interval, although less frequently than for total T4 (Shiel et al., 2007b, 2010), but this is not true of all sighthounds, such as Whippets.

In addition, free T4 is a less sensitive diagnostic test than total T4, particularly in the early stages of the illness (Dixon and Mooney, 1999). It is also susceptible to endogenous and exogenous sample effects (see above).

Total triiodothyronine: The measurement of serum total T3 offers no real advantage over the measurement of total or free T4 concentrations. It is a relatively poor predictor of thyroid function for the following reasons:

- There is a high prevalence of interfering T3AAs in hypothyroid dogs
- Upregulation of deiodinase activity may occur in animals with failing thyroid function, resulting in maintenance of circulating total T3 concentrations
- There is a suppressive effect of non-thyroidal illness, even when mild and not affecting total T4, which presumably is metabolically protective and a beneficial response to illness
- There is a suppressive effect of various drug therapies, including sulphonamides, aspirin, glucocorticoids, amiodarone and clomipramine.

In animals that are known to be TgAA negative, measurement of serum total T3 may be helpful in specific circumstances, e.g. in euthyroid sighthounds such as Greyhounds, total T3 concentrations tend to lie within the general canine all-breed reference interval (Shiel et al., 2007b).

Thyrotropin (TSH): Dogs with primary hypothyroidism are expected to have an increased serum cTSH concentration because of the loss of the negative feedback effect of the thyroid hormones. Unfortunately, not all cases of primary hypothyroidism exhibit increased values and some euthyroid (sick and healthy) dogs have been shown to have increased values. Clinical studies of cTSH measurement for the diagnosis of hypothyroidism report sensitivity between 58 and 87% and specificity between 82 and 100% (see Figure 17.7).

The poor diagnostic sensitivity of cTSH measurement could arise for several reasons, not all of which are well understood:

- The presence of concurrent non-thyroidal illness could potentially suppress a previously high cTSH into the reference interval in a dog with primary hypothyroidism
- Concurrent drug therapy, particularly with glucocorticoids, potentially suppresses cTSH concentrations into the reference interval in hypothyroid dogs

- Random fluctuation of cTSH into the reference interval in hypothyroid animals, particularly if only minimally elevated initially
- The existence of central rather than primary hypothyroidism
- The possible existence of various isomers of cTSH, not all of which are measured using current assay techniques
- Chronic decline in pituitary TSH production over time.

Elevated cTSH values in euthyroid dogs are less common but also not well understood. Possible explanations include:

- Recovery of thyroid function from the effects of previous non-thyroidal illness or drug use
- Treatment with sulphonamide-containing drugs or phenobarbital
- During the subclinical or compensating phase of lymphocytic thyroiditis, increased concentrations of TSH are generated to stimulate the decreasing thyroid mass and maintain normal thyroid hormone concentrations (see above).

The use of cTSH measurement alone is therefore not recommended; it should be interpreted in conjunction with other thyroid hormone results. However, interestingly, in euthyroid sighthounds, which are known to have lower thyroid hormone concentrations in health, cTSH concentrations typically remain within the general canine reference interval.

Thyroglobulin autoantibodies: A proportion of canine hypothyroidism is caused by lymphocytic thyroiditis. Measurement of TgAA provides evidence for an active inflammatory process in the thyroid glands. A positive TgAA status does not provide any information on thyroid function *per se* because thyroid dysfunction does not occur until at least approximately 75% of the gland is destroyed. Consequently, both lymphocytic thyroiditis and TgAAs can be present in dogs that are not yet functionally hypothyroid. It may take several months to years for hypothyroidism to develop and, in some cases, a functional problem never arises (see above).

Overall TgAA prevalence in hypothyroidism is approximately 50%, corresponding to the estimated prevalence of lymphocytic thyroiditis in this disorder. Limited studies have been published comparing TgAA results and histological examination of thyroid biopsy material. However, of those published, there is excellent diagnostic sensitivity and specificity (>90% in each case) for thyroiditis (see Figure 17.7).

Measurement of TgAA provides advantages in detecting thyroid pathology long before a change in thyroid function is apparent. This may allow timely institution of therapy without waiting for dramatic clinical signs to develop. Additionally, TgAA measurement may be used in breeding programmes. Breed predispositions and the familial nature of hypothyroidism have long been known and various genetic risk factors have been identified. A positive TgAA status provides an indirect measurement of at-risk individuals. A decision may be made not to breed from such animals in an attempt to decrease the prevalence of hypothyroidism in a particular breed.

Thyroid hormone antibodies: Autoantibodies to T4 and T3 only develop in a proportion of TgAA-positive dogs and are exceptionally rare, if they occur at all, in TgAA-negative dogs. T3AAs have an estimated prevalence of 37% in TgAA-positive dogs, compared with 11% for T4AAs (Graham *et al.*, 2007). Almost all dogs with T4AAs also have T3AAs. The high prevalence of T3AAs in the dog is one of the main reasons that measurement of T3 has limited value in the diagnosis of hypothyroidism. In most commonly used assay systems, autoantibodies cause falsely elevated values that can be extreme and easily identifiable as unusual in a dog undergoing investigation for hypothyroidism. However, they may also result in elevation of a low value into the reference interval. The presence of T4AAs potentially results in an underdiagnosis of hypothyroidism in approximately 10% of cases if the diagnosis is solely reliant on demonstration of low total T4 values, as T4AAs increase measured values into the reference interval. Their existence accounts for the less than perfect sensitivity of total T4 for diagnosing hypothyroidism and explains why a reference interval value cannot rule out hypothyroidism in all cases.

Putting it all together – thyroid profiles: The introduction of methods for free T4, cTSH and TgAA measurement has significantly improved the diagnostic capability for hypothyroidism compared with total T4 measurement alone; when they are used together the diagnostic shortcomings of each test are minimized. In most situations, a combined thyroid 'profile' is better for investigating hypothyroidism than serial individual tests. The minimum recommended thyroid profile is total T4 and cTSH. In combination, the gain from the high sensitivity of T4 and high specificity of cTSH measurements is maximized. Free T4 should be added or used instead of total T4 when the patient is known to have non-thyroidal illness or is receiving potentially interfering therapies (e.g. glucocorticoids and barbiturates), or when T4 cross-reacting TgAA are suspected. The addition of TgAA to the initial profile serves as a screen to determine whether the total T4 result can be believed to be free from interference by T4AA and helps define the pathogenesis of thyroid dysfunction. In addition, it may help with some equivocal cases and identify subclinical thyroid disease.

The most common diagnostic dilemma is finding a low total T4 and reference interval cTSH result in a dog. Apart from representing a breed-specific effect, this could indicate that:

- The animal is responding appropriately to a physiological stress (such as non-thyroidal illness)
- The animal is on medication that suppresses T4 concentrations
- It is one of the proportion of hypothyroid dogs (approximately 15% (or more)) in which an elevated TSH result is not detected.

In such cases, assessment of free T4 and TgAA may be warranted. Free T4 analysis serves to differentiate the non-thyroidal illness syndrome or the effect of drug therapies from true hypothyroidism in many cases. If a diagnosis remains unclear, retesting at a later date, instituting a therapeutic trial or embarking on a TSH stimulation test is recommended.

In interpreting the results of tests which have less than perfect diagnostic sensitivity and specificity, the effect of prevalence on the predictive value of positive and negative test results must be considered (see Chapter 2). In large thyroid diagnostic laboratories, a rough estimate can be made of the prevalence of hypothyroidism in the population being tested. Clear-cut diagnoses of hypothyroidism were made in approximately 8% of samples submitted to one laboratory (Diagnostic Center for Population and Animal Health, Michigan State University), and unclassified cases (low total or free T4 but reference interval cTSH) accounted for a further 17%. Figure 17.10 compares the predictive values of positive and negative test results for total T4 measured alone and for total T4 measured in combination with cTSH, and illustrates the enhanced diagnostic confidence for combined results.

Dynamic thyroid function tests: The ideal tools for investigating endocrine disorders are the dynamic function (stimulation and suppression) tests. Certainly, the TSH stimulation test is considered by many to be the closest to a 'gold standard' laboratory test of thyroid function. Unfortunately, pharmaceutical grade bovine TSH now has limited availability. More recently, a recombinant human β-subunit TSH has become available (Campos et al., 2012) but given its expense, it has not gained widespread use except in diagnostically equivocal cases.

The TRH response test gained some support after the availability of TSH decreased, but the results of this test are difficult to interpret and many euthyroid dogs are classified erroneously as hypothyroid. It may have some use in assessing the pituitary production of TSH in rare cases of suspected pituitary hypothyroidism. It may also be used to detect excess growth hormone production in chronic cases of hypothyroidism (Diaz-Espineira et al., 2008).

Monitoring thyroid hormone replacement therapy

The exogenous T4 used to treat hypothyroidism is immunologically identical to endogenous T4, so the same assays can be used to measure its circulating concentration. In addition, the negative feedback effect of exogenous T4 decreases production of cTSH. Thus, the measurement of both T4 and cTSH concentrations can provide a useful indication of the adequacy of thyroid hormone supplementation. Measurement of free T4 concentration is not required for therapeutic monitoring unless T4AA are confirmed or suspected. It is an additional expense and there are no published studies suggesting its superiority over total T4 measurement alone.

The measurement of serum total T4 concentration provides an indication of the adequacy of therapy on the day of the test; peak concentrations are usually achieved approximately 3 hours post pill. Common recommendations for therapeutic monitoring are to measure total T4 4–6 hours after medication. There are few studies specifically assessing target total T4 concentrations with once- or twice-daily dosing, leading to many anecdotal recommendations. Recommendations based on achieving concentrations within the reference interval for 24 hours do not take account of the extended biological half-life of T4 compared with its relatively short serum half-life of

between 6 and 10 hours. One study suggested that, following once-daily therapy, a serum total T4 concentration exceeding the upper half of the reference interval (>35 nmol/l; median 55 nmol/l) 6 hours post administration was adequate in most cases (Dixon et al., 2002).

Some manufacturers suggest measuring peak (at 3 hours) and trough (prior to next dose administration) concentrations, aiming for both values to be within the reference interval, but studies assessing the correlation with clinical outcome are lacking. Combining a 6–10-hour half-life with a 6-hour minimum of 35 nmol/l yields minimum 3-hour peak concentrations of 43–50 nmol/l. With twice-daily therapy, lower (28–42 nmol/l) minimum 3-hour peak concentrations may be adequate to achieve the same goal. Signs of hyperthyroidism may occur if circulating concentrations chronically exceed 100 nmol/l, and even if not noticed a lower dose is recommended. Therapeutic efficacy can first be assessed 2 weeks after commencing treatment. Although there is wide interindividual variation in absorption and therefore total T4 concentrations, a more important factor is to ensure that owners administer the medication in the usual way on the day of monitoring. This is because feeding at dosing times significantly decreases T4 absorption.

The serum concentration of cTSH takes several days to change and therefore the measurement of this hormone provides information on the adequacy of therapy in the preceding few days rather than just on the day of the test. Compared with the measurement of total T4 alone, combined total T4 and cTSH helps to identify long-term compliance failures and avoids unnecessary dose adjustment. A serum total T4 concentration within the therapeutic range for the respective interval post pill, with a corresponding high cTSH value, suggests adequate drug administration on that day but poor compliance in the immediate past. However, reference interval cTSH concentrations may occur in inadequately treated dogs with total T4 concentrations below the therapeutic target. The assay is incapable of detecting suppressed values indicative of hyperthyroidism, and dose reductions are usually based on total T4 concentrations alone (see above). Of course, cTSH measurement is unlikely to be of any additional value in therapeutic monitoring in the proportion of dogs that do not have elevated pretreatment values.

Feline hypothyroidism

Hypothyroidism also potentially occurs in cats. Usually this is iatrogenic following treatment for hyperthyroidism, but there have also been some spontaneous congenital and one adult case reported. The measurement of TSH using the widely available canine assay may be helpful in making a diagnosis of primary or iatrogenic hypothyroidism. Further information is given below.

Test			Pretest probability					
			10%		25%		50%	
	Sensitivity	Specificity	PPV	NPV	PPV	NPV	PPV	NPV
Low total T4 alone	89	75	28	98	54	95	78	87
Low total T4/high TSH	87	98	83	99	94	96	98	88

17.10 Positive (PPV) and negative (NPV) predictive values for the measurement of total T4 and the combination of total T4 and TSH at three different levels of pretest probability (or prevalence of hypothyroidism in tested group) at example levels of diagnostic sensitivity and specificity. The table shows that a pretest probability of 10% (similar to that experienced by diagnostic laboratories) means that less than 30% of dogs with a low total T4 result alone have hypothyroidism. Even at the relatively high pretest probability of 25%, a low total T4 still only has a positive predictive value of approximately 50%, similar to the clinician guessing whether hypothyroidism is present. The combination of total T4 and TSH measurement gives more useful PPV and NPV over a range of pretest probabilities consistent with clinical practice (10–25%). All values presented as percentages. See Chapter 2 for methods of calculation. T4 = thyroxine; TSH = thyroid-stimulating hormone (thyrotropin).

Hyperthyroidism

Hyperthyroidism is primarily a concern in cats. First definitively diagnosed in 1979, its incidence has increased dramatically since then. It is now the most common endocrine disorder of the cat and a disease frequently encountered in small animal practice. On the other hand, naturally occurring hyperthyroidism rarely requires investigation in dogs.

Feline hyperthyroidism

Hyperthyroidism is a multisystemic disorder arising from increased thyroid hormone production by an abnormally functioning thyroid gland. Histopathologically, the normal thyroid follicular architecture is replaced by multiple well defined hyperplastic nodules ranging from <1 mm to >2 cm in diameter and usually described as adenomatous hyperplasia (adenoma). This results in enlargement of either one (<30% of cases) or more commonly both (>70% of cases) thyroid lobes (goitre). Thyroid carcinoma is a rare cause of hyperthyroidism in the cat, accounting for less than 2% of cases at least at initial diagnosis.

Hyperthyroidism typically affects older cats (usually >10 years of age) of either sex and any breed. There has been a report of hyperthyroidism in a kitten but given that the histopathological appearance was different from that seen in older cats, it probably represented a distinct and rare clinical entity (Gordon et al., 2003).

The aetiology of the disorder remains unclear, and prevention is therefore not possible. However, because of the benign nature of the lesions in the majority of cases, the disease carries an excellent prognosis with effective therapy.

Laboratory diagnosis of feline hyperthyroidism

Classically, hyperthyroidism is associated with weight loss despite an increased or normal appetite, hyperactivity, tachycardia, intermittent gastrointestinal signs of vomiting and diarrhoea, cardiac murmur and goitre. However, cats are less highly symptomatic now than 15 years ago, presumably because of increased awareness and earlier diagnosis. This, coupled with the high prevalence, means that many older cats undergo testing for hyperthyroidism, some of which actually have the disease, but others may be suffering from a variety of non-thyroidal illnesses or may indeed be healthy. This affects the performance of the diagnostic tests used in confirming, but probably more importantly in refuting, a diagnosis of hyperthyroidism.

Routine clinicopathological features

Routine haematological and biochemical investigations are useful in providing supportive evidence of hyperthyroidism (Figure 17.11). However, they prove more useful in eliminating the diagnosis or diagnosing non-thyroidal illnesses in animals presenting with similar clinical signs, or in detecting concurrent disorders that may ultimately affect the prognosis.

Haematological changes are of limited clinical significance, although mild to moderate erythrocytosis (increased packed cell volume (PCV), red blood cell (RBC) count and haemoglobin concentration) and macrocytosis have been described, reflecting thyroid hormone-mediated stimulation of erythroid marrow and increased production

Abnormality	Percentage of hyperthyroid cats
Haematology	
Erythrocytosis	50
Macrocytosis	50
Stress leucogram	30
Serum biochemistry	
Increased liver enzyme activities	90
Azotaemia	20
Hyperphosphataemia	36–43
Hyperglycaemia	12–21
Decreased fructosamine	17–50

17.11 Common routine clinicopathological abnormalities in hyperthyroid cats.
(Data from Peterson et al., 1983; Thoday and Mooney, 1992; Broussard et al., 1995)

of erythropoietin resulting from increased oxygen consumption. Not surprisingly, a stress leucogram, as evidenced by mature neutrophilia usually accompanied by lymphopenia and eosinopenia, is common. Occasionally, there is a lymphocytosis and eosinophilia, which is thought to relate to a relative lack of cortisol induced by thyroid hormone excess.

By far the most striking biochemical abnormalities are the elevations in liver enzyme activities that occur in over 90% of hyperthyroid cats (Shiel and Mooney, 2007). The elevations in these enzymes can be dramatic (>500 IU/l) but are usually significantly correlated to total T4 concentrations. Liver enzyme elevation may be minimal, if present at all, in early or mild cases of hyperthyroidism, and concurrent hepatic disease should be suspected if there are marked elevations in these enzymes but only mildly elevated serum thyroid hormone concentrations. When elevated as a result of hyperthyroidism, liver enzyme concentrations decrease to within the reference interval with successful management of the thyrotoxicosis. The exact cause of these abnormalities is unknown but may be related to malnutrition, congestive cardiac failure, hepatic hypoxia, infections and direct toxic effects of thyroid hormones on the liver. However, histopathological examination of the liver usually reveals non-specific changes and there are no significant abnormalities found on hepatic ultrasonography or with tests of liver function (bile acid stimulation). It is known, however, that both liver and bone contribute to the increase in serum ALP activity.

The existence of azotaemia is worthy of particular note. Approximately 20% of hyperthyroid cats have evidence of azotaemia at diagnosis. Such a prevalence of renal dysfunction is not unexpected in a group of aged cats. The increase in urea concentration could be exacerbated by the increased protein intake and protein catabolism of hyperthyroidism. On the other hand, even when elevated, circulating creatinine concentrations may be lower because of a loss of muscle mass. Pre-existing azotaemia in hyperthyroid cats has a significant effect on prognosis. Cats that had a prior diagnosis of chronic kidney disease or were azotaemic at the time of diagnosis of hyperthyroidism had a survival time of only approximately 6 months, compared with approximately 20 months for those hyperthyroid cats with no evidence of renal dysfunction at the time of diagnosis (Williams et al., 2010b). The survival time for cats that develop azotaemia once hyperthyroidism is controlled does not differ from that for hyperthyroid cats that do not develop azotaemia with treatment.

Increased phosphate concentration without evidence of azotaemia occurs in approximately one-third of cats, usually in association with a mild ionized hypocalcaemia and hyperparathyroidism of unknown aetiology.

Blood glucose concentrations may be mildly increased, presumably reflecting a stress response. Circulating fructosamine concentration can be decreased in hyperthyroidism, probably as a result of increased protein turnover. As with hypothyroid dogs, caution is necessary when fructosamine is used to monitor diabetic cats with concurrent hyperthyroidism. Hypokalaemia has occasionally been associated with hyperthyroidism, although the pathogenesis remains unclear.

Assessment of thyroid function

Unlike the situation in canine hypothyroidism, there are no laboratory tests that depict the underlying thyroid pathology in hyperthyroid cats. Elevated circulating concentrations of the thyroid hormones serve as the biochemical hallmark of hyperthyroidism, irrespective of underlying pathology.

Thyroid hormones: For the diagnosis of hyperthyroidism, total T3, total T4 and free T4 can be measured, although the diagnostic performance of each varies. Although TSH measurement is frequently used in humans with hyperthyroidism, it has only recently been studied in cats.

Total thyroxine concentration: Most hyperthyroid cats exhibit an elevated circulating total T4 concentration, with values up to approximately 20 times the upper limit of the reference interval reported. Total T4 is considered a highly specific diagnostic test for hyperthyroidism. However, in recent years many laboratories have decreased the upper limit of the reference interval to improve their diagnostic sensitivity for hyperthyroidism and perhaps to account for the effects of age. Therefore, the specificity of this test now may be less than ideal, although it remains high. Measurement of total T4 is relatively inexpensive and readily accessible. However, approximately 10% of hyperthyroid cats have serum total T4 concentrations within the reference interval (Peterson *et al.*, 2001). This increases to 40% of cases if only those with mild clinical disease are selected. In most of these cats, total T4 values are within the mid to high end of the reference interval. Thus, hyperthyroidism cannot be excluded in cats by demonstration of a single high-end reference interval total T4 concentration alone. There are several explanations for reference interval total T4 values in hyperthyroid cats:

- Non-specific thyroid hormone fluctuation may result in reference interval total T4 values in cats with marginal elevations. A circadian rhythm does not exist in cats but circulating hormone concentrations vary both within and more pronouncedly between days (Shiel and Mooney, 2007). Increased thyroidal production and fluctuations in binding proteins or other undefined haemodynamic alterations possibly account for these changes. Serum total T4 concentrations will often increase into the thyrotoxic range on retesting 3–6 weeks later. However, in some cats, a longer interval is required and testing when more overt clinical signs develop may be more appropriate. In cats with markedly elevated circulating total T4 concentrations, the degree of fluctuation is of little diagnostic significance.
- Non-thyroidal illness has a suppressive effect on circulating total T4 concentration in cats (Figure 17.12), resulting in mid to high reference interval values in mild hyperthyroidism. The mechanisms remain unclear but are more likely to involve changes in peripheral thyroid hormone metabolism or protein binding than any effect

	Hormone			
	Total T3	Total T4	Free T4	TSH
Hyperthyroid	↔↑	↔↑	↑	U
Euthyroid with NTI	↔↓	↔↓	↔↑	D/U
Hyperthyroid with NTI	↔	↔↑	↑	U

17.12 The potential effect of hyperthyroidism and non-thyroidal illness (NTI) in both euthyroid and hyperthyroid cats on thyroid hormone concentrations. These effects are largely known for T3 and T4. There is growing evidence of the effect of hyperthyroidism and non-thyroidal illness on feline TSH but only as assessed by the canine assay. Suppressed values for TSH are difficult to measure and therefore usually indicated as being detectable or undetectable (i.e. at or below the lower limit of detection of the assay). D = detectable; T3 = triiodothyronine; T4 = thyroxine; TSH = thyroid-stimulating hormone (thyrotropin); U = undetectable; ↓ = concentrations decrease; ↔ = concentrations remain the same; ↑ = concentrations increase.

on the hypothalamic–pituitary axis. Similar to the phenomenon of fluctuation, the degree of suppression has little diagnostic significance in hyperthyroid cats with markedly elevated circulating total T4 concentrations. In euthyroid cats, non-thyroidal illness tends to suppress total T4 concentrations into the low end or below the reference interval, depending on the severity of the illness, and its measurement can be used as a prognostic indicator (Mooney *et al.*, 1996; Figure 17.13). Consequently, concurrent hyperthyroidism should always be suspected in cats with severe non-thyroidal illness and serum total T4 concentrations within the mid to high end of the reference interval. It is likely that serum total T4 concentrations would increase into the thyrotoxic range upon treatment or recovery from the non-thyroidal illness. Occasionally, serum total T4 concentrations are suppressed to the lower half of the reference interval in hyperthyroid cats that have extreme non-thyroidal illnesses. However, in these cases, the non-thyroidal illness dictates the prognosis and pursuing hyperthyroidism is of less clinical importance.

In large studies of hyperthyroid cats, approximately 20% of cats with total T4 values within the reference interval have an identifiable concurrent illness. The overwhelming majority are classified as mild or early cases.

Free thyroxine by equilibrium dialysis: In human thyrotoxicosis, assessment of free T4 is considered a better diagnostic test for hyperthyroidism because it is less affected by non-thyroidal factors than total T4 and provides

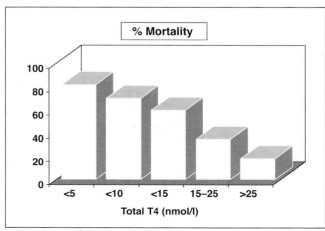

17.13 The relationship of mortality to serum total T4 concentrations in 107 cats with a variety of non-thyroidal illnesses.

a more accurate reflection of thyroid status. In addition, when serum total T4 concentration is increased, the concentration of free T4 is disproportionately increased. In hyperthyroid cats, serum free and total T4 concentrations are highly significantly correlated. In all cats with markedly elevated total T4 concentrations, free T4 concentration is concurrently elevated, adding little diagnostic information to that already obtained. However, as in humans, it is a more sensitive indicator of hyperthyroidism than total T4 measurement alone. Estimates suggest that up to 98% of hyperthyroid cats have an elevated circulating free T4 concentration. More significantly, approximately 95% of hyperthyroid cats with total T4 values in the reference interval, because of mild disease or the suppressive effects of concurrent non-thyroidal illness, have concurrent elevated free T4 concentrations (Shiel and Mooney, 2007).

Measurement of free T4 concentrations is more expensive and less readily available than total T4 and is more subject to sample handling errors. More importantly, it is a less specific diagnostic test for hyperthyroidism as elevated values have been demonstrated in up to 20% of sick euthyroid cats (Shiel and Mooney, 2007; see Figure 17.12). Most of these cats have serum total T4 concentrations in the lower end or below the reference interval. As a consequence, caution is advised in interpreting an elevated free T4 value alone. A stepwise approach is recommended: serum total T4 concentrations should be assessed first in cats suspected of hyperthyroidism. If values are found within the mid to high end of the reference interval, consideration should be given to measurement of the corresponding free T4 concentration. If it is elevated, hyperthyroidism is confirmed.

Total triiodothyronine concentration: Serum total T4 and T3 concentrations are highly correlated in hyperthyroid cats. However, over 30% of hyperthyroid cats have serum total T3 concentrations within the reference interval (Shiel and Mooney, 2007). The majority of cats with such values have serum total T4 concentrations either within the reference interval or only marginally elevated (usually <65 nmol/l, always <100 nmol/l). These cases are usually classified as early, or mildly affected, and it is likely that total T3 concentrations would increase into the diagnostic thyrotoxic range if the disorder were allowed to progress untreated. It is possible that this phenomenon reflects a compensatory decrease in peripheral conversion of T4 to the more active T3 as hyperthyroidism is developing, although in a small number of cases the suppressive effect of severe concurrent non-thyroidal illness may play a role. Owing to the poor diagnostic sensitivity of total T3 measurement, it is not recommended for the evaluation of hyperthyroidism.

Thyrotropin: In humans, measurement of TSH is considered a first-line diagnostic test for hyperthyroidism. Suppressed TSH values are easily demonstrated using the current assays that have a lower limit of detection that is up to 30 times lower than the lower limit of the reference interval. Additionally, there is a log–linear relationship between free T4 and TSH such that small and modest changes in free T4 result in much larger changes in TSH. A species-specific assay does not yet exist for cats (see above). However, regardless of the suitability of using the canine assay to measure feline TSH, it is gaining in popularity. The relatively high lower limit of detection of this assay curtails its usefulness in definitively diagnosing hyperthyroidism. This may be further compromised by the inability of this assay fully to detect feline TSH.

Various studies have shown that TSH, as measured by the canine assay, is below the limit of detection in almost all hyperthyroid cats, conferring a high diagnostic sensitivity (Wakeling *et al.*, 2008). Euthyroid cats with undetectable cTSH concentrations were more likely to have histopathological evidence of thyroid nodular hyperplasia than cats with detectable values (Wakeling *et al.*, 2007). Finally, older cats with undetectable cTSH concentrations were more likely to develop hyperthyroidism within a 9–14-month follow-up period than cats with detectable concentrations (Wakeling *et al.*, 2011).

Unfortunately, a known response to illness is suppression of TSH (see Figure 17.12) and undetectable cTSH concentrations have been reported in euthyroid cats with non-thyroidal illness (Wakeling *et al.*, 2008). This test is therefore of relatively poor specificity. Additionally, roughly 50% of cats with undetectable cTSH values do not develop hyperthyroidism. On the other hand, cats with detectable cTSH concentrations rarely develop hyperthyroidism in the short term. As such, measurement of cTSH in cats may be more useful in eliminating a possible diagnosis of hyperthyroidism if a value exceeds the lower limit of detection of the assay. Caution is advised, however, as detectable cTSH concentrations have been reported in hyperthyroid cats, albeit rarely.

Dynamic thyroid function tests: In the majority of hyperthyroid cats with total T4 concentrations within the reference interval, the diagnosis can be confirmed by consideration of the presence of concurrent non-thyroidal illness, retesting at a later date, or by simultaneous assessment of free T4 concentrations. Dynamic thyroid function tests, previously recommended for confirming hyperthyroidism in equivocal cases, are therefore almost obsolete. They should only be considered in cats with clinical signs of hyperthyroidism when repeated serum total T4 concentrations remain within the reference interval, or free T4 analysis is unavailable or diagnostically unhelpful. A brief description of these tests is given here and in Figure 17.4. Further details can be found elsewhere (Shiel and Mooney, 2007).

T3 suppression test: In healthy individuals, T3 has a suppressive effect on pituitary TSH secretion and subsequently on T4 production by the thyroid gland. In hyperthyroidism, because of autonomous production of thyroid hormones and chronic suppression of TSH, this suppressive effect is lost. Thus, serum total T4 concentrations show minimal or no decrease in hyperthyroid cats following exogenous T3 administration and values remain higher than approximately 20 nmol/l, with less than 35% suppression over the duration of the test. Simultaneous measurement of serum total T3 concentrations is required to ensure compliant administration and adequate absorption of the drug and thus avoid false positive results. Generally, the test is most useful in ruling out, rather than confirming, hyperthyroidism.

TSH stimulation test: As a result of its poor diagnostic performance this test has largely been superseded, despite the availability of rhTSH. Exogenous TSH is a potent stimulator of thyroid hormone secretion, usually causing at least a 100% increase in total T4 concentrations in healthy cats, but serum total T4 concentrations show little or no increase following exogenous TSH administration in hyperthyroid cats. This is presumably because the thyroid gland of affected cats secretes thyroid hormones independently of TSH control or because T4 is already being produced at a near maximal rate with limited reserve capacity. Cats with equivocally elevated serum total T4 concentrations tend to exhibit results indistinguishable from those in healthy animals, and thus the test has limited diagnostic value.

TRH stimulation test: TRH is less expensive and easier to obtain than TSH. Serum total T4 concentrations increase minimally (<50%) after TRH administration in mildly hyperthyroid cats, whereas in healthy cats there is an increase of >60%. Compared to the T3 suppression test, this test is quicker and avoids tablet administration. However, TRH is associated with transient adverse reactions such as salivation, vomiting, tachypnoea and defecation. In addition, results of the test are largely indistinguishable between euthyroid cats with non-thyroidal illness and hyperthyroid cats with concurrent disease and total T4 concentrations within or below the reference interval (Tomsa *et al.*, 2001).

Monitoring response to therapy

Irrespective of the therapeutic modality chosen, measurement of serum total T4 concentrations is of most value in monitoring efficacy. Few studies have specifically evaluated free T4 concentrations and clinical response. Of concern is the effect of non-thyroidal illness in causing not only decreased but, more importantly, increased free T4 concentrations. Although cTSH measurement has been used to assess the efficacy of therapy, particularly the development of hypothyroidism, no cut-off values are yet available for routine and widespread use (see below).

In cats treated with the antithyroid drug, methimazole and its prodrug carbimazole, assessment of total T4 concentration is recommended 2–3 weeks after commencing therapy or after each dose adjustment. Once cats are stable, serum total T4 concentrations should be checked every 3–6 months or more frequently if indicated clinically. Regular assessment is necessary because antithyroid drugs have no effect on the underlying lesions and the thyroid nodules continue to grow and enlarge, necessitating an increased dosage long term. It is generally accepted that the aim of therapy is to suppress serum total T4 concentrations to within the lower half of the reference interval in order to obtain adequate control of the disease (Daminet *et al.*, 2014). Previously, because clinical signs of hypothyroidism rarely developed, a more suppressed total T4 concentration was considered inconsequential, particularly as corresponding total T3 (the more metabolically active hormone) concentrations tended to remain within the reference interval (Mooney *et al.*, 1992). However, today the potential effect of hypothyroidism on decreasing glomerular filtration rate (GFR) has resulted in a revision of this recommendation (see below). Serum total T4 concentrations should not be maintained in the upper half of the reference interval because serum free T4 concentrations appear to remain relatively higher during antithyroid medication.

If medication is given on a daily or divided daily regime, the timing of blood sampling after antithyroid drug therapy is unimportant, whether the drug is administered orally or transdermally (Rutland *et al.*, 2009; Boretti *et al.*, 2013). If alternate-day dosing (occasionally used for the sustained-release formulation) is used, it may be prudent to take blood samples just before drug administration.

Serum total T4 concentrations are usually low for weeks to months after surgical thyroidectomy or radioactive iodine therapy but will eventually increase into the reference interval. There is a general concern regarding the effect of even transient hypothyroidism in these cats. Some veterinary surgeons (veterinarians) routinely supplement with thyroxine in the immediate postoperative or post-radioactive iodine phase. The necessity of this remains unproven but care should be taken if total T4 concentrations remain below the reference interval at 6 months.

Monitoring adverse reactions: Laboratory analysis may be required to assess adverse reactions specifically associated with antithyroid drug administration. Early in the course of therapy, mild and transient haematological abnormalities, including lymphocytosis, eosinophilia or leucopenia with a normal differential count, occur in up to approximately 15% of cases but without any apparent clinical effect (Mooney *et al.*, 1992). More serious haematological complications occur in less than 5% of cases, usually within the first 3 months of therapy, and include severe neutropenia and thrombocytopenia either alone or concurrently or, more rarely, immune-mediated haemolytic anaemia. Drug withdrawal is required. Fortnightly complete blood and platelet counts have been recommended in order to detect such reactions. However, because of their rarity and unpredictability, assessment of a complete blood count if clinical signs indicate is more cost effective. A hepatopathy characterized by marked increases in liver enzyme activities and bilirubin concentration occurs in less than 2% of treated cats. Serum antinuclear antibodies develop in approximately 50% of hyperthyroid cats treated with methimazole for longer than 6 months, usually in cats on high-dose therapy (>15 mg/day).

Assessment of renal function: Hyperthyroidism is known to increase GFR, decrease circulating creatinine concentration and mask underlying renal disease. All treatments for hyperthyroidism have been associated with a decrease in GFR capable of unmasking latent renal disease (Shiel and Mooney, 2007). Renal dysfunction should always be considered a potential adverse effect of treatment and assessed at each monitoring visit, or sooner if clinical signs develop. Several studies have attempted to predict those cats in which renal failure is likely to develop. However, the only successful methods have involved estimation of GFR, which is not readily applicable in practice.

Over one-third of treated hyperthyroid cats develop azotaemia. A decline in renal function is noticeable within 1 month of treatment but the condition remains stable for approximately 6 months thereafter. Although prognosis is guarded in hyperthyroid cats with pre-existing azotaemia (see above), the survival of hyperthyroid cats that develop azotaemia after treatment is not different from that of non-azotaemic cats. However, survival is adversely affected in treated hyperthyroid cats that develop azotaemia and iatrogenic hypothyroidism (Williams *et al.*, 2010a). Diagnosing hypothyroidism in cats is challenging given the effect of non-thyroidal illness (i.e. azotaemia) in suppressing total T4 values. Measurement of cTSH concentrations may help, and while a feline reference interval has been published with a lower upper limit than for dogs (0.15 ng/ml) (Williams *et al.* 2010a), defined cut-offs for diagnosing hypothyroidism are not yet available. An alternative, albeit expensive, method is to perform a TSH stimulation test using rhTSH (Campos *et al.*, 2012).

Canine hyperthyroidism

Hyperthyroidism is exceptionally rare in dogs and is almost always the result of thyroid carcinoma, with only sporadic reports associated with thyroid adenoma. However, hyperthyroidism only occurs in approximately 10–20% of dogs with thyroid carcinoma. Measurement of serum total T4 is adequate for diagnosis but elevations are usually modest compared with the marked increases often seen in hyperthyroid cats. Iatrogenic hyperthyroidism is also possible either as a result of thyroxine overdose or because of feeding raw meat diets or fresh or dried gullets (Kohler *et al.*, 2012). Elevated total T4 concentrations may also arise because of the effect of T4AAs in dogs with lymphocytic thyroiditis.

Case examples

CASE 1

SIGNALMENT

7-year-old male Japanese Spitz.

HISTORY

Increasing weight and exercise intolerance. Coat dry but no alopecia. On clinical examination there were no notable findings.

CLINICAL PATHOLOGY DATA

Haematology	Result	Reference interval
RBC (x 10^{12}/l)	6.09	5.5–8.5
Haemoglobin (g/dl)	13.8	12.0–18.0
Packed cell volume (l/l)	0.40	0.37–0.55
MCV (fl)	66.9	60–77
MCHC (g/dl)	33.8	31.0–36.2
WBC (x 10^9/l)	7.54	6.0–17.0
Neutrophils (x 10^9/l)	4.85	3.0–11.15
Band neutrophils (x 10^9/l)	0.00	0–0.54
Lymphocytes (x 10^9/l)	1.56	1.00–3.60
Monocytes (x 10^9/l)	0.55	0.1–1.35
Eosinophils (x 10^9/l)	0.54	0.10–1.47
Basophils (x 10^9/l)	0.01	0.0–0.1
Platelet count (x 10^9/l)	356	150–550

Film comment: Platelet numbers appear consistent with count. No morphological abnormalities observed.

Biochemistry	Result	Reference interval
ALP (IU/l)	**210**	0–82
AST (IU/l)	**38**	0–37
ALT (IU/l)	**160**	0–36
GGT (IU/l)	6	0–16
Glutamate dehydrogenase (IU/l)	**20**	0–16
Total bilirubin (µmol/l)	4.3	0.9–10
Total protein (g/l)	69	55–75
Albumin (g/l)	32	25–38
Globulin (g/l)	37	28–42
Albumin:globulin ratio	0.86	0.59–1.11
Urea (mmol/l)	8.2	3.6–8.6
Creatinine (µmol/l)	104	20–120
Calcium (mmol/l)	2.63	2.3–3.0
Phosphorus (mmol/l)	1.13	0.8–1.8 ▶

Abnormal results are in **bold**.

Biochemistry *continued*	Result	Reference interval
Creatine kinase (IU/l)	**147**	0–122
Cholesterol (mmol/l)	**13.6**	3.2–6.5
Amylase (IU/l)	389	400–2750
Lipase (IU/l)	230	230–550
Glucose (mmol/l)	5.3	3.0–6.5
Sodium (mmol/l)	146.1	137–150
Potassium (mmol/l)	4.3	3.7–5.8
Chloride (mmol/l)	112.8	105–117

Abnormal results are in **bold**.

WHAT ABNORMALITIES ARE PRESENT? WHAT ARE YOUR DIFFERENTIAL DIAGNOSES? WHAT FURTHER TESTS WOULD YOU LIKE TO PERFORM?

Haematology
- No clear abnormalities

Biochemistry
- Mild elevations in alkaline phosphatase (ALP), glutamate dehydrogenase (GLDH), alanine aminotransferase (ALT) and creatine kinase (CK)

The elevations in ALP, GLDH, ALT and CK are mild. Such a finding is non-specific and observed in many medically ill dogs and in some hypothyroid dogs. The increase in cholesterol is more marked and increases suspicion of hypothyroidism.

Total T4 and TSH measurement is practical because it is diagnostic in the majority of hypothyroid dogs and also is not too expensive.

Endocrinology	Result	Reference interval
Thyroxine (total T4) (nmol/l)	**<6.44**	15–50
TSH (ng/ml)	**3.23**	<0.68

Abnormal results are in **bold**.

HOW WOULD YOU INTERPRET THESE RESULTS?

The combination of low total T4 and moderately elevated TSH provides very strong support for the presence of primary hypothyroidism. One caveat to this interpretation would be the assumption that the animal has not recently received sulphonamide medications or other reversible thyroid inhibitors.

While the Japanese Spitz is not a breed typical for hypothyroidism, this disorder can affect any breed. Dermatological features, while frequently noted, may be subtle and are usually non-specific. It is worth noting that even in cases where a confident diagnosis of hypothyroidism can be made, some of the classically reported clinical pathology features (e.g. normocytic, normochromic anaemia) are absent. A positive clinical response to adequate thyroid replacement therapy would confirm the diagnosis further. If the elevations in ALP, GLDH and ALT continued, further investigation for hepatic disease may be warranted.

CASE 2

SIGNALMENT

8-year-old intact female Tibetan Terrier.

HISTORY

The owners presented the patient because of hair loss noted over the previous several months. Clinical examination was unremarkable, with the exception of ventral alopecia and thinning of the undercoat on the dorsum, with several areas of erythema and mild crusting consistent with superficial pyoderma.

CLINICAL PATHOLOGY DATA

Haematology	Result	Reference interval
RBC (x 10^{12}/l)	**5.01**	5.4–8.5
Haemoglobin (g/dl)	**10.7**	12–18
Packed cell volume (l/l)	**0.33**	0.37–0.56
MCV (fl)	65.4	65–75
MCHC (g/dl)	32	31–35
WBC (x 10^9/l)	**22.4**	5.0–18.0
Neutrophils (x 10^9/l)	**18.14**	3.7–13.32
Band neutrophils (x 10^9/l)	0.00	0–0.54
Lymphocytes (x 10^9/l)	2.69	1.00–3.60
Monocytes (x 10^9/l)	**1.34**	0.20–0.72
Eosinophils (x 10^9/l)	0.22	0.10–1.25
Basophils (x 10^9/l)	0.00	0.05–0.18
Platelet count (x 10^9/l)	472	200–550

Abnormal results are in **bold**.

Film comment: platelet numbers appear adequate on the smear. Red blood cells are normochromic, normocytic with no polychromasia. White blood cells show no morphological abnormalities.

Biochemistry	Result	Reference interval
ALP (IU/l)	**625**	0–135
AST (IU/l)	11	0–45
ALT (IU/l)	29	0–40
GGT (IU/l)	2	0–14
Glutamate dehydrogenase (IU/l)	3	0–9
Total bilirubin (μmol/l)	4.4	0–5.0
Total protein (g/l)	66	55–75
Albumin (g/l)	23	29–35
Globulin (g/l)	**43**	18–38
Albumin:globulin ratio	0.53	0.50–1.20
Urea (mmol/l)	**8.1**	3.5–7.0
Creatinine (μmol/l)	85	0–130
Calcium (mmol/l)	2.71	2.3–3.0
Phosphorus (mmol/l)	1.4	0.9–1.6

Abnormal results are in **bold**.

Biochemistry *continued*	Result	Reference interval
Creatine kinase (IU/l)	87	0–400
Cholesterol (mmol/l)	**11.3**	3.8–7.9
Amylase (IU/l)	427	400–2750
Lipase (IU/l)	496	0–500
Glucose (mmol/l)	4.6	3.0–5.5
Chloride (mmol/l)	102	95–124
Sodium (mmol/l)	140	135–150
Potassium (mmol/l)	**5.7**	3.5–5.6

Abnormal results are in **bold**.

Endocrinology	Result	Reference interval
Thyroxine (total T4) (nmol/l)	**54**	13–52

Abnormal results are in **bold**.

WHAT ABNORMALITIES ARE PRESENT?

Haematology
- Mild normocytic, normochromic anaemia
- No evidence of regeneration given absence of polychromasia

Biochemistry
- Moderate elevation in ALP and cholesterol
- Mild elevation in urea and globulin

Endocrinology
- Borderline high thyroxine

HOW WOULD YOU INTERPRET THESE RESULTS?

Mild non-regenerative anaemia can result from many chronic illnesses, bone marrow disease or may reflect pre-regeneration in cases of very recent haemorrhage or haemolysis. Mild elevation in ALP with no other evidence of hepatopathy is a common, non-specific finding in cases of medical illness. It may also result from glucocorticoid use, including topical treatments.

An elevation in urea without an elevation in creatinine suggests a prerenal origin. Correlation with hydration status and urine specific gravity would be required to understand the significance of this finding further. However, the mild elevation may not be significant.

Elevation in globulin suggests an inflammatory process and is not an uncommon finding in cases of chronic pyoderma.

On a fasted sample, hypercholesterolaemia has a limited range of differential diagnoses, including endocrinopathies (hypothyroidism, hyperadrenocorticism, diabetes mellitus), nephrotic syndrome, cholestasis, pancreatitis and primary hyperlipidaemia. Given the available results, diabetes mellitus is ruled out.

HAS HYPOTHYROIDISM BEEN RULED OUT? IF NOT, WHAT FURTHER TESTS WOULD YOU RECOMMEND?

Hypothyroidism has not been ruled out by this single total T4 result. In particular, in this case there is cause to be suspicious. In dogs with significant non-thyroidal illness a low or low-normal T4 concentration would be expected. In this patient, there is some evidence from both haematology and clinical chemistry that a medical illness may be present. The presence of T4

→ **CASE 2 CONTINUED**

cross-reacting anti-thyroglobulin antibodies (T4AA) causes false increases in reported total T4 concentrations. Such antibodies are observed in approximately 10% of hypothyroid dogs. In this suspicious case, further tests should be considered. Thyrotropin measurement would help identify primary hypothyroidism; free T4 by equilibrium dialysis is free from interference by T4AA; and TgAA (or direct measurement of T4AA) will help identify any potentially cross-reacting antibodies.

FURTHER RESULTS

The following further results were obtained by requesting a complete thyroid panel.

Endocrinology	Result	Reference interval
TSH (ng/ml)	**3.6**	<0.68
Free T4 by equilibrium dialysis (pmol/l)	**<2.0**	7–40
Total T3 (nmol/l)	**0.0**	0.8–2.1
Free T3 (pmol/l)	**>18.6**	1.2–8.2
TgAA (%)	**184**	<35
T4AA (%)	**57**	<20
T3AA (%)	**85**	<10

Abnormal results are in **bold**.

HOW WOULD YOU INTERPRET THIS FURTHER SET OF RESULTS?

The combination of elevated TSH and low free T4 confirms primary hypothyroidism. The positive TgAA result confirms lymphocytic thyroiditis as the underlying pathology and opens up the possibility of T4AA as a possible interfering factor in the total T4 result. The positive T4AA result confirms their presence and the reason behind the 'misleading' total T4. In this case, and in cases where the effect of T4AA is so great as to cause a result above the reference interval, there is reason to be suspicious and continue with further thyroid testing. However, not all hypothyroid dogs demonstrate anaemia or hypercholesterolaemia that might give a reason to continue investigation, and in many cases of T4AA the total T4 result is not clearly high. A minimum canine thyroid investigation, therefore, should include at least TSH (if not also TgAA) in addition to total T4.

In this larger additional panel including total T3, free T3 and T3AA, we can also see the impact of T3AA on total and free (by analogue assay) T3 results at this particular laboratory. In most but not all immunoassays, the presence of cross-reacting patient autoantibodies will cause a false elevation in the results (as seen for free T3). However, in the case of this particular laboratory the effect of T3AA is to cause a low total T3 result. T3AA are more common than T4AA and are a significant explanation for why total T3 is not considered a useful test for canine hypothyroidism.

CASE 3

SIGNALMENT

9-year-old neutered female Miniature Poodle.

HISTORY

2-month history of polydipsia and polyuria. On clinical examination, the dog was obese with a thin haircoat.

CLINICAL PATHOLOGY DATA

Haematology	Result	Reference interval
RBC (x 10¹²/l)	6.72	5.4–8.5
Haemoglobin (g/dl)	13.5	12–18
Packed cell volume (l/l)	0.45	0.37–0.56
MCV (fl)	66.4	65–75
MCHC (g/dl)	**30**	31–35
WBC (x 10⁹/l)	13.20	5.0–18.0
Neutrophils (x 10⁹/l)	12.28	3.7–13.32
Band neutrophils (x 10⁹/l)	0	0–0.54
Lymphocytes (x 10⁹/l)	**0.13**	1.00–3.60
Monocytes (x 10⁹/l)	**0.79**	0.20–0.72
Eosinophils (x 10⁹/l)	0	0.10–1.25
Basophils (x 10⁹/l)	0	0.05–0.18
Platelet count (x 10⁹/l)	**553**	200–550

Abnormal results are in **bold**.

Film comment: platelet numbers appear appropriate on the smear. Red blood cells are normocytic, normochromic. White blood cells show no morphological abnormalities.

Biochemistry	Result	Reference interval
ALP (IU/l)	**4505**	0–135
AST (IU/l)	38	0–45
ALT (IU/l)	**395**	0–40
GGT (IU/l)	**29**	0–14
Glutamate dehydrogenase (IU/l)	**94**	0–9
Total bilirubin (µmol/l)	3.0	0–5.0
Total protein (g/l)	66	55–75
Albumin (g/l)	29	29–35
Globulin (g/l)	37	18–38
Albumin:globulin ratio	0.78	0.50–1.20
Urea (mmol/l)	4.9	3.5–7.0
Creatinine (µmol/l)	83	0–130
Calcium (mmol/l)	2.4	2.3–3.0
Phosphorus (mmol/l)	1.5	0.9–1.6
Creatine kinase (IU/l)	143	0–400
Cholesterol (mmol/l)	**12.9**	3.8–7.9
Amylase (IU/l)	1232	400–2750
Lipase (IU/l)	473	0–500
Glucose (mmol/l)	5.8	3.0–5.5

Abnormal results are in **bold**.

→ CASE 3 CONTINUED

Following review of the haematology and biochemistry results, the following endocrine tests were requested by the clinician based on the combination of polydipsia and elevated ALP and the combination of elevated cholesterol and thin haircoat.

Endocrinology	Result	Reference interval
Thyroxine (total T4) (nmol/l)	**<6**	13–52
TSH (ng/ml)	0.29	<0.68
TgAA (%)	98	<200
Basal cortisol	201	28–250
Cortisol 1 h post-ACTH	**998**	220–550

Abnormal results are in **bold**.

WHAT ABNORMALITIES ARE PRESENT?

Haematology
- Lymphopenia, monocytosis and absolute eosinopenia

Biochemistry
- Marked elevations in ALP, ALT, gamma-glutamyl transferase (GGT) and moderate elevation in GLDH
- Moderately elevated cholesterol

Endocrinology
- Subnormal thyroxine
- Positive adrenocorticotropic hormone (ACTH) stimulation test

HOW WOULD YOU INTERPRET THESE RESULTS?

The dominating results are the liver enzyme changes, 'stress leucogram' and hypercholesterolaemia. In combination with the ACTH stimulation test result and the clinical features including signalment and presenting signs, the veterinary surgeon made the judgement that hyperadrenocorticism was present.

There is a subnormal total T4 but the TSH is normal. The negative TgAA rules out the presence of active immune-mediated thyroid pathology. It could be that this dog is also one of the proportion of hypothyroid dogs in which an elevated TSH is not detected. This proportion

is variably reported but may be as low as 13%. TgAA-negative cases account for only around half of this proportion, meaning that this dog could be one of as few as 7% of hypothyroid dogs that could give this pattern of test results. An alternative explanation is that this dog has a low total T4 as a physiological consequence of medical illness. In this case, where hyperadrenocorticism is suspected the chance of a low T4 resulting from the non-thyroidal illness syndrome is high.

The hypercholesterolaemia in this case cannot be used to provide support for a diagnosis of hypothyroidism because it would also be expected in cases of hyperadrenocorticism.

IS HYPOTHYROIDISM CONFIRMED? IF NOT, WHAT FURTHER TESTS WOULD YOU RECOMMEND?

No. To elucidate further whether hypothyroidism could be a contributing factor in this dog's obesity, it would be wise to wait until the non-thyroidal illness was controlled before repeating total T4 and TSH measurements. An alternative would be to measure free T4 by equilibrium dialysis, as it is less commonly affected by the presence of non-thyroidal illness than is total T4.

FOLLOW-UP RESULTS

After 2 months of trilostane therapy a repeat sample was taken.

Endocrinology	Result	Reference interval
Thyroxine (total T4) (nmol/l)	34	13–52
TSH (ng/ml)	0.24	<0.68

HOW WOULD YOU INTERPRET THESE ADDITIONAL RESULTS?

Taken along with the previous negative TgAA result, hypothyroidism has been conclusively ruled out.

Repeat TgAA testing was not necessary. The absence of immune-mediated thyroid disease had already been confirmed and the negative TgAA result ruled out T4AA, making it possible to be confident in the total T4 result within the reference interval in this further set of tests.

CASE 4

SIGNALMENT

4-year-old neutered female Cocker Spaniel weighing 15 kg.

HISTORY

A confirmed diagnosis of hypothyroidism was made, including a low T4 and elevated TSH, 3 months ago. TgAA was negative at the time of diagnosis. Since that time the dog had been receiving 0.3 mg L-thyroxine once daily. A monitoring sample was obtained according to the clinic's policy on repeat prescriptions. The owners felt that the dog was not as lively as it had been during the first month of treatment.

CLINICAL PATHOLOGY DATA

Endocrinology	Result	Reference interval
Thyroxine (total T4) (nmol/l)	28	13–52
TSH (ng/ml)	**0.95**	<0.68

Abnormal results are in **bold**.

HOW WOULD YOU INTERPRET THE TOTAL T4 RESULT?

The total T4 result can be believed because this patient was recently shown to be TgAA negative. It would be very unlikely that TgAA (including T4 cross-reacting subsets) would start to appear after diagnosis and the initiation of therapy. On the face of it, the total T4 value seems reasonable; it is well inside the reference interval for healthy dogs.

→ **CASE 4 CONTINUED**

WOULD YOU INTERPRET THE TOTAL T4 RESULT ANY DIFFERENTLY WITH THE INFORMATION THAT THE SAMPLE WAS OBTAINED 4 HOURS POST PILL?

At 4 hours post pill, the peak T4 concentration (at 3 hours) has been passed and values will continue to decline until the time of the next pill. The rate of decline will be equivalent to a half-life of between 6 and 10 hours. The next pill is due in 20 hours. At a half-life of 6 hours, we can expect more than three half-lives to pass and can predict a trough concentration less than 4 nmol/l (28, 14, 7, 3.5). Even with a half-life of 10 hours, the predicted trough concentration would be subnormal (7 nmol/l). Given the interval post pill, this total T4 concentration may reflect inadequate therapy.

WHAT IS YOUR OVERALL INTERPRETATION OF THE RESULTS?

The TSH value is elevated, confirming continued physiological hypothyroidism. The TSH concentration takes days to change and therefore additionally confirms that therapy has been suboptimal for some time and not just on the day of the test. What initially appear to be conflicting therapeutic monitoring results are in fact supporting one another when combined with knowledge of the interval post pill. To remedy this, one option is to increase the total daily dose. Moving to twice-daily dosing should not be required but would be an alternative strategy if it suited the owners and did not adversely affect compliance.

CASE 5

SIGNALMENT

11-year-old neutered female Domestic Shorthair cat.

HISTORY

The cat was presented with a history of polydipsia and weight loss. On clinical examination, the veterinary surgeon was unsure whether a thyroid nodule was palpable. The following results were obtained from a blood sample.

Haematology	Results	Reference interval
RBC (x 10¹²/l)	8.7	5.9–11.2
Haemoglobin (g/dl)	11.1	8–15
Haematocrit/PCV (l/l)	0.35	0.24–0.46
MCV (fl)	40.9	37.0–55.0
MCHC (g/dl)	32	26–36
WBC (x 10⁹/l)	12.4	7.7–19.0
Neutrophils (x 10⁹/l)	9.67	2.5–12.5
Band neutrophils (x 10⁹/l)	0	0–0.3
Lymphocytes (x 10⁹/l)	1.61	1.5–6.5
Monocytes (x 10⁹/l)	0.5	0–1.0
Eosinophils (x 10⁹/l)	0.62	0–1.5
Basophils (x 10⁹/l)	0	0–1.0
Platelet count (x 10⁹/l)	368	230–680

Abnormal results are in **bold**.

Film comment: platelet numbers appear appropriate on the smear. Red blood cells are normocytic, normochromic. White blood cells show no morphological abnormalities.

Biochemistry	Result	Reference interval
ALP (IU/l)	**150**	7–75
ALT (IU/l)	58	30–60
GGT (IU/l)	0	0–7
Total protein (g/l)	74	55–78
Albumin (g/l)	29	22–36
Globulin (g/l)	45	25–55
Albumin:globulin ratio	0.64	0.53–1.36
Urea (mmol/l)	7.6	3.5–8.0
Creatinine (µmol/l)	69	40–180
Calcium (mmol/l)	2.5	2.0–2.8
Phosphorus (mmol/l)	1.60	0.81–1.61
Cholesterol (mmol/l)	3.8	2.0–3.9
Glucose (mmol/l)	**18.2**	4.3–6.6
Fructosamine (µmol/l)	**621**	146–271
Chloride (mmol/l)	110	100–120
Sodium (mmol/l)	148	141–155
Potassium (mmol/l)	4.1	3.5–5.5
Sodium:potassium ratio	36	

Abnormal results are in **bold**.

Thyroid profile	Result	Reference interval
Thyroxine (total T4) (nmol/l)	**18**	19–65
Free T4 equilibrium dialysis (pmol/l)	**60**	10–50

Abnormal results are in **bold**.

WHAT ABNORMALITIES ARE PRESENT?

Haematology
- No abnormalities

Biochemistry
- Moderate elevation in ALP and glucose
- Marked elevation in fructosamine

Endocrinology
- Subnormal total thyroxine
- Elevated free thyroxine

→ CASE 5 CONTINUED

HOW WOULD YOU INTERPRET THESE RESULTS?

The combination of elevated glucose and markedly elevated fructosamine is consistent with a diagnosis of diabetes mellitus. The elevation in ALP is consistent with that diagnosis.

IS HYPERTHYROIDISM CONFIRMED?

The total and free T4 results present discordant findings concerning the likely presence of hyperthyroidism.

However, with knowledge of the diagnostic performance of these two tests, along with an understanding of what physiological responses to illness can be expected, the most likely explanation is straightforward.

In euthyroid cats with significant non-thyroidal illness, total T4 is expected to be suppressed and to lie either within the lower half of the reference interval or below the reference interval. This is likely to be what is happening in this case. Conversely, free T4 does not have perfect diagnostic specificity and is sometimes mildly elevated in cases of significant non-thyroidal illness. These results make a diagnosis of hyperthyroidism very unlikely.

References and further reading

Beale K and Torres S (1991) Thyroid pathology and serum antithyroglobulin antibodies in hypothyroid and healthy dogs. *Journal of Veterinary Internal Medicine* **5**, 128

Boretti FS and Reusch CE (2004) Endogenous TSH in the diagnosis of canine hypothyroidism. *Schweizer Archiv für Tierheilkunde* **146**, 183–188

Boretti FS, Sieber-Ruckstuhl NS, Schafer S et al. (2013) Duration of T4 suppression in hyperthyroid cats treated once and twice daily with transdermal methimazole. *Journal of Veterinary Internal Medicine* **27**, 377–381

Broussard JD, Peterson ME and Fox PR (1995) Changes in clinical and laboratory findings in cats with hyperthyroidism from 1983–1993. *Journal of the American Veterinary Medical Association* **206**, 302–305

Campos M, van Hoek I, Peremans K and Daminet S (2012) Recombinant human thyrotropin in veterinary medicine: current use and future perspectives. *Journal of Veterinary Internal Medicine* **26**, 853–862

Castillo VA, Lalia JC, Junco M et al. (2001) Changes in thyroid function in puppies fed a high iodine commercial diet. *Veterinary Journal* **161**, 80–84

Daminet S, Croubels S, Duchateau L et al. (2003) Influence of acetylsalicylic acid and ketoprofen on canine thyroid function tests. *The Veterinary Journal* **166**, 224–232

Daminet S and Ferguson DC (2003) Influence of drugs on thyroid function in dogs. *Journal of Veterinary Internal Medicine* **17**, 463–472

Daminet S, Kooistra HS, Fracassi F et al. (2014) Best practice for the pharmacological management of hyperthyroid cats with anti-thyroid drugs. *Journal of Small Animal Practice* **55**, 4–13

Diaz-Espineira MM, Galac S, Mol JA, Rijnberk A and Kooistra HS (2008) Thyrotropin-releasing hormone-stimulated growth hormone secretion in dogs with primary hypothyroidism. *Domestic Animal Endocrinology* **34**, 176–181

Dixon RM and Mooney CT (1999) Evaluation of serum free thyroxine and thyrotropin concentrations in the diagnosis of canine hypothyroidism. *Journal of Small Animal Practice* **40**, 72–78

Dixon RM, Reid SW and Mooney CT (1999) Epidemiological, clinical, haematological and biochemical characteristics of canine hypothyroidism. *Veterinary Record* **145**, 481–487

Dixon RM, Reid SW and Mooney CT (2002) Treatment and therapeutic monitoring of canine hypothyroidism. *Journal of Small Animal Practice* **43**, 334–340

Dodgson SE, Day R and Fyfe JC (2012) Congenital hypothyroidism with goiter in Tenterfield terriers. *Journal of Veterinary Internal Medicine* **26**, 1350–1357

Gordon JM, Ehrhart EJ, Sisson DD and Jones MA (2003) Juvenile hyperthyroidism in a cat. *Journal of the American Animal Hospital Association* **39**, 67–71

Graham PA, Refsal KR and Nachreiner RF (2007) Etiopathologic findings of canine hypothyroidism. *Veterinary Clinics of North America: Small Animal Practice* **37**, 617–631

Gulikers KP and Panciera DL (2003) Evaluation of the effects of clomipramine on canine thyroid function tests. *Journal of Veterinary Internal Medicine* **17**, 44–49

Iversen L, Jensen AL, Hoier R et al. (1998) Development and validation of an improved enzyme-linked immunosorbent assay for the detection of thyroglobulin autoantibodies in canine serum samples. *Domestic Animal Endocrinology* **15**, 525–536

Kohler B, Stengel C and Neiger R (2012) Dietary hyperthyroidism in dogs. *Journal of Small Animal Practice* **53**, 182–184

Mooney CT (2011) Canine hypothyroidism: a review of aetiology and diagnosis. *New Zealand Veterinary Journal* **59**, 105–114

Mooney CT, Little CJ and Macrae AW (1996) Effect of illness not associated with the thyroid gland on serum total and free thyroxine concentrations in cats. *Journal of the American Veterinary Medical Association* **208**, 2004–2008

Mooney CT and Peterson ME (2012) *BSAVA Manual of Canine and Feline Endocrinology, 4th edn*. BSAVA Publications, Gloucester

Mooney CT, Shiel RE and Dixon RM (2008) Thyroid hormone abnormalities and outcome in dogs with non-thyroidal illness. *Journal of Small Animal Practice* **49**, 11–16

Mooney CT, Thoday KL and Doxey DL (1992) Carbimazole therapy of feline hyperthyroidism. *Journal of Small Animal Practice* **33**, 228–235

Nachreiner RF, Refsal KR, Graham PA, Hauptman J and Watson GL (1998) Prevalence of autoantibodies to thyroglobulin in dogs with non-thyroidal illness. *American Journal of Veterinary Research* **59**, 951–955

Nelson RW, Ihle SL, Feldman EC and Bottoms GD (1991) Serum free thyroxine concentration in healthy dogs, dogs with hypothyroidism, and euthyroid dogs with concurrent illness. *Journal of the American Veterinary Medical Association* **198**, 1401–1407

Panciera DL (1994) Hypothyroidism in dogs: 66 cases (1987–1992). *Journal of the American Veterinary Medical Association* **204**, 761–767

Panciera DL, MacEwen EG, Atkins CE, Bosu WT, Refsal KR and Nachreiner RF (1990) Thyroid function tests in euthyroid dogs treated with L-thyroxine. *American Journal of Veterinary Research* **51**, 22–26

Panciera DL, Refsal KR, Sennello KA and Ward DL (2006) Effects of deracoxib and aspirin on serum concentrations of thyroxine, 3,5,3'-triiodothyronine, free thyroxine, and thyroid-stimulating hormone in healthy dogs. *American Journal of Veterinary Research* **67**, 599–603

Paradis M, Sauve F, Charest J, Refsal KR, Moreau M and Dupuis J (2003) Effects of moderate to severe osteoarthritis on canine thyroid function. *Canadian Veterinary Journal* **44**, 407–412

Peterson ME, Kintzer PP, Cavanagh PG et al. (1983) Feline hyperthyroidism: pretreatment clinical and laboratory evaluation of 131 cases. *Journal of the American Veterinary Medical Association* **183**, 103–110

Peterson ME, Melian C and Nichols R (1997) Measurement of serum total thyroxine, triiodothyronine, free thyroxine, and thyrotropin concentrations for diagnosis of hypothyroidism in dogs. *Journal of the American Veterinary Medical Association* **211**, 1396–1402

Peterson ME, Melian C and Nichols R (2001) Measurement of serum concentrations of free thyroxine, total thyroxine, and total triiodothyronine in cats with hyperthyroidism and cats with nonthyroidal disease. *Journal of the American Veterinary Medical Association* **218**, 529–536

Rayalam S, Eizenstat LD, Davis RR, Hoenig M and Ferguson DC (2006a) Expression and purification of feline thyrotropin (fTSH): Immunological detection and bioactivity of heterodimeric and yoked glycoproteins. *Domestic Animal Endocrinology* **30**, 185–202

Rayalam S, Eizenstat LD, Hoenog M and Ferguson DC (2006b) Cloning and sequencing of feline thyrotropin (fTSH): Heterodimeric and yoked constructs. *Domestic Animal Endocrinology* **30**, 203–217

Rutland BE, Nachreiner RF and Kruger JM (2009) Optimal testing for thyroid hormone concentration after treatment with methimazole in healthy and hyperthyroid cats. *Journal of Veterinary Internal Medicine* **23**, 1025–1030

Sauve F, Paradis M, Refsal KR, Moreau M, Beauchamp G and Dupuis J (2003) Effects of oral administration of meloxicam, carprofen, and a nutraceutical on thyroid function in dogs with osteoarthritis. *Canadian Veterinary Journal* **44**, 474–479

Scott-Moncrieff JC, Nelson RW, Bruner JM and Williams DA (1998) Comparison of serum concentrations of thyroid-stimulating hormone in healthy dogs, hypothyroid dogs, and euthyroid dogs with concurrent disease. *Journal of the American Veterinary Medical Association* **212**, 387–391

Shiel RE, Acke E, Puggioni A, Cassidy JP and Mooney CT (2007a) Tertiary hypothyroidism in a dog. *Irish Veterinary Journal* **60**, 88–93

Shiel RE, Brennan SF, Omodo-Eluk AJ and Mooney CT (2007b) Thyroid hormone concentrations in young, healthy, pretraining greyhounds. *Veterinary Record* **161**, 616–619

Shiel RE and Mooney CT (2007) Testing for hyperthyroidism in cats. *Veterinary Clinics of North America: Small Animal Practice* **37**, 671–691

Shiel RE, Sist M, Nachreiner RE, Ehrlich CP and Mooney CT (2010) Assessment of criteria used by veterinary practitioners to diagnose hypothyroidism in sighthounds and investigation of serum thyroid hormone concentrations in healthy Salukis. *Journal of the American Veterinary Medical Association* **236**, 302–308

Thoday KL and Mooney CT (1992) Historical, clinical and laboratory features of 126 hyperthyroid cats. *Veterinary Record* **131**, 257–264

Tomsa K, Glaus TM, Kacl GM, Pospischil A and Reusch CE (2001) Thyrotropin-releasing hormone stimulation test to assess thyroid function in severely sick cats. *Journal of Veterinary Internal Medicine* **15**, 89–93

Wakeling J, Elliott J and Syme H (2011) Evaluation of predictors for the diagnosis of hyperthyroidism in cats. *Journal of Veterinary Internal Medicine* **25**, 1057–1065

Wakeling J, Moore K, Elliott J and Syme H (2008) Diagnosis of hyperthyroidism in cats with mild chronic kidney disease. *Journal of Small Animal Practice* **49**, 287–294

Wakeling J, Smith K, Scase T, Kirkby R, Elliott J and Syme H (2007) Subclinical hyperthyroidism in cats: a spontaneous model of subclinical toxic nodular goiter in humans. *Thyroid* **17**, 1201–1209

Williams TL, Elliott J and Syme HM (2010a) Association of iatrogenic hypothyroidism with azotemia and reduced survival time in cats treated for hyperthyroidism. *Journal of Veterinary Internal Medicine* **24**, 1086–1092

Williams TL, Peak KJ, Brodbelt D, Elliott J and Syme HM (2010b) Survival and the development of azotemia after treatment of hyperthyroid cats. *Journal of Veterinary Internal Medicine* **24**, 863–869

Chapter 18

Laboratory evaluation of adrenal diseases

Ian Ramsey and Michael Herrtage

Each adrenal gland is composed of a cortex and a medulla, which are functionally separate endocrine glands. The cortex is essential for life, but the medulla is not. The most common disorders affect the adrenal cortex and cause either hyperadrenocorticism (HAC) or hypoadrenocorticism. Conditions affecting the adrenal medulla are rare, the most common being neoplasia (phaeochromocytoma).

The adrenal cortex produces about 30 different hormones, many of which have little or no clinical significance. The hormones can be divided into three groups based on their predominant actions:

- Mineralocorticoids are responsible for electrolyte and water homeostasis. Aldosterone, the most important, is produced by the zona glomerulosa
- Glucocorticoids promote gluconeogenesis, lipolysis and protein catabolism. They also antagonize the effect of insulin and are anti-inflammatory and immunosuppressive. Cortisol, the most important, is produced in the zonas fasciculata and reticularis
- Sex hormones, particularly male hormones that have weak androgenic activity, are produced in small quantities in the zonas fasciculata and reticularis.

Adrenal steroid synthesis and release

Glucocorticoid release is controlled almost entirely by adrenocorticotropic hormone (ACTH) secreted by the anterior pituitary gland, which, in turn, is regulated by corticotropin-releasing hormone (CRH) from the hypothalamus (Figure 18.1). ACTH causes cortisol release from the adrenal cortex, with serum concentrations rising almost immediately. Cortisol has direct negative feedback effects on:

- The hypothalamus, to decrease formation and release of CRH
- The anterior pituitary gland, to decrease formation and release of ACTH.

There is probably an internal or 'short loop' negative feedback control by ACTH on CRH. These feedback mechanisms help to regulate the plasma concentration of cortisol.

The principal mineralocorticoid released by the adrenal cortex is aldosterone. The secretion of aldosterone is mainly regulated by the renin–angiotensin system and the serum potassium concentration.

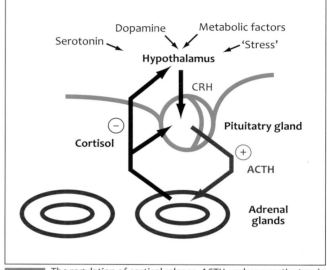

18.1 The regulation of cortisol release. ACTH = adrenocorticotropic hormone; CRH = corticotropin-releasing hormone.

ACTH has only a permissive effect on aldosterone secretion at physiological doses (Figure 18.2). Pharmacological doses of ACTH will, however, induce the secretion of aldosterone, e.g. when performing an ACTH stimulation test. Aldosterone primarily acts on the proximal

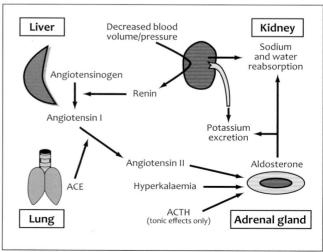

18.2 The regulation of aldosterone release. ACE = angiotensin converting enzyme; ACTH = adrenocorticotropic hormone.

convoluted tubule to increase sodium reabsorption and on the distal convoluted tubule to increase sodium reabsorption in exchange for potassium ions. Osmotic forces ensure that this results in an increase in water retention.

Further details on adrenal steroid synthesis and regulation of their release can be found in the *BSAVA Manual of Canine and Feline Endocrinology* (Herrtage and Ramsey, 2012).

Canine hyperadrenocorticism

Hyperadrenocorticism (HAC) results from a chronic excess of glucocorticoid secretion. The disease has two spontaneous forms and may also be produced iatrogenically by the administration of steroids. The most common cause of spontaneous HAC is the overproduction of ACTH by a small benign pituitary microadenoma (pituitary-dependent HAC (PD-HAC), or Cushing's disease). Excessive secretion of ACTH results in bilateral adrenocortical hyperplasia and overproduction of cortisol and its precursors. Other causes of PD-HAC include larger tumours (macroadenomas) and diffuse hyperplasia of the ACTH-secreting cells (corticotrophs). PD-HAC accounts for about 85% of all spontaneous canine HAC. Macroadenomas are seen in about 10% of these cases. Rarely, pituitary adenocarcinoma has been documented. The incidence of pituitary corticotroph hyperplasia is debated in the literature.

Adrenal-dependent HAC (AD-HAC) results from the overproduction of cortisol by an adrenal tumour. Adrenal tumours may show a range of biological (including metastatic) behaviour and the neoplastic cells release variable amounts of cortisol (and other precursor steroids). Approximately half these tumours are malignant. The release of cortisol from the tumour may, or may not, be influenced by ACTH. Moreover, the extent of the effect of ACTH on cortical secretion is variable. Therefore, adrenal tumours do not behave predictably in any endocrine test. The contralateral adrenal gland is usually atrophic.

Ectopic ACTH production would appear to be a very rare cause of HAC in the dog, with only one suspected case reported. However, in humans a number of tumours, for example oat cell carcinomas of the lung, are capable of synthesizing and secreting excessive quantities of ACTH. Moreover, hypercortisolism not associated with ACTH or tumours is also recognized in humans and there is one report of food-associated hypercortisolaemia in a dog.

The clinical signs of HAC are summarized in Figure 18.3. Signs of AD-HAC are indistinguishable from those of PD-HAC, but AD-HAC is more common in larger breeds than PD-HAC, and is more common in bitches (about 70% of cases are in females).

HAC is a chronic disease; often the changes develop slowly and therefore are not noticed by the owners. Clinical signs vary considerably between individual animals and a few cases may only show one or two signs.

Iatrogenic HAC may be produced by the administration of glucocorticoids. The clinical and clinicopathological presentations are similar to spontaneous HAC but the results of specific endocrine tests are different. The differences observed depend on the dose and type of glucocorticoid administered. There is also considerable individual variation in the response to different formulations of glucocorticoid. Even small doses of exogenous glucocorticoids administered for a short time can have a severe effect on some dogs. Obtaining a reliable history can prevent expensive and unnecessary testing.

Common signs of hyperadrenocorticism

• Polydipsia, polyuria, polyphagia
• Lethargy
• Dermatological changes
  • Symmetrical alopecia, poor hair regrowth, comedones, skin thinning
  • Hyperfragile skin (in cats)
• Abdominal distension ('pot belly')
• Excessive panting
• Muscle weakness
• Anoestrus and genital atrophy

Uncommon signs of hyperadrenocorticism

• Dermatological changes
  • Coat colour changes, hyperpigmentation, calcinosis cutis
  • Excessive bruising and poor wound healing
• Stiff hindlimb gait (due to pseudomyotonia)
• Dyspnoea (due to pulmonary thromboembolism)
• Neurological signs (due to rapid tumour growth)
  • Ataxia, depression, apparent blindness, inappetence, aimless walking, seizures, alteration in normal behaviour patterns

18.3 Clinical signs of canine hyperadrenocorticism. It is important to employ specific endocrine tests only in animals that have appropriate clinical signs.

Investigation of hyperadrenocorticism

The process of investigating and confirming canine HAC is summarized in Figure 18.4. Before performing any laboratory tests for HAC it is important to obtain an accurate history and perform a thorough clinical examination (Herrtage and Ramsey, 2012).

Full blood and urine profiles are obtained to:

- Identify any non-specific indicators of the disease
- Exclude other causes of polyuria/polydipsia (PU/PD), polyphagia, etc.
- Identify intercurrent disease that might affect subsequent therapy.

The more common laboratory changes that are seen in canine HAC are summarized in Figure 18.5 and below.

Blood profiles

Alkaline phosphatase (ALP): Serum ALP concentrations are increased in over 90% of cases of canine HAC. The concentration is commonly 5–40 times the upper end of the reference range, and this is perhaps the most sensitive biochemical indicator of HAC. Glucocorticoids, both endogenous and exogenous, induce a specific isoenzyme of ALP that is unique to the dog. However, increases in serum ALP occur in many other conditions and a normal serum ALP concentration does not exclude a diagnosis of HAC.

The steroid-induced alkaline phosphatase (SIALP) can be quantified (see Chapter 12) and initial studies suggested that SIALP measurement provided an accurate differentiation of the causes of increased ALP. However, subsequent studies have concluded that, while measurement of SIALP is quite sensitive, it is no more specific for spontaneous canine HAC than ALP: SIALP can be increased in primary hepatopathies, diabetes mellitus and with anticonvulsant and exogenous glucocorticoid therapy.

Alanine aminotransferase (ALT): ALT is commonly mildly increased in HAC, as a result of hepatocyte damage due to glycogen accumulation. Increases to more than five times the upper limit of the reference range warrant further investigation as they may affect subsequent therapy.

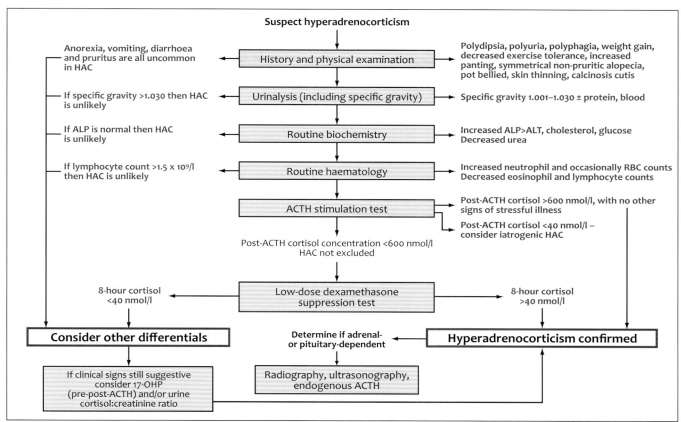

18.4 A summary of the investigation of canine hyperadrenocorticism (HAC). It is not necessary to perform all these investigations in every case. Text in blue refers to typical features of HAC; text in red refers to uncommon findings. ACTH = adrenocorticotropic hormone; ALP = alkaline phosphatase; ALT = alanine aminotransferase; 17-OHP = 17-hydroxyprogesterone; RBC = red blood cell.

Haematology
• Increased total WBC count
• Neutrophilia
• Eosinopenia
• Lymphopenia
• Monocytosis
• Thrombocytosis

Biochemistry
• Increased ALP: high proportion of dogs but only 30% of cats
• Increased ALT: less elevated than ALP
• Hypercholesterolaemia
• Hyperglycaemia: more pronounced in cats – overt diabetes mellitus is common
• Decreased circulating total T4 (normal endogenous TSH)

Urinalysis
• Specific gravity is generally low (<1.015), sometimes very low
• Proteinuria
• Glucosuria common in cats, less so in dogs
• Urinary tract infection (UTI): blood, protein, pH changes, active sediment or occult UTI

18.5 Summary of changes seen on routine haematology, biochemistry and urinalysis in HAC, in approximate order of frequency. ALP = alkaline phosphatase; ALT = alanine aminotransferase; T4 = thyroxine; TSH = thyroid-stimulating hormone; WBC = white blood cell.

Bile acid concentrations: Resting and postprandial serum bile acid concentrations may show mild to moderate increases (up to 100 µmol/l pre- and postprandially) in some cases of HAC, due to steroid hepatopathy. When abnormal results are obtained, HAC is best differentiated from primary liver disorders by the clinical history, physical examination and diagnostic imaging. If fine-needle aspiration (or biopsy) is performed on the liver of a dog with HAC then vacuolar hepatopathy would be expected; however, this investigation is not usually necessary.

Glucose: The glucose concentration is usually in the high-normal range. About 10% of cases develop overt diabetes mellitus, which is caused by antagonism to the action of insulin by the gluconeogenic effects of excess glucocorticoids. Initially, serum insulin concentrations increase to maintain normoglycaemia, but eventually the pancreatic islet cells become exhausted, giving rise to overt diabetes mellitus.

Urea and creatinine: Creatinine concentration usually tends to be in the low to normal range. This may reflect loss of muscle mass as well as the effects of glucocorticoid-induced polyuria. Urea is variable: increased protein catabolism and glucocorticoid-induced diuresis are conflicting factors and blood urea may be normal, increased or decreased.

Cholesterol and triglyceride: Cholesterol and triglyceride concentrations are usually increased owing to glucocorticoid stimulation of lipolysis. Cholesterol is usually >8 mmol/l but is also raised in hypothyroidism, diabetes mellitus, chronic pancreatitis, cholestatic liver disease and protein-losing nephropathy, all of which may be differential diagnoses. Increased triglyceride and consequent lipaemia can also occur, although less frequently than increased cholesterol.

Electrolytes: Sodium, potassium and calcium concentrations are usually in the reference range. Phosphate is often increased when compared with age-matched controls (Ramsey *et al.*, 2005). This probably reflects the increased bone metabolism in dogs with HAC.

Urinalysis

Urine specific gravity: Urine specific gravity (SG) is usually <1.015, and is often hyposthenuric (<1.008) as long as water has not been withheld. This is due to relative antagonism of antidiuretic hormone (ADH) leading to a secondary nephrogenic diabetes insipidus. Dogs with HAC can usually concentrate their urine to some extent if deprived of water, but their concentrating ability is frequently reduced. However, in some cases of PD-HAC due to a macroadenoma, compression of the posterior lobe of the pituitary and extension into the hypothalamus may cause complete disruption of ADH production and release. This will result in massive PU/PD, consistent with central diabetes insipidus (see Chapter 10). However, confirmation of this diagnosis using a water deprivation test can only be made after the HAC has been controlled.

Urinary tract infection: Urine (collected by cystocentesis) should be cultured, because urinary tract infections occur in about 50% of cases of HAC. Urinary tract infection occurs because voiding is never complete owing to muscle weakness. Immunosuppression may also play a role. There is often little evidence of inflammatory cells in the urine sediment and, indeed, there are often few clinical signs of urinary tract infection, owing to the immunosuppressive action of excess glucocorticoids. Lower urinary tract infections can ascend to the kidneys to cause pyelonephritis.

Urine protein: Most dogs with untreated HAC have proteinuria, defined as a urine protein:creatinine ratio (UPCR) >0.5, in the absence of urinary tract infection. Proteinuria is usually mild to moderate (UPCR <5.0), but can be severe (>10.0), and may be associated with systemic hypertension. Despite the severity of proteinuria in some cases, HAC has not been shown to produce the nephrotic syndrome or hypoalbuminaemia.

Urine glucose: Glucosuria occurs in 10% of dogs with HAC: these represent cases with overt diabetes mellitus.

Endocrine tests

Before performing endocrine tests: Specific endocrine tests should only be undertaken in animals with clinical evidence of HAC. Indiscriminate testing alters diagnostic efficiency and makes accurate interpretation difficult. False positive results can occur, leading to unnecessary treatment, which is also potentially dangerous and expensive.

Note on measurement of cortisol: It is important to understand the differences among the various techniques for measuring cortisol before undertaking specific endocrine tests. The diagnosis of adrenocortical disease is dependent on the accurate and sensitive measurement of concentrations of cortisol in urine, blood, saliva or even hair samples. There are several assays on the market and they use different antibodies which recognize different parts of the cortisol molecule because of the way that they are made (Zeugswetter *et al.*, 2013). As a result, cortisol metabolites, including glucuronidated forms that are common in urine (commonly called 'corticoids'), and glucocorticoid drugs will cross-react to differing extents depending on the method used to produce the antibody.

For example, one antibody used to measure cortisol in urine probably just measures cortisol and therefore the cut-off for the urine cortisol:creatinine ratio to exclude HAC can be set quite low (e.g. 8.3×10^{-6}) (Vonderen *et al.*, 1998), whereas another antibody may measure cortisol and corticoids and so measures a median of eight times more 'cortisol', and thus needs a higher cut-off to rule out HAC (e.g. 26×10^{-6}) and a much higher cut-off to make a positive diagnosis of HAC (e.g. 160×10^{-6}) (Zeugswetter *et al.*, 2010). These antibody differences may matter less in serum because cortisol is mostly free in serum rather than conjugated (Zeugswetter *et al.*, 2010, 2013).

In addition to how the antibody binds to the cortisol molecule, the method of detecting antibody binding to the cortisol molecule varies. Radioimmunoassays (RIAs) have long been held as the gold standard because they are least affected by sample quality, but they use radioactivity and are therefore not suitable for in-practice use. Chemiluminescent assays (CLAs) (such as those in the Immulite analysers used by some commercial laboratories) are more suitable for large sample numbers but are more affected by jaundice and tend to detect slightly less cortisol than RIAs (Russell *et al.*, 2007). Enzyme-linked immunosorbent assays (ELISAs) tend to be even less sensitive and suffer from a loss of accuracy at low cortisol concentrations (Ginel *et al.*, 1998). They are also affected by bilirubin and haemolysis. However, they can be adapted to run on individual samples and are therefore useful for in-practice, single-patient use (e.g. SNAP™ ELISA tests). These ELISAs tend to report lower cortisol concentrations than RIAs or CLAs. This has significant implications in the diagnosis of hypoadrenocorticism and HAC as the generally accepted concentration of 40 nmol/l may not be suitable as the cut-off value in ACTH stimulation tests for hypoadrenocorticism or for low-dose dexamethasone suppression tests (LDDSTs) for HAC. Similarly, monitoring trilostane therapy with ELISAs may be difficult.

In addition, there is emerging evidence from quality control schemes such as the one run by the European Society of Veterinary Endocrinology that there is also a small amount of variation among laboratories using the same assays. This manual, in common with other textbooks, is based on the authors' experiences with RIAs and CLAs and the published literature (of which there is very little on in-practice, single-patient ELISAs).

The implications to the practitioner are significant and can be summarized as follows:

- Know what method of cortisol measurement you are using and understand that this alters the interpretation. Try to stick to one method and, better still, one laboratory
- When using an external laboratory, ask which quality control schemes the laboratory participates in (see Chapter 2 for further information). Use the individual laboratory reference ranges rather than those supplied in a textbook. Ask for assistance from the laboratory in interpretation
- ELISAs should really be reserved for emergency cases, and any results that suggest a change in treatment, or which do not fit the clinical picture, should be checked using another method.

Basal cortisol: Basal cortisol measurements are of no value in the diagnosis of HAC because normal dogs, those with HAC and those stressed by another illness have cortisol concentrations that fluctuate widely and overlap to a considerable extent.

Standard endocrine tests

There are three long-established tests used for the diagnosis of canine HAC: the ACTH stimulation test; the LDDST; and the urine corticoid:creatinine ratio (UCCR). The test chosen depends on individual owner, dog and veterinary factors, including time constraints, cost, personal preference and the particular form of HAC that is suspected.

About 80% of all dogs with HAC are positive on the ACTH stimulation test, and 90–95% are positive on the LDDST. The sensitivity of ACTH stimulation testing in the diagnosis of adrenal-dependent disease is much lower (as low as 60%). Some dogs, particularly those with functional adrenal tumours, can give normal results on both tests. It should be noted that the reported sensitivity and specificity, and the positive and negative predictive values, for these two tests vary with the population sampled. For example, if dogs with clinical presentations not suggestive of HAC and final diagnoses of non-adrenal illnesses are examined then 14% are (falsely) positive on ACTH stimulation and 56% are (falsely) positive on the LDDST (Kaplan et al., 1995). False positive results may be seen, for example, with diabetes mellitus, renal failure or pyometra. However, this group of dogs is not normally tested for HAC. (See Chapter 2 for discussions of sensitivity, specificity and positive and negative predictive values.)

Some cases of HAC are presented with highly suggestive clinical signs but these two diagnostic tests prove equivocal or negative. In these circumstances it is sensible to check for other endocrine diseases (particularly hypothyroidism) and then to repeat the tests. If this approach is unsuccessful at determining the cause of the dog's presenting signs then the UCCR may sometimes be useful. However, this test is not a replacement for the ACTH stimulation test or LDDST in cases with suggestive clinical signs.

In some cases in which HAC is only a minor differential diagnosis, it is useful to exclude HAC as a cause of the clinical signs. For this purpose the UCCR is very useful as it has a high negative predictive value.

ACTH stimulation test: The test method is described in Figure 18.6.

Cortisol is stable for many weeks at 4°C. Interpretation of the ACTH stimulation test is summarized in Figure 18.7. In normal dogs, pre-ACTH cortisol concentrations are usually between 20 and 250 nmol/l and post-ACTH cortisol concentrations are between 200 and 450 nmol/l. Regardless of the pre-ACTH cortisol value, a diagnosis of HAC is confirmed by a post-ACTH cortisol concentration >600 nmol/l in dogs with compatible clinical signs and no evidence of acute stressful illnesses. Severe metabolic stress (such as that caused by diabetic ketoacidosis or haemorrhagic gastroenteritis) can lead to very marked elevations in post-ACTH cortisol concentrations. There is no absolute value above which HAC can be diagnosed with 100% accuracy. It is the combination of the clinical signs and abnormal ACTH stimulation test results which

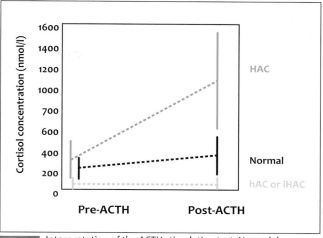

18.7 Interpretation of the ACTH stimulation test. Normal dogs show a 2–3-fold increase in cortisol concentrations but these remain <450 nmol/l. Most dogs with HAC have post-ACTH cortisol concentrations >600 nmol/l. False positive results occur with 'stressful' illnesses, such as unstable diabetes mellitus. The expected results in cases of iatrogenic HAC (iHAC) and hypoadrenocorticism (hAC) are also shown.

confirms the diagnosis. Values between 450 and 600 nmol/l should be regarded as indicative of an abnormal adrenal cortical response, but the cause (HAC or stress) cannot be determined. Post-ACTH cortisol concentrations <40 nmol/l in dogs with obvious clinical signs of HAC are consistent with the diagnosis of iatrogenic HAC.

When interpreting ACTH stimulation tests it is important to remember that other steroids will be detected in the cortisol assay. The degree of cross-reactivity between cortisol and pharmaceutical steroids varies; for example, prednisolone cross-reacts about 30% whereas dexamethasone does not cross-react. Prednisolone can be detected by a cortisol assay for up to 24 hours after administration.

Advantages of the ACTH stimulation test include:

- Simple, quick and specific
- Best screening test for distinguishing spontaneous and iatrogenic HAC
- Provides baseline information for monitoring trilostane and mitotane therapy (see below).

Disadvantages of the ACTH stimulation test include:

- Minimal value in differentiating pituitary from adrenal HAC
- False negative results (i.e. a normal response) may occur, especially in AD-HAC
- False positive results (i.e. an exaggerated response) may occur with chronic stress due to non-adrenal illness. The highest post-ACTH cortisol concentration recorded in one series of 59 dogs with non-adrenal illnesses was about 850 nmol/l (although 95% of the dogs had values <600 nmol/l) (Kaplan et al., 1995). The authors have occasionally seen post-ACTH cortisol concentrations even higher than this in dogs with severe non-adrenal illness.

Low-dose dexamethasone suppression test: The method for the LDDST is described in Figure 18.8.

The expected results of LDDSTs are shown in Figure 18.9. Interpretation must be based on the laboratory's reference range. As a guide, normal dogs show a marked (usually >50%) suppression of cortisol concentrations at

---

1. Obtain a 2 ml blood sample in a heparin or plain tube.
2. Administer synthetic ACTH intravenously (preferably) or intramuscularly (painful). Dose is 250 µg in dogs >5 kg or 125 µg in dogs <5 kg. Alternatively, a 5 µg/kg dose is more common.
3. Obtain another 2 ml blood sample 30–90 minutes (if ACTH given intravenously) or 1–2 hours (if ACTH given intramuscularly) later.

Serum or plasma should be separated before transport to laboratory.

18.6 Method for the ACTH stimulation test.

1. Obtain a 2 ml blood sample in a plain or heparin tube early in the morning.
2. Administer dexamethasone at a dose of 0.01–0.015 mg/kg i.v.
3. Collect blood samples 3–4 hours and 8 hours after administration of dexamethasone.
4. Serum or plasma should be separated before transport to laboratory.

The basal and 8-hour post-dexamethasone samples are the most important for interpretation of the test. The intermediate sample is not essential but may be useful in some cases.

18.8   Method for the low-dose dexamethasone suppression test.

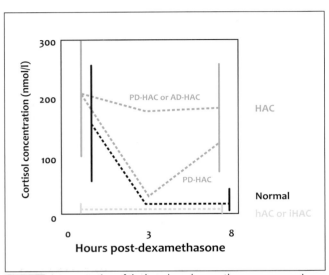

18.9   Interpretation of the low-dose dexamethasone suppression test. Normal dogs show >50% suppression of cortisol concentrations at 3 hours with values <40 nmol/l at 8 hours. Dogs with HAC show little or no suppression at 8 hours. Cases with PD-HAC may show an initial suppression at 3 hours. The effects of iatrogenic HAC (iHAC) and hypoadrenocorticism (hAC) are also shown.

3 hours, to an absolute value <40 nmol/l and stay suppressed to <40 nmol/l at 8 hours. If the dose of dexamethasone fails to suppress circulating cortisol concentrations adequately (i.e. the 8-hour cortisol is >40 nmol/l) in a dog with compatible clinical signs, a diagnosis of HAC is confirmed.

If the 3–4-hour sample is suppressed normally or near-normally (to <40 nmol/l), while the 8-hour sample shows escape from suppression (i.e. is >40 nmol/l), then a diagnosis of PD-HAC can be made. A failure to suppress plasma cortisol at both 3–4 hours and 8 hours is not helpful in determining the cause of the HAC (i.e. it could be pituitary or adrenal dependent).

Some cases show a pattern of low cortisol production that is not suppressed throughout the test. This abnormal pattern should prompt further investigation for an adrenal tumour, as some adrenal tumours may principally release cortisol precursors.

A few dogs with HAC confirmed by other methods may show an 'inverse' pattern of results, i.e. a failure of suppression at 4 hours but suppression at 8 hours (Mueller *et al.*, 2006). As the 4-hour result is not normal, these dogs cannot be described as false negatives. The importance and reliability of this pattern has still to be determined.

Advantages of the LDDST include:

- More sensitive than the ACTH stimulation test in confirming HAC
- May confirm the diagnosis of PD-HAC.

Disadvantages of the LDDST include:

- Not as specific as the ACTH stimulation test, i.e. it is more likely to produce false positives, especially if it is performed in a stressful environment. In chronically ill animals that do not have HAC it can be (falsely) positive in up to 56% of cases
- Takes longer to perform than ACTH stimulation
- Does not provide pretreatment information that may be used in monitoring the effects of therapy.

Urine corticoid:creatinine ratio: Cortisol and its metabolites (corticoids) are excreted in urine. By measuring urine corticoids in the morning sample, the concentration will reflect cortisol release over several hours, thereby adjusting for fluctuations in plasma cortisol concentrations. Urine corticoid concentration increases with increased plasma cortisol concentration. Relating the urine corticoid concentration to urine creatinine concentration provides a correction for any differences in urine concentration. Evaluation of UCCR, rather than the more laborious 24-hour urinary corticoid excretion, has been shown to be a simple and valuable screening test. However, urine corticoids may not always reflect plasma cortisol concentrations and the rate of cortisol breakdown can be influenced by other factors (e.g. hepatic disease, drug administration).

The owner should obtain a urine sample at home every morning for 3 days; these samples can either be analysed separately (preferred) or 1 ml aliquots can be mixed together before analysis (cheaper). Urine samples obtained in a clinical environment are unsuitable because the stress of being taken to the clinic is sufficient to increase the urine cortisol to concentrations that are suggestive of HAC. A single sample obtained at home is also unsuitable.

The UCCR is calculated as:

$$\frac{\text{Urine cortisol concentration } (\mu mol/l)}{\text{Urine creatinine concentration } (\mu mol/l)}$$

Before performing this calculation it may be necessary to convert from other units into $\mu mol/l$ (see Appendix 7).

Depending on the laboratory method for measuring cortisol (see above), the upper limit of the reference ratio for normal dogs may be as low as <8.3 x 10^{-6} or as high as <30 x 10^{-6}. The ratio is increased in dogs with HAC but also in many dogs with non-adrenal illness. Therefore, this test is not very specific, but is useful for screening for HAC because it is highly sensitive. Values in the reference range make a diagnosis of HAC highly unlikely, and the test is best used to exclude the diagnosis of HAC. The test cannot reliably differentiate PD- from AD-HAC unless the ratio exceeds 100 x 10^{-6}, when it becomes very likely that the dog is suffering from PD-HAC. It is of little value in monitoring the response to trilostane or mitotane therapy in dogs with HAC.

Additional tests for atypical HAC

There are breed-specific variations in clinical presentation and the response to diagnostic tests. Some cases of HAC have classical clinical signs and changes on routine haematology and biochemistry but equivocal results on the specific endocrine tests described above; these are termed atypical HAC. A recent paper has suggested that dogs with 'atypical HAC' have increased average cortisol concentrations compared with normal dogs but that these are less than 'typical' HAC (Frank *et al.*, 2015). Scottish Terriers seem particularly affected by this situation. If, on repetition of the standard tests outlined above, the results remain inconclusive and the clinical signs persist, then further tests for atypical forms of HAC can be undertaken.

ACTH stimulation of 17-hydroxyprogesterone (17-OHP): The measurement of 17-OHP before and after ACTH stimulation may be useful in helping to confirm the diagnosis of atypical HAC (Ristić *et al.*, 2002; Benitah *et al.*, 2005; Monroe *et al.*, 2012). In atypical HAC there may be derangement of the steroid production pathway, and some of the precursors of cortisol, such as 17-OHP, may be abnormally increased. Both pituitary-dependent and adrenal-dependent atypical HAC cases have been reported. However, this is a controversial area of endocrinology and other authors have argued against the use of this term and test (Behrend *et al.*, 2013).

The method is identical to that described in Figure 18.6 for the standard ACTH stimulation test and thus measurements of 17-OHP can be made on the same samples after cortisol concentrations have been measured. The 17-OHP concentrations are stable in plasma at 4°C for several weeks.

Figure 18.10 summarizes the interpretation. In normal dogs, post-ACTH 17-OHP concentrations are mostly between 1.0 and 8.0 nmol/l. In dogs with classical and atypical HAC, plasma 17-OHP concentrations show an exaggerated response to ACTH stimulation with concentrations increasing to between 6.5 and 38 nmol/l after stimulation (Ristić *et al.*, 2002). There is a degree of overlap between normal and affected animals and there is some controversy over the cut-off value for the diagnosis of HAC. One study suggested that a post-ACTH stimulation 17-OHP concentration of >8.5 nmol/l could be used as a cut-off with a sensitivity and specificity of about 70%, but a few normal dogs may have post-ACTH 17-OHP concentrations as high as 17 nmol/l and dogs with 'stressful' diseases may have values as high as 38 nmol/l (Chapman *et al.*, 2003). There are also sex differences in post-ACTH 17-OHP values, with entire bitches having the highest concentrations (Benitah *et al.*, 2005).

The test is best used to obtain confirmatory evidence of abnormalities of steroid metabolism in animals with considerable clinical evidence of such abnormalities. All

studies emphasize that the ACTH stimulation of 17-OHP is not superior to that of cortisol, but may be useful when the cortisol is not diagnostic. It is unlikely that the 17-OHP produces clinical signs on its own but, rather, it is serving as a marker for the abnormalities of steroid metabolism.

ACTH stimulation of other steroid hormones: ACTH will also stimulate other adrenal steroids such as the sex hormones produced in the zonas fasciculata and reticularis. Some laboratories provide assays for these hormones, including 17-OHP, progesterone, oestradiol, androstenedione and testosterone. These assays are valuable for the very rare cases of sex hormone-producing adrenal tumours that have been recorded in both dogs and cats (but are very common in ferrets). In such circumstances there is common agreement that the measurement of these sex hormones is useful; however, the interpretation of the results depends on the tests used and practitioners are advised to seek appropriate advice from the specialist laboratory. There is little value in measuring such hormones in dogs and cats in an attempt to diagnose HAC because they are less sensitive and less specific than 17-OHP alone (Hill *et al.*, 2005). The main indication for performing these tests is in dogs with clinical signs suggestive of HAC and a confirmed adrenal mass, but negative findings on a LDDST and an ACTH stimulation test measuring cortisol and 17-OHP (very rare). Since HAC is a slowly progressive disease in most cases, it is more appropriate to wait a few months and retest using a 'standard' ACTH stimulation test and LDDST.

Distinguishing pituitary- and adrenal-dependent HAC

Distinguishing the two major forms of HAC is useful in the management and essential for the prognosis of the condition, though it is not necessary to make the distinction in all cases. Both endocrine tests and adrenal ultrasonography are used (Herrtage and Ramsey, 2012). The best endocrinological test is the endogenous ACTH assay, although the low- and high-dose dexamethasone suppression tests may contribute. It is usually assumed that if an adrenal tumour is not detected the disease is pituitary in origin. It is only necessary to confirm the presence and size of a suspected pituitary tumour in dogs with HAC and neurological signs. Magnetic resonance imaging is the best method for examining the pituitary gland. In its absence, high resolution computed tomography (HRCT) is an acceptable alternative.

Sometimes conflicting results are obtained, such as a low ACTH concentration with evidence of mild bilateral adrenomegaly. In these cases the only solution is repeating some or all of the tests. In rare cases pituitary and adrenal tumours have been found in the same animal. This situation is identified after in-depth investigations of animals that have conflicting results from the investigations outlined in this section or after failure of conventional therapy.

Endogenous ACTH: The endogenous ACTH concentration is usually high or normal in PD-HAC (>25 pg/ml), but low in AD-HAC (<5 pg/ml). Equivocal results (5–25 pg/ml) are sometimes seen. The assay should be repeated in these circumstances, because some of these results are due to poor sample handling (see below). On rare occasions low ACTH values (<5 pg/ml) have been recorded in PD-HAC cases, but high ACTH values have never been recorded with adrenal tumours (Rodríguez Piñeiro *et al.*,

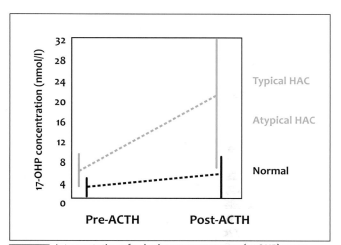

18.10 Interpretation of 17-hydroxyprogesterone (17-OHP) assay. Normal dogs show a 2–3-fold increase in 17-OHP concentrations but these remain <10 nmol/l. Most dogs with typical or atypical HAC have post-ACTH 17-OHP concentrations >8 nmol/l. False positive results may occur with 'stressful' illnesses, such as unstable diabetes mellitus, neoplasia and liver disease. False negatives can also occur but are uncommon.

2009). The assay is therefore less specific for the diagnosis of adrenal-dependent disease than for pituitary-dependent disease. The test is easy to perform but is less accurate than ultrasonography performed by an experienced operator in the exclusion of adrenal tumours.

Endogenous ACTH is measured (by RIA) after collecting a single blood sample into ethylediamine tetra-acetic acid (EDTA) and rapidly separating and freezing the plasma (within 15 minutes). The sample must be sent by a guaranteed express delivery service in a special freezer pack that can be borrowed from a specialist laboratory.

Low-dose dexamethasone suppression test: As discussed above, the LDDST may help in distinguishing between causes of HAC because some cases of PD-HAC show suppression of cortisol at 3 hours but not at 8 hours. However, if this does not occur, then PD-HAC cannot be excluded. Some cases of AD-HAC may show low concentrations of cortisol throughout the test without any suppression.

High-dose dexamethasone suppression test: The high-dose dexamethasone suppression test is probably now unnecessary in most situations, owing to the availability of other, more convenient, tests. The procedure is as outlined in Figure 18.8 for the LDDST except that the dose of dexamethasone used is increased to 0.1 mg/kg. Suppression of cortisol at 3 hours or at 3 and 8 hours is consistent with PD-HAC. However, if this does not occur, then PD-HAC cannot be excluded. Lack of adequate suppression (i.e. cortisol concentrations >40 nmol/l at 3–4 hours and at 8 hours) is seen not only in all AD-HAC cases, but also in 20–30% of PD-HAC cases. The high-dose dexamethasone suppression test cannot be used to distinguish between normal dogs and those with HAC (unlike the LDDST), because both normal dogs and those with PD-HAC can show suppression of cortisol at both 3 and 8 hours.

Effects on other endocrine tests

Thyroxine concentrations: Basal thyroxine (T4) concentrations are decreased in about 70% of dogs with HAC. This is thought to be due to inhibition of pituitary secretion of thyroid-stimulating hormone (TSH), and so TSH concentrations are usually low. The response of thyroxine to thyroid-releasing hormone (TRH) or TSH stimulation usually parallels a normal response, but thyroxine concentrations both pre and post TRH or TSH are subnormal. However, in some cases of spontaneous canine HAC, TSH concentrations are normal or even (paradoxically) increased; in these cases, the low T4 may be due to cortisol altering thyroid hormone binding to plasma proteins or enhancing the metabolism of thyroid hormone. Treatment of the HAC (with trilostane) results in an expected increase in both total T4 and TSH (Kenefick and Neiger, 2008). However, this study also showed that there was a decrease in the free thyroxine concentration (although most of the post-treatment concentrations were still within the reference range). The explanation for this observation is not clear.

Parathyroid hormone concentrations: Glucocorticoids are known to increase urinary calcium excretion in canine HAC. In order to maintain normal circulating concentrations of calcium, parathyroid hormone (PTH) concentrations are increased in over 80% of cases of HAC (Ramsey et al., 2005); this has been called adrenal secondary hyperparathyroidism. PTH concentrations decrease with treatment, but not usually to normal concentrations (Tebb et al., 2005).

Tests for monitoring therapy
Trilostane

Trilostane is a steroid synthesis inhibitor that is authorized for the treatment of HAC in Europe and the USA and is used in other countries as an alternative to mitotane (Neiger et al., 2002). It is recommended that ACTH stimulation tests are performed at 30 days and then every 90 days after starting therapy (Ramsey, 2010). An ACTH stimulation test can be performed 10–14 days after starting therapy; however, as the clinical signs and cortisol concentrations continue to improve in most dogs in the first month and very few cases indeed develop trilostane overdosage in the first 2 weeks of therapy, changing the dose at this stage would risk increasing the dose of trilostane too early. A review consultation at 10–14 days may be adequate and an ACTH stimulation test only performed if an overdose is suspected. This recommendation is independent of the method used to establish the original diagnosis. As trilostane has a short plasma half-life, the manufacturer recommends that ACTH stimulation tests are performed 4–6 hours after dosing to enable accurate interpretation of results. However, in accordance with other authorities, the authors' current preference is to start the ACTH stimulation test 2–4 hours after dosing because this is more likely to be the nadir of cortisol production following trilostane administration (Griebsch et al., 2014). A recent study did not find any significant difference between stimulation tests performed at 2 or 4 hours (Bonadio et al., 2014). Various target cortisol concentrations for the ACTH stimulation test have been used to monitor trilostane therapy. The lower the target range, the greater the possibility of the animal developing signs of hypoadrenocorticism. The interpretation of ACTH stimulation tests in dogs being treated with trilostane is summarized in Figure 18.11 and described below.

- If the post-ACTH cortisol concentration is <40 nmol/l and the dog is showing any clinical signs of hypocortisolism (typically a poor appetite) then electrolytes should be checked and appropriate treatment started. Trilostane should only be restarted (at a 30–50% lower dose) when the dog is better and post-ACTH stimulation cortisol is above 120 nmol/l.
- If the post-ACTH cortisol concentration is <40 nmol/l and the dog is **not** showing any clinical signs of hypocortisolism then the trilostane may be continued for a month. However, the owner should be warned of the signs of hypocortisolism and the dog re-examined in 1 month and a further ACTH stimulation test performed. If the post-ACTH cortisol concentration is still <40 nmol/l then a dose reduction of 30–50% is advisable.
- If the post-ACTH cortisol concentration is between 40 and 120 nmol/l and the patient appears to be clinically well controlled then the dose is not changed.
- If the post-ACTH cortisol is >120 nmol/l and the clinical signs appear poorly controlled then an increase in dose of approximately 50% is warranted. However, if dogs have a post-ACTH cortisol concentration of 120–200 nmol/l and are responding well to treatment, an increase in monitoring rather than dose may be more appropriate.
- If the post-ACTH cortisol is >200 nmol/l then a dose increase of approximately 50% is warranted.
- If the post-ACTH cortisol concentration is <120 nmol/l and the clinical signs appear poorly controlled then the dose of trilostane may need to be increased to twice-

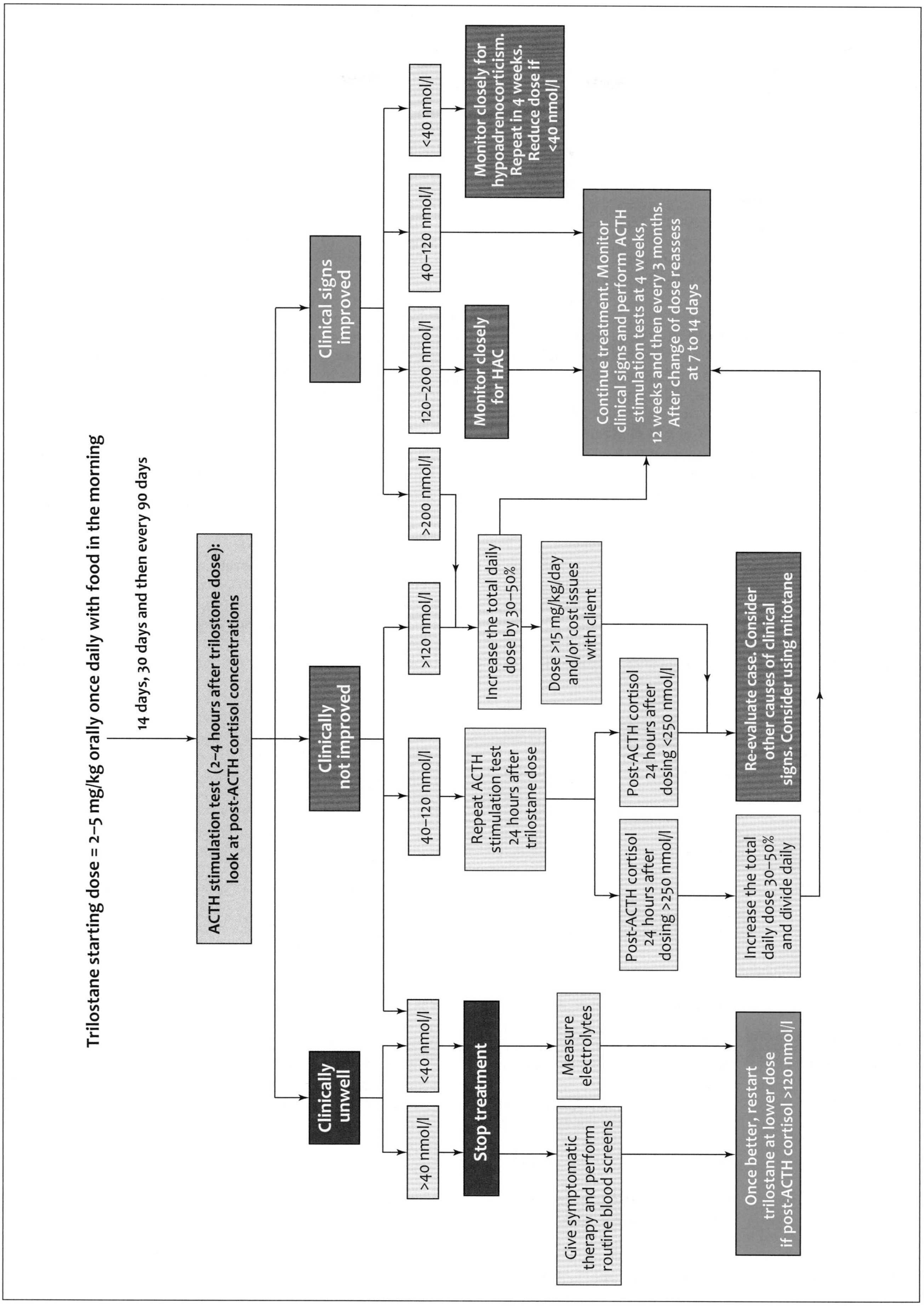

Trilostane starting dose = 2–5 mg/kg orally once daily with food in the morning

14 days, 30 days and then every 90 days

ACTH stimulation test (2–4 hours after trilostane dose): look at post-ACTH cortisol concentrations

Clinically unwell

- >40 nmol/l
  - Give symptomatic therapy and perform routine blood screens
  - Once better, restart trilostane at lower dose if post-ACTH cortisol >120 nmol/l
- <40 nmol/l
  - **Stop treatment**
  - Measure electrolytes
  - Once better, restart trilostane at lower dose if post-ACTH cortisol >120 nmol/l

Clinically not improved

- 40–120 nmol/l
  - Repeat ACTH stimulation test 24 hours after trilostane dose
    - Post-ACTH cortisol 24 hours after dosing >250 nmol/l
      - Increase the total daily dose 30–50% and divide daily
    - Post-ACTH cortisol 24 hours after dosing <250 nmol/l
      - Re-evaluate case. Consider other causes of clinical signs. Consider using mitotane
- >120 nmol/l
  - Increase the total daily dose by 30–50%
  - Dose >15 mg/kg/day and/or cost issues with client
    - Re-evaluate case. Consider other causes of clinical signs. Consider using mitotane

Clinical signs improved

- >200 nmol/l
- 120–200 nmol/l
  - Monitor closely for HAC
- 40–120 nmol/l
- <40 nmol/l
  - Monitor closely for hypoadrenocorticism. Repeat in 4 weeks. Reduce dose if <40 nmol/l

Continue treatment. Monitor clinical signs and perform ACTH stimulation tests at 4 weeks, 12 weeks and then every 3 months. After change of dose reassess at 7 to 14 days

18.11 Interpretation of ACTH stimulation tests in the monitoring of trilostane treatment of canine hyperadrenocorticism.

daily administration. An ACTH stimulation test can be performed 24 hours after trilostane administration (i.e. just before the next dose) to investigate this. If the post-ACTH cortisol concentration is >250 nmol/l at 24 hours after trilostane, but the post-ACTH cortisol concentration 4 hours after trilostane is <120 nmol/l then an increase to twice-daily dosing is justified.

- If an ACTH stimulation test is performed inadvertently at times other than 2–4 hours after dosing with trilostane, the post-ACTH cortisol concentration should be >20 nmol/l and <250 nmol/l.
- It is imperative that these results are interpreted in conjunction with the clinical signs. If the clinical signs have resolved but the post-ACTH cortisol is higher than ideal it may be sensible to continue the same dose and monitor closely.

Once the clinical condition of the animal and the dose rate have been stabilized, the dog should be examined and an ACTH stimulation test performed every 3–6 months. Serum biochemistry should be performed periodically to check for hyperkalaemia (which may reflect low aldosterone concentrations in some, but not all, cases).

In atypical HAC treated with trilostane, measurement of 17-OHP is not helpful in monitoring because the concentrations are massively increased. This is presumably due to cross-reactivity in the assay with 17-hydroxypregnenolone, which would be expected to increase because of inhibition of 3β-hydroxysteroid dehydrogenase by trilostane.

It should be noted that, despite its widespread use, the ACTH stimulation test has never been validated for trilostane therapy. If ACTH is not available or too expensive to use regularly then the manufacturers of trilostane currently recommend measurement of basal cortisol concentrations 4–6 hours after trilostane administration;

however, this tends to lead to undertreatment in the authors' experience. It is also possible to monitor trilostane therapy by measuring cortisol just before and 2–3 hours after the administration of trilostane (pre- and post-pill cortisol concentrations) (Ramsey et al. 2015). Good clinical control tends to be associated with pre-pill (peak) cortisol concentrations in the range 40–140 nmol/l. If pre-pill concentrations are *less* than 40 nmol/l then the dog is at risk of iatrogenic hypocortisolism; pre-pill concentrations *higher* than 140 nmol/l tend to be associated with clinical signs of poor control. If the dog is not well controlled then more frequent dosing (if the post-pill concentration is <40 nmol/l) or an increase in dose (if the post-pill concentration is >40 nmol/l) may be required.

As with ACTH stimulation tests, it is imperative that the results of pre- and post-pill cortisol measurements are interpreted in conjunction with the clinical signs. If the clinical signs have resolved but the peak and/or trough concentration is higher than ideal it may be sensible to continue the same dose and monitor closely. The suggested interpretation of pre- and post-pill cortisol is illustrated in Figure 18.12. These recommendations are made on the basis of a study of 70 dogs at various stages of control published in abstract form by one of the authors (IKR) and published papers of Bell et al. (2006) and Griebsch et al. (2014); further refinement may be necessary.

Mitotane

Mitotane is an effective alternative to trilostane in the medical management of PD-HAC and indeed may be considered the first choice in countries that do not have access to trilostane. It is a cytotoxic agent that principally causes necrosis of the zona fasciculata and zona reticularis of the adrenal glands.

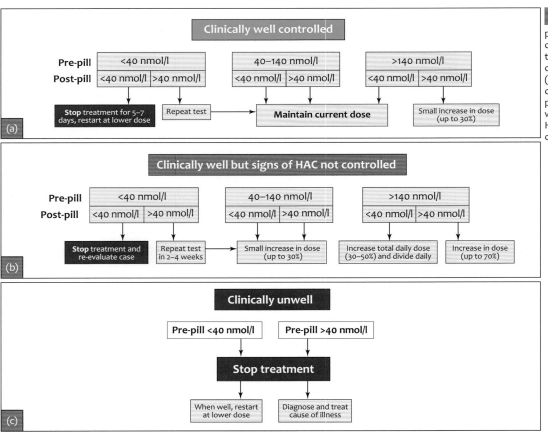

18.12 Suggested interpretation of pre- and 2–3 hour post-pill cortisol in the monitoring of trilostane treatment of canine hyperadrenocorticism (HAC). (a) The clinically well controlled patient. (b) The patient appears clinically well but there are signs that HAC is not controlled. (c) The clinically unwell patient.

Mitotane is initially given as an induction course, which results in suppression of the ACTH stimulation test. Generally a post-ACTH cortisol of between 20 and 120 nmol/l indicates satisfactory control. Maintenance therapy is then given and monitored by ACTH stimulation tests, initially monthly and then every 3–6 months. Further details on mitotane therapy are available in the *BSAVA Manual of Canine and Feline Endocrinology* (Herrtage and Ramsey, 2012).

Dogs treated with mitotane, particularly when they have been treated for several months, may develop acute signs of hypoadrenocorticism (see below). Occasionally, there may be evidence of hyperkalaemia and hyponatraemia. Should this occur, treatment should be stopped and an ACTH stimulation test should be performed: post-ACTH cortisol would be expected to be <20 nmol/l to confirm the diagnosis.

Plasma 17-OHP concentrations can be used to monitor treatment of atypical HAC cases when mitotane is used, although this offers no advantage over measuring cortisol using the criteria mentioned above.

Other medical therapy

In some countries, ketoconazole is used for the treatment of PD-HAC, particularly in those dogs that cannot tolerate mitotane and do not have access to trilostane. Ketoconazole therapy is monitored in a similar fashion to that described for trilostane. Ketoconazole can cause hepatotoxicity: increases in liver enzymes in dogs treated with this drug are a cause for concern and require withdrawal of the drug in most cases.

In the USA and some other countries, selegiline (L-deprenyl) is authorized for the treatment of PD-HAC. The current evidence indicates that there is minimal endocrinological improvement but some clinical improvement; no laboratory monitoring is recommended.

Feline hyperadrenocorticism

In the cat, HAC is far less common than in the dog. Although fewer studies have been published in the cat, it appears that PD-HAC accounts for a similar proportion of HAC cases to those seen in dogs. Primary hyperaldosteronism (or Conn's syndrome) is also reported in cats (see later). Most (80%) cats with confirmed HAC have concurrent diabetes mellitus, which means that weight loss may also be seen. As well as showing most of the same signs of HAC as dogs, including PU/PD, polyphagia and a pot-bellied appearance, many also have hyperfragile skin (Figure 18.13). Hyperglycaemia (about 90%) and hypercholesterolaemia (about 50%) are the most common serum biochemistry abnormalities. High serum ALP activity is uncommon, developing in only one-quarter of cats. Urine SG is variable with a third of cases being <1.030.

The best test for diagnosing feline HAC has not been established and there is some disagreement in the scientific literature. The best option is probably to perform both tests outlined below and seek the assistance of a specialist with experience in these cases. The ACTH stimulation test can be a useful test for the diagnosis of feline HAC. However, the peak response in cats is variable in both timing and magnitude. Samples should be obtained at 60 and 90 minutes after the intravenous injection of 5 μg/kg or 0.125 mg/cat ACTH (Schoeman *et al.*, 2000; DeClue *et al.*, 2011). The sensitivity of the test is variably reported to be

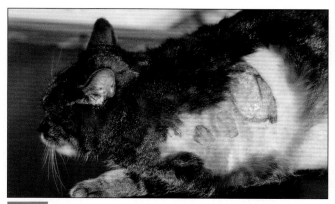

18.13 Hyperfragile skin in a cat with hyperadrenocorticism.

from 50 to 80%. Normal cats and cats with chronic diseases rarely have a post-ACTH cortisol of >400 nmol/l (Ramspott *et al.*, 2012). However, some stressful illnesses such as hyperthyroidism can increase the post-ACTH cortisol to as high as 600 nmol/l. As in the dog, values >600 nmol/l are very suggestive, and values between 400 and 600 nmol/l are supportive of HAC in the presence of appropriate clinical signs. However, overall values tend to be lower than in dogs, and cats with HAC rarely have a post-ACTH cortisol concentration greater than 800 nmol/l.

The LDDST uses a higher dexamethasone dosage (0.1 mg/kg) than in dogs. Serum cortisol values in all normal cats and most cats with non-adrenal illness are suppressed with this dose. Importantly, the results of the LDDST using 0.1 mg/kg dexamethasone are normal in non-Cushingoid cats with diabetes mellitus, independent of the quality of glycaemic control (Kley *et al.*, 2007). It is therefore a specific test; however, while in all cats with AD-HAC cortisol is not suppressed at either 3–4 or 8 hours, some cats with PD-HAC will suppress, and this reduces the sensitivity. Too few cases have been evaluated to assess the sensitivity and specificity accurately. Note that this higher dose dexamethasone suppression test used in cats is a screening test, and not for distinguishing between adrenal and pituitary forms of the disease.

A combined dexamethasone suppression/ACTH stimulation test protocol was suggested for use in cats; however, it has not been sufficiently investigated to recommend its routine use.

The value of any test for distinguishing reliably between pituitary- and adrenal-dependent forms of feline HAC has not been assessed. Measurement of basal endogenous ACTH concentration or a very high dose (1.0 mg/kg) dexamethasone suppression test can be used to differentiate cats with PD-HAC from those with AD-HAC. However, care should be taken when using the high dose dexamethasone suppression test in diabetic cases, and be mindful that the 1.0 mg/kg dose can cause diabetes. Normal to high plasma ACTH levels support a diagnosis of PD-HAC, whereas low concentrations are consistent with AD-HAC.

The UCCR is not widely used in cats because it is sensitive but non-specific. Urine should always be collected at home (not in the hospital environment) as all stressful situations will elevate the ratio. Almost all cats with HAC will be positive, but false positive test results may be seen frequently in cats with non-adrenal illness. Importantly, hyperthyroid cats have increased ratios. Recent results suggest that laboratory extraction of corticoids may improve the diagnostic efficiency but larger-scale studies are needed before this can be recommended.

There are no reliable reports of the use of ACTH stimulation tests to monitor the treatment of large numbers of cats with HAC, and therefore target values have to be extrapolated from dogs (see above). Cats have been successfully treated with trilostane using these extrapolated values (Neiger *et al.*, 2004).

Canine hypoadrenocorticism

Hypoadrenocorticism is defined as the absolute lack of adrenocortical steroids. This includes a lack of mineralocorticoids and glucocorticoids. Isolated deficiencies in glucocorticoids and mineralocorticoids have been reported as single case reports (Dunn and Herrtage, 1998; Lobetti, 1998). Canine hypoadrenocorticism can be classified according to the underlying cause, of which four are of importance:

* Spontaneous hypoadrenocorticism (= idiopathic primary hypoadrenocorticism)
* Trilostane-induced hypoadrenocorticism
* Mitotane-induced hypoadrenocorticism
* Iatrogenic secondary hypoadrenocorticism (due to sudden withdrawal of glucocorticoid therapy).

Different causes of hypoadrenocorticism are associated with varying degrees of mineralocorticoid and glucocorticoid deficiency.

Investigation of hypoadrenocorticism

Many cases are presented with signs that could be suggestive of hypoadrenocorticism, such as lethargy, weight loss, poor appetite, vomiting, diarrhoea or episodic collapse (Figure 18.14). Figure 18.15 summarizes the approach to a suspected case of canine hypoadrenocorticism.

Routine biochemistry, haematology and urinalysis

A routine blood profile often provides the first indication that hypoadrenocorticism may be present. The common biochemical, haematological and urinalysis findings in cases of hypoadrenocorticism are shown in Figure 18.16.

Biochemistry: In cases of canine hypoadrenocorticism, biochemistry will nearly always (>90%) demonstrate hyperkalaemia and hyponatraemia, with hypochloraemia being seen in about 80% of cases. While hypoadrenocorticism is the commonest cause of a combination of reduced sodium and increased potassium, individual changes are associated with a wider range of conditions (Figure 18.17; see also Chapter 8).

Many laboratories quote the sodium:potassium ratio. While a reduced sodium:potassium ratio (<27:1) is suggestive of hypoadrenocorticism, it is not diagnostic of the condition and the authors do not recommend its routine use. This is particularly true when one of the electrolytes is within its reference range. In one survey of 238 dogs with a low sodium:potassium ratio only 27 dogs actually had hypoadrenocorticism (Neilsen *et al.*, 2008). A ratio of <20:1 is very suggestive of hypoadrenocorticism but this is not very sensitive. At ratios between 20 and 27, the higher the lymphocyte count, the more likely it is that the dog has hypoadrenocorticism; however, this is still no substitute for an ACTH stimulation test (Seth *et al.*, 2011). Absolute electrolyte concentrations are more reliable indicators of

Body system/organ	Examples	Similarities in presenting signs
Kidney	Decompensated renal failure	Dehydration Polyuria/polydipsia Vomiting Anorexia
Exocrine pancreas	Acute pancreatitis	Abdominal pain Dehydration Anorexia Vomiting Diarrhoea
Gastrointestinal tract	Infectious enteritis (various)	Anorexia Vomiting Haemorrhagic diarrhoea
Hepatobiliary tract	Hepatitis (toxic, inflammatory)	Vomiting Diarrhoea
Neuromuscular system	Myasthenia gravis	Episodic weakness Regurgitation/vomiting
Endocrine system	Hypothyroidism	Bradycardia Dullness
Cardiovascular system	Third-degree heart block	Bradycardia Episodic collapse
Haemopoietic system	Anaemia	Pale mucous membranes Collapse
Multisystem disease	Neoplasia (e.g. lymphoma)	Many!

18.14 Conditions that may resemble canine hypoadrenocorticism in at least two major presenting signs.

hypoadrenocorticism. Artefactual changes in electrolytes should be excluded, for example, haemolysis can lead to marked elevations in potassium concentrations. Cases of hypoadrenocorticism with normal sodium and potassium concentrations are rare. In such cases, further testing (ACTH stimulation test) should always be performed before starting therapy.

Biochemistry commonly demonstrates azotaemia, hypercalcaemia and hypoglycaemia; hypoalbuminaemia and hypocholesterolemia may also be seen. Metabolic acidosis is often evident on blood gas analysis. None of these changes is as specific or as sensitive as the changes in electrolyte concentrations. Azotaemia may be very severe and is caused by prerenal factors (predominantly hypovolaemia; gastrointestinal haemorrhage may also contribute to the increased urea concentration). Dehydration may mask some of the changes noted above. See below and Chapter 11 for further discussion of how to make the important distinction between renal failure and hypoadrenocorticism.

Haematology: Haematology profiles of dogs with hypoadrenocorticism are characterized more by the absence of abnormalities than by their presence. In many ill (and therefore stressed) dogs, neutrophil numbers are high-normal to increased, whereas eosinophils and lymphocytes are low-normal to decreased. In hypoadrenocorticism there may be a lack of this 'stress leucogram' with normal white blood cell (particularly lymphocyte) counts. Occasionally there may be an overt 'reverse stress leucogram' (increased numbers of lymphocytes and/or eosinophils with low-normal or subnormal numbers of neutrophils).

Anaemia is present in about one-quarter of dogs with hypoadrenocorticism at presentation, but the actual prevalence may be much higher because it is often masked by concurrent dehydration. Usually this anaemia is mild,

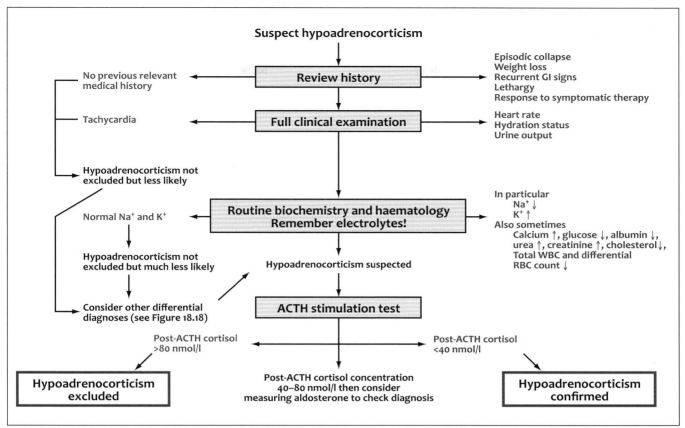

Suspect hypoadrenocorticism

Review history

No previous relevant medical history

Episodic collapse
Weight loss
Recurrent GI signs
Lethargy
Response to symptomatic therapy

Full clinical examination

Tachycardia

Heart rate
Hydration status
Urine output

Hypoadrenocorticism not excluded but less likely

Routine biochemistry and haematology
Remember electrolytes!

Normal Na⁺ and K⁺

In particular
Na⁺ ↓
K⁺ ↑
Also sometimes
Calcium ↑, glucose ↓, albumin ↓,
urea ↑, creatinine ↑, cholesterol ↓,
Total WBC and differential
RBC count ↓

Hypoadrenocorticism not excluded but much less likely

Hypoadrenocorticism suspected

Consider other differential diagnoses (see Figure 18.18)

ACTH stimulation test

Post-ACTH cortisol >80 nmol/l

Post-ACTH cortisol <40 nmol/l

Hypoadrenocorticism excluded

Post-ACTH cortisol concentration
40–80 nmol/l then consider
measuring aldosterone to check diagnosis

Hypoadrenocorticism confirmed

18.15 A summary of the investigation of canine hypoadrenocorticism. It is not necessary to perform all these investigations in every case. Text in blue refers to typical features of hypoadrenocorticism; text in red refers to uncommon findings. ACTH = adrenocorticotropic hormone; GI = gastrointestinal; RBC = red blood cell; WBC = white blood cell.

Test	Abnormality
Biochemistry	
Azotaemia	Increased urea, creatinine and phosphate (can be very high)
Electrolytes	Increased potassium Decreased sodium Decreased chloride Decreased sodium:potassium ratio (<27:1)
Calcium	May be increased (usually <4.0 mmol/l)
Glucose	May be decreased (rarely clinically significant)
Albumin	May be decreased
Haematology	
Red blood cells	Normally mild non-regenerative anaemia May be masked by haemoconcentration May be severe due to haemorrhage Occasionally severe due to concurrent immune-mediated haemolytic anaemia
White blood cells	Total count is normal to low Lymphocytes may be increased Neutrophil:lymphocyte ratio decreased Eosinophilia
Urinalysis	
Specific gravity	Usually low normal (1.015–1.030) May not increase in dehydrated dogs with hypoadrenocorticism and it can be difficult to distinguish prerenal azotaemia from intrinsic renal failure

18.16 Common abnormalities in routine laboratory profiles of dogs with hypoadrenocorticism.

Metabolic
• Hypoadrenocorticism • Severe gastrointestinal disease with haemorrhage into intestines • Renal disease • Chylothorax/pleural effusions • Pregnancy (+ vomiting)
Drugs/poisons
• Trilostane • Mitotane • Combination therapy for cardiac disease, especially if combined with sodium-restricted diet

18.17 Differential diagnosis of combined hyponatraemia and hyperkalaemia. Conditions that may cause isolated hyponatraemia or hyperkalaemia are listed in Appendix 3.

normocytic and normochromic. However, in some cases, gastrointestinal haemorrhage or concurrent immune-mediated haemolytic anaemia may produce a more severe anaemia with evidence of regeneration.

Urinalysis: Urinalysis may often demonstrate a normal to low normal SG. This can make the differentiation of hypo-adrenocorticism and renal failure difficult in the azotaemic patient. Clinical history and laboratory findings must be combined to make this distinction (Figure 18.18). Decompensated chronic renal failure will only rarely be associated with hyperkalaemia and/or hyponatraemia. Acute renal failure, while associated with electrolyte changes, can usually be distinguished from acute hypo-adrenocorticism by the reduction in urinary output and

	Acute (oliguric) renal failure	Chronic renal failure	Hypoadrenocorticism
History			
Weight loss	No	Yes	Yes
Polyuria/polydipsia	Can develop later	Yes – often severe	Uncommon and usually mild
Other: vomiting, diarrhoea, collapse, depression, recent 'stressful' incident	Yes	Yes	Yes
Clinical examination			
Urine output	Poor or none	Excessive	Normal or mildly increased
Uraemic glossitis	Uncommon	Rare	Never reported
Normal heart rate	Tachycardia more likely	Tachycardia more likely	Bradycardia possible
Pale mucous membranes	No	Likely	Likely
Clinical pathology			
Urine specific gravity	>1.030	Between 1.008 and 1.020	Variable but can be as low as 1.008
Hyperkalaemia	Possible	Normo- or hypokalaemic	Very common
Hyponatraemia	Possible	No	Very common
Increased urea	Yes	Yes	Yes
Urea >40 mmol/l	Rare	Common	Occasional
Increased creatinine	Yes	Yes	Yes
Increased calcium	Rare	Rare	About 30%
Increased phosphate	After 4 days	Very common	About 30%
'Stress' leucogram	Yes	Yes	No
Anaemia	No	Yes	Yes

18.18 Summary of the differences between hypoadrenocorticism and renal failure, one of its commonest differential diagnoses. This table presents only a general overview. In some clinical cases the distinction may be less clear than suggested. Some forms of each category have subtle differences, e.g. hypercalcaemia is relatively common in chronic renal failure due to juvenile nephropathies. The categories are also not mutually exclusive; for example, acute decompensation may occur with chronic renal failure.

the short clinical history. Moreover, with adequate fluid therapy, the increased urea and creatinine concentrations of a dog with hypoadrenocorticism will return to normal usually within 24 hours, whereas in renal failure the urea and creatinine concentrations will take longer to recover (if at all).

The most practical implication of this discussion is that any dog, but particularly younger dogs, should have their electrolytes measured when presented with signs that are suggestive of renal failure to avoid missing the alternative diagnosis of hypoadrenocorticism.

Specific endocrine tests

It is not acceptable to diagnose hypoadrenocorticism on the basis of a therapeutic trial of steroids. There are several conditions that may present with clinical signs similar to those seen in hypoadrenocorticism (and/or electrolyte changes) which will also improve significantly with glucocorticoid administration.

Basal cortisol: A basal cortisol concentration >55 nmol/l effectively excludes the diagnosis of hypoadrenocorticism in dogs that present with clinical signs suggestive of the condition, and only rarely do dogs that do not have hypoadrenocorticism have cortisol concentrations that are this low (Lennon *et al.*, 2007; Bovens *et al.*, 2014). However, the poor accuracy of many patient-side analysers at low cortisol concentrations prevents this information being applicable in many emergency situations, and a higher limit of 60 nmol/l is suggested as being safer. Using this cut-off, a significant number of dogs with a cortisol concentration <60 nmol/l will in fact not have hypoadrenocorticism. However, all those dogs with a cortisol concentration >60 nmol/l will not have hypoadrenocorticism. This information will considerably reduce the number

of ACTH stimulation tests that are necessary in practice. If a more accurate and robust method of measuring cortisol is available for less urgent cases then the lower limit may be used with increased diagnostic accuracy.

ACTH stimulation test: The ACTH stimulation test is a highly sensitive and specific test for hypoadrenocorticism (>95% in both cases) and should be performed in all suspected cases. It is not suggested that an ACTH stimulation test is performed on every case that is presented with recurrent vomiting and diarrhoea, but a routine haematology and biochemistry profile (including electrolyte analysis) should be obtained, looking for evidence of hypoadrenocorticism. For cases with a greater range of the clinical signs of hypoadrenocorticism (e.g. vomiting, diarrhoea, weight loss and episodic collapse) the clinician may elect to perform an ACTH stimulation test at the same time as the routine laboratory profiles. The test is performed as described in Figure 18.6.

Note that hypoadrenocorticism cannot be diagnosed using the LDDST. The diagnosis is confirmed if the post-ACTH cortisol concentration is <40 nmol/l. However, a small percentage of cases of hypoadrenocorticism with classical laboratory abnormalities and consistent clinical signs may have post-ACTH cortisol concentrations as high as 80 nmol/l (see Figure 18.7). Note that if a supranormal result (>500 nmol/l) is obtained this is unlikely to indicate *hyper*adrencorticism but rather the metabolic stress of another illness that more closely resembles hypoadrenocorticism in its presentation.

As discussed above, the test can be influenced by the administration of exogenous glucocorticoids. Hydrocortisone and prednisolone cross-react in the assay and therefore give false increases. Other glucocorticoids, such as dexamethasone, do not cross-react but may suppress the response. The duration and dose of such therapy will determine the degree of suppression of the response. Sometimes clinicians are presented with patients with suspected hypoadrenocorticism that have been given a single dose of dexamethasone the previous evening. In such circumstances, it is prudent to support the animal with fluid therapy for 24 hours before performing an ACTH stimulation test. It is highly unlikely that the ACTH stimulation test will be sufficiently suppressed to give a false positive result for hypoadrenocorticism 36 hours after a single dose of dexamethasone. Prednisolone should not be given during the 24 hours before an ACTH stimulation test as it may cross-react with cortisol in the assay.

If ACTH is unavailable, the diagnosis may have to rely on electrolyte concentrations, lymphocyte counts and basal cortisol as described above. In more chronic cases the measurement of basal cortisol over 2 or 3 days may help to increase diagnostic confidence, though no specific research has been published on this. Similarly, measuring ACTH may also be useful in primary hypoadrenocorticism, because ACTH concentrations would be expected to be high when compared with the cortisol concentration (whereas healthy dogs with low cortisol concentrations would normally have low ACTH concentrations). The ratio of cortisol to endogenous ACTH has been shown to be very useful in one recent study (Lathan *et al.*, 2014). In this study, if the ratio was less than 2.2 (when cortisol is measured in nmol/l and ACTH in pg/ml) then the diagnosis of hypoadrenocorticism was possible. However, this study had an unusual bias of cases with normal electrolyte concentrations and, although this did not appear to affect the results, more studies are needed.

Measurement of aldosterone: Some cases of hypoadrenocorticism (probably less than 10%) have normal electrolyte concentrations (sometimes referred to as having atypical hypoadrenocorticism). In these cases it is valuable to measure the response of aldosterone to ACTH stimulation to distinguish between isolated primary hypocortisolism and a mineralocorticoid deficiency that has not produced electrolyte abnormalities at the time of examination (Figure 18.19). Aldosterone should also be measured in cases of suspected hypoadrenocorticism with post-ACTH cortisol concentrations between 40 and 80 nmol/l. Normal aldosterone values post-ACTH stimulation may vary with the assay used; however, anything <100 pmol/l should be regarded as abnormal and values up to 1660 pmol/l have been reported in normal and non-Addisonian dogs (Baumstark *et al.*, 2014). Some cases of so-called atypical hypoadrenocorticism in fact have undetectably low aldosterone concentrations (Baumstark *et al.*, 2014) and can go on to develop electrolyte abnormalities with time. However, rare cases of spontaneous and trilostane-induced primary isolated hypocortisolism have been described, as has primary isolated mineralocorticoid deficiency (associated either with increased renin concentrations, suggesting a failure of aldosterone synthesis, or decreased renin concentrations, suggesting a failure to stimulate aldosterone production).

Measurement of endogenous ACTH: Secondary hypoadrenocorticism results from a lack of ACTH due to pituitary disease. It is very rare and is seen in dogs with clinical signs of hypoadrenocorticism but generally with normal serum electrolyte concentrations. Determination of endogenous plasma ACTH concentrations is valuable in differentiating this from primary hypocortisolism (see above). In secondary hypoadrenocorticism ACTH concentrations would be low or normal whereas primary hypoadrenocorticism (or hypocortisolism) is characterized by concentrations above (normally well above) the reference range (which for most laboratories is about 12–25 pmol/l). Secondary hypoadrenocorticism can also result from rapid withdrawal of exogenous corticosteroid therapy.

Tests for monitoring therapy

There is no point in performing an ACTH stimulation test to monitor dogs with naturally occurring hypoadrenocorticism: the post-ACTH cortisol is low at diagnosis and remains low. Urea and creatinine should be monitored initially to ensure adequate hydration status. Serum electrolytes should be checked weekly for the first month, then monthly. Once the regimen has been adapted to the individual patient the frequency of rechecks can be reduced to every 3 months. Many dogs require increasing doses of fludrocortisone during their lives and so some form of electrolyte monitoring is advisable. Relying on clinical signs is a relatively poor indicator of the quality of control achieved. It is useful to measure the electrolytes before and 4–6 hours after fludrocortisone administration to check both the dose and the duration of action. Quite a few dogs on once-daily fludrocortisone have low sodium and high potassium concentrations before dosing, and these are best managed with twice-daily therapy (Roberts *et al.*, 2013). Plasma renin activity has been used to monitor the efficacy of mineralocorticoid therapy in hypoadrenocorticism (Baumstark *et al.*, 2014), however, the renin assay is not widely available and stringent sample handling and expense are likely to restrict its use.

Condition	Cause	Electrolytes	Cortisol post-ACTH	Aldosterone post-ACTH	Endogenous ACTH
'Classical' primary hypoadrenocorticism	Destruction of adrenal glands	High K, low Na, Cl	Low	Low	High
'Atypical' primary hypoadrenocorticism	Early 'classical' hypoadrenocorticism	Normal	Low	Low	High
Isolated primary hypocortisolism	Trilostane and other causes as yet unknown	Normal	Low	Normal	High
Isolated primary hypoaldosteronism	Presumed destruction of the zona glomerulosa	High K, low Na, Cl	Normal	Low	Normal?
Secondary hypoadrenocorticism	Decreased production of ACTH from pituitary gland	Normal	Low	Normal or low	Low
	Sudden steroid withdrawal	Normal	Low	Normal	Low

18.19 Classification of hypoadrenocorticism. This figure provides a summary of the features of each type of hypoadrenocorticism. Note that in many cases of suspected primary hypoadrenocorticism measurement of electrolytes and a cortisol response to ACTH stimulation will be sufficient to make a diagnosis. For more complicated cases measurement of aldosterone and endogenous ACTH may be indicated.

Feline hypoadrenocorticism

Hypoadrenocorticism has been reported in fewer than 20 cats. The clinicopathological changes seen in cats with hypoadrenocorticism are similar to those in dogs. The sodium:potassium ratio is particularly unreliable in cats, and is decreased by several other conditions such as gastrointestinal diseases and body cavity effusions (Bell *et al.*, 2005). An ACTH stimulation test (see section on Feline hyperadrenocorticism for the specific protocol) is needed to confirm the diagnosis. The diagnosis is confirmed in cases with appropriate clinical signs and post-ACTH cortisol concentrations <40 nmol/l.

Other adrenal diseases

Hyperaldosteronism (Conn's syndrome)

Several examples of functional adrenal tumours and bilateral nodular hyperplasia that release aldosterone (primary hyperaldosteronism) have been reported in cats (Ash *et al.*, 2005), and similar tumours have been reported in dogs. The excessive aldosterone causes potassium excretion and sodium retention that in turn leads to hypertension. The condition has been increasingly diagnosed as more attention is paid to electrolyte concentrations in cats.

Clinical signs of hypokalaemia (severe weakness and depression) predominate, with cervical ventroflexion being seen in most of the affected cats. The major laboratory finding is hypokalaemia with high-normal, or even occasionally increased, sodium concentrations. Creatine kinase (CK) is increased as a consequence of the hypokalaemic polymyopathy. Metabolic alkalosis and hypertension may also be seen in these cases and should be monitored if they are present. Alkalosis rarely requires specific treatment, but hypertension, if found, should be treated with spironolactone, an aldosterone antagonist, and amlodipine to avoid end-organ damage. Electrolytes should continue to be monitored during treatment.

The diagnosis is confirmed by measuring basal aldosterone concentrations, which are usually increased to >600 pmol/l. In the presence of hypokalaemia, even a mildly elevated aldosterone concentration can be regarded as inappropriately high. In equivocal cases, ACTH stimulation tests should be used to demonstrate an inappropriate aldosterone response. Normal values have not been published for post-ACTH aldosterone concentrations in cats. However, by extrapolation from dogs a value of >600 pmol/l would be regarded as suggestive of hyperaldosteronism. Occasionally it is desirable to measure plasma renin activity and calculate the plasma aldosterone:renin ratio, as this is thought to be a more sensitive test for distinguishing primary from secondary hyperaldosteronism (Djajadiningrat-Laanan *et al.*, 2011). In primary hyperaldosteronism, renin is expected to be low or low normal (although that is not always the case). However, the sample requires special handling, and the renin assay is not widely available. It is also not well standardized among laboratories and is currently very expensive. Adrenal ultrasonography can be useful to identify an adrenal tumour (however, many cases have bilateral nodular hyperplasia and this may not be evident on ultrasonography).

Surgical removal of the adrenal gland should be regarded as the treatment of choice after correction of the electrolyte disturbance with spironolactone and potassium supplementation. Conservative management with spironolactone and potassium supplementation has been used as an alternative when surgery is not indicated or has been refused.

Phaeochromocytoma

These are tumours of the adrenal medulla that secrete a variety of vasoactive amines, principally adrenaline (epinephrine) and noradrenaline (norepinephrine). Secretion by phaeochromocytomas is typically pulsatile and results in a vague group of clinical signs which include weakness, episodic collapse, restlessness, panting, vomiting, diarrhoea, inappetence, PU/PD, hypertension, weight loss, tachycardia and cardiac arrhythmias. The diagnosis of a phaeochromocytoma requires a high level of clinical alertness.

Ante-mortem diagnosis is complicated by the rapid breakdown of the vasoactive amines by plasma enzymes. Tests for adrenaline metabolites in the urine have been validated by a Swiss group, but rapid urinary acidification and freezing are required and the samples need to be transported to the laboratory still frozen (Quante *et al.*, 2010). The measurement of free metanephrines in plasma has also recently been proposed (Gostelow *et al.*, 2013). Clinicians are advised to contact the relevant laboratories or authors for further details as interpretation is not always straightforward. The best method of presurgical diagnosis is by demonstration of an adrenal mass on ultrasonography and the documentation of severe systolic hypertension (>160 mmHg). The demonstration of hypertension may require repeated examination, because catecholamines may be released intermittently. Unfortunately, failure to demonstrate hypertension does not exclude the diagnosis of phaeochromocytoma.

The treatment of choice for phaeochromocytomas is surgical excision after preoperative control of hypertension. However, the anaesthesia of these patients is a significant challenge. Referral is recommended for treatment.

Case examples

CASE 1

SIGNALMENT

13-year-old female neutered Collie cross weighing 23 kg.

HISTORY

Started 7 months ago with gradual alopecia and coat colour change (Figure 18.20) then became hungrier, to the extent that she was stealing food from the owners' children, which she had never done before. In the last 3 months there had also been an increase in thirst until she was drinking 130 ml/kg/day. She panted more. Her weight had increased and her coat had become lighter in colour. There were no comedones or loss of skin elasticity.

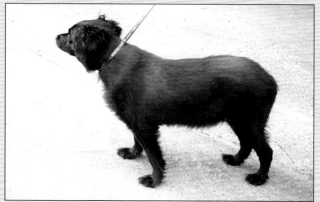

18.20 A 13-year-old female neutered Collie cross showing altered coat colour over the trunk and flank alopecia.

CLINICAL PATHOLOGY DATA

Biochemistry	Result	Reference interval
Total protein (g/l)	61	60–80
Albumin (g/l)	26	26–40
Globulin (g/l)	35	25–45
Glucose (mmol/l)	4.4	3.4–5.3
Sodium (mmol/l)	146	135–155
Potassium (mmol/l)	5.3	3.5–5.8
Chloride (mmol/l)	106	105–120
Calcium (mmol/l)	2.5	2.2–2.7
Phosphate (mmol/l)	**1.6**	0.6–1.3
Urea (mmol/l)	5.0	3.3–8.0
Creatinine (μmol/l)	67	45–150
Cholesterol (mmol/l)	**25.5**	2.3–6
Bilirubin (μmol/l)	2	0–10
ALT (IU/l)	**326**	21–59
ALP (IU/l)	**6401**	3–142
GGT (IU/l)	**21**	0–10
Bile acids (μmol/l)	**20**	0–5

Abnormal results are in **bold**.

Haematology	Result	Reference interval
RBC (x 10^{12}/l)	**8.55**	5.5–8.5
Haemoglobin (g/dl)	17.9	12–18
PCV (l/l)	0.55	0.37–0.55
MCV (fl)	64.3	60–77
MCHC (g/dl)	32.5	32–37
MCH (pg)	20.9	19.5–24.5
WBC (x 10^9/l)	8.0	6–17
Band neutrophils (x 10^9/l)	0	0–0.3
Segmented neutrophils (x 10^9/l)	6.19	3–11.5
Eosinophils (x 10^9/l)	**0**	0.1–1.3
Basophils (x 10^9/l)	0	0
Lymphocytes (x 10^9/l)	1.6	1–4.8
Monocytes (x 10^9/l)	0.27	0.2–1.5
Platelets (x 10^9/l)	202	175–500

Abnormal results are in **bold**.

Urinalysis	Result
Specific gravity	1.034
Dipstick analysis	Strongly positive (++++) for protein with a trace of blood; pH 8.5. Negative for glucose and ketones
UPCR	11.03
Sediment	Triple phosphate crystals, some red blood cells, occasional bacteria

WHAT ABNORMALITIES ARE PRESENT?

Haematology
- Eosinopenia.
- Erythrocytosis.

Biochemistry
- Significantly increased cholesterol, ALP and ALT.
- Mildly increased bile acids, gamma-glutamyl transferase (GGT) and phosphate.

HOW WOULD YOU INTERPRET THESE RESULTS AND WHAT ARE THE LIKELY DIFFERENTIAL DIAGNOSES?

The history and appearance of the dog are suggestive of an endocrinopathy, specifically HAC. Erythrocytosis and eosinopenia may be caused by exogenous or endogenous corticosteroids, although neutrophilia, lymphopenia and monocytosis are not present.

The most specific changes on routine biochemistry are the increased cholesterol and the disproportionately high ALP when compared with the ALT, which are consistent with a number of endocrinopathies (diabetes mellitus and HAC; hypothyroidism could cause the marked hypercholesterolaemia, but would not be associated with the high ALP). Diabetes can be ruled out by the normal blood glucose concentration. Postprandial effects might also cause an increase in cholesterol, but not as marked as in this case.

The mild increases in bile acids are very non-specific and could be due to almost any systemic metabolic,

→ CASE 1 CONTINUED

inflammatory, toxic or neoplastic condition as well as any hepatopathy. Postprandial bile acid measurement might be worthwhile to confirm that this is a non-specific finding. Similarly, the slightly high phosphate is probably not significant; however, this is seen in cases of HAC, renal failure (though the normal urea and creatinine make this unlikely) and hypoparathyroidism (but the calcium results make this unlikely).

The most likely differential diagnosis is HAC. An ACTH stimulation test was performed.

Endocrinology	Result	Reference interval
Cortisol (nmol/l) pre-ACTH	95	40–240
Cortisol (nmol/l) post-ACTH	275	80–450

The ACTH stimulation test is within reference limits.

WHAT FURTHER TESTS WOULD YOU RECOMMEND?

- Low-dose dexamethasone suppression test (as ACTH stimulation test negative).
- Combined T4 and TSH measurement.

Endocrinology	Result	Reference interval
Cortisol (nmol/l) pre-dexamethasone	81	40–240
Cortisol (nmol/l) 3 h post-dexamethasone	**53**	<40% baseline
Cortisol (nmol/l) 8 h post-dexamethasone	**98**	<40
Thyroxine (T4) (nmol/l)	22.5	15–50
TSH (ng/ml)	0.12	0–0.6

Abnormal results are in **bold**.

HOW WOULD YOU INTERPRET THESE RESULTS AND WHAT ARE THE LIKELY DIFFERENTIAL DIAGNOSES?

The low-dose dexamethasone suppression test shows that there is only mild suppression of cortisol following dexamethasone administration and there is escape from this suppression by 8 hours. This, with the clinical signs and laboratory data, is consistent with HAC, and the pattern may be consistent with an adrenal tumour but can also be seen with pituitary-dependent HAC.

The total T4 concentration and TSH concentration are normal. There is no evidence of the so-called sick euthyroid syndrome in this case (or low T4 state of medical illness; see Chapter 17).

WHAT FURTHER TESTS WOULD YOU RECOMMEND?

As this dog has been confirmed with HAC, endogenous ACTH measurement could be used to try to differentiate pituitary- and adrenal-dependent HAC. The concentration measured is consistent with pituitary-dependent disease.

Endocrinology	Result	Reference interval
Endogenous ACTH (pmol/l)	50	20–60

Performing urinalysis and in particular a urine culture would also be worthwhile.

FOLLOW UP

Medical therapy with trilostane is indicated. This was successful in controlling the clinical signs for 9 months. The biochemistry improved but was never normal during this time. At 9 months post diagnosis the ALT was 132 IU/l, ALP 3815 IU/l and cholesterol 14 mmol/l. Shortly afterwards the dog was euthanased for an unrelated cause (an extraskeletal osteosarcoma arising from the mammary gland).

CASE 2

SIGNALMENT

3-year-old male neutered Standard Poodle.

HISTORY

2-week history of lethargy, exercise intolerance and diarrhoea with a decreased appetite. Vomited 5 days previously and was semi-collapsed (Figure 18.21). On clinical examination the dog was thin, dehydrated and in shock. Mucous membranes were dry but pink, heart rate was 90 beats per minute. No other abnormalities were detected.

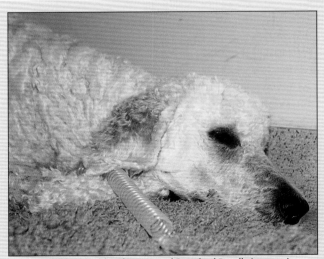

18.21 A 3-year-old male neutered Standard Poodle in a semi-collapsed state. Intravenous fluid therapy has been initiated.

→ CASE 2 CONTINUED

CLINICAL PATHOLOGY DATA

Biochemistry	Result	Reference interval
Total protein (g/l)	**55**	60–80
Albumin (g/l)	**22**	26–40
Globulin (g/l)	33	25–45
Glucose (mmol/l)	3.6	3.4–5.3
Sodium (mmol/l)	**134**	135–155
Potassium (mmol/l)	**7.8**	3.5–5.8
Sodium:potassium ratio	**17**	>27
Chloride (mmol/l)	111	105–120
Calcium (mmol/l)	**3.0**	2.2–2.7
Phosphate (mmol/l)	**2.2**	0.6–1.3
Urea (mmol/l)	**14.7**	3.3–8.0
Creatinine (μmol/l)	**242**	45–150
Cholesterol (mmol/l)	2.45	2.3–6
Bilirubin (μmol/l)	2	0–10
ALT (IU/l)	**160**	21–59
ALP (IU/l)	51	3–142
GGT (IU/l)	0	0–10

Abnormal results are in **bold**.

Haematology	Result	Reference interval
RBC (x 10¹²/l)	6.71	5.5–8.5
Haemoglobin (g/dl)	15.7	12–18
PCV (l/l)	0.44	0.37–0.55
MCV (fl)	65.6	60–77
MCHC (g/dl)	35.6	32–37
MCH (pg)	23.4	19.5–24.5
WBC (x 10⁹/l)	16.4	6–17
Band neutrophils (x 10⁹/l)	0	0–0.3
Segmented neutrophils (x 10⁹/l)	**12.0**	3–11.5
Eosinophils (x 10⁹/l)	0.4	0.1–1.3
Basophils (x 10⁹/l)	0	0
Lymphocytes (x 10⁹/l)	3.6	1–4.8
Monocytes (x 10⁹/l)	0.4	0.2–1.5
Platelets (x 10⁹/l)	202	175–500

Abnormal results are in **bold**.

Urinalysis	Result
Specific gravity	1.024
Dipstick analysis	No protein, blood, glucose or ketones; pH 6.5

WHAT ABNORMALITIES ARE PRESENT?

Haematology
- Relatively high lymphocyte count for a stressed and ill animal.
- Mild neutrophilia.

Biochemistry
- Hypoalbuminaemia.
- Azotaemia.
- Hyperkalaemia.
- Hyponatraemia.
- Hyperphosphataemia.
- Mild hypercalcaemia.

The calcium concentration is abnormal because the low albumin should lead to a lower total calcium; an ionized hypercalcaemia is suspected.

Urinalysis
- The SG suggests that concentrating ability is compromised.

HOW WOULD YOU INTERPRET THESE RESULTS AND WHAT ARE THE LIKELY DIFFERENTIAL DIAGNOSES?

There is hyperkalaemia and hyponatraemia, with a sodium:potassium ratio of 17. The hyperkalaemia can be seen with hypoadrenocorticism, metabolic acidosis, some forms of renal failure, liquorice poisoning and poor sample handling, e.g. contamination with potassium EDTA (which also gives a low calcium) or delayed separation. Hyponatraemia can be seen with severe diarrhoea, certain forms of renal failure, overhydration and lipaemia.

The azotaemia is significant, with relatively higher urea than creatinine concentration, which is common in prerenal azotaemia or where there is gastrointestinal haemorrhage. In prerenal azotaemia, increased urine SG is expected, unless there are other factors affecting the kidney's ability to concentrate urine, while in azotaemia of renal origin isosthenuria is expected. In this case the urine SG is intermediate, a common feature of hypoadrenocorticism. Assessment of the response to fluid therapy would be needed to evaluate renal function further.

Mild hypoalbuminaemia can be seen with hypoadrenocorticism, liver diseases and mild cases of protein-losing enteropathy and nephropathy (however, there is no significant proteinuria). Mild to moderate hypercalcaemia can also occur with hypoadrenocorticism. Lymphocytosis in a stressed animal is an unusual finding and suggests the absence of a cortisol response.

WHAT FURTHER TEST WOULD YOU PERFORM?

Since hypoadrenocorticism was suspected, an ACTH stimulation test was performed.

Endocrinology	Result	Reference interval
Cortisol (nmol/l) pre-ACTH	**<7**	40–240
Cortisol (nmol/l) post-ACTH	**<7**	80–450

Abnormal results are in **bold**.

The results of the ACTH stimulation test confirm this as a case of hypoadrenocorticism. The abnormal electrolytes indicate that mineralocorticoid output is also affected. There are some features of hypoadrenocorticism that are absent in this case, for example eosinophilia, low cholesterol and hypoglycaemia. Very few cases of hypoadrenocorticism have every single finding. In this case the electrolyte abnormalities and the azotaemia resolved within 24 hours of starting fluids.

References and further reading

Ash RA, Harvey AM and Tasker S (2005) Primary hyperaldosteronism in the cat: a series of 13 cases. Journal of Feline Medicine and Surgery **7**, 173–182

Baumstark ME, Nussberger J, Boretti FS et al. (2014) Use of plasma renin activity to monitor mineralocorticoid treatment in dogs with primary hypoadrenocorticism: desoxycorticosterone versus cortisone. Journal of Veterinary Internal Medicine **28**, 1471–1478

Baumstark ME, Sieber-Ruckstuhl NS, Müller C, Wenger M, Boretti FS and Reusch CE (2014) Evaluation of aldosterone concentrations in dogs with hypoadrenocorticism. Journal of Veterinary Internal Medicine **28**, 154–159

Behrend EN, Kooistra HS, Nelson R, Reusch CE and Scott-Moncrieff JC (2013) Diagnosis of spontaneous canine hyperadrenocorticism: 2012 ACVIM Consensus Statement (Small Animal). Journal of Veterinary Internal Medicine **27**, 1292–1304

Bell R, Mellor DJ, Ramsey I and Knottenbelt C (2005) Decreased sodium:potassium ratios in cats: 49 cases. Veterinary Clinical Pathology **34**, 110–114

Bell R., Neiger R., McGrotty Y and Ramsey IK (2006) Effects of once daily trilostane administration on cortisol concentrations and ACTH responsiveness in hyperadrenocorticoid dogs. Veterinary Record **159**, 277–281

Benitah N, Feldman EC, Kass PH and Nelson RW (2005) Evaluation of serum 17-hydroxyprogesterone concentration after administration of ACTH in dogs with hyperadrenocorticism. Journal of the American Veterinary Medical Association **227**, 1095–1101

Bonadio CM, Feldman EC, Cohen TA and Kass PH (2014) Comparison of adrenocorticotropic hormone stimulation test results started 2 versus 4 hours after trilostane administration in dogs with naturally occurring hyperadrenocorticism. Journal of Veterinary Internal Medicine **28**, 1239–1243

Bovens C, Tennant K, Reeve J and Murphy KF. (2014) Basal serum cortisol concentration as a screening test for hypoadrenocorticism in dogs. Journal of Veterinary Internal Medicine **28**, 1541-1545

Chapman PS, Mooney CT, Ede J et al. (2003) Evaluation of the basal and post-adrenocorticotrophic hormone serum concentrations of 17-hydroxyprogesterone for the diagnosis of hyperadrenocorticism in dogs. Veterinary Record **153**, 771–775

DeClue AE, Martin LG, Behrend EN, Cohn LA, Dismukes DI and Lee HP (2011) Cortisol and aldosterone response to various doses of cosyntropin in healthy cats. Journal of the American Veterinary Medical Association **238**, 176–182

Djajadiningrat-Laanen S, Galac S and Kooistra H (2011) Primary hyperaldosteronism: expanding the diagnostic net. Journal of Feline Medicine and Surgery **13**, 641–650

Dunn KJ and Herrtage ME (1998) Hypocortisolaemia in a Labrador retriever. Journal of Small Animal Practice **39**, 90–93

Frank LA, Henry GA, Whittemore JC, Enders BD, Mawby DI and Rohrbach BW (2015) Serum cortisol concentrations in dogs with pituitary-dependent hyperadrenocorticism and atypical hyperadrenocorticism. Journal of Veterinary Internal Medicine **29(1)**, 193–199

Ginel PJ, Pérez-Rico A, Moreno P and Lucena R (1998) Validation of a commercially available enzyme-linked immunosorbent assay (ELISA) for the determination of cortisol in canine plasma samples. Veterinary Research Communications **22**, 179–185

Gostelow R, Bridger N and Syme HM (2013) Plasma-free metanephrine and free normetanephrine measurement for the diagnosis of pheochromocytoma in dogs. Journal of Veterinary Internal Medicine **27**, 83–90

Griebsch C, Lehnert C, Williams GJ, Failing K and Neiger R (2014) Effect of trilostane on hormone and serum electrolyte concentrations in dogs with pituitary-dependent hyperadrenocorticism. Journal of Veterinary Internal Medicine **28**, 160–165

Herrtage ME and Ramsey IK (2012) Canine hyperadrenocorticism. In: BSAVA Manual of Canine and Feline Endocrinology, 4th edn, ed. CT Mooney and ME Peterson, pp. 167–189. BSAVA Publications, Gloucester

Hill KE, Scott-Moncrieff JC, Koshko MA et al. (2005) Secretion of sex hormones in dogs with adrenal dysfunction. Journal of the American Veterinary Medical Association **226**, 556–561

Kaplan AJ, Peterson ME and Kemppainen RJ (1995) Effects of disease on the results of diagnostic tests for use in detecting hyperadrenocorticism in dogs. Journal of the American Veterinary Medical Association **207**, 445–451

Kenefick SJ and Neiger R (2008) The effect of trilostane treatment on circulating thyroid hormone concentrations in dogs with pituitary-dependent hyperadrenocorticism. Journal of Small Animal Practice **49**, 139–143

Kley S, Alt M, Zimmer C, Hoerauf A and Reusch CE (2007) Evaluation of the low-dose dexamethasone suppression test and ultrasonographic measurements of the adrenal glands in cats with diabetes mellitus. Schweizer Archiv für Tierheilkunde **149**, 493–500

Lathan P, Scott-Moncrieff JC and Willls RW (2014) Use of the cortisol-to-ACTH ratio for diagnosis of primary hypoadrenocorticism in dogs Journal of Veterinary Internal Medicine **28**, 1546-1550

Lennon EM, Boyle TE, Hutchins RG et al. (2007) Use of basal serum or plasma cortisol concentrations to rule out a diagnosis of hypoadrenocorticism in dogs: 123 cases (2000-2005). Journal of the American Veterinary Medical Association **231**, 413–416

Lobetti RG (1998) Hyperreninaemia hypoaldosteronism in a dog. Journal of the South African Veterinary Association **69(1)**, 33–35

Monroe WE, Panciera DL and Zimmerman KL (2012) Concentrations of noncortisol adrenal steroids in response to ACTH in dogs with adrenal-dependent hyperadrenocorticism, pituitary-dependent hyperadrenocorticism, and nonadrenal illness. Journal of Veterinary Internal Medicine **26**, 945–952

Mueller C, Sieber-Ruckstuhl N, Wenger M, Kaser-Hotz B and Reusch CE (2006) Low-dose dexamethasone test with 'inverse' results a possible new pattern of cortisol response. Veterinary Record **159**, 489–491

Neiger R, Ramsey I, O'Connor J, Hurley KJ and Mooney CT (2002) Trilostane treatment of 78 dogs with pituitary dependent hyperadrenocorticism. Veterinary Record **150**, 799–804

Neiger R, Witt AL, Noble A and German AJ (2004) Trilostane therapy for treatment of pituitary-dependent hyperadrenocorticism in 5 cats. Journal of Veterinary Internal Medicine **18**, 160–164

Neilsen L, Bell R, Zoia A, Mellor D, Neiger R and Ramsey IK (2008) Decreased sodium:potassium ratios in dog: 238 cases. Veterinary Record **162**, 431–435

Quante S, Boretti FS, Kook PH et al. (2010) Urinary catecholamine and metanephrine to creatinine ratios in dogs with hyperadrenocorticism or pheochromocytoma, and in healthy dogs. Journal of Veterinary Internal Medicine **24**, 1093–1097

Ramsey I (2010) Trilostane: a review. Veterinary Clinics of North America: Small Animal Practice **40**, 269–283

Ramsey IK, Tebb AJ, Harris E, Evans H and Herrtage ME (2005) Hyperparathyroidism in dogs with hyperadrenocorticism. Journal of Small Animal Practice **46**, 531–536

Ramsey IK, Parkin T and Cosgrove L (2015) Assessment of novel methods of monitoring trilostane treatment of canine hyperadrenocorticism Proceedings of the British Small Animal Veterinary Association April 9-12, Birmingham

Ramspott S, Hartmann K, Sauter-Louis C, Weber K and Wehner A (2012) Adrenal function in cats with hyperthyroidism. Journal of Feline Medicine and Surgery **14**, 262–266

Ristić JME, Ramsey IK, Heath FM, Evans HJ and Herrtage ME (2002) The use of 17-hydroxyprogesterone in the diagnosis of canine hyperadrenocorticism. Journal of Veterinary Internal Medicine **16**, 433–439

Roberts E, Boden L and Ramsey I (2013) Stabilisation of dogs with primary hypoadrenocorticism, comparing once-daily versus twice-daily oral dosing of fludrocortisone acetate. Proceedings of the 23rd Congress of the European College of Veterinary Internal Medicine – Companion Animals, September 12–14, Liverpool

Rodríguez Piñeiro MI, Benchekroun G, de Fornel-Thibaud P, Maurey-Guenec C, Garnier F and Rosenberg D (2009) Accuracy of an adrenocorticotropic hormone (ACTH) immunoluminometric assay for differentiating ACTH-dependent from ACTH-independent hyperadrenocorticism in dogs. Journal of Veterinary Internal Medicine **23**, 850–855

Russell NJ, Foster S, Clark P, Robertson ID, Lewis D and Irwin PJ (2007) Comparison of radioimmunoassay and chemiluminescent assay methods to estimate canine blood cortisol concentrations. Australian Veterinary Journal **85**, 487–494

Schoeman JP, Evans HJ, Childs D and Herrtage ME (2000) Cortisol response to two different doses of intravenous synthetic ACTH (tetracosactrin) in overweight cats. Journal of Small Animal Practice **41**, 552–557

Seth M, Drobatz KJ, Church DB and Hess RS (2011) White blood cell count and the sodium to potassium ratio to screen for hypoadrenocorticism in dogs. Journal of Veterinary Internal Medicine **25**, 1351–1356

Tebb AJ, Arteaga A, Evans H and Ramsey IK (2005). Canine hyperadrenocorticism: effects of trilostane on parathyroid hormone, calcium and phosphate concentrations. Journal of Small Animal Practice **46**, 537–542

Vonderen IK, Kooistra HS and Rijnberk A (1998) Influence of veterinary care on the urinary corticoid:creatinine ratio in dogs. Journal of Veterinary Internal Medicine **12**, 431–435

Zeugswetter F, Bydzovsky N, Kampner D and Schwendenwein I (2010) Tailored reference limits for urine corticoid:creatinine ratio in dogs to answer distinct clinical questions. Veterinary Record **167**, 997–1001

Zeugswetter FK, Neffe F, Schwendenwein I, Tichy A and Möstl E (2013) Configuration of antibodies for assay of urinary cortisol in dogs influences analytic specificity. Domestic Animal Endocrinology **45**, 98–104

Chapter 19

Laboratory evaluation of the reproductive system

Gary C.W. England, Marco Russo and Sarah L. Freeman

Investigation of diseases of the reproductive tract requires a detailed breeding history and a thorough clinical examination, followed by careful application of a number of laboratory tests. The purpose of this chapter is to describe the logical application of laboratory testing to common clinical presentations met by veterinary surgeons (veterinarians) in first-opinion practice.

Female

The bitch

The bitch differs from the females of many domestic species (which are polyoestrous) in that she is mono-estrous, with a long obligatory period of anoestrus between successive oestrus periods, whether she is pregnant or not. There does not seem to be a seasonal cyclicity in most breeds and the average interval between oestrus periods is 7 months. Understanding the normal physiology is essential so that these normal, but unusual, features of reproductive function are not confused with pathology.

Reproductive physiology of the bitch

Puberty generally commences between 6 and 24 months of age, often within 1–6 months of the bitch attaining adult height and weight. Before puberty, and during each period of anoestrus, the ovaries appear quiescent. The onset of oestrus (or puberty) is initiated by increased secretion of gonadotrophin-releasing hormone (GnRH) from the hypothalamus and a subsequent release of follicle-stimulating hormone (FSH) and luteinizing hormone (LH) from the pituitary gland; these, in turn, stimulate follicular growth in the ovaries and the production of oestrogen. A raised plasma oestrogen concentration initiates the onset of pro-oestrus, when vulval oedema and a sanguineous discharge occur. The bitch is attractive to the male at this time, but will not accept mating. A subsequent decline in oestrogen and slight increase in plasma progesterone initiate oestrus, at which time the bitch will allow mating. During oestrus, the vulva becomes less oedematous and the discharge clearer and less sanguineous. The rise in plasma progesterone concentration is the result of preovulatory luteinization of follicles, and the low oestrogen:progesterone ratio causes a surge in LH from the pituitary gland. Most ovulations begin 48 hours after peak LH concentrations are reached. Formation of the corpus luteum occurs quickly after ovulation. High concentrations of progesterone occur approximately 7 days after ovulation and in many bitches this signifies the end of standing oestrus. In most species, progesterone concentrations increase after behavioural oestrus and this increase of progesterone is designated the onset of metoestrus (dioestrus). The terminology for the phases of the oestrous cycle is confusing in the bitch because progesterone concentrations increase during behavioural oestrus (Figure 19.1).

The non-pregnant luteal phase is termed metoestrus or dioestrus (these terms are used synonymously – see above). Unusually, when compared with other domestic species, progesterone secretion is similar in both the non-pregnant and the pregnant bitch (Figure 19.2). In both pregnancy and the non-pregnant luteal phase, progesterone is produced solely by the corpora lutea within the ovaries. Progesterone production during the luteal phase is maintained principally by the luteotrophic effects of the pituitary hormone prolactin.

During the non-pregnant luteal phase, progesterone causes mammary gland enlargement and, when combined with an increase in plasma prolactin (caused by a decline in plasma progesterone), this results in the secretion of milk and in behavioural changes that are typical of pregnancy. This latter condition, termed pseudopregnancy, is a normal event that is observed in all non-pregnant bitches. In some cases the changes are marked and produce obvious clinical signs, while in others the signs may be unnoticed by the owner. As previously mentioned, progesterone concentrations are similar in pregnancy and the non-pregnant luteal phase. Interestingly, progesterone concentrations decline rapidly prior to the onset of parturition (and this event can be used to predict the onset of parturition), but this does not occur in non-pregnant bitches, where the luteal phase is longer than that of pregnancy. Relaxin is a specific pregnancy-related hormone which is produced by placental tissues; raised concentrations can be detected from day 24 of pregnancy onwards.

Following pregnancy or the non-pregnant luteal phase, the quiescent anoestrus state resumes, and plasma progesterone concentrations return to baseline. The factors that result in cessation of progesterone secretion are unknown.

The queen

The queen is a polyoestrous breeder in which ovulation is induced by coitus. Cyclicity in the queen is influenced by photoperiod. In the northern hemisphere, periods of anoestrus are normally observed from November to January inclusive.

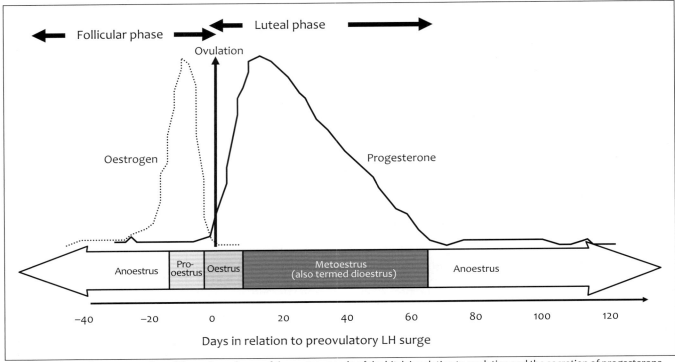

19.1 Schematic representation of the various phases of the oestrous cycle of the bitch in relation to ovulation and the secretion of progesterone. LH = luteinizing hormone.

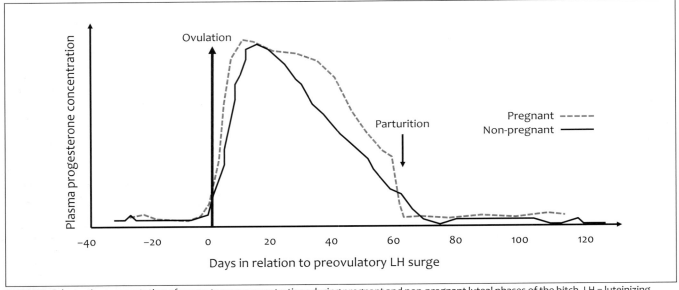

19.2 Schematic representation of progesterone concentrations during pregnant and non-pregnant luteal phases of the bitch. LH = luteinizing hormone.

Reproductive physiology of the queen

In queens, the secretion of pituitary hormones is upregulated as day length increases, and suppressed as day length decreases (most likely as a result of melatonin release from the pituitary gland). In this way queens have a classical 'long day' photoperiodic breeding season. In most queens, ovulation must be induced by coitus (or artificial stimulation), although it may occur in a small number of queens without an obvious stimulus. In the majority, copulation produces a rapid pituitary-mediated release of LH. Ovulation occurs once LH concentration exceeds a threshold value.

Multiple copulations within a short time are generally required to produce an LH surge of sufficient magnitude to induce ovulation. Progesterone concentration remains basal until after the mating-induced LH surge, and increases after ovulation; peak values are reached 3–4 weeks after mating. In pregnant queens, the progesterone concentration declines slowly until day 60 and remains relatively low for the last week, before declining abruptly at parturition; the duration of pregnancy is usually 64–68 days from mating. In a queen that has been mated but does not become pregnant, progesterone concentration is initially identical to that of early pregnancy but then returns to basal values, with the luteal phase lasting between 30 and 45 days (Figure 19.3), before the queen returns to oestrus. These queens are said to be pseudo-pregnant, although the only clinical sign is an absence of oestrus. Non-ovulating (non-mated or inadequately mated) queens do not have a luteal phase and return to oestrus after an interval of approximately 21 days. Throughout pregnancy the primary source of progesterone is the ovary, and there does not appear to be a significant contribution from the placenta.

Oestradiol concentration is elevated during the last week of pregnancy; prolactin concentration is elevated in the last third of pregnancy and throughout lactation. Prolactin has a luteotrophic action similar to that in the bitch. There are no significant changes in prolactin concentration during pseudopregnancy.

In the pregnant queen, relaxin is present in the plasma from approximately day 25 and, similarly to relaxin in the bitch, it increases to peak values at approximately day 50 and declines after parturition.

Laboratory techniques

Techniques available for the investigation of female reproductive tract disease include measurement of concentrations of the reproductive sex steroids (progesterone, oestrogen and testosterone) and LH, and cytological investigation of collected smears, fluids or aspirates. Endocrinological evaluation frequently requires radioimmunoassays (RIAs) performed in specialist laboratories, but enzyme-linked immunosorbent assays (ELISAs) are available for the measurement of both progesterone and LH. Hormone concentrations can be measured in either plasma or serum.

Failure to cycle

A common clinical presentation of bitches is a failure to cycle. In many cases this may be an apparent absence of oestrus or an apparent delay in puberty because the owner has not observed the signs of oestrus. Elevated plasma progesterone concentrations (>2.0 ng/ml (6.5 nmol/l)) demonstrate that ovulation has occurred within the last 60 days (i.e. the oestrus or puberty has been missed); clearly it is difficult to demonstrate a 'missed' oestrus more than 60 days previously.

In the queen there is a normal period of anoestrus during winter. This influences the timing of the onset of puberty because most queens reach puberty in the spring. Cyclicity may therefore commence at 6 months of age (or slightly less) for queens born in the autumn, but queens born in spring often do not reach puberty until the next spring, when they are 12 months old. Vaginal cytology will enable the documentation of normal cyclical activity.

In those cases where it is clear that lack of oestrus is not the result of failure of observation by the owner, failure to cycle may be primary (no oestrus before 24 months, i.e. delayed puberty) or secondary (no oestrous activity within 12 months of a previous cycle, i.e. prolonged anoestrus). In most cases a specific disease process is responsible, and careful investigation of the underlying cause is important for appropriate treatment and prognosis.

Delayed puberty: Bitches that do not reach puberty by 2.5 years of age are generally considered to have delayed puberty. Investigation involves evaluating housing and diet (poor environmental conditions and poor nutrition may be associated with failure to cycle), and clinical examination to rule out chronic disease. Chromosomal abnormalities may cause delayed puberty and establishing the karyotype is key to diagnosis. Ethylenediamine tetra-acetic acid (EDTA) blood samples need to be transported rapidly to the laboratory. Normally there are 78 chromosomes (77XX); common abnormalities include either absence (77XO) or additional chromosomes (79XXX, 79XXY) or, in some cases, mixed chromosome aberrations (78XX/78XY). Many of these bitches are phenotypically abnormal (with a small cranially positioned and some-times elongated vulva and developing clitoral enlargement at puberty). A smaller proportion of bitches are phenotypically normal but the abnormal complement of sex chromosomes results in ovarian hypoplasia or ovarian dysgenesis. Karyotyping is available at the Cytogenetics Laboratory, University of Pennsylvania School of Veterinary Medicine, USA.

There is little information available for queens, although it is clear that chromosomal abnormalities can influence the onset of puberty in the same manner as in the bitch.

Prolonged anoestrus: Prolonged anoestrus in the bitch represents an interoestrus interval greater than anticipated for that particular animal (usually more than 12 months

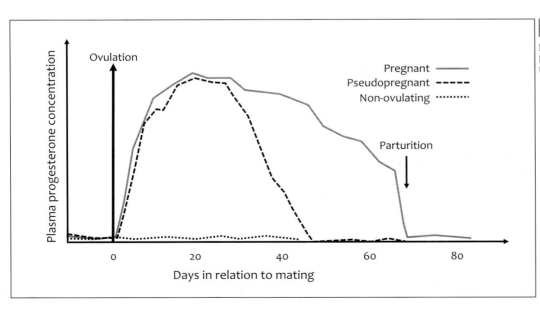

19.3 Schematic representation of progesterone concentrations in pregnant, pseudopregnant and non-ovulating queens.

from the previous cycle). In the queen it represents an animal that does not resume cyclical activity after the winter anoestrus.

There are several causes of failure to resume normal cyclicity, including chronic systemic disease, drug-induced anoestrus (glucocorticoids, anabolic steroids, androgens and progestagens) and hypothyroidism (see Chapters 17 and 18). Although hypothyroidism has been associated with prolonged anoestrus, the mechanism of this abnormality has not been fully established. Following replacement therapy most bitches return to oestrus within 6 months, although a consistent relationship between thyroid disease and reproductive function has yet to be established.

Progesterone-producing ovarian cysts have been described in the bitch and queen; they lead to prolonged interoestrus intervals and cystic endometrial hyperplasia. The ovarian cysts may be identified ultrasonographically and the diagnosis confirmed by persistently elevated plasma progesterone concentrations. Hormone concentrations that remain at an elevated plateau over a period of 6 weeks would be suspicious, because in the normal luteal phase progesterone concentrations decline during this time; elevated values of progesterone for >8 weeks would be diagnostic.

In some cases, ovarian neoplasms that produce either progesterone or androgens result in a failure to return to cyclical activity. They may be diagnosed by serial estimation of plasma progesterone and testosterone concentrations and by ultrasonographic examination of the ovaries.

Optimal time to breed

The most common cause of infertility in the bitch is mating at an inappropriate time. In the queen, on the other hand, coitus is the trigger for ovulation, and the optimal mating time is generally thought to be during the first few days of oestrus.

Bitches ovulate approximately 12 days after the onset of pro-oestrus; however, some normal bitches may ovulate as early as 5 days while others ovulate as late as 30 days after the onset of pro-oestrus. Many breeders try to impose standard mating regimes, for example mating on days 10 and 12, but for many bitches this is not appropriate. Careful monitoring of oestrus is important to establish the time of ovulation and therefore the most appropriate time for mating (Figure 19.4). Observation of

the behaviour of the bitch has limited value, and although there may be clear changes affecting the external genitalia (for example the onset of vulval softening occurs 1–2 days prior to ovulation), laboratory investigation can be extremely useful.

Hormone measurement: Measurement of the peripheral plasma concentration of LH is a potentially useful method to determine the optimum time for mating, although assay kits are not always readily available, and the LH surge occurs over a short period of time and may be missed even with daily blood sampling. Plasma progesterone concentrations begin to increase towards the end of pro-oestrus at the time of the LH surge, so serial monitoring of plasma progesterone concentration allows the anticipation of ovulation (Figure 19.5). Progesterone may be measured using ELISA test kits designed for in-practice use or in commercial laboratories using RIA and chemiluminescence. The in-house kits are semi-quantitative, using a colour change to assess progesterone concentration, whereas the laboratory methods provide a numerical result. Both methods have been shown to be useful for predicting the optimum mating time in the bitch.

Ovulation occurs when progesterone is approximately 6.5 ng/ml (20 nmol/l); oocytes mature for 48 hours and are then fertile for 2–4 days (i.e. day 3, 4 or 5 after ovulation). Sperm survival is very long for healthy, young males (survival up to 7 days), but much shorter for older males or when semen has been frozen and then thawed (survival 12–24 hours). Breeding or insemination should be planned between 4 and 6 days after progesterone concentrations exceed 2.0 ng/ml (6.5 nmol/l; the concentration typically observed at the time of the LH surge). Several reports suggest that breeding should commence 1 day after progesterone concentrations exceed 8.0–10.0 ng/ml (25.0–32.0 nmol/l), which is commonly seen 2 days after ovulation when oocytes become fertilizable.

Period	Days from LH surge	Days from ovulation
Period of potential fertility – the 'fertile period'	−3 to +7 (or later)	−5 to +5 (or later)
Period of potential fertilization of mature oocytes – the 'fertilization period'	+4 to +6 (or later)	+2 to +4 (or later)
Time of oocyte maturation	+ 4 to +5	+2 to +3
Period of peak fertility in normal bitches at natural mating	0 to +6	−2 to +4
Preferred time for managed breeding by natural mating or artificial insemination (AI) with fresh semen	+2 to +6	0 to +4
Time for managed breeding when bitch has subfertility (e.g. endometrial hyperplasia) or when semen quality is poor (e.g. frozen semen AI)	+4 to +6	+2 to +4

19.4 The timing of peak fertility in the bitch in relation to the day of the luteinizing hormone (LH) surge and the day of ovulation. Note that ovulation occurs 2 days after the LH surge.

Parameter	Progesterone concentration (nmol/l)	Interpretation
Interpretation of progesterone concentration for repeated sampling	<1.0–4.0	No luteinization Bitch is still in pro-oestrus or early oestrus Re-sample in 3–4 days
	4.0–10.0	Functional luteinization Bitch is close to ovulation or has just ovulated Re-sample in 2–3 days
	10.0–20.0	Ovulation has almost certainly occurred Re-sampling in 1 day will probably confirm ovulation
	>20.0	Ovulation has occurred Re-sampling not required
	>80.0	The end of the fertile period in most bitches Most bitches will not stand to be mated
Interpretation of progesterone concentration for mating	16.0–20.0	Mate, starting within 2–3 days
	20.0–38.0	Mate, starting within 1–2 days
	>38.0	Mate immediately

19.5 Interpretation of plasma progesterone concentration in the bitch for re-sampling and mating advice to owners. In most cases it is appropriate to commence measurement of progesterone approximately 7 days after the onset of pro-oestrus.

Queens are induced ovulators and therefore hormone measurement is not useful in determining the optimal time to breed. Ovulation occurs in response to a mating-induced increase in LH; the greatest magnitude LH surge in response to mating occurs when mating is on day 3 after the onset of oestrus, and therefore mating is best planned from this time onwards. Multiple matings (preferably more than two) within a short period of time (preferably 6 hours) are most likely to result in an LH surge of sufficient magnitude to induce ovulation.

Vaginal cytology: Examination of exfoliated vaginal epithelial cells is frequently used to monitor the oestrous cycle. During pro-oestrus, increased plasma oestrogen concentrations cause thickening of the vaginal mucosa, which becomes a keratinized squamous epithelium. Surface vaginal epithelial cells may be collected using a saline-moistened swab or by aspiration using an inseminating catheter and 5 ml syringe. The cotton swab technique requires a speculum to ensure that cells are not collected from the vulval lips or the vestibule. The swab is inserted into the vagina and rotated to collect cells from the vaginal wall; following removal, the swab is gently rolled on to a clean dry microscope slide to transfer the collected cells. The aspiration technique uses a 20 cm inseminating catheter attached to a syringe, which is gently inserted into the cranial vagina before gentle suction is applied; a small volume of vaginal fluid will be collected in the catheter and a drop of this fluid is then transferred to a microscope slide and smeared in the same way as a haematology smear.

The relative proportions of different types of epithelial cell can be used as a marker of the endocrine environment. The fertile period can be predicted from the proportion of cornified or anuclear epithelial cells, using a Romanowsky stain such as modified Wright–Giemsa stain or a rapid dunking stain. Breeding should be attempted throughout the period when >80% of epithelial cells are anuclear (Figures 19.6 and 19.7). While this is a useful guide, some bitches reach peak values of only 60% anuclear cells, while in others there may be two anuclear cell peaks and so this is a less accurate method of determining the optimum time to breed than measuring progesterone.

Neutrophils are generally absent from the vaginal smear during oestrus because the keratinized epithelium is impervious to these cells. Their reappearance during late oestrus occurs when there is sloughing of the vaginal epithelium; the associated cellular debris and thinner epithelium allows an influx of neutrophils, which appear in the lumen in large numbers. The return of neutrophils to the vaginal smear is sometimes used as an indicator of the time of optimum fertility. Typical changes in vaginal cytology are shown in Figure 19.8.

At the Guide Dogs for the Blind Association in the UK, mating on the basis of vaginal cytology was found to increase the pregnancy rate and litter size of bitches when compared with a similar group mated only on the basis of the onset of pro-oestrus (England, 1992). Whelping rates have been consistently maintained above 90% over a 20-year period since the introduction of this regime.

Parameter	Anoestrus	Early pro-oestrus	Pro-oestrus	Early oestrus	Oestrus	Early 'metoestrus'
Anuclear cells (%)	0	10	30	50	80	5
Large intermediate epithelial cells (%)	0	20	30	30	20	0
Small intermediate epithelial cells (%)	0	20	30	20	0	20
Parabasal cells (%)	100	50	10	0	0	75
Erythrocytes	–	+++	++	+	–	–
Neutrophils	++	+	–	–	+	++++
Debris and mucus	++	+++	++	–	–	+++

19.6 Periovulatory changes in vaginal smears from bitches.

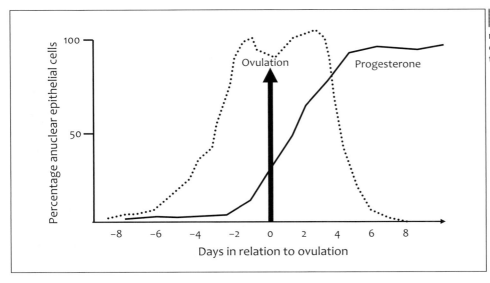

19.7 Changes in the percentage of anuclear vaginal epithelial cells in relation to ovulation and the periovulatory changes in progesterone concentration in the bitch.

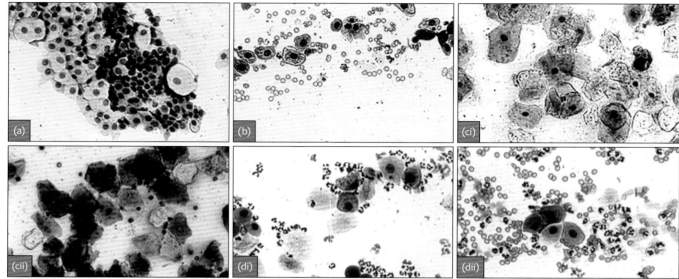

19.8 Exfoliative vaginal cytology from bitches. (a) Anoestrus. The predominant cell types are small parabasal epithelial cells, which have a small volume of cytoplasm compared with the size of the nucleus. The majority of cells are roughly circular in shape. Neutrophils may be present in small numbers but are not evident in this example. (b) Pro-oestrus. The predominant cell type is small intermediate epithelial cells, which have an increased volume of cytoplasm compared with the size of the nucleus. The cells are irregular in shape and appear somewhat flattened with sharp edges. Erythrocytes are present in large numbers. Neutrophils may be present in small numbers, as in this sample. (c) Oestrus. The predominant cell types are large intermediate epithelial cells and anuclear epithelial cells, which have a large volume of cytoplasm compared with the size of the nucleus, and no nucleus, respectively. The cells are two-dimensionally flattened and very irregular in shape (often referred to as 'cornflake cells'). Erythrocytes are present in small numbers. Neutrophils are absent from the smear. (d) Metoestrus. The predominant cell types are large and small intermediate epithelial cells. Large numbers of neutrophils are again present. Erythrocytes may be present in small numbers. (Diff-Quik® stain; original magnification X400)

Abnormal oestrous cycles

Oestrous cycles may be abnormal because of a shorter or longer interval between periods of oestrus. A shortened interval is most commonly associated with ovulation failure and an absence of the luteal phase, while a prolonged interval is prolonged anoestrus, as described above. The period of pro-oestrus and oestrus behaviour may also be abnormally short or long, as described below. Investigation of these cases involves careful monitoring of each cycle, using vaginal cytology and progesterone measurements to establish the particular aberration present.

Split oestrus: In bitches, a short period of attractiveness followed 2–12 weeks later by a return to signs of oestrus is described as a split oestrus. This occurs most frequently at puberty, but can occur at any age. After an initial phase of follicular growth and oestrogen secretion, the follicles regress and signs of oestrus cease. Vaginal cytology shows an initial (normal) progressive increase of anuclear cells, followed by a decline, usually before the anticipated maximum percentage of anuclear cells is reached. Often there is only a maximum of 50% anuclear cells. There is no increase in plasma progesterone. In some cases this may be repeated several times until finally the bitch ovulates normally. This syndrome is confusing and sometimes the return to oestrus is mistaken for a vulval discharge with a different cause; for example, the bitch may be thought to have become pregnant and then to have suffered embryonic resorption.

Ovulation failure: Ovulation failure is probably one of the most common causes of infertility in the queen. Several matings within a short period of time are necessary to ensure that the LH surge occurring after coitus is of sufficient magnitude to exceed the threshold necessary to stimulate ovulation. Frequent matings are likely to produce a larger LH surge if they occur on the second or third day of oestrus. Inappropriate mating regimes imposed by the breeder may result in a failure of ovulation. This can readily be detected by an absence of elevated plasma progesterone after the end of oestrus; queens that do not ovulate generally return to oestrus with a short interval, while ovulating queens either enter pseudopregnancy or become pregnant.

In cases of ovulation failure in the bitch, vaginal cytological changes are similar to those observed in a normal cycle, although there is a less rapid decline in anuclear cells and a smaller influx of neutrophils just prior to the end of the signs of oestrus, compared with a normal oestrus. The accurate diagnosis is made by detecting an absence of an increase in plasma progesterone concentration on serial samples.

Prolonged pro-oestrus or oestrus: Although unusual, some normal bitches may show pro-oestrus or oestrus behaviour lasting up to 30 days or more. These animals do not require treatment but careful assessment of the optimum mating time is necessary, usually by evaluation of vaginal cytology or measurement of plasma progesterone.

In some cases, however, there is an underlying pathology. Oestrogen-secreting follicular cysts may produce persistent oestrus. This is often inconvenient for the owner and may ultimately lead to bone marrow suppression with anaemia, leucopenia and thrombocytopenia. In these bitches, there is persistence of a large proportion of anuclear vaginal epithelial cells and no increase in plasma progesterone. In addition, large (8–12 mm diameter) fluid-filled follicles may be identified using ultrasonography. This syndrome is not recognized in the queen.

Ovarian neoplasia: Epithelial tumours are the most frequently identified ovarian neoplasms in bitches and queens, but are not common and account for approximately 1% of all neoplasms. Tumours that release oestrogen may produce signs of persistent oestrus and bone marrow suppression, although clinical signs are also often related to a mass effect or ascites (the latter is usually due to widespread metastasis throughout the abdominal cavity, often termed carcinomatosis). Signs of persistent oestrus relate to persistently elevated plasma oestrogen (>50 pg/ml (180 pmol/l)). There is thickening of the vaginal wall and an increase in the percentage of anuclear cells found on vaginal cytology. However, in some cases the principal hormone produced is either progesterone or testosterone. With progesterone production the common clinical feature is absence of oestrus, while with testosterone production it is absence of oestrus combined with virilization; in these cases serial estimation of these hormones may confirm the diagnosis.

Neoplasia may be suspected on the basis of an ultrasound examination, although confirmation requires cytological or histological investigation.

Retained ovarian tissue after ovariectomy or ovariohysterectomy

Apparent oestrus activity following a routine 'spay' is not an uncommon presentation. In some cases, owners observe mounting and/or thrusting behaviour and assume that this is a sign of oestrus (although it is commonly observed in both neutered and entire bitches). In other cases, males are attracted to the bitch because of a non-oestrus vulval discharge (e.g. vaginitis), or because of other odours (e.g. anal sac or skin disease). Clinical history and examination will distinguish these from a retained ovary or portion of an ovary. True remnant ovarian tissue is most simply detected by examination of the female during periods of apparent attractiveness to allow clinical and vaginal cytological examination (see later), while presentation of the female at other times usually requires measurement of plasma hormones or use of a hormonal stimulation test.

There is much confusion about the use of stimulation tests but these can simply be classified as those that cause an increase in oestrogen from an inactive ovary (here oestrogen is measured immediately before, and shortly after, administration), and those that stimulate ovulation in an ovary where there is existing follicular activity (here progesterone is measured some weeks after administration). The confusion is caused by the fact that both GnRH (buserelin) and human chorionic gonadotrophin (hCG) can be used to stimulate oestrogen production, GnRH because it causes a release of endogenous FSH and LH which act upon the ovary to stimulate oestrogen production, and hCG because it is LH-like in action and stimulates theca cells to produce androgens and androgen precursors which are converted to oestrogens. Furthermore, in the oestrus queen, both GnRH and hCG are able to stimulate ovulation (and therefore cause a subsequent rise in progesterone). A variety of different dose regimes and routes of administration are recommended by different diagnostic laboratories; values in this text are given as broad guidance and the reader should seek advice from their laboratory of choice.

In all species, when there is an absence of ovaries there will be elevated concentrations of FSH and LH (because of lack of negative feedback from the ovary), and basal concentrations of anti-Müllerian hormone (which is normally produced by growing follicles); however, these assays are not commonly run in veterinary laboratories. In the sections below, the diagnostic methods used are described according to when the animal is presented (see also Figures 19.9 and 19.10).

Bitch or queen presented during periods of attractiveness to males: In these cases the simplest diagnostic tool is clinical examination and collection of a vaginal smear, with evaluation for changes typical of pro-oestrus or oestrus. Clinical examination often demonstrates a swollen vulva (turgid or flaccid) and in some cases a mucoid vulval discharge; in the bitch there is rarely a red-coloured

Diagnosis	Clinical findings	Suggested order and findings of laboratory tests
Ovarian remnant; bitch presented during apparent oestrus	• Vulva swollen • Vulval discharge may be clear, mucoid or red-coloured if surgery has not removed entire uterus • Bitch may deviate tail if vulva and perineum stimulated	• Vaginal cytology reveals anuclear epithelial cells (percentage depends on exact time of presentation). Number of neutrophils will depend on the exact time of presentation. These features are diagnostic • Plasma oestrogen measurement may not be necessary but if measured it may be elevated or basal and is not reliable; only elevated oestrogen would be diagnostic • Plasma progesterone measurement is not warranted at this time. Progesterone will increase in late oestrus but the time the bitch presented may be uncertain; only elevated progesterone would be diagnostic • The oestrogen response to GnRH or hCG will depend upon the exact time of presentation in oestrus and is therefore not reliable; only a substantial increase after stimulation would be diagnostic
Ovarian remnant; bitch presented shortly after period of attractiveness (i.e. likely to be in luteal phase)	• Mammary gland enlargement likely • Behavioural manifestation of pseudopregnancy possible • Mucoid vulval discharge possible	• Plasma progesterone concentrations are elevated for 60 days after the period of attractiveness and detection of elevated progesterone is diagnostic • Vaginal smears are not indicated but if performed will reveal predominantly small intermediate (often vacuolated) and parabasal epithelial cells. Neutrophils are present in large numbers. Considerable background debris and mucus will be present. These features are, however, not diagnostic • GnRH or hCG stimulation test not warranted but if performed will show increase in plasma oestrogen post stimulation, which is diagnostic
Ovarian remnant; bitch presented some time remote from period of attractiveness (i.e. likely to be in anoestrus)	• No obvious clinical features	• Increased concentrations of oestrogen in response to administration of GnRH or hCG are diagnostic • Vaginal smears not indicated but if performed will reveal parabasal and small intermediate epithelial cells and scant neutrophils typical of anoestrus, although these features are not diagnostic • Plasma progesterone concentrations will be basal and this is not diagnostic because it would not differentiate the patient from a neutered female

19.9 Presenting features and laboratory diagnosis of retained ovarian tissue in bitches. GnRH = gonadotrophin-releasing hormone; hCG = human chorionic gonadotrophin. (continues) ▶

Diagnosis	Clinical findings	Suggested order and findings of laboratory tests
Mounting behaviour in neutered bitch	• No evidence of reproductive tract pathology	• Vaginal smear typical of anoestrus (parabasal epithelial cells), which is diagnostic if found at the time the bitch is thought to be attractive • Measurement of progesterone concentrations not warranted but if undertaken progesterone will be low; this is not diagnostic, as progesterone will also be low in a neutered female • Measurement of the response of oestrogen to GnRH or hCG stimulation is not warranted in most cases because of the clinical history but if undertaken there will be no increase of plasma oestrogen after either test (likely to be diagnostic although some oestrus bitches fail to respond)
Non-oestrus vulval discharge in neutered bitch	• Vulval discharge which may be mucoid, purulent or haemorrhagic • No behavioural changes in the bitch but interest from males	• Vaginal cytology will reveal absence of anuclear epithelial cells. Smear may be dominated by neutrophils and mucus, or erythrocytes. These features may be useful in reaching a diagnosis (e.g. neutrophils and bacteria in vaginitis) • Measurement of progesterone concentrations is not warranted if there has been no history of recent oestrus but if undertaken progesterone will be low • Measurement of the response of oestrogen to GnRH or hCG stimulation is not warranted if there has been no history of recent oestrus but if undertaken there will be no increase of plasma oestrogen after either test (likely to be diagnostic although some oestrus bitches fail to respond, which would give a false negative diagnosis)
Male attraction to unusual smell (anal sac or skin disease) in neutered bitch	• No behavioural manifestation in the bitch but interest from males • No evidence of reproductive tract pathology • Pathology of the anal sacs or skin likely to be apparent	• Vaginal cytology will reveal absence of anuclear vaginal epithelial cells. Smear may be dominated by neutrophils and mucus, indicating vaginitis • Measurement of progesterone concentrations not warranted but if undertaken progesterone will be low • Measurement of the response of oestrogen to GnRH or hCG stimulation is not warranted, but if undertaken there will be no increase of plasma oestrogen after either test (likely to be diagnostic although some oestrus bitches fail to respond, which would give a false negative diagnosis)

19.9 (continued) Presenting features and laboratory diagnosis of retained ovarian tissue in bitches. GnRH = gonadotrophin-releasing hormone; hCG = human chorionic gonadotrophin.

Diagnosis	Clinical findings	Suggested order and findings of laboratory tests
Ovarian remnant; queen presented during apparent oestrus	• Vulva may be swollen • Typical 'calling' behaviour may be present	• Vaginal cytology reveals large intermediate epithelial cells (percentage depends on exact time of presentation). Neutrophils are usually absent. These features are diagnostic • Administration of GnRH or hCG will cause the queen to ovulate, and blood sampling 2 weeks later will reveal increased concentration of progesterone, which is diagnostic • Plasma oestrogen may be elevated or basal and is not reliable; only elevated oestrogen is diagnostic • Oestrogen response to GnRH or hCG will depend upon exact time of presentation in the oestrous cycle and therefore is not reliable
Ovarian remnant; queen presented shortly after period of attractiveness (i.e. likely to be in interoestrus)	• No obvious features	• No diagnostic procedures are required as the queen is likely to return to signs of oestrus within 3 weeks and should be examined as described above • GnRH or hCG stimulation test not warranted but if performed will show an increase in plasma oestrogen, which is diagnostic • Measurement of plasma progesterone is not warranted. If measured, concentrations will be low as queens are induced ovulators, but this is not diagnostic. Values may be high if the queen has been mated • Vaginal smear not indicated but if performed will reveal small intermediate epithelial cells and moderate numbers of neutrophils, but these features are not diagnostic
Ovarian remnant; queen presented during winter (i.e. likely to be in anoestrus)	• No obvious clinical features	• Increased concentrations of oestrogen in response to administration of GnRH or hCG; this is diagnostic • Vaginal smear not indicated but if performed will reveal small intermediate and parabasal epithelial cells and scant neutrophils typical of anoestrus, but this is not diagnostic • Measurement of plasma progesterone is not warranted. If measured, concentrations will be low because queens are induced ovulators, but this is not diagnostic as low progesterone concentrations are also seen in neutered females
Non-oestrus vulval discharge in neutered queen	• Vulval discharge which may be mucoid, purulent or haemorrhagic	• Vaginal cytology will reveal absence of large intermediate epithelial cells. Smear may be dominated by neutrophils and mucus (e.g. with vaginitis) or erythrocytes. These features are diagnostic if observed at the time the queen is thought to be attractive • Measurement of plasma progesterone is not warranted but, if measured progesterone concentrations will be low; this is not diagnostic as it does not differentiate the queen from a neutered female • Measurement of the oestrogen response to GnRH or hCG stimulation is not warranted but if undertaken there will be no increase of plasma oestrogen after either test (likely to be diagnostic although some oestrus queens fail to respond, which would give a false negative diagnosis)

19.10 Presenting features and laboratory diagnosis of retained ovarian tissue in queens. GnRH = gonadotrophin-releasing hormone; hCG = human chorionic gonadotrophin.

discharge because red cells arise by uterine diapedesis and the uterus is removed in most 'spay' procedures. The appearance on vaginal cytology will vary depending upon exactly when the vaginal smear was taken. If the female is presented in pro-oestrus there will be a low percentage of cornified (in the bitch anucular) epithelial cells and small numbers of neutrophils, while if presented at maximum oestrus there will be a high percentage of cornified (in the bitch anuclear) epithelial cells and no neutrophils, and if presented in the early luteal phase there will be a low percentage of cornified (in the bitch anuclear) epithelial cells, large numbers of neutrophils and much cellular debris. However, by understanding the normal changes that occur during the course of the period of attractiveness, it is possible for these variable presentations to be recognized, allowing a clear diagnosis to be made.

Plasma hormone testing during the period of attractiveness may be useful, but requires consideration of the time at which the sample was taken. Plasma/serum oestrogen concentrations are elevated (25–50 pg/ml (90–180 pmol/l)) during late anoestrus, pro-oestrus and early oestrus. They decline to basal concentrations during mid and late oestrus, therefore oestrogen may not be elevated at the time a blood sample is taken even if the bitch or queen is attractive at that time. In the bitch, plasma progesterone measurement in late oestrus is very useful, because progressive luteinization of preovulatory follicles results in increased plasma progesterone (to values >2.0 ng/ml (6.5 nmol/l)) around the time of ovulation. Therefore, while the bitch is attractive to males it can be useful to measure plasma oestrogen concentrations and if these are not elevated also to measure plasma progesterone. Tests designed to stimulate oestrogen production (e.g. by the administration of GnRH or hCG) are best avoided when the bitch is attractive because oestrogen may already be elevated or have recently been elevated (such that response to stimulation is poor), making either test difficult to interpret. Furthermore, unlike the situation in the queen, the bitch is not an induced ovulator and it is not likely that a single dose of either GnRH or hCG given during oestrus will cause ovulation and a subsequent rise in progesterone.

In the queen there will be no increase in progesterone unless ovulation has been stimulated. Ovulation can be induced by the administration of either GnRH or hCG. Detection of elevated plasma progesterone between 7 and 30 days later is diagnostic of an ovarian remnant (i.e. the queen was in oestrus, the GnRH or hCG has stimulated ovulation and now there are corpora lutea secreting progesterone).

Bitch presented up to 60 days after a period of attractiveness to males: Bitches with an ovarian remnant usually have normal follicular tissue and therefore they will ovulate, and progesterone concentrations will increase after the period of attractiveness. Progesterone will then remain elevated for the normal luteal phase, which is approximately 60 days after the end of oestrus. A single blood sample demonstrating elevated progesterone during this period is diagnostic of remnant ovarian tissue (remember that, in the queen, there will be no elevated progesterone unless ovulation has been stimulated either by mating or by the administration of GnRH or hCG).

Bitch or queen presented remote from a period of attractiveness to males: In bitches that do not currently have signs of oestrus, or are not within 60 days of the last suspected oestrus, it is necessary to consider stimulation tests for the confirmation of remnant ovarian tissue. Gonadotrophins stimulate the release of 17β-oestradiol from theca interna cells within the ovarian remnant, and can be given directly in the form of hCG (which is LH-like in activity), or GnRH can be used to stimulate the release of endogenous gonadotrophin. The authors use a regime where a blood sample is taken for assay of basal oestrogen, and either hCG (44 IU/kg i.m.) or GnRH analogue/buserelin (2.0 μg/kg i.m.) is injected, and a second blood sample is taken 2 hours later. With both tests, oestrogen concentrations increase by a factor of 2–3 when there is ovarian tissue; it is feasible that the total amount of oestrogen produced is dependent upon the volume of ovarian tissue remaining. These tests are also applicable in the queen, using similar doses and routes of administration of hormones (see Figures 19.9 and 19.10).

Pregnancy diagnosis

There are a variety of methods for pregnancy diagnosis in both the bitch and queen. In many veterinary practices, transabdominal palpation and diagnostic real-time ultrasonography are widely used. Measurement of plasma relaxin, acute phase proteins, progesterone and prolactin may all be used for pregnancy diagnosis, although the plasma relaxin concentration is considered the most reliable.

Plasma relaxin: Relaxin is a pregnancy-specific protein that is produced by the placenta. Relaxin concentrations increase in pregnant bitches and queens from approximately 24 days after ovulation, and continue to increase progressively until the last 2 weeks prior to parturition, when there is a slight decrease. Relaxin may be measured using ELISA test kits designed for in-practice use; concentrations increase significantly from day 24 onwards and samples taken after this time have high accuracy and precision. Some studies suggest that higher concentrations of relaxin are present with a larger litter (presumably due to a greater volume of placental tissue), but other studies have disputed this relationship.

Acute phase proteins: Acute phase proteins (fibrinogen, C-reactive protein, haptoglobin) are elevated in pregnant bitches compared with concentrations in non-pregnant bitches. Pregnancy can be diagnosed as early as 20 days after ovulation by measuring fibrinogen or C-reactive protein, although false positive diagnoses may occur with other conditions that stimulate release of these proteins (e.g. some inflammatory conditions such as pyometra). Unlike the situation with plasma relaxin, there is no relationship between absolute concentration and the number of fetuses.

Plasma progesterone: In the bitch, there are great similarities in endocrinology between pregnancy and non-pregnancy (see Figure 19.2). Importantly, there is a long non-pregnant luteal phase. Similarly, in the queen there is a significant elevation of progesterone when ovulation occurs but pregnancy does not ensue. Thus, for both species, the measurement of plasma progesterone alone has no value in the diagnosis of pregnancy. However, in bitches the combination of plasma progesterone and acute phase protein concentrations is a more useful indicator, and some commercial diagnostic laboratories 'weight' the measure of acute phase proteins in blood (see above) according to the concentration of progesterone. In this method the laboratory would pay greater attention to a 'medium' concentration of acute phase proteins in the face of a 'high' concentration of progesterone than in the face of a 'medium' or 'low' concentration of progesterone. It is suggested that this algorithm improves the reliability of the acute phase protein assay. The combined assay can be used to diagnose pregnancy from 3 weeks after mating, but is most accurate from 28 days after mating.

Prolactin: Prolactin is produced in the pregnant and non-pregnant bitch, although prolactin concentrations are greater during pregnancy. Measurement of this hormone is not commonly used for pregnancy diagnosis.

Other changes that occur during pregnancy: Pregnant bitches normally develop a significant decrease in haematocrit; the decline commences on approximately day 20 of pregnancy and continues an almost linear decline, reaching minimum values by day 60 of pregnancy. This finding is attributed to a pregnancy-related increase in blood volume.

Vulval discharge

Vulval discharge is a relatively common problem in the bitch and queen. It is most frequently seen in prepubertal animals with prepubertal vaginitis, also called juvenile vaginitis. There are many causes of vulval discharge that may result in discharge from the urinary or reproductive tract (Figure 19.11).

Investigation of vulval discharge involves assessment of the breeding history and a full breeding soundness examination, including endoscopy of the caudal genitourinary tract and ultrasonography of the uterus, ovaries, bladder and kidneys. Laboratory investigation of any discharge should include routine cytology. In some specific cases, bacteriological and virological investigation may also be useful.

Cytology: Cytological examination of vulval discharge may be useful (Figure 19.11) to determine its aetiology, although cytology is only part of the investigation and clinical examination, radiography and ultrasonography also need to be employed.

Nature of discharge	Condition	History	Condition of the vulva	Cytological findings	Comments
Clear or mucoid discharge					
Clear or straw-coloured	Oestrus	Expected in 'heat'	Swollen or slightly soft	LIEC, AEC, RBC, no WBC	Attractive to male
Mucoid	Metoestrus	Recent oestrus	Large but soft	PBC, SIEC, VSIEC, WBC	No malaise
Mucoid	Normal pregnancy	Pregnant/recent oestrus	Large but soft	PBC, SIEC, WBC	No malaise, does not threaten pregnancy
Principally purulent discharge					
Purulent	Juvenile vaginitis	Before first 'heat'	Normal	PBC, SIEC, WBC	May respond to antibiotics but recurs. Recovery after puberty
Purulent	Vaginitis	Variable but often excessive licking, attractive to male	Depends on the stage of the cycle	Depends on the stage of the cycle. WBC and possible intracellular organisms	Specific causes include chemical irritation (urine), mechanical irritation (FB), neoplasia, anatomical abnormalities and certain bacterial or viral infections
Purulent/ haemorrhagic	Pyometra	Oestrus 2–8 weeks previously	Slightly swollen	WBC, SIEC, LIEC, RBC, bacteria, cell debris	Diagnosis using ultrasonography or radiography. Often malaise
Purulent/ haemorrhagic	Metritis	Recent parturition	Large	Multinucleated cells, LIEC, uterine cells (often short columnar epithelial cells)	Severe malaise
Haemorrhagic/coloured discharge					
Haemorrhagic	Pro-oestrus	Expected in 'heat'	Swollen	SIEC, LIEC, RBC, WBC	Attractive to male
Haemorrhagic	Oestrus	Expected in 'heat'	Swollen or slightly soft	LIEC, AEC, RBC, no WBC	Attractive to male
Haemorrhagic	Follicular cysts	Persistent discharge	Swollen	AEC, LIEC, RBC ± WBC	No malaise, attractive to male, may develop bone marrow suppression
Haemorrhagic	Vaginal ulceration	Recent trauma or mating	Depends on stage of cycle	RBC, depends on stage of cycle	Rare, may start up to 2 weeks after mating
Haemorrhagic	Placental separation	Pregnant	Normal or slightly swollen	RBC, mucus	Ultrasonography or radiography will confirm pregnancy
Haemorrhagic	Subinvolution of placental sites	Persistent discharge for more than 4 weeks after whelping	Normal or slightly swollen	RBC, large polynucleated vacuolated epithelial cells	No malaise, refractory to treatment
Haemorrhagic	Transmissible venereal tumour	Not all countries (not in UK)	Depends on stage of cycle	RBC ± neoplastic cells?	Identification of tumour on vulva or in vagina confirms diagnosis
Haemorrhagic	Cystitis	Frequent urination	Depends on stage of cycle	RBC, mucus	Small volumes of urine, dysuria
Haemorrhagic	Urinary tract neoplasia	Dysuria	Depends on stage of cycle	RBC ± neoplastic cells?	Endoscopy may show origin of haemorrhage; ultrasonography or contrast cystourethrography may be diagnostic
Haemorrhagic/ brown-coloured	Abortion	Pregnant	Slightly enlarged	RBC, mucus	Ultrasonography shows uterus with similar appearance to postpartum
Green/ brown-coloured	Parturition	Pregnant	Slightly swollen	RBC, SIEC, uterine cells	Panting, nest-making, milk production
Green/ brown-coloured	Dystocia, placental separation	Non-productive straining	Slightly swollen	RBC, SIEC, uterine cells	Ultrasonography will confirm pregnancy and fetal viability

19.11 Differential diagnosis of vulval discharge in the bitch. AEC = anuclear epithelial cells; FB = foreign body; LIEC = large intermediate epithelial cells; PBC = parabasal cells; RBC = red blood cells (erythrocytes); SIEC = small intermediate epithelial cells; VSIEC = vacuolated small intermediate epithelial cells ('metoestrus cells'); WBC = white blood cells (polymorphonuclear leucocytes).

Microbiology:

Bacteriology: In the UK there are no bacterial venereal pathogens, although *Brucella canis* is widely present in much of continental Europe. In both the bitch and queen, routine bacteriological screening of a vulval discharge normally results in the isolation of mixed bacterial commensal organisms, including *Escherichia coli*, staphylococci, streptococci (including beta-haemolytic streptococci) and others, such as *Pseudomonas* and *Proteus* spp. Rarely, a pure growth of bacteria is isolated, but even in these cases it is very unusual for the organism to be the primary pathogen; rather, it is an opportunistic invader secondary to an underlying disease. Currently in the UK there is no rationale for the routine bacteriological screening of bitches or stud dogs prior to breeding.

In countries where *Brucella canis* is present, it may be a recognized cause of infertility in bitches and be associated with a vulval discharge. There is the possibility of this organism entering the UK with the increased transportation of dogs to other countries for the purpose of breeding.

Virology: Canine herpesvirus is found with a low prevalence in the UK, and may be associated with a vulval discharge if it causes fetal resorption or abortion. In some cases small vesicles are identified within the vestibule and vagina, and virus may be isolated from these. In other cases paired serology samples are useful for documenting acute infection. Swabs taken of vesicles can be examined by polymerase chain reaction (PCR) for canine herpesvirus.

In the queen, serological screening (see Chapter 28) is used to test for organisms that may result in pregnancy failure and result in a vulval discharge (feline herpesvirus-1, feline panleucopenia virus, feline leukaemia virus, feline coronavirus). Care is required with interpretation in vaccinated cats. Multiplex PCR on swabs taken from the reproductive tract may be a useful option, although there are few published data on assay sensitivity from such swabs.

Male

The dog and tom cat

Reproductive dysfunction appears to be common in the male dog, with the authors observing increased referrals for male factor infertility over the last 10 years.

Reproductive physiology of the male

The control of testicular function is via the gonadotrophin system, as described above for the female. Luteinizing hormone (LH) (previously called interstitial cell stimulating hormone) stimulates the Leydig cells to produce testosterone, dihydrotestosterone and small quantities of oestradiol. LH secretion is regulated by a feedback mechanism involving testosterone and oestradiol. Androgens mediate the development and maintenance of primary and secondary sexual characteristics and normal sexual behaviour and potency, as well as playing an important role in the initiation and maintenance of spermatogenesis. Follicle-stimulating hormone (FSH) stimulates spermatogenesis indirectly by an action upon the Sertoli cells (which act as nurse cells for the developing spermatozoa). These cells also secrete inhibins (which act upon the pituitary to inhibit the secretion of FSH) and activins (which stimulate the production of FSH). Concentrations of testosterone, LH and FSH fluctuate throughout the day. Spermatozoa are produced in the seminiferous tubules and then transported into the epididymides for maturation and storage. Sperm acquire the ability to fertilize an ovum during the phase of epididymal maturation, and there is good evidence that dihydrotestosterone is pivotal in this event.

Breeding soundness

A breeding soundness examination involves collection of a breeding history, detailed clinical examination (including ultrasonography of the testes) and laboratory investigation of a semen sample. Methods of semen collection are described in standard texts.

The ejaculate of the dog has three distinct fractions, of which the first and third originate from the prostate gland. In the tom cat the ejaculate is relatively homogeneous. Normally only the second fraction of the dog's ejaculate, but the entire ejaculate of the tom, is evaluated for the purpose of investigating fertility. Cytological and bacteriological examination of the third fraction of the dog's ejaculate may be useful for demonstrating the cause of prostatic disease; for this purpose prostatic fluid may also be collected by urethral lavage after prostatic massage per rectum.

Assessment of semen quality: Evaluation of a semen sample can be useful for confirmation of normal fertility in an animal prior to breeding or artificial insemination, or when there is concern over infertility. Furthermore, detailed semen evaluation should be undertaken in potential stud dogs prior to purchase, before importation and before embarking upon semen preservation.

Spermatozoal number: Measurement of the total number of sperm within the ejaculate provides the most accurate assessment of sperm production. The total sperm output is calculated by multiplying the volume of the sperm-containing (second) fraction by the sperm concentration. Sperm concentration is conventionally measured using a haemocytometer counting chamber after dilution of the sample, usually with distilled water (samples are not diluted with saline because the objective is to kill the spermatozoa and prevent their movement so that they can be counted) at a ratio of 1 in 200. A traditional Neubauer counting chamber or C-chip disposable counting chamber (see Figure 25.3) is often used; the number of sperm in five of the large squares (each comprising 16 small squares) is counted and the total multiplied by 10×10^6 (which corrects for the dilution and the volume counted). For example, if, after a 1:200 dilution, 36 sperm are counted in this area, the sperm concentration will be 360 million sperm per ml (360×10^6/ml).

A relationship has been demonstrated between breed and the number of sperm ejaculated. Larger breeds produce more sperm. There is, however, a wide normal range of total sperm output for fertile dogs (Figure 19.12) and tom cats (Figure 19.13).

Spermatozoal morphology: Sperm morphology can be examined using a background stain such as Indian ink, or by staining with Giemsa, Spermac® or nigrosin–eosin. Spermac® is a dunking-style stain kit that facilitates evaluation of acrosomal morphology, while nigrosin–eosin allows assessment of live/dead ratios.

Nigrosin–eosin is the technique most commonly used: a drop of semen is mixed with five drops of stain and a smear is made immediately and allowed to dry. Examination with oil-immersion microscopy allows

Measurement	Progressive motility (%)	Sperm-rich volume (ml)	Sperm concentration (x 10⁶/ml)	Total sperm output (x 10⁶)	Live normal sperm (%)
Mean	82.1	1.2	328.6	410.8	73.5
Standard error of mean	0.9	0.05	15.3	21.3	2.1
Range	40–95	0.3–3.2	50–610	36–1550	50–92

19.12 Characteristics of semen from 121 fertile dogs (unpublished observations).

Measurement	Progressive motility (%)	Sperm-rich volume (ml)	Sperm concentration (x 10⁶/ml)	Total sperm output (x 10⁶)	Live normal sperm (%)
Mean	62.5	0.65	95.2	145.0	56.4
Standard error of mean	2.8	0.02	25.3	34.3	4.2
Range	40–65	0.25–1.10	52–120	32–178	39–69

19.13 Characteristics of semen from five fertile tom cats (semen collected by artificial vagina; unpublished observations).

determination of individual sperm morphology and distinguishes live sperm (which remain unstained) and dead or membrane-damaged sperm (which stain pink). One hundred sperm are examined and noted as being either dead (pink) or live (white) and their individual morphology is recorded. An example of a table for recording sperm morphology and vital staining is given in Figure 19.14.

For normal fertility there are usually >60% live normal spermatozoa; values <60% are associated with reduced fertility, although some fertile dogs and cats have values below this (see Figures 19.12 and 19.13). Normal and abnormal sperm morphology is demonstrated in Figure 19.15.

Morphology	Number of live sperm	Number of dead sperm
Normal		
Proximal droplets		
Distal droplets		
Coiled tail		
Detached head		
Other morphological abnormalities recorded here as a list when observed		

19.14 Example of a table used for recording the morphological and vital status of sperm stained with nigrosin–eosin.

Spermatozoal motility: Dog and cat sperm motility is conventionally evaluated by placing a drop of semen on a microscope slide under a coverslip and observing sperm movement at X200 and X400 magnification. Importantly, sperm motility is influenced by temperature, and samples should be examined at a standard temperature, commonly 38°C. Not all sperm that are motile have normal motility, and it is important to record the type of motility and the percentage of sperm with that motility. Sperm that have normal motility swim very quickly in straight lines across the field of view (they have good progression). An example of a table used for recording sperm motility is given in Figure 19.16.

For normal fertility there are usually >60% of sperm with normal motility, defined as rapid forward progression (category IV in Figure 19.16). Note that motile sperm in categories I–III do not have normal motility. The cut-off point for a reduction in fertility is when the percentage of sperm with rapid forward progression reduces below 60%, although some fertile dogs and tom cats have values slightly below this (see Figures 19.12 and 19.13).

Microbiological screening: In some countries, routine screening of dogs for *Brucella canis* is recommended. This organism is not currently present in the UK and therefore screening is unnecessary here. Dogs may harbour herpesvirus in small vesicles on the penis and the mucosa of the sheath, but clinical inspection usually reveals the lesions, and virological screening of the prepuce is unlikely to detect virus in the absence of lesions.

Absence of testicular tissue

Males with an absence of scrotal testes are either previously castrated or are bilateral cryptorchids. Anorchia is very rare in both the dog and tom cat. Tom cats that have no testes have an absence of penile spines.

In normal entire dogs and cats there is significant variation in testosterone production throughout the day, with testosterone concentrations of 0.5–1.5 ng/ml (1.7–5.2 nmol/l) at the trough of production, and 3.5–6.0 ng/ml (12.1–20.8 nmol/l) at the peak of production. In dogs with no testes, testosterone concentrations are <0.5 ng/ml (<1.7 nmol/l). Single samples could potentially be taken at the trough of production, resulting in a false diagnosis of absent testicular tissue. For this reason, stimulation tests are normally performed using either hCG or a GnRH analogue. A basal plasma/serum sample is obtained, hCG (44 IU/kg i.m.) or GnRH analogue (2.0 μg/kg i.m.) is injected and a second blood sample is taken 60–120 minutes later. In both cases a significant increase in testosterone concentration (to >5.0 ng/ml (17 nmol/l)) in the post-stimulation sample is diagnostic of testicular tissue. There should be no false positive diagnoses.

The infertile male

Males with presumed infertility should have semen collected and evaluated as described above. Such examination may reveal the cause of the infertility. In addition, it may also be prudent to undertake a more detailed examination of the seminal plasma.

Semen quality: Laboratory investigation of a semen sample in an alleged infertile male may reveal a number of different abnormalities, including abnormalities of sperm number, sperm morphology or sperm motility. These abnormalities may be identified concurrently.

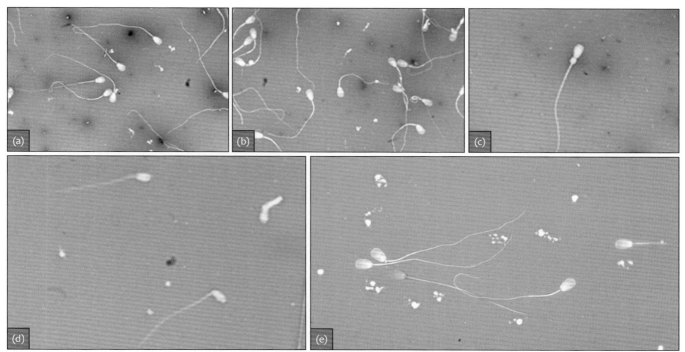

19.15 Dog semen stained with nigrosin–eosin. (a) Normal sperm morphology (one centrally positioned sperm has a coiled tail). Nigrosin provides the background colour and eosin stains dead sperm (none is present in this field). (b) A large number of sperm have significant bending of the tails and midpieces. These morphological changes are either secondary or tertiary sperm abnormalities. The sperm positioned in the top right corner has a distal cytoplasmic droplet. (c) Individual sperm with a spherical swelling in the neck region. This is a typical proximal cytoplasmic droplet. (d) Two sperm with broken/abnormal necks and a significant tail abnormality. (e) In the centre of the image two live sperm (white) and one dead sperm (pink). One of the live sperm has a neck abnormality, and the dead sperm has also lost the acrosomal cap. There are two further live sperm one of which has a bent tail.

Category	Description	Percentage of sperm
0	Immotile sperm	
I	Sperm that are motile but not progressive	
II	Sperm that have sluggish motility and poor progression	
III	Sperm with reasonable motility and moderate progression	
IV	Sperm with rapid forward progressive motility	

19.16 Example of a table used for recording estimated sperm motility in unstained sperm examined at body temperature.

Azoospermia: Azoospermia is an apparently normal ejaculation producing an ejaculate that contains no sperm. There are a number of causes, including incomplete ejaculation, obstructive azoospermia and gonadal dysfunction (which may be congenital or acquired). In the dog, measurement of alkaline phosphatase (ALP) concentration in seminal plasma may be helpful in differentiating these conditions (see Seminal plasma, below).

Oligozoospermia: Oligozoospermia is an ejaculate containing low numbers of morphologically normal sperm. This is rare in dogs but may occur for one of several reasons:

* Incomplete ejaculation
* Retrograde ejaculation
* Frequent ejaculation
* Recent testicular insult.

Confirmation of retrograde ejaculation can be obtained by preventing the dog from urinating prior to semen collection and then, after attempted semen collection, catheterizing the bladder, collecting the urine and lavaging the bladder with 10–20 ml of saline. The collected urine and flushings should be centrifuged to look for the presence of sperm. A large number of sperm (>10 per low power field) in a wet preparation of the centrifuged pellet is diagnostic.

Teratozoospermia: Teratozoospermia is an abnormal sperm morphology, which, in many cases, results in impaired sperm motility. When present in large numbers, abnormal midpiece droplets, other midpiece defects, and abnormalities of the base/midpiece region are associated with infertility (see Figure 19.15). Sperm with midpiece defects and deformed acrosomes have been found following experimental *B. canis* infection.

Primary spermatozoal abnormalities (abnormalities that occur during spermatogenesis, e.g. malformations of the sperm head) may result from orchitis, congenital defects of spermatogenesis, toxin exposure, administration of hormonal or chemotherapeutic agents or elevated scrotal temperature. Secondary spermatozoal abnormalities (abnormalities that occur after sperm formation but during sperm maturation, e.g. bending of the midpiece or tail) may occur with epididymal disorders or following the administration of agents that influence epididymal function. Tertiary abnormalities, such as broken tails, occur as a result of poor semen collection or handling.

Asthenozoospermia: Asthenozoospermia is normal sperm morphology but a reduction in motility. The condition is rare in the dog without concurrent oligozoospermia. Recognized causes include:

* Contamination of the ejaculate with toxic compounds (latex artificial vagina liners, lubricants, certain plastic syringes, urine, water, sterilizing agents)

- Agglutination of sperm in dogs that produce anti-sperm antibodies (seen in some dogs with *B. canis* infection).

Seminal plasma: Measurement of ALP concentration in the seminal plasma may be useful for the diagnosis of obstruction of the tubular genitalia in dogs. This enzyme originates from the epididymides, and therefore a low concentration may indicate either incomplete ejaculation or tubular obstruction. Normal concentrations (5000–40,000 IU/l) combined with an absence of sperm indicate azoospermia.

The ejaculate of the tom cat also contains significant concentrations of ALP.

Cytology: Standard haematology stains can be used for cytological examination of ejaculate. It is not uncommon for low numbers of inflammatory cells to be identified within the semen sample; most originate from the prepuce during semen collection. High numbers of inflammatory cells are seen in cases of epididymitis, orchitis and prostatitis. Red blood cells and prostatic cells are commonly identified in the prostatic fluid of dogs with benign prostatic hyperplasia, and multinucleate cells may be identified in dogs with prostatic neoplasia. Many dogs with significant prostatic disease will not ejaculate and therefore prostatic fluid needs to be collected from the sedated/anaesthetized animal via lavage of the prostatic urethra after massage of the gland per rectum, or via ultrasound-guided fine-needle aspiration (FNA).

Microbiology: There is little information available about normal microbiology in the tom cat, or on bacterial causes of disease.

Bacteriology: There has been considerable debate on the role of bacteria within the prostatic fluid and seminal plasma of dogs. However, many aerobic and anaerobic organisms are frequently isolated from the prepuce of the dog and the bacterial flora is usually mixed. These bacteria are similar to those identified in the bitch, including beta-haemolytic *Streptococcus*, and they are now considered normal commensal organisms. *Brucella canis* may cause epididymitis, orchitis and infertility and is a known venereal pathogen, but is not currently present in the UK. Recent data suggest that mycoplasmas and ureaplasmas are also commensal organisms, although some authors have suggested that they are implicated in cases of infertility.

Virology: Canine herpesvirus may cause vesicular lesions on the penis and prepuce. These lesions are usually asymptomatic, although in some cases there is secondary infection and pain at coitus. The main concern is potential of transmission to the bitch at coitus. Virus may be isolated from the vesicles, or exposure may be detected serologically.

Hormone measurement: There is little published information on the measurement of plasma hormones and their relationship to infertility in dogs and tom cats. In some infertile males there may be normal plasma concentrations of testosterone and LH, and elevated concentrations of FSH (presumably due to reduced production of inhibin by the Sertoli cells); however, there is no commercially available FSH assay so this technique is not clinically useful.

Low serum testosterone and LH concentrations indicate a possible hypothalamic, pituitary or testicular dysfunction. Pituitary or hypothalamic disease can be further demonstrated by persistently low LH concentrations following GnRH challenge (2.0 µg/kg i.m.), whereas increased LH following such administration confirms the problem to be testicular in origin.

Testicular disease

In males with known testicular disease (small testes or testes of abnormal texture), the primary diagnostic tool is testicular ultrasonography. In addition, it may be helpful to collect a semen sample (see above), or to perform FNA for cytological evaluation.

Ultrasonography is useful in the evaluation of suspected testicular tumours. Oestrogen-secreting tumours (usually Sertoli cell tumours) can be diagnosed by documenting a higher basal concentration of oestradiol or an increased concentration after stimulation with GnRH or hCG. Although the latter is more reliable, the diagnostic efficiency of ultrasonography is very high, making this the method of choice.

Testicular biopsy is widely recommended in standard texts for the investigation of a wide range of disease processes. It is now clear, however, that testicular biopsy may itself result in severe testicular pathology. While the sample collected may be diagnostic, the benefit of reaching a diagnosis rarely justifies the risk to future fertility, in the authors' opinion. However, FNA is clinically useful, especially for examining cases of suspected neoplasia. FNA has a limited risk of complications, although this may include dissemination of infection, seeding of tumour cells or haemorrhage. Ultrasonographic guidance for FNA of testicular lesions is helpful. In cases of bacterial infection, neutrophilic inflammation is pronounced, while in cases of neoplasia characteristic features of the tumour type are observed. Sertoli cell tumours are often characterized by round cells with a moderate to high nuclear:cytoplasmic ratio, lightly basophilic foamy cytoplasm and stippled nuclear chromatin, while interstitial cell tumours consist of smaller cells with a moderate amount of vacuolated basophilic cytoplasm. Seminomas are characterized by large round cells with a high nuclear:cytoplasmic ratio and a prominent nucleolus within a nucleus of finely stippled chromatin. Apart from the differentiation of tumour type and of inflammation, haemorrhage and necrosis, FNA has little use in the assessment of other causes of infertility.

Case examples

CASE 1

SIGNALMENT

4-year-old entire female Labrador Retriever.

HISTORY

Mated once previously 14 months ago, producing 8 normal puppies at term. Presented to the stud dog at this current oestrus on day 12 after the onset of vulval swelling but would not stand to be mated.

CLINICAL PATHOLOGY DATA

Vaginal cytology of sample collected on the morning of presentation is shown in Figure 19.17.

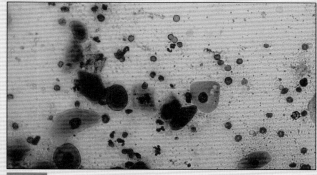

19.17 Vaginal cytology smear.

Plasma progesterone concentrations measured using an ELISA were 28.5 nmol/l (refer to Figure 19.5 for interpretation).

HOW WOULD YOU INTERPRET THESE RESULTS AND WHAT ARE THE POSSIBLE DIFFERENTIAL DIAGNOSES?

The vaginal smear shows a predominance of small intermediate epithelial cells, neutrophils and erythrocytes. The large number of neutrophils is characteristic of early metoestrus (dioestrus). This is confirmed by the plasma progesterone concentrations, which are elevated. The diagnosis in this case is that the bitch has already ovulated and passed into the luteal phase. Many owners and veterinary surgeons are confused about the day on which ovulation occurs: while this is commonly day 12, ovulation may also occur as early as day 5 or as late as day 30. Early ovulation, as in this case, means that the bitch needs to be mated earlier, and the optimal time can best be detected by serial vaginal cytology or measurement of plasma progesterone commencing on day 7 after the onset of pro-oestrus. It is also possible that in this case there is a split oestrus, although while in such a circumstance the appearance on vaginal cytology would be similar, plasma progesterone concentrations would be low, indicating an absence of ovulation.

CASE 2

SIGNALMENT

2.5-year-old entire female Golden Retriever.

HISTORY

The bitch underwent an apparently uncomplicated ovariohysterectomy 4 months previously. Five days after surgery there was substantial mammary gland development with lactation, which was treated symptomatically. At the time of suture removal the bitch had significant mastitis. This was managed by the administration of a depot progestagen (proligestone) and oral clavulanic acid-potentiated amoxicillin (co-amoxiclav). The clinical signs regressed over the subsequent 2 weeks and the bitch was asymptomatic until 4 days ago, when mammary enlargement, lactation and behavioural changes typical of pseudopregnancy were apparent.

CLINICAL PATHOLOGY DATA

Plasma progesterone concentrations are 1.0 nmol/l (refer to Figure 19.5 for interpretation). A GnRH stimulation test showed that plasma oestradiol concentrations before stimulation were 2.0 pmol/l and after stimulation were 3.0 pmol/l). (Note that values <10.0 pmol/l are considered basal.)

HOW WOULD YOU INTERPRET THESE RESULTS AND WHAT ARE THE POSSIBLE DIFFERENTIAL DIAGNOSES?

A common concern in these cases is that there is remnant ovarian tissue. In this case remnant tissue was not present, as confirmed by the lack of oestradiol response to GnRH stimulation. The basal levels of oestrogen were probably of adrenal origin. Furthermore, there is no luteal tissue, demonstrated by basal concentrations of progesterone. This case is an example of an iatrogenic pseudopregnancy. Removal of the ovaries during the luteal phase results in an abrupt decrease in plasma progesterone concentration and a subsequent increase in prolactin. The prolactin produces the clinical signs of pseudopregnancy. In this case, treatment with a depot progesterone-like drug (progestagen) resulted in suppression of prolactin secretion and resolution of clinical signs, but a rebound of prolactin occurred when progestagen concentrations decreased, resulting in a return of the clinical signs. Signs of pseudopregnancy are not diagnostic for an ovarian remnant unless there has been an intervening period of oestrus.

References and further reading

England GCW (1992) Vaginal cytology and cervicovaginal mucus arborisation in the breeding management of bitches. *Journal of Small Animal Practice* **33**, 577–582

England GCW (1999) Semen quality in dogs and the influence of a short-interval second ejaculation. *Theriogenology* **52**, 981–986

England GCW (2010a) Physiology and endocrinology of the female. In: *BSAVA Manual of Reproduction and Neonatology*, ed. GCW England and A von Heimendahl, pp. 1–12. BSAVA Publications, Gloucester

England GCW (2010b) Physiology and endocrinology of the male. In: *BSAVA Manual of Reproduction and Neonatology*, ed. GCW England and A von Heimendahl, pp. 13–22. BSAVA Publications, Gloucester

Moxon R, Copley D and England GCW (2010a) Quality assurance of canine vaginal cytology: a preliminary study. *Theriogenology* **74**, 479–485

Moxon R, Copley D and England GCW (2010b) Technical and financial evaluation of assays for progesterone in canine practice in the UK. *Veterinary Record* **167**, 528–531

von Heimendahl A and England GCW (2010) Determining breeding status. In: *BSAVA Manual of Reproduction and Neonatology*, ed. GCW England and A von Heimendahl, pp. 44–50. BSAVA Publications, Gloucester

Chapter 20

Laboratory evaluation of cardiac disease

Melanie Hezzell

Cardiac disease is commonly encountered in small animal practice. However, deciding whether an animal's clinical signs are due to underlying cardiac disease or another process can be difficult. For example, determining whether an older small-breed dog is coughing because of congestive heart failure, compression of the left mainstem bronchus by an enlarged left atrium, or primary respiratory disease (or a combination of these processes) can be particularly challenging. Thoracic radiography is usually helpful in these cases, as the heart size can be assessed and the lung fields examined for evidence of respiratory disease or pulmonary oedema. However, radiographic changes do not always allow a conclusive diagnosis to be made. Echocardiography is a valuable tool in the diagnosis of heart disease, but does not allow a diagnosis of congestive heart failure to be made and is not available in all cases. A number of laboratory tests are available to help the clinician make accurate diagnoses and thereby provide the most appropriate therapy. This chapter will review these tests and describe the clinical circumstances in which they are most likely to be useful. In general, it should be remembered that indiscriminate testing of animals at low risk for disease is more likely to result in false positives. Careful patient selection, such as animals with clinical findings consistent with cardiac disease, will improve the accuracy and usefulness of any of the tests discussed below. The various diagnostic cut-off values discussed in the text are summarized in Figures 20.1 and 20.2.

Test	Disease	Cut-off	Indication
NT-proBNP	DMVD	>740 pmol/l	Increased risk of death
		>1500 pmol/l	High risk of CHF in the next 6 months
	Dyspnoea	<900 pmol/l	Likelihood of CHF low
		>1800 pmol/l	Increased likelihood of CHF
	Occult DCM in Dobermanns	>457 pmol/l	In combination with abnormal Holter findings, occult DCM is likely to be present
cTnI	DMVD	>0.025 ng/ml	Increased risk of death
Plasma taurine	Taurine deficiency	>25 nmol/ml	Normal

20.1 Diagnostic recommendations for the use of laboratory tests in dogs with suspected cardiac disease. CHF = congestive heart failure; cTnI = cardiac troponin I; DCM = dilated cardiomyopathy; DMVD = degenerative mitral valve disease; NT-proBNP = amino-terminal fragment of proB-type natriuretic peptide.

Test	Disease	Cut-off	Indication
NT-proBNP	Dyspnoea	>270 pmol/l	Cause of dyspnoea is likely to be cardiac
	Occult cardiomyopathies	>100 pmol/l	Observed clinical findings are likely to be due to significant cardiac disease
cTnI	HCM	>0.2 ng/ml	Animals are likely to have moderate or severe HCM
Plasma taurine	Taurine deficiency	<30 nmol/ml	At risk
Whole blood taurine	Taurine deficiency	275–701 nmol/ml	Normal

20.2 Diagnostic recommendations for the use of laboratory tests in cats with suspected cardiac disease. cTnI = cardiac troponin I; HCM = hypertrophic cardiomyopathy; NT-proBNP = amino-terminal fragment of proB-type natriuretic peptide.

B-type natriuretic peptide

B-type natriuretic peptide (BNP) is produced by the cardiomyocytes in response to stretch; it is, therefore, a marker of cardiac volume loading. The neurohormonal effects of BNP (natriuresis, diuresis and vasodilatation) oppose those of the renin–angiotensin–aldosterone system. BNP, therefore, has important homeostatic actions in healthy animals. However, the half-life of circulating BNP is only 90 seconds in the dog, which makes its measurement clinically impractical. The amino-terminal fragment of proBNP (NT-proBNP) remains in the circulation longer and so its measurement is preferred.

Available assays and sample requirements

The structure of NT-proBNP differs considerably among species, meaning that only assays specific for the species of the patient can be used. Enzyme-linked immunosorbent assays (ELISAs) for both canine and feline NT-proBNP are commercially available. A point-of-care ELISA test is also available for feline, but not canine, samples. Ethylenediamine tetra-acetic acid (EDTA) plasma samples should be collected for NT-proBNP testing. NT-proBNP may also be measured in feline pleural fluid samples which have been collected into EDTA.

A number of additional factors need to be taken into account when interpreting the results of plasma NT-proBNP tests:

* NT-proBNP is increased in patients with compromised renal function
* NT-proBNP is increased in cats with systemic hypertension
* NT-proBNP is increased in dogs with pulmonary hypertension.

As with any clinical test, careful patient selection will improve the clinical usefulness of NT-proBNP measurements (Oyama et al., 2013).

NT-proBNP in canine heart disease

NT-proBNP in degenerative mitral valve disease

The diagnosis of degenerative mitral valve disease (DMVD) in an older, small or medium-sized dog can be made on the basis of careful auscultation and therefore does not require NT-proBNP measurement. However, increasing circulating NT-proBNP concentrations are associated with increasing severity of DMVD, and with more rapid disease progression. Dogs with NT-proBNP concentrations >740 pmol/l have been shown to have decreased survival times, independent of the eventual cause of death (Moonarmart et al., 2010). In dogs with compensated DMVD, plasma NT-proBNP concentrations >1500 pmol/l indicate that the risk of onset of congestive heart failure (CHF) in the next 6 months is high (Reynolds et al., 2012).

NT-proBNP in canine cardiomyopathies

Canine cardiomyopathies frequently involve a protracted occult phase, during which physical examination findings may be unremarkable. Identification of dogs at high risk of sudden death or congestive heart failure would be of considerable clinical benefit. At present, the gold standard for diagnosis remains a combination of echocardiography and 24-hour Holter electrocardiography (ECG), although cost is often prohibitive. In Dobermanns, plasma NT-proBNP measurements >457 pmol/l, when measured in combination with Holter monitoring for arrhythmias, identify dogs at high risk for subclinical dilated cardiomyopathy (DCM) (Singletary et al., 2012a).

Differentiation of cardiac from non-cardiac causes of dyspnoea in dogs

Measurements of circulating NT-proBNP can be used to distinguish respiratory distress as a result of congestive heart failure from primary pulmonary disease. This test is best used as a way to rule out heart failure as the cause of signs. In dogs with respiratory distress, measurements of NT-proBNP <900 pmol/l mean that congestive heart failure is highly unlikely (Oyama et al., 2009). Measurements of NT-proBNP >1800 pmol/l are suggestive of congestive heart failure. However, a wide 'grey zone' exists between these two cut-offs in which the measurements are difficult to interpret. Unfortunately, no point-of-care assay is currently available for use in the emergency setting.

NT-proBNP in feline heart disease

NT-proBNP in feline cardiomyopathies

Measurement of circulating NT-proBNP can be used to distinguish cats with subclinical cardiomyopathies from both healthy cats and those with CHF. In cats with physical examination findings or history consistent with possible heart disease (murmur, gallop, arrhythmia, radiographic cardiomegaly or cardiomyopathy in a sibling), plasma NT-proBNP >100 pmol/l distinguished cats with occult cardiomyopathy from healthy animals with excellent specificity (100%) but only moderate sensitivity (70.8%) (Fox et al., 2011). In other words, NT-proBNP >100 pmol/l can be used to rule in the disease, but NT-proBNP <100 pmol/l is less reliable for ruling out the disease. However, this test has not been found to be useful to distinguish mildly affected cats from healthy controls.

Differentiation of cardiac from non-cardiac causes of dyspnoea in cats

This clinical situation can be very challenging, as there can be much overlap in the history, physical examination and radiographic findings in these cases. The cause of respiratory signs is likely to be cardiac in cats if NT-proBNP concentrations are >270 pmol/l (Fox et al., 2009). As discussed above, measurements <100 pmol/l are unlikely to be associated with clinically significant heart disease. However, a 'grey zone' exists from 100 to 270 pmol/l within which both cardiac and respiratory causes of dyspnoea must be considered. If pleural fluid samples are used, the cause of respiratory signs is likely to be cardiac if NT-proBNP concentrations are >240 pmol/l. It has been shown that, when NT-proBNP measurements were provided in addition to standard clinical information (history, physical examination, thoracic radiographs, ECG traces and biochemical analysis), general practitioners were able to distinguish cardiac and respiratory disease in cats more accurately (Singletary et al. 2012b). The availability of a point-of-care ELISA allows rapid differentiation of cardiac and respiratory causes of dyspnoea in feline emergency patients, increasing the clinical utility of this test.

Troponins

Cardiac troponins I, T and C are involved in the regulation of myocyte contraction. Unlike BNP, they are intracellular proteins that are only found in the circulation if cardiomyocytes have been damaged or destroyed. They are, therefore, considered markers of cardiac injury. It is possible to use assays designed for human samples to measure cardiac troponins in dogs and cats. The use of cardiac troponin I (cTnI) has been most extensively described.

Available assays

A variety of cTnI assays are available, with differences in their lower limits of detection. These differences can have an impact on the clinical usefulness of the test. For example, an assay with a lower limit of detection of 0.2 ng/ml (e.g. the Immulite® Troponin ELISA) might be useful for detection of myocarditis, but is not low enough to detect the more subtle increases in cTnI in dogs with DMVD. An assay with a lower limit of detection of 0.01 ng/ml (e.g. the AccuTnI ELISA) would be more appropriate for these cases.

A number of factors need to be taken into account when interpreting the results of serum cTnI tests:

- cTnI can increase as a consequence of cardiac injury secondary to non-cardiac disease (e.g. renal failure, pyometritis or gastric dilatation–volvulus). It should not be considered a marker specific for primary cardiac disease
- cTnI concentrations increase with age (Ljungvall et al., 2010). Healthy older animals will therefore have higher measurements than young animals, although age-specific reference intervals have not been published
- cTnI concentrations might be increased in animals with pulmonary hypertension, although studies have not provided conclusive evidence.

cTnI in canine heart disease

cTnI in degenerative mitral valve disease

As discussed above, measurement of circulating markers is not necessary for the diagnosis of DMVD in dogs. However, circulating cTnI concentrations increase with increasing disease severity. Dogs with cTnI concentrations >0.025 ng/ml have decreased survival times (Hezzell et al., 2012).

cTnI in canine cardiomyopathies

cTnI is higher in Dobermanns with DCM and Boxers with arrhythmogenic right ventricular cardiomyopathy (ARVC) than in healthy dogs (Baumwart et al., 2007; Wess et al., 2010); however, the test has not been shown to identify dogs with occult disease and clinically useful cut-offs have not been found (Oyama et al., 2007).

cTnI in pericardial disease

Preliminary studies suggest that measurement of cTnI in serum, plasma or pericardial fluid might be useful to differentiate neoplastic from non-neoplastic causes of pericardial effusion (Shaw et al., 2004; Linde et al., 2006; Chun et al., 2010). However, further studies are required before clinically useful cut-off values can be suggested.

Differentiation of cardiac from non-cardiac causes of dyspnoea

cTnI has not been found to be useful in differentiating cardiac from non-cardiac causes of respiratory distress in dogs.

cTnI in feline heart disease

cTnI in feline cardiomyopathies

cTnI is higher in cats with hypertrophic cardiomyopathy (HCM) than in healthy control cats. Cats with cTnI >0.2 ng/ml (measured using the Immulite® ELISA) are more likely to have moderate or severe HCM, although this test has a sensitivity of 87% and therefore a negative result does not rule out the presence of significant disease (Connolly et al., 2003). Cats with HCM that have cTnI >0.14 ng/ml have shorter survival times (Langhorn et al., 2014).

Differentiation of cardiac from non-cardiac causes of dyspnoea

Measurement of cTnI has not been found to be clinically useful in the differentiation of cardiac from non-cardiac causes of respiratory distress in cats.

cTnI in myocarditis

cTnI is increased as a result of myocardial injury secondary to inflammation and necrosis. Underlying causes include:

- Physical insults (e.g. trauma)
- Chemical insults (e.g. doxorubicin toxicity)
- Infectious causes (e.g. parvovirus, *Toxoplasma gondii*, *Neospora caninum*, *Borrelia burgdorferi*, *Trypanosoma cruzi*, *Leishmania* spp.).

Appropriate aberrant ancillary tests are indicated if the history is suggestive of an infectious myocarditis.

Combined measurements of NT-proBNP and cTnI

Measurement of both serum NT-proBNP and cTnI has been shown to provide superior prognostic information to measurement of either marker alone in dogs with DMVD. Dogs with both NT-proBNP >524 pmol/l and cTnI >0.025 ng/ml had significantly shorter survival times than those with either one or neither marker above these cut-offs (Hezzell et al., 2012). It remains unknown whether combining measurements in other clinical scenarios, such as cats with occult cardiomyopathies, would be of benefit.

Monitoring of digoxin therapy

The use of cardiac glycosides has declined in veterinary medicine since the positive inotrope pimobendan became available. However, digoxin is still commonly used to reduce the ventricular response rate in atrial fibrillation. Monitoring of serum digoxin concentrations is important owing to its narrow therapeutic index, i.e. the toxic dose is close to the therapeutic dose. The therapeutic range quoted varies among laboratories: a commonly used range is 0.65–2.55 nmol/l, although some cardiologists recommend aiming for a concentration ≤1.28 nmol/l. Indeed, control of ventricular rate can be achieved with levels this low in some patients. Clinical signs of toxicity can sometimes occur when the serum digoxin level is within the therapeutic range. Serum concentrations should be measured 6–8 hours post drug administration (Nagashima et al., 2001) 7 days post initiation of therapy. If necessary, the dose is adjusted and the test repeated at 7–14 days until an appropriate, stable serum concentration has been attained. Once the digoxin concentration is within the desired range, further tests should be conducted at 3-monthly intervals; early retesting is recommended if clinical signs compatible with digoxin toxicity are observed (e.g. vomiting, diarrhoea, anorexia or weight loss).

Assessment of nutritional deficiencies

Taurine

Dietary deficiencies in taurine lead to the development of myocardial failure in cats (Sisson et al., 1991) as well as central retinal degeneration. The echocardiographic changes are similar to those seen in idiopathic DCM. Cats cannot synthesize taurine and therefore require a dietary source. A similar syndrome is seen occasionally in dogs, although this species is much less prone to developing plasma taurine deficiency. However, taurine deficiency should be suspected if DCM is diagnosed in an atypical breed, particularly the American Cocker Spaniel (Kittleson *et al.*, 1997).

Sample requirements

Taurine concentrations can be measured in either heparinized plasma or heparinized whole blood (Kramer *et al.*, 1995). In feline plasma samples, taurine concentrations decrease significantly in response to fasting; this is not the case for whole blood samples, which are therefore preferred in this species (Pion *et al.*, 1991; Heinze *et al.*, 2009). In dogs, heparinized plasma is most commonly used. Samples for both species should be acquired prior to the initiation of dietary taurine supplementation owing to rapid increases in circulating concentrations. There is some variation in the reference intervals for taurine given in the literature; the concentrations given in Figures 20.1 (Kramer *et al.*, 1995) and 20.2 (Heinze *et al.*, 2009) are intended as a guide and it is important to check with the laboratory performing the test.

Carnitine

Myocardial carnitine deficiency has been associated with dilated cardiomyopathy in dogs. However, plasma carnitine concentrations do not correlate well with myocardial concentrations and so its measurement is not clinically useful.

Genetic tests

Numerous mutations which cause an HCM, ARVC or DCM phenotype have been identified in human patients; it is unlikely that all the possible causative mutations have yet been discovered in dogs and cats. Additionally, not all animals with the same genotype go on to develop a clinical cardiomyopathy or, if they do, the same severity of disease. Caution should therefore be exercised in interpreting the results of genetic tests. These tests are therefore probably more useful for breeders wishing to decrease the proportion of affected animals in the population than they are in predicting whether an individual animal will develop a clinical cardiomyopathy. It is currently recommended by those who offer the genetic tests that heterozygotes be mated with unaffected animals to decrease the prevalence of the mutations in the population, as eliminating all heterozygotes from the gene pool would limit genetic diversity to an undesirable degree. It is, however, recommended that homozygotes are not used for breeding purposes.

Sample acquisition

EDTA blood or oral swabs can be submitted for testing.

Hypertrophic cardiomyopathy in cats

Two mutations associated with HCM have been identified in cats. Tests for both of these mutations are commercially available.

Myosin binding protein C mutation in Maine Coon cats

In some Maine Coon cats, HCM is caused by a single base-pair change (G to C) in exon 3 of the myosin binding protein C gene (Meurs *et al.*, 2005). The prevalence of this mutation in Maine Coon cats is 34%; the incidence of HCM in this breed remains unclear (Fries *et al.*, 2008). This mutation has not been identified in other breeds.

Myosin binding protein C mutation in Ragdoll cats

In some Ragdoll cats, HCM is caused by a single base-pair change (C to T) in codon 820 of the myosin binding protein C gene (Meurs *et al.* 2007). This mutation is distinct from that observed in Maine Coon cats and no overlap of mutations between the breeds has been found to date.

Arrhythmogenic right ventricular cardiomyopathy in Boxers

A deletion in the 3' untranslated region of striatin has been identified in Boxers with ARVC in the USA (Meurs *et al.*, 2010). A test for this mutation is commercially available. Anecdotally, however, many dogs in Europe with an ARVC phenotype appear to be negative for this mutation, suggesting that other, as yet undiscovered, mutations might exist.

Dilated cardiomyopathy in Dobermanns

A splice site mutation in a gene on chromosome 14 encoding pyruvate dehydrogenase kinase 4 (a mitochondrial protein) has been identified in some Dobermanns with DCM (Meurs *et al.*, 2012). A test for this mutation is commercially available. However, a study in Europe identified a region on chromosome 5, suggesting that more than one causative mutation exists (Mausberg *et al.*, 2011).

Case examples

CASE 1

SIGNALMENT

8-week-old male entire Rottweiler puppy.

HISTORY

2-day history of progressive lethargy and diarrhoea, and two puppies from the same litter had died. History of coccidiosis. A tick had been removed 4 weeks prior to presentation.

PHYSICAL EXAMINATION

The heart rate was 260 bpm with a regular rhythm. Capillary refill time was 3–4 seconds. On auscultation a grade II/VI systolic murmur and a gallop were detected. Other auscultatory and physical examination findings were unremarkable.

ELECTROCARDIOGRAPHY

The ECG trace is shown in Figure 20.3. Normal sinus complexes are seen intermittently. Four paroxysms of wide, bizarre complexes with no associated P waves and a rapid heart rate (approximately 300 bpm), consistent with ventricular tachycardia, are also seen.

ECHOCARDIOGRAPHY

Echocardiography revealed moderate left ventricular dilatation and mild left atrial enlargement. Left ventricular

systolic motion was decreased and dyssynchronous. Evidence of moderate mitral regurgitation was seen (Figure 20.4). The velocity of the mitral regurgitant jet was decreased (3.49 m/s), which is consistent with left ventricular systolic dysfunction.

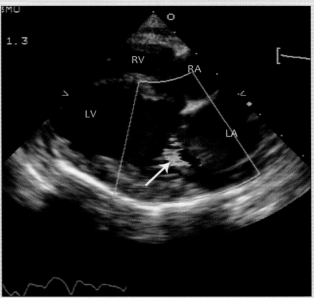

20.4 Right parasternal long-axis view of the heart of the puppy. The left atrium (LA) is enlarged and the left ventricle (LV) appears dilated, while the right atrium (RA) and right ventricle (RV) are more normal in appearance. Turbulent retrograde flow across the mitral valve, consistent with regurgitation, is also visible (arrowed).

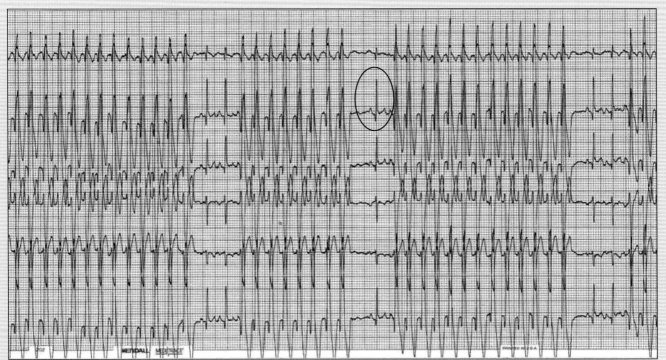

20.3 A six-lead ECG trace from the puppy. Normal sinus complexes are visible, such as the example circled. Multiple paroxysms of wide, bizarre complexes with a rapid heart rate, consistent with ventricular tachycardia, are also seen.

→ **CASE 1 CONTINUED**

CLINICAL PATHOLOGY DATA

Biochemistry	Result	Reference interval
Glucose (mmol/l)	4.6	3.6–7.0
Urea (mmol/l)	3.8	2.5–6.7
Creatinine (µmol/l)	**18.7**	20.0–150.0
Inorganic phosphate (mmol/l)	**1.8**	0.80–1.60
Sodium (mmol/l)	**139**	140–150
Potassium (mmol/l)	5.1	4.0–5.2
Chloride (mmol/l)	117	109–120
Total protein (g/l)	**36**	54–71
Albumin (g/l)	**14**	25–37
Globulin (g/l)	**22**	24–40
Albumin:globulin ratio	**0.6**	0.7–1.5
ALT (IU/l)	**13**	16–91
ALP (IU/l)	134	20–155
Cholesterol (mmol/l)	4.4	3.2–6.2

Abnormal results are in **bold**.

Haematology	Result	Reference interval
RBC (x 10^{12}/l)	3.95	3.8–5.2
Haemoglobin (g/dl)	**8.47**	8.7–12.6
Haematocrit (l/l)	**0.25**	0.28–0.35
MCV (fl)	62.1	58.0–72.0
MCH (pg)	21.4	17.5–27.3
MCHC (g/dl)	34.5	28.8–37.7
Platelets (x 10^9/l)	379	177–398
WBC (x 10^9/l)	8.60	5.3–19.8
Segmented neutrophils (x 10^9/l)	4.39	3.1–14.4
Lymphocytes (x 10^9/l)	2.67	0.9–5.5
Monocytes (x 10^9/l)	0.60	0.1–1.4
Eosinophils (x 10^9/l)	0.86	0.0–1.6
Basophils (x 10^9/l)	0.09	0.0–0.2
Platelet morphology	Few enlarged platelets	
Other RBC changes	None noted	
WBC morphology	No abnormality noted	
Reticulocytes – absolute (x 10^9/l)	0	<104.2

Abnormal results are in **bold**.

Serum cTnI: 5.06 ng/ml (reference range 0–0.07 ng/ml).

WHAT ABNORMALITIES ARE PRESENT AND WHAT ARE THE DIFFERENTIAL DIAGNOSES?

The hypoproteinaemia may be due to liver failure, renal loss, malassimilation or malnutrition, or a protein-losing enteropathy (PLE). Given the history of coccidiosis and diarrhoea and the unremarkable liver and renal parameters, PLE was considered to be the most likely differential. The degree of hypoproteinaemia was too severe to be solely attributable to the dog's age.

Similarly, the mild non-regenerative anaemia may be due to chronic disease (the reference range for haematocrit in a puppy of this age is 0.28–0.35 l/l). However, the raised phosphorus is most likely to be age-related, as this parameter is normally higher in puppies.

Echocardiography revealed asymmetrical systolic dysfunction of the left ventricle, with mitral regurgitation and left atrial enlargement. ECG revealed frequent paroxysms of ventricular tachycardia. Differential diagnoses include:

- Myocarditis
- Myocardial infarction
- Primary arrhythmia
- Mitral valve dysplasia
- Mitral regurgitation secondary to left ventricular dilatation and stretching of the valve annulus.

The serum cTnI is very high, consistent with significant myocardial injury. However, this injury is non-specific and could be caused by myocarditis, myocardial infarction or primary ventricular tachycardia. It is unlikely to be the result of mitral valve dysplasia.

WHAT FURTHER TESTS WOULD YOU PERFORM?

Faecal analysis is warranted to investigate further the history of diarrhoea and finding of hypoproteinaemia. Serological testing for *Borrelia burgdorferi* is warranted to rule out Lyme myocarditis, given the history of possible tick exposure.

CASE OUTCOME

Treatment of the ventricular tachycardia with intravenous lidocaine was initiated and transitioned to oral sotalol (2 mg/kg q12h). Given the history of coccidiosis and possible tick exposure, antiparasitic therapy and treatment with doxycycline were started empirically while awaiting results of the faecal analysis and tick panel. However, the puppy died suddenly at home 3 days later.

POST-MORTEM FINDINGS

Gross pathology
• Heart: pericardial effusion • Abdomen: mild ascites • Liver: hepatomegaly
Histopathology
• Pericardium: multifocal fibrin deposits • Heart, right: mild multifocal interstitial fibroplasia and oedema • Heart, left and septum: severe multifocal to regionally extensive chronic lymphoplasmacytic, neutrophilic and histiocytic myocarditis with multifocal myocardial necrosis, loss and mineralization; moderate multifocal fibroplasia and Anitschkow cell hyperplasia • Otherwise unremarkable
Diagnosis
• Severe multifocal chronic myocarditis • Right- and left-sided heart failure
Comments
The cause of the myocarditis is not evident in the sections examined

→ CASE 1 CONTINUED

The ventricular tachycardia, systolic dysfunction and mitral regurgitation seen in this puppy were therefore the result of myocarditis. Definitive ante-mortem diagnosis would have required endomyocardial biopsy, which was not considered advisable in an unstable patient because general anaesthesia is required.

Serology was negative for *Ehrlichia canis*, *Borelia burgdorferi*, *Anaplasma* spp., *Babesia canis*, Rocky Mountain spotted fever, *Bartonella hensalae* and *Bartonella vinsonii*. Faecal analysis revealed oocysts of *Isospora canis* and *Isospora ohiohensis*.

(Case 1 courtesy of DJ Trafny)

CASE 2

SIGNALMENT

15-year-old female neutered Domestic Shorthair cat.

HISTORY

3-day history of increased respiratory rate and effort with sudden onset. Inspiratory wheezes were audible when sleeping. The cat had a history of potential food hypersensitivity and had been vomiting every other day for 2 weeks.

PHYSICAL EXAMINATION

The heart rate was 160 bpm and the respiratory rate was 38 bpm with a moderate increase in respiratory effort. A grade III/VI parasternal heart murmur was heard on auscultation. Other auscultatory and physical examination findings were unremarkable.

RADIOGRAPHY

Radiographs taken at presentation are shown in Figure 20.5.

CLINICAL PATHOLOGY DATA

The results of serum biochemistry and haematology were unremarkable. Plasma NT-proBNP was <24 pmol/l (see Figure 20.2).

WHAT ABNORMALITIES ARE PRESENT AND WHAT ARE THE DIFFERENTIAL DIAGNOSES?

The radiographs show evidence of mild cardiomegaly. Thin pleural fissure lines are visible. A diffuse bronchial pattern can be seen throughout the lungs, with an interstitial to mild alveolar pattern visible ventrally. Differential diagnoses include:

- Left-sided congestive heart failure with cardiogenic oedema and scant pleural effusion
- Pneumonia and pleural thickening or scant effusion
- Age-related increase in bronchial pattern
- Chronic lower airway disease.

Differential diagnoses for a newly detected heart murmur in an aged cat include:

- Dynamic left ventricular outflow tract obstruction (e.g. systolic anterior motion of the mitral valve secondary to hypertrophic obstructive cardiomyopathy)
- Flow murmur (e.g. fever, anaemia, hyperthyroidism, increased sympathetic tone)
- Previously undetected congenital heart disease (e.g. ventral septal defect or mitral dysplasia).

However, a plasma NT-proBNP below the lower limit of detection means that heart failure is unlikely in this patient, making pneumonia the most likely differential diagnosis.

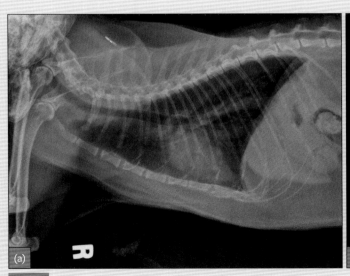
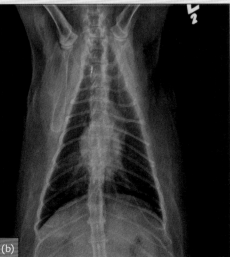

20.5   (a) Right lateral and (b) dorsoventral views of the thorax of the cat.

→ CASE 2 CONTINUED

WHAT FURTHER TESTS WOULD YOU PERFORM?

A bronchoalveolar lavage (BAL) should be performed if the patient is clinically stable enough to be anaesthetized.

RESULTS OF FURTHER TESTS

The BAL revealed the presence of large numbers of neutrophils, many of which appeared degenerate. Some neutrophils contained intracellular bacteria. Culture of the BAL fluid yielded a heavy pure growth of *Enterococcus faecium*, which was sensitive to chloramphenicol, erythromycin and vancomycin and resistant to ampicillin, gentamicin, penicillin, rifampin and tetracycline.

HOW WOULD YOU INTERPRET THESE RESULTS?

The results of the BAL are consistent with a bacterial bronchopneumonia or bacterial bronchitis. The presence of intracellular bacteria suggests that the bacteria seen are not contaminants introduced during sample acquisition.

CASE OUTCOME

Azithromycin at a dose of 8.5 mg/kg was administered once daily for 10 days. The clinical signs and radiographic changes consistent with bronchopneumonia resolved (Figure 20.6), and the cat continued to do well at home.

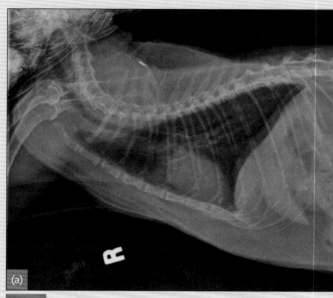
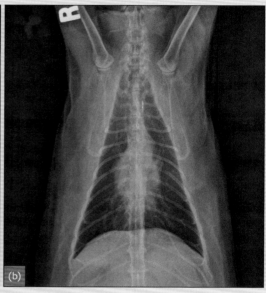

20.6 (a) Right lateral and (b) dorsoventral views of the thorax of the cat following administration of azithromycin for 10 days.

(Case 2 courtesy of MA Oyama)

References and further reading

Baumwart RD, Orvalho J and Meurs KM (2007) Evaluation of serum cardiac troponin I concentration in Boxers with arrhythmogenic right ventricular cardiomyopathy. *American Journal of Veterinary Research* **68**, 524–528

Chun R, Kellihan HB, Henik RA and Stepien RL (2010) Comparison of plasma cardiac troponin I concentrations among dogs with cardiac hemangiosarcoma, noncardiac hemangiosarcoma, other neoplasms, and pericardial effusion of nonhemangiosarcoma origin. *Journal of the American Veterinary Medical Association* **237**, 806–811

Connolly DJ, Cannata J, Boswood A, Archer J, Groves EA and Neiger R (2003) Cardiac troponin I in cats with hypertrophic cardiomyopathy. *Journal of Feline Medicine and Surgery* **5**, 209–216

Fox PR, Oyama MA, Reynolds C *et al.* (2009) Utility of plasma N-terminal pro-brain natriuretic peptide (NT-proBNP) to distinguish between congestive heart failure and non-cardiac causes of acute dyspnea in cats. *Journal of Veterinary Cardiology* **11** (Suppl 1), S51–S61

Fox PR, Rush JE, Reynolds CA *et al.*(2011) Multicenter evaluation of plasma N-terminal probrain natriuretic peptide (NT-pro BNP) as a biochemical screening test for asymptomatic (occult) cardiomyopathy in cats. *Journal of Veterinary Internal Medicine* **25**, 1010–1016

Fries R, Heaney AM and Meurs KM (2008) Prevalence of the myosin-binding protein C mutation in Maine Coon cats. *Journal of Veterinary Internal Medicine* **22**, 893–896

Heinze CR, Larsen JA, Kass PH and Fascetti AJ (2009) Plasma amino acid and whole blood taurine concentrations in cats eating commercially prepared diets. *American Journal of Veterinary Research* **70**, 1374–1382

Hezzell MJ *et al.* (2015) Differentiating Cardiac *vs* Non-Cardiac Causes of Pleural Effusion in: *Cats Using Plasma and Pleural Fluid with a Point-of-Care NT-proBNP Test*, ACVIM Forum

Hezzell MJ, Boswood A, Chang YM, Moonarmart W, Souttar K and Elliott J (2012) The combined prognostic potential of serum high-sensitivity cardiac troponin I and N-terminal pro-B-type natriuretic peptide concentrations in dogs with degenerative mitral valve disease. *Journal of Veterinary Internal Medicine* **26**, 302–311

Kittleson MD, Keene B, Pion PD and Loyer CG (1997) Results of the multicenter spaniel trial (MUST): taurine- and carnitine-responsive dilated cardiomyopathy in American cocker spaniels with decreased plasma taurine concentration. *Journal of Veterinary Internal Medicine* **11**, 204–211

Kramer GA, Kittleson MD, Fox PR, Lewis J and Pion PD (1995) Plasma taurine concentrations in normal dogs and in dogs with heart disease. *Journal of Veterinary Internal Medicine* **9**, 253–258

Langhorn R, Tarnow I, Willesen JL, Kjelgaard-Hansen M, Skovgaard IM and Koch J. (2014) Cardiac troponin I and T as prognostic markers in cats with hypertrophic cardiomyopathy. *Journal of Veterinary Internal Medicine Sep-Oct* **28(5)**, 1485–1491

Linde A, Summerfield NJ, Sleeper MM *et al.* (2006) Pilot study on cardiac troponin I levels in dogs with pericardial effusion. *Journal of Veterinary Cardiology* **8**, 19–23

Ljungvall I, Hoglund K, Tidholm A *et al.* (2010) Cardiac troponin I is associated with severity of myxomatous mitral valve disease, age, and C-reactive protein in dogs. *Journal of Veterinary Internal Medicine* **24**, 153–159

Mausberg TB, Wess G, Simak J *et al.* (2011) A locus on chromosome 5 is associated with dilated cardiomyopathy in Doberman Pinschers. *PLoS One* **6**, e20042

Meurs KM, Lahmers S, Keene BW *et al.* (2012) A splice site mutation in a gene encoding for PDK4, a mitochondrial protein, is associated with the development of dilated cardiomyopathy in the Doberman pinscher. *Human Genetics* **131**, 1319–1325

Meurs KM, Mauceli E, Lahmers S, Acland GM, White SN and Lindblad-Toh K (2010) Genome-wide association identifies a deletion in the 3' untranslated region of striatin in a canine model of arrhythmogenic right ventricular cardiomyopathy. *Human Genetics* **128**, 315–324

Meurs KM, Norgard MM, Ederer MM, Hendrix KP and Kittleson MD (2007) A substitution mutation in the myosin binding protein C gene in ragdoll hypertrophic cardiomyopathy. *Genomics* **90**, 261–264

Meurs KM, Sanchez X, David RM *et al.* (2005) A cardiac myosin binding protein C mutation in the Maine Coon cat with familial hypertrophic cardiomyopathy. *Human Molecular Genetics* **14**, 3587–3593

Moonarmart W, Boswood A, Luis Fuentes V, Brodbelt D, Souttar K and Elliott J (2010) N-terminal pro B-type natriuretic peptide and left ventricular diameter independently predict mortality in dogs with mitral valve disease. *Journal of Small Animal Practice* **51**, 84–96

Nagashima Y, Hirao H, Furukawa S *et al.* (2001) Plasma digoxin concentration in dogs with mitral regurgitation. *Journal of Veterinary Medical Science* **63**, 1199–1202

Oyama MA, Boswood A, Connolly DJ *et al.* (2013) Clinical usefulness of an assay for measurement of circulating N-terminal pro-B-type natriuretic peptide concentration in dogs and cats with heart disease. *Journal of the American Veterinary Medical Association* **243**, 71–82

Oyama MA, Rush JE, Rozanski EA *et al.* (2009) Assessment of serum N-terminal pro-B-type natriuretic peptide concentration for differentiation of congestive heart failure from primary respiratory tract disease as the cause of respiratory signs in dogs. *Journal of the American Veterinary Medical Association* **235**, 1319–1325

Oyama MA, Sisson DD and Solter PF (2007) Prospective screening for occult cardiomyopathy in dogs by measurement of plasma atrial natriuretic peptide, B-type natriuretic peptide, and cardiac troponin-I concentrations. *American Journal of Veterinary Research* **68**, 42–47

Pion PD, Lewis J, Greene K, Rogers QR, Morris JG and Kittleson MD (1991) Effect of meal-feeding and food deprivation on plasma and whole blood taurine concentrations in cats. *Journal of Nutrition* **121**, S177–S178

Reynolds CA, Brown DC, Rush JE *et al.* (2012) Prediction of first onset of congestive heart failure in dogs with degenerative mitral valve disease: the PREDICT cohort study. *Journal of Veterinary Cardiology* **14**, 193–202

Shaw SP, Rozanski EA and Rush JE (2004) Cardiac troponins I and T in dogs with pericardial effusion. *Journal of Veterinary Internal Medicine* **18**, 322–324

Singletary GE, Morris NA, Lynne O'Sullivan M, Gordon SG and Oyama MA (2012a) Prospective evaluation of NT-proBNP assay to detect occult dilated cardiomyopathy and predict survival in Doberman Pinschers. *Journal of Veterinary Internal Medicine* **26**, 1330–1336

Singletary GE, Rush JE, Fox PR, Stepien RL and Oyama MA (2012b) Effect of NT-pro-BNP assay on accuracy and confidence of general practitioners in diagnosing heart failure or respiratory disease in cats with respiratory signs. *Journal of Veterinary Internal Medicine* **26**, 542–546

Sisson DD, Knight DH, Helinski C *et al.*1991) Plasma taurine concentrations and M-mode echocardiographic measures in healthy cats and in cats with dilated cardiomyopathy. *Journal of Veterinary Internal Medicine* **5**, 232–238

Wess G, Simak J, Mahling M and Hartmann K (2010) Cardiac troponin I in Doberman Pinschers with cardiomyopathy. *Journal of Veterinary Internal Medicine* **24**, 843–849

Chapter 21

Diagnostic cytology

Paola Monti and Francesco Cian

Cytopathology, often abbreviated to cytology, is the micro-scopic examination of individual cells or groups of cells to identify their origin and any changes characteristic of disease. It is a quick and safe diagnostic tool that can be used to investigate superficial or internal masses, internal organs, lymph nodes and fluids (effusions, joint fluids, cerebrospinal fluid (CSF), bronchoalveolar lavages (BALs), urine, prostatic washes).

In clinical situations, cytology has several advantages over histopathology; most importantly it has a relatively low risk of complications for the patient and has a rapid turnaround time. Additionally, cytology may provide an initial diagnosis that allows planning of the diagnostic and surgical approaches. However, there are also limitations that are usually associated with the quality of the sample (low cellularity or artefacts) and absence of an architec-tural arrangement. A more extensive list of the advantages and disadvantages of cytology is presented in Figure 21.1.

The accuracy of the cytological examination from any body site depends greatly on:

- Quality of collection
- Staining
- Interpretation of the material.

Inadequacy in any of these steps will adversely affect the quality of diagnostic cytology.

In the literature there are many papers describing the agreement of cytology with the gold standard histo-pathology. This agreement varies from the 90% found in cytology of cutaneous and subcutaneous tumours to 30%

Advantages
• Non-invasiveness
• No need for general anaesthesia
• Low risk of complications
• Rapid results
• Low costs
• Basic interpretation can be made in clinic
• Can be applied to anatomical locations that are not readily accessible to a biopsy needle or scalpel

Disadvantages
• Inconclusive results due to low cellularity or artefacts
• Misinterpretation may be caused by absence of architectural context
• Relies on accuracy of localization of the sampling
• Often provides only a broad diagnosis of neoplasia and histopathology is required for grading and further classification

21.1 Advantages and disadvantages of cytopathology.

agreement for liver cytology in dogs. Cytology is helpful in the diagnosis of neoplasia (benign or malignant), infection (bacterial, fungal, parasitic), inflammation and infiltration (e.g. amyloidosis).

When an inflammatory process is recognized, cytology aids in the identification of the underlying cause or helps in listing the most probable differential diagnoses guiding the diagnostic process.

Tumour cytology can sometimes be challenging. While some neoplasms are easy to recognize and diagnose, sometimes tumour diagnosis can be difficult. This is mainly due to the poorly exfoliative nature of some lesions or the concurrent presence of inflammatory cells. In this case, the challenge is to differentiate a primary neoplasm with secondary inflammation from a cellular dysplasia or fibro-plasia caused by the inflammatory process. In these situa-tions, a biopsy sample is often obtained to evaluate the architecture of the tissue.

The intent of this chapter is to provide the reader with a good basic knowledge of cytopathology, including the different sampling techniques, the most common staining procedures and a simple practical approach to slide exam-ination. Attention will be focused mainly on the lesions or organs that are more frequently aspirated in general prac-tice, such as cutaneous masses and lymph nodes.

General sampling guidelines

The efficacy of sample acquisition for cytological examin-ation depends primarily on the characteristics of the lesion being investigated and its tendency to exfoliate cells during aspiration. However, the quality of the sample and the cytological diagnosis is dependent on use of an appro-priate sampling technique. Errors in sampling technique may irreversibly affect the quality of the sample, making it non-diagnostic. The following sections explain how to collect diagnostic samples for:

- Aspiration cytology
- Impression smear cytology
- Scraping cytology
- Exfoliative cytology.

Aspiration cytology

Fine-needle aspiration (FNA) is the most common approach for skin masses, lymph nodes and internal organs. Samples

BSAVA Manual of Canine and Feline Clinical Pathology, 3rd edition. Edited by Elizabeth Villiers and Jelena Ristić. ©BSAVA 2016

may be achieved with different techniques, depending on the nature of the lesion.

- **Needle-only method:** this method has the advantage that delicate and fragile cells are not damaged by suction and haemodilution is minimized. It is commonly used for aspiration of soft masses and lymph nodes. These are immobilized with one hand while a 21–23 G, 16–25 mm needle is inserted into the lesion (without the syringe). The needle is then moved to and fro within the mass, while redirecting it in many directions (Figure 21.2). Thus, the sample will be representative of the entire lesion and not of only a part of it. This is particularly important for lymph nodes, where selective aspiration of cells from the centre of a follicle might lead to an erroneous diagnosis of lymphoma, or in large tumours where the centre may often be necrotic and inflamed, thus misclassifying the lesion as inflammatory rather than neoplastic (Figure 21.3). Care must be taken to ensure the needle is not pushed through the mass into the surrounding tissues. Accidental aspiration of adipose tissue is a common sequela of this. The needle-only method leads to the accumulation of the sample in the hub of the needle.

- **Continuous suction method:** this method is useful for aspirating firm and poorly exfoliative masses (e.g. fibrosarcomas). A 21–23 G, 16–25 mm needle attached to a 2.5–5 ml syringe is inserted into the lesion, and suction is applied by withdrawing the plunger. While the suction is maintained, the needle is moved to and fro within the lesion, redirecting it each time, and taking care to avoid pushing it through the mass into the surrounding tissues. Suction is then released before removing the needle from the lesion.

- **Intermittent suction:** this method is used for small lesions where the needle cannot be moved. The needle with syringe attached is inserted into the lesion and then the plunger withdrawn and released intermittently, keeping the needle still. Suction is then released before removing the needle from the lesion.

Aspiration from internal organs (liver, spleen, lungs, etc.) is usually performed under ultrasound guidance. If there is a reason to suspect a coagulopathy, haematology and a coagulation profile should be performed prior to the aspiration. Once the lesion has been identified on ultrasonography, the site should be prepared for aspiration by cleaning the surface of the skin with antiseptic, taking care to remove the ultrasound gel (Figure 21.4).

Once the aspiration has been performed, an air-filled syringe is attached to the needle. If a suction technique was used, the syringe should be disconnected, filled with air and then reattached to the needle. Holding the tip of the needle over a clean glass slide, the plunger is briskly depressed and the contents of the needle are expelled on to the slide. The sample is then smeared by one of the following methods.

- **Squash preparation:** slide 1 is held in the left hand (for right-handed people). A second slide (now referred to as slide 2) is held in the right hand and placed flat on to slide 1 at right angles to it. Slide 2 is then used to spread the sample. The pressure applied should be adequate to spread the cells on the slide, obtaining a monolayer, but at the same time it should be sufficiently gentle to avoid cell rupture. Some cell types (e.g. lymphoid cells) are particularly fragile and their preservation is highly technique dependent. Slide 2 is then slid quickly and smoothly across slide 1 (Figure 21.5). This procedure should produce a monolayer of cells. If excessive material is used, the resulting smear is too thick, hampering examination of the cells (Figure 21.6).

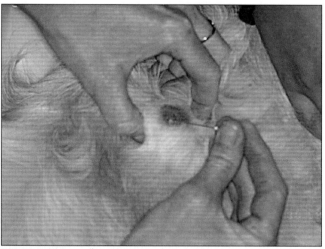

21.2 Fine-needle aspiration technique. The mass is immobilized with one hand while the needle is inserted into the lesion and moved to and fro.

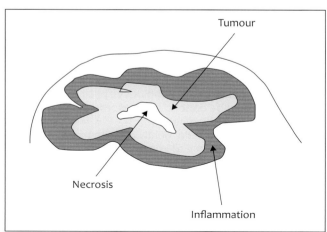

Tumour

Necrosis

Inflammation

21.3 The centre of large masses is frequently necrotic and inflamed. Hence, during sampling, aspiration from peripheral areas of the mass should guarantee a more representative sample.
(© D Berlato, AHT)

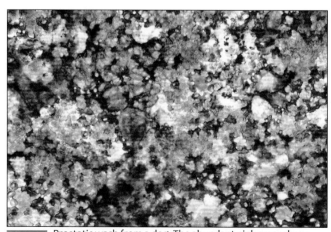

21.4 Prostatic wash from a dog. The abundant pink amorphous material is lubricant gel, which hampers visualization of cellular details. (Wright–Giemsa stain; original magnification X500)

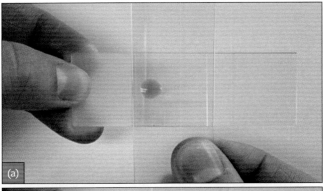

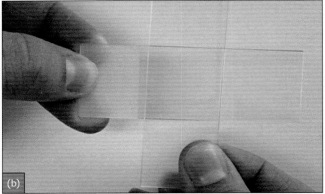

21.5 Squash smear preparation. (a) A drop of specimen is placed on one edge of the bottom side. (b) A second slide is gently applied on top and drawn across at right angles.

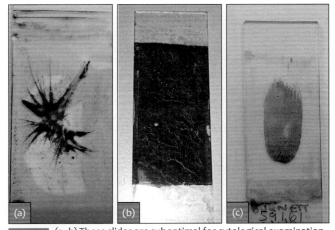

21.6 (a–b) These slides are suboptimal for cytological examination. (a) The specimen is insufficiently smeared. (b) The slide contains an excessive amount of material and the smer is too thick. (c) The slide shows an ideal cytological preparation. (Stained with Wright–Giemsa)

- **Blood smear technique:** this is based on the technique routinely used for making peripheral blood smears and described in Chapter 3. This method should reduce cell damage and may be useful in the absence of sufficient confidence in making squash preparations (although it may lead to streak artefacts).
- **Line concentration technique:** the sample is smeared as for the blood smear technique, but when the spreader slide has been advanced about two-thirds of the way, it is abruptly lifted upwards. This technique is useful for fluid samples (e.g. cystic masses or haemodiluted samples), although centrifugation techniques, especially using a cytospin centrifuge, give superior smears (Figure 21.7).

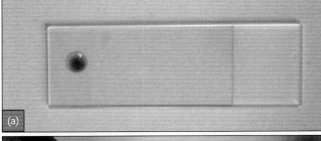

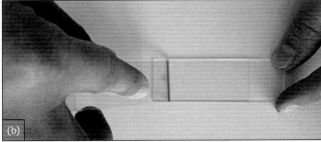

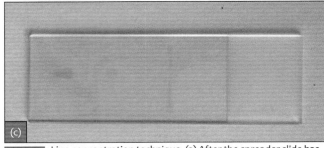

21.7 Line concentration technique. (a) After the spreader slide has been advanced two-thirds of the way along the bottom slide, (b–c) it is lifted upwards in order to concentrate cells at the end of the smear.

Impression smear cytology

This procedure is used for superficial ulcerated lesions or to perform intraoperative cytology on solid tissue biopsy samples. Cells may exfoliate well during this technique and architectural evaluation may also be maintained. However, the sample is frequently not representative of the entire lesion and may reflect only the superficial part of it. A classical example is the squamous cell carcinoma (SCC). This tumour is frequently ulcerated, and impression smears may sometimes exfoliate only inflammatory cells, leading to an erroneous misdiagnosis of inflammation.

The procedure for taking a correct impression smear is described below (Figure 21.8).

1. Clean the surface of the ulcerated mass with a saline-moistened gauze swab. For biopsy specimens the sample should be dabbed into absorbent tissue to absorb surface blood/serum.
2. Take a clean glass slide, gently appose this to the surface of the lesion and immediately lift it off without smearing the slide across the lesion.
3. Repeat the procedure to obtain several imprints on one slide.

Scraping cytology

There are two main types of scraping technique, superficial and deep. Superficial scraping provides information on the surface of the epidermis. It can be used for the identification of specific superficial parasites such as

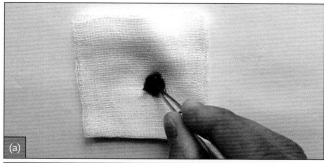

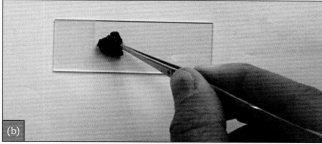

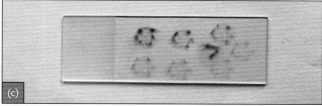

21.8 Impression smear technique for a surgical biopsy specimen. (a) Excess blood is firstly removed from the lesion by blotting the cut surface with a clean swab. (b–c) Several imprints from the mass are obtained by apposing the sample to the slide.

Cheyletiella. Deep scraping collects material from within the hair follicle and usually causes minimal bleeding. It is usually performed to evaluate the presence of mites that live deep in the hair follicles, such as *Demodex*. Scrapings are usually performed using a surgical size 10 or 15 scalpel blade. Squeezing the skin to 'milk' mites from the hair follicles during sampling may increase the chance of finding mites.

1. Scrape a scalpel blade across the surface of the lesion several times.
2. Transfer the material collected on the blade on to a slide using the blade like a paintbrush to gently smear the sample.
3. If the material is thickly spread, a squash preparation is made as previously described.

Exfoliative cytology

This relies on the spontaneous exfoliation of cells into fluids or on to swabs. Typical examples of exfoliative cytology are:

- CSF, urine and fluid cytology (pleural, abdominal, pericardial and synovial fluids): cytology smears are prepared from the spun sediment or using a cytospin centrifuge, or for cellular samples a direct smear or line concentration smear is made
- Vaginal and ear cytology: this is performed by rolling a cotton bud on the surface to be examined and then rolling this along the surface of a slide.

Routine stains

The staining method used should guarantee rapid and good quality results to facilitate the visualization of structures by increasing the contrast between them. Several staining techniques have been used in cytopathology, although they can all be placed into two main categories:

- **Romanowsky-based stains:** these include May–Grünwald–Giemsa (MGG), Wright–Giemsa and Diff-Quik® (which is a modified Wright–Giemsa stain). Samples are air-dried before staining. These stains adequately stain nuclei and they are superior for the evaluation of cytoplasmic details and extracellular material
- **Trichrome Papanicolaou (Pap) and bichrome haematoxylin and eosin (H&E) stains:** these are based on wet-fixation by the use of a 95% ethanol solution. They are less commonly used in cytopathology, although they are considered to provide better nuclear and nucleolar detail (Figure 21.9).

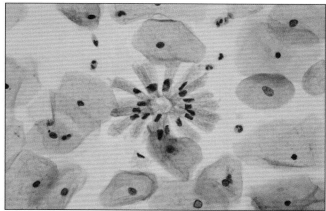

21.9 Cytological sample stained with Papanicolaou. (Papanicolaou stain; original magnification X600)
(Courtesy of Paul Elgert, New York University School of Medicine)

Romanowsky stains

Romanowsky stains are a combination of basic dyes (methylene blue, azure), which bind to acidic cellular structures such as DNA and RNA, and acidic dyes (eosin), which bind to basic cellular structures such as basic proteins and haemoglobin. These stains impart the characteristic basophilic and eosinophilic tinctorial properties usually observed on blood films. Wright's or Wright–Giemsa are commonly used Romanowsky methanolic stains which allow accurate evaluation of the nuclear detail (chromatin pattern, nucleoli), especially important when a neoplastic process is suspected. These stains are also recommended for certain specimens such as bone marrow, splenic and lymph node aspirates where the nuclear features of the cells are crucial in making a cytological diagnosis. Diff-Quik® stain is an aqueous Romanowsky stain, commonly used in veterinary practices because it is easy and quick to use, although it gives poorer cellular and nuclear definition. Diff-Quik® staining is considered sufficient for the evaluation of an inflammatory process and for some basic cytological procedures (e.g. ear and vaginal cytology), although it may not be optimal for the evaluation and classification of neoplastic processes. In general practice the majority of veterinary surgeons (veterinarians) use Diff-Quik® or similar stains, although if the technique is frequently used, Giemsa or MGG staining should be considered (Jorundsson *et al.*, 1999).

Mast cell granules sometimes may not stain well with Diff-Quik®; therefore, if a round cell tumour of unclear origin is suspected, Giemsa or Wright–Giemsa stain should be used to demonstrate the possible presence of these granules (Figure 21.10). Similarly, granules of large granular lymphocytes (LGL) and granules of basophils are also more difficult to visualize with Diff-Quik®. Conversely, intracytoplasmic distemper virus inclusions are better visualized with this stain.

Staining procedures are usually provided with the stain kit, although they can be modified depending on the thickness of the cytological preparation. A thick aspirate from lymph node or bone marrow may require more prolonged staining than a poorly cellular aspirate. Other factors that may influence the staining times are the freshness and the status of preservation of the staining solutions. At the end of the staining process, the smears are usually washed with running water and dried (manually or with an air-dryer) in a vertical position.

Stains must be changed periodically, according to the manufacturer's indications, and cleaned (by filtration) in order to avoid the formation of stain precipitates, which may interfere with cytological examination and interpretation.

Staining quality can be compromised by exposure of the sample to formalin fumes before fixation. This leads to loss of cellular and nuclear detail that often hampers interpretation. Hence, cytology and histopathology samples should be submitted separately to the reference laboratory.

Cytochemical stains

Special chemical stains routinely used in histopathology can also be easily performed on cytology samples. They may be very useful to confirm the origin of cells and the nature of extracellular/intracellular materials. They are usually run by specialized laboratories and can be performed on unstained regular slides. However, pre-stained slides can also be used, commonly after a destaining process (with alcohol, acid or microwave). This has been reported not to alter the quality of the sample and may be a valuable diagnostic strategy when only a few slides or only stained slides are available. Figure 21.11 lists the special stains most commonly used in veterinary cytopathology.

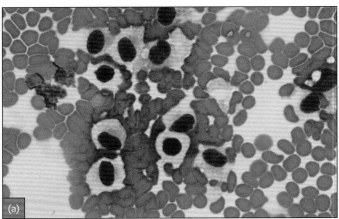
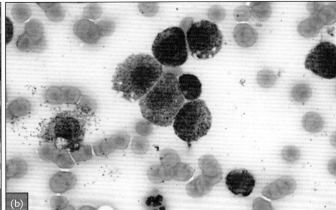

21.10 Fine-needle aspirates from a mediastinal mass in a dog. Some slides were stained with (a) Diff-Quik® and others with (b) Wright–Giemsa. Diff-Quik® failed to stain the mast cell granules, making the cytological interpretation more difficult. (Original magnification X500)

Cytochemical stain	Substance	Appearance (colour)	Main applications
Periodic acid–Schiff	Glycogen, mucin	Magenta	Fungal infection (cell wall), hepatic glycogenosis
Alcian blue	Mucin	Blue	Myxoma/myxosarcoma
Oil red O	Lipid	Red	Lipoma/liposarcoma, hepatic lipidosis
Sudan black	Lipid	Black	Lipoma/liposarcoma, hepatic lipidosis
Rhodanine	Copper	Golden brown to orange	Copper storage
Rubeanic acid	Copper	Black	Copper storage
Ziehl–Neelsen	Acid-fast bacilli (*Mycobacterium* spp.)	Red	Mycobacterial infection
Congo red	Amyloid	Red	Amyloidosis
Mucicarmine	Fungi (glycoprotein coat)	Purple	Fungal infection
Grocott–Gomori	Fungi (glycoprotein coat)	Black	Fungal infection
Von Kossa	Phosphate	Black	Calcinosis cutis
Masson–Fontana	Melanin	Dark brown	Melanocytic tumour
Toluidine blue	Polysaccharides and nucleic acids	Blue (nucleic acids) and purple (polysaccharides)	Mast cell tumour
Prussian blue	Iron	Black	Haemosiderin
Luxol fast blue	Myelin	Blue	Central nervous system

21.11 Common histochemical stains used in veterinary cytopathology.

Immunocytochemistry

Immunocytochemistry (ICC) is used to detect the presence of specific surface cellular proteins on cytological preparations by the use of specific antibodies and is performed by specialized laboratories. Guidelines for sampling for ICC include the following:

- The material obtained by the FNA should be placed on polylysine-coated slides, which enhance the adhesion of cells to the glass surface. These slides are usually provided by the laboratory performing the staining
- Since a panel of antibodies may be used, multiple smears should be submitted (one for each antibody required plus one additional slide for the negative control). Four smears are usually considered sufficient for a basic protocol.

There are two types of immunocytochemical technique (Figure 21.12):

- **Direct technique:** the primary antibody binds to the specific antigen on the cell surface
- **Indirect technique:** a primary antibody binds to the cell antigen. A secondary antibody is then added, which binds to the primary antibody. The secondary antibody is conjugated to a linker molecule such as biotin. Finally, a tertiary reagent is added. This contains an enzymatic substance that reacts with the linker molecule leading to a colour change, showing that the antibody has bound.

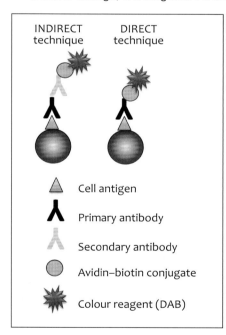

21.12 Direct and indirect techniques for immunocytochemistry. Refer to text for more details. DAB = diaminobenzidine.

INDIRECT technique
DIRECT technique

△ Cell antigen

Y Primary antibody

Y Secondary antibody

◯ Avidin–biotin conjugate

✦ Colour reagent (DAB)

Most methods use biotin conjugated to the secondary antibody. The bound antibody is then exposed to an avidin–biotin conjugate that contains several molecules of biotin bound to horseradish peroxidase. The biotin on the secondary antibody binds to this complex and is detected by the addition of a colour reagent, usually diaminobenzidine (DAB), that is converted into a brown precipitate by peroxidase, which may be observed on microscopic examination. Immunocytochemical staining can be carried out manually or using automated strainers. An example of ICC is shown in Figure 21.13.

Figure 21.14 lists the most common immunocytochemical stains used in veterinary cytopathology.

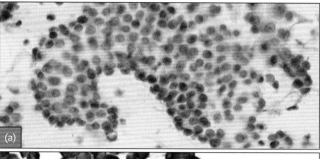

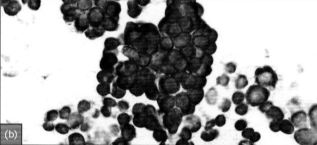

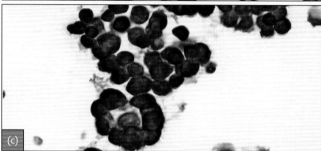

21.13 Immunocytochemistry on a canine pleural mesothelioma. (a) Negative control. (b–c) The plasma membrane of the neoplastic mesothelial cells reacted positively (brown colour) with (b) cytokeratin and (c) vimentin. (Original magnification X500)

Immunocyto-chemical stain	Target	Main applications
Cytokeratin	Epithelial cells	Confirming the epithelial origin of a neoplasm, especially when poorly differentiated
Vimentin	Mesenchymal cells Lymphoid cells	Confirming the mesenchymal origin of a neoplasm, especially when poorly differentiated
CD3	T-lymphoid cells	Immunophenotyping lymphoma/leukaemia
CD79a, CD20	B-lymphoid cells	Immunophenotyping lymphoma/leukaemia
CD18	Lymphoid and histiocytic cells	Confirming the histiocytic origin of a neoplasm
Melan A	Melanocytes	Confirming the diagnosis of melanoma
Desmin	Skeletal and smooth muscle	Confirming the diagnosis of smooth or skeletal muscle (leiomyosarcoma, rhabdomyosarcoma)
Myoglobin	Skeletal and cardiac muscle	Confirming the skeletal muscle origin (rhabdomyosarcoma)
Chromogranin or synaptophysin	Neuroendocrine cells	Confirming the diagnosis of neuroendocrine tumour

21.14 Common immunocytochemical stains used in veterinary cytopathology. CD = cluster of differentiation.

Complications and contraindications of cytology

Complications associated with FNA are infrequent and usually minor. The most common complications during aspirations from superficial masses are minor bleeding and haematoma formation or, less frequently, bacterial infection. Applying manual pressure to the site can prevent or control the bleeding.

FNA of internal organs can lead to complications such as bleeding, pneumothorax, infections and tumour seeding. However, various studies have shown a low rate of complications.

In some specific cases, FNA may be contraindicated. The most common contraindications for FNA, especially of internal organs, are:

- Aspiration from internal organs/lesions of patients with severe thrombocytopenia (platelet count <50 × 10^9/l) (see Chapter 6 for further detail) or a coagulopathy. For this reason, a complete blood count and coagulation times are recommended for patients at high risk of coagulopathy, such as those with liver disease
- Aspiration of highly vascular masses
- Suspected abscesses in internal organs such as the prostate gland
- Percutaneous prostatic or bladder aspiration when a transitional cell carcinoma is suspected.

In human medicine, needle tract seeding of neoplastic cells after aspiration has been associated with a variety of tumours. In veterinary medicine, a few case reports of tumour implantation into the needle tract have been described (bladder transitional cell carcinoma in dogs and pulmonary adenocarcinoma in a dog and a cat; Vignoli *et al.*, 2007). An assessment of risk *versus* benefit should be performed before embarking on aspiration of 'at risk' tumours.

Cytological cell types

Cytology is used to classify the nature of the aspirated lesions into inflammatory, hyperplastic, neoplastic (benign or malignant) or response to tissue injury. The distinction among these categories is simple when the lesion consists of either inflammatory *or* tissue cells, but is more difficult when both inflammatory and tissue cells are aspirated.

Cytology of inflammation

As a general rule, a lesion is classified as inflammatory when all or most of the intact cells are inflammatory cells. Once inflammation has been recognized, the next step is to subclassify the process on the basis of the predominant cell type (e.g. neutrophilic, macrophagic, eosinophilic inflammation) because this provides important clues to the underlying aetiology.

Neutrophilic inflammation

Neutrophilic inflammation is diagnosed when the sample contains more than 85% neutrophils and this is the most common inflammatory pattern seen on cytology. It may be caused by bacterial infection, trauma, or tissue necrosis, e.g. associated with a solid tumour or with pancreatitis.

Once neutrophilic inflammation is recognized, it is very important to evaluate the morphology of the neutrophils, classifying them as degenerate or non-degenerate, because this provides valuable information on the underlying cause of the inflammation.

Non-degenerate neutrophils maintain their typical nuclear lobulation with dense dark purple chromatin (Figure 21.15). These are mostly seen in non-septic inflammation, e.g. caused by immune-mediated diseases, neoplasia or irritants. An exception to this rule is septic arthritis, in which neutrophils often do not show signs of degeneration (see Chapter 23). Prior antibiotic treatment may also mask degenerative change in septic lesions.

Degenerate neutrophils are often associated with bacterial infections or necrosis. Neutrophilic degeneration is caused by the detrimental effect of the bacterial endotoxins (often produced by Gram-negative bacteria) on the nuclear and cytoplasmic membranes, which causes nuclear and cell swelling. Nuclear swelling, also defined as karyolysis, is morphologically recognized by the loss of segmentation and less darkly stained chromatin (Figure 21.16).

Degenerate neutrophils should trigger a careful examination of the slide, searching for bacteria. However, bacteria are not always found in septic inflammation, either

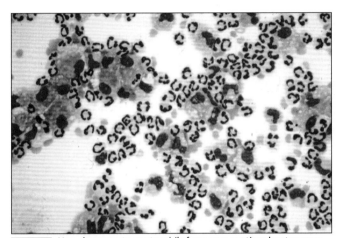

21.15 Non-degenerate neutrophils from non-septic subcutaneous neutrophilic inflammation in a dog. The nuclei of the neutrophils are lobulated and the chromatin is dense and darkly stained. Low numbers of macrophages are also present in the photograph. (Wright–Giemsa stain; original magnification X500)

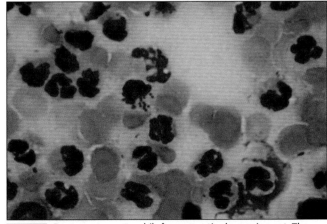

21.16 Degenerate neutrophils from a septic abscess in a cat. The nuclei of the neutrophils are swollen (karyolytic) and have lost the typical lobulation. The chromatin is paler and less condensed. A few intracytoplasmic cocci are seen in a neutrophil. (Wright–Giemsa stain; original magnification X500)

because they are present in low numbers or because the patient has received antibiotics prior to FNA. To confirm septic inflammation, bacteria should be found phagocytosed by neutrophils (see Figure 21.16). If only extracellular bacteria are seen, these could be due to contamination of the sample (depending on the sample site) rather than a true infection.

Other types of neutrophilic degeneration are pyknosis and karyorrhexis. These degenerative cell forms represent cell death due to the ageing of the cells in the tissue. Pyknosis reflects the condensation of the nucleus (apoptosis), which becomes round and very darkly stained. This can fragment, leading to karyorrhexis, which forms small dense nuclear particles (Figure 21.17).

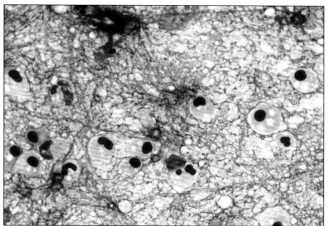

21.17 Pyknotic and karyorrhectic neutrophils from a sterile abscess in a dog. Pyknotic nuclei are round and the chromatin is condensed and deeply basophilic. The fragmentation of pyknotic nuclei is defined as karyorrhexis. (Wright–Giemsa stain; original magnification X500)

Macrophagic inflammation

This type of inflammation is characterized by a predominance of macrophages, which are often activated (Figure 21.18). They have abundant and foamy cytoplasm that may contain amorphous phagosomes (cell fragments, debris or infectious agents). Causes of macrophagic inflammation include foreign body reactions and mycobacterial or fungal infections.

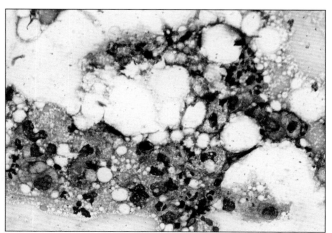

21.18 Fine-needle aspirate from a subcutaneous nodule of a dog with steatitis. Numerous foamy activated macrophages are seen in a background of clear (lipid) vacuoles. Macrophages have abundant cytoplasm containing small clear vacuoles. (Wright–Giemsa stain; original magnification X500)

In chronic macrophagic inflammation, epithelioid and giant multinucleated cells are usually found. This is often referred to as granulomatous inflammation. Formation of granulomas is often the consequence of the inability of the host to eliminate the cause of the inflammation, leading instead to its segregation into a granuloma.

Inflammation composed of a mixture of neutrophils and macrophages is defined as pyogranulomatous inflammation (see Figure 21.15). The differential diagnoses for pyogranulomatous inflammation are similar to those causing a granulomatous inflammation. In more chronic forms, lymphocytes and plasma cells may also be present.

Eosinophilic inflammation

Inflammation is defined as eosinophilic when more than approximately 10% of eosinophils are counted among other inflammatory cells (Figure 21.19). Increased numbers of eosinophils, with or without the concurrent presence of a few mast cells, usually accompany hypersensitivity, parasitic or fungal diseases. A predominance of eosinophils is often found in aspirates from eosinophilic granulomas/plaques and in BAL samples from cats with feline asthma or from dogs with an eosinophilic bronchopneumopathy. Eosinophilic infiltration is also commonly found as a paraneoplastic condition in which the tumour produces specific cytokines such as interleukin (IL)-5. Common causes of paraneoplastic eosinophilic inflammation are mast cell tumours and lymphomas (mainly of T-cell phenotype). Morphologically, these cells are similar to the eosinophils found in the circulation.

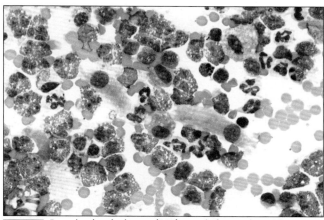

21.19 Bronchoalveolar lavage (BAL) sample from a dog with an eosinophilic bronchopneumopathy (EBP). High numbers of eosinophils and a few columnar respiratory epithelial cells are seen in the preparation. (Wright–Giemsa stain; original magnification X500)

Lymphocytic and lymphocytic–plasmacytic inflammation

In this type of inflammation, a predominance of small lymphocytes is present with varying numbers of plasma cells. Differential diagnoses for this inflammatory pattern include insect bites, recent vaccination and antigenic stimulation (delayed or type IV hypersensitivity). When a pure lymphocytic infiltration is found, the interpretation is more challenging, because small cell lymphoma should be included in the differential diagnosis list.

Cytology of infectious agents

Infectious agents are frequently encountered during the cytological examination of canine and feline samples. They can be broadly classified into bacterial, protozoal, fungal and parasitic infections. The scope of this chapter is to describe the morphological features of the most common aetiological agents found in Europe, and especially in the UK. For the clinical implications of these agents, the reader should refer to specific textbooks.

Bacterial infections

Bacterial infections usually cause a neutrophilic response. With routine staining, bacteria can be classified as rods or cocci, based on their shape (elongated *versus* round) (Figure 21.20). As previously mentioned, the key feature to differentiate a true bacterial infection from sample contamination is the presence of bacteria within the cytoplasm of neutrophils. Most bacteria stain deeply basophilic (whether they are Gram-positive or Gram-negative) with the exception of *Mycobacterium* spp., which typically appear as negatively stained rods within the macrophages (Figure 21.21a). *Nocardia* spp. and *Actinomyces* spp. infections have a characteristic cytological appearance with long branching chains of thin filamentous beaded bacteria (Figure 21.22). These infections may be seen in bite wounds and in cats with pyothorax. *Actinomyces* are anaerobic Gram-positive bacteria that are difficult to culture. *Nocardia* are aerobes and are less fastidious.

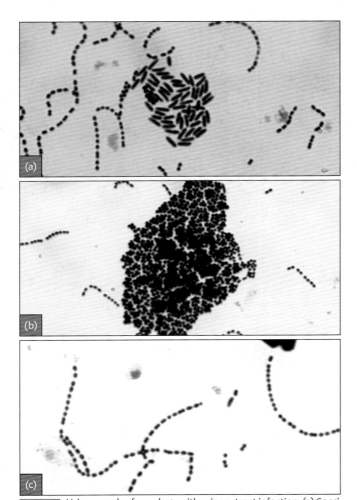

21.20 Urine samples from dogs with urinary tract infection. (a) Cocci and rod-shaped bacteria (bacilli) are visible. (b–c) Round bacteria (cocci) are visible. (b) The bacteria are arranged in a large group, sugggesting *Staphylococcus* spp. (c) The bacteria form chains of variable length, suggesting *Streptococcus* spp. (Wright–Giemsa stain; original magnification X500)

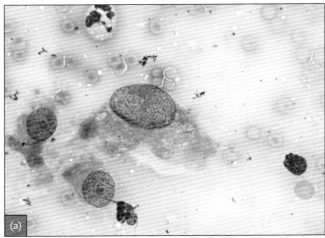

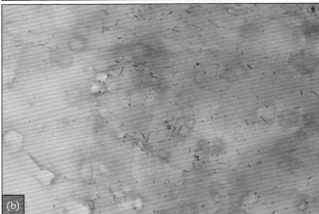

21.21 Sample from a mass on the cheek of a cat. (a) Numerous fine negatively stained rods of mycobacteria are seen within the cytoplasm of a macrophage. (Wright–Giemsa stain; original magnification X500). (b) With acid-fast staining, mycobacteria appear as fine purple rods. (Ziehl–Neelsen; original magnfication X500)

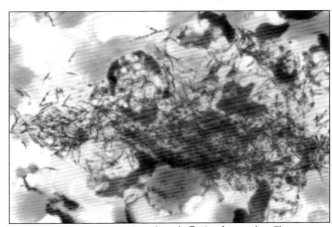

21.22 *Actinomyces* spp. in a pleural effusion from a dog. The filamentous bacterial rods stain lightly basophilic with small purple dots. (Wright–Giemsa stain; original magnification X1000)

Special stains may be used to obtain a preliminary broad subclassification of bacteria:

- **Gram stain:** this may be used prior to culture to aid in the preliminary choice of an antibiotic. This differentiates Gram-positive (e.g. *Clostridium* spp., *Staphylococcus* spp., *Streptococcus* spp.) from Gram-negative bacteria (e.g. *Escherichia coli*, *Salmonella* spp., *Pseudomonas* spp., *Proteus* spp.)

- **Ziehl–Neelsen (ZN; acid-fast):** this is used to confirm a mycobacterial infection (see Figure 21.21b) and may help in the differentiation between *Actinomyces* and *Nocardia* because *Actinomyces* is non-acid-fast, while *Nocardia* is acid-fast when stained using the Fite–Faraco modified ZN stain (Greene *et al.*, 2012).

Fungal and yeast infections

Fungal infections usually elicit a pyogranulomatous or granulomatous inflammation with a variable eosinophilic component. Depending on the specific fungal species, systemic or localized infection can occur.

Different fungal maturation stages can be observed on cytology, but most commonly hyphae and yeast forms are found (Figure 21.23 and Figure 21.24). Hyphae are filamentous structures characterized by a regular width and no constrictions around the septae (Figure 21.23b). Depending on the fungal species, hyphae can variably stain with Romanowsky stains. Some fungi do not stain with routine stains, making their identification more challenging, and histochemical stains such as periodic acid–Schiff (PAS) or Grocott–Gomori stain may be used to facilitate their identification.

Yeasts are unicellular fungi and do not grow as hyphae although some, such as *Candida* spp., may become multicellular when the yeast cells undergo cell division without becoming detached from adjacent cells, and form pseudohyphae. These are elongated chains of cells with clear constriction at septation sites (Figure 21.23a). Unicellular yeasts appear as spherical or oval structures surrounded by a variably thick capsule (Figure 21.23cd).

Recently, *Pneumocystis* spp. has been classified as a fungus. This pathogen is responsible for causing a pneumomycosis in immune-compromised dogs and is reported in Cavalier King Charles Spaniels and Dachshunds with an inherited immunodeficiency. Small trophozoites and cysts are seen in BAL smears (Figure 21.25).

Protozoal and parasitic infections

The most common protozoal infections are toxoplasmosis (Figure 21.26), neosporosis, cytauxzoonosis and leishmaniosis (Figure 21.27). These infectious agents most commonly elicit a mixed but predominantly macrophagic inflammatory response.

Examples of parasites that may be found on cytological preparations include *Dirofilaria immitis* (Figure 21.28a) and *D. repens* (Figure 21.28b), *Angiostrongylus* (Figure 21.29) and *Aelurostrongylus* spp. The inflammation caused by these parasites is variable but is usually mixed, with or without an eosinophilic component.

Response to injury

Haemorrhage within tissues must be distinguished from blood contamination caused by the sampling process (Figure 21.30). In both situations there are numerous red blood cells in the background. Platelets are not observed in true haemorrhage, because they rapidly disintegrate, but they are usually identified with blood contamination. Moreover, macrophages are observed in true haemorrhage and these often display erythrophagia (engulfed intact red blood cells; Figure 21.31a). In time, the macrophages degrade the erythrocytes, leading to the formation of haemosiderin and then later haematoidin crystals in the cytoplasm (Figure 21.31bc).

Another example of the tissue response to injury is scar tissue formation. This is seen as proliferation of spindle cells (fibroblasts and fibrovascular cells) as part of the wound healing process (Figure 21.32). Cytologically, these cells may be difficult to distinguish from dysplastic/neoplastic mesenchymal cells because these display similar morphological features. In this situation, clinical history plays an important role in the interpretation.

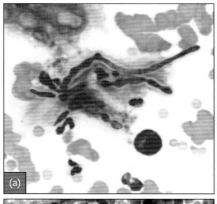
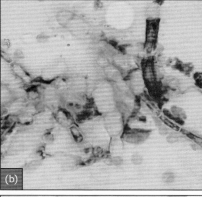
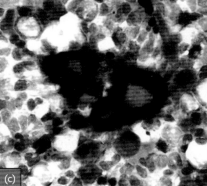
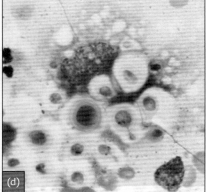
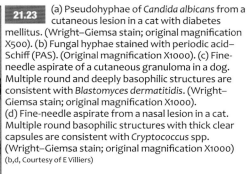

21.23 (a) Pseudohyphae of *Candida albicans* from a cutaneous lesion in a cat with diabetes mellitus. (Wright–Giemsa stain; original magnification X500). (b) Fungal hyphae stained with periodic acid–Schiff (PAS). (Original magnification X1000). (c) Fine-needle aspirate of a cutaneous granuloma in a dog. Multiple round and deeply basophilic structures are consistent with *Blastomyces dermatitidis*. (Wright–Giemsa stain; original magnification X1000). (d) Fine-needle aspirate from a nasal lesion in a cat. Multiple round basophilic structures with thick clear capsules are consistent with *Cryptococcus* spp. (Wright–Giemsa stain; original magnification X1000)
(b,d, Courtesy of E Villiers)

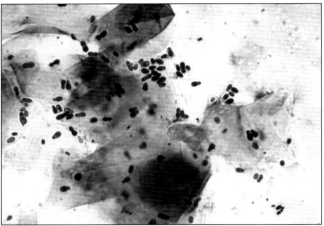

21.24 Ear swab preparation from a dog with otitis externa. Numerous peanut-shaped basophilic yeasts consistent with *Malassezia* spp. are seen in this sample. (Wright–Giemsa stain; original magnification X500)

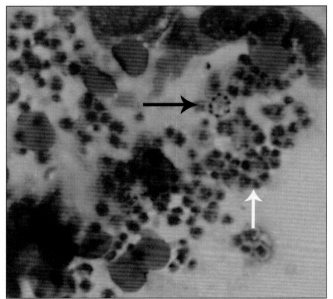

21.25 BAL sample from a young Cavalier King Charles Spaniel with interstitial pneumonia secondary to *Pneumocystis* spp. Multiple trophozoites (white arrow) and a cyst (black arrow) are present. Inexperienced cytologists can easily confuse the trophozoites with platelets. (Wright–Giemsa stain; original magnification X500)

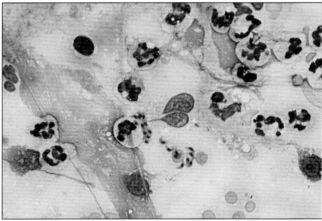

21.26 BAL sample from a cat with respiratory signs. *Toxoplasma* tachyzoites are seen in the centre of the picture. These are 'banana-shaped' bodies with a lightly basophilic cytoplasm and a deeply staining nucleus. (Wright–Giemsa stain; original magnification X1000)

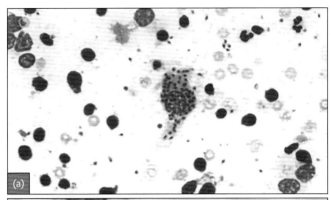

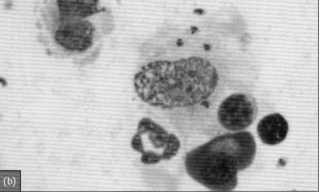

21.27 *Leishmania* organisms in (a) lymph node and (b) bone marrow aspirates from a dog. *Leishmania* amastigotes are seen within the macrophages or free in the background. They measure approximately 2–4 μm and are oval with a small purple nucleus and a small rod-shaped kinetoplast. (Wright–Giemsa stain; original magnification (a) X500 and (b) X1000)

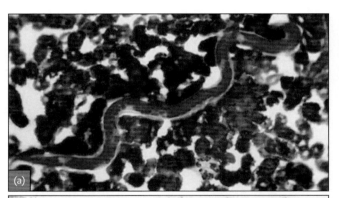

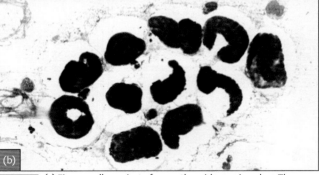

21.28 (a) Fine-needle aspirate from a thyroid mass in a dog. The background is heavily haemodiluted and contains a blood-derived microfilarium (*Dirofilaria immitis*). No thyroid tissue is present in this image. (b) Fine-needle aspirate from a skin nodule in a dog. Several round structures containing small larvae are consistent with *Dirofilaria repens* 'egg cells'. (Wright–Giemsa stain; original magnification (a) X500 and (b) X1000)

(a, Courtesy of I Lloverals, CV AMVET)

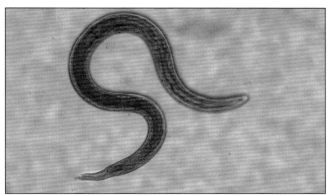

21.29 Wet faecal preparation from a dog with lungworm infection (*Angiostrongylus vasorum*). Note the kinked tail typical of this parasite (extremity on the left). (Original magnification X1000)

Pre-existing haemorrhage
• Numerous red blood cells
• No platelets
• Acute haemorrhage:
• Macrophages showing erythrophagia
• Chronic haemorrhage:
• Macrophages containing haemosiderin
• Macrophages containing haematoidin crystals

Blood contamination at sampling
• Numerous red blood cells
• Platelets
• No erythrophagia, haemosiderin or haematoidin

21.30 The main characteristics that help to differentiate between blood contamination and pre-existing haemorrhage.

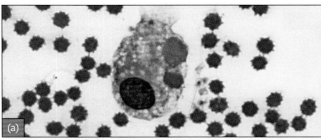

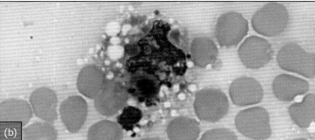

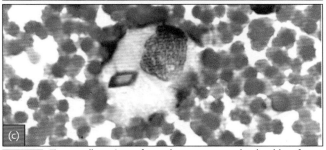

21.31 Fine-needle aspirates from a haematoma on the shoulder of a dog. Macrophages display (a) erythrophagia, or (b) contain basophilic amorphous material (haemosiderin) or (c) rhomboid orange crystals (haematoidin). (Wright–Giemsa stain; original magnification X500)

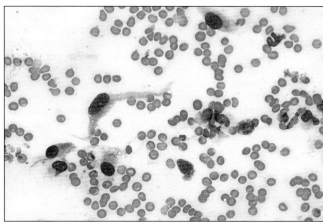

21.32 Fine-needle aspirate from a surgical scar of a dog. Fusiform mesenchymal cells represent reactive fibroblasts involved in the wound healing process. (Wright–Giemsa stain; original magnification X1000)

Cytology of non-inflammatory lesions

When cells other than inflammatory cells are aspirated, the cytologist should try to categorize them into the three major cytological groups, epithelial, mesenchymal and round cells, and then to subclassify the lesion as benign or malignant, or possibly hyperplastic (hyperplasia can be difficult to distinguish from benign neoplasia). When doing so, signalment, history and clinical presentation should always be considered, as these can give vital clues.

There are significant morphological and architectural differences among these three cell types, and knowing their typical features helps in recognizing the tissue of origin (Figure 21.33).

Cell type	Features	Morphology
Epithelial tumours	• High cellularity • Cohesive sheets	• Cuboidal, polygonal, columnar • Well defined margins • Round nuclei
Mesenchymal tumours	• Often poor cellularity • Individual cells or non-cohesive aggregates	• Spindle, plump-oval, stellate • Often poorly defined cell borders • Round to oval nuclei
Round cell tumours	• High cellularity • Individual cells	• Round or oval • Well defined cell borders • Generally round nuclei

21.33 The main morphological features of the three cytological tumour cell types: epithelial, mesenchymal and round cells.

Epithelial cells

Epithelia usually exfoliate cells in sheets or cohesive clusters and the cellularity of the sample is usually moderate to high. A feature of all epithelial lesions is the cell-to-cell adhesion. Cell borders are usually well defined and the junction between contiguous cells may appear as a thin and light line (tight junction; Figure 21.34). Nuclei are generally round. Depending on the organ or tissue of origin, epithelial cells are arranged in different architectural patterns and have different morphology.

Epithelial cells are subdivided into squamous, cuboidal, columnar (ciliated or non-ciliated; Figure 21.35) or transitional cells. The most typical cell arrangements are pavement, acinar, honeycomb, papillary, palisade and trabecular (Figure 21.36).

It is important to keep in mind that in less differentiated tumours these classical features may be lost, making it more difficult to recognize the cell type.

Aspirates from endocrine and neuroendocrine tumours usually exfoliate numerous cells. These cells are characterized by having poorly defined cytoplasmic borders and often appear as bare nuclei embedded in a lightly basophilic background of cytoplasmic material. This typical feature is associated with the particular fragility of these

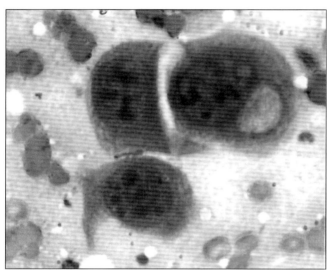

21.34 Fine-needle aspirate from a lymph node with a metastatic prostatic carcinoma. Malignant neoplastic epithelial cells are intimately cohesive. The clear line separating the two contiguous epithelial cells represents the tight junction. (Wright–Giemsa stain; original magnification X1000)

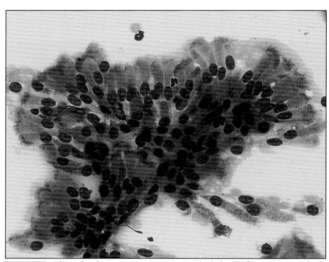

21.35 Ciliated columnar respiratory epithelial cells from the nasal mucosa of a cat. (Wright–Giemsa stain; original magnification X1000)

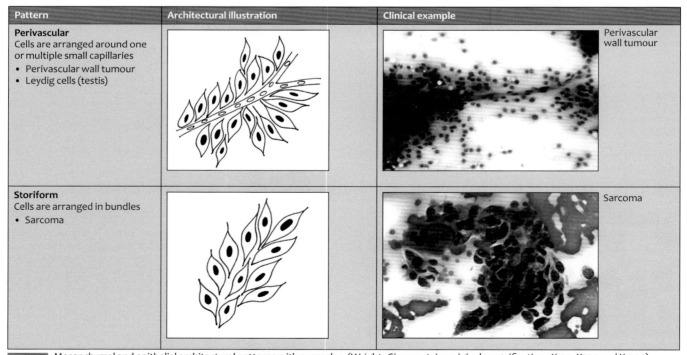

Pattern	Architectural illustration	Clinical example
Perivascular Cells are arranged around one or multiple small capillaries • Perivascular wall tumour • Leydig cells (testis)		Perivascular wall tumour
Storiform Cells are arranged in bundles • Sarcoma		Sarcoma

21.36 Mesenchymal and epithelial architectural patterns with examples. (Wright–Giemsa stain; original magnifications X100, X500 and X1000) (continues)

(Illustrations by Paola Monti)

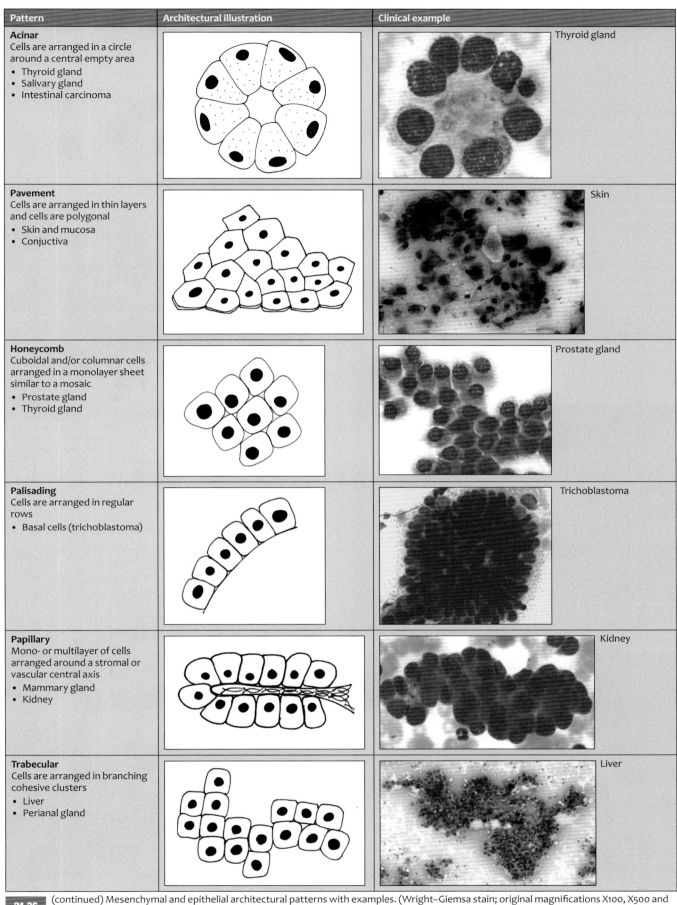

Pattern	Architectural illustration	Clinical example
Acinar Cells are arranged in a circle around a central empty area • Thyroid gland • Salivary gland • Intestinal carcinoma		Thyroid gland
Pavement Cells are arranged in thin layers and cells are polygonal • Skin and mucosa • Conjuctiva		Skin
Honeycomb Cuboidal and/or columnar cells arranged in a monolayer sheet similar to a mosaic • Prostate gland • Thyroid gland		Prostate gland
Palisading Cells are arranged in regular rows • Basal cells (trichoblastoma)		Trichoblastoma
Papillary Mono- or multilayer of cells arranged around a stromal or vascular central axis • Mammary gland • Kidney		Kidney
Trabecular Cells are arranged in branching cohesive clusters • Liver • Perianal gland		Liver

21.36 (continued) Mesenchymal and epithelial architectural patterns with examples. (Wright–Giemsa stain; original magnifications X100, X500 and X1000)

(Illustrations by Paola Monti)

cells, which tend to be disrupted upon aspiration and smearing (Figure 21.37). In spite of having a malignant behaviour, tumours such as thyroid carcinoma or phaeochromocytoma do not usually display many features of malignancy and the cells appear bland and generally uniform (Figure 21.38).

Mesenchymal cells

In contrast to epithelial cells, mesenchymal cells tend not to form cohesive clusters, although they can be found in variably dense aggregates or individually. The classical mesenchymal architectural arrangements are storiform and perivascular (see Figure 21.36). The presence of abundant extracellular matrix within the aspirated tissue can lead to cell aggregation but also reduces cell exfoliation. Mesenchymal lesions are in fact characterized by a small to moderate cell harvest, although cellularity is higher in malignant mesenchymal tumours. Mesenchymal cells have different morphology depending on the tissue of origin. Some mesenchymal cells are spindle shaped, fusiform or stellate (e.g. fibroblasts/fibrocytes) and have oval nuclei and two cytoplasmic tails extending from each pole of the nucleus (Figure 21.39a). Others are oval (e.g. osteoblasts, chrondroblasts) and have round to oval eccentric nuclei. Cytoplasmic borders are often fuzzy and poorly defined. In poorly differentiated malignant mesenchymal tumours the cells may become larger and rounded (Figure 21.39b).

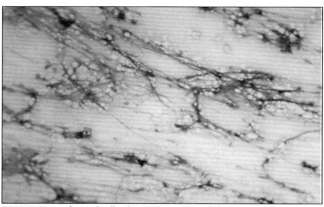

21.37 Artefactual cells: disruption occurred during smearing. (Wright–Giemsa stain; original magnification X200)

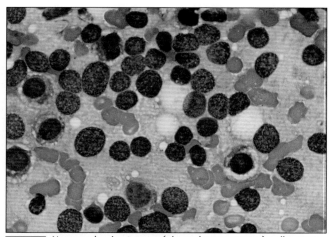

21.38 Neuroendocrine tumour (phaeochromocytoma): cells occur as bare nuclei embedded in a lightly basophilic background of cytoplasmic material. (Wright–Giemsa stain; original magnification X1000)

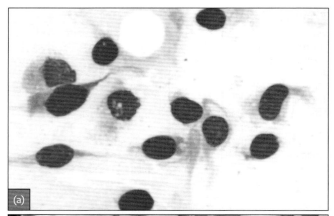

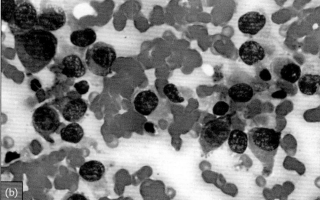

21.39 (a) Fine-needle aspirate from a well differentiated soft tissue sarcoma in a dog. Cells are fusiform with two slim cytoplasmic tails and do not display atypical features. (b) Poorly differentiated sarcoma in a dog. Cells are oval, plump and display moderate anisokaryosis, a high nuclear:cytoplasmic (N:C) ratio and prominent nucleoli. (Wright–Giemsa stain; original magnification X500)

Round cells (discrete cells)

Examples of round cells are lymphocytes, plasma cells, histiocytes and mast cells. These cells are not cohesive, so they exfoliate well and smears are usually very cellular, consisting of numerous individual round or oval cells with round to oval, occasionally convoluted nuclei. Cell margins are very distinct (Figure 21.40). These tumour types are discussed in more detail later in the chapter.

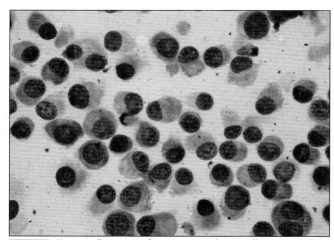

21.40 Fine-needle aspirate from a canine plasma cell tumour. Cells are discrete with an eccentric nucleus and basophilic cytoplasm. (Wright–Giemsa stain; original magnification X500)
(Courtesy of E Villiers)

Hyperplasia

Hyperplasia of an organ or tissue is associated with increased numbers of cells due to increased mitotic division and is usually caused by excessive hormonal stimulation or chronic irritation. Hyperplastic tissues are difficult to recognize on cytology because hyperplastic cells are morphologically similar to normal cells. The diagnosis is often obtained by integrating the cytology results with the clinical history and signalment.

A few subtle features may be observed in hyperplastic cells, such as slightly increased nuclear:cytoplasmic (N:C) ratio and slightly more basophilic cytoplasm. The most common example of hormone-dependent hyperplasia is benign prostatic hyperplasia (BPH) in entire male dogs. Aspirates show sheets of epithelial cells arranged in a honeycomb pattern (see Figure 21.36). The cells are similar in size and have uniform nuclei. They are columnar but may appear cuboidal when observed in a transverse plane. Their nuclei are medium sized, round and basal. The chromatin is stippled and one small round nucleolus may occasionally be seen. The cytoplasm is lightly basophilic and may contain small clear punctate vacuoles (Figure 21.41).

thought to be associated with a loss of contact inhibition by neoplastic cells. Decreased cohesiveness is usually caused by downregulation of the cellular adhesion molecules. Cytologically, crowded cells are characterized by having less cytoplasm visible between the nuclei or by displaying nuclear moulding (the nucleus of a cell being deformed by the nucleus of another cell; Figure 21.42).

Loss of cell cohesion (Figure 21.43a) is usually associated with the increased exfoliative nature of some malignant tumours (hypercellularity). Additionally, while normal cells tend to form very uniform and tidy clusters, neoplastic cells often display haphazard and irregular arrangements (Figure 21.43b). Other general criteria of malignancy are pleomorphism (increased variation in cell morphology) and cytomegaly (the presence of cells that are significantly larger than other cells from the same population).

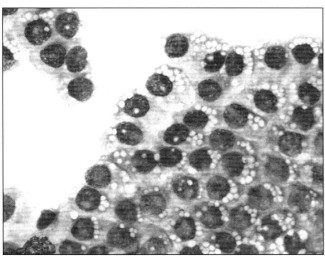

21.41 Fine-needle aspirate from an enlarged prostate gland in an entire adult dog. Numerous uniform epithelial cells with small round nuclei and granular chromatin are seen. The cytoplasm contains many clear punctate vacuoles. (Wright–Giemsa stain; original magnification X500)

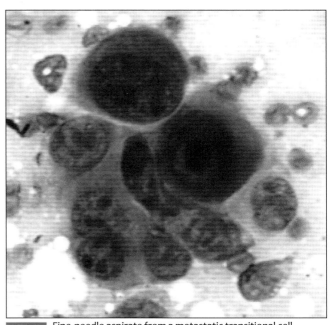

21.42 Fine-needle aspirate from a metastatic transitional cell carcinoma in a dog. Nuclear moulding is displayed in the centre of the picture where the nucleus of a cell is deforming the nucleus of a contiguous cell. (Wright–Giemsa stain; original magnification X1000)

Criteria of malignancy

On light microscopy, neoplastic cells often, but not always, display morphological alterations if compared with the 'normal' cells from which they derive. These morphological features are referred to as criteria of malignancy and include abnormal architectural features as well as nuclear or cytoplasmic abnormalities.

Tissue architectural abnormalities and general criteria of malignancy

In histopathology, but also in cytology, extremely important information can be obtained by closely examining the cell arrangement. The alterations in tissue organization that are most easily identified on cytology include cell crowding and loss of cell cohesion. Cell crowding is

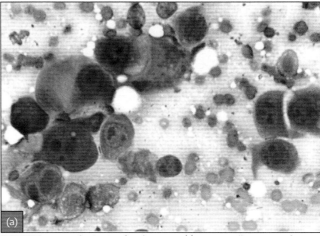

21.43 General criteria of malignancy. (a) Fine-needle aspirate from a transitional cell carcinoma. The neoplastic epithelial cells are arranged in loosely cohesive clusters. (Wright–Giemsa stain; original magnification X500) (continues) ▶

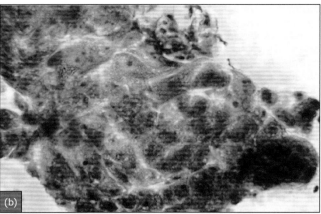

21.43 (continued) General criteria of malignancy. (b) Fine-needle aspirate from a hepatocellular carcinoma. Atypical cells are arranged in disorganized clusters. (Wright–Giemsa stain; original magnification X500)
(Courtesy of E Villiers)

Nuclear criteria of malignancy

Malignant features at a nuclear level are considered to be more reliable because these are less likely to be influenced by non-neoplastic processes such as inflammation. The nuclear criteria of malignancy include:

- Anisokaryosis (nuclear size variation)
- Variable to high N:C ratio
- Multinucleation
- Karyomegaly (enlarged nuclei)
- Increased and/or abnormal mitotic figures (Figure 21.44)
- Irregular or thickened nuclear membrane with blebbing
- Coarse and/or variable chromatin pattern
- Large, single or multiple, irregular, variably sized, and angular nucleoli. One small nucleolus may be visible in some non-neoplastic cells such as hepatocytes.

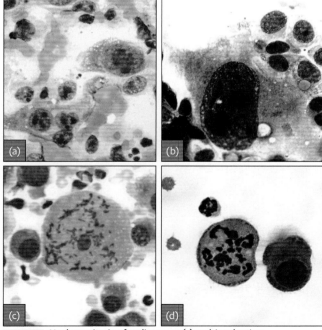

21.44 Nuclear criteria of malignancy: (a) multinucleation, (a–b) anisokaryosis and prominent multiple nucleoli, (c–d) atypical mitotic figures. (Wright–Giemsa stain; original magnification X500)

Cytoplasmic criteria of malignancy

These include:

- Increased cytoplasmic basophilia
- Asynchronous nuclear and cytoplasmic maturation
- Loss of characteristic features of that cell line
- Abnormal vacuolation.

Neoplastic cells usually have basophilic cytoplasm. This reflects an increased amount of rough endoplasmic reticulum and ribosomes as a consequence of the active protein synthesis necessary for rapid cell growth.

Asynchronous nuclear and cytoplasmic maturation is commonly seen in SCC. In this tumour, cells often have an immature and relatively large nucleus with immature chromatin and a mature cytoplasm characterized by being abundant and lightly basophilic (partially keratinized cytoplasm). In other types of tumour, the cytoplasm exhibits loss of the characteristic features of that cell line. For example, poorly differentiated mast cell tumours contain fewer magenta granules.

Increased cytoplasmic vacuolation is observed in some degenerating neoplastic cells as a result of hydropic or lipid degeneration. Occasionally, malignant epithelial tumours of glandular origin can have a large single vacuole deforming the nucleus (signet ring; Figure 21.45), which probably forms as a consequence of the coalescence of intracytoplasmic vacuoles.

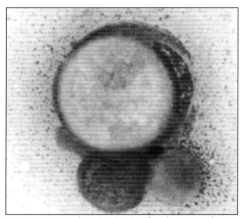

21.45 Cytoplasmic criteria of malignancy: the cytoplasm contains a large vacuole of secretory material, which deforms and displaces the nucleus to the periphery (signet ring). Canine prostatic carcinoma. (Wright–Giemsa stain; original magnification X1000)

The approach to slide examination

These steps should be followed when examining a cytological slide:

- Look at the slide with the naked eye: aim for the blue areas (this is where the cells are)
- Scan the slide at low power (X100) first; this helps in finding the cells and appreciating their organization
- Establish whether cellularity and preservation are adequate; if there are only a few cells or they are all disrupted, an accurate cytological interpretation is often prevented
- Evaluate the background (haematic, proteinaceous)
- Identify the cell types present. Follow a logical approach as outlined in Figure 21.46.

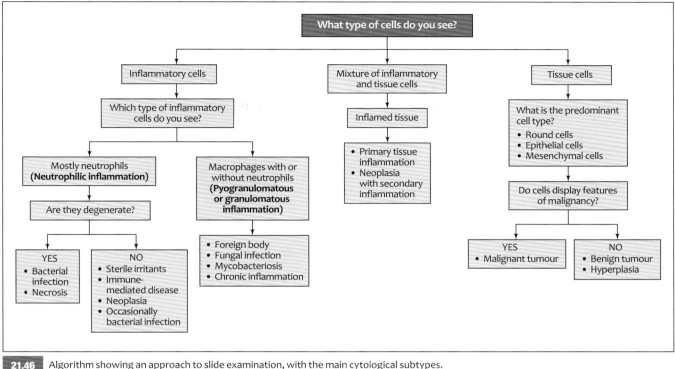

21.46 Algorithm showing an approach to slide examination, with the main cytological subtypes.

Skin cytology

The skin is the largest organ in the body. There are three different skin layers, the epidermis, dermis and subcutis. The epidermis is composed of squamous epithelium at different maturation stages, from the deeper basal stratum to the most superficial keratinized layer. Basal cells are characterized by being relatively small with a high N:C ratio. As the cells mature and move to the surface of the skin, the volume of cytoplasm progressively increases and the size of the nucleus decreases. Mature squamous epithelial cells (also known as keratinocytes) are polygonal/angular and have abundant lightly basophilic cytoplasm. They contain a small central nucleus, which progressively becomes pyknotic. When fully keratinized, these cells become anucleated.

The dermis is made of connective tissue and contains blood and lymphatic vessels, nerves and skin appendages. The skin adnexal structures are hair follicles and sweat and sebaceous glands. The subcutis is composed of adipose tissue and collagen.

Non-neoplastic skin lesions
Epidermal inclusion cyst

These are single or multiple cutaneous lesions that consist of an accumulation of keratin material with a cystic wall. Older animals are more prone to developing these lesions. Cytologically they are easily recognized by an abundance of anucleated squamous epithelial cells (Figure 21.47), keratin shards and cholesterol crystals (Figure 21.48). Nucleated cells are generally absent. These are benign lesions and do not cause clinical problems unless the cyst wall ruptures, causing the exposure of keratin to the surrounding tissue and leading to a localized chronic pyogranulomatous response. In this case, surgical excision is required and is curative.

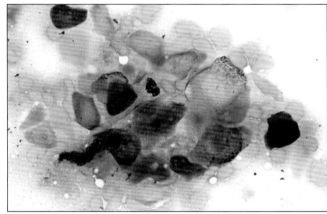

21.47 Fine-needle aspirate from an epidermal inclusion cyst on the back of a dog. Numerous anucleate squamous epithelial cells are present. (Wright–Giemsa stain; original magnification X1000)

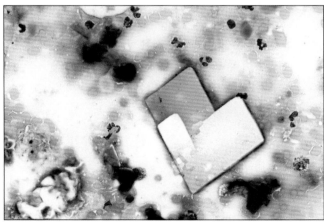

21.48 Epidermal inclusion cyst. A large polygonal negatively stained structure consistent with a cholesterol crystal is present. (Wright–Giemsa stain; original magnification X1000)

Apocrine cyst

The formation is caused by the occlusion of the pore of a sweat gland. Aspirates from these lesions are usually acellular or may be slightly haemodiluted. The prognosis is very good after surgical removal.

Neoplasia

The tumours that can be found in the skin of domestic animals are classified as epithelial, mesenchymal and round cell tumours.

Epithelial tumours

Squamous cell carcinoma: SCC is a common tumour in domestic animals and accounts for 5% of skin tumours in dogs and 15% in cats. The anatomical location varies between these two species. In dogs, common sites include the nail bed, scrotum, nasal planum, anus and legs. In cats, SCCs arise more frequently in lightly pigmented, poorly haired areas such as the nasal planum, eyelids and pinnae, and progress within areas of actinic keratosis (skin thickening), which is associated with sun exposure.

Macroscopically, SCCs may present as ulcerative or proliferative lesions (Figure 21.49a). FNA or scraping of these tumours yields a population of epithelial cells in variably cohesive sheets, or individual cells. Care should be taken to obtain a representative sample of the deep tissue because aspiration of superficial layers may yield only neutrophils and other inflammatory cells, sometimes with bacteria, reflecting superficial inflammation/infection.

Depending on the degree of differentiation of the tumour, neoplastic cells are variably large and show a variable N:C ratio. Well differentiated SCCs exfoliate a predominance of mature keratinocytes that are usually large and have a variable amount of dense and lightly to moderately basophilic cytoplasm with clearly defined borders (Figure 21.49b). Fully keratinized squames lacking nuclei are also seen. Nuclei are pleomorphic and often have irregular contours. They may undergo degeneration and become pyknotic. Nucleoli are poorly visible.

In less differentiated SCCs, most of the cells are round to oval and have an increased N:C ratio (Figure 21.50). Bizarre shapes can be found such as tadpole-shaped cells (Figure 21.51). The cytoplasm is scant to moderate and generally moderately basophilic. The nuclei are larger

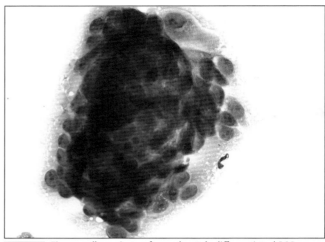

21.50 Fine-needle aspirate of a moderately differentiated SCC. Compared with the cells shown in Figure 21.49b, these cells display a higher N:C ratio and the cytoplasm is more deeply basophilic. Nucleoli are prominent. (Wright–Giemsa stain; original magnification X500)

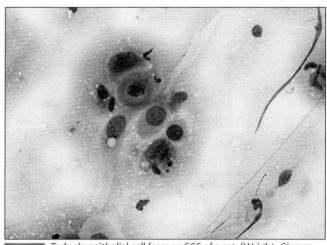

21.51 Tadpole epithelial cell from an SCC of a cat. (Wright–Giemsa stain; original magnification X500)

and the chromatin is irregular. In these cells, nucleoli are often multiple, prominent and variably sized. Asynchrony of the nuclear and cytoplasmic maturation can also be found (large active nuclei in a mature abundant cytoplasm).

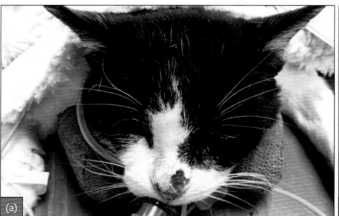

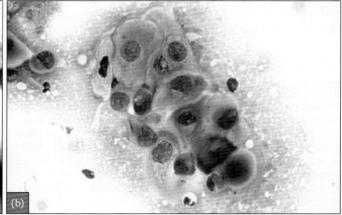

21.49 (a) Squamous cell carcinoma on the nose of a cat. (b) The neoplastic cells appear well differentiated and have abundant lightly basophilic cytoplasm. Small punctate perinuclear keratohyaline vacuoles can be observed in most of these cells. (Wright–Giemsa stain; original magnification X1000)
(a, ©D Berlato, AHT)

Squamous epithelial cells may also contain small punctate and clear perinuclear vacuoles, which represent keratohyalin accumulation. Cellular aggregates of concentric layers of cells are occasionally found in aspirates from SCCs (pearls). Emperipolesis is another common finding. This consists of the passive penetration of one cell (usually a neutrophil) within a neoplastic epithelial cell (Figure 21.52).

The diagnosis of SCCs can sometimes be difficult. False positive results may occur with non-neoplastic inflammatory cutaneous lesions, because dysplastic changes in squamous cells caused by the inflammatory process may be erroneously interpreted as neoplastic features. Epidermal ulceration or necrosis of the centre of a SCC may cause neutrophilic inflammation, leading to a similar cytological picture. Hence, the combination of inflammatory cells and atypical squamous cells should be interpreted cautiously. Well differentiated SCCs can be difficult to identify cytologically because the squamous cells appear only mildly atypical, leading to false negative results.

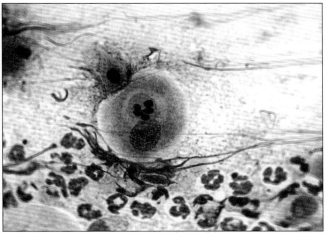

21.52 Emperipolesis in an aspirate from a feline SCC. A neutrophil is transiting within the cytoplasm of a squamous epithelial cell. (Wright–Giemsa stain; original magnification X500)

Trichoblastoma (basal cell tumour): Trichoblastoma is a benign tumour of the follicular germinative cells, previously classified as basal cell tumour. This is the most common cutaneous neoplasm in cats (15–26% of all skin tumours) and is less frequent in dogs (4–12%). Adult dogs and older cats are predisposed. Trichoblastomas are usually small and solitary well circumscribed masses, which have a predilection for the head, neck and shoulders.

Cytologically, trichoblastomas are characterized by exfoliating variably sized and highly cohesive sheets of cuboidal epithelial cells, which often show a typical palisading arrangement in rows (see Figure 21.36). These epithelial cells are uniform in size and shape, showing minimal anisokaryosis and anisocytosis. The nuclei are small to medium sized and are round and centrally placed. The chromatin is condensed and nucleoli are generally indistinct. Only occasionally, a small central and poorly visible, round nucleolus may be seen. The cytoplasm is scant and is lightly to moderately basophilic (Figure 21.53). Occasionally, fine dark granules are seen in the cytoplasm (melanin). The vast majority of these tumours are benign and surgical excision is generally curative. However, the malignant counterpart has rarely been described.

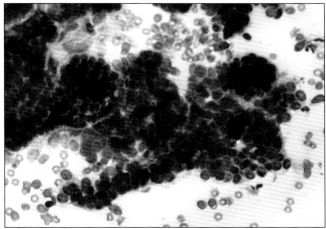

21.53 Cohesive cluster of uniform basal cells from a trichoblastoma on the neck of a dog. At the edges of these clusters, cells are arranged in rows (palisades). (Wright–Giemsa stain; original magnification X500)

Histopathology is required to confirm the origin of these cutaneous tumours and to differentiate them from other less common neoplasms such as trichoepithelioma or pilomatricoma.

Sebaceous glands tumours: Sebaceous glands are present in the skin of mammals and are associated with the hair follicle, where they release sebum. Tumours arising from these glands are sebaceous gland hyperplasia, sebaceous gland adenoma or carcinoma and sebaceous epithelioma. Sebaceous gland tumours are common in dogs (6.8–7.9% of all skin tumours) and less frequent in cats (2.3–4.4%). Sebaceous hyperplasia and adenoma macroscopically appear as single or multiple masses, often raised and multilobulated (Figure 21.54a).

Cytologically, sebaceous hyperplasia cannot be differentiated from sebaceous adenoma but this differentiation is not clinically significant, as both carry a good prognosis with surgical excision being considered curative. Sebaceous epithelial cells often exfoliate in tridimensional clusters and are very cohesive (Figure 21.54b). The cells typically have a low N:C ratio and cell boundaries are well demarcated. The nuclei are small, round and central. The chromatin is often dense or sometimes finely stippled. Occasionally, a small central and round nucleolus can be appreciated. The cytoplasm is abundant and is heavily vacuolated. The vacuoles are discrete, often small and clear. On histological examination, sebaceous hyperplasia appears more common than sebaceous adenoma. In dogs, both can be found anywhere on the body but they are more frequent on the limbs, thorax and eyelids, and some breeds, including Cocker Spaniel, Miniature Schnauzer and Poodle, are over-represented.

Sebaceous epithelioma is a benign sebaceous gland tumour classified by the World Health Organization as a low grade malignant neoplasm. It has a predilection for the head and is more frequently seen in breeds such as the Shih Tzu, Lhasa Apso, Alaskan Malamute, Siberian Husky and Irish Setter. On aspiration, this tumour yields a predominance of reserve germinal epithelial cells and fewer mature sebocytes. Germinal cells exfoliate in cohesive clusters and are morphologically similar to basal cells. They are often uniform in size and are cuboidal. Their N:C ratio is high and nuclei are small and centrally placed. The cytoplasm is scant and lightly to moderately basophilic. Germinal cells may contain melanin. Recurrence is uncommon after surgical excision.

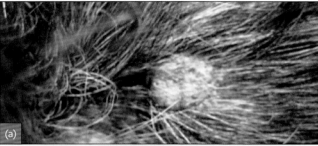

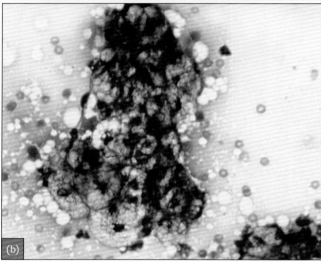

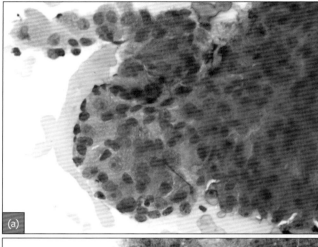

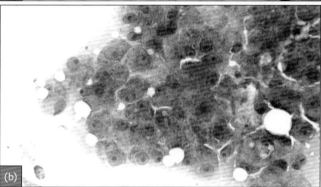

21.54 (a) Macroscopic appearance of a sebaceous adenoma. These tumours are often raised, multilobulated and hairless. (b) Microscopic appearance of a sebaceous adenoma. Epithelial cells have abundant and heavily vacuolated cytoplasm. Vacuoles are discrete and clear. These cells often exfoliate in tridimensional balls. (Wright–Giemsa stain; original magnification X500) (a, © D Berlato, AHT)

21.55 (a) Fine-needle aspirate of a perianal gland tumour from a mass on the tail base of an entire male Labrador Retriever. Cells have exfoliated in uniform sheets and display minimal cell size variation. These cells are also known as hepatoid cells given their similarity to (b) hepatocytes. (Wright–Giemsa stain; original magnification X500)

Sebaceous adenocarcinomas are rare and are usually solitary masses, often poorly circumscribed and ulcerated. On cytology, they display morphological features typical of the tissue of origin but the cells show nuclear atypia such as anisokaryosis, prominent nucleoli and frequent mitoses. These tumours are locally invasive but rarely metastasize.

Perianal gland tumours: Perianal glands are modified sebaceous glands that are also known as hepatoid glands because of the morphological similarity of these cells to hepatocytes (Figure 21.55). These glands are exclusively found in dogs. Their primary location is in the perianal area but they may also be found on the tail, hindlimbs, ventral abdomen, prepuce and lumbar area.

Perianal glands may undergo hyperplasia or become neoplastic. Benign tumours are more frequent than the malignant counterpart. Entire males are more susceptible, suggesting an androgen dependency. In entire male dogs, an increased incidence of these tumours has been proposed in association with the presence of androgen-secreting testicular tumours such as interstitial cell tumour and seminoma. Perianal gland tumours have also been described in neutered male dogs and females, especially if spayed.

On cytology, sheets of cohesive epithelial cells, often uniform in size, are seen. These cells have abundant cytoplasm so that the N:C ratio is typically low. The cytoplasm is lightly to moderately basophilic or amphophilic and finely granular. The nuclei are small to medium sized and are round and central. The chromatin is often reticular,

and one small round central nucleolus may be seen (Figure 21.55a). Occasionally, low numbers of smaller cuboidal cells (reserve cells) may be seen.

The prognosis for perianal gland adenomas is good and surgical excision is often curative. Castration is also recommended given the suspected hormonal dependency of this tumour.

Perianal gland adenocarcinomas are infrequent but have been described. Cells often exfoliate in more disorganized sheets and display increased morphological variability. Nuclear atypia and increased or variable N:C ratio is observed. Histopathology is recommended for confirmation of the diagnosis.

Anal sac tumours (apocrine anal sac adenocarcinoma): Tumours of the anal sac are uncommon in dogs and rare in cats. Anal sac adenocarcinomas (ASCs) account for 2% of canine skin tumours, but their importance should not be underestimated, considering the extremely locally invasive behaviour and the metastatic rate of up to 95%. Additionally, approximately 25–50% of ASCs are associated with paraneoplastic hypercalcaemia and consequent clinical signs of polydipsia and polyuria. Hypercalcaemia can lead to renal failure.

On FNA, these tumours exfoliate large sheets of epithelial cells that are often arranged in papillary or occasionally acinar structures. The cells often lyse during aspiration and smearing and therefore the cells commonly occur as bare nuclei embedded in a lightly basophilic background of cytoplasmic material. The nuclei are round, medium sized and generally show minimal anisokaryosis, although there are usually a few much larger nuclei scattered around. The chromatin is finely to coarsely stippled and nucleoli are single to multiple, small and variably visible. When intact, the cytoplasm is lightly basophilic and finely granular and may contain small clear vacuoles (Figure 21.56). In spite of its aggressive behaviour, this tumour does not show many criteria of malignancy. The most common malignant features are nuclear moulding, variable chromatin pattern and the presence of large and hyperchromic nuclei. Occasional mitoses may be observed.

Once this tumour is diagnosed, further recommended testing includes investigation for distant and nodal metastases and measurement of calcium.

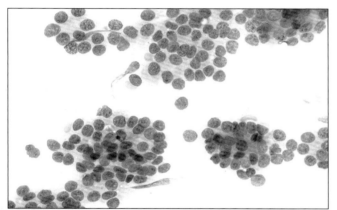

21.56 Fine-needle aspirate of an anal sac mass in a dog. The mass has yielded a population of uniform epithelial cells with indistinct cytoplasmic margins. An acinoid arrangement is present in the top left corner of the photograph. (Wright–Giemsa stain; original magnification X500

Mesenchymal tumours

Cytology of mesenchymal tumours is challenging. In the skin, both benign and malignant mesenchymal tumours are described. Soft tissue sarcomas (STSs) represent 7% of all cutaneous and subcutaneous tumours in cats and 15% in dogs. The term 'soft tissue sarcoma' is used to describe different types of mesenchymal tumours with similar pathological features and biological behaviour and includes fibrosarcoma, peripheral nerve sheath tumour, perivascular wall tumour (PWT), myxosarcoma and liposarcoma (Figure 21.57). Cytomorphology alone is not always sufficient to identify the cell type of origin, leading to a general diagnosis of soft tissue sarcoma. However, because of their similar biological behaviour and treat-ment, the identification of the precise histotype is probably not clinically relevant. The most common anatomical locations in dogs are the limbs, trunk and head.

Fibroma: Fibromas are poorly exfoliative tumours, and therefore aspirates from these masses are often poorly cellular. Fibromas are found uncommonly in adult and older dogs and rarely in cats. They arise from cutaneous or subcutaneous fibrocytes. They often present as solitary round masses of variable size, usually on the limbs or head. As expected for benign tumours, the cells are uniform and well differentiated. They are spindle shaped, often fusate, and may be found embedded in a lightly eosinophilic fibrillar material (collagen).

Fibrosarcoma: Fibrosarcoma is most common in cats (17.8% of skin tumours) and less common in dogs (5.4%). Older dogs and cats are more at risk but no breed or sex predilection have been observed.

In cats, the occurrence of fibrosarcoma has been associated with the injection of vaccines or other drugs and also with the insertion of microchips, hence the name 'injection-site sarcoma'. A virus-associated fibrosarcoma (feline sarcoma virus) has also been recognized. This form is more common in younger cats (<5 years of age) and usually presents as a multicentric form, but is very rare.

In dogs, most fibrosarcomas are low grade, being locally invasive but with a low metastatic rate.

On aspiration, these tumours usually give a variable cell harvest. The cellularity of the sample is inversely proportional to the degree of collagenization. In less differentiated forms, collagen is scant and therefore the cell harvest is high. Cells usually occur singly or in non-cohesive aggregates.

In well differentiated fibrosarcomas, the cells are spindle shaped and have lightly to moderately basophilic cytoplasm and oval nuclei. The less differentiated the tumour, the plumper and more oval shaped the cells become. The N:C ratio increases and anisokaryosis and anisocytosis become more prominent. Cytoplasm appears more basophilic, and eosinophilic to purple granules may be seen in a few cells. Nuclei are round to oval and the chromatin is coarsely stippled and occasionally hyperchromic. One or more prominent nucleoli are present and these may vary in size and shape. Admixed with the cells, there may also be a small amount of extracellular amorphous pink to eosinophilic material (collagen). Multinucleated cells and mitoses can be found in variable numbers (Figure 21.58).

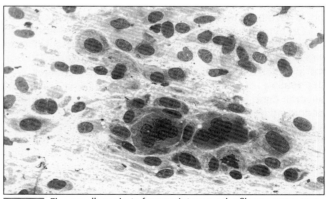

21.58 Fine-needle aspirate from an interscapular fibrosarcoma on a cat. Cells are spindle shaped and loosely arranged. They display multiple criteria of malignancy (anisokaryosis, coarse chromatin, prominent nucleoli, multinucleation and mitoses). (Wright–Giemsa stain; original magnification X500)

Type of sarcoma	Tumours
Soft tissue sarcoma	• Fibrosarcoma • PNST/PWT • Liposarcoma • Myxosarcoma
Other soft tissue sarcoma	• Leiomyosarcoma • Rhabdomyosarcoma • Synovial cell sarcoma • Lymphangiosarcoma
Other sarcomas with more aggressive clinical behaviour	• Histiocytic sarcoma • Haemangiosarcoma • Osteosarcoma • Chondrosarcoma • Melanoma

21.57 Types of soft tissue sarcoma. PNST = peripheral nerve sheath tumour; PWT = perivascular wall tumour.
(Data from Withrow and Vail, 2012)

As a general rule, fibrosarcomas in dogs and cats are locally invasive but the metastatic rate is low to moderate and depends largely on the histological grade.

Lipoma: Lipoma is a benign tumour arising from the adipocytes of the subcutaneous adipose tissue. This is a very common neoplasm found especially in older dogs. Grossly, aspirates appear greasy and usually contain low numbers of adipocytes and a large amount of free fat globules. Cells can occur singly or in variably sized aggregates. They typically have voluminous clear cytoplasm containing a large lipid-filled vacuole and small to medium sized and round nuclei, often displaced by the cytoplasmic content. Small capillaries may be seen associated with the adipocytes. Cytologically, the adipocytes originating from a lipoma cannot be distinguished from those present in the normal subcutaneous adipose tissue (Figure 21.59).

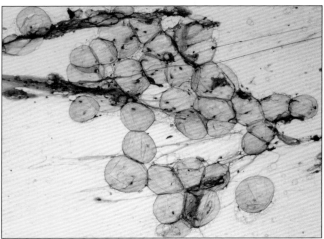

21.59 Fine-needle aspirate from a lipoma in a dog. The adipocytes have large cytoplasmic lipid vacuoles and small nuclei. Two small capillaries are seen crossing this aggregate. (Wright–Giemsa stain; original magnification X500)

Liposarcoma: This is a rare malignant tumour originating from the lipoblasts of the subcutaneous adipose tissue. It is probably more common in dogs than in cats. There is no sex or breed predisposition but the incidence increases with age.

These tumours are described as firm and poorly defined masses more commonly reported along the ventrum and limbs. They tend to be locally invasive but the metastatic rate is low. Metastases to lung, spleen, liver and bone have been reported.

On cytology, the cells are ovoid to spindle shaped and have small to large lipid globules in the cytoplasm (Figure 21.60a). Multinucleated cells may be found (Figure 21.60b). As in other sarcomas, cell pleomorphism increases with the degree of undifferentiation of the tumour. Recently, several case reports of lingual liposarcoma have been described (Piseddu et al., 2011).

Perivascular wall tumour: Perivascular wall tumours (PWTs) are neoplasms that arise from the different cellular components of the vascular wall, such as pericytes and myopericytes, but excluding the endothelial lining. These tumours are commonly found in dogs and are rare in cats. They often occur on the extremities but may occur in any other location such as the trunk and abdomen.

FNA usually yields numerous neoplastic cells, occurring either individually or in aggregates, with or without small

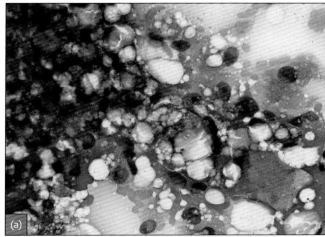

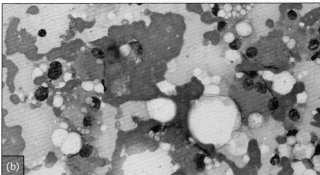

21.60 Fine-needle aspirates from a liposarcoma on the hindlimb of a dog. (a) The background of this aspirate contains abundant fat globules. The atypical mesenchymal cells display features of malignancy and are characterized by numerous cytoplasmic lipid droplets. (b) Less vacuolated neoplastic cells often have a pink, finely granular cytoplasm. (Wright–Giemsa stain; original magnification X500)

capillaries. Usually, these cells exhibit a perivascular arrangement. Cell morphology ranges between spindle shaped, wispy, stellate and occasionally plump oval (Figure 21.61a). Nuclei are medium to large in size and are round to oval. The chromatin is finely to coarsely stippled and nucleoli are usually small, round and variably distinct. The cytoplasm has indistinct borders and is lightly to moderately basophilic. It often contains small clear punctate vacuoles. Cell margins are often frayed. The cells are mostly mononucleated but binucleated cells are often encountered; these have their two nuclei bulging from one end of the cell (similar to insect heads). Multinucleated cells with three or more nuclei arranged at the periphery of the cytoplasm and forming a circle can be found (crown cells; Figure 21.61b). Although crown cells and 'insect head' cells are not pathognomonic for PWTs, their presence significantly increases suspicion for this tumour.

PWTs are locally invasive and have a high tendency to recur after incomplete surgical excision. However, the metastatic rate is low. Cytologically and histologically, PWTs are difficult to differentiate from peripheral nerve sheath tumours (PNSTs) and immunohistochemistry is often required.

Haemangiosarcoma: Haemangiosarcoma (HSA) of the skin is a malignant tumour that arises from endothelial cells. Canine cutaneous HSAs can be classified as dermal (stage I), subcutaneous (stage II), and a deep form involving the underlying muscle (stage III). This differentiation is clinically important given that surgery alone is usually effective for dermal HSAs whereas subcutaneous HSAs

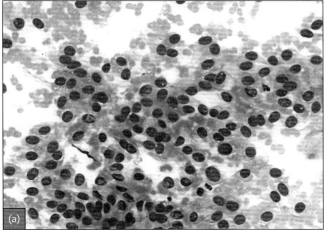

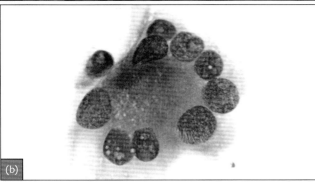

21.61 Fine-needle aspirates from a perivascular wall tumour (PWT) on the leg of a dog. (a) The cells are arranged in loose aggregates. The cytoplasm has poorly defined and fringed borders giving a veil-like appearance. (b) Crown cell: this is a multinucleated cell, characterized by nuclei arranged in a circle at the periphery of the cytoplasm. This typical cell is frequently seen in PWTs. (Wright–Giemsa stain; original magnification (a) X500, (b) X1000)

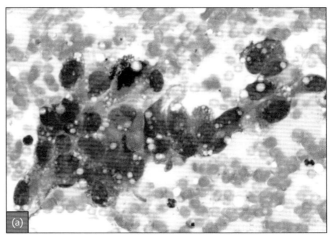

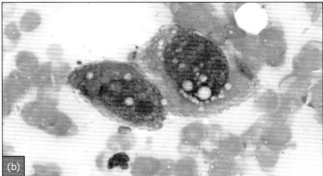

21.62 Fine-needle aspirates from a cutaneous haemangiosarcoma (HSA) in a dog. (a) The background is heavily haemodiluted. Neoplastic cells are large, plump, spindle shaped and have a high N:C ratio and prominent nucleoli. (b) One of the neoplastic cells contains an engulfed red blood cell (erythrophagia). (Wright–Giemsa stain; original magnification (a) X500, (b) X1000)

require adjuvant chemotherapy after wide surgical excision and bear a poor prognosis. Stage II and stage III tumours have a metastatic rate of 60% and usually spread to the lungs, draining lymph node and distant cutaneous locations. In cats, HSAs are locally invasive and bear a recurrence rate of 50–80%. The reported metastatic rate ranges from 33 to 50%.

In both dogs and cats, cutaneous HSAs occur more frequently in lightly pigmented and less haired areas such as the ventral abdomen, head and prepuce, and it seems that they may be sun induced.

Cytological preparations are characterized by abundant haemodilution and low cellularity. Not infrequently, only blood is aspirated and no intact tissue cells are harvested, and so histopathology is often required. The cells are generally pleomorphic and display criteria of malignancy. They may vary from spindle shaped to a plump oval. Anisokaryosis and anisocytosis may be prominent and the N:C ratio is variable to high. Nuclei are medium sized to large, round to oval and are often folded. The chromatin is coarse and multiple prominent nucleoli are present, which may vary in size and shape (round, angular or irregular). The cytoplasm is moderately basophilic and can contain clear punctate vacuoles (Figure 21.62a). The neoplastic cells can sometimes display erythrophagia (Figure 21.62b). In cutaneous forms, as with splenic haemangiosarcomas, concurrent extramedullary haemopoiesis has been described.

Histopathology and immunohistochemistry are used to confirm the cytological diagnosis and to grade this tumour.

Rhabdomyosarcoma: This is a rare malignant tumour that originates from the skeletal muscle precursor cells. Rhabdomyosarcomas are divided into four subtypes depending on the histological findings: embryonal; alveolar; pleomorphic; and botryoid. Several case reports of canine subcutaneous embryonal (Figure 21.63) and alveolar rhabdomyosarcomas have been published (Avallone *et al.*, 2010; Murakami *et al.*, 2010).

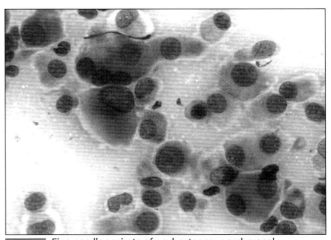

21.63 Fine-needle aspirate of a subcutaneous embryonal rhabdomyosarcoma on the antebrachium of a dog. The cells are large and polygonal and have abundant basophilic cytoplasm, large eccentric nuclei and prominent nucleoli. A few multinucleated cells are also present. (Wright–Giemsa stain; original magnification X500)
(Courtesy of G Avallone, University of Milan)

Neoplastic cells from the alveolar subtype exfoliate singly and are large and round, resembling lymphoid cells. Their nuclei are round to oval and display minimal size variation. The cytoplasm is scant to moderate and lightly basophilic. Several cells may contain small clear vacuoles.

The cells from the embryonal subtype appear more variable, displaying marked anisokaryosis and anisocytosis. They are large, individual and round to polygonal. Mostly mononucleated cells are present but binucleated and multinucleated cells can be found. The nuclei are large and eccentric and the cytoplasm is often abundant. Admixed with these cells, a distinct cell population has been described consisting of smaller round cells with a high N:C ratio and condensed chromatin (germinal cells).

For a definitive diagnosis, immunohistochemistry is often required. The main cytological differential diagnoses that have been proposed for subcutaneous rhabdomyosarcoma are lymphoma, plasmacytoma, amelanotic melanoma and anaplastic carcinoma and sarcoma.

Myxoma/myxosarcoma: Subcutaneous myxoma (benign form) and myxosarcoma (malignant form) are uncommon tumours of fibroblast origin. They usually occur on the trunk or the extremities. On aspiration, these tumours exfoliate variable numbers of individual mesenchymal cells. The cells are often spindle shaped and, depending on their clinical behaviour, may display variable features of malignancy (Figure 21.64). Typical of myxomas/myxosarcomas is the presence of abundant lightly basophilic extracellular material in the background. This has a typical viscous consistency that often causes the cells to line up in rows and which stains with Alcian blue.

Melanoma: Benign and malignant cutaneous melanocytic tumours are relatively common in dogs (5–7% of skin tumours) and rare in cats (<3%) and are characterized by a variable presentation and biological behaviour. They are most common in older animals, especially those with dark skin pigmentation. Some canine breeds such as Dobermanns and Miniature Schnauzers are more likely to have benign melanomas, while Miniature Poodles are more at risk of developing malignant forms.

Macroscopically, a cutaneous melanoma appears as a single dome-shaped mass. Benign forms are usually smaller, mobile and heavily pigmented. Malignant melanomas are larger, with irregular margins, variably pigmented and often ulcerated.

In dogs, the majority of the melanomas originating from the haired skin are benign, whereas the majority of melanomas arising in the oral cavity, nailbed and mucocutaneous junctions are malignant.

Cytology of benign melanocytic tumours (occasionally referred to as melanocytomas) is generally rewarding because they tend to exfoliate high numbers of cells that usually show minimal size variation and are well differentiated, containing numerous dark green–black cytoplasmic melanin granules. Nuclei are small to medium sized and the cytoplasm is abundant (Figure 21.65).

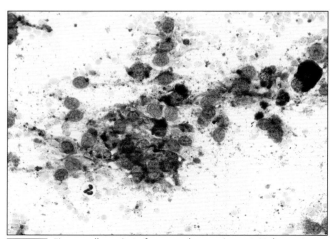

21.65 Fine-needle aspirate from a melanoma in a cat. Melanocytes contain numerous intracytoplasmic dark green–black pigment (melanin) granules. (Wright–Giemsa stain; original magnification X500)

More challenging is the cytology of less differentiated and amelanotic melanomas because the cell arrangement and morphology can be extremely variable. Neoplastic cells may appear similar to those in benign melanomas and do not always exhibit criteria of malignancy. Others can be pleomorphic, varying from round to spindle shaped or epithelioid cells, sometimes in aggregates, or as single cells. Malignant morphological features such as prominent anisokaryosis and anisocytosis, variable N:C ratio and large nuclei, coarse chromatin and multiple prominent nucleoli are common. Additionally, less differentiated cells contain scant melanin pigment, making the cytological diagnosis more challenging (Figure 21.66). However, even

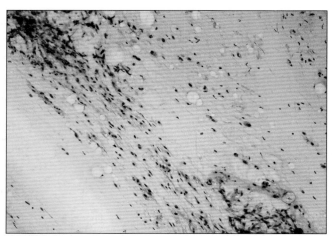

21.64 Fine-needle aspirate from a subcutaneous myxosarcoma in a dog. The cells are typically aligned in rows owing to the viscosity of the mucinous secretory material. (Wright–Giemsa stain; original magnification X100)

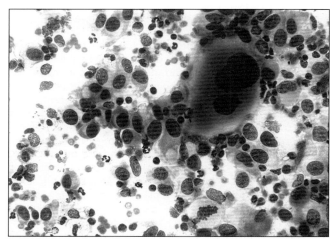

21.66 Fine-needle aspirate from an oral amelanotic melanoma in a dog. Large atypical cells display marked criteria of malignancy and a lack of cytoplasmic melanin granules. The diagnosis was confirmed by immunohistochemical staining (Melan A). (Wright–Giemsa stain; original magnification X500)

in these cases, it is almost always possible to find a few cells containing a fine dust-like cytoplasmic pigmentation. There is sometimes an overlapping of cytological features between benign and malignant forms and the clinical presentation and localization of the mass are very important for the cytological interpretation.

Histopathology is always recommended for a definitive diagnosis because the histological mitotic activity is the best predictive indicator of malignancy. In dogs, benign forms carry a good prognosis after surgical excision while malignant forms bear a guarded to poor prognosis with a high metastatic rate. In cats, dermal melanomas have a fair prognosis and the reported metastatic rate is 5–50%.

Histiocytic sarcoma: Histiocytic sarcomas can occur in a localized form in cutaneous and subcutaneous sites, usually on a distal limb in close proximity to a joint. They appear as rapidly growing solid masses, often ulcerated. Over-represented breeds are Flat Coated, Golden and Labrador Retrievers and Rottweilers. Adult and older dogs are predisposed. These tumours may also arise in the spleen, liver, lymph nodes, lung and bone marrow.

Upon aspiration, these tumours exfoliate high numbers of discrete pleomorphic cells. They are often round to oval shaped but occasionally plump spindle cells are seen. The majority of these cells are mononucleated but multinucleated forms are common. Moderate to marked criteria of malignancy are displayed, such as prominent anisokaryosis and anisocytosis, karyomegaly and coarse chromatin. Nuclei are variably sized, round to oval, indented and irregular. Prominent multiple nucleoli are seen, which vary in size, shape and number. The cytoplasm is moderate to abundant, moderately basophilic and has distinct borders. It often contains clear vacuoles or amorphous phagosomes. Mitoses are frequent and include atypical forms (Figure 21.67).

Histopathology and immunocyto/histochemistry may be required to differentiate this tumour from other types of sarcoma. Given the high metastatic rate, full staging is recommended including draining lymph node cytology and thoracic and abdominal imaging.

Round cell tumours

Round cell tumours are among the most common skin tumours in dogs. Cytology is a powerful tool in their diagnosis, given their tendency to exfoliate very well upon aspiration and their distinctive features. As a group, they exfoliate as individual cells which are round to oval with discrete cytoplasmic borders.

Round cell tumours include lymphoma, histiocytoma, plasma cell tumour or plasmacytoma, mast cell tumour and transmissible venereal tumour (TVT). The latter is uncommon in the UK and in most parts of Europe, and is usually observed only in dogs from tropical areas.

Each of these tumours presents specific morphological features which make them identifiable on cytology. However, when a poorly differentiated form is present, histochemical or immunohistochemical staining is necessary to achieve a specific diagnosis.

Histiocytoma: Histiocytoma is a benign tumour that originates from the epidermal dendritic cells (also called Langerhans cells). It is the most common skin tumour in young dogs, although it can also arise in older animals. It usually appears as a solitary lesion on any part of the body, with a predilection for the pinna, the head and the limbs. Multiple histiocytomas occur very rarely. Histiocytoma has a benign behaviour and usually undergoes spontaneous regression within a few weeks to months. A tumour showing lack of regression warrants surgical excision.

Aspirates from cutaneous histiocytomas are usually highly cellular, with high numbers of round discrete cells seen dispersed in a basophilic background. Histiocytic cells have abundant lightly to moderately basophilic cytoplasm with defined borders and a round, frequently indented paracentral nucleus, with granular chromatin and with or without a prominent round nucleolus. Anisocytosis and anisokaryosis may be moderate and binucleated cells may be seen (Figure 21.68). The presence of a concurrent infiltrate of small lymphocytes may suggest ongoing regression.

Mast cell tumour: Mast cell tumour (MCT) is one of the most common round cell neoplasms in small animals, together with lymphoma, and it accounts for 20% of all cutaneous tumours in both dogs and cats.

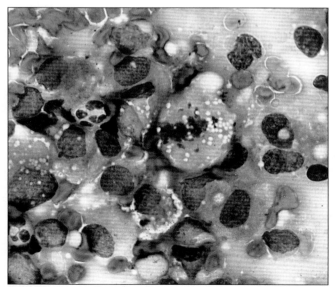

21.67 Fine-needle aspirate from a periarticular mass in a Flat Coated Retriever consistent with a histiocytic sarcoma. Neoplastic cells are discrete and display features of malignancy (anisokaryosis, irregular mitosis). (Wright–Giemsa stain; original magnification X1000)

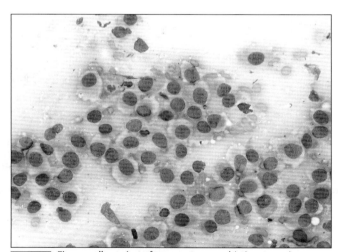

21.68 Fine-needle aspirate from a cutaneous histiocytoma in a young dog. Discrete cells show mild size variation and have abundant lightly basophilic cytoplasm, often lighter than the surrounding background. The cells are often compared to fried eggs. (Wright–Giemsa stain; original magnification X500)

Canine mast cell tumour: This has variable clinical appearance and for this reason is sometimes referred to as the 'great pretender'. Mast cell tumours in dogs are usually solitary with no predilection site, although multiple forms have been reported. They are more common in older dogs, with no gender predilection. Boxers and Retrievers are over-represented. Aspirates are usually highly cellular, consisting of numerous mast cells which have moderate amounts of lightly basophilic cytoplasm usually containing numerous purple granules, frequently obscuring the nucleus. Nuclei may be obscured by granules but, when visible, are round, central to paracentral, with granular chromatin and have poorly distinct nucleoli (Figure 21.69). In well differentiated mast cell tumours, anisocytosis and anisokaryosis are minimal and cytoplasmic granules are numerous and evenly distributed. In poorly differentiated forms there may be binucleated (or rarely multinucleated) cells and the mast cells may show marked features of atypia. There may be low numbers of cytoplasmic granules, which are finer and less densely staining and may be unevenly distributed (Figure 21.70). Histochemical stains are recommended in these cases (toluidine blue).

Eosinophils and reactive fibroblasts are frequently seen in all types of mast cell tumours and are secondary to the release of histamine and chemokines from the granules of the mast cells. The degranulation of these cells may also cause collagenolysis, which is represented cytologically by the presence of pink fibrillar structures (Figure 21.71). Occasionally, mast cell granules do not stain with Diff-Quik®, making identification of the mast cells difficult. Romanowsky stains such as Wright–Giemsa are preferable.

Even though, in the majority of cases, cytology provides a definitive diagnosis of mast cell tumour, histopathology is always required to grade the tumour and for evaluation of the surgical margins after excision.

Aspiration of regional lymph nodes and full staging (ultrasonography of the liver and spleen) are recommended, especially for the cytologically less well differentiated forms. Metastases are not uncommon with grade II and III MCTs. However, interpretation of lymph node involvement may be challenging because mast cells in a reactive process or a well granulated mast cell tumour are morphologically indistinguishable and an increased number of mast cells may be difficult to interpret. One of the main criteria used to define the presence of metastatic disease is the presence of mast cells in groups (Krick *et al.*, 2009).

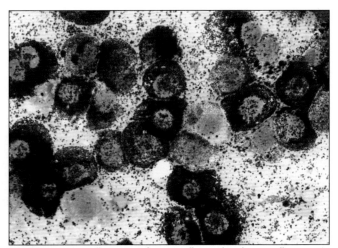

21.69 Fine-needle aspirate from a well granulated mast cell tumour in a dog. Mast cells contain numerous fine purple granules, often obscuring the nuclei. (Wright–Giemsa stain; original magnification X500)

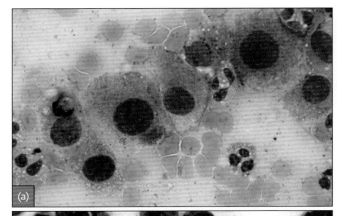

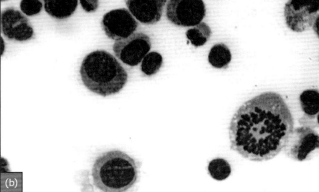

21.70 Fine-needle aspirates from a poorly granulated mast cell tumour in a dog. (a) Mast cells contain low numbers of dust-like purple granules, often grouped together on one side of the cytoplasm. (b) Mitotic mast cell. (Wright–Giemsa stain; original magnification X500)

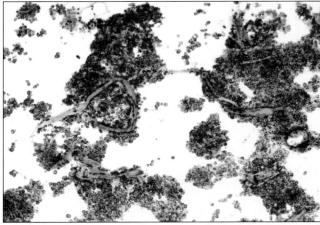

21.71 Fine-needle aspirate from a mast cell tumour in a dog. Several eosinophilic elongated structures are present in the aspirate. These are collagen fibrils and suggest collagenolysis caused by the degranulation of the mast cells. (Wright–Giemsa stain; original magnification X100)

Identification of mast cells in the buffy coat is no longer routinely used to diagnose metastatic disease because it is considered non-specific. Several disorders (e.g. inflammatory status, regenerative anaemia, neoplasia other than mast cell tumours) may be associated with mastocytaemia.

Feline mast cell tumour: Cutaneous mast cell tumours in cats are usually solitary lesions, frequently located on the head (Figure 21.72a) or the neck, although they have been reported anywhere in the body. In cats, visceral MCTs are much more common than in dogs, accounting for up to

50% of cases; the preferential sites are the spleen and intestine. There is no sex and age predilection, although there is a predisposition in Siamese cats, which may develop an atypical form of mast cell tumour (see below).

Feline mast cell tumours are not histologically graded in the same way as canine tumours, but have different subtypes, some features of which can also be recognized cytologically. They are classified as either well differentiated (resembling normal mast cells) or poorly differentiated, and either type may have a histologically diffuse or compact form. Most feline mast cell tumours are composed of well differentiated cells. Uncommonly, both well and poorly differentiated tumours may show pleomorphism (variation in cellular and nuclear size, with eccentric nuclei, prominent nucleoli, possible giant or multinucleate cells), which alone does not imply a poor prognosis (Johnson *et al.*, 2002; Rodriguez-Carino *et al.*, 2014). However, well differentiated but pleomorphic tumours with a high mitotic index may carry a poorer prognosis, and poorly differentiated tumours with pleomorphism are referred to as anaplastic and are clinically aggressive. Cats may also develop an atypical form of mast cell tumour (previously referred to as histiocytic). This is rare, and is reported mainly in young Siamese cats, which may develop multiple tumours that spontaneously regress. These mast cells are large with abundant cytoplasm containing very few granules, resembling histiocytes (Figure 21.72b).

Plasma cell tumour: Plasma cell tumours, also called plasmacytomas, are benign tumours, which are relatively common in old dogs and rare in cats. They present mostly as solitary masses, often on the digits, ears and mouth. They usually have an excellent prognosis after surgical excision. Cytological samples from plasma cell tumours are highly cellular and contain many plasma cells, which are often moderately pleomorphic. They are round, discrete cells with moderate amounts of deeply basophilic cytoplasm, frequently containing a clear perinuclear halo (Golgi zone) (Figure 21.73). The nucleus is eccentric and round, with granular chromatin and indistinct nucleoli. Binucleated cells and moderate anisocytosis and anisokaryosis are frequently observed. Amorphous eosinophilic material (amyloid) may be seen in a small proportion of cases. Sometimes poorly differentiated forms lack these peculiar cytological features or may display more pronounced malignant features (Figure 21.74) and immunohistochemical staining may be required (CD79a, CD21, MUM1). Although plasmacytomas can exhibit marked cytological criteria of malignancy, they usually have benign biological behaviour and carry a good prognosis following excision.

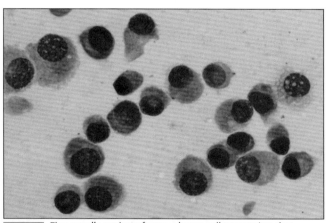

21.73 Fine-needle aspirate from a plasma cell tumour in a dog. Plasma cells have eccentric nuclei with clumped chromatin and a moderate amount of deeply basophilic cytoplasm, often showing a perinuclear halo. (Wright–Giemsa stain; original magnification X500) (Courtesy of E Villiers)

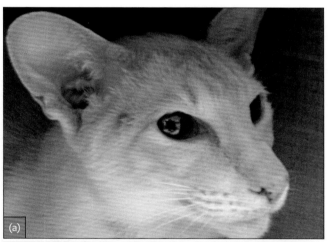

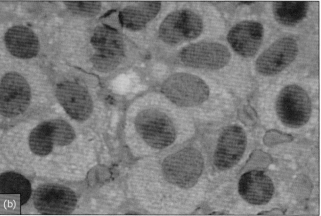

21.72 (a) Mast cell tumour in the temporal area of a Siamese cat. (b) Mast cells contain rare intracytoplasmic purple granules and have a vacuolated appearance (atypical subtype, previously classified as histiocytic type). (Wright–Giemsa stain; original magnification X1000) (a, © D Berlato, AHT; b, © R Powell, PTDS)

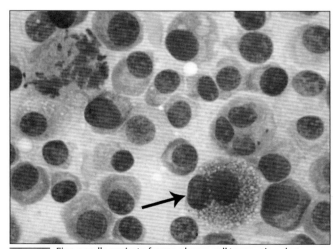

21.74 Fine-needle aspirate from a plasma cell tumour in a dog. Plasma cells display marked features of atypia (multinucleation, anisokaryosis, atypical mitosis). One Mott cell containing multiple Russell bodies (immunoglobulins) is also seen (arrowed). (Wright–Giemsa stain; original magnification X500) (Courtesy of E Villiers)

Cutaneous lymphoma: Cutaneous lymphoma is reported in both dogs and cats and is more common in older animals. It may occur as a primary disease or may be a manifestation of generalized lymphoma and leukaemia. The appearance of skin lesions is very variable although plaque-like lesions are observed more frequently. The prognosis is poor. Aspirates usually yield high numbers of lymphoid cells, which may be either small or large (Figure 21.75). When large lymphoid cells predominate, the diagnosis of lymphoma is straightforward. When most of the lymphoid cells are small and resemble small lymphocytes, the differentiation from lymphocytic inflammation is challenging and histological examination is recommended. Histologically, cutaneous lymphoma is divided into epitheliotropic and non-epitheliotropic forms, with the latter being more common in dogs. Cutaneous lymphomas usually have a T-cell phenotype.

Transmissible venereal tumour: Transmissible venereal tumour (TVT) is a sexually transmitted neoplasm commonly affecting the external genitalia in dogs. This tumour is uncommon in the UK and in most parts of Europe and is usually endemic in tropical and subtropical areas. It primarily arises in the mucous membranes of the external genitalia of dogs of either sex, although it can occur anywhere in the body. Young and free-roaming dogs are more at risk. FNAs are usually highly cellular with high numbers of discrete round cells. The cells have moderate amounts of lightly basophilic cytoplasm, frequently containing multiple clear punctate vacuoles (which are a distinctive feature of this tumour; Figure 21.76). Nuclei are round, paracentral to eccentric and have granular chromatin. Occasionally, a single small round and central nucleolus is seen. Anisokaryosis and anisocytosis are usually moderate and mitoses are frequently observed. TVT is considered a benign tumour and spontaneous regression usually occurs within 6 months. Metastasis to the local lymph node has occasionally been reported.

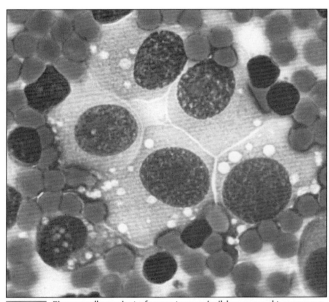

21.76 Fine-needle aspirate from a transmissible venereal tumour on the prepuce of a stray dog. The neoplastic cells have large round nuclei with granular chromatin and a small round nucleolus. The cytoplasm contains typical punctate clear vacuoles. (Wright–Giemsa stain; original magnification X1000)

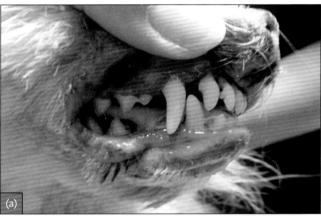

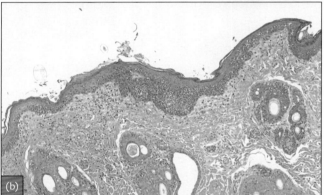

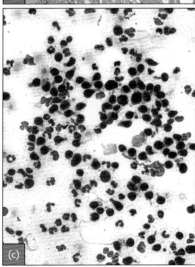

21.75 (a) Lymphoma in the buccal mucocutaneous junction of a Maltese. (b) Histological examination shows extensive neoplastic lymphoid cells infiltrating the epidermis and dermis. (Haematoxylin and eosin-stain; original magnification X40). (c) Cytological examination of the lesion shows high numbers of small lymphoid cells and small numbers of neutrophils. These lesions are frequently ulcerated and concurrent inflammation is common. (Wright–Giemsa stain; original magnification X500)

Cytology of lymph nodes

FNA cytology is a useful step in the identification of the causes of lymphadenopathy in patients that present with one or multiple enlarged lymph nodes. When aspirating lymph nodes, the needle-only method is preferred over the suction techniques because lymphoid cells are fragile and the negative pressure created by the suction may easily rupture the cells. This cell disruption manifests as naked lymphoid nuclei, which are larger and have looser and lighter chromatin than intact lymphoid cells and which hamper accurate interpretation.

In animals with generalized lymphadenopathy when lymphoma is suspected, aspiration from multiple lymph nodes is recommended, although lymph nodes draining reactive areas (e.g. the submandibular lymph nodes which drain the oral cavity) should be avoided, because con-current reactive hyperplasia may mask an underlying lymphoma.

Accidental aspiration of non-lymphoid tissue may occasionally happen when attempting to obtain a lymph node aspirate. Aspiration of perinodal fat is common, especially when lymph nodes are not enlarged or when the patient is overweight. Moreover, aspiration of salivary gland epithelial cells is common when attempting to aspirate submandibular lymph nodes (Figure 21.77).

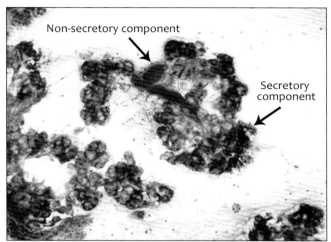

Non-secretory component

Secretory component

21.77 Incidental aspiration of a submandibular salivary gland is not uncommon while attempting aspiration of the submandibular lymph node. Both secretory and non-secretory salivary epithelial cells are present in the smear. Secretory cells have abundant and heavily vacuolated cytoplasm. Non-secretory cells are cuboidal. (Wright–Giemsa stain; original magnification X100)

Normal lymph node structure and cytology

FNA of normal lymph node is usually not performed, although an understanding of the cytological findings of aspirates from normal organs is considered crucial in the correct interpretation of pathological conditions. A normal lymph node (Figure 21.78) is characterized by:

- Prevalence of small lymphocytes (>90% of the nucleated cells), which are small cells with a basophilic cytoplasmic rim and a small round condensed nucleus, similar in size to a canine red blood cell. Nucleoli are not visible
- Occasional intermediate to large lymphoid cells (<10%), which are medium-sized to large cells with increased amounts of basophilic cytoplasm. The nucleus is round and paracentral and measures 2–3 times the diameter of a canine red blood cell. The chromatin is coarsely granular and up to three prominent nucleoli are seen
- Very rare macrophages and plasma cells.

Lymphadenitis

Lymphadenitis is defined as inflammation of the lymph node. It is classified according to the prevalent inflammatory cell type. Lymphadenitis is usually accompanied by a reactive lymphoid population with predominantly small lymphocytes and with variably increased proportions of intermediate and large forms and plasma cells (see later).

Neutrophilic lymphadenitis

This is characterized by the presence of more than 5% neutrophils and is usually associated with bacterial, neoplastic or immune-mediated conditions (Raskin and Meyer, 2010).

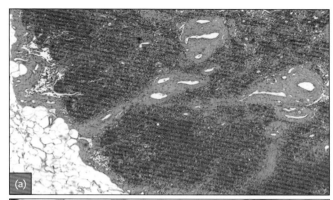

(a)

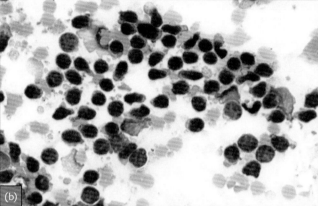

(b)

21.78 Normal lymph node in a dog. (a) Tissue section. Cortical area containing lymphoid nodules composed mostly of small lymphocytes. (Haematoxylin and eosin stain; original magnification X40). (b) The fine-needle aspirate from the same lymph node is characterized by the prevalence of small lymphocytes. (Wright–Giemsa stain; original magnification X500)
(a, Courtesy of L Aresu, University of Padua)

Eosinophilic lymphadenitis

This is diagnosed when eosinophils make up more than 3% of all nucleated cells (Figure 21.79; Raskin and Meyer, 2010). Primary differentials include type I hypersensitivity, parasitic infections, feline eosinophilic skin diseases, hypereosinophilic syndrome and paraneoplastic syndromes (usually associated with mast cell tumour, T-cell lymphoma and rarely carcinomas).

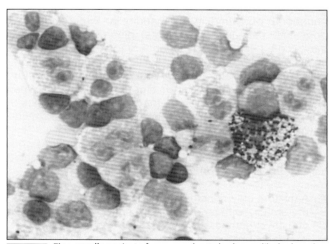

21.79 Fine-needle aspirate from an enlarged submandibular lymph node from a cat with hypereosinophilic syndrome. Increased numbers of eosinophils and one granulated mast cell are seen together with small lymphocytes. (Wright–Giemsa stain; original magnification X500)

Granulomatous lymphadenitis

This is associated with an increased number of macrophages (>3% of all nucleated cells; Raskin and Meyer, 2010).

Pyogranulomatous lymphadenitis

This is the term used when both neutrophils and macrophages are increased (Figure 21.80). This type of inflammation is frequently associated with either fungal or mycobacterial infections and special stains may help identify these (e.g. Ziehl–Neelsen for the identification of mycobacteria, PAS for fungal hyphae or spores). Other differentials for granulomatous lymphadenitis include leishmaniosis, protothecosis, bartonellosis, juvenile cellulitis, vasculitis and idiopathic/steroid-responsive lymphadenitis.

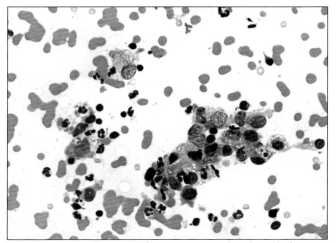

21.80 Fine-needle aspirate from a mesenteric lymph node of a cat with feline infectious peritonitis (FIP). Increased numbers of macrophages and neutrophils are seen in this preparation, supporting a diagnosis of pyogranulomatous lymphadenitis. (Wright–Giemsa stain; original magnification X500)

Lymphoid hyperplasia/reactive hyperplasia

Lymphoid hyperplasia is defined as a benign and reversible enlargement of lymphoid tissue secondary to antigenic stimulation. It may affect a single lymph node, usually in response to a localized inflammation, as commonly observed in submandibular lymph nodes of dogs and cats with periodontal disorders. However, it may also be generalized, secondary to systemic antigenic stimulation, as observed in association with feline leukaemia virus (FeLV) and feline immunodeficiency virus (FIV) infections, bartonellosis or in chronic ehrlichiosis. When a generalized lymphadenopathy occurs, the distinction from lymphoma can be clinically challenging and cytology is required.

Aspirates from reactive/hyperplastic lymph nodes consist of a heterogeneous and mixed population of lymphoid cells (Figure 21.81 and Figure 21.82a), characterized by:

- A mixture of lymphoid cells at different stages of maturation, with a prevalence of small lymphocytes and lower numbers of intermediate and large forms
- A variable number of plasma cells (Figure 21.82b). Mott cells containing packets of immunoglobulin (Russell bodies) may be seen
- Rare macrophages, eosinophils and mast cells may also be observed.

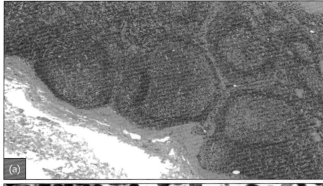

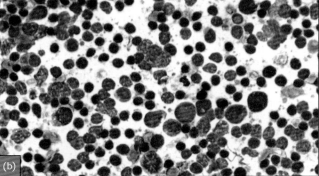

21.81 Hyperplastic lymph node. (a) Tissue section. Cortical area containing multiple reactive lymphoid follicles composed of two zones: a dark zone with a thin rim of small lymphocytes, and a light middle zone composed of larger lymphoid cells. (Haematoxylin and eosin stain; original magnification X40). (b) Fine-needle aspirate from the same lymph node. The majority of the cells are small lymphocytes with a lower but significant percentage of intermediate to large forms. (Wright–Giemsa stain; original magnification X500)
(a, Courtesy of L Aresu, University of Padua)

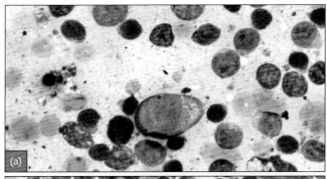

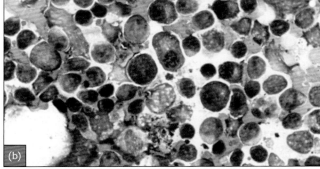

21.82 (a) Fine-needle aspirate from an enlarged lymph node from a dog with reactive lymphoid hyperplasia. The majority of the cells are small lymphocytes with a lower percentage of intermediate forms and a large lymphoid cell in the centre of the picture. (b) Fine-needle aspirate from an enlarged lymph node from a dog with plasma cell hyperplasia. Increased numbers of plasma cells are present in the aspirate. This is usually associated with antigen stimulation. (Wright–Giemsa stain; original magnification X500)

Sometimes, it can be difficult on cytology to differentiate reactive hyperplasia from early lymphoma, especially when the percentage of intermediate to large lymphoid cells is significantly increased. In these instances, whole lymph node excision and histopathological examination of the lymph node with evaluation of its architecture are recommended in order to classify the disorder properly.

Lymphoma

Lymphoma is the most common haemopoietic tumour affecting dogs and cats. It is defined as a neoplastic malignant proliferation of lymphoid cells arising in peripheral lymphoid tissues (e.g. lymph node, spleen, lymphoid tissue associated with the mucosa). Cytological examination of samples from these organs is usually the first step in the diagnosis of lymphoma and, in dogs, this is diagnostic most of the time, although in cats there is a higher frequency of intermediate to low-grade lymphoma, which can be more challenging to diagnose cytologically and often requires histopathology.

Several classifications have been proposed in recent decades with the intent of categorizing the different subtypes and associating them with a clinical prognosis. The main principles used by these classifications are based on the anatomical location, cellular morphology, tissue architecture, immunophenotype and genetics. In cytology, lymphoma is usually classified into high-grade and low-grade forms; each category is then further distinguished according to the phenotype (T and B phenotype) (Figure 21.83).

Parameter	Lymphoma type
Cell size [a]	Small cells (1–1.5x RBC) Intermediate cells (2–2.5x RBC) Large cells (>3x RBC)
Mitotic index [b]	Low grade (0–1 mitoses per 5 hpf) Intermediate grade (2–3 mitoses per 5 hpf) High grade (>3 mitoses per 5 hpf)

21.83 Cytological specifications for lymphoid cell size and mitotic index. [a] Nuclear size is compared with the size of a canine red blood cell (RBC). [b] Mitotic index is evaluated by counting the number of mitoses in five high power fields (hpf) (X500).
(Data from Raskin and Meyer, 2010)

High-grade lymphoma

High-grade lymphomas are the most common forms of lymphoma in dogs. They are characterized by the predominance of a homogeneous population of intermediate and/or large lymphoid cells. Nuclei are medium-sized to large and are generally round, although irregular or convoluted forms may be observed. The chromatin is finely stippled or finely clumped and one or multiple small to medium-sized, round and prominent nucleoli are present. The cytoplasm is generally moderate in amount and varies from lightly to deeply basophilic (Figure 21.84). In a subtype known as large granular lymphoma (LGL), small pink granules may be seen in the cytoplasm, clustered together on one side of the nucleus (Figure 21.85). Additional support for high-grade lymphoma is provided by abnormal nuclear, nucleolar or cytoplasmic features such as pleomorphic nuclei, binucleation or clear punctate cytoplasmic vacuoles. There is a moderate to high mitotic rate (>3 mitotic figures in five high-power (X500) fields), and often there are numerous tingible body macrophages containing phagocytosed apoptotic lymphoid cells (Figure 21.86). High-grade lymphomas have a rapid onset and progression, although they usually respond well to chemotherapy.

Disseminated lightly basophilic cytoplasmic fragments of lymphocytes, called lymphoglandular bodies, are frequently observed in the background of lymphoma aspirates and reflect increased '*in vivo*' and '*in vitro*' cell fragility. They are frequently observed in association with high-grade lymphomas although their presence is not pathognomonic of lymphoma, and they are observed in several other conditions characterized by rapidly dividing lymphoid populations (e.g. reactive lymphoid hyperplasia).

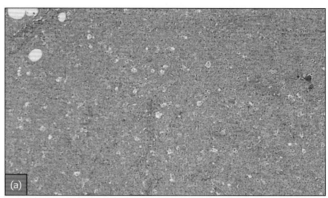

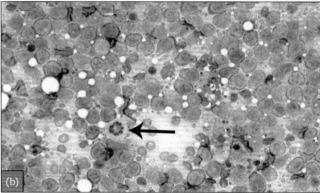

21.84 Lymph node from a dog with lymphoma. (a) Tissue section. Dense and diffuse infiltration of neoplastic lymphoid cells effacing the normal architecture. No appreciable difference between cortex and medulla is present. (Haematoxylin and eosin stain; original magnification X100). (b) The fine-needle aspirate shows that the majority of the lymphoid cells are intermediate to large in size. A mitotic figure is present (arrowed). Frequent lymphoglandular bodies are seen in the background. (Wright–Giemsa stain; original magnification X500)
(a, Courtesy of L Aresu, University of Padua)

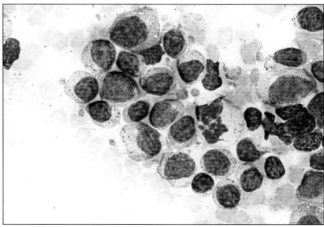

21.85 Fine-needle aspirate of a mediastinal mass in a dog with lymphoma. Lymphoid cells are intermediate to large in size and have a moderate amount of lightly basophilic cyotplasm containing small intracytoplasmic purple granules. This is consistent with large granular lymphoma. (Wright–Giemsa stain; original magnification X500)

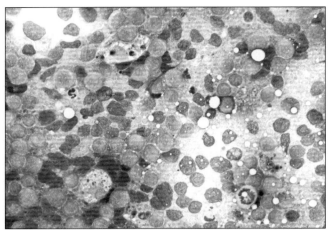

21.86 Fine-needle aspirate of a lymph node from a dog with large B-cell lymphoma. There are a few macrophages containing amorphous phagosomes (tingible body: phagocytosed cellular debris). Tingible body macrophages are frequently seen in high-grade lymphoma. They may also be observed in hyperplastic and reactive processes. (Wright–Giemsa stain; original magnification X500)

Low-grade lymphoma

This is characterized by the predominance of a homogeneous population of small mature lymphoid cells. The diagnosis of small cell lymphoma is more challenging because the neoplastic cells may resemble normal small lymphocytes, but it is suspected if an aspirate from an enlarged lymph node yields a monomorphic population of small lymphoid cells. However, in these cases histopathological examination should be performed for confirmation, because evaluation of the architecture helps to confirm the diagnosis. Flow cytometry and PARR (polymerase chain reaction for antigen receptor rearrangement) are other tests which can be used in the confirmation of lymphoma (see Chapter 5). Lymphocytes in low-grade lymphoma are small and have a small to medium-sized, round and eccentric nucleus whose chromatin is slightly less condensed than that of mature lymphocytes. Nucleoli are indistinct or absent. Additionally, these cells have scant to moderate amounts of moderately basophilic cytoplasm, which often protrudes to one side of the nucleus, giving the cell the typical appearance known as a 'hand mirror' cell (Figure 21.87). This morphological feature is helpful in identifying

small cell lymphoma because it is not seen in normal or reactive lymphoid populations. This feature differs from an artefactual smearing of the cells because the cytoplasmic tails extend in different directions rather than only in the direction of the smear. Low-grade lymphomas are less sensitive to chemotherapy but have a slow onset and patients show longer survival times than with high-grade lymphomas.

Immunophenotyping in lymphoma

Immunophenotyping is considered a crucial step in the diagnosis of canine lymphoma, because in high-grade canine multicentric lymphoma the T phenotype is a negative prognostic factor, although this is not the case for low-grade/indolent canine T-cell lymphomas. The prognostic role of the immunophenotype in feline lymphoma is controversial and requires further investigation.

Further important prognostic factors for canine and feline lymphomas are the clinical stage, with the possible involvement of non-lymphoid tissues such as bone marrow, central nervous system (CNS) and kidneys (stage V lymphoma), and the presence of paraneoplastic syndromes (e.g. hypercalcaemia of malignancy, anaemia). A complete blood count (CBC), full biochemistry profile (with total and ionized calcium), abdominal ultrasonography and aspirates from the liver and spleen are always recommended in patients with lymphoma. In cats, evaluation of the retroviral status (FeLV, FIV) is also considered important.

Metastatic tumours

Cytology is a useful and sensitive technique for tumour staging and in the identification of metastasis, with sensitivity of 100% and specificity of 96% in one study (Langenbach et al., 2001). FNA of lymph nodes draining a tumour is always recommended, in particular when there is a malignant tumour with high metastatic index. Lymph nodes are frequently enlarged and may be firm, although lymph node size has been shown to be an unreliable indicator of the presence of metastatic disease. Carcinomas frequently metastasize to the lymph node and are easy to identify given the tendency of epithelial cells to exfoliate in large clusters (Figure 21.88). Metastatic sarcomas are usually characterized by the presence of individual atypical mesenchymal spindle cells admixed with the lymphoid cells (Figure 21.89). Metastatic mast cell tumours can be

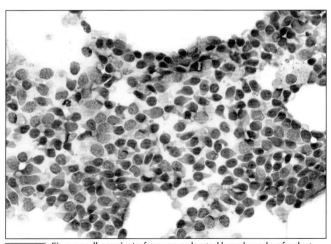

21.87 Fine-needle aspirate from an enlarged lymph node of a dog with a small cell lymphoma. The lymphoid cells are small, with a small amount of basophilic cytoplasm, often extending away from the nucleus (hand mirror cells). (Wright–Giemsa stain; original magnification X500)

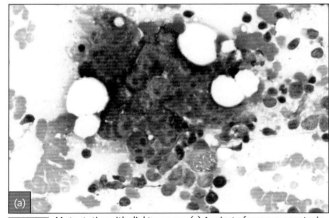

(a)

21.88 Metastatic epithelial tumours. (a) Aspirate from a mesenteric lymph node from a dog with metastatic intestinal adenocarcinoma. A cluster of epithelial cells with large nuclei is present. (Wright–Giemsa stain; original magnification X500). (continues) ▶
(Courtesy of E Villiers)

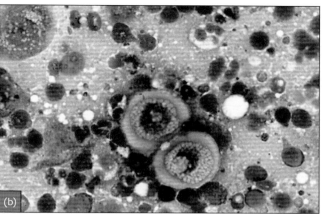

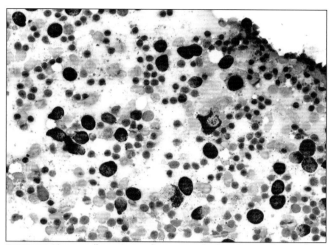

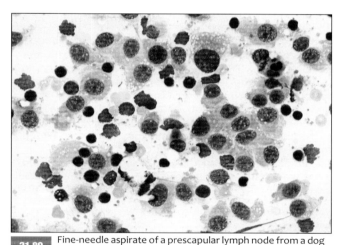

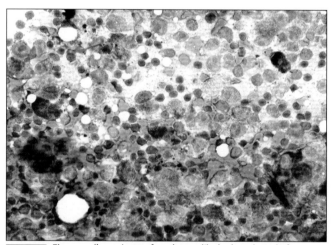

21.88 (continued) Metastatic epithelial tumours. (b) Aspirate from a submandibular lymph node from a cat with metastatic squamous cell carcinoma. Three large atypical squamous epithelial cells with vacuolated cytoplasm are present. (Wright–Giemsa stain; original magnification X500)
(Courtesy of E Villiers)

21.90 Fine-needle aspirate of a prescapular lymph node from a dog with a metastatic mast cell tumour. Numerous mast cells with heavily granulated cytoplasm are present. (Wright–Giemsa stain; original magnification X200)

21.89 Fine-needle aspirate of a prescapular lymph node from a dog with metastatic soft tissue sarcoma. Neoplastic cells are plump and spindle shaped. Only low numbers of residual small lymphocytes are seen scattered around in the slide. (Wright–Giemsa stain; original magnification X500)

21.91 Fine-needle aspirate of a submandibular lymph node from a dog with a metastatic oral melanoma. Note the presence of cells containing green-black melanin granules. (Wright–Giemsa stain; original magnification X500)

difficult to recognize, given that low numbers of normal mast cells can be present in normal lymph nodes (Figure 21.90). Atypical morphological features in the mast cells, and mast cells arranged in groups more than individually, are supportive of metastasis rather than a reactive process. Figure 21.91 illustrates a metastatic lymph node with neoplastic infiltration by a melanoma. In well pigmented

melanomas, cytological identification is simple and the cells contain numerous intracytoplasmic green–black pigmented granules of melanin, but poorly granulated melanocytes are more difficult to identify. Melanocytes can sometimes be confused with haemosiderin-laden macrophages. If this is suspected, histochemical stains may be helpful (Fontana–Masson).

Case examples

CASE 1

SIGNALMENT

8-year-old neutered male Golden Retriever.

HISTORY

Evidence of a distinct mass in the ventral region of the neck over recent weeks.

CLINICAL PATHOLOGY DATA

Haematology and biochemistry profile data are all within the reference intervals.

Fine-needle aspiration was performed on the ventral neck swelling (Figure 21.92).

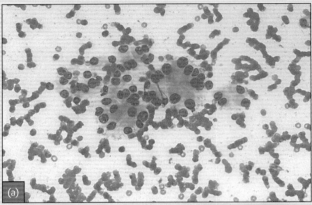

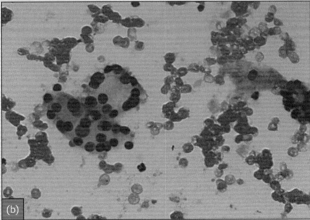

21.92 (a–b) Fine-needle aspirates from the mass in the ventral region of the neck. In (b) note the extracellular pinkish colloid between the cells. (Wright–Giemsa stain; original magnification (a) X1000, (b) X500)

BASED ON THE MORPHOLOGY AND ARRANGEMENT OF THESE CELLS, IS THIS AN EPITHELIAL, MESENCHYMAL OR ROUND CELL POPULATION?

The cells appear cuboidal to columnar and are arranged in small clusters, which is supportive of an epithelial origin. Moreover, the evidence of an acinar arrangement reflects a glandular origin (thyroid gland).

IS THERE ANY SPECIFIC CYTOLOGICAL FEATURE THAT MAY SUGGEST A THYROID GLAND ORIGIN?

Between the clusters of cells, there is variable amount of amorphous pink material, which is colloid. This is the material produced by thyroid follicular cells and contains the precursors of thyroid hormones.

CAN YOU IDENTIFY ANY CRITERIA OF MALIGNANCY DISPLAYED BY THESE CELLS?

These cells do not display marked criteria of atypia, with the exception of a mild to moderate anisocytosis and anisokaryosis. This may suggest a benign origin (adenoma) of the lesion. However, malignant thyroidal tumours (carcinoma) are much more common in dogs and frequently do not show marked features of malignancy. Given this, the correct cytological diagnosis is thyroid tumour, and histopathology is recommended to characterize the lesion further.

Surgical excision and histopathology were performed a few weeks after the diagnosis. The histological diagnosis was well differentiated thyroidal follicular carcinoma.

ARE THERE ANY METABOLIC/ENDOCRINE ABNORMALITIES EXPECTED WITH THESE TUMOURS IN DOGS?

The majority of the canine thyroid tumours are not functional. Total thyroxine was measured and was within the reference range.

CASE 2

SIGNALMENT

4-year-old entire female Labrador Retriever.

HISTORY

The bitch had had a litter 6 months previously and had been in season 3 weeks prior to presentation. She was inappetent, lethargic and had lost weight. On examination there was a cloudy vaginal discharge. Antibiotic therapy failed to improve the clinical signs, and therefore haematology, biochemistry, urinalysis and cytological evaluation of the vaginal discharge were performed.

CLINICAL PATHOLOGY DATA

The most significant changes observed on routine haematology and biochemistry included an inflammatory leucogram with mild neutrophilia and monocytosis and low numbers of circulating reactive lymphocytes, and a mild hyperglobulinaemia.

Dipstick testing of the urine showed mild proteinuria and haematuria. Figure 21.93 shows the wet preparation of the urine sediment.

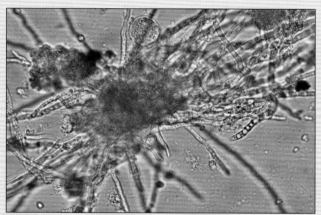

21.93 Wet preparation of the urine sediment. (Original magnification X400)

WHAT STRUCTURES ARE PRESENT?

There is a large bundle of elongated septate structures consistent with fungal hyphae. Low numbers of leucocytes are also present.

WHAT TYPES OF CELL ARE SEEN IN THE VAGINAL SMEAR (FIGURE 21.94): INFLAMMATORY CELLS, TISSUE CELLS OR BOTH? WHAT ELSE DO YOU SEE?

Numerous neutrophils are seen and they display moderate karyolysis. In the centre of the image, there is a fungal hypha with two other small fragments above this (arrowed). This is consistent with neutrophilic inflammation and fungal infection.

FURTHER INVESTIGATIONS

On abdominal imaging, the uterine horns appeared enlarged and fluid filled. The left medial iliac lymph node was enlarged. A lymph node aspirate was taken for cytological examination (Figure 21.95).

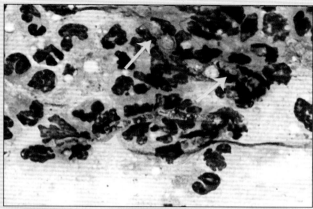

21.94 Vaginal smear showing a fungal hypha and associated fragments (arrowed). (Wright–Giemsa stain; original magnification X500)

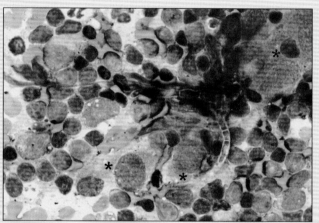

21.95 Fine-needle aspirate from the left medial iliac lymph node showing lymphocytes and macrophages (*). (Wright–Giemsa stain; original magnification X500)

WHAT DO YOU SEE IN THE LYMPH NODE ASPIRATE (FIGURE 21.95)?

There is a mixed lymphoid cell population with a predominance of small lymphocytes and a few larger forms. In this sample there are also low numbers of macrophages (indicated by asterisks). Low numbers of fungal hyphae were also seen in the lymph node (in the centre of the image). This indicates macrophagic lymphadenitis caused by a fungal infection.

CULTURE

Aspergillus terreus was isolated on fungal culture of the urine. This organism was sensitive to itraconazole and amphotericin B.

FOLLOW-UP

Ovariohysterectomy was performed and the iliac lymph node was removed. Both tissues were submitted for histopathology and culture, which confirmed a fungal pyogranulomatous endometritis and lymphadenitis. Treatment was commenced with antifungal agents but the dog developed severe intractable neck pain and hip pain. This was assumed to be due to systemic aspergillosis, although magnetic resonance imaging (MRI) and a CSF tap were unremarkable and the cause was not confirmed. The owners requested euthanasia.

References and further reading

Avallone G, Pinto da Cunha N, Palmieri C *et al.* (2010) Subcutaneous embryonal rhabdomyosarcoma in a dog: cytologic, immunocytochemical, histologic, and ultrastructural features. *Veterinary Clinical Pathology* **39**, 499–504

Cowell RL, Tyler RD and Meinkoth JH (2008) *Diagnostic Cytology and Hematology of the Dog and Cat, 3rd edn*. Mosby Elsevier, St Louis, Missouri

Greene C (2012) *Infectious Diseases of the Dog and Cat, 4th edn*. Saunders Elsevier, St. Louis, Missouri

Johnson TO, Schulman FY, Lipscomb TP *et al.* (2002) Histopathology and biological behavior of pleomorphic cutaneous mast cell tumours in fifteen cats. *Veterinary Pathology* **39**, 452–457

Jorundsson E, Orosz SE, Richman LK *et al.* (1999) Rapid staining techniques in cytopathology: a review and comparison of modified protocols for hematoxylin and eosin, Papanicolaou and Romanowsky stains. *Veterinary Clinical Pathology* **28**, 100–108

Krick EL, Billings AP, Shofer FS *et al.* (2009) Cytological lymph node evaluation in dogs with mast cell tumours: association with grade and survival. *Veterinary and Comparative Oncology* **7**, 130–138

Langenbach A, Mcmanus PM, Hendrick MJ *et al.* (2001) Sensitivity and specificity of methods of assessing the regional lymph nodes for evidence of metastasis in dogs and cats with solid tumours. *Journal of the American Veterinary Medical Association* **218**, 1424–1428

Maxie GM (2007) *Jubb, Kennedy and Palmer's Pathology of Domestic Animals, 5th edn*. Saunders Elsevier, St. Louis, Missouri

Meuten DJ (2002) *Tumors in Domestic Animals, 4th edn*. Iowa State University Press, Blackwell Publishing Company, Ames, Iowa

Murakami M, Sakai H, Iwatani N *et al.* (2010) Cytologic, histologic, and immunohistochemical features of maxillofacial alveolar rhabdomyosarcoma in a juvenile dog. *Veterinary Clinical Pathology* **39**, 113–118

Piseddu E, De Lorenzi D, Freeman K *et al.* (2011) Cytologic, histologic and immunohistochemical features of lingual liposarcoma in a dog. *Veterinary Clinical Pathology* **40**, 393–397

Raskin RE and Meyer DJ (2010) *Canine and Feline Cytology, A Color Atlas and Interpretaion Guide, 2nd edn*. Saunders Elsevier, St. Louis, Missouri

Rodríguez-Cariño C, Fondevila D, Segalés J and Rabanal RM (2014) Expression of KIT receptor in feline cutaneous mast cell tumors. *Veterinary Pathology* **46**, 878–883

Sabbatini S and Bettini G (2010) Prognostic value, histologic and immunohistochemical features in feline cutaneous mast cell tumours. *Veterinary Pathology* **47**, 643–653

Sharkey LC, Dial SM and Matz ME (2007) Maximizing the diagnostic value of cytology in small animal practice. *Veterinary Clinics of North America: Small Animal Practice* **37**, 351–372

Vignoli M, Rossi F, Chierici C *et al.* (2007) Needle tract implantation after fine needle aspiration biopsy (FNAB) of transitional cell carcinoma of the urinary bladder and adenocarcinoma. *Schweizer Archiv für Tierheilkunde* **149**, 314–318

Withrow SJ and Vail DM (2012) *Withrow and MacEwen's Small Animal Clinical Oncology, 5th edn*. Saunders Elsevier, St. Louis, Missouri

Chapter 22

Body cavity effusions

Emma Dewhurst

Body cavity effusions occur when there is abnormal accumulation of fluid in a body cavity. In dogs and cats, effusions commonly occur in the pleural, peritoneal or pericardial spaces. Clinical signs, such as dyspnoea, lethargy, exercise intolerance and abdominal distension, can be due to the presence of the effusion, the disease responsible for producing the effusion or both. Analysis of effusions is an important component of diagnosis: it can identify the pathological process responsible for the fluid accumulation and lead to a specific diagnosis, or it can indicate further investigative procedures which may be helpful.

Pathophysiology of effusion formation

In healthy animals, the body cavities are lined by a single continuous layer of mesothelium that covers the inner body wall, the mediastinum and the viscera. Interstitial fluid (i.e. lymph) constantly permeates into the thoracic cavity through the pleural capillaries and into the abdominal cavity through the intestinal capillaries. This movement out of the capillary is favoured by the fact that the capillary hydraulic pressure (dependent on the blood pressure; hydraulic pressure is the pressure of a fluid in motion) exceeds the oncotic pressure (dependent on the blood albumin concentration). However, most of the fluid is rapidly absorbed through the lymphatic capillaries, so that only a small amount remains in the cavities, where it acts to lubricate the abdominal and thoracic organs. The amount of fluid present in the cavity at any one time is determined by equilibration between the mechanisms governing the production (hydraulic pressure, oncotic pressure) and resorption (lymphatic drainage) of the fluid.

In summary, effusions can be formed as a result of one or more of the following primary pathophysiological mechanisms:

- Decreased plasma colloid oncotic pressure. Effusions occur because there is a loss (i.e. hypoalbuminaemia) of the oncotic pull that keeps fluid within the vasculature. As a result, fluid is lost from the capillaries at a rate that exceeds the absorptive capacity of the lymphatics
- Increased hydraulic pressure (the pressure of a fluid in motion). Effusions occur because fluid is forced into the body cavity. Fluid production is increased, exceeding the transport capacity of the lymphatics
- Increased vascular permeability. Effusions occur because there is an excessive loss of fluid from abnormal vasculature into the body cavity
- Compromised lymphatic flow, e.g. rupture. Effusions occur because removal of fluid from the body cavity is impaired.

Certain effusions can also occur through other mechanisms or a combination of the mechanisms above, such as haemorrhagic effusions, effusions secondary to viscus rupture and also with neoplasia. Classification of these effusions is more complicated owing to the variability in mechanism of formation.

Collection of body cavity effusions

Equipment

Equipment for collection of body cavity effusions includes:

- Clippers
- Surgical scrub and alcohol spray
- Local anaesthetic (optional)
- Sterile needle, butterfly needle, or over-the-needle catheter
- Sterile syringe
- Extension tube and three-way tap
- Scalpel blade and suture (for over-the-needle catheter only)
- Gloves
- Kidney dish or measuring jug (if collecting large volume of fluid for therapeutic reasons)
- Three sample tubes (ethylenediamine tetra-acetic acid (EDTA, plain, plain sterile).

Pleural effusion

Thoracocentesis is best performed with the patient standing or in sternal recumbency because this is safer than lateral recumbency, especially for severely dyspnoeic patients. The patient is restrained manually and the lateral thorax is clipped (either side) and surgically prepared from the fifth to the eleventh intercostal space. Drainage is generally carried out through the seventh or eighth intercostal space, just above the costochondral junction (Figure 22.1a). If local anaesthetic is used, it should be injected in the appropriate rib space, infiltrating not only the subcutaneous tissue but also the pleura to avoid discomfort during thoracocentesis.

A needle, butterfly needle or over-the-needle catheter (18–20 G; ideally fenestrated) is then advanced at an angle of 45 degrees next to the cranial aspect of the rib, to avoid the intercostal vessels and nerve which are located parallel to the caudal aspect of the rib. If a catheter is used, a small stab incision through the skin can be made first, using a scalpel blade. Drawing the skin forwards before penetrating the chest reduces the risk of pneumothorax, because after the needle is withdrawn the hole in the skin is not directly over the hole in the pleural cavity. Once the pleural cavity is penetrated, an extension tube and three-way tap are placed between the needle (or catheter) and a 20–60 ml syringe. Pleural effusions are usually bilateral but occasionally can be unilateral and/or pocketed. In these situations, radiography or ultrasonography should be used to identify the site for thoracocentesis. If a large quantity of fluid is to be drained or the fluid is viscid, full of debris or fibrin clots then it may be necessary to place a chest drain (Figure 22.1b).

Pericardial effusion

For pericardiocentesis, the patient is allowed to adopt a comfortable position, usually sternal recumbency, although some operators prefer the patient to be in lateral recumbency so that the heart falls away from the uppermost chest wall and puncture site. Manual restraint or light sedation may be required to minimize movement. A large area of the right or left hemithorax (sternum to mid-thorax, third to eighth rib) is prepared surgically. Examination of thoracic radiographs may indicate where the heart is most closely associated with the body wall and thus determine the puncture site. The most common site is between the fourth and sixth ribs at the level of the costochondral junction, but can also be determined by identifying the point at which the cardiac impulse feels strongest by palpation (Figure 22.1c).

The area is infiltrated with local anaesthetic in the same manner as for thoracocentesis. A skin incision is made with a scalpel blade and an over-the-needle catheter is passed into the chest. Medium-sized to large dogs may require a 14–16 G (7–20 cm long) catheter, while smaller dogs and cats usually require an 18–20 G (5–8 cm long) catheter. Alternatively, an over-the-needle catheter can be

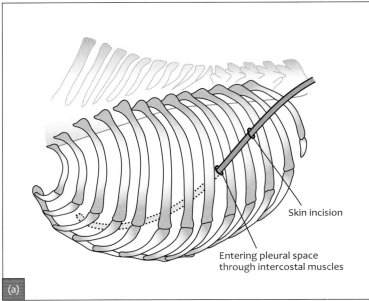

Skin incision

Entering pleural space through intercostal muscles

(a)

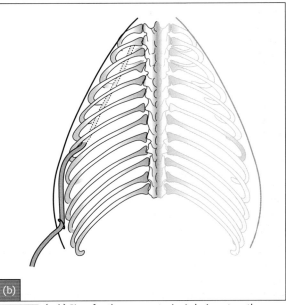

(b)

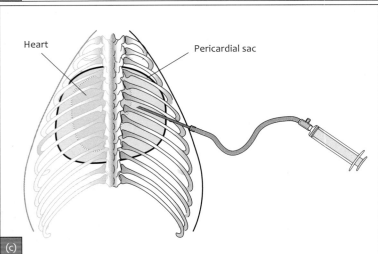

Heart

Pericardial sac

(c)

22.1 (a–b) Sites for thoracocentesis. A drain enters the pleural cavity through the eighth intercostal space, just above the costochondral junction. The drain is tunnelled subcutaneously (only required for an indwelling drain). (c) Site for pericardiocentesis. In this case the sixth intercostal space is being used (see text).

used and a suitably sized urinary catheter fed through the cannula after withdrawal of the stylet. This avoids kinking of the catheter, especially where large volumes are involved. Specialized pericardiocentesis catheters can be purchased.

The catheter is attached to a three-way tap and a 20–60 ml syringe; extension tubing can also be used. The catheter is advanced into the chest towards the heart. As the needle contacts the pericardium a scratching sensation may be noticed, before the catheter penetrates the tense pericardial sac. Once fluid is present the catheter is advanced over the needle and the three-way tap and syringe attached. Fluid can then be aspirated from the pericardium. Haemorrhagic pericardial effusion does not clot (except where haemorrhage has occurred acutely), while blood collected directly from the heart does.

Peritoneal effusion

Abdominocentesis can be performed with the patient standing or in lateral recumbency. If standing, an area of 5 x 5 cm at the point of maximal dependency (fluid accumulation) should be clipped and surgically prepared. If the patient is in lateral recumbency, an area between the bladder and umbilicus, either in the midline or slightly to the right of midline, should be clipped and surgically prepared. Emptying the bladder before attempting peritoneal drainage will reduce the risk of accidental cystocentesis. Some authors do not advocate performing abdominocentesis with the patient standing because this can increase the risk of omentum occluding the needle, resulting in a dry tap. It has also been suggested that collection from the point of maximal dependency may increase the risk of seroma formation post drainage.

In most cases, sedation or local anaesthesia is not needed and the patient is restrained manually in order to minimize movement and avoid accidental bowel puncture. The usual site for abdominocentesis is on the ventral midline, or slightly to the right to avoid the falciform fat and spleen, 1–2 cm caudal to the umbilicus, where an 18 or 20 G needle is inserted. Collection of fluid is more effective with the needle only, so a syringe is not usually attached. If a syringe is attached, only slight negative pressure (up to 3 ml) should be applied, to minimize blockage of the needle by omentum. A fenestrated catheter can also be used for abdominocentesis. A 'dry' tap can occur when the effusion is localized or pocketed, and it does not mean that there is no fluid present. In these situations, ultrasonography should be used to identify the site for abdominocentesis. Other approaches include performing abdominocentesis from each quadrant of the abdomen but this blind procedure is unlikely to harvest localized fluid.

Historically, diagnostic peritoneal lavage (DPL) was often recommended; it is very rarely indicated in small animals (the only indication being suspected diffuse peritonitis and a dry tap). DPL is absolutely contraindicated where neoplasia is suspected, and may result in extension of a localized peritonitis. It is generally carried out with the animal in lateral recumbency. The area around the umbilicus is clipped and aseptically prepared and a small 'nick' incision is made 1–2 cm caudal to the umbilicus. A large-bore (10–14 G) over-the-needle catheter which has been fenestrated, or a trocar peritoneal catheter if available, is placed through the incision and into the peritoneal cavity in a caudal direction. The catheter is advanced and the trocar/stylet removed. The catheter is then sutured in place and 20 ml/kg of warm normal saline or Hartmann's solution instilled. The patient is rolled from side to side, and a few minutes later fluid is harvested (only a small proportion of the instilled fluid will be drained). Identification of fluid by ultrasonography often allows sampling without recourse to DPL.

Handling of samples

Fluid samples should be placed in EDTA and sterile plain tubes. The EDTA tube is used for total nucleated cell count (TNCC) and cytology. EDTA anticoagulant is required to prevent the sample from clotting, which can lead to disruption of cell morphology and decreased TNCC (Conner et al., 2003). It can also be used for polymerase chain reaction (PCR) assays to detect infectious organisms. The sterile plain sample is used for measurement of total protein concentration (TP) and other biochemical tests and may also be submitted for bacterial culture if necessary (prior to any other testing). Serological testing, including coronavirus antibody titres, can also be performed using plain samples, and effusions collected in plain tubes are also generally suitable for in-house biochemistry analysers.

Formalin is often added to samples that are submitted to diagnostic laboratories for cytology. Formalin is generally inappropriate for cytological samples as it interferes with the routine stains used for cytological preparations. However, some laboratories can perform specialized staining procedures which allow them to process some fluid samples with added formalin (e.g. cerebrospinal fluid, in which EDTA does not provide adequate preservation of cells). It is therefore advisable to contact the laboratory and check these procedures are available before submitting samples with added formalin for cytological examination.

Samples should preferably be submitted to the laboratory directly. If there is likelihood of delay, e.g. collection on a Saturday, then storage in the refrigerator with preparation of a smear (which should not be stored in the refrigerator) should be performed. Different smears can be made depending on the gross quality of the fluid recovered. A direct smear is similar to one prepared from peripheral blood. A line smear can be made if the fluid is clear and colourless; here the slide is abruptly halted such that a line of fluid is formed in which any cells are concentrated. Both types of smear should be rapidly air-dried (using either a cool hair-dryer or by gently waving the slide in the air).

It has been reported that there are changes in the cellular composition of fluids over time (Maher et al. 2010). In this study, it was found that, in body cavity effusions kept at room temperature for either 24 or 48 hours, there were significant decreases in TNCC, and in absolute numbers of neutrophils, macrophages and small lymphocytes. The changes in TNCC would have changed the classification of 4 of the 47 samples examined.

Laboratory evaluation

Gross examination

Gross examination of an effusion is as important as any other examination procedure but is often overlooked. Colour, consistency and smell may all provide information on the possible pathological process. Septic effusions may have an opaque green/brown colour and be foul smelling, particularly if anaerobes are present. Blood contamination at the time of sampling may be evident from the presence of blood strands through the sample, or there may be fibrin strands running through the sample. Flocculent material is suggestive of high-protein content. A white milky lactescent fluid is pathognomonic for chylous effusion (Figure 22.2, Tube A). The white milky appearance is due to the high concentration of triglycerides; this can be seen grossly with a triglyceride concentration >1 mmol/l.

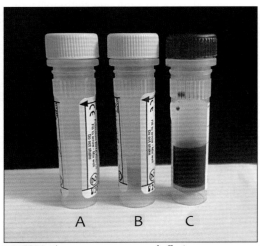

A   B   C

22.2 The gross appearance of effusions can vary markedly and may provide additional information. Tube A: this thoracic effusion is lactescent in appearance and is chylous. Tube B: this abdominal effusion is bright yellow with a small red cell sediment; the protein findings were suggestive of feline infectious peritonitis. Tube C: this abdominal effusion appears haemorrhagic.

Total protein concentration

The TP is used with TNCC to classify body cavity effusions as a:

- Transudate, protein-poor
- Transudate, protein-rich
- Exudate.

(After Stockham and Scott, 2008; see Classification of effusions below and Figure 22.3.) Very bloody or turbid fluids should be centrifuged (at 150–350xg for 5 minutes) and the supernatant used for TP measurement. Bloody fluids can also be centrifuged in a capillary tube using a microhaematocrit centrifuge (e.g. Hawksley microhaematocrit, StatSpin centrifuge). This will allow the determination of packed cell volume (PCV), while the supernatant fluid can be used for TP estimation by refractometry.

The TP can be measured using a refractometer, urine test strips (negative, 0.3–1, 1–3, 3–20, >20 g/l), and various in-house dry chemistry analysers (Hetzel et al., 2012). Peritoneal and pleural fluids from dogs and cats can be efficiently differentiated into a transudate, protein-poor or a transudate, protein-rich/exudate on the basis of TP ≤20 g/l, or >20 g/l, respectively. In the author's experience, dry chemistry analysers provide the most accurate in-house measurement of TP in body cavity effusions. TP measured on a refractometer can be falsely elevated if the fluid is chylous because a high concentration of triglycerides will affect the refractive index, and will also affect the measurement in wet chemistry analysers, but not in dry chemistry methods. In order to clear lipaemia for protein measurement, the sample can be centrifuged at very high speed (ultracentrifugation) or refrigerated for several hours. A lipid layer forms above the supernatant; the latter is harvested with a pipette but there may be some lipid contamination of the sample as the pipette passes through this lipid layer on collection.

In feline patients, in addition to TP measurement, albumin and globulin concentrations should always be determined because this can be helpful in diagnosing or ruling out certain diseases, especially feline infectious peritonitis (FIP) (see below and Chapter 28).

Total nucleated cell count

The combination of TP and TNCC is used to classify fluids as transudate, protein-poor, transudate, protein-rich, or exudate (Figure 22.3). TNCC can be performed using a haematology cell counter or a haemocytometer. The TNCC includes the mesothelial cells, macrophages, white blood cells and any other nucleated cells in the effusion.

Cytological examination

For rewarding cytological examination of effusion samples, good quality preparations are essential. Direct smears from the collected fluid should always be prepared as for peripheral blood smears. Fluid samples that do not appear turbid or purulent should be centrifuged (150–350xg for 5 minutes) and smears prepared from the resuspended pellet. Centrifugation of samples using microhaematocrit (PCV) or StatSpin centrifuges should be avoided because the generated speed is much higher than 350xg and causes cell damage. However, in an emergency situation it is often possible to gain diagnostically useful information (for example, to visualize debris from ingesta, degenerate neutrophils and intracellular bacteria in suspected peritonitis after intestinal surgery). Samples should always be submitted to the laboratory for confirmation.

Effusion	Appearance	TP (g/l)	TNCC (x 10⁹/l)	Cytology	Some common causes
Transudate, protein-poor	Clear, colourless or pale straw colour	<20 (often <15)	<1.5	Neutrophils and macrophages with some mesothelial cells	Hypoalbuminaemia, e.g. chronic hepatic disease, protein-losing nephropathy and enteropathy
Transudate, protein-rich	Often yellow, blood-tinged, turbid	Usually >20	<5	Macrophages and mesothelial cells, increasing numbers of neutrophils and small lymphocytes	Congestive heart failure, chronic hepatic disease, portal venous hypertension
Exudate	Typically turbid, various colours	>20	>5	Neutrophils, or neutrophils and macrophages	Septic: due to gut penetration and leakage, e.g. foreign body, post surgery, pyothorax. Sterile: secondary to bile or urine leakage

22.3 Criteria employed for the classification of effusions as transudate, protein-poor; transudate, protein-rich; or exudate. TNCC = total nucleated cell count; TP = total protein.
(Data from Stockham and Scott, 2008)

Samples can also be processed using cytocentrifuges (e.g. Cytospin). These are cell preparation systems, distinct from a general purpose centrifuge, which use centrifugal force to deposit cells directly on to a microscope slide. Although Cytospins are routinely employed by commercial diagnostic laboratories, the expense may not be justifiable for general practice.

Cytological examination should always be performed, irrespective of the TNCC. However, although a low TNCC does not exclude the possibility of the presence of diagnostically significant cells, such as neoplastic cells, cytological evaluation of samples with moderate to high TNCC is generally most rewarding.

Normal body cavities contain a very small amount of fluid. The cells usually present in this fluid include a mixture of mature neutrophils, monocytes/macrophages in various stages of activation and mesothelial cells, with much lower numbers of small lymphocytes and very occasional eosinophils and mast cells.

The mesothelial cells line the pleural and peritoneal cavities and cover the visceral surfaces from where they are naturally exfoliated into the body cavity fluids. These cells are typically large (25–35 µm (3–5 canine erythrocytes) in diameter), mononuclear or binuclear, with uniformly sized round to oval nuclei and pale basophilic cytoplasm. Recently exfoliated mesothelial cells may have small cytoplasmic projections or a pink cytoplasmic brush border (glycocalyx halo) (Figure 22.4). Mesothelial cells can be problematic to evaluate owing to their propensity to exhibit cytological criteria of malignancy in response to any inflammatory process.

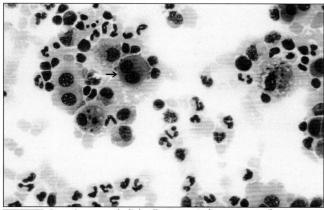

22.4 Reactive mesothelial cells. Cytospin (concentrated) preparation of a pleural effusion from a dog. Moderate numbers of red blood cells are present. The nucleated cells consist of neutrophils, small morphologically normal lymphocytes, occasional macrophages and low numbers of reactive mesothelial cells. The reactive mesothelial cells have a basophilic cytoplasm, glycocalyx halo and may also be multinucleate (a binucleate form is seen here). (Romanowsky stain; original magnification X500)

Classification of effusions

The most commonly used classification system in veterinary medicine for effusions originates from material published over 40 years ago. Classification of effusions in this system is generally based on TP, TNCC and cytological findings. Initially, effusions were differentiated into transudates and exudates (Gilmore and Munson, 1968). In 1971, Perman introduced the category 'modified transudate' to describe fluids that could not easily be differentiated into either a transudate or an exudate.

Modified transudates are not a category of effusion described in human medicine. Modified transudates are only rarely transudates that have subsequently been modified by the addition of protein and nucleated cells; the term is in fact a misnomer and rarely illuminates the pathological mechanism. It is only recently that this classification system has been re-evaluated in the veterinary field (Stockham and Scott, 2008; Dempsey and Ewing, 2011). Zoia et al. (2009) stated that the lactate dehydrogenase concentration in feline pleural fluid and the pleural fluid:serum total protein ratio best categorized feline pleural effusions into transudates or exudates. As defined by the pathophysiology, transudates are due to congestive heart failure or hypoalbuminaemia and exudates are seen with neoplasia, pyothorax and FIP. Stockham and Scott (2008) proposed a system based on pathogenesis, which the author has adopted in this chapter and which is presented in the following text.

Using the effusion classification system published by Stockham and Scott, the most common general categories of effusions with their physical, biochemical and cytological characteristics are presented in Figure 22.3. However, some types of effusion do not fall into any of these general categories:

- Haemorrhagic effusions
- Effusions that are lymphatic in origin
- Those due to viscus rupture
- Effusions secondary to neoplasia.

These will be discussed individually later in the chapter. It is important to remember that different factors (e.g. sample ageing, chronicity of disease and repeated drainage of the effusion) can change these characteristics. Therefore, this information should be treated as general guidelines, not as absolutes. Common underlying causes of canine and feline body cavity effusions are summarized in Figure 22.5.

Transudate, protein-poor

Transudate, protein-poor, effusions are usually the result of altered fluid dynamics: changes in fluid hydraulic pressure occur, often in association with hypoalbuminaemia, which decreases the plasma colloid oncotic pressure, thus allowing fluid to accumulate in body cavities. The serum albumin concentration must fall below at least 15 g/l (in

Body cavity effusions	Dogs		Cats	
	Pleural (n = 168) (%)	Peritoneal (n = 240) (%)	Pleural (n = 216) (%)	Peritoneal (n = 239) (%)
Neoplastic process	44	28	32	24
Cardiac disease	18	38	20	10
Feline infectious peritonitis	–	–	19	42
Bacterial infection	13	8	13	6
Haemorrhage	6	9	2	1
Hypoalbuminaemia	4	10	0	6
Tissue/organ inflammation	7	2	0.5	3

22.5 Common underlying causes of canine and feline body cavity effusions. Not all causes are given and therefore percentages do not total 100.
(Data from Else and Simpson, 1988; Hirschberger and Koch 1995, 1996; Davies and Forrester, 1996; Hirschberger et al., 1999; Wright et al., 1999; Mellanby et al., 2002)

many cases <10 g/l) for spontaneous transudation to occur due to hypoalbuminaemia alone. Transudate, protein-poor, can also be seen with cirrhosis, lymphatic obstruction and presinusoidal or sinusoidal portal hypertension.

The most common causes of transudates due to hypoalbuminaemia are protein-losing nephropathy (e.g. glomerulonephropathy), hepatic failure and protein-losing enteropathy (e.g. primary intestinal lymphangiectasia). Severe malnutrition can also result in transudate effusion.

Grossly, transudates are typically clear colourless fluids. Cytological findings are generally non-specific with low numbers (TNCC <1.5 x 10^9/l) of macrophages, meso-thelial cells, neutrophils and occasional lymphocytes.

Transudate, protein-rich

The TP is the most important parameter in differentiating protein-rich from protein-poor transudates, because the TNCC is relatively low in both categories and counts may overlap: in protein-poor fluids the TP is <20 g/l (often <15 g/l), while in protein-rich fluids it is ≥20 g/l. It should be remembered that long-standing transudates may irritate the mesothelium, resulting in exfoliation of mesothelial cells and secondary inflammation, which will result in increased TP and TNCC.

Protein-rich transudates are usually the result of increased hydraulic pressure within the blood and/or lymphatic circulation, typically within the lungs or liver. The protein-rich effusion develops because the capillaries in the lungs and liver sinuses are more permeable to plasma proteins than those in other parts of the body. Portal hypertension leads to the accumulation of protein-rich fluid in the space of Disse (the space between the hepa-tocyte and a sinusoid). This fluid is absorbed by regional lymphatics, but when their resorptive capacity is over-whelmed ascites develops. Disorders that commonly result in transudate, protein-rich, are cardiovascular disease, neoplasia, thrombosis and chronic liver disease.

Grossly, transudate, protein-rich, is often yellow/amber (see Figure 22.2, Tube B). Cytological findings are gener-ally non-specific unless overtly neoplastic cells are seen. Cell types identified can include macrophages, mesothelial cells, neutrophils, small morphologically normal lympho-cytes and the occasional eosinophil. A small number of red cells may also be seen and there may be erythro-phagia (Figure 22.6).

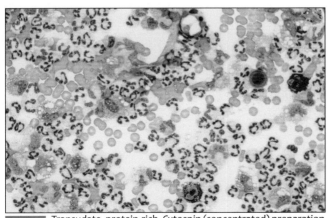

22.6 Transudate, protein-rich. Cytospin (concentrated) preparation of an abdominal effusion from a dog with hepatic dysfunction. A mixed population of cells, including macrophages, neutrophils and small morphologically normal lymphocytes, is commonly seen in this type of effusion. Note that this appears very cellular owing to the cytocentrifugation technique, although the cell count was low at 1.2 x 10^9/l. (Romanowsky stain; original magnification X200)

Effusions in liver disease

Ascites in liver disease can develop for two main reasons, either hypoalbuminaemia or portal hypertension, or a com-bination of both. Ascites that develops predominantly as a result of hypoalbuminaemia will be a transudate, protein-poor, whereas an effusion that develops as a result of portal hypertension may be a protein-poor or protein-rich transudate, depending on where exactly the pathology lies.

Portal hypertension can be subdivided into prehepatic (luminal or extraluminal obstruction of portal vein/hepatic portal vein, e.g. due to portal vein hypoplasia), hepatic and posthepatic (pathology in hepatic vein, vena cava or right heart). Posthepatic portal hypertension causes a transu-date, protein-rich, as fluid is forced from the sinusoids into the space of Disse. Prehepatic portal hypertension causes a transudate, protein-poor. Portal hypertension of hepatic origin may lead to either protein-poor or protein-rich transudates. Furthermore, once an effusion has been present for some time, or if the gastrointestinal (GI) tract becomes congested, the amount of protein in the effusion can increase.

Exudates

Exudates are formed as the result of an inflammatory process. During inflammation, there is release of chemo-tactants and vasoactive substances which attract inflam-matory cells into the cavity and also cause increased vascular permeability. The result is the leakage of a high-protein fluid which can be rich in neutrophils and other phagocytic/inflammatory cells. The TNCC is the most important parameter in differentiating transudate, protein- rich, from an exudate, because the TP in these categories may overlap: in transudates TNCC is <5 x 10^9/l, while in exudates it is >5 x 10^9/l. Exudates can be classified as septic or non-septic. Septic exudates can be caused by aerobic or anaerobic bacteria, fungi or mycoplasmas.

Septic exudates

Septic exudates may arise from penetrating wounds, secondary to surgery, extension or rupture of an adjacent infected lesion and, uncommonly, from bacteraemia. One of the most common causes of a septic abdominal effu-sion is rupture or leakage from the GI tract; this can occur secondary to neoplasia, an ulcer, or necrosis due to tissue death after an intussusception. Septic exudates usually contain numerous degenerate neutrophils; cell counts are typically >13 x 10^9/l (Dempsey and Ewing, 2011) and intracellular and/or extracellular bacteria are present (Figure 22.7). Cytology cannot reliably identify the bacterial species or predict antimicrobial sensitivities. Occasionally, effusions from body cavities infected by bacteria contain a high number of neutrophils but no bac-teria can be identified microscopically. This may be due to recent/ongoing antimicrobial treatment, the presence of a very low number of bacteria or bacteria that are not visible because they are too small and/or poorly stained.

When bacteria are identified cytologically, or where there is suspicion of sepsis even in the absence of obvious bacteria or degenerate neutrophils, a fluid sample (avoid swabs) should be submitted for culture and antibiotic sensitivity testing (see Chapter 27). The most commonly isolated species of bacteria are anaerobes or facultative anaerobes (e.g. *Clostridium* spp., *Bacteroides* spp., *Fuso-bacterium* spp., *Pasteurella* spp., filamentous bacteria

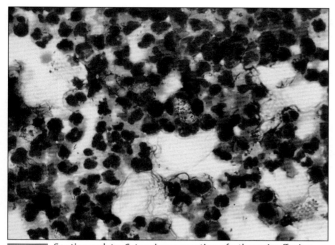

22.7 Septic exudate. Cytospin preparation of a thoracic effusion from a cat, in which intracellular bacteria can be seen. (Romanowsky stain; original magnification X1000)

(*Nocardia* spp., *Actinomyces* spp.)). Some of these bacteria are fastidious and difficult to grow, so a negative culture does not exclude bacterial infection if cytological findings are compatible. If only extracellular bacteria are seen and the neutrophils are low in number or appear non-degenerate, a possibility of *in vitro* contamination during collection of the sample or a peracute inflammatory process should be considered.

Apart from cytology and culture, it may be possible to identify septic exudates by simultaneous measurement of other analyte concentrations in plasma and fluid. One study (Bonczynski *et al.*, 2003) concluded that, in dogs, a difference between blood and effusion glucose concentrations of >1 mmol/l was 100% sensitive and 100% specific for septic peritoneal effusion. All blood and effusion samples were collected into heparinized tubes and analysed for glucose within 15 minutes of collection using an in-house dry chemistry analyser. It should be stated that the fluid comparisons were made between sterile fluids with very low TNCC and septic ones with very high TNCC. Using glucose as a sole differentiator when all fluids investigated have a high TNCC may be more problematic because the cells within the effusion could also consume glucose, leading to a lower glucose concentration in the effusion, rather than bacteria being present which consume the glucose. Hence, cytology should remain the mainstay for the diagnosis of septic exudates. This study also evaluated feline cases, in which it was reported that a difference between blood and effusion glucose concentrations of >1 mmol/l was 86% sensitive and 100% specific for a diagnosis of septic peritonitis.

Lactate has also been used as a diagnostic test for septic peritoneal effusions (Levin *et al.*, 2004). In this study it was found that all dogs had higher lactate levels in the effusion than in the blood. In dogs, the diagnostic accuracy of peritoneal fluid lactate concentration was found to be 95%. Peritoneal lactate concentration was not, however, accurate for diagnosis of septic effusions in cats. Although measurement of lactate may be useful as an ancillary test, there will be occasions when sterile exudates can occur, such as with a necrotic tumour or splenic torsion, in which lactate may be elevated, and therefore cytology should remain the gold standard for diagnosis of a septic exudate.

A more recent study (Szabo *et al.*, 2011) suggested that there are limitations to the measurement of both lactate and glucose when categorizing effusions post coeliotomy.

In a study involving 10 healthy Beagles it was found that the ratio of blood:peritoneal fluid glucose and lactate concentrations collected from a closed suction drain 4 days post coeliotomy would categorize the fluid as a septic effusion in all dogs (glucose) or 70% of dogs (lactate) when sepsis was not present.

Non-septic exudates

Non-septic exudates may develop from organ inflammation or neoplasia. Cytologically, non-septic exudates are characterized by a predominance of non-degenerate neutrophils and an absence of bacteria, although the neutrophils may appear aged (i.e. hypersegmented, pyknotic) and the macrophages may exhibit neutrophilic phagocytosis (Figure 22.8).

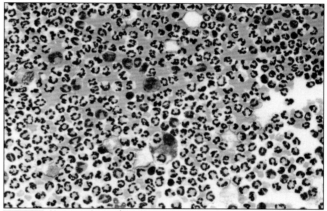

22.8 Non-septic exudate. Cytospin preparation of a thoracic effusion from a cat. Note the markedly increased neutrophils (confirmed by an automated TNCC) consistent with an inflammatory process. There is no cytological evidence of a septic process (i.e. there is an absence of pathogenic microorganisms and their toxins). (Romanowsky stain; original magnification X200)

Leakage of sterile irritants (urine, bile) can also cause non-septic exudates, which are diagnosed by biochemical tests (Figure 22.9).

Uroperitoneum: Uroperitoneum is easily diagnosed because it is characterized by higher concentrations of urea, potassium and creatinine in the fluid than in blood. Uroperitoneum may initially be a transudate, protein-poor, but over time there is often an increase in cellularity and protein concentration, leading to an exudate. However, urea equilibrates rapidly (hours) between the effusion and blood as postrenal azotaemia develops, and for this reason measurement of creatinine is a more reliable way to detect uroperitoneum, because the creatinine concentration remains elevated in the fluid for a longer period of time (days). These animals are commonly hyperkalaemic and may be hyponatraemic (see Chapter 8; Schmiedt *et al.*, 2001).

Bile peritonitis: Bile peritonitis is a non-septic inflammatory response to bile in the peritoneal cavity. Typically, bile in abdominal fluid appears as a green–gold material which may be found intra- and extracellularly within an inflammatory cell background. A case series has also been reported describing 'white bile' in the dog (Owens *et al.*, 2003), in which the bile pigment was found as a fibrillar mucinous basophilic material. It was also found in these cases that the fluid bilirubin concentration was greater than twice the serum bilirubin concentration.

Analyte	Effusion	Finding	Additional notes
Bilirubin	Bile peritonitis; exudate	Fluid bilirubin is typically twice the concentration of serum bilirubin	May detect intracellular yellow or brown bile pigment
Cholesterol and triglycerides	Chylous	Fluid triglycerides >1 mmol/l. Fluid cholesterol:triglyceride ratio <1 (convert into mg/dl before calculating ratio) (Waddle and Giger, 1990)	
Glucose	Exudate; septic	Fluid glucose lower than serum glucose in all dogs and 70% of cats. A difference of −1 mmol/l supports a septic exudate (Bonczynski et al., 2003) but is not specific for sepsis	Fluids with the greatest difference from serum also have the highest TNCC, so this may be cell consumption related, rather than due to the presence of bacteria
Urea, creatinine and potassium	Uroperitoneum	Blood:effusion urea can normalize within 45 hours. Creatinine concentration is typically at least twice that of the blood (Schmiedt et al., 2001). Potassium increases in peritoneal fluid in cats (Aumann et al., 1998) and in dogs (Schmiedt et al., 2001)	Effusion creatinine concentration depends on duration of uroperitoneum. Effusion may require dilution to achieve a measurable value

22.9 Readily available analyses that may aid in identification of the aetiopathogenesis of fluid formation. TNCC = total nucleated cell count.

Feline infectious peritonitis: Effusions due to FIP are the result of a non-septic inflammatory process which is characterized by deposition of immune complexes within vessels, resulting in increased vascular permeability and chemotaxis of neutrophils. For this reason, an FIP-associated effusion is typically a non-septic exudate, although some patients may have a transudate, protein-rich, effusion. These effusions are viscid and straw to golden in colour with fibrin strands or flecks (see Figure 22.2, Tube B). The TP is high (>35 g/l) and TNCC is typically <10 x 10⁹/l, although counts >25 × 10⁹/l have also been reported. Cytologically, FIP effusions are characterized by a protein-rich pink granular background with non degenerate neutrophils, lymphocytes, macrophages, mesothelial cells and, occasionally, plasma cells. Protein analysis of effusions has proven to be the most valuable of the laboratory tests for diagnosing FIP. Fluid electrophoresis may also be considered and typically reveals a gamma-globulin concentration of >32% and an albumin:globulin (A:G) ratio of <0.81; these are highly suggestive of FIP (Shelley et al., 1988). Duthie et al. (1997) reported effusion albumin:globulin ratios of <0.81 in 42 out of 43 FIP cases, and in 19 of these cases the ratio was <0.4.

In addition, TP of >35 g/l with ≥50% globulins in feline effusions has been shown to have a sensitivity of 100% for FIP (Sparkes et al., 1994). However, effusions due to lymphocytic–plasmacytic cholangiohepatitis may also have high globulins. It should be noted that estimation of globulin concentration (globulins = TP – albumin) by in-house dry chemistry analysers in feline effusions can be inaccurate as albumin concentration can be underestimated.

The Rivalta test has also been used as a means of assessing the protein content of effusions. The Rivalta test is based on precipitation of protein by the addition of an acid (Figure 22.10). This test has been said to be useful as part of the diagnostic work-up for suspected cases of FIP (Hartmann et al., 2003). A recent study has suggested that, although a good screening test (sensitivity 91.3%), this test should not be used for diagnosis because the specificity is suboptimal at 65.5% (Fischer et al., 2012).

1. Mix one drop of 98% acetic acid with 5 ml of distilled water.
2. Gently place one drop of the *effusion* on the surface of the *mixture*; both liquids should be at room temperature.
3. Positive: a layer of gel forms at the surface, or the drop slowly floats to the bottom.
4. Negative: the drop disperses.

22.10 The Rivalta test is used to assess the protein content of effusions.

The potential value of increased levels of alpha-1-acid glycoprotein (AGP) in the diagnosis of FIP has also been studied. Although AGP concentrations can be increased in a variety of diseases, Duthie et al. (1997) have shown that effusion AGP concentrations >1.5 g/l (serum AGP reference interval: 0.1–0.48 g/l) can differentiate cats with FIP from cats with clinically similar conditions (sensitivity 85%, specificity 100%).

Feline coronavirus (FCoV) antibody titres can be measured by immunofluorescence or enzyme-linked immunosorbent assay (ELISA) among other methods. Analysis is typically performed on serum, although titres can also be measured in effusions (Hartmann et al., 2003). A cat with a positive FCoV serum titre will also have a positive effusion titre, so there may be little additional diagnostic information obtained with measurement of effusion titre (Hartmann, 2013). FCoV titres cannot be used as a diagnostic test because the overlap in titre between healthy cats and cats subsequently diagnosed with FIP is too great (Sparkes et al., 1991). A negative titre makes FIP less likely, although does not exclude it (Pedersen, 2008). It was found in one study that 10% of the cats diagnosed with FIP were FCoV serology negative (Hartmann et al., 2003).

Reverse transcriptase (rt)PCR has been developed for identification of FCoV, although commerically available rtPCR currently does not differentiate FCoV from FIP virus. A group working in Utrecht has identified the possible mutant gene which codes for a putative fusion peptide of the spike protein, which enables the mutant virus to enter macrophages. rtPCR is being developed to identify this mutant form of the virus but is not currently commercially available (Chang et al., 2012; Hartmann, 2013). Recent work has suggested that the mutation which this PCR detects, specifically an S protein mutation, is actually a marker of systemic FCoV1 infection and can therefore be found in cats which do not have FIP but do have systemic FCoV infection. Although these cats are not commonly seen, this PCR cannot currently be used to definitively diagnose FIP (Porter et al., 2014). Given this lack of specificity, currently a positive rtPCR result from either serum or effusion must be interpreted in the light of the presentation (German, 2012). In one study, the rtPCR primer was directed against a highly conserved section of the FCoV genome and was found to have a positive predictive value of 0.90 for diagnosis of FIP (Hartmann et al., 2003).

Immunocytological detection of intracellular virus within macrophages from effusions has also been described and has been purported to provide a definitive ante-mortem diagnosis of FIP (Kipar et al., 1998). The presence of the virus within macrophages is important because it suggests the virus has the spike gene mutation, which means that the virus is no longer able to enter enterocytes but can enter macrophages. It is this property that allows the virus to spread around the body. It would still be suggested that absolute confirmation of FIP requires histopathological examination.

An excellent summary of the laboratory findings useful in the diagnosis of wet FIP is provided on the website 'Feline Infectious Peritonitis and Coronavirus', associated with the University of Glasgow, written by Dr Diane Addie. This can be found at http://www.dr-addie.com/WhatIsFIP.htm#PCReffn. It states: 'A cat with wet FIP should be FCoV seropositive, the total protein of the effusion must be over 35 g/l and the albumin:globulin less than 0.4 (or at least less than 0.8), the AGP should be high (over 1500 mg/ml) and the cytology should reveal few nucleated cells which are mainly neutrophils and macrophages. A Rivalta test should be positive. Diagnosis can be confirmed by detecting FCoV in the macrophages in the effusion.'

Other effusions

Effusions secondary to compromise to the lymphatic system

Stockham and Scott (2008) suggest the term 'lymphorrhagic' for leakage of lymph into a body cavity. This term is accurate but may be rather a mouthful, so here these effusions are described as chylous or lymphoid-rich non-chylous effusions. Pathology leading to such effusions can include trauma, with rupture of lymphatics, and any mechanism which alters lymphatic flow, e.g. changes in pressure and flow of lymph.

Chylous effusions: Chylous effusions can result from any disorder that causes obstruction or destruction of lymphatics leading to leakage of chyle (lymph and lipids) into the body cavity. Because the major lipid in chyle is derived from triglyceride-rich chylomicrons, chylous effusions have a unique characteristic: the triglyceride concentration is higher and the cholesterol concentration lower than those of serum.

It has been suggested that most chylous effusions form a thick, white layer at the top of the tube on standing in the refrigerator, owing to the presence of the triglyceride-rich chylomicrons. This has been disputed by a report which suggested that, after a 16-hour stand in the fridge, only 20% of samples which had chylomicrons detected by electrophoresis were positive (McNeely *et al.*, 1981). Another way to identify chyle is by centrifuging a microhaematocrit tube filled with the chylous fluid: the triglycerides create a white plug at the top of the fluid or a diffuse turbidity above the packed cells.

Chylous effusions occur most frequently in the thoracic cavity but occasionally can occur in the abdomen. Causes of chylothorax include (Dunn and Villiers, 1998):

- Idiopathic
- Secondary to heart disease (believed to be the most common cause in cats)
- Neoplasia
- Thoracic trauma
- Thrombosis of the thoracic duct
- Diaphragmatic hernia
- Congenital defects in the lymphatic system
- Mediastinal fungal granulomas.

Causes of chylous abdominal effusions include:

- Cardiac disease
- Hepatic disease
- Neoplasia (e.g. lymphoma)
- Steatitis.

Cytological examination typically reveals a predominance of morphologically normal small lymphocytes (Figure 22.11). However, lipid material can act as a significant irritant, causing an increase of neutrophils and macrophages over time (days to weeks) such that neutrophils can eventually outnumber lymphocytes in the fluid. Macrophages, neutrophils and lymphocytes may also have small, clear cytoplasmic vacuoles which are most likely associated with lipid accumulation by the cells (Figure 22.12).

Non-chylous lymphoid-rich effusions: These effusions typically form within the pleural cavity of cats as a consequence of increased hydraulic pressure, e.g. due to cardiac disease or intrathoracic masses. These effusions lack chylomicrons, and so do not have a grossly lactescent appearance; typically they are pale yellow–pink in colour

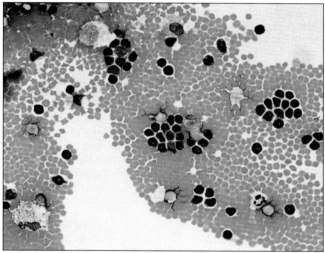

22.11 Chylous effusion. Cytospin preparation of a thoracic effusion from a cat. The nucleated cells are predominantly small morphologically normal lymphocytes. (Romanowsky stain; original magnification X500)

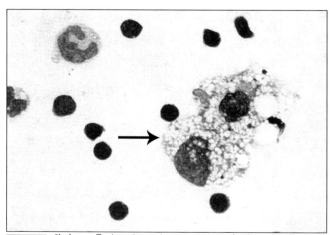

22.12 Chylous effusion. Cytospin preparation of a thoracic effusion from a cat. The macrophages contain large numbers of small vacuoles consistent with ingestion of lipid (arrowed). (Romanowsky stain; original magnification X1000)

and clear to mildly turbid. Cytologically, these effusions are rich in small lymphocytes with lower numbers of non-degenerate neutrophils and macrophages seen. In the author's experience this is a pattern often seen in cats with hypertrophic cardiomyopathy (HCM), often secondary to hyperthyroidism but possibly also due to idiopathic HCM. As with chylous effusions, the cytological pattern can change over time.

Haemorrhagic effusions: Haemorrhagic effusions (see Figure 22.2, Tube C) occur with many disorders, including surgical and non-surgical trauma, haemostatic defects, neoplasia (especially haeman-giosarcoma), vascular mal-formations and infections. Typically, haemorrhagic effu-sions have a significant PCV (≥3%) while the TP is variable depending on the fluid dilution of the haemorrhage. In the majority of acute haemorrhagic effusions the PCV is comparable to that of peripheral blood, while the PCV is often reduced by dilution in more chronic effusions.

Cytological examination can be useful in differentiating chronic from acute haemorrhage. Chronic haemorrhagic fluids typically reveal cytological evidence of erythrocyte and haemoglobin breakdown, such as erythrophago-cytosis (Figure 22.13), the presence of haemosiderophages and haematoidin crystals. Haemosiderophages are macro-phages which contain dark brown–black–green haemo-siderin pigments (a breakdown product of haemoglobin). Haematoidin crystals are rhomboid, yellow crystals which do not contain iron and represent anaerobic haemoglobin breakdown. In contrast, acute haemorrhagic fluids reveal no evidence of erythrocyte or haemoglobin breakdown.

In some cases, differentiation between true haemor-rhage and iatrogenic blood contamination during sample collection may prove difficult. Once blood enters a body cavity, the platelets aggregate, degranulate and disappear very quickly (<6 hours). Therefore, the presence of clumped platelets will indicate intravascular sampling (or peracute haemorrhage) rather than true haemorrhage.

Neoplastic effusions

Neoplastic effusions are the most complicated of all categories of effusions. They occur due to any (or any combination) of the primary mechanisms of effusion for-mation, and for this reason have variable appearance, TP and TNCC. Neoplastic effusions are typically transudates,

protein-rich, or exudates, although primary and metastatic neoplastic diseases of the kidney or liver can result in marked hypoalbuminaemia and formation of a transudate, protein-poor. Neoplasms affecting the intestines can cause septic exudates through leakage or rupture. Obstruction of lymphatic drainage due to a space-occupy-ing neoplasm can result in a chylous effusion. In addition, invasion of neoplasms into vessels or tissues can cause a haemorrhagic effusion.

Neoplastic cells are difficult to find in haemorrhagic fluids, especially those with a PCV of >20%. In these cases, cytological examination should be performed on a buffy coat smear following centrifugation of the fluid in a microhaematocrit tube (as for measurement of PCV in blood). Cytology is essential for the detection of neoplastic cells but their presence or absence depends on the loca-tion and type of the neoplasm, and an apparent absence of neoplastic cells does not rule out neoplasia. However, cytological examination of body cavity effusions is a mod-erately sensitive tool for diagnosing malignant tumours. Hirschberger et al. (1999) reported 64% sensitivity in dogs and 61% in cats with malignant effusions. In general, lymphoma (Figure 22.14), carcinoma (Figure 22.15) and mesothelioma (Figure 22.16) are the neoplasms most commonly identified in body cavity fluids. Carcinomas and round cell tumours tend to exfoliate more readily than mesenchymal tumours. Most effusions associated with carcinomas are due to metastatic disease. It has been suggested that an underlying neoplastic process should be suspected in body cavity effusions where eosinophils

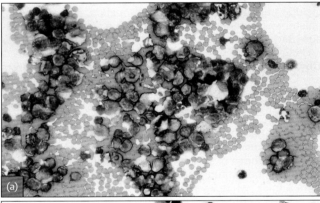
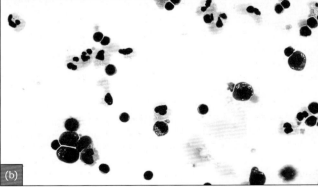

22.14 Neoplastic effusion, lymphoma. (a) Cytospin preparation of a thoracic effusion from a cat. Moderate numbers of red blood cells are present. The nucleated cells consist of a population of large atypical lymphoid cells. These cells are approximately 30–50 μm in diameter, with high nuclear:cytoplasmic (N:C) ratio, fine chromatin and multiple large, prominent abnormally shaped nucleoli. (Romanowsky stain; original magnification X200). (b) Higher magnification of (a). Note that some of the bizarre nuclear morphologies can be due to the cytospin preparation. (Romanowsky stain; original magnification X500)

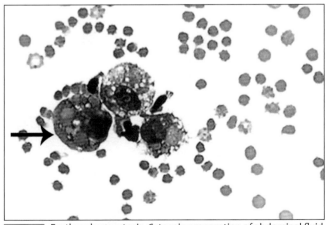

22.13 Erythrophagocytosis. Cytospin preparation of abdominal fluid from a dog. Red blood cells have been phagocytosed by macrophased (arrowed), suggesting that red cells are less likely to be due to blood contamination at the time of sampling. (Romanowsky stain; original magnification X200)
(Courtesy of JK Dunn)

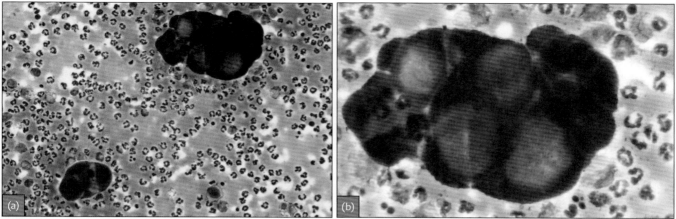

22.15 Neoplastic effusion, carcinoma. (a) Cytospin preparation of a thoracic effusion from a dog. Abundant red blood cells and neutrophils are present. Two cohesive clusters of very large mononuclear cells are seen; these cells appear pleomorphic. Detailed examination is hampered by the extremely basophilic nature of these cells. This animal was found to have a carcinoma on histopathology from lung tissue collected via a thoracotomy. Differentiation from mesothelioma is not always possible on cytology alone. (Romanowsky stain; original magnification X200). (b) Higher magnification of (a). Atypical large round mononuclear cells are present in a cohesive cluster which has an acinus-like formation. High N:C ratio is also discernible at this magnification. (Romanowsky stain; original magnification X500)

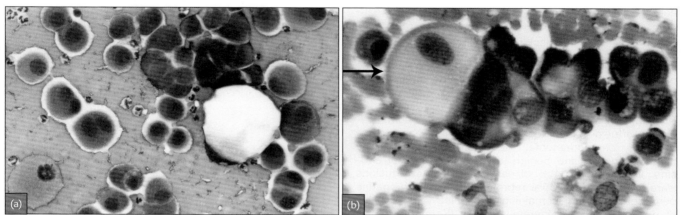

22.16 Neoplastic effusion, mesothelioma. (a) Cytospin preparation of a thoracic effusion from a dog. Moderate numbers of red blood cells are present, but there is no cytological evidence of inflammation. The nucleated cells consist of a pleomorphic population of large atypical mesothelial cells. Anisokaryosis is also present, and a prominent nucleolus is visible. (Romanowsky stain; original magnification X200). (b) Higher magnification of (a). Note the bizarre signet ring form on the far left of the cohesive cluster of mononuclear cells (arrowed). No cytological evidence of inflammation. (Romanowsky stain; original magnification X500)

are ≥10% of the TNCC. In a retrospective study of 14 cases of eosinophilic effusion in dogs and cats, over half of the cases had lymphoma or disseminated mast cell tumours (Fossum *et al.*, 1993). Eosinophilic effusions have also been associated with parasitic migration or disease, hypersensitivity and lymphomatoid granulomatosis.

Determining the origin of the neoplastic cells present in effusions is not always straightforward because the cells tend to appear round irrespective of their origin; for example, epithelial and mesothelial cells appear round, though they are not of round cell origin (Figure 22.17). In addition, clumping of cells (a feature associated with epithelial tumours) tends to occur, not only with carcinoma and adenocarcinoma, but with mesothelioma as well. Another important problem in diagnosing neoplastic effusions occurs when there is significant inflammation present. The mesothelial surfaces of body cavities react by producing dysplastic/hyperplastic mesothelial cells, which can exhibit cytological characteristics similar to those of malignant cells: increased cell numbers, anisocytosis, anisokaryosis, variation in nuclear:cytoplasmic (N:C) ratio and presence of prominent multiple nucleoli (see Chapter 21). Despite these limitations, it has been

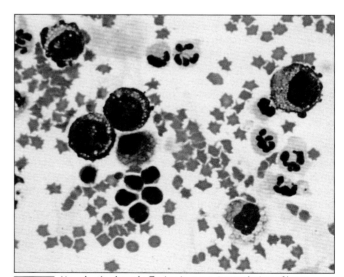

22.17 Neoplastic pleural effusion in a cat. A population of large atypical mononuclear cells is seen, which have morphological characteristics of both lymphoid and epithelial cells. This cat was found to have a carcinoma on histopathology. (Romanowsky stain; original magnification X500)

shown that the specificity of cytology in diagnosing neoplastic effusions can be excellent (99% in dogs and 100% in cats) (Hirschberger *et al.*, 1999), although sensitivity is more limited. It is recommended that fluid cytology is carried out, or verified, by an experienced cytologist.

Advances in diagnostic techniques to aid in the diagnosis of neoplastic effusions have included PCR for antigen receptor rearrangement (PARR), which is used for characterization of suspected lymphoma effusions. This is especially useful in the assessment of populations of small morphologically unremarkable lymphocytes for which further evaluation is not possible by examination of morphology alone (Avery and Avery, 2004). Flow cytometry has also been employed with effusion samples to identify their lymphoid origin when morphological evaluation is inconclusive. Immunocytochemistry can be used to distinguish epithelial from mesothelial populations.

Pericardial effusions

Pericardial effusions are the most common type of pericardial abnormality in dogs but are uncommon in cats. They are typically haemorrhagic in appearance and classification although, less frequently, they may be septic exudates or transudates, protein-rich.

In some haemorrhagic effusions the PCV of the pericardial fluid can exceed that of peripheral blood. Additional localized haemorrhage and increased pressure within the pericardial sac (the development of tamponade), forcing fluid egress at a more rapid rate than red blood cells (RBCs), may explain this observation.

Common diagnoses in cases of haemorrhagic pericardial effusions include neoplasia (mainly haemangiosarcoma, chemodectoma, mesothelioma and ectopic thyroid tumours) and benign idiopathic pericardial effusion. In one study, 41% of canine pericardial effusions were neoplastic and 45% represented benign idiopathic pericarditis, with the remaining 14% being various forms of non-neoplastic pericardial disease (Kerstetter *et al.*, 1997). Other causes include infection (e.g. *Actinomyces* spp., *Mycobacterium* spp., *Bacteroides* spp.), trauma and haemostatic disorders. Hypoproteinaemia, congestive heart failure, uraemia and FIP can cause non-haemorrhagic pericardial effusions but are reported infrequently.

A retrospective study of pericardial effusions in the cat (Hall *et al.*, 2007) found that congestive heart failure was the most common cause, accounting for 75% of the cases seen. It was not stated in this paper whether these were haemorrhagic or non-haemorrhagic pericardial effusions. In only one of the cases seen was FIP suspected; this contrasts with a previous publication which attributed 17% of the pericardial effusions seen in cats to FIP (Rush *et al.*, 1990).

Haemorrhagic pericardial effusions: On cytology, erythrocytes predominate, with variable numbers of neutrophils, macrophages exhibiting erythrophagocytosis, reactive mesothelial cells, lymphocytes and, rarely, neoplastic cells. Cytological evaluation may be an unreliable means of distinguishing between neoplastic and non-neoplastic pericardial effusions owing to the difficulty in interpreting morphological changes associated with reactive mesothelial cells which can be very marked in pericardial effusions (Figure 22.18). Therefore, the most important objective for cytological evaluation of pericardial fluid is to rule out infection or inflammation. The other causes should be investigated further using diagnostic modalities such as coagulation assessment

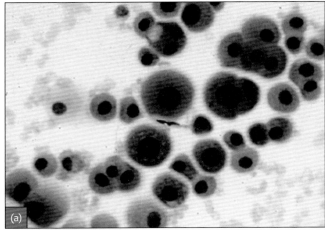

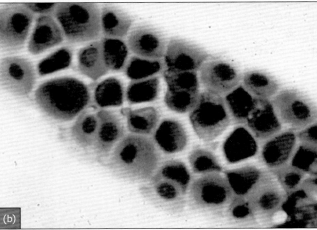

22.18 Pericardial effusion. (a) Cytospin preparation of pericardial effusion from a dog. Abundant red blood cells are present. The mononuclear cells consist of a population of mesothelial cells showing moderate variation in cell and nuclear size. This animal was believed to have an idiopathic pericardial effusion. (Romanowsky stain; original magnification X200). (b) Pericardial effusion. Further example of reactive mesothelial cells (same case as in (a)). (Romanowsky stain; original magnification X400)
(Courtesy of JK Dunn)

(see Chapter 6), radiography, ultrasonography, pericardiectomy and histopathology.

The pH of the pericardial effusion has been used to try to differentiate neoplastic from non-neoplastic effusions. One study reported that non-inflammatory (usually neoplastic) pericardial effusions typically had a pH >7.3 when measured using a calibrated pH meter and a pH >7.0 using a urine strip (Edwards, 1996). However, a more recent study concluded that the discriminatory ability of pH to differentiate neoplastic from non-neoplastic pericardial effusions is not as great as previously perceived, and reported that 87% of effusions had overlapping pH values between the two groups (Fine *et al.*, 2003), so measurement of pH is not recommended as a screening technique.

Evaluation of cardiac troponin I (cTnI) may also be useful for differentiating idiopathic pericardial effusions from those secondary to haemangiosarcoma (Shaw *et al.*, 2004). cTnI was significantly greater in pericardial effusions where a diagnosis of haemangiosarcoma was made (median 2.77 ng/dl, range 0.09–47.18 ng/dl) than in idiopathic pericardial effusions (median 0.05 ng/dl, range 0.03–0.09 ng/dl). cTnI is expressed in cardiac myocytes, and blood levels are found to increase in cases of cardiac ischaemia and necrosis (see Chapter 20). A recent study (Chun *et al.*, 2010) found that a plasma concentration of cTnI >0.25 ng/ml could be used to identify cardiac haemangiosarcoma in dogs with pericardial effusion, with a sensitivity of 81% and specificity of 100%.

In some cases, patient factors, such as time to recurrence of clinical signs post pericardectomy and survival time, may help differentiate a non-neoplastic (idiopathic) from a neoplastic (mesothelioma) pericardial effusion (Stepien *et al.*, 2000); this study did not include cases with haemangiosarcoma.

Conclusion

Figure 22.19 is a schematic showing the decision-making process which can be employed in a practice situation to evaluate a cavity effusion. The decision-making process is based on the macroscopic appearance of the effusion and also measurement of the effusion protein concentration. The effusion protein concentration may be measured using a refractometer or an in-house chemistry analyser.

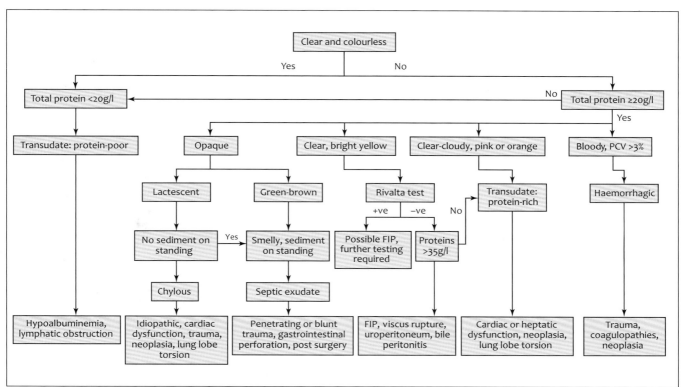

22.19 Schematic of clinical decision-making process which can be performed in practice in association with effusion total protein assessment. FIP = feline infectious peritonitis; PCV = packed cell volume.

Case examples

CASE 1

SIGNALMENT

5-year-old neutered male Domestic Shorthair cat.

HISTORY

Recent history reported lack of appetite and lethargy. In the last 24 hours there had been acute deterioration and dyspnoea. On clinical examination the cat was in good body condition. Breathing was laboured, and on auscultation the heart and respiratory sounds were muffled. Thoracocentesis harvested a slightly turbid fluid.

CLINICAL PATHOLOGY DATA

Fluid analysis	Result
Total protein (g/l)	38
Albumin (g/l)	18
Globulin (g/l)	20
Albumin:globulin ratio	0.9
RBC (x 10^{12}/l)	0.5
WBC (x 10^9/l)	5.0
FCoV antibodies	Negative

→ **CASE 1 CONTINUED**

EXAMINE FIGURE 22.20, A CYTOSPIN PREPARATION AT 1:10 DILUTION; WHAT ARE YOUR FINDINGS?

Scant red cells are seen. Moderate numbers of eosinophils are seen, with rare intermediate lymphoid cells.

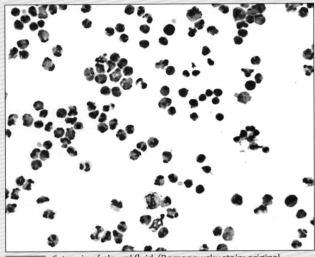

22.20 Cytospin of pleural fluid. (Romanowsky stain; original magnification X400)

HOW WOULD YOU CLASSIFY THE EFFUSION, AND WHAT ARE THE MOST LIKELY CAUSES?

The proteins here are consistent with a transudate, protein-rich. The A:G ratio is not suggestive of FIP and FCoV antibodies were negative. Differentials for a transudate, protein-rich, may include cardiac dysfunction, neoplasia and lung lobe torsion, among other causes. The effusion here is eosinophil-rich; eosinophils may be associated with primary eosinophilic pathology, e.g. hypereosinophilic syndrome, hypersensitivity and parasitism as well as a paraneoplastic process secondary to lymphoma and mast cell tumours.

WHAT FURTHER TESTS WOULD YOU RECOMMEND?

Imaging is essential in this case, with aspiration or biopsy of any possible thoracic masses seen.

CASE OUTCOME

The cat was very distressed and was initially stabilized with a combination of steroids, antimicrobials and diuretics. His condition improved overnight. The following day, echocardiography and radiography were performed. There were no abnormalities detected on echocardiography. On radiography, there was an interstitial pattern throughout the lungs with evidence of some pleural fluid remaining. On further discussion with the owners it became known that in the previous 24 hours the cat had been exposed to significant paint fumes. It was felt that, given the lack of abnormalities on imaging and the response to therapy, this may have been an acute allergic reaction to paint fumes.

CASE 2

SIGNALMENT

9-year-old neutered female Domestic Shorthair cat.

HISTORY

Acute-onset dyspnoea. On clinical examination the cat was clearly distressed, heart sounds were muffled with a heart rate of 240 bpm and a murmur was auscultated. Biochemistry and haematology were run in-house. There was a mild elevation in urea (11 mmol/l; reference interval (RI) 6–10 mmol/l) and a mild elevation in alanine aminotransferase (ALT) (134 IU/l; RI 30–75 IU/l). There was a mildly elevated RBC count (10.16 x 10^{12}/l; RI 5.5–10.0 x 10^{12}/l) and marginal eosinophilia (1.8 x 10^9/l; RI 0.0–1.5 x 10^9/l). Thoracocentesis harvested the fluid seen in Figure 22.21.

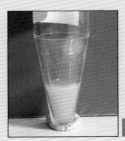

22.21 Gross appearance of pleural fluid.

CLINICAL PATHOLOGY DATA FOR EFFUSION

Fluid analysis	Result
Total protein (g/l)	43.6
Albumin (g/l)	23.4
Globulin (g/l)	20.2
Albumin:globulin ratio	1.2
RBC (x 10^{12}/l)	0.03
WBC (x 10^9/l)	3.58
Triglycerides (mmol/l)	12.8
Cholesterol (mmol/l)	2.3
Cholesterol:triglyceride ratio (calculated after converting cholesterol and triglycerides to mg/dl)	0.1

CYTOSPIN PREPARATION: DESCRIBE THE CELLS SEEN IN FIGURE 22.22.

A mixed population of non-degenerate neutrophils, small lymphocytes and macrophages is seen. Many of the macrophages contain a moderate number of small clear vacuoles.

→ CASE 2 CONTINUED

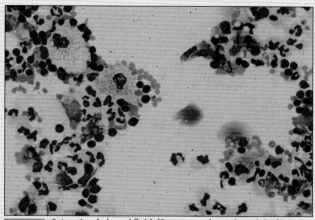

22.22 Cytospin of pleural fluid. (Romanowsky stain; original magnification X1000)

HOW WOULD YOU DESCRIBE AND CLASSIFY THE EFFUSION? WHAT ARE YOUR DIFFERENTIAL DIAGNOSES?

The gross appearance (see Figure 22.21), together with the triglyceride (>1.13 mmol/l) and cholesterol concentrations (cholesterol:triglyceride ratio <1), in association with the microscopic findings, is consistent with a chylous effusion. Lymphocytes often predominate in these effusions, but there may be a mix of lymphocytes with neutrophils and macrophages, as seen here. The vacuoles in the macrophage cytoplasm suggest ingestion of lipid. Chylous effusion can be idiopathic but may also be secondary to any interruption to lymphatic drainage, including cardiac failure, neoplasia or thoracic duct trauma.

WHAT FURTHER TESTS WOULD YOU RECOMMEND?

- Thyroxine (T4) measurement.
- Imaging: echocardiography may be more useful than radiography because effusions can obscure the cardiac silhouette. In addition, echocardiography can be used to assess cardiac chamber size and wall thickness.

CASE OUTCOME

T4 was evaluated and was elevated at 125 nmol/l (RI 15–40 nmol/l), which supported a diagnosis of hyperthyroidism. On echocardiography the cat was found to have hypertrophic cardiomyopathy. Methimazole therapy was instituted along with furosemide and benazepril, and the cat responded well to treatment.

CASE 3

SIGNALMENT

3-year-old male neutered English Bull Terrier.

HISTORY

The dog was presented with a 48-hour history of vomiting. He had a history of scavenging and prior surgery had been performed because of ingestion of both tea towels and socks. On clinical examination the dog was very subdued; there was pain on cranial abdominal palpation and a suspected fluid thrill. He was pyrexic. Given the previous history, ultrasonography was immediately performed. A small amount of peritoneal fluid was detected and a jagged-appearing hyperechoic object was visible in the proximal small intestine. Fluid was collected and found to be orange in colour and moderately opaque; the fluid was analysed as a priority.

CLINICAL PATHOLOGY DATA FOR EFFUSION

Fluid analysis	Result
Total protein (g/l)	58
Albumin (g/l)	24
Globulin (g/l)	34
Albumin:globulin ratio	0.7
RBC (x 10¹²/l)	1.3
WBC (x 10⁹/l)	37

CYTOSPIN PREPARATION AT 1:100 DILUTION: EXAMINE FIGURE 22.23 AND DESCRIBE YOUR FINDINGS

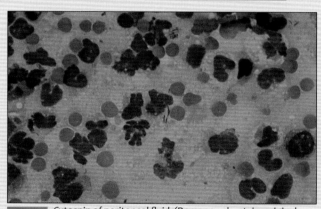

22.23 Cytospin of peritoneal fluid. (Romanowsky stain; original magnification X1000)

Low numbers of red cells are seen. Abundant degenerate neutrophils are seen, with intracellular bacteria evident.

HOW WOULD YOU CLASSIFY THE EFFUSION AND WHAT ARE THE MOST LIKELY CAUSES?

The elevated proteins with markedly increased white cell count are consistent with an exudate. Exudates can be septic or non-septic. The presence of intracellular bacteria here is consistent with a septic process.

→ **CASE 3 CONTINUED**

Differentials may include viscus rupture secondary to neoplasia or a penetrating foreign body. A septic process may also occur secondary to blunt trauma, e.g. a kick, which can lead to viscus rupture. The presence of bacteria makes bile peritonitis or uroperitoneum less likely here.

CASE OUTCOME

Given the fluid and imaging findings in association with the previous history, it was strongly suspected that there was a penetrating foreign body. Exploratory laparotomy revealed that a chicken bone had punctured the proximal small intestine. The bone was removed and the portion of associated necrotic gut dissected away. Repair of the intestine was followed by thorough peritoneal lavage with sterile saline. Empirical antimicrobial therapy was commenced with amoxicillin/clavulanic acid (co-amoxiclav) and metronidazole. Culture of the fluid isolated an extended-spectrum beta lactamase-producing *Escherichia coli* so the antimicrobials were changed to marbofloxacin and metronidazole on the basis of sensitivity testing. The dog recovered well.

Acknowledgement

The author would like to thank Kostas Papasouliotis for his kind help with the chapter.

References and further reading

Aumann M, Worth LT and Drobatz KJ (1998) Uroperitoneum in cats; 26 cases (1986–1995. *Journal of the American Animal Hospital Association* **34**, 315–324

Avery AL and Avery PR (2004) Molecular methods to distinguish reactive and neoplastic lymphocyte expansions and their importance in transitional neoplastic states. *Veterinary Clinical Pathology* **33**, 196–207

Bonczynski JJ, Ludwig LL, Barton LJ et al. (2003) Comparison of peritoneal fluid and peripheral blood pH, bicarbonate, glucose, and lactate concentration as a diagnostic tool for septic peritonitis in dogs and cats. *Veterinary Surgery* **32**, 161–166

Chang HW, Egberink HF, Halpin R et al. (2012) Spike protein fusion peptide and feline coronavirus virulence. *Emerging Infectious Diseases* **18**, 1089–1095

Chun R, Kellihan HB, Henik RA and Stepien RL (2010) Comparison of plasma cardiac troponin I concentrations among dogs with cardiac haemangiosarcoma, non-cardiac haemangiosarcoma, other neoplasms, and pericardial effusion of non-haemorrhagic origin. *Journal of the American Veterinary Medical Association* **237**, 806–811

Conner BD, Lee YCG, Branca P et al. (2003) Variations in pleural fluid WBC count and differential counts with different sample containers and different methods. *Chest* **123**, 1181–1187

Davies C and Forrester SD (1996) Pleural effusions in cats: 82 cases (1987–1995). *Journal of Small Animal Practice* **37**, 217–224

Dempsey SM and Ewing PJ (2011) A review of the pathophysiology, classification and analysis of canine and feline cavitary effusions. *Journal of the American Animal Hospital Association* **47**, 1–11

Dunn J and Villiers E (1998) Cytological and biochemical assessment of pleural and peritoneal effusions. *In Practice* **20**, 501–505

Duthie S, Eckersall PD, Addie DD, Lawrence CE and Jarrett O (1997) Value of α1-acid glycoprotein in the diagnosis of feline infectious peritonitis. *Veterinary Record* **141**, 299–303

Edwards NJ (1996) The diagnostic value of pericardial fluid pH determination. *Journal of the American Animal Hospital Association* **32**, 63–67

Else RW and Simpson JW (1988) Diagnostic value of exfoliative cytology of body fluids in dogs and cats. *Veterinary Record* **123**, 70–76

Fine DM, Tobias AH and Jacob KA (2003) Use of pericardial fluid pH to distinguish between idiopathic and neoplastic effusions. *Journal of Veterinary Internal Medicine* **17**, 525–529

Fischer Y, Sauter-Louis C and Hartmann K (2012) Diagnostic accuracy of the Rivalta test for feline infectious peritonitis. *Veterinary Clinical Pathology* **41**, 558–567

Fossum TW, Wellman M, Relford RL and Slater MR (1993) Eosinophilic pleural or peritoneal effusions in dogs and cats: 14 cases (1986–1992). *Journal of the American Veterinary Medical Association* **202**, 1873–1876

German A (2012) Update on feline infectious peritonitis. *In Practice* **34**, 282–291

Gilmore CH and Munson TO (1968) Abnormal chest fluid including chylothorax. In: *Current Veterinary Therapy III Small Animal Practice, 3rd edn*, ed. RW Kirk, pp. 174–177. WB Saunders, Philadelphia

Hall DJ, Shofer F, Meier CK et al. (2007) Pericardial effusion in cats: A retrospective study of clinical findings and outcome in 146 cats. *Journal of Veterinary Medicine* **21**, 1002–1007

Hartmann K (2013) Diagnosing feline infectious peritonitis and other feline virus diseases. *Proceedings of the European College of Veterinary Clinical Pathology*, Berlin, pp. 61–67

Hartmann K, Binder C, Hirschberger J et al. (2003) Comparison of different tests to diagnose feline infectious peritonitis. *Journal of Veterinary Internal Medicine* **17**, 781–790

Hetzel N, Papasouliotis K, Dodkin S et al. (2012) Biochemical assessment of canine body cavity effusions using three bench-top analysers. *Journal of Small Animal Practice* **53**, 459–464

Hirschberger J, DeNicola DB, Hermanns W et al. (1999) Sensitivity and specificity of cytological evaluation in the diagnosis of neoplasia in body fluids from cats and dogs. *Veterinary Clinical Pathology* **28**, 142–146

Hirschberger J and Koch S (1995) Validation of the determination of the activity of adenosine deaminase in the body effusions of cats. *Research in Veterinary Science* **59**, 226–229

Hirschberger J and Koch S (1996) Validation of an adenosine deaminase assay and its use in the evaluation of body fluid in dogs. *Veterinary Clinical Pathology* **25**, 100–104

Kerstetter KK, Krahwinkel DJ, Millis DL et al. (1997) Pericardiectomy in dogs: 22 cases (1978–1994). *Journal of the American Veterinary Medical Association* **211**, 736–740

Kipar A, Bellmann S, Kremendahl J et al. (1998) Cellular composition, coronavirus antigen expression and production of specific antibodies in lesions in feline infectious peritonitis. *Veterinary Immunology and Immunopathology* **65**, 243–257

Levin GM, Bonczynski JJ, Ludwig LL et al. (2004) Lactate as a diagnostic test for septic peritoneal effusion in dogs and cats. *Journal of the American Animal Hospital Association* **40**, 364–371

Maher I, Tennant KV and Papasouliotis K (2010) Effect of storage time on automated cell count and cytological interpretation of body cavity effusions. *Veterinary Record* **167**, 519–522

Mellanby RJ, Villiers E and Herrtage ME (2002) Canine pleural and mediastinal effusions: a retrospective study of 81 cases. *Journal of Small Animal Practice* **43**, 446–451

McNeely S, Seatter K, Yuhaniak J et al. (1981) The 16-hour-standing test and lipoprotein electrophoresis compared for detection of chylomicrons in plasma. *Clinical Chemistry* **27**, 731–732

Owens SD, Gossett R, McElhaney MR et al. (2003) Three cases of canine bile peritonitis with mucinous material in abdominal fluid as a prominent cytological finding. *Veterinary Clinical Pathology* **32**, 114–120

Pedersen NC (2008) A review of feline infectious peritonitis virus infection, 1963–2008. *Journal of Feline Medicine and Surgery* **11**, 225–258

Perman P (1971) Transudates and exudates. In: *Clinical Biochemistry of Domestic Animals, 2nd edn*. ed. JJ Kaneko and CE Cornelius, pp. 157–160. Academic Press, New York and London

Porter E, Tasker S and Day MJ et al. (2014) Amino acid changes in the spike protein of feline coronavirus with systemic spread of virus from the intestine and not with feline infectious peritonitis. *Veterinary Research* **45**, 4

Rush JE, Keene BW and Fox PR (1990) Pericardial disease in the cat: a retrospective evaluation of 66 cases. *Journal of the American Animal Hospital Association* **26**, 39–46

Schmiedt C, Tobias KM and Otto CM (2001) Evaluation of abdominal fluid; peripheral blood creatinine and potassium for diagnosis of uroperitoneum in dogs. *Journal of Veterinary Emergency and Critical Care* **11**, 275–280

Shaw SP, Rozanski EA and Rush JE (2004) Cardiac troponins I and T in dogs with pericardial effusion. *Journal of Veterinary Internal Medicine* **18**, 322–324

Shelley SM, Scarlett-Kranz J and Blue JT (1988) Protein electrophoresis on effusions from cats as a diagnostic test for feline infectious peritonitis. *Journal of the American Animal Hospital Association* **24**, 495–500

Sparkes AH, Gruffydd-Jones TJ and Harbour DA (1991) Feline infectious peritonitis: a review of clinicopathological changes in 65 cases, and a critical assessment of their diagnostic value. *Veterinary Record* **129**, 209–212

Sparkes AH, Gruffydd-Jones TJ and Harbour DA (1994) An appraisal of the value of laboratory tests in the diagnosis of feline infectious peritonitis. *Journal of the American Animal Hospital Association* **30**, 345–350

Stepien RL, Whitley NT and Dubielzig RR (2000) Idiopathic or mesothelioma-related pericardial effusion: clinical findings and survival in 17 dogs studied retrospectively. *Journal of Small Animal Practice* **41**, 342–347

Stockham SL and Scott MA (2008) *Fundamentals of Veterinary Clinical Pathology, 2nd edn*. Blackwell Publishing, Oxford

Szabo SD, Jermyn K, Neel J *et al.* (2011) Evaluation of postceliotomy peritoneal drain fluid volume, cytology and blood-to-peritoneal fluid lactate and glucose differences in normal dogs. *Veterinary Surgery* **40**, 444–449

Waddle JR and Giger U (1990) Lipoprotein electrophoresis differentiation of chylous and nonchylous pleural effusions in dogs and cats and its correlation with pleural effusion triglyceride concentration. *Veterinary Clinical Pathology* **19**, 80–85

Wright KN, Gompf RE and DeNovo RC (1999) Peritoneal effusion in cats: 65 cases (1981–1997). *Journal of the American Veterinary Medical Association* **214**, 375–381

Zoia A, Slater LA, Heller J *et al.* (2009) A new approach to pleural effusion in cats: Markers for distinguishing transudates from exudates. *Journal of Feline Medicine and Surgery* **11**, 847–855

Chapter 23

Laboratory evaluation of joint disease

Martina Piviani

Laboratory evaluation of joint disease is based on the examination of synovial fluid. Synovial fluid analysis rarely yields a definitive aetiological diagnosis but it does help to confirm the presence of an arthropathy, to discriminate between broad categories of joint disease, and to guide the choice of further tests (e.g. serology, culture, polymerase chain reaction (PCR), antinuclear antibody titre, rheumatoid factor titre, etc.). The results should, however, be interpreted in the context of the whole clinical picture, and the initial medical database should also include clinical history, physical examination, radiography, complete blood cell count, biochemical profile and urinalysis.

Physiology and composition

Synovial fluid is an ultrafiltrate of blood from synovial vessels supplemented by molecules produced by adjacent tissues. It is contained within the space delimited by the synovium, which lines the inner surface of the articular capsule, and the cartilage, which covers two bone ends (Figure 23.1). The joint fluid can actually be considered a semi-liquid, avascular, hypocellular connective tissue, rather than a true body cavity fluid, because synovium and cartilage do not have an intact cellular layer seated on a basement membrane (Figures 23.2 and 23.3). Thus, the matrix of both tissues is in direct contact, allowing a more homogeneous chemical and biological environment to develop within the joint (Denton, 2012).

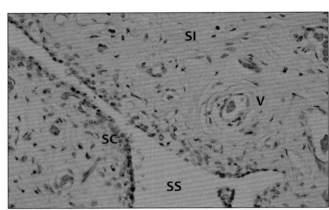

23.2 Histology of normal synovium showing the synovial space (SS) limited by a sparse layer of synovial cells (SC) embedded among a fibrous subintima (SI) with vessels (V). (Haematoxylin and eosin stain; original magnification X200)
(Courtesy of Joelle Pinard)

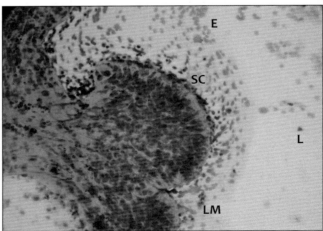

23.3 Cytology specimen with a fragment of synovial membrane showing a membrane lined by synovial cells (SC) and small numbers of large mononuclear cells (LM), small lymphocytes (L) and moderate numbers of erythrocytes (E). (Wright–Giemsa stain; original magnification X200)

23.1 Schematic representation of a joint.
(Reproduced from the BSAVA Textbook of Veterinary Nursing, 5th edition)

Labels in Figure 23.1: Periosteum, Ligament, Synovial membrane, Fibrous capsule, Articular cartilage, Synovial (joint) cavity (contains synovial fluid), Articulating bone

Synovial fluid has three major functions: supplying nutrients and oxygen to articular chondrocytes; removal of waste products and carbon dioxide; and lubrication of joint surfaces. Under non-loadbearing motion the last function depends greatly on the interaction of the mucinous glycoprotein lubricin and the glycosaminoglycan hyaluronan, which is also responsible for the fluid viscosity. These molecules are produced mainly by type B fibroblast-like synovial cells, while type A cells are phagocytes that remove debris from the synovial fluid (Carlson and Weisbrode, 2012). Type C synoviocytes have recently been described as transitional or stem cell-like with properties of type A and B cells (Vasanjee *et al.*, 2008).

Pathogenesis of joint effusion

A joint effusion may result from haemorrhage within the joint space (e.g. due to trauma or coagulopathy) or extravasation of fluid from synovial vessels as a result of increased vascular permeability (Berembaum, 2013). Vascular injury and inflammation are the triggers leading to leakage of plasma and protein from capillaries (Carlson and Weisbrode, 2012). Depending on the stimulus, the composition of the fluid varies, allowing a crude discrimination among different categories of joint disease. Historically, arthropathies have been classified as *inflammatory* and *non-inflammatory* *arthropathies*. However, the latter term may be rather misleading because some degree of inflammation, although with a different cytological pattern, is present in joint diseases belonging to both groups, whenever there is joint swelling due to either effusion or thickening of the synovium.

Indications and contraindications for arthrocentesis

In general, arthrocentesis should be performed on joints that appear swollen on clinical examination. At least four joints should be sampled whenever there is a suspicion of immune-mediated polyarthritis, favouring tarsal and carpal joints, even in the absence of detectable swelling or pain.

There are only a few possible contraindications to synovial fluid aspiration and complications are very rare. Diagnostic imaging investigations should ideally be performed before arthrocentesis to avoid potential confounding factors such as procedure-related haematomas. Other possible risks related to arthrocentesis are cartilage injury and iatrogenic infection. Indications and contraindications for arthrocentesis are listed in Figure 23.4.

Indications
• Joint effusion or swelling • Periodic shifting lameness • Stiff or altered limb function associated with fever • Joint deformity associated with lameness • Pyrexia or leucocytosis of unknown origin even if joint disease is not apparent • Monitoring response to therapy in infective and immune-mediated arthritis
Contraindications (arthrocentesis should be avoided or performed with caution in these cases)
• Cellulitis or dermatitis overlying the joint of interest • Bacteraemia • Severe coagulopathy • Before imaging investigations

23.4 Indications and contraindications for arthrocentesis.

Arthrocentesis technique

It is important that an animal does not struggle during arthrocentesis, therefore, general anaesthesia or heavy sedation is usually required. All materials needed should be prepared in advance; they include:

- Hair clippers and sterile scrub solution and alcohol
- Sterile gloves
- 5 or 2.5 ml syringes depending on the size of the patient
- 21 G (most dogs) or 23 G (smaller joints or smaller dogs and cats) needles, long enough to reach the joint cavity (1 or 1.5 inches); 3 inch spinal needle for hip joint aspiration in larger breeds (see Appendix 7 for metric sizes)
- Glass slides
- Blood culture bottle
- Collection tubes:
  - Ethylenediamine tetra-acetic acid (EDTA) tubes: preferred for preservation of cellular morphology and if fluid is contaminated with peripheral blood. Unsuitable for mucin clot test, culture and protein determination by refractometry if markedly under-filled
  - Heparin tubes: preferred for mucin clot test
  - Plain tubes: preferred for evaluation of the presence of crystals and, if sterile, acceptable (but not ideal) for culture; may allow clot formation in cases of inflammation or blood contamination of the sample.

The area over the joint to be aspirated should be prepared aseptically after clipping the overlying hair. With the patient appropriately positioned and restrained, sterile gloves should be worn and the anatomical landmarks palpated to identify the appropriate insertion site. The needle attached to the syringe is then passed gently through the joint and aspiration should begin only once the correct position is reached. Once the desired amount of fluid has been obtained, the suction should be released before the needle and syringe are withdrawn from the joint to minimize the risk of blood contamination of the sample. Usually only small amounts of synovial fluid are collected from each joint and tests need to be prioritized (Figure 23.5 The techniques most commonly used for arthrocentesis of different joints are shown in Figure 23.6.

Cytology is the most useful part of the laboratory examination of joint fluid, thus glass slides need to be prepared first. Slides may be prepared using a blood smear technique or a squash technique. The former is adequate for synovial fluid with reduced viscosity while the latter

Amount	Medium	Test
If >1 ml of synovial fluid available, split the sample four ways:		
One drop	Direct smear on slide	Cytology
0.5–1.3 ml	EDTA tube (0.5, 1, 1.3 ml)	Cell counts, total protein, PCR
± 0.5–1.3 ml	Heparin tube	Mucin clot test, total protein, PCR
Remaining amount	Blood culture tube/bottle	Bacterial culture and sensitivity
If <1 ml of synovial fluid available:		
One drop	Direct smear on slide	Cytology
Remaining amount	Blood culture tube/bottle	Bacterial culture and sensitivity

23.5 Test priorities and appropriate sample medium for synovial fluid analysis.

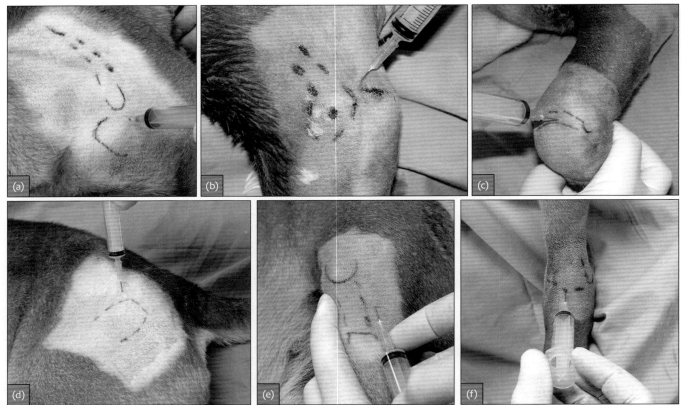

23.6 Sites for arthrocentesis. (a) Lateral view of the shoulder. The needle is inserted distal to the acromion at the end of the scapular spine (dotted line) and slightly caudal to the greater tubercle of the humerus (solid line). (b) Lateral view of the elbow. With the elbow extended, the needle is inserted between the olecranon (solid line) and the medial aspect of the lateral epicondyle (dotted line) into the olecranon fossa. (c) Craniolateral view of the carpus. To perform an antebrachial carpal bone arthrocentesis, the joint is flexed and the needle is inserted between the distal aspect of the radius (dotted line) and the cranioproximal aspect of the radial carpal bone (solid line), either medial or lateral to the midline in order to avoid vascular structures. (d) Lateral view of the hip. The needle is inserted cranial and proximal to the greater trochanter (dotted line) and directed ventrally and caudally. (e) Craniolateral view of the stifle. With the stifle partially flexed, the needle is inserted medial or lateral to the patellar tendon (dotted line) midway between the tibial tuberosity and the patella and directed medially and proximally towards the patella. (f) Cranial view of the left hock. With the hock slightly flexed, palpate the space between the tibia and the tibiotarsal bone adjacent to the flexor tendons and insert the needle perpendicular to the long axis of the tibia.

(Reproduced from How to... collected articles from BSAVA companion)

may be superior for fluids with normal viscosity. Both methods are described in Chapter 21. Priority should be given to culture if there is a strong suspicion of septic arthritis but it is advisable to proceed with microbiology testing only if there are compatible cytological findings. Caution should be taken to avoid under-filling the EDTA tube whenever possible because this anticoagulant may interfere with total protein reading by refractometry.

Synovial fluid analysis

Normal synovial fluid is:

- Colourless to pale yellow
- Clear
- Viscous
- Unable to clot
- Hypocellular
- Aparticulate.

Changes in these characteristics are usually secondary to inflammation, haemorrhage or iatrogenic blood contamination and may be detected by a combination of macroscopic and microscopic examination. The major synovial fluid alterations found in the most common joint diseases are outlined in Figure 23.7.

Macroscopic evaluation

Macroscopic evaluation should include assessment of volume, colour, turbidity, viscosity and the presence of clots or other particulates. When sending the sample to an external laboratory these findings should always be reported on the laboratory submission form.

Volume

The volume of joint fluid usually correlates with the distension of the joint capsule, which may be estimated subjectively by physical examination. The amount of fluid that can be obtained by arthrocentesis in healthy patients ranges from one drop to 0.25 ml in cats and one drop to 1 ml in dogs, depending upon the joint sampled and the animal's size. Higher volumes may be collected in diseases characterized by joint effusion.

Colour

Pink or red colour indicates the presence of erythrocytes or free haemoglobin. This may be due to haemorrhage within the joint or blood contamination at sampling. The presence of platelets should be noted on microscopic evaluation in the latter case. The sudden appearance and uneven distribution of blood in the synovial fluid during

Disease	Colour	Turbidity	Viscosity	Total protein	Mucin clot quality	Nucleated cellularity	Predominant cell type	Comments
Osteoarthritis	Colourless to straw	Clear	Normal to slightly decreased	Normal	Good to fair	Normal to mildly increased	Large mononuclear cells Neutrophils <12%	Often increased vacuolated cells (>10%)
Trauma	Colourless, or yellow to red if also haemorrhage	Clear to hazy	High to mildly reduced	Normal to increased	Good to fair	Normal to mildly increased	Variable	Erythrocytes if haemorrhagic component; erythrophagia and haemosiderophages may be seen
Haemorrhage	Red to orange (xanthochromic)	Hazy to opaque	Mildly to markedly reduced	Increased proportionally to amount of blood	Fair to poor	Normal to mildly increased	Large mononuclear cells and haemosiderophages if chronic. Differential similar to peripheral blood if acute	Platelets may be seen if peracute. Erythrophagia if acute or ongoing. Haemosiderin if long-standing
Septic arthritis	Yellow to white or pink	Hazy, cloudy or opaque	Mildly to markedly reduced	Increased	Fair to poor	Increased, often markedly	Neutrophils, degenerate or non-degenerate	Intracellular bacteria may be seen but this is rare
Immune-mediated arthritis	Yellow to white or pink	Hazy, cloudy or opaque	Mildly to markedly reduced	Increased	Fair to poor	Increased, often markedly	Non-degenerate neutrophils	LE cells supportive of SLE; ragocytes can be seen with both erosive and non-erosive forms of IMPA and rheumatoid arthritis

23.7 Synovial fluid findings in the most common joint diseases of the dog and cat. IMPA = immune-mediated polyarthritis; SLE = systemic lupus erythematosus.

aspiration are reliable indicators of a traumatic tap. A gold–yellow discoloration (xanthochromia) is usually associated with prior haemorrhage and the presence of haemoglobin breakdown products. A white or opaque light yellow colour suggests increased cellularity.

Turbidity

Normal synovial fluid is clear, similar to raw egg white. If print cannot be read through a sample it is considered turbid or cloudy. Increased turbidity is usually due to increased cellularity, or the presence of fibrin or other debris, including crystals.

Viscosity

Viscosity correlates with the concentration and quality of mucinous proteins within the fluid. Synovial fluid viscosity is most commonly assessed subjectively. This can be done directly at the moment of fluid collection by expelling one or two drops of fluid from the syringe into the container or on to a glass slide. At the laboratory, a small amount of fluid is pulled from the tube with a wooden stick. Normal synovial fluid forms a long string (2.5–5 cm) before breaking (Figure 23.8). If the fluid flows with the ease of water and no string forms, viscosity is markedly decreased. Reduced viscosity is most often associated with an inflammatory process secondary to the action of bacterial enzymes (e.g. hyaluronidase) on synovial fluid constituents, dilution by increased leakage of serum or joint lavage, and decreased synthesis of hyaluronan and lubricin by injured synovial cells. Samples stored in EDTA may have slightly decreased viscosity due to *in vitro* degradation of hyaluronan. The mucin clot test is discussed later in the chapter.

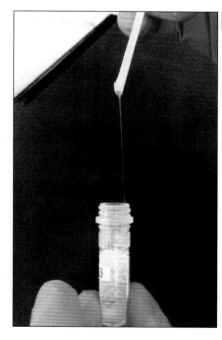

23.8 Macroscopic evaluation of synovial fluid viscosity. If viscosity is normal a string at least 2.5 cm long should form when a small amount of the fluid is pulled from the tube with a stick.

Clotting

Under normal conditions joint fluid is devoid of coagulation factors. Joint fluid becomes a gel under static conditions, mimicking the formation of a clot. However, if shaken, it becomes thin and less viscous. This property is called *thixotropy*. True clots can form if there is blood contamination or in cases of inflammation, when there is leakage of proteins including fibrinogen and other coagulation factors from synovial vessels.

Cell counts

Erythrocyte and total nucleated cell counts may be performed using a manual haemocytometer or C-Chip (see Chapter 25), or an automated analyser. The latter method has the limitation of having a relatively higher limit of detection for erythrocyte count (usually 10,000 RBC/μl) than manual methods, but obtaining an accurate erythrocyte count is rather irrelevant in synovial fluid analysis. Nucleated cell counting may be significantly affected by fluid viscosity and cell clumping with both methods. Incubation for 5–30 minutes with hyaluronidase (one or two drops of a 150 IU/ml solution) usually improves accuracy and is recommended (Ekmann et al., 2010), although this may not be required when analysing samples stored in EDTA for 24 hours or more. Dilution with saline is advisable when counting with a manual haemocytometer if the sample is expected to be hypercellular (e.g. a turbid sample). Grossly, blood contaminated samples may also be mixed with a hypotonic solution to cause erythrocyte lysis and facilitate counting of nucleated cells. In that case the number obtained should then be multiplied by the appropriate dilution factor. Normal canine joint fluids are expected to have <3000 nucleated cells/μl (MacWilliams and Friedrichs, 2003) but cellularity is often lower, and in several laboratories the upper reference limit is set at 1000 nucleated cells/μl.

Cell counts should, however, be compared with a subjective estimation made on a direct smear, whenever available (see below).

Cytology

Direct smears should be prepared immediately after sample collection and submitted along with the fluid. Slides should be kept away from sources of cold to avoid artefacts due to freezing (Figure 23.9). At the laboratory additional slides will be prepared, including direct and concentrated preparations, and all slides will be routinely stained using Romanowsky-type stains, air-dried and examined.

Guidelines for the examination of direct smears of synovial fluid are summarized in Figure 23.10.

The density of the pink granular background on the slide should be noted because it correlates with the fluid viscosity (Figure 23.11). In thicker areas of the smear this layer may appear folded (Figure 23.12). The degree of

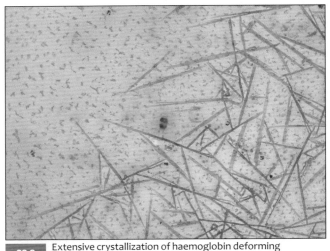

23.9 Extensive crystallization of haemoglobin deforming erythrocytes, probably due to thermal shock caused by storage of the slide in the fridge before staining. (Wright–Giemsa stain; original magnification X100)

Low magnification (X40–200)
• Assessment of the density and distribution of nucleated cellularity • Appearance of the background • Presence of crystals, bone or cartilage fragments • Presence of erythrocytes and platelet clumps

Higher magnification (X400–1000)
• Estimation of cell count: each nucleated cell per field at X400 magnification is considered equivalent to 1000 cells/μl (Gibson et al., 1999) • Nucleated cell differential: large mononuclear cells, lymphocytes, neutrophils, eosinophils and 'other cells' • Percentage of 'vacuolated cells' • Presence of platelets

23.10 Guidelines for the evaluation of direct smears of synovial fluid.

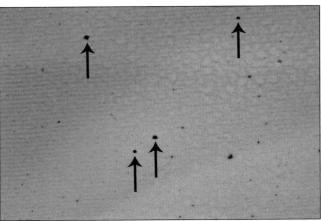

23.11 Direct smear of normal synovial fluid. Note the characteristic pink homogeneous background in which rare small mononuclear cells (arrowed) are embedded. (Wright–Giemsa stain; original magnification X100)

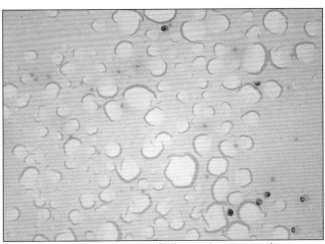

23.12 Direct smear of synovial fluid. Note the crescents due to folding of the mucoproteinaceous material with scattered large mononuclear cells and few erythrocytes. (Wright–Giemsa stain; original magnification X200)

separation between granules is an indirect estimation of the concentration of glycosaminoglycan (hyaluronan) in the fluid (Figure 23.13). Cell windrowing (a linear alignment of cells on the fluid smear) is commonly suggested as an indication of normal viscosity. However, cell windrowing may not be obvious in normal joint fluid with low cellularity, whereas it may still be seen in hypercellular inflammatory fluids when fluid viscosity and the glycosaminoglycan concentration are likely to be reduced (Figure 23.14). Cell and

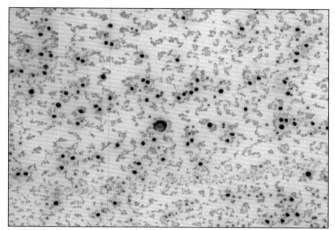

23.13 Direct smear of synovial fluid from a cat with an inflammatory arthropathy. Many neutrophils, one multinucleated large mononuclear cell and a few erythrocytes are present. Note the clear spaces separating the pink granules. This finding suggests a decreased concentration of glycosaminoglycans. (Wright–Giemsa stain; original magnification X200)

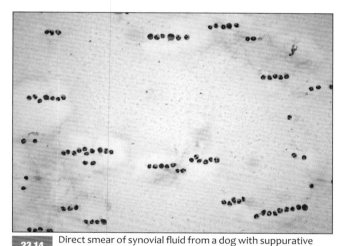

23.14 Direct smear of synovial fluid from a dog with suppurative arthritis, containing many neutrophils and fewer large mononuclear cells. Note the decreased density of pink granules in the background but persistence of cell windrowing. (Wright–Giemsa stain; original magnification X200)
(Courtesy of Roger Powell)

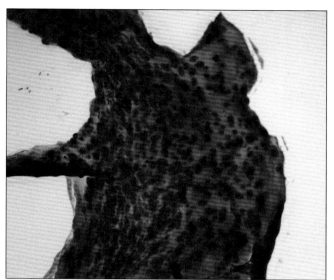

23.15 Fragment of cartilage appearing as dense bright pink material in which chondrocytes are embedded. (Wright–Giemsa stain; original magnification X200)

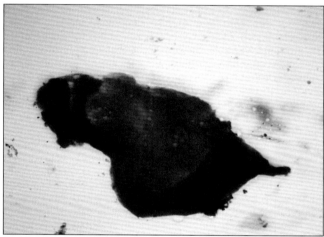

23.16 Fragment of bone appearing as a spicule of dense acellular pink material. (Wright–Giemsa stain; original magnification X100)

erythrocyte windrowing in those cases may be due to the addition of fibrinogen to the fluid secondary to inflammation.

All slides should also be scanned to detect any particulate material, including crystals and fragments of denser matrix compatible with bone or cartilage, which could suggest erosion of cartilage or subchondral bone (Figures 23.15 and 23.16).

The type and number of leucocytes that infiltrate the synovium and migrate into the synovial fluid define the cellular components of the joint effusion. Nucleated cells should be classified as:

- Large mononuclear cells
- Lymphocytes
- Neutrophils
- Eosinophils
- Other cells.

'Other cells' may be other inflammatory cells usually not encountered in synovial fluid (e.g. mast cells), lymphoid blasts, osteoclasts (Figure 23.17), osteoblasts (Figure 23.18) or other atypical discrete cells. Large mononuclear cells have an oval shape with a slightly eccentric round to

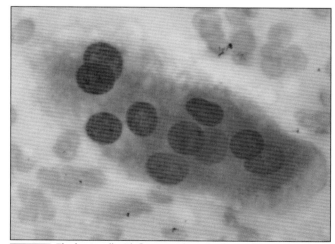

23.17 The large cell with fine granular cytoplasm with square edges and multiple oval nuclei is an osteoclast. This cell is seen rarely in joint fluid. Its presence may indicate erosion of cartilage and subchondral bone. (Wright–Giemsa stain; original magnification X1000)
(Courtesy of Roger Powell)

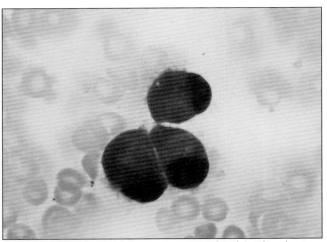

23.18 Cells with an oval shape, eccentric oval nuclei and moderate amounts of deeply basophilic cytoplasm are compatible with osteoblasts. Their presence indicates bone remodelling. Compared with plasma cells they are larger and have less prominent paranuclear clearing. The major axis of their nuclei is orthogonal to the major axis of the cell. (Wright–Giemsa stain; original magnification X1000)
(Courtesy of Roger Powell)

oval nucleus with fine mature chromatin and indistinct nucleoli (Figure 23.19). Cytoplasm is scant to moderate in amount and variably basophilic, occasionally with a few fine pink granules (Figure 23.20). Large mononuclear cells encompass blood-derived monocytes, tissue macrophages and synovial lining cells. Moderate to marked procedural blood contamination may significantly affect the differential count, leading to a spurious increase in the neutrophil percentage, especially if the fluid has low nucleated cellularity. Hypercellular fluids are less affected. Thus, it is important to evaluate the differential count in the context of the overall cellularity.

The proportion of large mononuclear cells with foamy vacuolated cytoplasm and/or phagocytosed material or cell debris should be recorded (Figure 23.21). These cells are interpreted as macrophages or phagocytic synoviocytes. Osteoclasts and osteoblasts may be seen with osteolysis and bone remodelling.

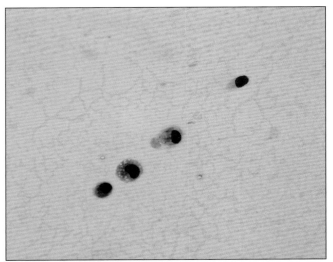

23.19 Normal canine joint fluid with a finely stippled eosinophilic background and small numbers of large mononuclear cells lined up in a row (cell windrowing). Large mononuclear cells have an oval shape and a slightly eccentric round to oval nucleus with fine mature chromatin and indistinct nucleoli. (Wright–Giemsa stain; original magnification X200)

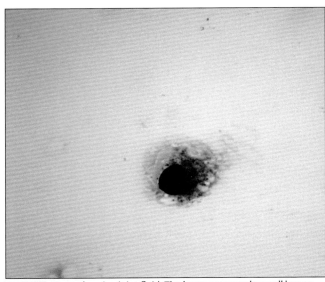

23.20 Normal canine joint fluid. The large mononuclear cell has an oval shape and a scant to moderate amount of light blue cytoplasm, with a few fine pink granules and rare vacuoles. (Wright–Giemsa stain, original magnification X1000)

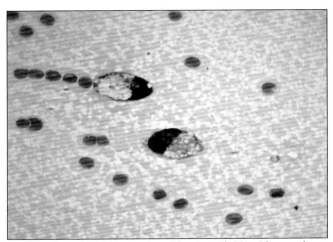

23.21 Synovial fluid from a dog with osteoarthritis, with more than 10% of large mononuclear cells appearing 'vacuolated'. (Wright–Giemsa stain; original magnification X500)

Joint diseases manifest with a rather limited number of cytological patterns and these tend to correlate with the clinical features of the underlying arthropathy (Figure 23.22).

Absence of cytological abnormalities

The body of a direct smear made from normal synovial fluid should contain an average of two cells at X400 magnification (Fernandes, 2013) or fewer than 2–3 cells at X1000 (Innes, 2005; see Figure 23.19). Large mononuclear cells predominate while neutrophils account for less than 5–12% in non-haemodiluted samples, depending on the reference used (Center, 2012; Fernandes, 2013).

Red blood cells may be seen in normal synovial fluid in cases of traumatic arthrocentesis. Platelets are expected with procedural bleeding or other causes of peracute haemorrhage. Cells are embedded, and occasionally windrowing (lining up in a row), in a thin layer of homogeneous to finely granular pink material consistent with mucoproteins.

It is important to bear in mind that absence of cytological abnormalities may be compatible with normal synovial

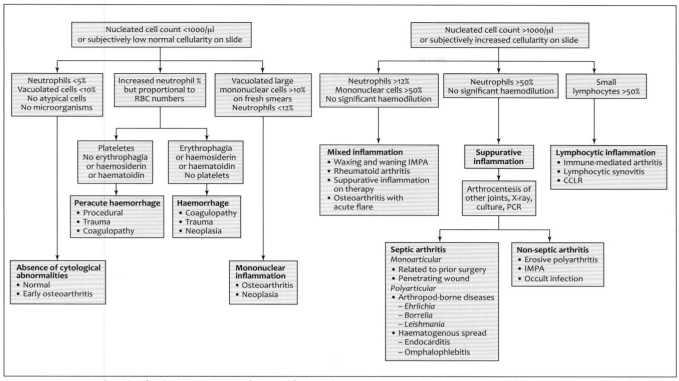

23.22 Diagnostic algorithm for the interpretation of synovial fluid cytology. CCLR = cranial cruciate ligament rupture; IMPA = immune-mediated polyarthritis; PCR = polymerase chain reaction; RBC = red blood cell.

fluid but does not rule out the possibility of a degenerative arthropathy. Some degree of inflammation is expected, although not always detectable cytologically, whenever there is a joint effusion.

Suppurative inflammation

Suppurative inflammation is characterized by an increase in nucleated cells (often marked) in the synovial fluid, with a predominance of neutrophils (Figure 23.23). Suppurative inflammation may be due to infectious arthritis or an immune-mediated disorder. A mild neutrophilic component, with neutrophils usually accounting for <12% of all

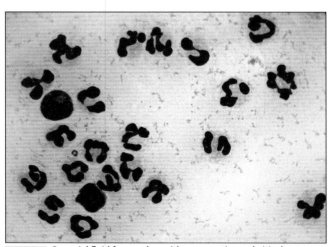

23.23 Synovial fluid from a dog with suppurative arthritis due to immune-mediated polyarthropathy. The nucleated cellularity is markedly increased and predominated by neutrophils. The granular background appears less dense, consistent with reduced glycosaminoglycan content. (Wright–Giemsa stain; original magnification X1000)

nucleated cells, may be seen in some cases of osteo-arthritis (Innes, 2005), crystal deposition, neoplasia, joint trauma and secondarily to haemodilution. The background pink staining is less homogeneous and may appear 'diluted', with clear spaces separating the pink granules (see Figure 23.13), correlating with variably reduced viscosity on gross evaluation and often reduced mucin clot quality. Erythrocytes may enter synovial fluid by diapedesis facilitated by increased vascular permeability due to inflammation.

Septic arthritis: Septic arthritis is joint inflammation due to an intra-articular infectious aetiology. Septic suppurative inflammation defines a cytological pattern characterized by a predominance of neutrophils, accompanied by intralesional (and intracellular) microorganisms (Figures 23.24–23.28), and this is diagnostic of septic arthritis. Stain precipitate and the granular mucoproteinaceous background material should be discriminated from true bacteria (see Figure 23.29). Markedly increased nucleated cellularity and a very high neutrophil percentage (usually >75–90%) are expected in bacterial arthritis but the inflammatory pattern may be characterized by a more pronounced mononuclear component in chronic or treated bacterial arthritis, and in mycobacterial, fungal and protozoal infections. Neutrophil degeneration, characterized by swollen chromatin and loss of definition of nuclear and cytoplasmic contours, is highly suspicious for bacterial infection but it is an insensitive marker of infectious aetiology in synovial fluid (Figure 23.25). Thinner areas of the smear where neutrophils are well spread out should be scanned at X400. The lateral edges of the smear often provide the best conditions for this purpose. Slides can also be destained to apply Gram stain in order to facilitate the identification of Gram-positive bacteria (Marcos *et al.*, 2009), but experience with this stain is

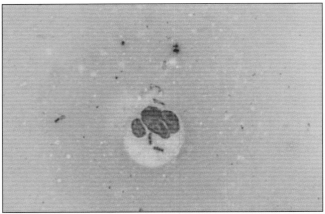

23.24 Synovial fluid from the stifle of a dog with septic arthritis. One degenerate neutrophil is seen, with an intracellular chain of bacterial cocci. Rare chains of cocci are also noted extracellularly, scattered in the mucoproteinaceous background. Culture was positive for beta-haemolytic *Streptococcus*. (Wright–Giemsa stain; original magnification X1000)
(Courtesy of Roger Powell)

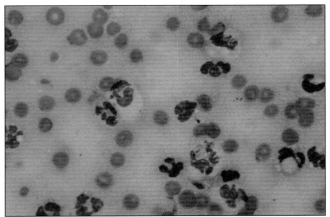

23.25 Elbow synovial fluid from a 4-month-old German Shepherd Dog with septic arthritis due to *Pasteurella multocida* infection. Increased cellularity is seen, predominated by neutrophils admixed with many erythrocytes scattered amid a pink granular background. Several neutrophils appear degenerate with swollen chromatin and vacuolated cytoplasm. Two neutrophils contain several phagocytosed coccobacilli. (Wright–Giemsa stain; original magnification X1000)
(Courtesy of Marta Dell'Orco)

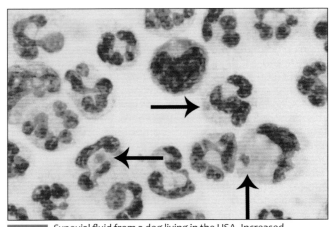

23.26 Synovial fluid from a dog living in the USA. Increased cellularity is observed, predominated by non-degenerate neutrophils and rare mononuclear cells. The lightly basophilic round slightly granular structures within the neutrophil cytoplasm (arrowed) are compatible with morulae of *Anaplasma phagocytophilum* or *Ehrlichia ewingii*. (Wright–Giemsa stain; original magnification X1000)
(Courtesy of Raquel Walton)

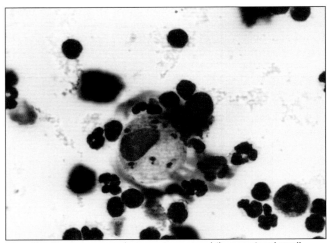

23.27 Numerous non-degenerate neutrophils, occasional small lymphocytes and one large macrophage with intracellular organisms, compatible with amastigotes of *Leishmania infantum*, in synovial fluid from a dog with arthritis. (Diff-Quik® stain; original magnification X1000)

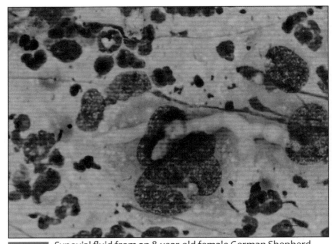

23.28 Synovial fluid from an 8-year-old female German Shepherd Dog with fungal osteomyelitis of the patella due to *Aspergillus fumigatus* infection. Note the negative-staining branched structure surrounded by multinucleated macrophages and degenerate neutrophils. (Wright–Giemsa stain; original magnification X1000)

required for interpretation and the false negative rate of Gram-stain microscopy for diagnosis of septic arthritis is reported to be between 25 and 78% (Stirling *et al.*, 2014).

It is important to bear in mind that an absence of detectable microorganisms on cytology or even a negative culture does not rule out a septic process. Clinical experience and experimental studies indicate that direct culture of joint fluid on blood agar produces false negative results in roughly 50% of cases that are clinically consistent with septic arthritis (Clements *et al.*, 2005), and microorganisms are seen in fewer than 50% of culture-positive synovial specimens (MacWilliams and Friedrichs, 2003). Thus, septic arthritis is most often a clinical diagnosis based on clinical presentation, the presence of suppurative inflammation on synovial fluid cytology and compatible history. Arthritis due to bacterial infection is usually monoarticular, has an acute onset, and most often follows an infected penetrating wound or joint surgery. In dogs without a history of prior surgery, the organisms most commonly cultured are skin commensals, including *Staphylococcus pseudintermedius*, *Staphylococcus aureus* and beta-haemolytic *Streptococcus* spp. The stifle and the elbow are the most common joints affected (Clements *et al.*, 2005). Infections due to meticillin-resistant forms of *S. aureus* and *S. pseudintermedius* (MRSA/MRSP) have also been reported.

Septic arthritis due to haematogenous spread is also possible and may be polyarticular in immunocompromised patients. Potential causes include omphalophlebitis in neonates and bacterial endocarditis or urinary tract infection in adults, although the latter conditions may also trigger reactive immune-mediated polyarthritis. Investigations to rule out these possibilities (e.g. urine and blood culture, echocardiography) are therefore advisable in cases of suspected or confirmed septic arthritis, especially if polyarticular involvement is present. In cats, bacterial arthritis most often results from bite wounds, and the micro-organisms isolated are components of the oral flora (*Pasteurella multocida*, *Bacteroides* spp. and *Escherichia coli*). Bacterial L-forms (cell wall deficient bacteria) have been described in cats presenting with cellulitis, synovitis, bacteraemic spread and secondary polyarthritis. One case of polyarthritis secondary to the L-form of *Nocardia asteroides* has also been reported in a dog. The source of infection is often a penetrating wound or surgical incisions. These organisms are difficult to demonstrate by light microscopy and do not grow in available culture media. Electron microscopy may be required for definitive identification (Greene and Chalker, 2012).

Other potential causative agents that can also be difficult or impossible to detect with standard cultures are *Bartonella* spp., *Mycoplasma* spp., spirochaetes such as *Borrelia burgdorferi*, rickettsiales such as *Ehrlichia canis*, *E. ewingii* (not present in Great Britain) and *Anaplasma phagocytophilum*, and protozoa (e.g. *Leishmania infantum*). Arthropod-borne diseases may lead to polyarthritis or pauciarthritis. Dogs infected by *B. burgdorferi* most often present with monoarthritis or pauciarthritis. PCR and serology may help to identify these microorganisms (see Chapters 27 and 29). Fungal arthritides (*Aspergillus* spp., *Cryptococcus neoformans*) are uncommon and usually secondary to osteomyelitis (Figure 23.28) or disseminated infection. Feline calicivirus has been reported to cause lameness and acute arthritis in cats (Dawson *et al.*, 1994). Polyarthritis is also occasionally seen after vaccination against feline calicivirus; this may rarely represent an immune-mediated form but it is mainly due to co-infection with field virus or vaccine virus itself (Scherk *et al.*, 2013).

Immune-mediated arthritis: Cases of suppurative arthritis not associated with intra-articular infectious agents and with a polyarticular presentation are most often due to immune-mediated disease (Figure 23.29). Based on the presence or absence of radiographic evidence of cartilage erosion, these are further characterized as non-erosive (most common) and erosive arthritis. Clinical entities are listed in Figure 23.30. These diseases are generally due to a type III hypersensitivity reaction with deposition of antigen–antibody complexes in the synovial blood vessel wall and a secondary inflammatory response. Multiple joints are usually affected, concurrently or consecutively, with more severe signs in the distal joints (tarsi and carpi). Arthrocentesis of four or more joints may be necessary to establish the clinical diagnosis of pauciarthritis (>2 joints affected) or polyarthritis (≥5 joints affected). The hock appeared to be the most reliable joint for the diagnosis of immune-mediated polyarthritis in a recent review of cases (Stull *et al.*, 2008).

Similarly to septic arthritis, immune-mediated arthropathies typically cause joint effusions with high cellularity

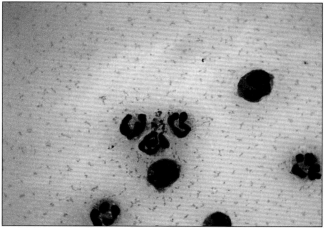

23.29 Synovial fluid from a dog with immune-mediated polyarthritis. The increased nucleated cellularity is predominated by non-degenerate neutrophils and a few large mononuclear cells. The extracellular, variably sized and shaped, deep purple granules are stain precipitate and not microorganisms. (Wright–Giemsa stain; original magnification X1000)

Non-erosive immune-mediated arthritis

• Idiopathic immune-mediated polyarthritis
  • Type I – idiopathic
  • Type II – reactive to inflammation or infection in distant site
  • Type III – associated with gastroenteritis or hepatopathy
  • Type IV – associated with malignancy remote from joint
• Drug-associated
• Vaccine reaction
• Polyarthritis–meningitis syndrome
• Polyarthritis–polymyositis syndrome
• Systemic lupus erythematosus
• Lymphoplasmacytic gonitis
• Juvenile-onset polyarthritis of Akitas
• Synovitis–amyloidosis of Shar Peis

Erosive arthritis
• Canine rheumatoid arthritis • Feline progressive polyarthritis (erosive and proliferative forms) • Greyhound polyarthritis

23.30 Causes of non-septic suppurative arthritis in dogs and cats.

predominated by neutrophils, although cellularity can occasionally be more mixed or rarely mostly mononuclear. Cytological findings may also differ among different joints, be partially masked by concurrent immuno-suppressive therapy and fluctuate during the disease. The finding of dark purple irregular granular intracytoplasmic inclusions in neutrophils is considered strongly supportive of immune-mediated arthritis and can be seen in both non-erosive and erosive forms. These inclusions are thought to be fragments of phagocytosed immune complexes, including rheumatoid factors (Figure 23.31). Neutrophils with these inclusions are called ragocytes by most veterinary pathologists, although this term referred originally to cells of any lineage (granulocytes in particular) with intracytoplasmic refractile granules appearing apple-green to black in unstained wet preparations examined with a partially closed condensed diaphragm (Denton, 2012).

Systemic signs may be present, including fever, lymphadenopathy, proteinuria, generalized stiffness and pain that is difficult to localize. The diagnosis of immune-mediated arthritis relies on compatible clinical presentation, suggestive cytological findings and exclusion of intra-articular infection via culture, PCR or empirical therapy.

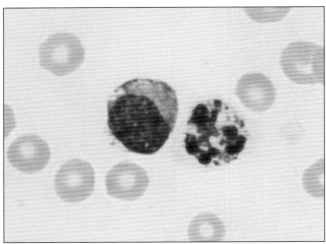

23.31 Synovial fluid from a dog with rheumatoid arthritis. A large mononuclear cell and a neutrophil containing variably sized deep purple granules are seen. Neutrophils with these inclusions are often called ragocytes. (Wright–Giemsa stain; original magnification X500) (Courtesy of Roger Powell)

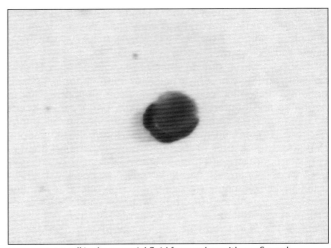

23.32 LE cell in the synovial fluid from a dog with confirmed systemic lupus erythematosus. Note the large intracytoplasmic pink glassy round inclusion displacing the nucleus to the periphery. (Wright–Giemsa stain; original magnification X1000) (Courtesy of Marta Dell'Orco)

- **Idiopathic immune-mediated polyarthropathies** are the most common forms of non-erosive immune-mediated arthritis and may be a primary (idiopathic) condition or triggered by underlying inflammatory/ infectious or neoplastic disease (see Figure 23.30). Therefore, once a diagnosis of inflammatory polyarthritis has been established, additional diagnostic work-up should be undertaken to classify the polyarthritis and identify any underlying cause. It is important to rule out infection in distant sites (e.g. urogenital or gastrointestinal tract, lungs, skin) and vector-borne diseases (anaplasmosis, ehrlichiosis, rickettsiosis, borreliosis, leishmaniosis) before starting immunosuppressive therapy because these can also cause an immune-mediated polyarthritis (type II or reactive).
- **Systemic lupus erythematosus (SLE)** is a rare disease but a non-erosive immune-mediated polyarthritis is its most common manifestation in dogs. The detection of neutrophils or other leucocytes containing a variably sized light purple to pink homogeneous inclusion (LE cells) in synovial fluid preparations is considered highly supportive of the disease but its sensitivity is low (Figure 23.32). The inclusion in LE cells is nuclear material from ruptured cells that has been denatured and phagocytosed following binding of circulating antibodies to nuclear antigens. SLE is likely when the patient shows three or more separate manifestations of autoimmunity (Figure 23.33), as well as a high positive antinuclear antibody titre (ANA test). SLE should not be diagnosed or excluded on the basis of the result of this single test, and its low specificity (positive results can be seen in various infectious and inflammatory conditions) and sensitivity limit its value in veterinary patients.
- **Juvenile-onset polyarthritis of Akitas** typically affects young dogs and is characterized by suppurative inflammation within multiple joints, cyclical pain, generalized lymphadenopathy and fever. Diagnosis is usually made by exclusion of other potential causes. A positive ANA test or rheumatoid factor has been reported. Occasionally, concurrent meningitis may be present.

Systemic lupus erythematosus

- ANA test positivity not associated with drugs, infections, neoplasia
- Non-erosive, non-septic suppurative inflammatory arthritis in two or more peripheral joints
- Mucocutaneous lesions (depigmentation, erythema, erosions/ ulcerations, crusts, scales)
- Renal disorders (glomerulonephritis or persistent proteinuria in the absence of urine infection)
- Immune-mediated haemolytic anaemia and/or thrombocytopenia
- Leucopenia
- Polymyositis or myocarditis
- Serositis
- Neurological disorders (seizures)
- Antiphospholipid antibodies (lupus anticoagulant) causing prolongation of activated partial thromboplastin time that fails to correct with a 1:1 mixture of patient and normal plasma

23.33 Proposed criteria for the diagnosis of SLE. A diagnosis of SLE is established if the patient manifests three or more criteria simultaneously or over any period of time.

- **Shar Pei dogs** with familial amyloidosis may also present with lameness and arthritis, which may be monoarticular or pauciarticular, affecting mostly the tarsal joints.
- **Chronic progressive polyarthritis** has been described in cats, including a periosteal proliferative form and an erosive form. Synovial fluid analysis usually reveals suppurative inflammation but the pattern may be predominantly mononuclear in the erosive form. Affected cats are usually young adult male cats and may be co-infected by feline syncytia-forming virus and feline leukaemia virus. Hocks and carpi are most commonly affected.
- **Rheumatoid arthritis** is the most notable form of immune-mediated erosive polyarthritis in dogs. It is very rare in small animals and occurs predominantly in small-breed middle-aged dogs (Johnson and Mackin, 2012). Tarsal, carpal and phalangeal joints are most commonly involved. Diagnostic criteria for rheumatoid arthritis in dogs and cats are adapted from those defined for humans, and are outlined in Figure 23.34.

Canine and feline rheumatoid arthritis

- Radiographic evidence of bony destruction
- Seropositivity for rheumatoid factor
- Compatible cytological findings in synovial fluid (suppurative inflammation or mixed mononuclear and suppurative with high cell count)
- Stiffness after inactivity
- Swelling and/or pain in at least one joint
- Involvement of at least another joint within 3 months
- Symmetrical joint swelling
- Compatible histological findings in synovial membrane

Progressive feline polyarthritis

- Young adult male cat
- Two forms: periosteal proliferative or erosive
- Concurrent infection with feline leukaemia virus and foamy viruses

23.34 Clinical features for the diagnosis of erosive arthritides in dogs and cats.

Mononuclear inflammation

Mononuclear inflammation is characterized by a variable (usually mild) increase in nucleated cellularity with a predominance of large mononuclear cells (Figure 23.35). An increased number of vacuolated cells (>10% of large mononuclear cells) with or without a concurrent absolute increase in cellularity also reflects some degree of increased phagocytic activity and suggests some degree of chronic inflammation (Fernandez et al., 1983). Viscosity, mucin quality and the appearance of the mucinous background on cytology are usually within normal limits.

This cytological pattern is most commonly associated with the so-called *non-inflammatory arthropathies*. These include osteoarthritis, traumatic arthropathy, haemarthrosis, changes secondary to neoplasia, crystal-induced arthropathy and some virus-induced arthritides (MacWilliams and Friedrichs, 2003).

Osteoarthritis: Osteoarthritis is often referred to as *degenerative joint disease*. Degenerative joint disease and non-inflammatory arthropathies are actually misnomers. Degenerative joint disease has long been considered a 'wear and tear' process due to any cause leading to increased pressure on the joint (e.g. joint instability) or fragility of extracellular matrix with consequent loss of cartilage. Diseases that may cause osteoarthritis are listed in Figure 23.36. This process was considered

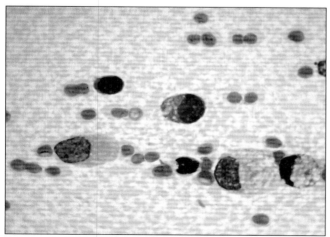

23.35 Synovial fluid from a dog with osteoarthritis, characterized by mildly increased nucleated cellularity. In this field there are a few large vacuolated mononuclear cells admixed with a small lymphocyte and a neutrophil. (Wright–Giemsa stain; original magnification X500)

Potential causes of osteoarthritis

- Primary osteoarthritis
- Osteochondrosis dissecans
- Elbow dysplasia
- Avascular necrosis of the femoral head
- Hip dysplasia
- Chronic patellar luxation
- Joint instabilities caused by ligament damage
- Trauma
- Nutritional disorders
- Neoplasia

23.36 Diseases that can lead to osteoarthritis.

non-inflammatory, but recent studies have shown that inflammation of the synovium plays an important role in its pathogenesis (Loeser et al., 2012; Berembaum, 2013). Synovial inflammation is a frequently observed phenomenon in osteoarthritic joints and contributes to alteration of the balance of cartilage matrix degradation and repair through the production of catabolic and proinflammatory mediators. The pathological changes seen in osteoarthritis include:

- Degradation of the articular cartilage
- Thickening of the subchondral bone
- Formation of osteophytes
- Variable degrees of inflammation of the synovium
- Degeneration of ligaments.

The cytological change most commonly seen in synovial fluid aspirated from joints with osteoarthritis is a low-grade mononuclear inflammatory response with a normal or mildly elevated nucleated cell count and increased percentage of vacuolated large mononuclear cells.

Other causes: A predominantly mononuclear inflammatory response may also be seen in some forms of rheumatoid arthritis, in septic suppurative arthritis treated chronically or with suboptimal doses of antimicrobials, and in waxing and waning immune-mediated polyarthritis, although this is usually associated with a concurrent increase of neutrophils (usually >20% of all nucleated cells).

Moderately to markedly increased cellularity with a predominance of macrophages with leucophagocytosis has also been seen in a kitten with feline calicivirus infection (Levy and Marsh, 1992). Low-grade mononuclear inflammation can also be seen with trauma, haemarthrosis and secondary to neoplasia or crystal deposition (see later in the chapter).

Lymphocytic inflammation

Small lymphocytes may be difficult to differentiate from small synoviocytes, although the former tend to be smaller and have a higher nuclear:cytoplasmic ratio with only a scant rim of cytoplasm. A clear predominance of small lymphocytes, usually accompanied by moderately to markedly increased cellularity and a neutrophilic component, indicates an inflammatory arthropathy and is most often seen with immune-mediated disease.

In humans, this pattern is seen in 10% of cases of inflammatory arthritis, may suggest tuberculosis if lymphocytes are >60%, is strongly suggestive of SLE when accompanied by LE cells, and in rheumatoid arthritis is linked with a better long-term prognosis (Denton, 2012).

Lymphocytic gonitis: In dogs, lymphocytic inflammation has been reported to be associated with cranial cruciate ligament rupture and lymphoplasmacytic gonitis (Muir *et al.*, 2011). The causative relationship between these two entities is undetermined but the initial trigger seems to be immune-mediated (Hayashi *et al.*, 2004).

Eosinophilic inflammation

Eosinophilic inflammation in synovial fluid has been reported only very rarely (Christopher and Wallace, 1986; Silverstein *et al.*, 2000). The underlying cause appears to be idiopathic and immune-mediated, although differentials should include parasitic disease, a paraneoplastic phenomenon and reaction to foreign substances.

Haemorrhage

The presence of many erythrocytes within synovial fluid indicates haemorrhage or blood contamination during the sampling procedure. The presence of platelets is supportive of the latter, although very recent intra-articular haemorrhage may lead to a similar cytological pattern (Figure 23.37).

History, clinical findings, and the gross appearance of the fluid at sampling may help differentiate between these two possibilities.

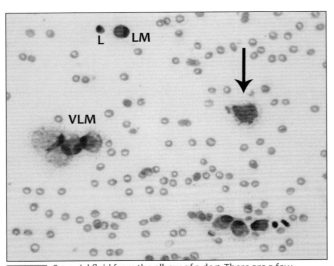

23.37 Synovial fluid from the elbow of a dog. There are a few windrowing large mononuclear cells (LM) including a group of vacuolated cells (VLM) and rare small lymphocytes (L), amid a background of many erythrocytes. Platelets are also present in a small clump (arrowed). The presence of platelets is indicative of very recent haemorrhage or contamination of the fluid with peripheral blood at sampling. (Wright–Giemsa stain; original magnification X200)

Trauma: Haemorrhage due to trauma is usually accompanied by some degree of inflammation. Initially this may be predominantly neutrophilic, whereas macrophages with erythrophagocytosis and intracellular haemoglobin breakdown products (haemosiderin and haematoidin) are usually seen with more long-standing haemorrhage (Figure 23.38). When not iatrogenic, other causes of haemorrhage within the synovial space include coagulopathies (e.g. intoxication with vitamin K antagonists, haemophilia A, especially if haemarthrosis is recurrent) and neoplasia.

Neoplasia

Neoplastic cells are found uncommonly in joint fluid. They may exfoliate from primary joint tumours such as synovial cell sarcomas (Figure 23.39) or result from invasion or metastasis from other primary sites.

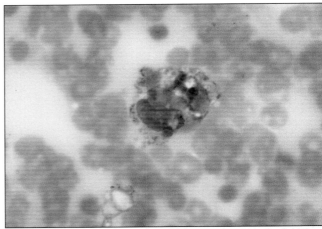

23.38 Synovial fluid from a dog with haemarthrosis. In the field there is a macrophage with erythrophagocytosis and globular gold–green pigment, consistent with haemosiderin breakdown products. (Wright–Giemsa stain; original magnification X1000)
(Courtesy of Roger Powell)

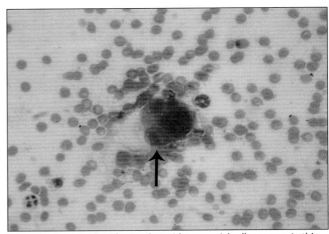

23.39 Synovial fluid from a dog with a synovial cell sarcoma. In this field there is a large atypical spindleoid cell and one neutrophil admixed with many erythrocytes. The atypical cell is extremely large compared with the neutrophil, has very high nuclear:cytoplasmic ratio and contains multiple giant nucleoli (arrowed). The cell population has many features of atypia, including an increased nuclear:cytoplasmic ratio, multinucleation, the presence of multiple often giant nucleoli, and anisokaryosis. (Wright–Giemsa stain; original magnification X200)

Primary neoplasia: Primary tumours of joints can cause lameness with bony lysis and proliferation on both sides of the joint. The most common types are:

- Histiocytic sarcoma (Figure 23.40), which has the worst prognosis and highest potential for metastasis
- Synovial cell sarcoma, which is a locally aggressive tumour that less commonly metastasizes (Craig et *al.*, 2002)
- Synovial myxoma, which consists of myxomatous nodules and sometimes infiltrative growth. It may require amputation, but does not metastasize and the prognosis is good (Craig *et al.*, 2010).

Differentiation requires histopathology and immunohistochemistry.

Metastatic neoplasia: A metastatic carcinoma with presumed prostatic or urothelial origin was diagnosed in a dog on the basis of cytomorphology and was confirmed by histopathology and immunohistochemistry (Colledge et *al.*, 2013).

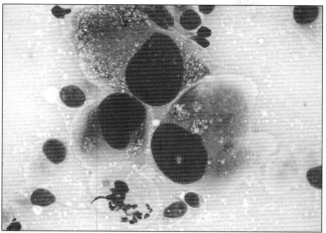

23.40 Synovial fluid from a dog with a periarticular histiocytic sarcoma. The neoplastic cells have oval to spindleoid discrete morphology and prominent criteria of malignancy including marked anisocytosis and anisokaryosis, angular nucleoli and atypical mitoses. (Wright–Giemsa stain; original magnification X1000)
(Courtesy of Roger Powell)

Deposition of mineral

Deposition of urates causes inflammatory arthritis and is common in birds and humans, but not reported in dogs and cats. Urates form thin tapering needle-shaped crystals that are negatively birefringent on examination under polarized light. Pseudogout, an acute arthritic form in which calcium pyrophosphate crystals are shed into the synovial fluid, is reported in dogs, although rarely (Forsyth et al., 2007).

Many of the presenting signs are similar to those of common gout, in which uric acid crystals are deposited into joints, and include acute pain involving one or more joints, with or without a low-grade fever. Calcium pyrophosphate crystals are usually elongated rhomboids that show positive birefringence, although rare crystals can appear to be negatively birefringent.

Chemical evaluation

Biochemical analysis of joint fluid has low priority in the laboratory evaluation of joint disease because the results do not usually provide discriminatory information. Also, in small patients it may not be possible to collect enough synovial fluid for these tests.

Mucin clot quality

The mucin clot test is a qualitative assessment of the degree of polymerization of synovial fluid hyaluronate. Synovial fluid is mixed with a solution of 2% glacial acetic acid (1 part synovial fluid:4 parts glacial acetic acid) in a glass tube with a glass stirring stick. Failure to form a tight mass in a clear fluid is considered abnormal and is associated with degradation of hyaluronan (e.g. by bacterial enzymes) or its dilution; a soft, less compact mass in a cloudy solution is defined as a fair mucin clot, while a friable mass which breaks up easily when shaken is considered poor. Inflammatory arthropathy is usually associated with fair to poor mucin clot formation, whereas in degenerative joint disease this test and the viscosity of the fluid may be normal.

This test is unlikely to alter clinical decision-making, and therefore is given low priority and is not routinely performed in dogs and cats.

Total protein

Total protein is routinely measured via refractometry, although this method is affected by the presence of other solutes. Quantitative biochemical assays are considered more accurate, but the sample viscosity may pose technical pitfalls. Reported reference intervals vary from 18–48 g/l (Fernandez et al., 1983) to 15–30 g/l (MacWilliams and Friedrichs, 2003).

Total protein tends to increase in cases of inflammation because of leakage of high molecular weight proteins (especially fibrinogen) from synovial vessels, due to increased vascular permeability, and intralesional immunoglobulin production by inflammatory cells. In cases of haemorrhage, both iatrogenic/procedural and pathological total protein increase owing to the contribution of plasma components.

Biomarkers

Topics of major interest in the research field include the identification of biomarkers that may aid in the distinction between septic and non-septic arthritis and the detection of early stages of osteoarthritis.

- Glucose and pH tend to decrease in cases of sepsis but a fasting sample should be used (Mundt and Shanahan, 2010). Disparity between fasting levels of glucose in synovial fluid and serum in infectious arthritis is due to the glycolytic activities of bacteria. However, marked suppurative inflammation in the absence of bacteria, such as seen in immune-mediated articular disease, can also account for decreased synovial fluid glucose, owing to glucose utilization by the white cells.
- Hyaluronic acid concentration correlates with disease severity in dogs with different stages of osteoarthritis but it is not suitable for staging disease owing to values overlapping between stages (Plickert et al., 2013).
- The complement system and proteins involved in lipid and cholesterol metabolism are increased in dogs with osteoarthritis secondary to cranial cruciate ligament disease, when compared with controls (Garner et al., 2013).
- Pro-inflammatory and anti-inflammatory cytokines, neuropeptides and matrix metalloproteinases are involved in osteoarthritis (Sutton et al., 2009; El-Hadi et al., 2012) and can lead to increased proteoglycan catabolism with consequent alteration of the content of glycosaminoglycans (Innes et al., 1998), keratan sulphate and chondroitin sulfate (Nganvongpanit et al., 2008).
- C-reactive protein has been evaluated as a potential marker to monitor the response to non-steroidal anti-inflammatory drugs in dogs with osteoarthritis (Bennett et al., 2013).

The use of these biochemical determinations is still limited to the research setting and their relevance in clinical decision-making is as yet undetermined in small animals.

Culture and sensitivity testing

Whenever there is a suspicion of septic arthritis an aliquot of the fluid should be sent for culture. Specimens should be collected before administration of antimicrobials. If this is not possible, collection should be performed immediately before the next dose is given. Samples submitted in EDTA tubes are not acceptable because they are not sterile and the anticoagulant may affect bacterial growth. Often swabs do not lead to adequate inoculation of culture plates. Blood culture bottles (Figure 23.41) are considered superior to plain tubes or swabs (Montgomery *et al.*, 1989). Liquid blood culture medium is thought to prevent sample coagulation, dilute bacterial growth inhibitors, inactivate or dilute antibiotics and curtail *in vitro* leucocytic phagocytosis of bacteria. Paediatric bottles and tubes are preferable, given the small amount of sample that can be harvested from small animal joints. For blood culture a 1:10 ratio of blood to blood culture medium is recommended (see Chapter 27). For synovial fluid there is no minimum amount established to obtain a meaningful result because this is dependent on the concentration of organisms in the fluid. After sterile collection, the sample is inoculated into the bottle using a new needle through the rubber diaphragm that has been previously disinfected with alcohol or povidone iodine solution. Air should not be allowed to enter vacuum bottles. The bottle is then gently inverted 2–3 times to disperse the fluid in the culture medium. The bottle may be maintained at room temperature but will be incubated for 24 hours at 37°C once in the laboratory and subcultured for aerobic and anaerobic bacteria. Specific transport and culture media are required for culture of *Mycoplasma* spp.

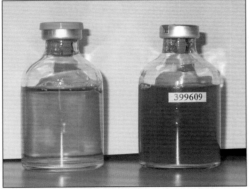

23.41 Blood culture bottles. The bottle on the right was inoculated with synovial fluid from a patient with septic arthritis. Note the cloudy appearance of the medium due to bacterial growth after 24 hours incubation at 37°C.
(Courtesy of Marta Dell'Orco)

Molecular detection of infectious agents

Polymerase chain reaction (PCR) may help detect or rule out infectious agents for which culture is difficult, slow or requires special sample handling. This test targets a specific sequence of the DNA of a specific agent or group and does not require viable organisms (air-dried and stained slides of synovial fluid, samples preserved in EDTA or frozen and plain swabs may also be used). PCR testing is currently available in the UK for *Anaplasma phagocytophilum*, *Ehrlichia* spp., *Borrelia* spp., *Bartonella henselae* and *Bartonella* spp., *Leishmania* spp., *Aspergillus fumigatus*, *Mycobacterium tuberculosis* and *M. avium* complex, among others (see Chapter 29).

Further tests

Depending on the case, in addition to serology for arthropod-borne diseases, testing for immune-mediated disease may be considered.

ANA test

Serum antinuclear antibody (ANA) is a hallmark of human, canine and feline SLE. The ANA test detects the presence of these antibodies in serum by indirect immunofluorescence or immunoperoxidase staining. The antibodies, once bound to the nuclei of a substrate tissue, are visualized with a fluorescein-conjugated or enzyme-linked polyvalent secondary antibody. Today, the most commonly used methods to detect ANA specificities are enzyme-linked immunosorbent assay (ELISA) and line blot techniques (Hansson-Hamlin and Rönnelid, 2010). Patient serum is usually screened at dilutions of 1 in 10 to 1 in 40 depending on the laboratory and, if positive, an end dilution is reported. Titres in excess of 1 in 160 are considered positive (Paul *et al.*, 2005) and an ANA titre greater than 1 in 640 was found to be a good predictor of immune-mediated disease in a recent study (Smee *et al.*, 2007). The titre may decrease significantly and even become negative after chronic treatment (Gershwin, 2010). ANA testing is indicated only when SLE is suspected on the basis of compatible clinicopathological abnormalities (see Figure 23.33). The results must be interpreted with caution: positive ANA results have been recorded in various canine diseases other than SLE, and up to 20% of healthy dogs and 10% of normal cats may show low titres of ANA (Gershwin, 2005). High titres have occasionally been observed in healthy German Shepherd Dogs and other breeds. Given its low specificity this test should be used to rule out SLE rather than confirm the disease.

Rheumatoid factor

Rheumatoid factor (RF) is an autoantibody to the Fc region of an immunoglobulin (IgG) molecule which may be found at low titre in 5–10% of healthy dogs and in both dogs and cats with a range of infectious, inflammatory and neoplastic diseases. Higher titres, usually >1:40, are demonstrated in the majority of dogs and cats with rheumatoid arthritis, but may also be found in the serum of both canine and feline patients with non-erosive joint disease. Cats with chronic progressive polyarthritis (periosteal proliferative polyarthritis) are usually seronegative for RF. Rheumatoid factor may be assayed by ELISA or by the Rose–Waaler test, which utilizes the ability of RF to agglutinate IgG-coated ovine substrate erythrocytes. Not all animals with rheumatoid arthritis will be RF positive and the titre may vary on a weekly basis. Serum RF is a non-sensitive and non-specific marker of erosive or immune-mediated arthritis in dogs, making its clinical utility highly questionable. RF may also be assessed in synovial fluid with increased sensitivity but decreased specificity.

Case examples

CASE 1

SIGNALMENT

7-year-old male neutered English Staffordshire Bull Terrier.

HISTORY

There was a 5-week history of lethargy, 1 week of reduced appetite, and hindlimb weakness during the previous few days. Treated with multiple courses of amoxicillin–clavulanate (co-amoxiclav) by the referring veterinary surgeon (veterinarian) for a suppurative laryngitis. The dog was imported to the UK 6 months previously from Spain. No history of recent vaccination. On physical examination the carpal and tarsal joints were swollen and flexion of the right carpus was painful. The prescapular and popliteal lymph nodes were mildly enlarged. No other abnormalities were found.

CLINICAL PATHOLOGY DATA

Arthrocentesis of the right stifle and both carpi and tarsi was performed.

Synovial fluid analysis	Reference interval	Right carpus	Left carpus	Right tarsus	Left tarsus	Right stifle
Total protein (g/l)	<40	**45**	**44**	**43**	**45**	38
RBC (x 10¹²/l)	–	0.01	0.01	0.02	0.01	0.2
Total nucleated cells (TNC) (x 10⁹/l)	<1.0	**14.5**	**12.2**	**9.6**	**11.4**	**4.7**
Neutrophils (%)	–	89	76	63	90	30
Large mononuclear cells (%)	–	5	17	10	6	60
Lymphocytes (%)	–	6	7	27	4	10

Abnormal results are in **bold**.

A smear of synovial fluid from the right carpus is shown in Figure 23.42.

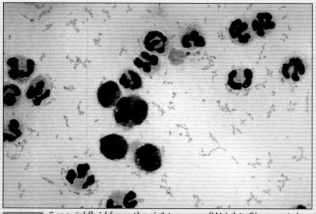

23.42 Synovial fluid from the right carpus. (Wright–Giemsa stain; original magnification X1000)

HOW WOULD YOU INTERPRET THESE RESULTS AND WHAT WOULD YOU INCLUDE IN THE DIFFERENTIAL DIAGNOSIS?

The smear shows increased numbers of neutrophils, a few large mononuclear cells and one erythrocyte amid a slightly granular background. The neutrophils appear non-degenerate and no bacteria are seen. Synovial fluid from all joints sampled has increased nucleated cellularity with mild haemodilution, increased total protein and a predominance of neutrophils in four joints and >12% neutrophils in one joint. The laboratory analysis of the joint fluids from the carpi and tarsi reveals suppurative inflammation while the synovial fluid from the right stifle has mixed inflammation. No microorganisms are identified and neutrophils are non-degenerate. The involvement of at least five joints indicates a suppurative polyarthropathy. The differential diagnoses would include immune-mediated polyarthropathy and rheumatoid arthritis and a haematogenous septic polyarthritis, e.g. due to a vector-borne infection.

WHAT FURTHER TESTS WOULD YOU RECOMMEND?

Haematology, serum biochemistry and complete urinalysis should be performed to rule out other concurrent diseases: cytopenias or glomerulonephropathy suggestive of systemic immune-mediated disease (e.g. SLE) or vector-borne disease, hepatopathy, enteropathy, evidence of urinary tract infection, endocarditis, etc. Radiographs of the swollen joints are indicated to rule out erosive changes. Thoracic radiography and abdominal ultrasonography are also recommended to rule out internal organ abnormalities or possible neoplasia.

Microorganisms were not found and a septic polyarthritis in an adult animal is unlikely, but culture of the synovial fluid should still be considered.

Fine-needle aspiration of the enlarged lymph nodes is indicated to rule out lymphoma as a possible cause of type IV immune-mediated polyarthritis and to characterize the lymphadenopathy.

Serology and/or PCR for vector-borne agents (*Borrelia* spp., *Leishmania* spp., *Ehrlichia* spp., *Anaplasma* spp.) is also advisable because these infectious agents are present in the country of origin of this dog.

If these tests lead to a strong suspicion of SLE or erosive polyarthritis, testing for antinuclear antibodies and rheumatoid factor could be considered, respectively.

RESULTS OF FURTHER TESTS PERFORMED

Haematology, biochemistry and urinalysis are unremarkable. Radiographs of both carpi reveal moderate soft tissue swelling but no evidence of bone lytic or proliferative lesions. Abdominal ultrasonography reveals a mild enlargement of the medial iliac lymph nodes. Cytology of the fine-needle aspirates from the prescapular and popliteal lymph nodes is compatible with reactive lymphoid hyperplasia. Serology for *Borrelia* spp., *Ehrlichia* spp. and *Anaplasma* spp. is negative. Serology for *Leishmania* spp. is positive with a low titre, indicating prior exposure but not diagnostic of active infection. PCR was then performed on lymph node aspirates and was negative, making leishmaniosis unlikely.

→ **CASE 1 CONTINUED**

WHAT WOULD BE THE MOST LIKELY DIAGNOSIS?

Based on these results a tentative diagnosis of immune-mediated polyarthritis, likely to be idiopathic (type I), was made.

OUTCOME

Prednisone was administered at 1.5 mg/kg q24h. Initially, while waiting for the serology results, doxycycline was administered at 5 mg/kg q12h. At reassessment 10 days later the dog had markedly improved but stiffness and a mild tarsal and carpal effusion persisted. Doxycycline was stopped while prednisone was continued at the same dose. Ten days later, the patient had further improved clinically but shifting lameness and a mild degree of joint effusion persisted. Arthrocentesis was repeated and showed persistence of suppurative inflammation with a variable mononuclear component. Another immunosuppressive drug (chlorambucil) was added, with a better clinical response.

CASE 2

SIGNALMENT

5-year-old male neutered Bull Mastiff.

HISTORY

The dog was presented with a few weeks' history of shifting lameness and weakness in all four limbs, worsening during the last few days. The dog had a surgical repair of a cranial cruciate ligament rupture of the right stifle 3 months previously (a tibial plateau levelling osteotomy was performed). On physical examination, the dog was tachypnoeic and tachycardic. The right stifle was markedly swollen and the carpal and tarsal joints were slightly swollen and painful on flexion. Pain was elicited on palpation of the spinal column at several points of the dorsal spine. Most palpable lymph nodes were enlarged, markedly in the case of the right popliteal lymph node (the size of a satsuma). The temperature was 40°C and there was a mild heart murmur.

CLINICAL PATHOLOGY DATA

The results of a full blood count, biochemistry and urinalysis are listed below.

Haematology	Result	Reference interval
RBC (x 10¹²/l)	**4.89**	5.4–8.0
Haemoglobin (g/dl)	**11.5**	12–18
Haematocrit (l/l)	**0.33**	0.35–0.55
MCV (fl)	67.5	65–75
MCH (pg)	23.6	19.5–24.5
MCHC (g/dl)	35.0	32–37
Reticulocytes (x 10⁹/l)	10	0–60
WBC (x 10⁹/l)	**33.6**	6.0–18.0
Neutrophils (x 10⁹/l)	**28.6**	6–18
Band (x 10⁹/l)	**1.7**	0–0.1
Monocytes (x 10⁹/l)	**3.0**	0–1.2
Lymphocytes (x 10⁹/l)	**0.3**	1.2–3.8
Eosinophils (x 10⁹/l)	**0.0**	0.1–1.3
Basophils (x 10⁹/l)	0.0	0–0.1
Platelets (x 10⁹/l)	**100**	150–400

Abnormal results are in **bold**.

Biochemistry	Result	Reference interval
Total protein (g/l)	57	57–78
Albumin (g/l)	23	23–31
Globulin (g/l)	**50**	23–45
Glucose (mmol/l)	4.0	3.3–6.7
Urea (mmol/l)	9.0	3.5–9.0
Creatinine (µmol/l)	100	20–110
ALP (IU/l)	**650**	0–100
ALT (IU/l)	**140**	0–50
Creatine kinase (IU/l)	**1180**	10–200
Sodium (mmol/l)	145	140–153
Chloride (mmol/l)	110	99–115
Potassium (mmol/l)	4.1	3.8–5.3
Calcium (mmol/l)	2.2	2.2–2.7
Phosphorus (mmol/l)	1.0	0.8–2.0
Serum quality	Icteric +	

Abnormal results are in **bold**.

Urinalysis was unremarkable.

Arthrocentesis of the right stifle and both carpi and tarsi was performed. A smear of the synovial fluid from the right stifle is shown in Figure 23.43.

Synovial fluid analysis	Reference interval	Right stifle	Right carpus	Left carpus	Right tarsus	Left tarsus
Total protein (g/l)	<40	**48**	**48**	**44**	**43**	**45**
RBC (x 10¹²/l)	–	0.01	0.01	0.01	0.02	0.01
Total nucleated cells (x 10⁹/l)	<1.0	**44.2**	**4.2**	**4.8**	**5.6**	**3.0**
Neutrophils (%)	–	99	97	86	93	60
Large mononuclear cells (%)	–	1	2	17	3	25
Lymphocytes (%)	–	0	1	17	4	15

Abnormal results are in **bold**.

→ **CASE 2 CONTINUED**

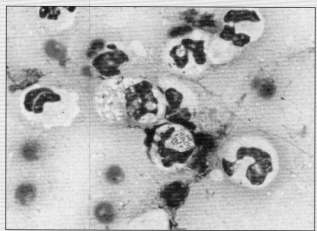

23.43 Synovial fluid from the right stifle. (Diff-Quik® stain; original magnification X1000)

HOW WOULD YOU INTERPRET THESE RESULTS AND WHAT WOULD YOU INCLUDE IN THE DIFFERENTIAL DIAGNOSIS?

The smear shows several neutrophils, one macrophage and a few erythrocytes amid a pink granular background with nuclear debris. The neutrophils appear degenerate with swollen nuclei and vacuolated cytoplasm. Bacterial cocci are well visible within the cytoplasm of the neutrophil in the centre of the image.

There is moderate neutrophilic leucocytosis with left shift and monocytosis consistent with an inflammatory leucogram, mild lymphopenia reflecting a combined stress component, mild non-regenerative normocytic, normochromic anaemia consistent with anaemia of chronic disease and mild thrombocytopenia, possibly related to consumption or immune-mediated destruction. Biochemistry changes are suggestive of a cholestatic hepatopathy and muscle damage. The increased globulin is most likely due to the inflammatory process.

Synovial fluid from all joints sampled has increased nucleated cellularity, particularly marked in the stifle, with mild, insignificant haemodilution, increased total protein and a predominance of neutrophils in all joints, consistent with suppurative polyarthritis. Bacteria were found in the synovial fluid from the right stifle, indicating septic arthritis. The involvement of the other joints could be due to haematogenous spread of the septic process or represent a type II (reactive) immune-mediated polyarthritis.

The patient was hospitalized and administered fluid therapy, analgesia and broad-spectrum antibiotics.

WHAT FURTHER TESTS WOULD YOU RECOMMEND?

Bacterial culture of the synovial fluid is indicated to identify the bacterial agent involved and for sensitivity testing. Blood culture is also advisable to rule out potential bacteraemia. Echocardiography is indicated to check for possible endocarditis, given the murmur detected on physical examination. Thoracic radiography and abdominal ultrasonography are indicated to evaluate for the presence of other potential septic foci (pneumonia, visceral abscesses) or other morphological abnormalities of internal organs. Radiographs of joints and the spine would be indicated to rule out areas of osteomyelitis. A cerebrospinal fluid tap could also be considered because of the pain elicited on palpation of the spine and to rule out concurrent meningitis, but this was not performed initially owing to the unstable condition of the patient.

RESULTS OF FURTHER TESTS PERFORMED

Culture of synovial fluid from the right stifle is positive for *Streptococcus canis*; culture of synovial fluid from other joints and the blood culture are negative. The echocardiogram reveals changes suggestive of endocarditis. Unfortunately the dog died suddenly as a result of cardiorespiratory arrest while hospitalized.

WHAT WOULD BE THE MOST LIKELY DIAGNOSIS?

This dog presented with polyarthritis, suggestive of an immune-mediated process. However, arthrocentesis of the stifle revealed suppurative inflammation with bacterial infection. It is possible that the infection had developed from the prior surgery, also causing the endocarditis. The suppurative inflammation within the other joints could be due to immune-mediated arthritis secondary to the septic process in distant sites (type II immune-mediated polyarthritis), although the negative cultures would not completely rule out the possibility of haematogenous spread of the infection to the joints. That would not necessarily have changed the case management because antibiotic therapy had already been instituted, based on the results of the culture and sensitivity testing performed on the stifle synovial fluid.

Acknowledgements

The author would like to thank John Innes for his kind help with the chapter.

References and further reading

Bennett D, Eckersall DP, Waterston M *et al.* (2013) The effect of robenacoxib on the concentration of C-reactive protein in synovial fluid from dogs with osteoarthritis. *BMC Veterinary Research* **9**, 42

Berembaum F (2013) Osteoarthritis as an inflammatory disease (osteoarthritis is not osteoarthrosis!). *Osteoarthritis and Cartilage* **21**, 16–21

Carlson CS and Weisbrode SE (2012) Bone, joints, tendons, and ligaments. In: *Pathologic Basis of Veterinary Disease, 5th edn*, ed. JF Zachary and MC McGavin, pp. 920–971. Elsevier, St Louis

Center S (2012) Fluid accumulation disorders. In: *Small Animal Clinical Diagnosis by Laboratory Methods, 5th edn*, ed. MD Willard and H Tvedten, pp. 226–259. Elsevier, St Louis

Christopher MM and Wallace LJ (1986) Synovial fluid eosinophilia: a case report and review of the literature. *Veterinary Clinical Pathology* **15**, 25–31

Clements DN, Owen MR, Mosley JR *et al.* (2005) Retrospective study of bacterial infective arthritis in 31 dogs. *Journal of Small Animal Practice* **46**, 171–176

Colledge SL, Raskin RE, Messick JB *et al.* (2013) Multiple joint metastasis of a transitional cell carcinoma in a dog. *Veterinary Clinical Pathology* **42**, 216–220

Craig L, Julian M and Ferracone J (2002) The diagnosis and prognosis of synovial tumors in dogs: 35 cases. *Veterinary Patholology* **39**, 66–73

Craig LE, Krimer PM and Cooley AJ (2010) Canine synovial myxoma: 39 cases. *Veterinary Pathology* **47**, 931–936

Dawson S, Bennett D, Carter SD *et al.* (1994) Acute arthritis of cats associated with feline calicivirus infection. *Research in Veterinary Science* **56**, 133–143

Denton J (2012) Synovial fluid analysis in the diagnosis of joint disease. *Diagnostic Histopathology* **18**, 159–168

Ekmann A, Rigdal ML and Gröndahl G (2010) Automated counting of nucleated cells in equine synovial fluid without and with hyaluronidase pretreatment. *Veterinary Clinical Pathology* **39**, 83–89

El-Hadi M, Charavaryamath C, Aebischer A *et al.* (2012) Expression of interleukin-8 and intercellular cell adhesion molecule-1 in the synovial membrane and cranial cruciate ligament of dogs after rupture of the ligament. *Canadian Journal of Veterinary Research* **76**, 8–15

Fernandes PJ (2013) Synovial fluid analysis. In: *Cowell and Tyler's Diagnostic Cytology and Haematology of the Dog and Cat, 4th edn*, ed. AC Valenciano and RL Cowell, pp. 195–215. Mosby Elsevier, St Louis

Fernandez FR, Grindem CB and Lipowitz AJ (1983) Synovial fluid analysis: preparation of smears for cytologic examination of canine synovial fluid. *Journal of the American Animal Hospital Association* **19**, 727–734

Forsyth SF, Thompson KG and Donald JJ (2007) Possible pseudogout in two dogs. *Journal of Small Animal Practice* **48**, 174–176

Garner BC, Kuroki K, Stoker AM *et al.* (2013) Expression of proteins in serum, synovial fluid, synovial membrane, and articular cartilage samples obtained from dogs with stifle joint osteoarthritis secondary to cranial cruciate ligament disease and dogs without stifle joint arthritis. *American Journal of Veterinary Research* **74**, 386–394

Gershwin LJ (2005) Antinuclear antibodies in domestic animals. *Annals of the New York Academy of Sciences* **1050**, 364–370

Gershwin LJ (2010) Autoimmune diseases in small animals. *Veterinary Clinics of North America: Small Animal Practice* **40**, 439–457

Gibson R, Carmichael S, Li A *et al.* (1999). Value of direct smears of synovial fluid in the diagnosis of canine joint disease. *Veterinary Record* **144**, 463–465

Greene CE and Chalker VJ (2012) Nonhemotropic mycoplasmal, ureaplasmal, and L-form infections. In: *Infectious Diseases of the Dog and Cat, 4th edn*, ed. CE Greene, pp. 324–325. Saunders Elsevier, St Louis

Hansson-Hamlin H, Lilliehöök I and Trowald-Wigh G (2006) Subgroups of canine antinuclear antibodies in relation to laboratory and clinical findings in immune-mediated disease. *Veterinary Clinical Pathology* **35**, 397–404

Hannson-Hamnlin H and Rönneld J (2010) Detection of antinuclear antibodies by the Inno-Lia ANA update test in canine systemic rheumatic disease. *Veterinary Clinical Pathology* **39**, 215–220

Hayashi K, Manley PA and Muir P (2004) Cranial cruciate ligament pathophysiology in dogs with cruciate disease: a review. *Journal of the American Animal Hospital Association* **40**, 385–390

Innes JF (2005) Laboratory evaluation of joint disease. In: *BSAVA Manual of Canine and Feline Clinical Pathology, 2nd edn*, ed. E Villiers and L Blackwood, pp. 355–363. BSAVA Publications, Gloucester

Innes JF, Sharif M and Barr A (1998) Relations between biochemical markers of osteoarthritis and other disease parameters in a population of dogs with naturally acquired osteoarthritis in the genual joint. *American Journal of Veterinary Research* **59**, 1530–1536

Johnson KC and Mackin A (2012) Canine immune-mediated polyarthritis: Part 1: pathophysiology. *Journal of the American Animal Hospital Association* **48**, 12–17

Levy JK and Marsh A (1992) Isolation of calicivirus from the joint of a kitten with arthritis. *Journal of the American Veterinary Medical Association* **201**, 735–753

Loeser RF, Goldring SR, Scanzello CR *et al.* (2012) Osteoarthritis: a disease of the joint as an organ. *Arthritis & Rheumatism* **6**, 1697–1707

MacWilliams PS and Friedrichs KR (2003) Laboratory evaluation and interpretation of synovial fluid. *Veterinary Clinics of North America: Small Animal Practice* **33**, 153–178

Marcos R, Santos M, Santos N *et al.* (2009) Use of destained cytology slides for the application of routine special stains. *Veterinary Clinical Pathology* **38**, 94–102

Montgomery R, Long I, Milton J *et al.* (1989) Comparison of aerobic culturette, synovial membrane biopsy, and blood culture medium in detection of canine bacterial arthritis. *Veterinary Surgery* **18**, 300–303

Muir P, Kelly JL, Marvel SJ *et al.* (2011) Lymphocyte populations in joint tissues from dogs with inflammatory stifle arthritis and associated degenerative cranial cruciate ligament rupture. *Veterinary Surgery* **40**, 753–761

Mundt M and Shanahan K (2010) Synovial fluid. In: *Graff's Textbook of Routine Urinalysis and Body Fluids, 2nd edn*, ed. M Mundt and K Shanahan, pp. 253–262. Lippincott Williams & Wilkins, Philadelphia

Nganvongpanit K, Itthiarbha A, Ong-Chai S *et al.* (2008) Evaluation of serum chondroitin sulfate and hyaluronan: biomarkers for osteoarthritis in canine hip dysplasia. *Journal of Veterinary Science* **9**, 317–325

Paul S, Wilkerson MJ, Shuman W *et al.* (2005) Development and evaluation of a flow cytometry microsphere assay to detect antihistone antibody in dogs. *Veterinary Immunology and Immunopathology* **107**, 315–325

Plickert HD, Bondzio A, Einspanier R, *et al.* (2013) Hyaluronic acid concentrations in synovial fluid of dogs with different stages of osteoarthritis. *Research in Veterinary Science* **94**, 728–734

Renwick A (2013) How to... perform a successful joint tap. In: *How to... collected articles from BSAVA Companion*, ed. M Goodfellow, pp. 174–179 BSAVA Publications, Gloucester

Scherk MA, Ford RB, Gaskell RM *et al.* (2013) 2013 AAFP Feline Vaccination Advisory Panel Report. *Journal of Feline Medicine and Surgery* **15**, 785–808

Silverstein DC, Almy FS, Zinkl JG *et al.* (2000) Idiopathic localized eosinophilic synovitis in a cat. *Veterinary Clinical Pathology* **29**, 90–92

Stirling P, Faroug R, Amanat S *et al.* (2014) False-negative rate of Gram-stain microscopy for diagnosis of septic arthritis: suggestions for improvement. *International Journal of Microbiology* **2014**, 830857

Smee NM, Harkin KR and Wilkerson MJ (2007) Measurement of serum antinuclear antibody titer in dogs with and without systemic lupus erythematosus: 120 cases (1997–2005). *Journal of the American Veterinary Medical Association* **230**, 1180–1183

Stone M (2010) Systemic lupus erythematosus. In: *Textbook of Veterinary Internal Medicine – Diseases of the dog and the cat, 7th edn*, ed. SJ Ettinger and ED Feldman, pp. 783–787. Elsevier Saunders, St Louis

Stull JW, Evason M, Carr AP *et al.* (2008) Canine immune-mediated polyarthritis: clinical and laboratory findings in 83 cases in western Canada (1991–2001). *Canadian Veterinary Journal* **49**, 1195–1203

Sutton S, Clutterbuck A, Harris P *et al.* (2009) The contribution of the synovium, synovial derived inflammatory cytokines and neuropeptides to the pathogenesis of osteoarthritis. *The Veterinary Journal* **179**, 10–24

Vasanjee S, Paulsen D, Hosgood G *et al.* (2008) Characterization of normal canine anterior cruciate ligament associated synoviocytes. *Journal of Orthopaedic Research* **26**, 809–815

Chapter 24

Laboratory evaluation of muscle disorders

Natasha Olby

Muscle disease can affect skeletal (striated), cardiac and, more rarely, smooth muscle. It can be primary or secondary to other systemic disorders (Figures 24.1 and 24.2) but can be difficult to recognize clinically owing to its non-specific signs. Even when muscle disease is suspected, the appropriate diagnostic work-up is often poorly understood and test results can be misinterpreted.

Disease process	Aetiology	Common causes
Degenerative	Hereditary structural disorders Endocrine disease	Muscular dystrophy Hypo- and hyperadrenocorticism Hypo- and hyperthyroidism
Metabolic	Hereditary errors of metabolism Endocrine disease	No common causes Hyper- and hypoadrenocorticism Hyper- and hypothyroidism
Neoplastic	Primary neoplasia Infiltrative or metastatic neoplasia Paraneoplastic diseases	No common causes
Nutritional	Anorexia Vitamin E deficiency	No common causes
Inflammatory	Immune-mediated Infectious	Myasthenia gravis, masticatory myositis Toxoplasmosis, neosporosis
Toxic		No common causes
Traumatic		
Vascular	Embolic disease Bleeding disorder Hypotension	Iliac thrombosis No common causes

24.1 Categories of muscle disease.

Systemic disorder	Myopathy
Hyperadrenocorticism	Profound muscle weakness and atrophy, pseudomyotonia
Hypoadrenocortism	Profound muscle weakness, megaoesophagus

24.2 Systemic diseases that can cause muscle disease. (continues)

Systemic disorder	Myopathy
Hypothyroidism	Muscle weakness
Hyperthyroidism	Muscle weakness and elevated creatine kinase
Renal disease and hyperaldosteronism	Hypokalaemic myopathy
Sepsis/shock/disseminated intravascular coagulation	Muscle weakness, elevated creatine kinase
Thromboembolic disease	Painful, oedematous extremity, markedly elevated creatine kinase

24.2 (continued) Systemic diseases that can cause muscle disease.

Clinical signs of muscle disorders

Classical signs of muscle disease include: weakness, characterized by exercise intolerance and/or a stiff, stilted gait; muscle atrophy or hypertrophy; muscle contractures (with associated skeletal deformities in growing animals); regurgitation and aspiration pneumonia (due to megaoesophagus); and myalgia (muscle pain). Dysphagia may be present if there is involvement of the pharyngeal muscles, and dysphonia can occur if laryngeal muscles are severely affected. Stertor and stridor can also be present with involvement of these muscle groups.

Weakness due to muscle disease can be profound and even cause recumbency, but can be differentiated from disease of the nervous system by the presence of intact myotactic reflexes (in the majority of cases) and intact proprioceptive placing. However, in very weak animals, the bodyweight must be supported carefully in order to evaluate proprioceptive placing accurately. A distinction should be drawn between myotactic reflexes, such as the patellar reflex, and withdrawal (flexor) reflexes. To evaluate the flexor reflex, the leg is extended and both the presence and the strength of the animal's ability to flex the leg is assessed in response to pinching its toes (see the *BSAVA Manual of Canine and Feline Neurology*). Animals with myopathies severe enough to cause recumbency tend to have reduced withdrawal reflexes because these reflect muscle strength, but their myotactic reflexes are usually intact. Involvement of cardiac muscle may lead to heart failure or cardiac arrhythmias with resultant weakness.

Laboratory evaluation of muscle disorders

Laboratory evaluation of muscle focuses on skeletal and cardiac muscle; although smooth muscle disorders exist they are poorly characterized at present. Routine markers of muscle disease are primarily limited to indicators of myocyte necrosis, which support the presence of muscle disease but are not specific, and measurement of antibody titres specific to muscle and its receptors. Specific diagnosis of a primary myopathy usually requires histological evaluation of a muscle biopsy specimen and may then require additional specialized testing to characterize the disease more fully. However, myopathies can occur secondary to other systemic diseases, such as renal disease and hyperadrenocorticism, and therefore routine haematology and biochemistry and endocrine testing can play an important role. Cardiomyopathies can result from dietary deficiencies, and the plasma concentrations of various substances should, therefore, be measured in cardiomyopathic animals (see Chapter 20). Finally, the genetic basis of many primary muscle diseases is now defined and, as a result, there are genetic tests available for increasing numbers of canine and feline myopathies (see Chapter 30). These tests play an important role both in diagnosing inherited diseases and in identifying carriers of such diseases.

Tests used in the investigation of skeletal (striated) muscle disorders

Enzymes

Creatine kinase

Creatine kinase (CK) is a very sensitive indicator of muscle disease and should be a part of any serum biochemistry panel owing to the non-specific nature of the signs of muscle disease in dogs and cats. It catalyses the reaction of phosphocreatine and adenosine diphosphate (ADP) that results in production of adenosine triphosphate (ATP) and creatine. The enzyme is made up of two subunits, denoted M (muscle) and B (brain). The various combinations of these subunits give rise to three different isoenzymes, found in the nervous system (BB or CK_1), cardiac muscle (MB or CK_2) and skeletal muscle (MM or CK_3). There is also a mitochondrial form of CK and, rarely, the enzyme can exist in one of two macro forms that can confound testing. CK activity is much lower elsewhere in the body, but can be detected in the kidney, intestinal tract, uterus, thyroid gland and urinary bladder. In practice, CK activity is much higher in skeletal muscle and it is a relatively specific marker of skeletal muscle injury. The isoenzymes can be separated by electrophoresis, but this is not routinely used.

CK is a cytosolic enzyme that is released into the interstitium when the sarcolemma (muscle cell membrane) becomes permeable. From there it passes via the lymphatic system to the venous system, causing an elevation in blood CK activity. The half-life of CK in blood is in the region of 2–4 hours. Plasma concentrations start to increase 4–6 hours after muscle injury, peak 12 hours after enzyme release into the circulation and decrease back to normal within 24–48 hours (unless muscle damage is ongoing). An elevation in CK therefore reflects a recent process and persistent elevations imply that there is ongoing muscle damage occurring.

CK activity can be influenced by a variety of non-pathological circumstances (Figure 24.3). In addition, it is a very sensitive test and in general it is only taken as clinically significant if:

* There are elevations >5–10-fold in its activity
* The elevation is persistent, even if it is lower
* There are accompanying compatible clinical signs.

* **Spurious:** in haemolysed samples, substances released from erythrocytes affect the assay, causing spurious increases
* **Age:** CK activity is up to 5 times higher in day-old puppies than in adult dogs. It decreases to the adult level by 7 months of age. As dogs age their CK activity gradually decreases but not enough to change the reference range
* **Recent surgery**
* **Intramuscular injection**
* **Exercise**
* **Recumbency** is frequently cited as a cause of elevations in CK activity. While this is undoubtedly true in large animals such as cows, it is unusual to see a significant or persistent elevation in CK in recumbent dogs and cats

24.3 Non-pathological causes of creatine kinase (CK) elevation.

If analysis is delayed, storage of plasma at room temperature can give spuriously low results. CK is stable for a week at −4°C and for a month at −20°C.

Diseases that cause an increase in CK activity are listed in Figure 24.4; these can be primary or secondary. Increased CK must be interpreted with the presenting clinical signs in mind. Only diseases that cause an increase in sarcolemmal permeability cause elevations in CK activity; normal CK values do not rule out muscle disease. In addition, CK activity may be reduced in end-stage disease associated with severe destruction of muscle, simply because there is little muscle mass left.

Disease	CK elevation
Degenerative myopathy e.g. X-linked muscular dystrophy Centronuclear myopathy	Marked elevation Mild to no elevation
Myositis: immune-mediated or infectious	Value depends on extent of injury
Excessive muscular activity: • Exertional rhabdomyolysis • Limber tail • Seizures • Tetanus • Malignant hyperthermia • Myokymia • Myotonia	Value depends on extent of injury
Metabolic myopathies: • Hypokalaemic myopathy • Mitochondrial myopathy • Lipid storage myopathy	Value depends on the disease
Endocrine myopathies: • Hyper- and hypothyroidism • Hyper- and hypoadrenocorticism	Value depends on the disease
Toxic and drug-induced myopathies e.g. monensin	Value depends on extent of injury
Trauma	Value depends on extent of injury
Vascular: • Hypotension • Arterial thromboembolism	Marked elevation

24.4 Pathological causes of an elevation in creatine kinase (CK).

Aspartate aminotransferase

Aspartate aminotransferase (AST) is found in the cytoplasm and mitochondria of many tissues and is therefore not a specific marker of disease. However, the highest concentrations are present in liver and in cardiac and skeletal muscle, and serum elevations usually reflect either a hepatic or a skeletal myopathic disease process in small animals. As AST has a much longer half-life than CK (approximately 12 hours) it will remain elevated for longer after an incident. Sample haemolysis leads to spurious elevations in AST because it is released from red blood cells.

Alanine aminotransferase

Alanine aminotransferase (ALT) is present at high concentrations in hepatocyte cytoplasm in small animals and it is generally considered to be a sensitive marker of hepatocellular damage. However, severe myonecrosis, such as that seen in X-linked muscular dystrophy, can cause an elevation in ALT in dogs concurrent with increases in CK and AST (Valentine et al., 1990). The half-life is approximately 2.5 days, so concentrations remain elevated much longer than those of CK.

Others

Lactate dehydrogenase (LDH) and aldolase are rarely measured in small animals because they lack specificity and sensitivity, and LDH is artefactually elevated in even slight haemolysis.

Myoglobin

Myoglobin is a haem protein that transports and stores oxygen in muscle. Severe skeletal muscle necrosis, such as that seen after arterial thromboembolism and exertional rhabdomyolysis, a rare condition that has been reported in Greyhounds and other breeds, results in release of myoglobin into the blood. This is a very specific indicator of severe muscle damage. At plasma concentrations >15–20 mg/dl (86–114 nmol/l), myoglobin is readily filtered at the glomerulus and is excreted in the urine. Myoglobinaemia can be differentiated from haemoglobinaemia by centrifuging a plasma sample. As myoglobin is cleared rapidly, the plasma is clear, in contrast to the pink appearance imparted by haemoglobin, which persists for longer in the blood. Myoglobin produces a brown coloration of urine and is detected by standard urine dipsticks as blood. It can be differentiated from haemoglobin by the addition of ammonium sulphate to precipitate haemoglobin and leave myoglobin in solution, and from haematuria by the absence of red cells in the sediment (see Figure 10.17). Unfortunately, this is not a reliable test; more accurate detection of myoglobin can be accomplished by immunodiffusion. Myoglobinuria is always a serious finding because myoglobinaemia can cause acute renal failure.

Potassium concentration

Potassium ions play an important role in the maintenance of a polarized membrane in the nervous system and muscle, and are found at high concentrations intracellularly throughout the body. Muscle contains approximately 95% of the total body potassium. If extensive muscle necrosis occurs, such as that seen after arterial thromboembolism in cats, a dangerous elevation in serum potassium concentration can occur (see Chapter 8).

Conversely, hypokalaemia can cause a myopathy associated with generalized weakness and an increase in CK. This is a well established phenomenon in cats as a result of renal loss, anorexia, primary hyperaldosteronism, diuretics, hyperthyroidism (rarely) and diabetic ketoacidosis, and occurs as an inherited disease in Burmese cats (Dow et al., 1989). This syndrome is rare in dogs but has been reported in one dog treated with furosemide for congestive heart failure (Harrington et al., 1996). Signs of weakness may occur with mild hypokalaemia, although rhabdomyolysis does not usually develop until potassium concentrations are <3.0 mmol/l. Conversely, marked hyperkalaemia with the associated hyponatraemia seen in Addison's disease can result in profound muscle weakness, in addition to the potentially fatal effects on cardiac muscle function. A syndrome of muscle cramping has also been recognized with the electrolyte imbalances and volume depletion seen in Addison's disease in Standard Poodles (Saito et al., 2002).

Antibody titres
Anti-type 2M antibodies

Masticatory myositis is an immune-mediated disease of the muscles of mastication in dogs (Shelton et al., 1987). These muscles (temporal, masseter and digastricus) have a different embryonic origin from other skeletal muscles and have a unique isoform of myosin that can be detected in a subset of myofibres, termed type 2M fibres. In masticatory myositis, antibodies are produced specifically to the heavy and light chain myosins and myosin-binding protein C unique to masticatory muscles (Shelton et al., 1987; Wu et al., 2007). Serum samples can be sent to the Comparative Neuromuscular Laboratory at the University of California, San Diego, USA, for measurement of antibody titres to this myofibre type in dogs using an enzyme-linked immunosorbent assay (ELISA). This test is highly specific (100%) and sensitive (85–90%) (Shelton and Cardinet, 1989). Immunosuppression will result in a decrease in this titre, and if the titre is negative in dogs with a high suspicion for masticatory myositis, further evaluation by muscle biopsy should be pursued. Low titres can be seen in end-stage disease when the muscles have atrophied.

Infectious disease titres

Myositis can be caused by the protozoal organisms Neospora caninum (dogs), Toxoplasma gondii (dogs and cats), Leishmania infantum (dogs), Sarcocystis spp. (dogs) and Trypanosoma cruzi (dogs). Less common causes of myositis include Hepatozoon canis and H. americanum, feline immunodeficiency virus (FIV), Ehrlichia canis, Leptospira australis, L. icterohaemorrhagiae, and clostridial infections. Many of these diseases are geographically specific, and rarely encountered. However, if a diagnosis of myositis is made on muscle biopsy, antibodies to protozoa should be measured and additional infectious diseases should be considered depending on the clinical picture (see Chapters 28 and 29).

Anti-acetylcholine receptor antibodies

There are acquired and congenital forms of myasthenia gravis (MG) but the acquired forms are more prevalent. Acquired MG is caused by production of antibodies to the nicotinic acetylcholine receptor (ACHR). Clinical syndromes include generalized exercise intolerance, with or without regurgitation, or a more specific form involving just the oesophageal and pharyngeal muscles, causing mega-oesophagus, regurgitation and aspiration. There is also a rare fulminant form that causes generalized lower motor neurone paralysis and is usually rapidly fatal. Concurrent diseases can include thymoma, immune-mediated myo-sitis and hypothyroidism, and therefore these diseases should also be considered during the diagnostic work-up of myasthenic cases. Antibody titres can be measured sensitively and specifically by immunoprecipitation radio-immunoassay and this test is recommended in patients with clinical signs consistent with unexplained regurgita-tion and megaesophagus, and/or exercise intolerance.

ACHR labelled with ^{125}I-α-bungarotoxin is used to quantitate circulating antibodies to these receptors in a serum sample (Comparative Neuromuscular Laboratory, University of California, San Diego, USA). Antibody con-centrations >0.6 nmol/l and >0.3 nmol/l are considered diagnostic of acquired MG in dogs and cats, respectively (Shelton, 2002). Approximately 2% of affected dogs are seronegative on this test. Possible explanations include a low circulating concentration of high-affinity antibodies, antibodies directed to a different region of the end-plate from the receptor, e.g. muscle-specific kinase (MuSK) (Evoli et al., 2003), and damage to the test receptors used in the assay during their preparation. Affected dogs may also express antibodies to titin and the ryanodine receptor, in particular dogs with thymoma and older dogs with more severe forms of the disease (Shelton et al., 2001). However, routine testing for these antibodies is not avail-able. An ELISA has been developed based on a subunit of the canine ACHR (Yoshioka et al., 1999). However, the sen-sitivity and specificity of this test remain to be established and it is not offered as a diagnostic test.

Endocrine testing

Muscle disease can result from hypothyroidism, hyper-thyroidism, hyperadrenocorticism and hypoadrenocorti-cism. In these diseases there are usually other clinical signs referable to the underlying cause. Appropriate test-ing for these diseases is indicated if there are compatible clinical signs (see Chapters 17 and 18).

Metabolic testing

Inborn errors of metabolism are a rare but important cause of exercise intolerance, weakness and collapse. Such dis-eases cause progressive signs and can be fatal. If a meta-bolic myopathy is suspected, it is standard for a complete work-up to include an evaluation of plasma lactate con-centration. Further metabolic testing is undertaken on the basis of the results of muscle biopsy (which may show characteristic changes in mitochondrial shape, size, distri-bution and numbers; see below) and measurement of lactate concentrations.

Lactate and pyruvate concentrations

Lactic acid is produced by anaerobic metabolism of pyru-vate in a process dedicated to glucose metabolism, known as glycolysis. Lactic acidaemia can be a secondary conse-quence of extreme muscular activity (e.g. heavy anaerobic exercise, malignant hyperthermia, seizures) or the result of a primary enzyme defect (e.g. pyruvate dehydrogenase phosphatase 1 deficiency in Clumber and Sussex Spaniels, pyruvate decarboxylase, enzymes of the respiratory chain or enzymes of the Krebs cycle). New hereditary disorders are described on a regular basis, and so it is appropriate to do a literature search for a newly described breed-specific myopathy when one is suspected. Lactic acidaemia can also result from generalized systemic disturbances, such as sepsis or hypovolaemia, leading to severe hypotension and causing failure of perfusion and hence anaerobic metabolism. Measurement of serum lactate concentration is indicated in the evaluation of exercise intolerance in which an underlying metabolic myopathy is suspected. Resting samples may be useful, but frequently lactic acid-aemia is only apparent when clinical signs are present. For optimal testing, the animal is exercised and blood samples are obtained both before and immediately after clinical signs appear. The exercise should be undertaken carefully, and ideally with an intravenous catheter in place in case of the need for emergency treatment. In general, having the owner exercise their pet is most effective, as they are familiar with the clinical course and dogs are usu-ally much more willing to exercise freely for their owners.

In the past, lactate was measured on chemistry analys-ers using blood samples collected in a specific anticoagu-lant tube containing a combined sodium fluoride/potassium oxalate anticoagulant (to halt glycolysis in red blood cells), cooled and centrifuged within 15 minutes. Using this method, immediate analysis is preferable, but the plasma can be stored at –20°C for up to 30 days. This has largely been superseded by the use of blood gas ana-lysers and point-of-care lactate analysers. Some blood gas analysers can measure lactate in addition to standard blood gas parameters. Hand-held point-of-care lactate devices that can measure lactate levels rapidly and accu-rately have become very popular, in large part because the prognostic importance of plasma lactate levels in critical care settings has driven the need for point- of-care meas-urements. These devices are cost effective and have the advantage of producing immediate results from whole blood. Comparisons with traditional techniques have vali-dated the accuracy and reliability of these devices in dogs, and have shown that the packed cell volume (PCV) does not affect the measurements (Acierno and Mitchell, 2007; Karagiannis et al., 2013). Commercially available devices that have been validated for dogs include the i-STAT (Abbott Laboratories, USA), Lactate Pro (now Lactate Pro 2; Cycle Classics Imports, Australia), Lactate Scout (SensLab GmbH, Germany) and Accutrend (Roche Diagnostics, Switzerland). All use drops of whole blood placed on test strips. The i-STAT, Lactate Pro and Scout devices measure lactate amperometrically, while the Accutrend uses a colorimetric reaction to generate a numerical value using reverse photometry. While all the devices listed have been validated for clinical use in dogs, there is some variability in the measurements, particularly if machines that use different methodology are compared, and therefore results from different devices should not be used interchangeably. Inaccuracies can also arise in sam-ples with PCVs >53% when using the Accutrend device, as the reduced volume of plasma can result in erroneously low lactate values (Karagiannis et al., 2013).

Lactate concentration will increase in normal animals in proportion to the amount and type of exercise that they do: normal values of pre- and post-exercise lactate con-centration have been reported for Labrador Retrievers (Figure 24.5; Matwichuk et al., 1999).

In order to determine the nature of lactic acidaemia, it is useful to measure pyruvate concentrations concurrently and to compute the ratio of these two substances. Pyruvate is produced from glucose during aerobic glycol-ysis. Following entry into mitochondria, it is normally

Lactate concentration (mmol/l)		Pyruvate concentration(mmol/l)		Lactate:pyruvate ratio	
Pre-exercise	Post-exercise	Pre-exercise	Post-exercise	Pre-exercise	Post-exercise
1.31 (0.53–3.07)	3.57 (0.8–9.86)	0.082 (0.5–0.12)	0.192 (0.05–0.32)	17	20.5

24.5 Mean pre- and post-exercise plasma lactate and pyruvate concentrations (the reference range is given in parentheses) in healthy working Labrador Retrievers, measured on a biochemistry analyser (Matwichuk et al., 1999). The dogs were exercised for 10 minutes doing retrieval work. The plasma lactate concentration returned to baseline in 60 minutes. The lactate:pyruvate ratio did not change significantly.

metabolized to acetyl-coenzyme (Co)A (catalysed by pyruvate dehydrogenase), which then enters the Krebs cycle. In the absence of oxygen, pyruvate is reduced to lactate in a reversible reaction. Different enzyme defects produce characteristic changes in the ratio of lactate to pyruvate concentrations. For example, if both lactate and pyruvate concentrations are elevated while maintaining a normal ratio, there is a defect in pyruvate dehydrogenase. Conversely, pyruvate carboxylase deficiency is associated with lactic acidaemia and an increased lactate:pyruvate ratio; defects in the mitochondrial electron transport chain or other mitochondrial abnormalities can also produce this change. Pyruvate is difficult to measure because samples must be diluted with an equal volume of 10% perchloric acid prior to centrifugation. The plasma should be removed and frozen at –20°C until analysis, although, as for lactate, prompt analysis is preferable. Normal pre- and post-exercise pyruvate concentrations have been reported for Labrador Retrievers (see Figure 24.5; Matwichuk et al., 1999).

Organic acid, amino acid and carnitine

Metabolic myopathies can result from a range of enzyme defects of oxidative phosphorylation and β-oxidation. Dysfunction of an enzyme can result in accumulation of fatty acids and amino acids. These can be measured in urine and plasma by specialist laboratories using gas chromatography–mass spectrometry. Appropriate samples must be frozen immediately after they are obtained and shipped to the laboratory on dry ice. Many metabolic disorders are a result of carnitine deficiency. Total, free and esterified muscle, plasma and urine carnitine levels can be measured by some laboratories (hospital laboratories and the Comparative Neuromuscular Laboratory, University of California, San Diego, USA). Indications for such tests include unexplained exercise intolerance, lactic acidaemia and pathological changes consistent with a metabolic myopathy on biopsy examination.

Genetic tests

Tests that detect mutant alleles associated with a variety of diseases are emerging and are a sensitive and specific method of identifying carriers and affected animals (see Chapter 30). The number of tests available and the laboratories offering them are constantly changing and so readers are referred to a searchable website for up-to-date global information on the genetic tests available (http://www.akcchf.org/canine-health/health-testing/; see also Figure 30.5). Testing laboratories will provide a summary of the correct interpretation of the results, as this varies with the mode of inheritance and penetrance of different diseases. Typically, DNA samples can be submitted in the form of a cheek swab (often mailed to the owner in a kit by the laboratory), saliva or an ethylenediamine tetra-acetic acid (EDTA) blood sample. Many laboratories will also accept sperm samples. Instructions on how to obtain the optimal sample will accompany any test kit. If submitting a cheek swab, it is important to ensure the patient has not eaten for at least 2 hours prior to sampling, to reduce the risk of contamination. Some laboratories require veterinary surgeons (veterinarians) to confirm the identity of the patient on laboratory-specific paperwork.

Muscle and nerve biopsy

Definitive diagnosis of primary myopathies and neuropathies usually requires evaluation of a biopsy specimen of the affected tissue. Muscle biopsy is a straightforward procedure that is minimally invasive. However, a specialist laboratory that can process frozen muscle is necessary to allow full interpretation of the sample. Nerve biopsy is technically more challenging and there is greater potential for causing permanent damage. It is also beneficial to have electrodiagnostic confirmation of nerve involvement prior to performing a biopsy, so this procedure is more appropriately performed by a specialist. As for muscle, it is preferable to use a laboratory experienced in the processing and interpretation of peripheral nerve biopsy specimens.

Muscle biopsy

Muscle biopsy is indicated in animals with unexplained muscle atrophy or hypertrophy, weakness or exercise intolerance, persistent or dramatic elevations in CK, or electromyographic evidence of myopathy. It is important to rule out other causes of weakness or exercise intolerance before proceeding to a muscle biopsy. Before performing biopsies it is advisable to liaise with the laboratory to ensure they are able to process the samples. Although core biopsy can be performed under sedation and local anaesthesia, these specimens are difficult to interpret and it is preferable to use an open dissection under general anaesthesia. In general it is prudent to harvest samples from more than one muscle. Sampling a muscle from both the thoracic and pelvic limbs and a proximal and distal site is desirable. The muscle to be sampled should not be at an end-stage, because this will often only reveal fibrosis and the underlying disease may not be apparent. Appropriate muscles to sample include the biceps femoris, quadriceps femoris, cranial tibial and gastrocnemius muscles in the pelvic limb, and the triceps brachii and extensor carpi radialis in the thoracic limb, although nearly any muscle can be sampled.

The technique is as follows:

1. Following surgical preparation, an incision approximately 2 cm long is made over the muscle.
2. The subcutaneous tissues are dissected to reveal the muscle to be sampled.
3. The direction of the myofibres is identified and the sample is taken parallel to them. The myotendinous junction should be avoided.
4. Parallel incisions about 1.5 cm long and 1 cm apart are made along the myofibres. These are joined at their proximal end by a transverse incision. The fibres are grasped with forceps just distal to this transverse incision and carefully dissected free from the muscle belly (Figure 24.6).
5. If possible, the sample is only handled at one end.
6. The incision is closed routinely.

Performing a muscle biopsy should not cause lameness; if this occurs the sample is either too large or has

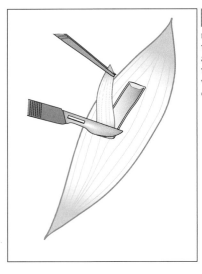

24.6 A diagram to illustrate taking a muscle biopsy sample. The tissue is grasped at one end and carefully dissected away from the rest of the muscle without touching the body of the sample.

been taken traumatically or from an inappropriate site. The sample can be frozen by immersion in pre-cooled (using liquid nitrogen) isopentane but this is not available to the majority of practitioners. If pre-cooled isopentane is not available, the sample can be placed in saline-moistened gauze and shipped on ice immediately to arrive at an appropriate laboratory within 24–48 hours. Alternatively, if analysis of frozen muscle is not an option, the sample can be placed in 10% buffered formalin following fixation to a tongue depressor, with needles, holding the muscle at normal length.

Muscle biopsy specimens are frozen and sections are cut with a cryostat. Processing includes (Figure 24.7):

- Haematoxylin and eosin staining to evaluate general histopathological features
- ATPases preincubated at acid and alkaline pHs (4.3, 4.6 and 9.8) to identify myofibre subtypes
- Periodic acid–Schiff (PAS) staining to identify glycogen

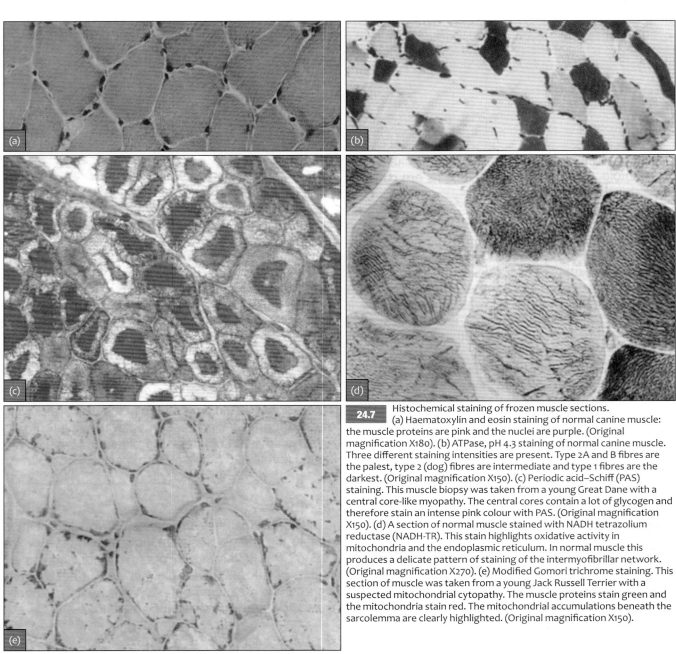

24.7 Histochemical staining of frozen muscle sections.
(a) Haematoxylin and eosin staining of normal canine muscle: the muscle proteins are pink and the nuclei are purple. (Original magnification X180). (b) ATPase, pH 4.3 staining of normal canine muscle. Three different staining intensities are present. Type 2A and B fibres are the palest, type 2 (dog) fibres are intermediate and type 1 fibres are the darkest. (Original magnification X150). (c) Periodic acid–Schiff (PAS) staining. This muscle biopsy was taken from a young Great Dane with a central core-like myopathy. The central cores contain a lot of glycogen and therefore stain an intense pink colour with PAS. (Original magnification X150). (d) A section of normal muscle stained with NADH tetrazolium reductase (NADH-TR). This stain highlights oxidative activity in mitochondria and the endoplasmic reticulum. In normal muscle this produces a delicate pattern of staining of the intermyofibrillar network. (Original magnification X270). (e) Modified Gomori trichrome staining. This section of muscle was taken from a young Jack Russell Terrier with a suspected mitochondrial cytopathy. The muscle proteins stain green and the mitochondria stain red. The mitochondrial accumulations beneath the sarcolemma are clearly highlighted. (Original magnification X150).

- Oil Red O staining to identify lipids
- NADH tetrazolium reductase (NADH-TR) to identify oxidative activity
- Modified Gomori trichrome staining to identify general histopathological features and to highlight myelin and connective tissues.

Further histochemical and immunohistochemical staining can be performed depending on the initial findings. For example, if X-linked muscular dystrophy is suspected, immunostaining for the rod and C-terminus of the dystrophin molecule can be undertaken.

Case examples

CASE 1

SIGNALMENT

5-month-old entire female Labrador Retriever.

HISTORY

The dog presented for evaluation of poor body condition and exercise intolerance first noted at around 4 months of age. After only 3–5 minutes of exercise, she would lie down and refuse to move for several minutes. She was always bright and alert during these episodes.

PHYSICAL EXAMINATION

General physical examination revealed a dog with poor body condition and generalized muscle atrophy (Figure 24.8). She had tarsal valgus bilaterally but was otherwise normal. On neurological examination the dog was exercise intolerant, choosing to lie down after walking for only a few minutes. When walking, she tended to bunny hop with her hindlimbs, but had normal postural reactions and no evidence of spinal ataxia that could indicate a primary problem affecting the central nervous system. Her patellar reflexes were absent bilaterally, and her withdrawal reflexes were present but reduced in strength in all four legs. Apart from her absent patellar reflexes, her neurological examination indicated a generalized myopathy (muscle atrophy, exercise intolerance and normal postural reactions with no ataxia).

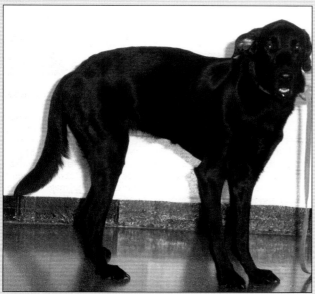

24.8 Labrador Retriever demonstrating poor body condition with a generalized lack of muscle mass.

WHAT ARE YOUR DIFFERENTIAL DIAGNOSES AND WHICH TESTS WOULD YOU LIKE TO PERFORM?

A hereditary myopathy was suspected based on the early onset of signs in an otherwise apparently healthy Labrador Retriever, but an infectious or parasitic disease such as neosporosis was also considered.

CLINICAL PATHOLOGY DATA

Haematology	Result	Reference interval
RBC (x 10¹²/l)	6.59	5.5–8.5
Hb (g/dl)	15.7	12–18
HCT (l/l)	46.6	35–56
MCV (fl)	71	60–77
WBC (x 10⁹/l)	11.2	6.0–17
Neutrophils (segmented) (x 10⁹/l)	6.0	3.0–11.5
Neutrophils (band) (x 10⁹/l)	0.0	
Lymphocytes (x 10⁹/l)	3.2	1.0–4.8
Monocytes (x 10⁹/l)	0.9	0.2–1.4
Eosinophils (x 10⁹/l)	0.9	0.1–1.3
Basophils (x 10⁹/l)	0.1	0–0.1
Platelets (x 10⁹/l)	192	181–350

Biochemistry	Result	Reference interval
Sodium (mmol/l)	156	141–156
Potassium (mmol/l)	4.6	3.8–5.6
Glucose (mmol/l)	5.8	3.3–6.9
Urea (mmol/l)	6.1	2.5–11.1
Creatinine (μmol/l)	53	8.8–159
Calcium (mmol/l)	2.8	2.25–2.9
Inorganic phosphate (mmol/l)	**2.5**	0.9–1.8
Total protein (g/l)	62	49–96
Albumin (g/l)	33	21–40
Globulin (g/l)	29	22–39
ALT (IU/l)	**146**	10–75
ALP (IU/l)	**319**	20–200
Creatine kinase (IU/l)	**233**	0–160

Abnormal results are in **bold**.

Urinalysis

Specific gravity: 1.041. No active sediment or bacteria.

→ **CASE 1 CONTINUED**

WHAT ABNORMALITIES ARE PRESENT?

- Elevated CK.
- Elevated ALT.
- Elevated phosphorus and alkaline phosphatase (ALP).

HOW WOULD YOU INTERPRET THESE RESULTS AND WHAT ARE THE LIKELY DIFFERENTIAL DIAGNOSES? WHAT FURTHER TESTS WOULD YOU PERFORM?

The ALT elevation and CK elevation are significant in light of the clinical presentation. While slight increases in CK are common and often not significant, persistent elevations, and small elevations in a patient showing signs of muscle disease, should be investigated. The elevated phosphorus and ALP probably reflect the age of the dog.

RESULTS OF FURTHER TESTS

Bile acid stimulation test

In light of the poor body condition, a bile acid stimulation test was performed to rule out a portosystemic shunt, and the results were within normal limits.

Electromyography and nerve conduction study

The electromyogram revealed marked spontaneous activity (fibrillation potentials and complex repetitive discharges) in all skeletal muscles. Nerve conduction studies of the ulnar and tibial nerve were normal.

Muscle biopsy

A muscle biopsy was performed on the biceps femoris of the left pelvic limb. Pathological changes in the muscle included marked variation in myofibre size with clusters of small fibres lying between much larger myofibres (Figure 24.9a). Hyalinized fibres and fibres with central nuclei were also visible. Immunohistochemistry confirmed normal expression and distribution of dystrophin, ruling out a dystrophinopathy (Figure 24.9b). A diagnosis of centronuclear myopathy was made.

Genetic testing

Genetic testing of DNA from this dog confirmed the diagnosis of centronuclear myopathy also known as hereditary myopathy of the Labrador Retriever.

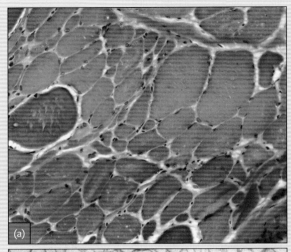
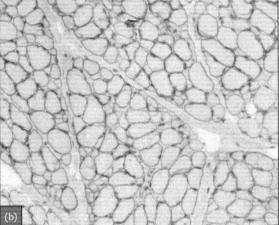

24.9 Frozen sections of the biceps femoris muscle (a) stained with haematoxylin and eosin and (b) stained immunohistochemically for dystrophin. There is marked variation in myofibre size and normal subsarcolemmal distribution of dystrophin.

TREATMENT AND CASE OUTCOME

There is no definitive treatment for this condition, although corticosteroids have been used. In many cases, the signs stabilize with time, and this was true of this dog. She was spayed (there is some association with crises when bitches come into season), and the owners managed her disorder by restricting exercise so that she did not collapse. She survived until the age of 13 years, when she died of an unrelated cause.

CASE 2

SIGNALMENT

13-year-old male neutered Miniature Pinscher.

HISTORY

The patient presented for evaluation of chronic progressive hindlimb gait abnormality, most notable in the last 2 months. The owners had obtained the dog 1 year previously as a rescue and so there was no previous medical history available. They reported ongoing problems with alopecia, but no other medical issues. The dog was not receiving any medications.

PHYSICAL EXAMINATION

The patient had a pot-bellied appearance with a thin haircoat and focal areas of alopecia surrounding patches of thickened and crusting skin lesions consistent with calcinosis cutis (Figure 24.10). Skin elasticity was poor. Abdominal palpation was suspicious for an

➜ CASE 2 CONTINUED

enlarged liver. While in the hospital the dog was noted to drink excessively. Orthopaedic examination was unremarkable apart from increased range of motion in both carpi. Neurologically the patient was alert and appropriate with a normal cranial nerve examination. He had a palmigrade stance and hyperextended pelvic limbs. He had a stiff, stilted gait in all four limbs, but his hindlimbs were most profoundly affected and appeared spastic with markedly reduced joint flexion when advancing the limbs. There was no spinal ataxia and myotactic reflexes were normal, but the withdrawal reflexes were reduced in all four limbs. His postural reactions were normal when he was supported carefully. His neurological signs localized to a generalized hypertonic myopathy. The palmigrade stance was felt to reflect breakdown of palmar ligamentous support.

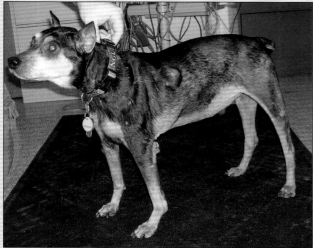

24.10 Miniature Pinscher at the time of presentation, showing the thin haircoat, the palmigrade stance and hyperextended hindlimbs. The dog also had a lipoma in the left thoracic region that is visible in this image.

CLINICAL PATHOLOGY DATA

Haematology	Result	Reference interval
RBC (x 10¹²/l)	**8.88**	5.7–8.01
Hb (g/dl)	20.1	13.8–20.3
HCT (l/l)	**56.1**	39.2–55.9
MCV (fl)	63.2	64–75.2
WBC (x 10⁹/l)	**17.0**	4.39–11.61
Neutrophils (segmented) (x 10⁹/l)	**16.56**	2.84–9.11
Neutrophils (band) (x 10⁹/l)	0	
Lymphocytes (x 10⁹/l)	**0.1**	0.59–3.31
Monocytes (x 10⁹/l)	0.34	0.08–0.85
Eosinophils (x 10⁹/l)	**0.0**	0.03–1.26
Basophils (x 10⁹/l)	0.0	0–0.19
Platelets (x 10⁹/l)	Marked clumping, numbers appear adequate on smear	

Abnormal results are in **bold**.

Biochemistry	Result	Reference interval
Sodium (mmol/l)	147	140–156
Potassium (mmol/l)	4.8	4–5.3
Glucose (mmol/l)	6.1	3.9–7.3
Urea (mmol/l)	4.3	2.1–9.3
Creatinine (μmol/l)	**35**	62–132
Calcium (mmol/l)	2.5	2.3–2.9
Inorganic phosphate (mmol/l)	1.7	0.8–1.8
Total protein (g/l)	60	52–73
Albumin (g/l)	35	30–39
Globulin (g/l)	26	17–38
ALT (IU/l)	**477**	12–54
ALP (IU/l)	**3167**	16–140
Creatine kinase (IU/l)	**314**	43–234
GGT (IU/l)	**219**	0–6

Abnormal results are in **bold**.

Urinalysis

Specific gravity: 1.008; pH: 7. No active sediment or bacteria.

WHAT ABNORMALITIES ARE PRESENT?

- Neutrophilia.
- Elevated liver enzymes, in particular ALP.
- Mild elevation in CK.
- Hyposthenuria.
- Mild erythrocytosis.

HOW WOULD YOU INTERPRET THESE RESULTS AND WHAT ARE THE LIKELY DIFFERENTIAL DIAGNOSES?

The neutrophilia and lymphopenia are consistent with a stress leucogram that could result from exogenous administration of corticosteroids, excessive endogenous production of corticosteroids or medical stress from other causes. Mild erythrocytosis can be seen with hyperadrenocorticism.

The elevated liver enzymes with most dramatic elevation of ALP are consistent with a steroid hepatopathy or a cholestatic hepatopathy.

The CK elevation is mild but if persistent could indicate muscle pathology.

The dilute urine together with the biochemical changes could be caused by hyperadrenocorticism.

The combination of the clinical pathological findings, coupled with the history, signalment, physical and neurological findings, make a diagnosis of hyperadrenocorticism with Cushing's myopathy the most likely differential.

RESULTS OF FURTHER TESTS

Electromyography and nerve conduction study

The electromyogram revealed marked spontaneous activity characterized by complex repetitive discharges in all skeletal muscles. Nerve conduction studies of the ulnar and tibial nerve were normal.

→ **CASE 2 CONTINUED**

Abdominal ultrasonography

An enlarged liver with a diffuse increase in echogenicity and bilaterally enlarged adrenal glands were identified.

Adrenocorticotropic hormone (ACTH) stimulation test

Pre-ACTH: 190 nmol/l (reference range: 50–250 nmol/l).
Post-ACTH: **1352** nmol/l (reference range: 150–550 nmol/l).
All of the above findings are consistent with hyperadrenocorticism with Cushing's myopathy.

TREATMENT AND CASE OUTCOME

The most effective way to treat the gait abnormality is to treat the metabolic cause. The dog was treated twice daily with mitotane until the ACTH stimulation test normalized (this occurred after 7 days of treatment) and then maintained with dosing 3 times a week. Trilostane was not available at the time the dog was treated, but would also be an appropriate choice. Intermittent ACTH stimulation testing and monitoring of the daily water intake were used to monitor progress. The dog's gait did not normalize but improved in character in the first 6 months of treatment, after which time the dog was lost to follow-up.

References and further reading

Acierno MJ and Mitchell MA (2007) Evaluation of four point-of-care meters for rapid determination of blood lactate concentrations in dogs. *Journal of the American Veterinary Medical Association* **230(9)**, 1315–1318

Bhalerao DP, Rajpurohit Y, Vite CH and Giger U (2002) Detection of a genetic mutation for myotonia congenita among Miniature Schnauzers and identification of a common carrier ancestor. *American Journal of Veterinary Research* **63**, 1443–1447

Dow SW, Fettman MJ, Curtis CR and LeCouteur RA (1989) Hypokalemia in cats: 186 cases (1984–1987). *Journal of the American Veterinary Medical Association* **194**, 1604–1608

Evoli A, Tonali PA, Padua L *et al.* (2003) Clinical correlates with anti-MuSK antibodies in generalized seronegative myasthenia gravis. *Brain* **126**, 2304–2311

Fyfe JC (2002) Molecular diagnosis of inherited neuromuscular disease. *Veterinary Clinics of North America: Small Animal Practice* **32**, 287–300

Guyton AC and Hall JE (2000) Contraction of skeletal muscle. In: *Textbook of Medical Physiology, 10th edn*, pp. 67–72. WB Saunders, Philadelphia

Harrington ML, Bagley RS and Braund KG (1996) Suspect hypokalemic myopathy in a dog. *Progress in Veterinary Neurology* **7**, 130–132

Karagiannis MH, Mann FA, Madsen RW, Berent LM and Greer R (2013) Comparison of two portable lactate meters in dogs. *Journal of the American Animal Hospital Association* **49(1)**, 8–15

Matwichuk CL, Taylor S, Shmon CL, Kass PH and Shelton GD (1999) Changes in rectal temperature and hematologic, biochemical, blood gas, and acid–base values in healthy Labrador Retrievers before and after strenuous exercise. *American Journal of Veterinary Research* **60**, 88–92

Pelé M, Tiret L, Kessler JL, Blot S and Panthier JJ (2005) SINE exonic insertion in the PTPLA gene leads to multiple splicing defects and segregates with the autosomal recessive centronuclear myopathy in dogs. *Human Molecular Genetics* **14(11)**, 1417–1427

Platt S and Olby N (2013) *BSAVA Manual of Canine and Feline Neurology, 4th edn*. BSAVA Publications, Gloucester

Saito M, Olby NJ, Obledo L and Gookin JL (2002) Muscle cramps in two standard poodles with hypoadrenocorticism. *Journal of the American Animal Hospital Association* **38(5)**, 437–443

Shelton GD (2002) Myasthenia gravis and disorders of neuromuscular transmission. *Veterinary Clinics of North America: Small Animal Practice* **32(1)**, 189–206

Shelton GD and Cardinet G (1989) Canine masticatory muscle disorders. In: *Current Veterinary Therapy, vol X*, ed. R Kirk, pp. 816–819. WB Saunders, Philadelphia

Shelton GD, Cardinet GH III and Bandman E (1987) Canine masticatory muscle disorders: a study of 29 cases. *Muscle and Nerve* **10**, 753–766

Shelton GD, Skeie GO, Kass PH and Aarli JA (2001) Titin and ryanodine receptor autoantibodies in dogs with thymoma and late-onset myasthenia gravis. *Veterinary Immunology and Immunopathology* **78(1)**, 97–105

Smith BF, Stedman H, Rajpurohit Y *et al.* (1996) Molecular basis of canine muscle type phosphofructokinase deficiency. *Journal of Biological Chemistry* **271**, 20070–20074

Tiret L, Blot S, Kessler JL, Guillot H, Breen M and Panthier JJ (2003) The CNM locus, a canine homologue of human autosomal forms of centronuclear myopathy, maps to chromosome 2. *Human Genetics* **112**, 297–306

Valentine BA, Blue JT, Shelley SM and Cooper BJ (1990) Increased serum alanine aminotransferase activity associated with muscle necrosis in the dog. *Journal of Veterinary Internal Medicine* **4**, 140–143

Wilson JS (1980) Toxic myopathy in a dog associated with the presence of monensin in dry food. *Canadian Veterinary Journal* **21**, 30–31

Wu X, Li ZF, Brooks R *et al.* (2007) Autoantibodies in canine masticatory muscle myositis recognize a novel myosin binding protein-C family member. *Journal of Immunology* **179(7)**, 4939–4944

Yoshioka T, Uzuka Y, Tanabe S *et al.* (1999) Molecular cloning of the canine nicotinic acetylcholine receptor alpha-subunit gene and development of the ELISA method to diagnose myasthenia gravis. *Veterinary Immunology and Immunopathology* **72**, 315–324

Laboratories providing testing for muscle disease

Animal Health Trust, Genetic Services, Lanwades Park, Kentford, Newmarket, Suffolk CB8 7UU UK
Email: dnatesting@aht.org.uk
Website: www.aht.org.uk

Antagene UK (HQ located in France and branches in Italy and Belgium)
Winchester House, 259–269 Old Marylebone Road,
London NW1 5RA, UK
Phone : +44 (0)20 7112 8522
Email : dnatest@ antagene.com
Website: http://www.antagene.com/

Comparative Neuromuscular Laboratory
Basic Science Building, Room 2095,
University of California, San Diego
La Jolla, CA 92093-0612 USA
Phone: +1 858 534 1537
Fax: +1 858 534 7319
Website: http://medicine.ucsd.edu

Orthopedic Foundation for Animals
2300 E Nifong Blvd.
Columbia, MO 65201-3806, USA
Phone: +1 573 442 0418
Email: ofa@offa.org
Website: http://www.offa.org

PennGenn Laboratories
3850 Spruce Street
Philadelphia, PA 19104-6010 USA
Phone: +1 215 898 3375
Fax: +1 215 573 2162
Email: penngen@vet.upenn.edu
Website: http:www.vet.upenn.edu

Chapter 25

Laboratory evaluation of cerebrospinal fluid

Kathleen Freeman

Cerebrospinal fluid (CSF) collection and laboratory analysis are recommended as part of the investigation of central nervous system (CNS) disease. A definitive diagnosis on the basis of CSF laboratory evaluation alone is rare, but the laboratory evaluation of CSF may provide documentation of normal or abnormal findings and help make distinctions among various differential diagnoses.

CSF collection

Indications and contraindications

Collection and laboratory evaluation of CSF is indicated in the investigation of any CNS disease of unknown cause.

General anaesthesia is required for collection, so any condition that would contraindicate anaesthesia precludes collection of CSF. Other contraindications include causes of increased intracranial pressure (ICP), such as acute head trauma, active or decompensated hydrocephalus, cerebral oedema and expansile masses. These conditions may result in herniation of the cerebellum, cerebrum or brainstem during collection, causing severe compromise of brain function, coma and/or death. Physical and neurological examination, history, presentation and imaging procedures may help to determine whether any conditions that would contraindicate CSF collection are present. A variety of clinical signs can be associated with increased ICP, including anisocoria, papilloedema, circling, head pressing and obtundation.

The risk of herniation may be reduced by administration of mannitol or hypertonic saline prior to induction of anaesthesia, and by hyperventilation with oxygen to reduce the partial pressure of carbon dioxide (PCO_2) during the procedure, as hypercarbia predisposes to herniation. Ketamine should not be used for anaesthesia for CSF collection because it causes an increase in ICP and may induce seizures.

Repeated CSF evaluations have been shown to be of benefit when initial therapy has been ineffective or when there is relapsing disease. Abnormal CSF findings at a 3-month check following diagnosis of steroid-responsive meningitis–arteritis have been found to be associated with increased risk of relapsing disease (Lowrie *et al.*, 2013).

Requirements

Sterile preparation of the site of collection is required, with clipping of the hair, scrubbing and maintenance of a sterile field. Sterile gloves should be worn.

A sterile disposable or resterilizable spinal needle with a stylet is used. Usually a 20–22 G, 1.5 inch needle is recommended, although smaller needles may be needed for very small dogs and cats, and longer needles may be needed for large or giant breeds of dog. Several needles should be available because replacement may be needed if there is blood contamination.

Several plain tubes should be reserved for collection of CSF. If the sample is bloody, collection into an ethylene-diamine tetra-acetic acid (EDTA) tube may help prevent clotting of the specimen. A paediatric EDTA tube should be used, because the volume of CSF may be quite small and there may be significant dilution by EDTA if the volume does not fill the tube to the recommended level.

Sites

If the neurological examination localizes the CNS lesion to the head and/or neck, collection from the cisterna magna (cerebellomedullary cistern) is recommended. Lumbar puncture may be preferred in cases with spinal disease localized to the thoracolumbar spine because it may be more likely to confirm abnormality than a cerebellomedullary collection. However, lumbar cistern collections are more difficult than those from the cerebellomedullary cistern, may be of smaller volume and are more likely to be contaminated with blood.

Volume and rate

- Approximately 1 ml of CSF per 5 kg bodyweight can be collected safely.
- Collection of approximately 1 ml per 30 seconds is safe.
- The volume of CSF collected should not exceed 4–5 ml from a dog, 0.5–1.0 ml from an adult cat, or 10–20 drops from a kitten or puppy.

Techniques

Cerebellomedullary cistern

For collection from the cisterna magna, the animal is placed in lateral recumbency and the neck is flexed such that the head and vertebral column are positioned at a 90-degree angle. Excessive flexion of the neck may result in elevation of ICP and increased potential for brain herniation, or may result in occlusion of the endotracheal tube. The nose should be supported so that its long axis is parallel to the table (Figure 25.1).

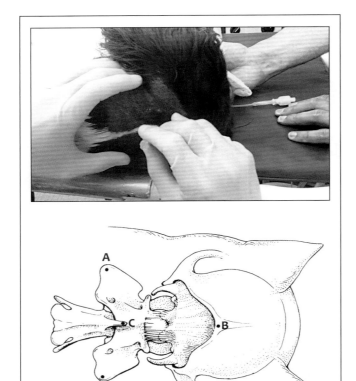

25.1 The correct site for collection of CSF from the cisterna magna is shown in the photograph. The drawing shows the important landmarks of the wings of the atlas vertebra (A) and the occipital protuberance (B), and the craniodorsal tip of the dorsal spine of the axis (C).
(Reproduced from the BSAVA Guide to Procedures in Small Animal Practice)

To locate the correct position for sampling, the area enclosed within a triangle of landmarks formed by the occipital protuberance and the most prominent points of the lateral wings of the atlas is palpated. The needle should be inserted on the midline, approximately one-third to halfway between the external occipital protuberance and the palpated lateral wings of the atlas. An 18 G needle or scalpel blade can be used for initial puncture of the skin, or the skin can be pinched and lifted so that the needle can be pushed through the skin with a twisting motion. The needle should be inserted with the bevel orientated cranially. It should be held perpendicular to the skin surface and gradually advanced, with the stylet in place. Periodically the needle can be stabilized and the stylet withdrawn to determine whether CSF is present.

A sudden loss of resistance may signal entry into the subarachnoid space due to penetrance of the dorsal atlanto-occipital membrane, which is very close to the subarachnoid space, but may not be recognized in all cases. It is very important that the needle is not inserted too far, because passage of the needle into the spinal cord will cause significant damage. If the needle hits bone during insertion, slight redirection cranially or caudally may be attempted. CSF may be collected directly from the spinal needle hub by allowing it to drip into a collecting tube or by gentle aspiration of drops as they form at the hub, using a syringe held adjacent to (but not attached to) the hub. Direct aspiration of CSF with an attached syringe should not be performed because this may result in spinal cord damage as well as blood contamination.

Lumbar cistern

For collection of CSF from the lumbar cistern, the animal is placed in lateral recumbency, with the back flexed to open the spaces between the dorsal laminae of the vertebrae. The L5–6 space is most commonly used in dogs because the subarachnoid space rarely extends to the lumbosacral junction. In cats, collection can be made from the L6–7 space.

To collect from the L5–6 space, the needle is inserted just off the midline at the caudal aspect of the L6 dorsal spinous process and advanced at an angle cranioventrally and slightly medially, to enter the spinal canal between the dorsal laminae of L5 and L6. Misdirection laterally into the paralumbar muscles or underestimation of the length of needle required may result in advancement of the needle to the hub without encountering bone. The needle may be passed into the dorsal subarachnoid space or advanced through the caudal nervous structures to the floor of the spinal canal for collection from the ventral subarachnoid space. A leg or tail twitch is often observed as the needle passes through the cauda equina/caudal spinal cord. The stylet is removed and the needle may be withdrawn carefully to encourage fluid flow. The rate of flow is usually slower than from the cerebellomedullary cistern.

Minimizing blood contamination

If the CSF appears to be bloody at the onset of collection, replacement of the stylet for 30–60 seconds may result in clearing of the CSF. If the first few drops are bloody, they can be collected separately from the following drops, which are often clear. If the rate of flow of CSF is slow, slight rotation of the needle may be helpful. If abundant blood is present, venous sinus puncture should be suspected and a new approach with a fresh needle is recommended.

Handling CSF specimens

CSF is normally a low-protein fluid with rapid turnover. Cells lyse rapidly in CSF once it is removed, and unfixed fluid should be processed within 30–60 minutes of collection. Addition of an equal volume of 40–90% ethanol or 2 drops of 10% buffered formalin per ml of specimen may be used for fixation of fluids that cannot be delivered immediately to a laboratory or cannot be processed immediately. Some laboratories are prepared to use special techniques for cytological evaluation of fixed CSF. It is advisable to check with the laboratory regarding their requirements prior to CSF submission. Cell counts may be affected by slight dilution when formalin fixation is used, but this is not usually clinically significant. Other techniques that may help retard cellular degeneration and/or increase cell stability include refrigeration, addition of fresh, frozen or thawed fetal calf or autologous serum, addition of 20% albumin or addition of hetastarch. Hetastarch does not interfere with measurement of CSF protein, while other additives do. Submission of a plain CSF sample for total protein and nucleated cell counts and a sample with additive (20% fetal calf serum or 1:1 hetastarch) for differential cell counts and morphological evaluation, with storage at 4°C, has been recommended for all CSF specimens that cannot be analysed within 1 hour of collection (Fry et al., 2006).

Protein and enzyme concentrations in CSF are relatively stable and submission using routine methods is usually sufficient for accurate determinations.

Laboratory analysis of CSF

Usually 1–2 ml of CSF is available from dogs or cats. Routine analysis of CSF should include:

- Macroscopic evaluation (colour and transparency)
- Cell counts: red blood cells (RBCs), nucleated cell count (NCC)
- Total protein (laboratory microprotein assay or commercial dipstick)
- Cytological evaluation.

General characteristics of normal and abnormal CSF are summarized in Figure 25.2.

Component of CSF evaluation	Normal	Abnormal
Colour	Colourless	Pink, red or xanthochromic, occasionally green to grey (slight, moderate or marked)
Transparency	Clear	Cloudy or turbid (slight, moderate or marked)
Erythrocyte count	Zero is considered to be normal but red cells are often present in small numbers (<250 per microlitre)	Variable
Nucleated cell count	Dogs: 0–6 cells per microlitre Cats: 0–8 cells per microlitre	Variable
Total protein	Microprotein (chemical determination): cerebellomedullary <0.30 g/l; lumbar <0.45 g/l	Microprotein (chemical determination): cerebellomedullary >0.30 g/l; lumbar >0.45 g/l

25.2 General characteristics of normal and abnormal CSF.

Macroscopic evaluation

Macroscopic evaluation should include evaluation of colour and transparency. Visible cloudiness or turbidity usually reflects a markedly elevated cell count, although moderate elevations in cellularity cannot be detected grossly. Yellow or orange discoloration is termed xanthochromia and indicates previous haemorrhage into the CSF, with resultant formation of haem pigments producing the colour change. Red discoloration indicates recent or current haemorrhage. Green to grey discoloration may result from various cellular and/or bacterial contents and is rarely observed. The macroscopic evaluation is aided by good natural non-fluorescent lighting and examining the tube containing the fluid against a piece of white paper.

Cell counts

Cell counts can be conducted using a standard haemocytometer (Figure 25.3a) or a C-Chip disposable haemocytometer (Figure 25.3b). The latter is a precision-engineered surface-patterned plastic disposable haemocytometer with two counting chambers and two ports for sample introduction. The chamber includes an integrated coverslip. It has an imprinted improved Neubauer grid (Figure 25.3c). Advantages of this haemocytometer over conventional reusable glass haemocytometers include:

- It is a disposable unit, eliminating the need for cleaning
- Unbreakable
- Integrated coverslip, eliminating the need for separate coverslips and incorrect coverslip placement that may cause errors in sample volume and/or counting of cells
- Reduced exposure to potentially infectious materials
- Requires 10 µl per chamber, suitable for small volume collections
- Precision-engineered chambers for accuracy and repeatability.

The haemocytometer should be fully loaded on both sides, so that duplicate counts can be made. If a traditional haemocytometer is used, the coverslip should be cleaned so that debris will not be confused with cells. The haemocytometer can be filled using well mixed CSF in a glass capillary tube. The cells should be allowed to settle for 5–10 minutes prior to counting. The cells in all nine large squares of the haemocytometer should be counted (Figure 25.3c). The condenser of the microscope should be lowered to provide contrast.

Erythrocytes are recognized as small clear refractile discs without nuclei, while nucleated cells are larger, more refractile or appear granular (Figure 25.3d). The total number of cells of each type (RBC and nucleated cells) should be divided by 9 (the number of squares counted) and multiplied by 10 (depth of the haemocytometer) in order to obtain the cell count per microlitre. Cell counts obtained from each side of the haemocytometer should be within 10–20% of each other. If there is larger variation than this, a repeat count should be considered. Reference intervals for nucleated cell counts in normal CSF may vary with the laboratory, but as a general guideline are <7 cells/µl in dogs and <9 cells/µl in cats. When the nucleated cell count is elevated, this is referred to as *pleocytosis*.

Various formulae have been applied to try to determine the possible contribution of blood contamination to the CSF nucleated cell count. These formulae have been shown to be unreliable in 'correcting' for blood contamination and are not recommended (Vernau *et al.*, 2008). If the specimen contains a large amount of blood suspected to be due to contamination, repeat collection is recommended. RBC counts as high as 15,000/ml may occur with minimal elevation in nucleated cell counts. Protein concentrations are higher in blood-contaminated specimens: approximately 1200 RBC/ml have been shown to be required to increase CSF protein by 0.01 g/l. Proportions of neutrophils are higher in blood-contaminated specimens than in those without blood contamination. However, the presence of activated macrophages and/or reactive lymphocytes is not expected with blood contamination and these are indications of likely CNS abnormalities when blood contamination is present (Doyle and Solano-Gallego, 2009).

Automated cell counts in CSF

Automated cell counts for CSF have been investigated and generally been found to compare well with haemocytometer cell counts. Accurate results (within 30%) were achievable for total nucleated cell counts up to 4000 cells/µl. Intra-assay coefficients of variation ranged from 4.19 to 25.94% (Becker *et al.*, 2008). The cost of quality control materials for automated CSF cell counts may be high if only small numbers of CSF samples are assayed. Therefore, each laboratory must weigh-up the advantages and disadvantages of the use of automated cell counts or haemocytometer cell counts for CSF.

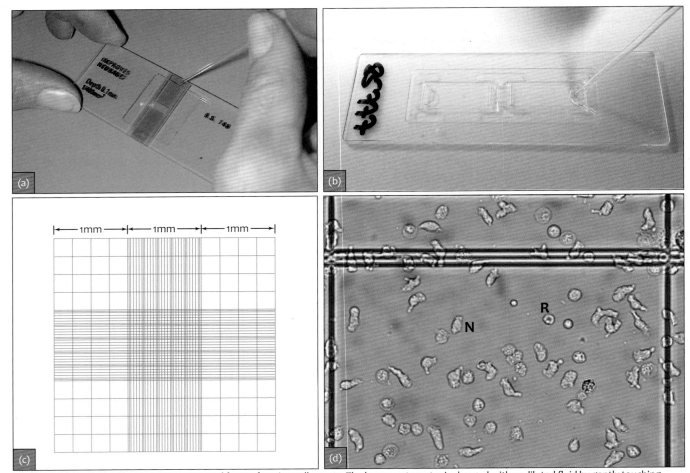

25.3 (a) A standard haemocytometer used for performing cell counts. The haemocytometer is charged with undiluted fluid by gently touching the tip of a capillary tube containing CSF to the end of the coverslip. (b) A disposable C-Chip haemocytometer is loaded by touching the tip of the charged capillary tube to the semicircular groove. (c) Diagrammatic representation of the grid lines seen microscopically. (d) The grid is viewed at X400 magnification with the condenser lowered. Red cells have a doughnut appearance (R); nucleated cells have a textured appearance and are slightly larger (N).
(Courtesy of Elizabeth Villiers)

Total protein (microprotein assay)

Albumin makes up approximately 80–95% of the total protein in normal CSF. Reference intervals for total protein may vary slightly with the laboratory and/or method used. Protein concentrations in cerebellomedullary CSF samples are usually <0.25–0.30 g/l and in lumbar cistern samples <0.45 g/l.

Reference laboratories use dye-binding spectrophotometric methods for quantitation of CSF protein levels, which are designed to measure very low amounts of protein (often referred to as microprotein assays). Standard chemistry methods for measuring serum protein, including in-house analysers, are not suitable for measuring CSF protein because they cannot measure the very low amounts of protein present in CSF. Likewise, refractometry is not suitable.

In practice, the use of urine dipsticks for estimation of CSF protein provides a rapid assessment of protein levels. Ames Multistix urine dipsticks have been validated for this purpose. Figure 25.4 summarizes the estimation of CSF protein using Ames Multistix urine dipsticks. The dipsticks are most sensitive to albumin, and good correlation has been shown with standard dye-binding microprotein determinations.

Previously, Pandy's or Nonne–Apelt tests were used to determine whether globulins were present in CSF. These tests have fallen out of favour and are not now routinely used because of difficulties in interpretation of

Ames Multistix urine dipstick result	Estimated total protein	Interpretation
Trace	<0.30 g/l (<30 mg/dl)	Within normal limits
1+	0.30 g/l (30 mg/dl)	Within normal limits
2+	1.0 g/l (100 mg/dl)	Abnormal
3+	3.0 g/l (300 mg/dl)	Abnormal
4+	>20.0 g/l (>2000 mg/dl)	Abnormal

25.4 Estimation of CSF protein using Ames Multistix urine dipsticks.

the significance of globulins and the semiquantitative nature of the tests.

Sometimes there will be elevation in the total protein of CSF but no abnormalities are detected cytologically. This is referred to as 'albuminocytological dissociation'. This is a relatively common finding and is non-specific, because it can occur with inflammatory, degenerative, compressive or neoplastic diseases. Elevated total protein may occur with increased permeability of the blood–brain barrier, interruption of normal CSF flow or absorption and/or intrathecal globulin production.

Cytological preparations

Cytocentrifugation is commonly used for cytology preparations because CSF is of very low cellularity compared with other body fluids. Chamber sedimentation or membrane-filter techniques may also be used. Staining of air-dried preparations is usually by Romanowsky stains (Diff-Quik®, Wright–Giemsa, May–Grünwald–Giemsa or others), while wet-fixed specimens may be stained using trichrome, Papanicolaou or haematoxylin and eosin (H&E).

Cytocentrifugation may be available at referral laboratories or specialized veterinary referral practices where extensive in-house laboratory facilities are justified by a high caseload. For in-practice use, a simple sedimentation chamber may be made using a 2.5 ml syringe (Figure 25.5). This method has the disadvantage that cells tend to shrink as they slowly dry. The technique is as follows:

1. The barrel of a syringe is cut in half.
2. A circular hole is cut into a piece of filter paper, which is then wrapped around a microscope slide.
3. The barrel of the syringe is aligned over the hole and attached using a small amount of petroleum jelly around its edge.
4. The filter paper and syringe are clipped to the slide using bulldog clips.
5. An aliquot of well mixed CSF is placed in the cylinder and the cells allowed to settle on the slide for 30 minutes.
6. The excess fluid is wicked away by the filter paper and the cells settle on the slide in the circle defined by the hole in the filter paper.

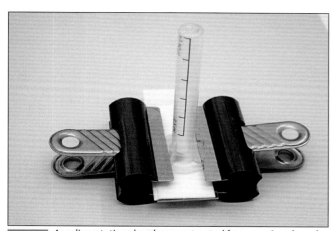

25.5 A sedimentation chamber constructed from a syringe barrel, filter paper, a slide and sticky tape.
(Courtesy of Roger Powell)

New methylene blue staining

The new methylene blue (NMB) staining method deserves separate mention as a rapid and easy method for the cytological evaluation of CSF. Addition of 1–2 drops of NMB to 1–2 drops of CSF can provide contrast that helps in identification of erythrocytes and nucleated cells. If used to perform a count, the dilution factor would need to be corrected. It is most commonly used as a wet-mount (1 drop of NMB–CSF mixture placed beneath a coverslip and examined under a microscope at low (25–40X) and intermediate (100–400X) magnification.

It is also possible to identify infectious agents easily with this stain, particularly when other types of air-dried preparations may have granular background material that could be confused with bacteria. NMB can also be used with air-dried cytological preparations as a wet-mount preparation beneath a coverslip. NMB is prone to precipitation, so care should be taken to eliminate precipitate that

may obscure or confuse the contents of the cytological preparation. One method is to use a dropper bottle and handle the bottle carefully so any sediment at the bottom of the bottle is not disturbed. The stain can be periodically filtered and should be stored away from light.

Other assays

Creatine kinase (CK) assay has been recommended in the past, because damage to nervous tissue may result in elevation of the isoenzyme found in the CNS. CK activity <38 IU/l has been reported to indicate a better prognosis for long-term functional recovery in dogs with intervertebral disc disease (Witsberger et al., 2012). However, there is difficulty in interpretation of elevated levels, particularly when blood contamination is present. CSF may also become contaminated with CK from skeletal muscle during collection. The difficulty in interpretation of the significance of elevated CK has resulted in discontinuance of its use in most laboratories.

Special stains or immunocytochemistry may be used to demonstrate bacteria, fungi, intracellular material or myelin (Srugo et al., 2011). Specialized analyses, including electrophoresis, immunoelectrophoresis, antibody titres, fungal antigen tests, microbiological cultures or polymerase chain reaction (PCR) amplification assays, may be used when particular conditions are suspected. An extensive review of all of these applications is beyond the scope of this chapter, but various ancillary tests may be of benefit with specific conditions.

When infectious disease is suspected, demonstration of increased antibody titres in CSF compared with serum may be helpful in the diagnosis of viral encephalopathies, and amplification of DNA from infectious agents by PCR may provide a definitive diagnosis with high sensitivity and specificity. Failure to demonstrate organisms by PCR may occur in the absence of organisms or as a result of their sequestration in various sites, DNA degradation or other factors. Negative antibody titres may occur in CSF in the presence of positive antibody titres in serum, complicating the interpretation. Therefore, combinations of serology and PCR may be of benefit in some cases (Tyler and Cullor, 1989; Jäderlund et al., 2009; Ishigaki et al., 2012).

Increased total IgA concentrations in serum and spinal fluid provide support for steroid-responsive meningitis–arteritis with high sensitivity but low specificity (Maiolini et al., 2012). CSF D-dimers were shown to be significantly elevated in dogs with steroid-responsive meningitis–arteritis compared with dogs with other inflammatory neurological diseases. Cerebrospinal fluid C-reactive protein (CRP) levels have been reported to be significantly elevated in dogs with a variety of types of inflammatory neurological disease and may be helpful in diagnosis of relapsing steroid-responsive meningitis–arteritis when other CSF abnormalities may have resolved but overt clinical signs are present (Martínez-Subiela et al., 2011).

PCR for antigen receptor rearrangements (PARR) to provide support for lymphoid malignancy and immunophenotyping for T- and B-lymphoid cells may be of benefit in distinguishing reactive from neoplastic conditions and in their classification, respectively (Turek et al., 2008). Various techniques for support of, or primary diagnosis of, specific conditions will continue to evolve as such tests become more widely available and as genetic tests specific for various conditions continue to be developed and validated for use in veterinary diagnostics and monitoring.

Normal and abnormal CSF

Cellular and non-cellular features of normal CSF

- **Small lymphocytes:** these are the predominant cell type in CSF from healthy dogs and cats. The appearance is similar to that of lymphocytes in peripheral blood: cells are usually 9–15 μm in diameter (canine and feline red blood cells have diameters of 7 and 5.5 μm, respectively), with a round to ovoid or slightly cleaved nucleus and a thin rim of palely basophilic cytoplasm. Reactive lymphocytes are an abnormal finding – these have slightly enlarged nuclei and more abundant basophilic cytoplasm (Doyle and Solano-Gallego, 2009).
- **Monocytoid cells:** these may be present in low numbers and are often slightly larger than small lymphocytes (12–15 μm diameter) with variable nuclear shape, open chromatin and moderate amounts of lightly basophilic cytoplasm that varies from homogeneous to finely vacuolated. Activated macrophages with abundant vacuolated cytoplasm are an abnormal finding.
- **Neutrophils and eosinophils:** a few neutrophils may be seen in normal CSF and these can constitute up to 20% of cells when the nucleated cell count is within the reference interval, although >10% neutrophils are considered abnormal when the nucleated cell count is elevated. Eosinophils are seen occasionally in very low numbers in CSF from healthy animals. In the absence of excessive blood contamination, neutrophil percentages >10–20% and eosinophils >1%, with or without elevations in total nucleated cell count, are considered abnormal and deserve further investigation.
- **Plasma cells:** these are not present in normal CSF, but may be seen with reactive or inflammatory processes as a response to antigenic stimulation.

Contaminants and unusual findings

Occasionally, ependymal or choroid plexus cells may be seen in CSF (Figure 25.6). These are round to cuboidal mononuclear cells, often occurring in cohesive groups. Subarachnoid (leptomeningeal) cells may be recognized as mononuclear cells with oval nuclei, delicate chromatin and elongated or indistinct cytoplasmic margins, and may be single or in small clusters. All of these cells are collectively referred to as 'surface epithelial cells' and are thought most often to be incidental findings, unrelated to specific diseases (Wessmann et al., 2010).

Haemopoietic precursor cells (immature cells of myeloid or erythroid origin; megakaryocytes) may occasionally be seen if bone marrow is accidentally punctured: they are most often seen in CSF from lumbar collections.

Mitotic figures are occasionally seen in CSF from healthy animals, but their presence is more often associated with proliferative conditions, particularly neoplasia (Wamsley and Alleman, 2004).

Coiled 'ribbons' of basophilic non-cellular material have been reported in CSF obtained during post-mortem examination, and have been hypothesized to represent denatured myelin or myelin fragments. Myelin-like material may also be seen in CSF samples from animals with a variety of neurological diseases (Figure 25.7). It is more frequently observed in lumbar than cerebellomedullary samples and in small dogs (<10 kg) compared with dogs >10 kg. Larger amounts of myelin-like material are seen more often in CSF from dogs with intervertebral disc disease than that from dogs with other diseases. However, no association has been found between myelin-like material and outcome, and it is thought to be more often an artefact of collection rather than due to the presence of neurological disease (Zabolotzky et al., 2010).

Silica particles can be seen as refractile crystalline material in CSF specimens as a result of specimen transport in silica-coated plastic tubes (Snyder et al., 2007).

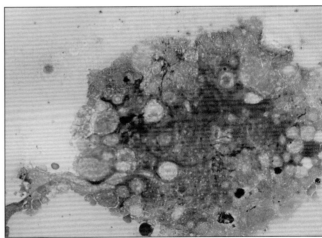

25.7 Myelin-like material seen in CSF obtained by lumbar puncture from a Border Terrier with intervertebral disc disease. (Modified Wright's stain; original magnification X1000)
(Courtesy of Elizabeth Villiers)

Cellular findings in neurological disease

'Normal' CSF in the presence of disease

In many patients with neurological disease no abnormalities of CSF are detected. The majority of cases of idiopathic epilepsy, congenital hydrocephalus, intoxication, metabolic or functional disorders, vertebral disease and myelomalacia have normal CSF, although intervertebral disc disease has also been reported to present with pleocytosis (Snyder et al., 2007). A significant proportion of cases with neurological disease due to feline infectious peritonitis (FIP), distemper encephalitis, neoplasia or granulomatous meningoencephalitis may also have CSF that is within normal limits.

25.6 A small cluster of surface epithelial cells with small round nuclei and abundant pinkish cytoplasm. (Modified Wright's stain; original magnification X1000)
(Courtesy of Paola Monti)

Slight to moderate neutrophilic inflammation

Slight to moderate neutrophilic inflammation (25–50% neutrophils, with or without elevated microprotein, with or without pleocytosis) may occur with bacterial, fungal, protozoal, parasitic, rickettsial or viral infections, as well as with neoplasia or non-infectious conditions. Non-infectious conditions that may result in this appearance include traumatic, degenerative, immune-mediated, metabolic or ischaemic conditions.

Marked neutrophilic inflammation

Marked neutrophilic inflammation (>50% neutrophils, with pleocytosis, often with increased microprotein) can be seen with bacterial meningitis and severe viral encephalitis, including FIP. It may also occur with acute steroid-responsive meningitis–arteritis (also known as meningitis of unknown origin), following myelography, with trauma, haemorrhage, acquired hydrocephalus or with neoplasia, especially meningioma.

Mixed cellular inflammation without a predominant type

Mixed cellular inflammation (mixed macrophages, lymphocytes and neutrophils, with or without plasma cells; with or without elevated microprotein) may occur with fungal, protozoal, parasitic or rickettsial infection, FIP, granulomatous meningoencephalitis (GME), degenerative diseases

and inadequately treated chronic bacterial infections. In addition, a mixed inflammatory response may be found in the early stages of therapy for bacterial meningitis or with chronic or relapsing steroid-responsive meningitis–arteritis.

Mononuclear inflammation

Mononuclear inflammation (predominantly monocytes, especially lymphocytes, usually with pleocytosis) can occur with GME, and in necrotizing encephalitis of small-breed dogs. It may occur with neoplasia, canine distemper virus infection and in a variety of non-infectious and degenerative conditions.

Eosinophilic inflammation

Eosinophilic inflammation (predominantly eosinophils, usually with pleocytosis) may occur with parasitic, protozoal, fungal, bacterial, viral and rickettsial infections. It has also been reported with neoplasia, steroid-responsive eosinophilic meningitis, hypersensitivity reactions and as part of non-specific inflammatory reactions.

CSF findings in selected clinical conditions

Findings in CSF in selected clinical conditions are summarized in Figure 25.8.

Condition	CSF characteristics	Clinical features	Comments and differential diagnoses
Feline infectious peritonitis (FIP)	• Frequently see neutrophilic pleocytosis • TP usually >2.0 g/l • NCC usually >100 cells/µl • Neutrophils often >50% • Mixed cell pleocytosis often present late in the course of disease	Often <4 years of age. Multifocal neurological signs referable to cerebellum and/or brainstem. Protracted course of illness	Need to rule out bacterial meningoencephalitis, non-FIP viral encephalomyelitis and other inflammatory conditions
Canine distemper	• Usually lymphocytic pleocytosis; may see mixed cell pleocytosis • NCC variable, but usually >60% lymphocytes • TP usually increased	Usually young dog. History of absence of vaccination and/or exposure to other dogs with illness and/or death	Occasionally viral inclusions may be identified. Serum and CSF antibodies to distemper virus in the absence of vaccination is supportive
Granulomatous meningoencephalitis (GME)	• Usually slight to moderate, lymphocytic or mixed cell pleocytosis; occasionally neutrophilic pleocytosis • NCC usually >100 cells/µl; wide range reported, including 'within normal limits' • TP usually >1.0 g/l (variable)	Usually young to middle-aged bitch. Toy and terrier breeds predisposed. Fever, ataxia, tetraparesis, seizures. May be localized as multifocal or focal (better prognosis)	Need to rule out necrotizing meningoencephalitis of small-breed dogs
Steroid-responsive suppurative meningitis–arteritis	• Neutrophilic pleocytosis • NCC often >500 cells/µl • Usually >75% non-degenerate neutrophils	Usually young to middle-aged dogs. Fever, cervical pain, hyperaesthesia, paresis	Improvement usually seen within 72 h of glucocorticoid treatment. Need to rule out bacterial and ehrlichial meningoencephalitis
Steroid-responsive eosinophilic meningitis	• Eosinophilic pleocytosis with >80% eosinophils • Slight to marked elevation in NCC	Reported in dogs and one cat. Golden Retrievers predisposed. Usually respond to glucocorticoid therapy. Type I hypersensitivity reaction suspected	Need to rule out fungal, parasitic, protozoal and neoplastic conditions
Necrotizing encephalitis of small-breed dogs	Lymphocytic pleocytosis; usually >200 cells/µl; lymphocytes usually >70% TP often >0.5 g/l	Pugs, Maltese and Yorkshire Terriers, usually >4 years old. Seizures, depression, ataxia. Lack of response to steroids. Possibly immune-mediated	Multifocal to massive necrosis and non-suppurative inflammation. Fatal or leading to euthanasia. Need to rule out GME. Histology may be required to detect necrosis
Neoplasia	Variable NCC, TP and cytological findings	Lymphoma is the most common neoplasm found in CSF	Well differentiated or small cell lymphoma may be difficult to differentiate from lymphocytic pleocytosis. Other tumour types, including primary brain tumours, rarely exfoliate into CSF; may require aspiration, crush preparations or imprint from biopsy sample for cytology

25.8 Characteristics of CSF in selected clinical conditions. NCC = nucleated cell count; TP = total protein.

Feline infectious peritonitis

Feline infectious peritonitis (FIP) is a common cause of neutrophilic pleocytosis in the cat, although this disease can also lead to a lymphocytic pleocytosis, sometimes with plasma cells, or a monocytic or mixed pleocytosis. Microprotein is often markedly elevated (>2.0 g/l). Cats with neurological disease due to FIP infection usually have multifocal neurological signs and often have a history of a protracted course of illness. Common neurological signs include seizures, behavioural changes, cranial nerve deficits, abnormal postural reactions, ataxia and spinal hyperaesthesia (see also Chapter 28). Immunocytochemistry has been used to demonstrate the FIP virus within CSF macrophages (Ives *et al.*, 2013).

Canine distemper virus infection

Canine distemper virus often results in a lymphocytic pleocytosis. Cell counts may vary from within normal limits to >50 cells/µl. Lymphocytes usually account for >60% of the nucleated cells. Some cases have an increase in macrophages and increased microprotein. Intracellular viral inclusions are rarely seen. Positive CSF titres for canine distemper virus may be helpful in providing support for a diagnosis of distemper viral encephalomyelitis (see Chapter 28). Dogs with canine distemper virus are often young and are usually unvaccinated. The neurological signs can be acute or chronic and include involuntary twitches, incoordination, circling, paresis to paralysis, distemper myoclonus (chewing-gum fits) or grand mal seizures.

Granulomatous meningoencephalitis

GME is most often seen in young to middle-aged, small and medium-sized dogs, especially of toy or terrier breeds, and occurs more often in females. Clinical signs include fever, ataxia, tetraparesis, cervical hyperaesthesia and seizures. The CSF may have slight to moderate lymphocytic inflammation, mixed cell pleocytosis (Figure 25.9) and/or occasionally neutrophilic pleocytosis. The majority of cases have nucleated cell counts >100 cells/µl. Microprotein levels are variable.

Steroid-responsive suppurative meningitis–arteritis

Steroid-responsive meningitis–artheritis (SRMA) is usually a condition of young to middle-aged large-breed dogs. Breed predilections include Beagles, Boxers, Weimaraners, Nova Scotia Duck Tolling Retrievers and Bernese Mountain Dogs. Clinical signs include fever, cervical pain, hyperaesthesia and paresis. The CSF is hypercellular, often containing >500 cells/µl, usually with >75% non-degenerate neutrophils and elevated microprotein (Figure 25.10) when acute disease is present. Bacteria are not present cytologically or on culture. A rapid response (improvement within 72 hours) is typically observed with glucocorticoid administration. A more mixed or mononuclear pleocytosis may be seen in chronic cases. Monitoring of acute phase proteins may be helpful in this disease. Serum concentrations of CRP decline in parallel with CSF nucleated cell counts in response to prednisolone therapy, and in patients that discontinue therapy following successful treatment, CRP and serum amyloid A (SAA) concentrations fall to within the reference range (Lowrie *et al.*, 2009a). In patients that suffer a relapse of SRMA, serum CRP and SAA concentrations may increase (Lowrie *et al.*, 2009b). Monitoring of serum levels avoids additional collection of CSF, which is a higher risk procedure and requires general anaesthesia. (See Chapter 7 for additional information on acute phase proteins.) *Anaplasma phagocytophilum* and *Ehrlichia canis* infections can result in similar clinical signs and cytological findings (see Chapter 29).

Steroid-responsive eosinophilic meningitis

Steroid-responsive eosinophilic meningitis has been reported in dogs and cats. This has been hypothesized to be the result of an allergic (type I hypersensitivity) reaction. Slight to marked pleocytosis may be present, but usually >80% of the nucleated cells are eosinophils. Protozoal, parasitic or fungal infections need to be ruled out. Golden Retrievers may be predisposed to this condition. There is usually a good response to glucocorticoid treatment.

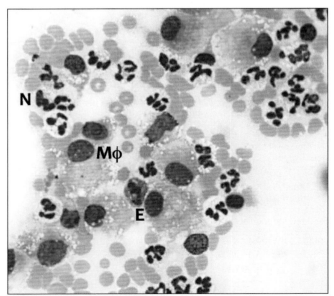

25.9 CSF from a dog with granulomatous meningoencephalitis. There is a mixed cell pleocytosis with moderate neutrophils (N) and macropahges (Mφ). A single eosinophil (E) is seen. (Wright–Giemsa stain; original magnification X1000)

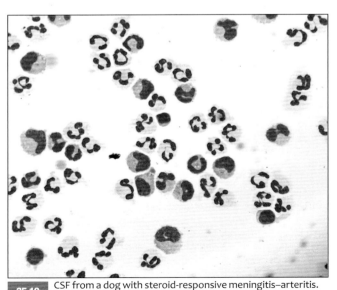

25.10 CSF from a dog with steroid-responsive meningitis–arteritis. There are numerous non-degenerate neutrophils as well as a moderate number of monocytes and a few small lymphocytes. Compare with Figure 25.11 showing degenerate and distorted neutrophils. (Modified Wright's stain; original magnification X500)
(Courtesy of Francesco Cian)

Necrotizing encephalitis in small-breed dogs

Necrotizing encephalitis in small-breed dogs has been primarily reported in young (<4 years old) Pugs and Maltese and Yorkshire Terriers. This condition has been hypothesized to be an immune-mediated disease with autoantibodies directed against astrocytes. Multifocal to massive necrosis and non-suppurative inflammation of the cerebrum and meninges occurs and may be fatal. Seizures, depression and ataxia are common presenting signs. Usually there is a moderate pleocytosis, sometimes with >200 cells/μl, with lymphocytes predominating (usually >70%). Microprotein is often >0.5 g/l.

Bacterial meningoencephalomyelitis

This appears to be uncommon in dogs and cats. It is also characterized by marked pleocytosis (usually >200 cells/μl, often >500 cells/μl) and is frequently accompanied by elevated microprotein. Neutrophils predominate (>70% of total nucleated cells) and may be degenerate. When intracellular bacteria are seen, this provides strong support for the presence of sepsis (Figure 25.11). Bacteria are not seen in all cases and correlation with the results of bacterial culture is important.

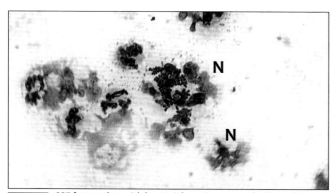

25.11 CSF from a dog with bacterial meningoencephalitis and sepsis. There are degenerate, smudged and distorted neutrophils (N) with blue-staining intracellular bacterial cocci. Compare with Figure 25.10. (Wright–Giemsa stain; original magnification X1000)

Neoplasia

Primary or metastatic neoplasia may result in clinical neurological signs. These are often localized or focal signs, but may be more generalized. Findings on CSF evaluation are variable, and neoplastic cells in CSF, although rarely present, may enable a positive diagnosis. Lymphoma is the most commonly identified neoplasm in CSF (Figure 25.12). Well differentiated or small cell lymphoma may be difficult to differentiate from lymphocytic pleocytosis. A positive PCR for antigen receptor rearrangements (PARR) provides support for differentiation of lymphoid malignancy from reactive lymphoid proliferation, although a negative PARR does not completely rule out underlying malignancy. Cells from plasma cell tumours and histiocytic sarcoma have been identified in CSF. Metastatic carcinoma may exfoliate clusters of cohesive cells with a classical epithelial appearance, but individual cells may be present, mimicking 'round cell' tumours. In such cases, immunocytochemistry is helpful in identifying the cells (Behling-Kelly et al., 2010). Other tumour types, including primary brain tumours, rarely exfoliate into CSF and may require aspiration, crush preparations or imprint from a biopsy specimen for cytological evaluation.

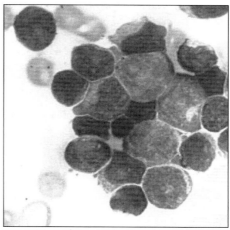

25.12 CSF from a dog with multicentric lymphoma and neurological signs. There are numerous large lymphoid cells with prominent nucleoli. (Wright–Giemsa stain; original magnification X1000)

Case examples

CASE 1

SIGNALMENT

10-month-old entire male Boxer.

HISTORY

Acute development of pyrexia and reluctance to move for 2 days. Low head carriage with kyphosis and cervical pain on palpation. No abnormalities of the vertebrae were detected on radiography of the head and spine.

CEREBROSPINAL FLUID ANALYSIS

Cerebrospinal fluid description: 1.0 ml of slightly opalescent, colourless fluid.

Parameter	Result	Reference interval
Erythrocyte count (cells/μl)	20	<2
Nucleated cell count (cells/μl)	75	<7
Microprotein (g/l)	0.50	<0.35

Abnormal results are in **bold**.

Microbiological culture of CSF: Negative.

→ CASE 1 CONTINUED

WHAT IS YOUR ASSESSMENT OF THESE CSF FINDINGS AND WHAT ARE THE DIFFERENTIAL DIAGNOSES?

There is a slight increase in the erythrocyte count that may be due to haemorrhage and/or contamination with blood during collection, with moderate to marked neutrophilic pleocytosis and a slight elevation in CSF protein. No infectious agents are recognized in the cytological preparations (Figure 25.13) or on microbiological culture. Differential diagnoses for this CSF appearance include discospondylitis, trauma (fracture), atlanto-occipital instability and steroid-responsive meningitis–arteritis. Given the absence of abnormalities on radiographic studies, steroid-responsive meningitis–arteritis is the primary consideration. Trial immunosuppressive steroid therapy should be considered, with continued monitoring.

FOLLOW-UP INFORMATION

The patient responded within 48 hours to immunosuppressive corticosteroid treatment, with resolution of pyrexia and cervical pain and improvement in locomotion. There was normalization of gait and return to normal activities within 10 days. A protocol of gradual reduction in steroid dose over a 6-month period was followed and no relapsing disease was noted over the next year, during which follow-up information was obtained.

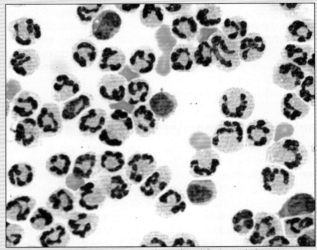

25.13 Cytospin preparation of CSF. (Modified Wright's stain; original magnification X1000)

CASE 2

SIGNALMENT

10-year-old entire female Border Collie.

HISTORY

Mammary gland carcinoma removed 6 months previously. Presented with repeated seizures and decreased awareness of surroundings. A mass was identified in the frontal lobe by magnetic resonance imaging (MRI). Cerebrospinal fluid was collected from the cerebellomedullary cistern.

CEREBROSPINAL FLUID ANALYSIS

Cerebrospinal fluid description: 0.5 ml, colourless, slightly cloudy.

Parameter	Result	Reference interval
Erythrocyte count (cells/µl)	**10**	<2
Nucleated cell count (cells/µl)	**100**	<7
Microprotein (g/l)	**0.60**	<0.35

Abnormal results are in **bold**.

Microbiological culture of CSF: Negative.

WHAT IS YOUR ASSESSMENT OF THESE CSF FINDINGS?

There is slight haemorrhage and/or contamination with blood, with a moderate increase in total protein. There is marked pleocytosis with a population of poorly differentiated cells with features of malignancy. These have oval to round nuclei with one or more round to angular nucleoli. The cytoplasm is scant to moderate and varies from pale to medium blue. The cytoplasm is usually ovoid, but sometimes elongated. A few small lymphocytes are present (Figure 25.14).

Given the history of previous removal of a mammary carcinoma and the finding of a discrete mass within the brain on MRI, metastatic mammary carcinoma is the primary concern. Other cell types of origin cannot be completely ruled out on the basis of the poorly differentiated features in the cytological preparation. Immunocytochemistry could be performed to classify these cells further.

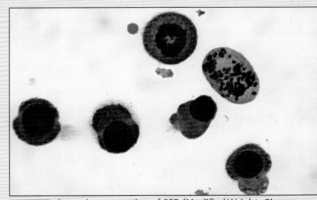

25.14 Cytospin preparation of CSF. (Modified Wright–Giemsa stain; original magnification X1000)
(Courtesy of Francesco Cian)

FOLLOW-UP INFORMATION

The dog was euthanased because of the poor prognosis associated with this malignancy. At post-mortem examination, there were multiple masses within the lungs and liver. These masses and the mass within the frontal lobe had features of poorly differentiated carcinoma consistent with metastatic mammary carcinoma.

References and further reading

Bailey CS and Higgins RJ (1986) Characteristics of cerebrospinal fluid associated with canine granulomatous meningoencephalomyelitis: a retrospective study. *Journal of the American Veterinary Medical Association* **188**, 418–421

Baroni M and Heinold Y (1995) A review of the clinical diagnosis of feline infectious peritonitis viral meningoencephalomyelitis. *Progress in Veterinary Neurology* **6**, 88–94

Becker M, Bauer N and Moritz A (2008) Automated flow cytometric cell count and differentiation of canine cerebrospinal fluid cells using the ADVIA 2120. *Veterinary Clinical Pathology* **37(3)**, 344–352

Behling-Kelly E, Petersen S, Muthuswamy A, Webb JL and Young KM (2010) Neoplastic pleocytosis in a dog with metastatic mammary carcinoma and meningeal carcinomatosis. *Veterinary Clinical Pathology* **39(2)**, 247–252

Bexfield N and Lee K (2014) *BSAVA Guide to Procedures in Small Animal Practice, 2nd edn.* BSAVA Publications, Gloucester

Bienzle D, McDonnell JJ and Stanton JB (2000) Analysis of cerebrospinal fluid from dogs and cats after 24 and 48 hours of storage. *Journal of the American Veterinary Medical Association* **216(11)**, 1761–1764

Chrisman CL (1992) Cerebrospinal fluid analysis. *Veterinary Clinics of North America: Small Animal Practice* **22**, 781–810

Cook JR and Denicola DB (1988) Cerebrospinal fluid. *Veterinary Clinics of North America: Small Animal Practice* **18**, 475–499

Dewey CW (2008) Encephalopathies: disorders of the brain. In: *A Practical Guide to Canine and Feline Neurology, 2nd edn*, ed. C Dewey, pp. 180–185. Blackwell Publishing (John Wiley & Sons), London.

Dewey CW and Ducote JM (2008) Neurodiagnostics In: *A Practical Guide to Canine and Feline Neurology, 2nd edn*, ed. C Dewey, pp. 80–81. Blackwell Publishing (John Wiley & Sons), London

Doyle C and Solano-Gallego L (2009) Cytologic interpretation of canine cerebrospinal fluid samples with low total nucleated cell concentration, with and without blood contamination. *Veterinary Clinical Pathology* **38(3)**, 392–396

Freeman KP and Raskin RE (2001) Cytology of the central nervous system. In: *Atlas of Canine and Feline Cytology,* ed. RE Raskin and DJ Meyer, pp. 325–365. WB Saunders, London

Fry MM, Vernau W, Kass PH and Vernau KM (2006). Effects of time, initial composition, and stabilizing agents on the results of canine cerebrospinal fluid analysis. *Veterinary Clinical Pathology* **35(1)**, 72–77

Galgut BI, Janardhan KS, Grondin TM, Harkin KR and Wight-Carter MT (2010) Detection of *Neospora caninum* tachyzoites in cerebrospinal fluid of a dog following prednisone and cyclosporine therapy. *Veterinary Clinical Pathology* **39(3)**, 386–390

Ishigaki K, Noya M, Kagawa Y, Ike K, Orima H and Imai S (2012) Detection of *Nesopora caninum*-specific DNA from cerebrospinal fluid by polymerase chain reaction in a dog with confirmed neosporosis. *Journal of Veterinary Medical Science* **74(8)**, 1051–1055

Ives EJ, Vanhaesebrouck AE and Cian F (2013). Immunocytochemical demonstration of feline infectious peritonitis virus within cerebrospinal fluid macrophages. *Journal of Feline Medicine and Surgery* **15(12)**, 1149–1153

Jäderlund KH, Bergström K, Egenvall A and Hedhammar A (2009) Cerebrospinal fluid PCR and antibody concentrations against *Anaplasma phagocytophilum* and *Borrelia burgdorferi* sensu lato in dogs with neurological signs. *Journal of Veterinary Internal Medicine* **23(3)**, 669–672

Jamison EM and Lumsden JH (1988) Cerebrospinal fluid analysis in the dog: methodology and interpretation. *Seminars in Veterinary Medicine and Surgery (Small Animal)* **3**, 122–132

Lowrie M (2012) Steroid responsive meningitis–arteritis in dogs – a pain in the neck? *Irish Veterinary Journal* **63(11)**, 695–700

Lowrie M, Penderis J, Eckersall PD, McLaughlin M, Mellor D and Anderson TJ (2009a) The role of acute phase proteins in the diagnosis and management of steroid-responsive meningitis-arteritis in dogs. *The Veterinary Journal* **182(1)**, 125–130

Lowrie M, Penderis J, Eckersall PD, McLaughlin M, Mellor D and Anderson TJ (2009b) Steroid responsive meningitis-arteritis: a prospective study of potential disease markers, prednisolone treatment, and long-term outcome in 20 dogs (2006-2008). *Journal of Veterinary Internal Medicine* **23(4)**, 862–870

Lowrie M, Smith PM and Garosi L (2013) Meningoencephalitis of unknown origin: investigation of prognostic factors and outcome using a standard treatment protocol. *Veterinary Record* **172**, 527–533

Maiolini A, Carlson R, Schwartz M, Gandini G and Tipold A (2012) Determination of immunoglobulin A concentrations in the serum and cerebrospinal fluid of dogs: an estimation of its diagnostic value in canine steroid-responsive meningitis–arteritis. *Veterinary Journal* **191(2)**, 219–224

Martínez-Subiela S, Caldin M, Parra MD *et al.* (2011) Canine C-reactive protein measurements in cerebrospinal fluid by a time-resolved immunofluorimetric assay. *Journal of Veterinary Diagnostic Investigation* **23(1)**, 63–67

Meinkoth JH and Crystal MA (1999) Cerebrospinal fluid analysis. In: *Diagnostic Cytology and Hematology of the Dog and Cat*, ed. RL Cowell, RD Tyler and JH Meinkoth, pp. 125–141. Mosby, St Louis

Oji T, Kamishina H, Cheeseman JA and Clemmons RM (2007) Measurement of myelin basic protein in the cerebrospinal fluid of dogs with degenerative myelopathy. *Veterinary Clinical Pathology* **36(3)**, 281–284

Parent JM and Rand JS (1994) Cerebrospinal fluid collection and analysis. In: *Consultations in Feline Internal Medicine 2*, ed. JR August, pp. 385–392. WB Saunders, Philadelphia

Ruotsalo K, Poma R, da Costa RC and Bienzle D (2008) Evaluation of the ADVIA 120 for analysis of canine cerebrospinal fluid. *Veterinary Clinical Pathology* **37(2)**, 242–248

Shibuya M, Matsuki N, Fujiwara K *et al.* (2007). Autoantibodies against glial fibrillary acidic protein (GFAP) in cerebrospinal fluids from Pug dogs with necrotizing meningoencephalitis. *Journal of Veterinary Medical Science* **69(3)**, 241–245

Snyder LA, Tarigo JL and Neel JA (2007). Cerebrospinal fluid from a dog with hind limb ataxia. *Veterinary Clinical Pathology* **36(4)**, 379–381

Srugo I, Aroch I, Christopher MM *et al.* (2011) Association of cerebrospinal fluid analysis findings with clinical signs and outcome in acute nonambulatory thoracolumbar disc disease in dogs. *Journal of Veterinary Internal Medicine* **25(4)**, 846–855

Tipold A, Vandevelde M and Zurbriggen A (1995) Neuroimmunological studies in steroid-responsive meningitis-arteritis in dogs. *Research in Veterinary Science* **58**, 103–108

Turek MM, Saba C, Paolini M and Argyle DJ (2008) Canine lymphoma and leukaemia. In: *Decision Making in Small Animal Oncology*, ed. DJ Argyle, MJ Brearerly and MM Turek, pp. 171–197. Wiley-Blackwell, Ames

Tyler JW and Cullor JS (1989) Titers, tests and truisms: rational interpretation of diagnostic serologic testing. *Journal of the American Veterinary Medical Association* **194**, 1550–1558

Vernau W, Vernau KM and Bailey CS (2008) Cerebrospinal fluid. In: *Clinical Biochemistry of Domestic Animals, 6th edn*, ed. JJ Kaneko, JW Harvey and ML Bruss, pp. 769–820. Academic Press, Elsevier, London

Wamsley H and Alleman AR (2004) Clinical pathology. In: *BSAVA Manual of Canine and Feline Neurology, 3rd edn*, ed. S Platt and NJ Olby, pp. 35–53. BSAVA Publications, Gloucester

Wessmann A, Volk HA, Chandler K, Brodbelt D and Szladovits B (2010) Significance of surface epithelial cells in canine cerebrospinal fluid and relationship to central nervous system disease. *Veterinary Clinical Pathology* **39(3)**, 358–364

Windsor RC, Sturges BK, Vernau KM and Vernau W (2009) Cerebrospinal fluid eosinophilia in dogs. *Journal of Veterinary Internal Medicine* **23(2)**, 275–281

Witsberger TH, Levine JM, Fosgate GT *et al.* (2012) Associations between cerebrospinal fluid biomarkers and long-term neurologic outcome in dogs with acute intervertebral disk herniation. *Journal of the American Veterinary Medical Association* **240(5)**, 555–562

Zabolotzky SM, Vernau KM, Kass PH and Vernau W (2010) Prevalence and significance of extracellular myelin-like material in canine cerebrospinal fluid. *Veterinary Clinical Pathology* **39(1)**, 90–95

Chapter 26

Laboratory evaluation of skin and ear disease

Tim Nuttall

Very few skin disorders have an unequivocally pathognomonic appearance and almost all require some form of laboratory investigation to confirm the diagnosis. Fortunately, the skin is readily accessible. Most tests are straightforward and can be assessed in a practice laboratory. However, any samples sent to external laboratories should be properly packaged with full clinical information, clearly labelling any samples that are potentially zoonotic. It is now easy to send digital images of skin lesions by email, and this can be of particular help to pathologists looking at skin biopsy samples.

Good light is essential for proper examination of the skin, lesions and collected material. Good fluorescent room lighting is a minimal requirement and a high-intensity spotlight is necessary for any serious examination. A hand lens is very useful for examining skin lesions and coat brushings for large parasites such as fleas, lice, *Cheyletiella*, *Otodectes* and *Neotrombicula* spp. Large illuminated lenses (e.g. those used for map reading) are best (Figure 26.1).

- Good light
- Flea comb
- Hand lens
- Otoscope
- Wood's lamp
- Curved scissors and electric clippers
- Fine-tipped curved forceps
- Liquid paraffin and potassium hydroxide
- No. 10 and No. 15 scalpel blades
- Spatula
- Cotton buds
- Bacteriology swabs
- Microscope slides
- Coverslips
- Modified Wright–Giemsa stain
- Lactophenol cotton blue
- Light microscope
- Toothbrushes
- Dermatophyte test medium
- A range of 4–8 mm biopsy punches (plus basic surgical kit and suture material)
- 10% neutral buffered formalin

26.1 Equipment required for examining and sampling the skin and ears.

Modified Wright–Giemsa stains

There are several modified Wright–Giemsa type stains available (Diff-Quik®, Rapi-Diff II®, etc.). They are the stains most commonly used in practice by virtue of their ease of use and interpretation. These all consist of three pots: fixer (pale blue to green), stain 1 (red eosinophilic) and stain 2 (purple basophilic). Samples should be air-dried before staining. Hair dryers on a cool setting are very useful for drying slides before and after staining without damaging the preparation. This works even for waxy or oily preparations, and there is no advantage to heat fixing (which can easily damage the preparation).

The standard 'two-stain' method:

1. Once air-dried, dip the slides in each pot 5–10 times for about 1 second each time (thicker and/or waxy preparations will need longer staining).
2. Adhesive tape preparations should be dipped in the two stains only, as the fixative destroys the adhesive layer and the sample.
3. Once stained, rinse the slide or tape under a tap or with distilled water (directing the flow against the back of the slide stops the preparation being washed down the sink).
4. Gently blot dry using textured paper towel without damaging the stained preparation.
5. Check the staining under low power, and if necessary repeat the staining steps.

The alternative 'one-stain' method:

1. Place a drop of the purple basophilic stain (pot 3) directly on the sample and place a coverslip over the stained sample.
2. For adhesive tape preparations, place one drop on a slide, fix the tape directly to the slide and then blot the excess stain away.

This technique gives a very intense stain that is particularly effective for microorganisms, but it is a very monochromatic stain compared with the 'two-stain' method (Figure 26.2).

Staining efficiency declines over time and the pots will accumulate skin debris, *Malassezia* and bacteria that can contaminate slides. The pots should be rinsed and replenished from the stock solutions every 1–2 weeks.

Light microscope

No piece of equipment is so vital or subject to so much abuse as a microscope. Robust and inexpensive models with binocular lenses and integral light sources are easily mastered and give good results. The use and abuse of microscopes is discussed in Appendix 1.

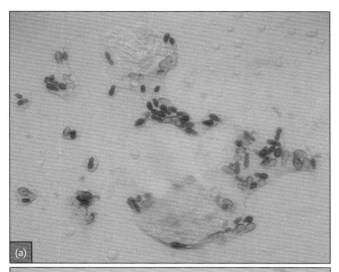

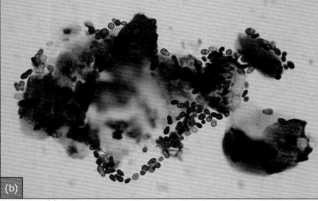

Finding	Description	Significance
Anagen hairs (Figure 26.4)	Fat, active, moist bulbs	Growing phase
Telogen hairs (Figure 26.5)	Tapered, slightly frayed bulbs	Resting phase. Excess is suggestive of an endocrine or metabolic disorder. The majority of hairs in most dog and cat breeds are normally in telogen. Poodles and similar breeds have more hairs in anagen
Shaft abnormalities	Twisted hairs, swellings, nodules, fractures, large melanin aggregates (macromelanosomes)	Hereditary shaft abnormalities, deficiency diseases, trauma, colour dilution alopecia, follicular dysplasias
Tapered tips	Hair tips smoothly taper to a point	Normal hairs
Fractured tips	Blunt, frayed ends	Fractured hairs: self-trauma, dermatophytes
Follicular casts (Figure 26.6)	Collars of scale tightly adherent to the proximal hair shaft	Follicular hyperkeratosis, follicular dysplasias, sebaceous adenitis, keratinization disorders, demodicosis, dermatophytosis
Demodex	Adults, larvae, nymphs and eggs often associated with hair bulbs	Demodicosis; this is a particularly useful technique in pedal demodicosis, especially if there is heavy scarring. One or two *Demodex* mites may be normal; demodicosis is associated with large numbers of adult mites, immature forms and eggs (see later)
Dermatophytes (Figure 26.7)	Disrupted and fractured hair shafts, small, bubble-like ectothrix spores surrounding affected hair shafts	Dermatophytosis; confirm with culture

(a) Adhesive tape strip preparation from a dog with *Malassezia* dermatitis stained with the 'one-stain' method. (Rapi-Diff II® stain; original magnification X400). (b) Adhesive tape strip preparation from the same dog as (a) stained with the 'two-stain' method. (Rapi-Diff II® stain; original magnification X400)

26.3 Trichogram findings and their significance.

Investigation of skin disease

Coat brushings

Surface debris can be collected with a flea comb or stiff brush. The material can be brushed on to dark card or a petri dish for examination with a hand lens. Alternatively, adhesive tape can be used to mount it on a microscope slide for examination under low power. Flea dirt, which is largely partly digested blood, leaves a reddish-brown stain on moistened white paper or cotton wool.

Hair plucks and trichograms

1. Grasp the hairs with a pair of fine forceps (using rubber sleeves over the tips can reduce damage to the hair shaft).
2. Pull in the direction of hair growth with a firm even pressure.
3. Place the hairs in some liquid paraffin on a microscope slide and apply a coverslip. Aligning the hairs makes interpretation easier.
4. Scan under low power and use high power to examine areas of interest in more detail (Figure 26.3).

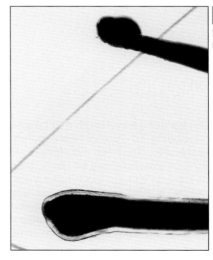

26.4 Anagen hairs from a German Shepherd Dog. (Original magnification X40)

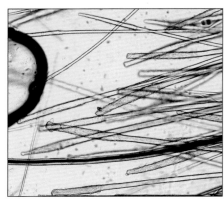

26.5 Telogen hairs from a crossbred dog with hyperadrenocorticism. (Original magnification X40)

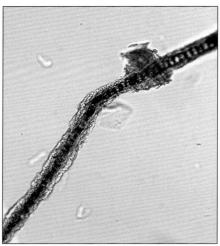

26.6 Follicular casts from a dog with sebaceous adenitis.
(Courtesy of Dr Bob Kennis)

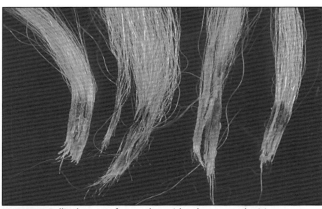

26.7 Ectothrix spores on a damaged hair from a cat with a *Microsporum canis* infection.

Fungal examination
Wood's lamp

These emit ultraviolet (UV) light of a wavelength that causes certain dermatophytes (including 50–70% of *Microsporum canis* strains) to fluoresce *in vivo*. They are therefore more useful for cats, where 95% of infections are *M. canis*, than for dogs. The best lamps have an integral magnifying glass. The examiner should allow a few minutes to become adapted to the dark, and then look for bright apple-green fluorescence of the hairs. Crusts and topical medications glow a dull yellow–green. Scale and fibres often shine blue–white.

Hair plucks

Ectothrix spores (see Figure 26.7) appear as tiny beads, particularly after clearing the hairs with potassium hydroxide (see Skin scrapes). Endothrix spores and hyphae may be visible inside cleared hairs.

Fungal culture

Dermatophytes grow on two media:

- Sabouraud's agar is the best medium, but culture can take 3–4 weeks. Samples are usually sent away, although plates can be incubated at room temperature in practice laboratories
- Dermatophyte test medium (DTM) (Dermafyt®, Fungassay®) is a quick and easy in-practice alternative but it is not as reliable as Sabouraud's agar and other techniques, and both false negative and false positive results are seen (see Chapter 27). Dermatophytes utilize protein in the agar, turning the indicator red as they grow (Figure 26.8). Saprophytes only use protein once the carbohydrate is exhausted and turn the agar red after profuse growth has already occurred. These plates should be incubated in the dark at room temperature and checked daily to detect when the colour change occurs relative to fungal growth. Dermatophytes are usually evident by 5–7 days, but growth can take up to 14 days. They form fluffy whitish colonies, but unfortunately DTM inhibits normal colony morphology, pigmentation and macroconidia production, which makes species identification more difficult than on Sabouraud's agar.

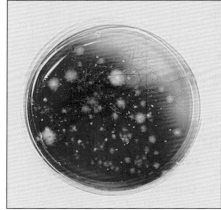

26.8 *Microsporum canis* on dermatophyte test medium. Note that the red colour change coincides with early fungal growth.

To obtain samples, the colony should be gently touched with adhesive tape and then attached to a microscope slide over a drop of lactophenol cotton blue. Identification is based on macroconidia morphology: *M. canis* forms thick walled slightly roughened macroconidia with more than six cells (Figure 26.9) whereas *Trichophyton* spp. tend to form smooth, cigar-shaped macroconidia with fewer cells.

Sample collection for fungal culture:

- **Hair plucks:** pick fluorescing hairs or hairs from the edge of lesions.
- **Mackenzie brush technique:** allows sampling of many more hairs. The coat should be vigorously combed with a new toothbrush or plastic grooming brush and sample directly inoculated on to DTM or sent away.

Samples should be sent for culture in sealed but not airtight containers (e.g. a universal container with the lid loosely closed), because bacteria will swamp fungi in moist, anaerobic environments.

Note that macroconidia (Figure 26.9) are frequently found on skin scrapes and cytology. These are from saprophytes; dermatophytes only produce macroconidia in culture.

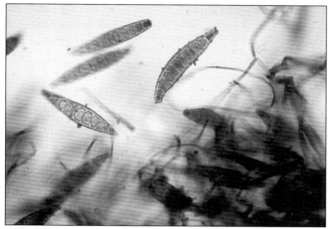

26.9 *Microsporum canis* macroconidia from *in vitro* culture; these are not produced *in vivo*. (New methylene blue stain; original magnification X400)
(Courtesy of Professor Susan Dawson)

Deep fungal infections

Careful examination of cytology smears from sinus tracts and ulcerated lesions can reveal fungal elements, but infection should be confirmed by fungal culture. This is best achieved by submitting a biopsy sample (see below) of the affected tissues to a recognized mycology laboratory (see Chapter 27). Swabbing the skin with alcohol prior to biopsy will reduce bacterial contamination.

Bacterial culture

Bacterial culture and sensitivity testing (see Chapter 27) is not necessary in every case. Staphylococci, which cause 95% of canine and feline pyodermas, have predictable antibiotic sensitivity so an empirical choice of antibiotic can be made (Figure 26.10). However, there are situations in which bacterial culture and antimicrobial sensitivity testing are appropriate.

Samples should be taken from intact or freshly ruptured lesions, avoiding chronic and excoriated lesions wherever possible. Pustules can be ruptured using a sterile needle and the pus absorbed on to a sterile swab. Material can also be expressed from furuncles and sinus tracts. Biopsies are more likely to recover representative organisms from deep pyodermas, especially heavily scarred lesions. Taking swabs from both the nares and the perineum when screening animals for staphylococcal carriage will reduce the chance of false negative findings. Swabs should be submitted in transport medium.

Ongoing antibiotic treatment may result in false negative cultures. If appropriate withdrawal times are not possible but cytology indicates the presence of bacteria, prolonged and/or enriched cultures may be necessary to decrease the chance of false negative cultures. It is therefore important to note recent or ongoing antibiotic therapy on the microbiology laboratory submission form.

Criteria for empirical systemic antimicrobial therapy; ALL of these should apply
• Non-life-threatening infection • First episode of a skin infection within 3 months • Clinical lesions consistent with a surface or superficial pyoderma • Cytology consistent with a staphylococcal infection • No reason to suspect antibiotic resistance
Bacterial culture and antimicrobial sensitivity testing is appropriate if any ONE of the following apply

• Life-threatening infections, as the first-choice antibiotic must be effective
• Clinical lesions consistent with a deep pyoderma
• The clinical signs and cytology are not consistent with each other
• Rod-shaped bacteria seen on cytology, as their antibiotic sensitivity is not predictable and may be limited
• Empirical antibiotic therapy does not resolve the infection as expected
• Where antibiotic resistance is more likely:
  • After one or more broad-spectrum antibiotic courses
  • Non-healing wounds
  • Postoperative and other nosocomial infections
  • The owner or animal has recent healthcare contacts

26.10 Criteria for empirical systemic antimicrobial therapy, and indications for when to undertake bacterial culture and antimicrobial sensitivity testing.

Swabbing the skin with alcohol will reduce the risk of contamination from surface organisms. This can, however, result in false negative cultures from superficial lesions if the alcohol penetrates the pustule or contacts the swab. Sufficient time should be allowed for the alcohol to evaporate prior to sampling.

It is helpful to perform cytology as well as taking material for culture, because cultured organisms may or may not be involved in the infection, particularly if they are normal commensal organisms. Cytology is useful to indicate the number of organisms involved, whether they have been phagocytosed by white blood cells, and their relationship to cutaneous cells and structures. The relative abundance of different organisms revealed by cytology can be useful to decide which organisms are likely to be significant when culture detects multiple species with differing antimicrobial sensitivity patterns.

Sensitivity testing techniques and interpretation

Kirby–Bauer disc diffusion tests use antibiotic-impregnated paper discs. The diameter of the clear halo around each disc, where bacterial growth is inhibited, is compared with agreed standards to determine whether the bacteria are susceptible or resistant to a particular antibiotic. In contrast, the minimum inhibitory concentration (MIC) is the lowest concentration of an antibiotic that completely inhibits growth of a microorganism. MICs are usually tested and reported in µg/ml ranges as the tests assume that the antimicrobial will be administered systemically. The isolate will be reported as susceptible, intermediate or resistant to the antimicrobials on the basis of accepted breakpoints. If the isolate is reported as susceptible then it is likely that if the antibiotic is administered systemically it will exceed the MIC in the target tissue. A low MIC by itself does not correlate with increased efficacy, as the susceptibility range for each organism–drug combination varies. Nevertheless, the more dilutions of a drug that still inhibit bacterial growth (i.e. the lower the MIC compared with the breakpoint), the more sensitive that bacterial isolate is to the drug.

Care should be taken with antibiotics where the susceptibilities are close to the breakpoint, as they may not achieve therapeutic concentrations in the target tissues.

Isolates with intermediate susceptibilities should be regarded as resistant, because it is unlikely that the MIC will be exceeded at the target tissue. However, using topical therapy, which delivers mg/ml antibiotic concentrations, can overcome apparent *in vitro* resistance.

In-house *in vitro* culture and antimicrobial sensitivity tests are not advised. Few practice laboratories can identify the bacteria or perform antimicrobial susceptibility tests to accepted standards (Clinical and Laboratory Standards Institute (CLSI) or European Committee on Antimicrobial Susceptibility Testing (EUCAST)).

Well-based tests (e.g. Speed® Biogram; Virbac Animal Health) can identify up to six bacteria and two yeast organisms to genus level, and give some indication of susceptibility or resistance to 13 antibiotics. However, these do not adhere to CLSI or EUCAST guidelines and interpreting antibiotic sensitivity tests can be difficult for inexperienced clinicians. Culture and antimicrobial sensitivity testing at a fully equipped laboratory working to CLSI or EUCAST standards, including regular validation and quality control, is therefore preferred. Discussing the results with experienced microbiologists can be particularly helpful when considering treatment of mixed and/or antimicrobial-resistant infections.

Other tests

Further testing may be necessary to confirm the identity, characteristics and antimicrobial susceptibility of bacterial isolates where simple culture and biochemical methods may be inadequate or misleading (see Chapter 27). These may include penicillin-binding protein A2 (PBPA2) latex bead agglutination tests, *mecA* polymerase chain reaction (PCR) and staphylococcal chromosomal cassette (SCCmec) typing for meticillin-resistant staphylococci (MRS) and PCR for extended-spectrum beta-lactamase (ESBL) *Escherichia coli* or mycobacteria. The results of these tests must be taken into account when considering therapy; for example, MRS and ESBL *E. coli* will be resistant to penicillins and cephalosporins even when *in vitro* tests suggest that they will be sensitive. Meticillin-resistant *Staphylococcus aureus* (MRSA), furthermore, may exhibit inducible clindamycin resistance *in vivo* despite apparent *in vitro* sensitivity. This is associated with the presence of *erm* genes, which can be tested for using D-zone tests (where the zone of inhibition around a clindamycin/erythromycin disc is smaller than that around a clindamycin disc) or PCR.

Why doesn't the clinical response match the *in vitro* test?

It is important to realise that *in vitro* susceptibility tests do not necessarily predict the clinical outcome. In human medicine there is a '90–60' rule: 90% of infections with susceptible bacteria respond to therapy, but infections with resistant isolates will respond to an 'inappropriate' antibiotic about 60% of the time. This can be explained by flaws and limitations in susceptibility tests, variations in pharmacodynamics and tissue distribution, dosing or other compliance errors, underlying diseases and/or immune status. In addition to the MIC, understanding the nature of the infection, the pharmacokinetic properties of the antibiotic and patient factors will help achieve a successful outcome.

Skin scrapes

Skin scrapes are usually performed to find ectoparasites (Figure 26.11). Samples should be taken from primary lesions at the predilection sites and excoriated skin avoided. Different parasites live at different levels within the skin and it is important to collect material from each layer.

1. Clip any hair with scissors but do not disrupt the skin surface.
2. Apply liquid paraffin to the skin and scrape with a No. 10 blade (No. 15 blades are useful for difficult sites such as the feet and ears).
3. Scrape until capillary oozing appears but do not collect too much blood; it obscures the view, making parasites very difficult to see. Too much hair and debris also makes it difficult to find anything, so divide the collected material if necessary.
4. Evenly mix the material into more liquid paraffin and apply a coverslip.
5. All ectoparasites are visible with the X4 lens, which makes for quick scanning. Look for movement and check any suspicious objects with the X10 lens if unsure.

Potassium hydroxide *versus* liquid paraffin

Potassium hydroxide (KOH) is an alternative to liquid paraffin. It clears keratinaceous debris, making parasites easier to see, but it is caustic to the animal, the user and the microscope, and should be used with care. Nothing stronger than a 5% solution should be used on the skin but a drop of 10% or 20% KOH can be placed on the slide and gently warmed for 30–60 seconds to enhance clearing. This is lethal to mites, however, and the lack of movement can be a drawback. Mites will be alive and moving in a 5% solution but this takes up to 30 minutes to clear debris. KOH should never be used near mucous membranes or delicate structures and the skin should be rinsed with water immediately after use.

Demodex

Finding *Demodex* is usually straightforward provided that clinicians scrape down to the dermis (i.e. capillary bleeding occurs). Squeezing the skin prior to scraping can force the mites out of the follicles on to the surface, where they can be collected by skin scrapes or adhesive tape. Chronically inflamed, thickened skin can be difficult to scrape, and hair plucks, material expressed from furuncles or even punch biopsies are more rewarding.

In clinical demodicosis there are usually large numbers of mites representing all stages of the life cycle. Because they are commensals, however, one or two adults occasionally turn up as incidental findings. Clinical judgement is important, but if necessary clinicians should treat for demodicosis, repeat the skin scrapes and carefully evaluate any clinical improvement.

Repeated scrapes will help assess the response to therapy. There should be an increasing ratio of dead and adult mites to live and immature mites. If not, the treatment regime should be re-evaluated and steps taken to diagnose any underlying conditions.

Sarcoptes

Sarcoptes are not commensals, therefore any mites, eggs or faecal pellets are significant. Finding them can be very difficult, however. Multiple scrapes should be taken from unexcoriated primary lesions (crusted papules) at the predilection sites (pinnal margins, elbows, hocks and ventral chest).

An enzyme-linked immunosorbent assay (ELISA) for serum-specific *Sarcoptes* immunoglobulin (Ig)G is a good

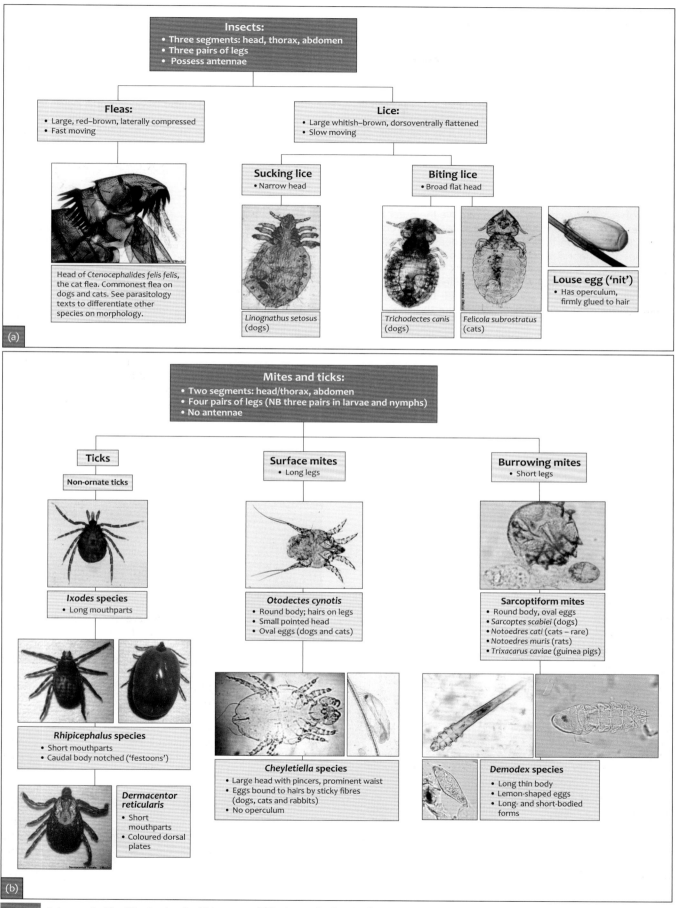

26.11 Ectoparasite identification key for (a) insects and (b) mites and ticks. This figure was produced with the assistance of Merial Animal Health.

alternative. The assay is very accurate, with sensitivity and specificity >90%. The negative predictive value is usually very high, although false negatives can occur early in the course of the disease. However, the positive predictive value can be low if *Sarcoptes* is uncommon in the tested population because false positives can occur (particularly in atopic dogs sensitized to *Dermatophagoides* house dust mites). The pinnal scratch reflex (eliciting hindlimb movements by rubbing the pinna against itself) has been shown to have good sensitivity and specificity. If all else fails, trial therapy with selamectin, imidacloprid/moxidectin or amitraz should be prescribed.

Tape strips

Clear adhesive tape can be used to remove the outer layers of the stratum corneum and ectoparasites or microorganisms. Clear adhesive tape should be repeatedly applied to the skin until debris is clearly stuck to it. If looking for ectoparasites, the tape should be stuck to a microscope slide and examined with the X4 lens. Flea faeces (Figure 26.12), lice, *Cheyletiella*, *Otodectes* and their eggs are easily seen. *Demodex* can also be found if the lesions are first squeezed. Adhesive tape samples (3M Scotch Tape is best, in the author's experience) can also be stained with modified Wright–Giemsa stains as described above (Figure 26.13). This is an excellent way to detect *Malassezia*, bacteria, inflammatory cells and exfoliated cells from eroded lesions such as squamous cell carcinoma.

Cytology

Impression smears

Direct or indirect impression smears are especially useful for moist or seborrhoeic lesions that will not stick to adhesive tape, but the surface should be gently debrided

to reveal representative cells first. For direct smears, a microscope slide can be firmly pressed on to the lesion (ulcers, erosions, crusts, pustules, plaques, papules, nodules, sinus tracts). Direct impression smears can also be made from the cut surfaces of excised lesions for quick identification of suspected tumours or inflammatory lesions (see Chapter 21).

Indirect smears are made using material collected by a swab or curette (Figure 26.14). The surface should be gently debrided before gently rolling the swab or curette on to the slide to leave a thin layer, taking great care to avoid rupturing the cells. Indirect smears are useful for more moist material and inaccessible areas of the skin (ears, feet).

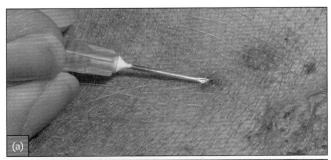

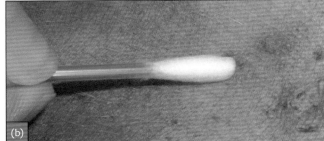

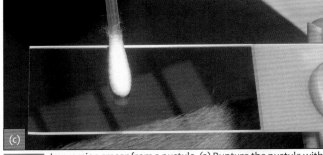

26.14 Impression smear from a pustule. (a) Rupture the pustule with a sterile needle. (b) Absorb the contents on to a swab. (c) Gently make a thin impression by rolling the swab on a microscope slide. Too much smearing will rupture the cells.

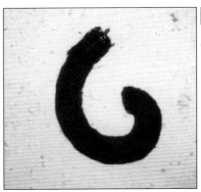

26.12 Flea faecal pellet. (Original magnification X100) (Courtesy of Peter Forsythe)

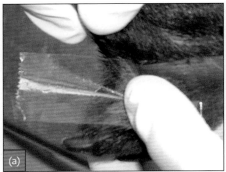

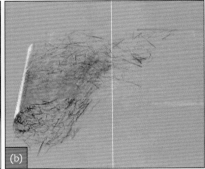

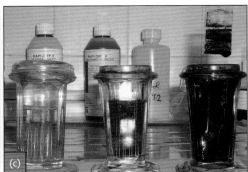

26.13 Tape strip cytology. (a) Tape-stripping from the skin. (b) Forming a loop on a microscope slide. (c) Staining in a Diff-Quik® stain.

Fine-needle aspirates

Fine-needle aspirates are a quick, cheap and minimally invasive way of investigating cutaneous masses and enlarged lymph nodes. See Chapter 21 for further details.

Interpretation of cutaneous cytology preparations

See Chapter 21 and Figure 26.15 for details.

Inflammatory lesions (Figure 26.16) are characterized by:

- Mixed populations of neutrophils, eosinophils, lymphoid cells, monocytes/macrophages, epithelial cells and fibroblasts
- 70% or more neutrophils is suggestive of acute inflammation; 50% or more monocytes suggests chronic inflammation
- Reactive fibroblasts and epithelial cells may appear neoplastic, and it is important to look at the whole picture
- It is important to look carefully for microorganisms. Free bacteria may be contaminants; phagocytosed bacteria are more significant. Mature degenerate neutrophils (karyorrhexis; large open fragmenting nuclei) suggest infection, whereas mature non-degenerate neutrophils (pyknosis; dark shrunken nuclei) suggest sterile inflammation (Figure 26.17). All apparently non-infectious lesions should still be cultured
- Pyogranulomatous inflammation can be associated with less common bacterial and fungal infections: bluish-staining hyphae suggest filamentous bacteria or a fungal mycetoma; thick-walled basophilic bodies suggest *Blastomyces* or *Cryptococcus* (with clear capsule); small, basophilic bodies with clear walls could be *Leishmania*, *Histoplasma* or *Sporothrix*. Mycobacteria rarely stain but can appear as clear

rod-shaped vacuoles in macrophages. Their presence should be confirmed with a Ziehl–Neelsen stain (see Chapter 27) and samples treated as potentially zoonotic
- Eosinophils suggest parasites, allergy, eosinophilic granuloma complex or foreign bodies (including free keratin and hair shafts in furunculosis), although a few can be found in almost any inflammatory dermatosis
- A few lymphocytes and plasma cells are often found in any inflammatory dermatosis but large numbers suggest neoplasia or lymphocytic/plasmacytic pododermatitis
- Acanthocytes are large round nucleated epidermal cells that are consistent with pemphigus foliaceus (Figure 26.18), although they can also (less commonly) occur in bacterial and fungal infections.

Skin biopsy

Skin biopsies are usually performed to obtain samples for histopathology or culture. Indications for biopsy include:

- Nodules and other possible neoplasms
- Ulcers
- Keratinization disorders
- Symmetrical alopecia with no obvious endocrine or metabolic cause
- Multifocal alopecia if cytology, skin scrapes and fungal culture are non-diagnostic
- Unexplained pigment changes
- Any suspected dermatosis that is most readily diagnosed by biopsy (e.g. sebaceous adenitis, follicular dysplasia or immune-mediated diseases)
- Unusual lesions or dermatoses
- Where a precise diagnosis is required for an accurate prognosis, suspected zoonosis or where treatment is expensive, long term or potentially hazardous.

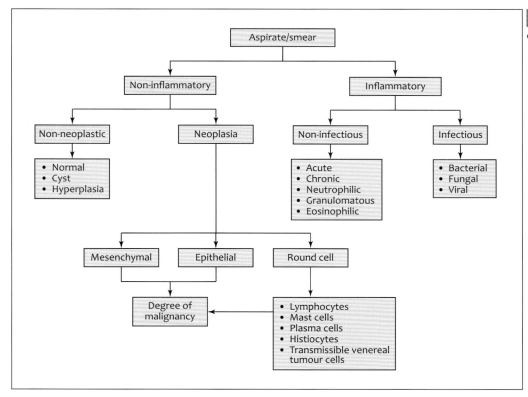

26.15 Algorithm for interpreting cutaneous cytology preparations.

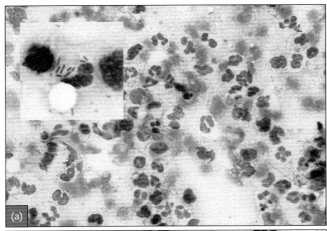

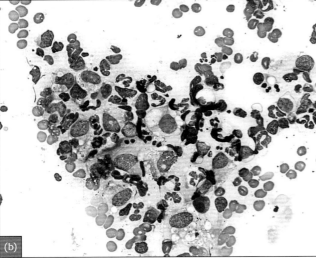

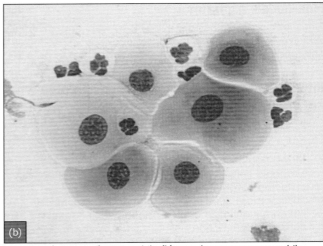

26.17 (continued) Neutrophils. (b) Non-degenerate neutrophils admixed with squamous epithelial cells; note the shrunken, hypersegmented intact nuclei. (Diff-Quik® stain; original magnification X1000)

(b, © Tim Nuttall)

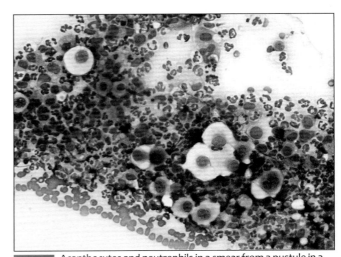

26.18 Acanthocytes and neutrophils in a smear from a pustule in a dog with pemphigus foliaceus. (Diff-Quik® stain; original magnification X400)

26.16 Inflammation. (a) Acute inflammation in a sample from a dog with otitis externa; note the preponderance of degenerate neutrophils. The insert shows a close-up of degenerate neutrophils containing phagocytosed rod-shaped bacteria. (Diff-Quik® stain; original magnification X400; inset X1000). (b) Chronic inflammation in a dog with deep pyoderma; there is a mixture of neutrophils and macrophages. (Diff-Quik® stain; original magnification X400)

Glucocorticoid and other immunosuppressive therapy should be withdrawn and any secondary infection controlled prior to biopsy to avoid masking the pathological changes. In most inflammatory dermatoses early lesions, such as pustules, vesicles, the leading edge of ulcers, etc., should be biopsied, avoiding chronic changes, infection, necrosis and excoriation. In contrast, endocrine or atrophic changes are most obvious in fully developed lesions. Selecting the right lesion takes some experience and, if unsure, a range of lesions including apparently healthy skin should be biopsied. There are a number of techniques that are used for different lesions and areas of the skin.

Punch biopsy

Punch biopsies are the quickest and easiest to perform. They are well suited to diffuse dermatoses but less so to ulcers and nodules as it is difficult to straddle the margin or encompass the lesion. Lesions such as pustules or papules should be centred, because during processing the biopsy specimen is sectioned through the centre. Punch biopsies only include the epidermis and dermis, not the subcutis.

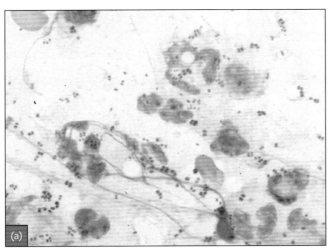

26.17 Neutrophils. (a) Degenerate cells in a staphylococcal pyoderma; note the swollen, fragmented nuclei (karyorrhexis), nuclear rupture and streaming, and swollen cytoplasm. There are numerous bacteria seen associated with neutrophils and extracellularly. (Diff-Quik® stain; original magnification X1000) (continues) ▶

Biopsy punches range from 4 to 8 mm in diameter; 6 mm is most commonly used but 4 mm may be better in restricted sites such as the face and feet. However, 4 mm punches only yield a small amount of skin and are more prone to shearing damage. Most animals can be biopsied under light sedation and local anaesthesia as follows:

1. Clip any hair with scissors but do not disturb the skin surface. Some dermatologists advocate lightly swabbing the site with alcohol. Others prefer not to disturb the skin at all, although an alcohol swab should be used before performing a biopsy for culture.
2. Draw a circle around the biopsy site in indelible pen and then bisect the circle with a line in the direction of hair growth (Figure 26.19a). Indicating the direction of hair growth helps the pathologist to orientate the biopsy specimen to section it in line with and not across the hair follicles.
3. Infiltrate the subcutis with 1 ml of 2% lidocaine (without adrenaline (epinephrine) to avoid inducing changes in the cutaneous bloodflow). Inserting the needle outside the circle (Figure 26.19b) will ensure that the specimen will not have a needle tract through it.
4. Press the biopsy punch firmly against the skin over the bisecting line and rotate in one direction (Figure 26.19c). Rotating the punch from side to side can cause separation of the epidermis and dermis.
5. Use a cocktail stick, bent needle or fine forceps to lift the base clear and cut it free (Figure 26.19d). Grasping the biopsy specimen itself will cause crush artefacts. If the specimen is firmly attached to the underlying tissues (e.g. on the ear pinna) grasp one end and carefully dissect it free.
6. Place the biopsy sample in 10% formalin as quickly as possible and close the skin with tissue adhesive or a single suture (Figure 26.19e). Where there is a risk of deforming the tissues (e.g. ear pinna) control any haemorrhage and allow the site to heal by secondary intention.
7. Biopsy specimens for culture should be submitted fresh or with a single drop of saline to prevent drying in transit; check the laboratory's preference.
8. Submit each specimen in a separate, clearly labelled pot to avoid any confusion.

Full clinical details, differential diagnoses and the biopsy sites should all be included on the submission form.

Sending digital images of the lesions can also be helpful. Most pathologists will read the biopsy specimen first, then the clinical history, and re-evaluate their findings if the two are incompatible.

Complications are rare, although care should be exercised in animals with bleeding disorders, poor wound healing or immunosuppression. Use lignocaine with caution in very small or young animals and those with cardiac disease or seizures, or patients receiving monoamine oxidase inhibitors (e.g. amitraz).

Wedge (incisional or excisional) biopsy

Scalpel blades can be used to take wedge-shaped biopsy specimens of varying size. In many situations, especially soft tissue sarcomas, attempting excisional biopsy (in which the whole lesion is excised) can make future therapy more difficult, and have a detrimental effect on prognosis. If the subsequent histology report indicates that the tumour is incompletely excised it can be very difficult to excise a surgical scar fully and achieve clean margins. Incisional biopsies (in which a small part of the mass is excised) are therefore recommended for suspected sarcomas. This leaves the tumour *in situ*, allowing for planning of future definitive surgical margins based on the original area of growth.

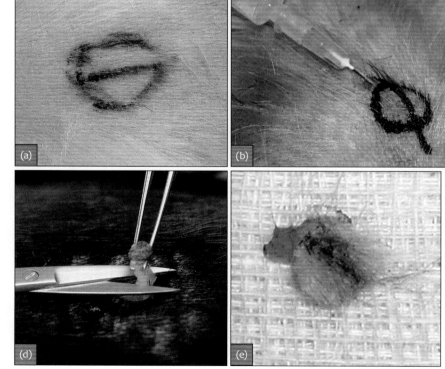

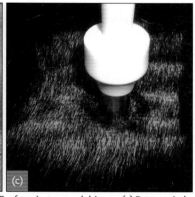

26.19 Performing a punch biopsy. (a) Draw a circle around the biopsy site and then bisect the circle with a line in the direction of hair growth. (b) Infiltrate the skin with local anaesthetic, introducing the needle outside the circle to avoid trauma to the biopsy site. (c) Press a 6 mm biopsy punch against the skin and rotate in one direction. (d) Dissect free from the underlying tissues, taking care not to damage the biopsy specimen. (e) Blot any excess blood away using a swab and fix in a 10X volume of 10% neutral buffered formalin. Note the line indicating the direction of hair growth.

Wedge biopsies are useful for deeper lesions (e.g. subcutaneous fat, pads), where closure of a circular punch could deform the tissues (e.g. nasal planum) and focal lesions such as ulcers where the active margin is of interest. The principles are otherwise similar to performing a punch biopsy except that it is often difficult to block these sites and local anaesthetic injected into subcutaneous tissues will distort them. A ring block, regional nerve block or general anaesthesia is preferable.

Phalanx III amputation

Most non-traumatic claw diseases (e.g. lupoid onychitis, vasculitis, neoplasia) are caused by lesions in the germinal tissues (nailbed) deep to the claw fold. This is impossible to biopsy by conventional means. Phalanx III (PIII) amputation is an invasive but effective technique that heals with minimal effect on function and appearance. It is a surgical procedure involving entry into a joint, however, and requires full asepsis. Dew claws (digit I) are preferred if present but if not, digits II and V are the least weightbearing. However, the chosen digit should be one that is likely to yield a diagnosis; affected claws without sloughing or secondary infection are preferred.

Allergy tests

Allergy tests should only be used to identify allergens for avoidance or specific immunotherapy in animals that have a clinical diagnosis of atopic dermatitis or rhinitis based on the history, clinical signs and elimination of other differential diagnoses. They are not diagnostic for atopic disease because positive tests can occur in healthy animals, and clinically atopic animals (i.e. that have atopic-like dermatitis) can be persistently negative. The diagnosis of allergic skin disease and allergy testing is discussed in more detail in the *BSAVA Manual of Canine and Feline Dermatology* (Jackson and Marsella, 2012).

Allergy tests are based around the detection of IgE, which is crucial in allergen capture and presentation, as well as allergen-specific mast cell degranulation and inflammation. IgE bound to mast cells in the skin can be demonstrated using intradermal tests (IDTs), whereas serological tests detect circulating IgE. IDTs and serology both have a number of advantages and disadvantages. Most veterinary dermatologists prefer intradermal allergen tests (IDTs), which test the capacity of allergens to trigger a reaction in the skin. Serum IgE, in contrast, does not necessarily correlate with IgE levels in the skin. However, IDTs are time consuming, require sedation and clipping, and cannot be performed on lichenified, hyperpigmented or inflamed skin. The test allergens are also expensive to maintain.

Whichever test is used, the clinical significance of any reactions must be carefully assessed; for example, is the animal likely to be exposed to the allergen, and does exposure correlate with the seasonality of clinical signs? Not all potential allergens can be included in a test but a broad spread of important allergens should be selected. Locally relevant allergens can be selected by consulting botany books, pollen charts, the internet, and local dermatologists and allergists. Reviews of the geographical distribution of potential allergens are widely available and European pollen data are regularly updated at www.polleninfo.org. Key allergen groups include: house dust (e.g. *Dermatophagoides farinae* and *D. pteronyssinus*) and storage (e.g. *Tyrophagus putrescentiae*, *Acarus siro* and *Lepidoglyphus destructor*) mites; animal epidermals and fibres; tree, weed

and grass pollens; and moulds. There is conflicting evidence as to whether IDT or serology reactivity declines outside the allergen season. Until further data are available, therefore, it is sensible to test animals no more than 6–8 weeks after the end of their allergy season.

Allergy tests may not be reliable in young animals. Animals less than 1 year old may not have been exposed to the full range of allergens. Testing can either be delayed or they can be retested at a later date. Very young animals (<3 months of age) do not respond to intradermal allergens and histamine, and may not have adequate IgE titres.

Intradermal allergen tests

Allergens should be obtained from a reputable supplier that standardizes and validates its product. Allergens can be obtained in concentrated form that requires regular dilution to testing strength or ready diluted, although the latter have a shorter shelf-life. Experience with one source is important, as there are differences between allergen extracts. Sedation or anaesthesia will prevent struggling and reduce stress. Most dermatologists use medetomidine, dexmedetomidine, butorphanol or propofol, although these should be used with care in animals with concurrent disease, especially cardiovascular disease. Acepromazine, benzodiazepines and other opiates can interfere with the test. Once the patient is sedated:

1. Place the animal in lateral recumbency.
2. Gently clip a patch on the chest but do not prepare the skin in any way.
3. Inject 0.05 ml of the positive control (0.01% histamine), negative control (buffered saline) and each allergen solution into the dermis. Positive reactions, marked by erythema and swelling, are evident by 15–20 minutes (Figure 26.20). There are two ways to assess these:

- Assigning scores of 0 and 4 to the negative and positive control sites, respectively. The test sites are subjectively compared to the two controls; a 2+ reaction or greater is considered positive
- Measuring the diameters of the negative and positive control sites to calculate the mean. A positive reaction is one with a diameter greater than the mean of the negative and positive controls.

The clinical significance of late phase (4–6 hours) and delayed (24 hours) reactions is unclear. However, these can be assessed by the owner or using digital images, and

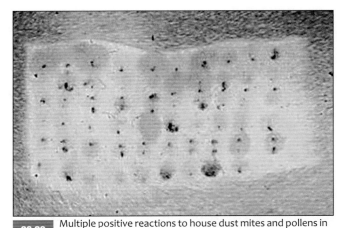

26.20 Multiple positive reactions to house dust mites and pollens in an atopic Shar Pei. Positive reactions are identified by erythema and swelling.

allergens can be included in allergen-specific immuno-therapy if exposure is thought to be clinically relevant. Pruritus at the test sites can be managed with topical emollients or glucocorticoids. Angioedema or anaphylaxis is very rare.

False positive reactions can occur with irritant or contaminated allergen solutions, poor technique and trauma, dermatographism or urticaria. False negative reactions may result from out-of-date allergens, subcutaneous injections, stress and recent administration of anti-inflammatory drugs. Suggested withdrawal times prior to IDT are:

- Antihistamines: 1 week
- Topical, oral or short-acting glucocorticoids: 2–4 weeks
- Depot glucocorticoids: 6–8 weeks
- Progestagens: 6–8 weeks.

Animals that have been on prolonged treatment may need considerably longer withdrawal times. Ciclosporin, oclacitinib, essential fatty acids (EFAs) and high-EFA diets do not appear to have a significant effect.

IDTs obviously require some experience in technique and interpretation. In particular, IDTs are more difficult to perform in cats than in dogs, because their skin is thinner and the reactions less obvious.

Serology

Serology is quicker and easier to perform than IDT. It is also less affected by prior anti-inflammatory therapy. Responses to allergen-specific immunotherapy following IDTs and serology appear to be similar, although the studies have been small and/or equivocal. Serological tests evaluate allergen-specific IgE, which is the key immuno-globulin involved in type I (immediate) hypersensitivity reactions. IgE will bind to high-affinity receptors on mast cells and Langerhans cells in sensitized individuals. Crosslinking of surface IgE by the appropriate allergen will induce mast cell degranulation with the release of pro-inflammatory mediators, resulting in a cascade of immediate, late phase and more chronic inflammatory reactions. Binding of IgE to Langerhans cells increases the efficiency of allergen capture, processing and presentation, which furthers ongoing allergic sensitization.

ELISAs are used to quantify allergen-specific IgE in a patient (Figure 26.21a). Briefly, the wells of the ELISA plate are coated with a specific allergen before incubation with the patient's serum. Specific immunoglobulin bound to the allergen can be detected using a detection reagent (usually an anti-IgE antibody coupled to an enzyme). The detection reagent is usually bound to an enzyme that catalyses a colour change when specific agents are added to the wells. The degree of colour change is therefore proportional to the amount of bound IgE, provided that the background is accounted for and known standards are used to address assay variation. The results may be expressed as the absolute optical density value or a corrected class score.

Most detection reagents are IgE-specific antibodies. IgE molecules have several antibody binding sites or epitopes, not all of which are present on all IgE molecules and some of which may be shared with other immunoglobulins. Polyclonal anti-IgE reagents recognize a range of epitopes whereas monoclonal antibodies are specific for a single epitope. Polyclonal antibodies could therefore potentially bind to IgG as well as IgE, affecting the reliability of an assay. Monoclonal antibodies are potentially more specific than polyclonal reagents. They could, however, be less sensitive because IgE molecules that do not bear the

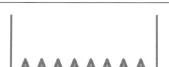
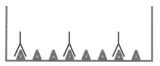
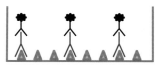
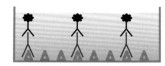

| An ELISA plate well, coated with a specific allergen | IgE from a sensitized patient binds to the allergen-coated well | A detection reagent coupled to an enzyme binds to the IgE | The enzyme catalyses a colour change in the dye; the degree is proportional to the amount of IgE |

(a)

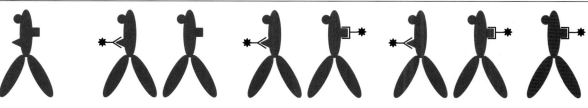

| IgE molecules bear multiple antibody binding sites (epitopes) | Monoclonal anti-IgE antibodies specific for individual epitopes will bind to IgE but not IgG molecules; however, they may miss IgE molecules without the specific epitope | Mixtures of monoclonal anti-IgE antibodies ('oligoclonal') specific for different epitopes can increase the sensitivity of IgE detection; polyclonal antibodies will also recognize multiple epitopes and could have greater sensitivity | However, use of oligoclonal or polyclonal anti-IgE that bind to epitopes that are shared with IgG (blue) can lead to false positive results and poor specificity; it is vital to screen IgE detection reagents for any cross-reaction with IgG |

(b)

26.21 (a) Schematic representation of a typical ELISA test for allergen-specific serum IgE. The sensitivity and specificity of the test depends on the efficiency with which the IgE detection reagent detects the allergen-bound IgE. (b) Monoclonal anti-IgE antibodies specific for certain IgE epitopes are highly specific (i.e. there are few false positives) but may be less sensitive if they fail to detect allergen-specific IgE without that particular epitope (i.e. there may be more false negatives). Polyclonal antibodies or oligoclonal antibody mixes recognize a greater range of epitopes and may therefore be more sensitive. However, if some epitopes are shared with IgG these tests may be less specific, with more false positive results.

relevant epitope may not be detected. Oligoclonal tests use a mixture of monoclonal antibodies, which may avoid these problems (Figure 26.21b). An alternative approach is to use the recombinant form of the α-chain of the high-affinity mast cell IgE receptor (FcεRI) to detect IgE. FcεRI should be absolutely specific for IgE but any other antibody that it recognizes is in theory capable of binding to mast cells.

There is, however, still some question over the specificity and sensitivity of these tests compared with IDTs. A blinded test of three laboratories using an FcεRIα ELISA showed some variation, but discrepancies in reporting positive/negative results were <4.2% and unlikely to affect the choice of allergens for immunotherapy (Thom *et al.*, 2008). However, a recent blinded test of four independent US laboratories using different serological tests revealed very poor correlation, with a major effect on the choice of allergens (Plant *et al.*, 2013). Clinicians should choose reputable laboratories that regularly review and validate their tests and publish their methodology, including the use of known standards, calculation of scores and cut-offs between positives and negatives. Laboratories should also be able to provide support and specialist advice on diagnosis, allergen relevance and therapy.

Adverse food reactions

Serological tests for food allergens are also available. The principle is similar to the detection of environmental allergen-specifc IgE (see above). Despite the commercial availability of these tests, little information has been published about their usefulness, and data comparing the results of commercially available tests to properly controlled food trials and provocation are lacking. Food trials with novel ingredients for at least 6 weeks followed by provocative testing remains the only reliable way to diagnose adverse food reactions (see the *BSAVA Manual of Canine and Feline Dermatology* for more details). However, food allergen serology may help in selecting foods suitable for a food trial. A recent study of the Avacta IgG/IgE food allergen serology test reported negative predictive values of 80.7/83.7% but the positive predictive values were only 15.4/34.8% (Bethlehem *et al.*, 2012). In other words, negative serology would correctly identify foods suitable for a diet trial in about four out of every five dogs. Positive serology, in contrast, cannot be used to make a diagnosis; no more than one-third of dogs with food-specific IgG or IgE actually have a food allergy.

Allergic contact dermatitis and patch tests

Allergic contact dermatitis is uncommon and difficult to diagnose. Suspected cases can be hospitalized for 5–10 days on plain cotton or newspaper, thoroughly rinsing the kennel with water after cleaning, using ceramic bowls and exercising on paved areas. If there is an improvement, patch testing can be used to identify the offending allergens.

Dogs should be sedated to allow clipping of the lateral chest and application of suspect allergens. These can be fixed in place using Opsite® adhesive dressing or Finn chambers. Liquids can be absorbed on to gauze swabs or suspended in petroleum jelly. Blanks should be included as negative controls. The site should be covered for 48–72 hours. It is usually necessary to hospitalize the animal, bandage the feet and fit an Elizabethan collar to prevent self-trauma of the test sites. Positive reactions are marked by erythema and swelling (Figure 26.22). Patch testing kits for humans contain a wide variety of potential allergens but these have not been validated in small animals.

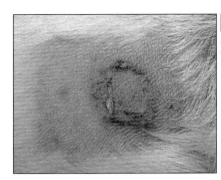

26.22 Contact reaction to an adhesive bandage in a dog.

Miscellaneous tests

Tests used in the diagnosis of immune-mediated skin disease

Antinuclear antibody (ANA) tests are immunofluorescent assays that evaluate antibodies raised against components of the cell nucleus. Nearly 100% of systemic lupus erythematosus (SLE) cases have positive ANA titres. Various ANA subtypes have been defined in both dogs and humans, including antibodies that recognize single- or double-stranded DNA, extractable nuclear antigens and histone proteins. In humans, different ANA subtypes are associated with different clinical phenotypes, but this has not been described in dogs. Anti-histone antibodies are the most common form in dogs. Antibodies directed against hnRNPG protein (heterogeneous nuclear ribonucleoprotein G) are particularly seen in German Shepherd Dogs. ANA tests involve incubating serum on a substrate of nucleated cells, such as liver or cell lines. Antibodies adherent to the cell monolayer are visualized with a species-specific anti-immunoglobulin reagent that has been conjugated to a fluorescent tag. Human Hep2 cell line monolayers are most commonly used. In addition to measuring the titre, the pattern of staining is assessed. There are four recognized patterns of staining (nuclear rim, homogeneous, speckled and nucleolar), which are known to have clinical relevance in humans, but this has not been proven in animals.

Positive titres, however, only support a clinical diagnosis of SLE because they are also seen in neoplasia, infectious diseases (especially leishmaniosis), other immune-mediated or inflammatory diseases and in healthy animals.

Other tests that may be used in evaluation of SLE cases to demonstrate systemic involvement include Coombs' tests (in anaemic animals), rheumatoid factor (in animals with erosive polyarthropathy) and urinary protein assays (where glomerulonephropathy is suspected). Cold agglutinin titres can be found in cases of cold-associated inflammation of the extremities.

Immunohistochemistry on skin biopsy samples can be used to reveal patterns of antibody deposition and/or distribution of T-cell subsets that can be used to support the diagnosis of immune-mediated diseases such as pemphigus, subepidermal blistering diseases, SLE, vasculitis, alopecia areata and others. Certain direct immunofluorescence studies can be performed on formalin-fixed sections, while others require Michel's medium or frozen tissues; the laboratory's requirements should be checked if these tests are considered. Indirect immunofluorescence tests using the patient's serum are rarely performed in veterinary medicine except for research purposes, but may become more widely available in the future.

Analysis of blood and urine

Routine haematology, biochemistry and urinalysis are not indicated in most dermatological conditions but may show:

- Abnormalities in certain endocrinopathies and metabolic conditions (see Chapters 17 and 18)
- Neutrophilia indicating infection and inflammation (see Chapter 5)
- Eosinophilia in hypersensitivity and parasitism (see Chapter 5).

Haematology and biochemistry may also be required for monitoring of animals undergoing immunosuppressive treatment. Other useful tests include:

- Feline immunodeficiency virus (FIV) and feline leukaemia virus (FeLV) testing in cats with recurrent pyoderma and other unusual dermatoses (see Chapter 28)
- Total and free thyroxine (TT4, FT4) and thyroid-stimulating hormone (TSH) (see Chapter 17)
- Serology to detect antibodies to *Sarcoptes*, *Leishmania*, *Cryptococcus* and *Aspergillus* (see Chapters 27 and 29)
- *Toxoplasma* serology can be performed prior to ciclosporin treatment in cats (see Chapter 29).

Antibodies to infectious organisms do not necessarily indicate active infection unless rising titres are demonstrated. Polymerase chain reactions (PCRs) to amplify and detect microbial DNA are a specific and sensitive method to detect mycobacteria, *Leishmania*, *Bartonella*, *Ehrlichia* and *Babesia* species in certain circumstances (see Chapters 27, 28 and 29). DNA can be detected in affected tissues, bone marrow aspirates and ethylenediamine tetra-acetic acid (EDTA) blood. However, the presence of DNA does not necessarily equate to the presence of intact organisms and infection. DNA, moreover, may not be present in tissue samples, particularly blood samples, from infected animals, leading to false negative results. The results of PCR tests must therefore be interpreted with caution and do not replace the need for other investigations, including serology. Virus isolation is not commonly performed in dermatology but may be helpful if herpesviruses, caliciviruses, poxviruses (cowpox or guinea pig orthopoxviruses) or papillomaviruses are suspected. PCR can also be used to identify these viruses (see Chapter 28).

Sex hormone assays

Assays are available for a variety of sex hormones but the wide variation in normal ranges means that baseline levels are unhelpful in diagnosing sex hormone dermatoses. Skin changes associated with Sertoli cell tumours, hyperandrogenism and hyperoestrogenism are best diagnosed by demonstrating neoplastic or hyperplastic changes in the gonads. However, there are a number of follicular dysplasia-like alopecic conditions that have been associated with abnormal gonad–adrenal steroid hormone metabolism, which may result in altered levels of sex hormones and/or steroid precursors. Alopecia X has been associated with increased 17-hydroxyprogesterone, particularly after administration of adrenocorticotropic hormone (ACTH), and other adrenal steroid hormones (including progesterone, 17-hydroxyprogesterone, oestrodiol, androstenedione and aldosterone), and has appeared to respond to treatment with deslorelin and trilostane. Despite this, the interpretation of these results is complex and their relationship to skin and other conditions is controversial (see Chapters 18 and 19). Values vary with gender and may vary with breed, and there is no clear causal association with alopecia. In addition, while 17-hydroxyprogesterone assays are widely available, the full adrenal panel is currently only available through the University of Tenessee College of Veterinary Medicine. Clinicians should therefore use the results of these tests with care. Dermatologists do not rely on these tests to achieve a diagnosis, looking instead at the whole picture including signalment, history, clinical signs and histopathology before considering these assays (see the *BSAVA Manual of Canine and Feline Dermatology* for further detail).

Faecal examination

Faecal examination is not commonly performed for skin cases. It may, however, reveal fleas, lice and *Cheyletiella* that may have been ingested by pruritic animals, hookworms in hookworm pododermatitis, or other endoparasites. Forage mites contaminating foodstuffs may also be ingested. Undigested food may be present in malabsorption syndromes associated with adverse food reactions and keratinization disorders. Identifying pollen grains in faeces may be useful in determining pollen exposure.

Diascopy

To differentiate macular erythema from petechiae or ecchymoses, a glass slide can be pressed firmly against the skin. Erythema, caused by hyperaemia, will blanch, while haemorrhaged red blood cells will not.

Otoscopes and examination of the ears

Otoscopic examination is mandatory for any animal with otitis. Gently pulling the pinna laterally and ventrally straightens the ear canals and allows access to the horizontal ear canal. Care should be taken in fractious animals, as struggling prevents a proper examination and can lead to injury. It is much better to sedate or anaesthetize the patient and flush out any obstructing debris if necessary. Careful examination will identify foreign bodies, *Otodectes*, inflammatory changes, ulceration, stenosis, the condition of the tympanic membrane, the amount and type of exudate and chronic changes.

Probing with a urinary catheter or feeding tube (with care) can assess the integrity of the tympanic membrane. The tympanic membrane can heal, trapping infection in the middle ear. A taut, translucent grey–white appearance (Figure 26.23) is normal, but myringotomy (the deliberate

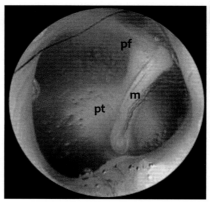

26.23 A normal tympanic membrane seen through a video otoscope. Note the taut and translucent pars tensa (pt), the dorsal, fleshy pars faccida (pf) and the C-shaped manubrium (m) of the malleus.
(© Karl Storz Endoscopy UK Ltd, Dundee, UK)

rupture of the tympanic membrane) should be considered if it appears opaque, discoloured or bulging. This should be performed under anaesthesia, first cleaning the external ear canal before changing the otoscope cone and piercing the caudoventral portion of the membrane with a sterile spinal needle. Ear, nose and throat (ENT) swabs (with small tips mounted on wire) can be used to collect samples, the first for bacterial culture and sensitivity and the second for cytology. If the ear is kept free from infection the tympanic membrane should heal within 21–35 days.

Otic cytology

Samples are usually taken from the ears to identify parasites or cells and microorganisms. Samples should be collected after an initial otoscopic examination, but before cleaning. A cotton bud is inserted down to the junction between the vertical and horizontal ear canals and rotated to collect debris, which is transferred on to a slide for cytology. The debris can be mixed with liquid paraffin, a coverslip applied and the slide examined. Under low power (X4 objective), *Otodectes*, *Demodex*, their eggs and plant debris are easily visible, but a higher magnification (the X40 or X100 lens) is required to see yeasts or bacteria clearly. Sterile swabs used to collect material can be submitted in transport medium for bacterial culture (Figures 26.24 to 26.26).

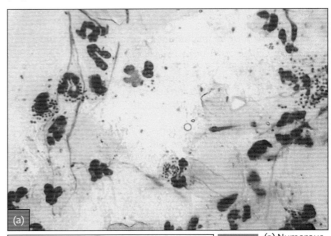

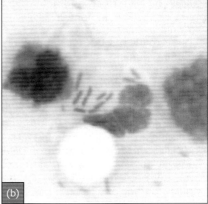

26.26 (a) Numerous extracellular and intracellular staphylococci, (b) *Pseudomonas aeruginosa* and degenerate neutrophils. Note the nuclear streaming from ruptured nuclei. (Diff-Quik® stain; original magnification (a) X400, (b) X1000)

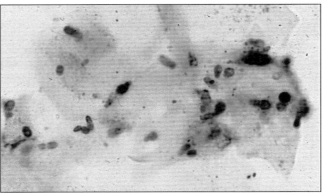

26.24 Oval and budding *Malassezia* yeasts overlying pale-staining, angular keratinocytes. (Diff-Quik® stain; original magnification X400)

Finding	Description	Significance
Keratinocytes (Figure 26.24)	Large, flat and angular. Stain pale blue to pale purple. May have melanin or keratohyaline granules. Occasionally nucleated	Shed keratinocytes; normal
	Large trapezoid to cigar shapes. Stain deep purple–blue	Shed keratinocytes; normal
	Large flat, angular to round, nucleated cells. Stain deep purple–blue	Acanthocytes; pemphigus foliaceus but also seen in severe bacterial infections
Neutrophils (Figure 26.26)	Polymorphic nucleus and pale cytoplasm	Associated with infection, inflammation and ulceration (see also red blood cells)
	Large nucleus, open and disrupted chromatin pattern (karyorrhexis). Often see nuclear streaming	Degenerate (or toxic) neutrophils; a good indication of infection
	Dark, shrunken nucleus (pyknosis). Nuclear streaming uncommon	Non-degenerate neutrophils; an indication of sterile inflammation
	Intracytoplasmic bacteria	Definite indicator of infection rather than bacterial contamination
Malassezia (Figure 26.24)	Large ovoid to budding yeasts	Low numbers (<5 per high power field) probably normal in most dogs; larger numbers suggest *Malassezia* otitis
Bacteria (Figure 26.26)	Small cocci, often in groups. Blue to purple stain	Staphylococci; low numbers probably normal in most dogs, larger numbers suggest bacterial overgrowth and otitis. More serious infections associated with neutrophils
	Small, short rods; blue to purple stain. Usually with degenerate neutrophils	Gram-negative rods, usually *Pseudomonas*; these are not seen in healthy ears and are therefore clinically significant
Red blood cells	Small, round anucleate cells	Haemorrhage, associated with trauma and ulceration

26.25 Otic cytology findings and their significance.

Case examples

CASE 1

SIGNALMENT

3-year-old male crossbred dog.

HISTORY

6-month history of slowly progressive pruritus and hair loss. This initially affected the muzzle, ventral neck and feet, but has now spread to include the ventral body, flanks and medial limbs (Figures 26.27 to 26.29). There had been a partial response to 5–7-day courses of 0.5 mg/kg prednisolone and various systemic antimicrobials. The dog was initially well, but is now dull, has a decreased appetite and is reluctant to exercise. On clinical examination the popliteal lymph nodes are enlarged, but otherwise abnormalities are restricted to the skin.

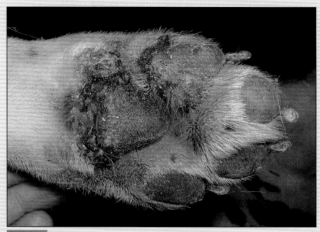

26.29 Palmar aspect of an affected forefoot.

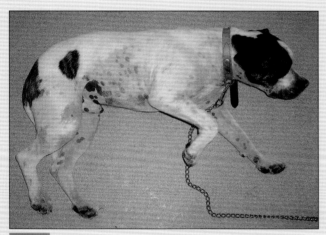

26.27 3-year-old crossbred dog exhibiting pruritus and alopecia.

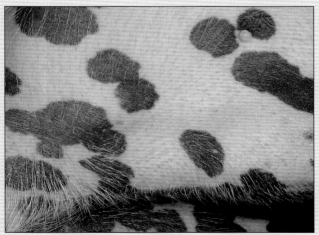

26.28 Close-up of the affected skin on the ventrolateral abdomen.

WHAT LESIONS ARE PRESENT?

There is widespread erythema and alopecia affecting the face, muzzle, medial limbs, ventral body, feet and flanks. Closer inspection reveals a macular–papular erythema centred on the hair follicles. There is a severe pododermatitis with swelling, a bloody to purulent discharge and crusting.

WHAT ARE YOUR DIFFERENTIAL DIAGNOSES?

There is obviously an inflammatory dermatosis. The alopecia may be primary or secondary to the pruritus. The distribution of lesions matches atopic dermatitis or an adverse food reaction, but the macular–papular nature of the erythema is more typical of an ectoparasite or a secondary infection such as staphylococcal pyoderma or *Malassezia* dermatitis. The follicular orientation suggests a follicular disease, such as *Demodex* or dermatophytosis. The pododermatitis could be secondary to allergic skin disease, *Demodex* or lymphocytic–plasmacytic pododermatitis with or without a secondary bacterial infection. The systemic signs could be due to pain and inflammation and/or an underlying endocrinopathy or metabolic condition. However, the latter would be unusual in a young dog and the systemic signs started after the skin lesions developed.

WHAT TESTS WOULD YOU LIKE TO PERFORM?

Appropriate initial tests include cytology, hair plucks and skin scrapes to identify the cause of the dermatitis, followed by further investigation as appropriate.

INITIAL FINDINGS

Look at the stained adhesive tape cytology from the ventral abdomen (Figure 26.30), stained indirect impression smear cytology from an affected foot (Figure 26.31), stained fine-needle aspirate cytology smear from a popliteal lymph node (Figure 26.32), and a hair pluck from the ventral neck (Figure 26.33).

→ **CASE 1 CONTINUED**

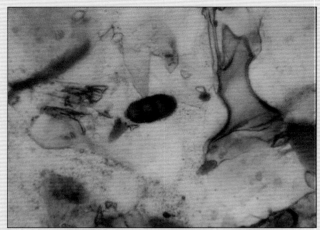

26.30 Adhesive tape cytology from the ventral abdomen. (Modified Wright–Giemsa stain; original magnification X400)

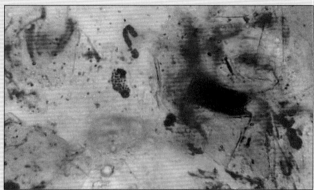

26.31 Indirect impression smear cytology from an affected foot. (Modified Wright–Giemsa stain; original magnification X400)

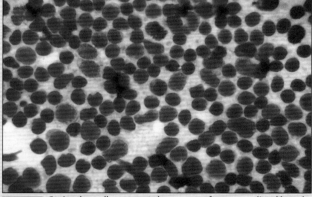

26.32 Stained needle core cytology smear from a popliteal lymph node. (Modified Wright–Giemsa stain; original magnification X400)

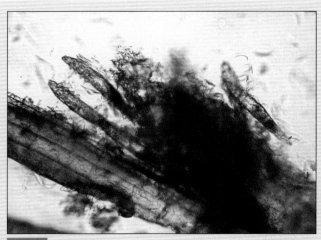

26.33 Hair pluck from ventral neck. (Original magnification X100)

WHAT IS YOUR DIAGNOSIS?

The adhesive tape strip cytology (see Figure 26.30) is unremarkable. The fungal arthroconidium is likely to be a contaminating saprophyte, as dermatophytes only produce arthroconidia in culture. The impression smear cytology from the foot (see Figure 26.31) reveals mature degenerate neutrophils with intracellular and extracellular cocci typical of a staphylococcal infection. The lymph node cytology (see Figure 26.32) shows mostly small lymphocytes with only a few large lymphoid cells and plasma cells, consistent with reactive hyperplasia. The hair pluck (see Figure 26.33) reveals numerous adult *Demodex* mites.

The diagnosis is adult-onset, generalized demodicosis with a secondary staphylococcal pyoderma.

WHAT FURTHER TESTS SHOULD BE PERFORMED?

Routine haematology, biochemistry and urinalysis are appropriate to screen for an underlying condition that may be associated with the demodicosis. These were unremarkable, apart from a low total thyroxine (TT4) (**9.6** nmol/l; reference range 13–45 nmol/l). However, the thyroid-stimulating hormone was normal (0.1 pmol/l; normal <0.41 pmol/l), suggesting that the low T4 is associated with the underlying disease (i.e. sick euthyroid syndrome).

Bacterial culture and antibiotic sensitivity testing is appropriate because the dog has a deep pyoderma and has received multiple antibiotic courses. In this case, a *Staphylcoccus pseudintermedius* sensitive to cephalosporins, clindamycin, clavulanate–amoxicillin (co-amoxiclav) and fluoroquinolones was cultured from fresh material expressed from a sinus tract.

CASE 2

SIGNALMENT

9-year-old male Bichon Frise.

HISTORY

6-month history of slowly progressive alopecia, polyuria and polydipsia. The dog is otherwise bright and well. On clinical examination, abnormalities were restricted to the skin (Figures 26.34 to 26.36).

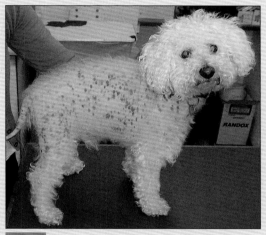

26.34 9-year old Bichon Frise exhibiting alopecia.

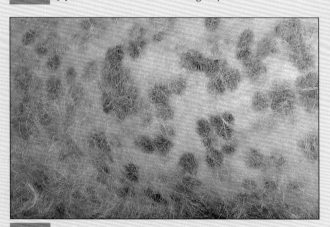

26.35 Close-up of the flank skin.

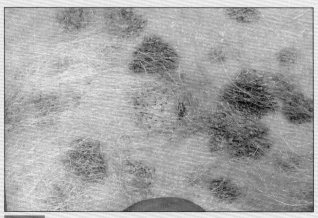

26.36 Close-up of lesional skin from the flank.

WHAT CLINICAL ABNORMALITIES ARE PRESENT?

The dog has marked alopecia of the trunk, sparing the head and distal limbs. The remaining hairs are abnormally thin and straight compared with the normal coat in this breed. There are numerous hyperpigmented macules but no other signs of inflammation. The skin is also atrophic, with some evidence of telangiectasia and comedones.

WHAT ARE THE MOST LIKELY DIFFERENTIAL DIAGNOSES?

These findings are most consistent with an atrophic dermatosis, particularly hyperadrenocorticism or a hyperoestrogenism, for example due to Sertoli cell tumour. Hypothyroidism could cause the symmetrical alopecia, but is less likely to be associated with cutaneous atrophy. Other causes of symmetrical alopecia (e.g. follicular dysplasia, cyclical flank alopecia, colour dilution alopecia, pattern baldness and alopecia X) normally start in younger dogs and are not usually associated with cutaneous atrophy. There is no evidence of stress, concurrent illness or drug exposure consistent with telogen effluvium. The lack of inflammation and the symmetrical diffuse nature of the alopecia make an infectious or inflammatory disease less likely.

WHAT ARE THE MOST APPROPRIATE INITIAL TESTS?

Haematology, serum biochemistry and urinalysis.

CLINICAL PATHOLOGY DATA

Haematology	Result	Reference interval
RBC (x 10^{12}/l)	**8.55**	5.40–8.50
Haematocrit (l/l)	**0.60**	0.35–0.55
Haemoglobin (g/dl)	**18.2**	12.0–18.0
MCV (fl)	70.0	65.0–75.0
MCHC (g/dl)	35.3	32.0–37.0
Reticulocytes (%)	0.8	0.0–1.0
WBC (x 10^9/l)	13.5	6.0–18.0
Neutrophils (segmented) (x 10^9/l)	**12.8**	3.0–12.0
Neutrophils (band) (x 10^9/l)	0.1	0–0.3
Lymphocytes (x 10^9/l)	**0.6**	1.2–3.8
Monocytes (x 10^9/l)	0	0.0–1.2
Eosinophils (x 10^9/l)	0	0.0–1.0
Platelets (x 10^9/l)	353	150–400

Abnormal results are in **bold**.

Biochemistry	Result	Reference interval
Total protein (g/l)	57	55–78
Albumin (g/l)	22	20–30
Globulin (g/l)	35	26–51
ALP (IU/l)	**1248**	0–100
ALT (IU/l)	**244**	7–50
Creatinine (µmol/l)	113	40–120

Abnormal results are in **bold**.

→ CASE 2 CONTINUED

Biochemistry *continued*	Result	Reference interval
Urea (mmol/l)	4.8	2.5–7.5
Cholesterol (μmol/l)	**6.8**	1.9–3.9
Glucose (mmol/l)	**8.9**	3.5–6.5
Calcium (mmol/l)	2.6	2.1–2.6
Phosphate (mmol/l)	2.1	1.1–2.3
Sodium (mmol/l)	154	145–156
Potassium (mmol/l)	4.4	3.80–5.30
Chloride (mmol/l)	127	117–140

Abnormal results are in **bold**.

Urine specific gravity: 1.012 (reference interval 1.015–1.045).

HOW WOULD YOU INTERPRET THESE RESULTS?

The haematology shows a mild erythrocytosis and a stress leucogram, which could be consistent with hyperadrenocorticism. This suspicion is supported by the marked elevation in alkaline phosphatase (ALP). The less marked increase in alanine aminotransferase (ALT) is consistent with a steroid hepatopathy. Mild to moderate increases in glucose and cholesterol are less specific and may be seen with a variety of endocrinopathies and metabolic conditions. Hyperadrenocorticism interferes with the action of antidiuretic hormone (ADH), leading to the production of dilute urine even with otherwise normal renal function.

WHAT FURTHER TESTS WOULD YOU LIKE TO PERFORM?

The clinical findings and screening tests are suggestive of hyperadrenocorticism, but are not diagnostic. Some form of dynamic adrenal function test is required to confirm the diagnosis. An ACTH stimulation test is the quickest and simplest to perform, but a low-dose dexamethasone suppression test would also be appropriate.

DYNAMIC ADRENAL FUNCTION TESTS

ACTH stimulation test

Pre-ACTH: 234 nmol/l (reference range 20–250 nmol/l).
Post-ACTH: **707** nmol/l (normal <600 nmol/l).

WHAT IS YOUR DIAGNOSIS? ARE THERE ANY OTHER TESTS THAT YOU WOULD CONSIDER?

The ACTH stimulation test is consistent with hyperadrenocorticism. This test, together with the clinical findings and screening tests, confirms the diagnosis of hyperadrenocorticism. Adrenal ultrasonography or an endogenous ACTH assay could be used to differentiate pituitary-dependent disease from an adrenal tumour.

References and further reading

Beco L, Guaguère E, Lorente Mendez C et al. (2013) Suggested guidelines for using systemic antimicrobials in bacterial skin infections: part one – diagnosis based on clinical presentation, cytology and culture. *Veterinary Record* **172**, 72–78

Behrend EN and Kennis R (2010) Atypical Cushing's syndrome in dogs: arguments for and against. *Veterinary Clinics of North America: Small Animal Practice* **40**, 285–297

Bethlehem S, Bexley J and Mueller RS (2012) Patch testing and allergen-specific serum IgE and IgG antibodies in the diagnosis of canine adverse food reactions. *Veterinary Immunology and Immunopathology* **145**, 582–589

Bowman DD (2006) *Georgi's Parasitology for Veterinarians, 9th edn*. WB Saunders, Philadelphia

Fondati A, De Lucia M, Furiani N et al. (2010) Prevalence of *Demodex canis* positive dogs at trichoscopic examination. *Veterinary Dermatology* **21**, 146–151

Frank LA, Hnilica KA, Rohrbach BW et al. (2010) Retrospective evaluation of sex hormones and steroid hormone intermediates in dogs with alopecia. *Veterinary Dermatology* **14**, 91–97

Gunn-Moore D, Dean R and Shaw S (2010) Mycobacterial infections in cats and dogs. *In Practice* **32**, 444–452

Jackson HA and Marsella R (2012) *BSAVA Manual of Canine and Feline Dermatology, 3rd edn*. BSAVA Publications, Gloucester

MacNeill AL (2011) Cytology of canine and feline cutaneous and subcutaneous lesions and lymph nodes. *Topics in Companion Animal Medicine* **26**, 62–76

Mendelsohn C, Rosenkrantz W and Griffin CE (2006) Practical cytology for inflammatory skin diseases. *Clinical Techniques in Small Animal Practice* **21**, 117–127

Miller WH, Griffin CE and Campbell KL (2013) Diagnostic methods. In: *Muller and Kirk's Small Animal Dermatology, 7th edn*, pp. 57–107. WB Saunders, Philadelphia

Noli C, Foster AP and Rosenkrantz WA (2013) *Allergic Diseases of Animals*. Wiley-Blackwell, Oxford.

Nuttall TJ (2013) Choosing the best antimicrobial for the job. *Veterinary Record* **172**, 12–13

Pereira AV, Pereira SA, Gremiao IDF et al. (2012) Comparison of acetate tape impression with squeezing versus skin scraping for the diagnosis of canine demodicosis. *Australian Veterinary Journal* **90**, 448–450

Plant J, Neradilek MB, Polissar NL et al. (2013) Agreement between allergen-specific IgE assays and ensuing immunotherapy recommendations from four commercial laboratories in the USA. *Veterinary Dermatology* **25**, 15–e16

Sharkey LC, Dial SM and Matz ME (2007) Maximizing the diagnostic value of cytology in small animal practice. *Veterinary Clinics of North America: Small Animal Practice* **37**, 351–372

Solano-Gallego L, Koutinas A, Miro G et al. (2009) Directions for the diagnosis, clinical staging, treatment and prevention of canine leishmaniosis. *Veterinary Parasitology* **165**, 1–18

Thom S, Favrot C, Failing K et al. (2008) Fc-ε receptor tests for atopic dogs: evaluation of inter- and intra-laboratory variability in three laboratories. *Veterinary Dermatology* **19(s1)**, 34

Toma S, Cornegliani L, Persico P et al. (2006) Comparison of 4 fixation and staining methods for the cytologic evaluation of ear canals with clinical evidence of ceruminous otitis externa. *Veterinary Clinical Pathology* **35**, 194–198

Chapter 27

Diagnosis of bacterial, fungal and mycobacterial diseases

Tim Jagger

Microorganisms interact continuously with animal hosts. Occasionally this leads to infection and disease in the host. Detection and identification of an infecting microorganism depends on good sampling technique, competent laboratory methodology and an understanding of the pathogenicity of specific microorganisms. Culture results should be correlated with other evidence of infection and with evidence of a host response. Antimicrobial susceptibility testing has an important role in directing therapy for successful resolution of bacterial infections. Veterinary practices face challenges in providing a safe and high-quality bacterial culture and antimicrobial susceptibility testing service. Multidrug-resistant bacterial pathogens are an emerging problem in veterinary practice.

Collection and storage of samples for culture

Samples for bacterial culture are ideally processed within 1–2 hours of collection, but this is rarely achieved. Delays in processing, temperature changes, exposure to atmospheric oxygen and desiccation can combine to reduce bacterial survival. Rapidly growing contaminants readily overgrow more fastidious pathogenic species. Sampling materials, sampling techniques and sample storage must be selected to optimize bacterial survival.

Principles of sampling

- Sample as early in the disease process as possible.
- Sample before antimicrobial treatment or wait a minimum of 3–5 days after cessation of treatment.
- Take all possible steps to minimize contamination.
- Do not use dry plain swabs; place inoculated swabs into bacterial or other transport medium to prevent desiccation and to maintain the viability of microorganisms.
- Always prepare the skin as for surgery if taking biopsy or fine-needle aspirate samples for culture.
- Pack samples for external laboratories safely and according to the carrier's regulations.

Sampling materials

- Swabs are made of non-inhibitory materials such as viscose, come in a sterile transport container and are marked with a use-by date. Swabs are supplied with transport medium in a separate tube.
- Transport media are buffered, non-nutritive materials formulated to limit the rate of replication of bacteria, preventing overgrowth by rapidly growing species. This helps to preserve the viability of more fastidious bacterial species. The most common example is Amies medium with or without charcoal. Transport media are suitable for aerobic and anaerobic bacteria, yeasts and some fungi. Occasional fastidious species will not survive in these nutritionally poor media.
- Boric acid preservative is a crystalline material in a sterile universal tube. It is used for urine culture samples only.
- Blood culture medium is a nutrient broth that supports both aerobic and anaerobic bacterial growth. It can only be used for fluid aspirated from a sterile site – most commonly blood or synovial fluid.
- Anaerobic transport devices contain pre-reduced transport media with reducing agents and are designed to transport material containing obligate anaerobes (bacteria unable to grow in the presence of oxygen). They are also suitable for aerobes, facultative anaerobes (bacteria able to grow in the presence or absence of oxygen), and microaerophilic bacteria (bacteria that require reduced oxygen tension to grow).
- Sterile universal containers are suitable for a range of materials including fluids, large pieces of fresh tissue, faeces and plain urine.

Sample collection: aerobic bacteria and yeasts

Aerobic bacterial cultures are indicated in all cases where bacterial infection is suspected. Yeast cultures are indicated when samples are collected from relevant sites, including the skin, ear and respiratory tract. The type of sample is determined by the site of infection (Figure 27.1).

Where tissue or fluid samples are available, these are always preferred to swabs. Further considerations depend upon the site and nature of the material sampled, for example:

- Conjunctival swabs should be inoculated prior to instillation of local anaesthetic
- Rectal swabs should only be used for neonatal animals or animals acutely ill with diarrhoea. Fresh faeces,

Sample type	Site
Swab in bacterial transport medium	Mucosal surfaces (ear canal, conjunctiva, nasal cavity, oral cavity, prepuce, vagina), skin (surface, superficial and deep pyodermas), wounds and abscesses
Fluid	Abscesses, cerebrospinal fluid (CSF), pleural and peritoneal fluid, synovial fluid, respiratory washes, prostatic washes, urine
Tissue aspirate (absorbed on to a swab in bacterial transport medium)	Lymph nodes, other fine-needle aspirates
Tissue biopsy or surgically curetted material (in a sterile tube with a small volume of sterile saline or wrapped in saline-soaked sterile surgical swabs)	Lymph nodes, skin biopsy samples, granulomas, other surgical biopsy samples, abscess wall, synovial membrane
Surgical implant or bone sequestrum (bone sequestrum as for tissue biopsy above; implants usually submitted in a dry sterile tube)	Non-healing surgical wounds

27.1 Preferred sample types for aerobic and yeast cultures.

collected per rectum and submitted in a sterile universal container, are always preferred to rectal swabs
- Vaginal swabs should be collected from the anterior vagina using a speculum or guarded swab where possible.

Sample collection: anaerobic bacteria

Anaerobic bacterial infection should be suspected in the following clinical conditions:

- Abscesses
- Anal sacculitis
- Bacterial peritonitis
- Bacteraemia
- Cellulitis
- Endometritis
- Fractures involving trauma to soft tissue
- Osteomyelitis
- Periodontal disease
- Postsurgical infection
- Pyothorax
- Skin granulomas
- Wounds.

Obligate anaerobic bacteria are unable to grow in the presence of oxygen and do not survive for more than 20 minutes in air. Recovery is enhanced by avoiding all contact with atmospheric oxygen.

- Collect samples that are large enough to maintain anaerobic conditions (>2 ml of fluid or >2 cm³ of tissue).
- Place tissue samples in a sterile tube. Add a small volume of sterile saline or wrap in saline-soaked sterile surgical swabs if sample desiccation is a concern.
- Exclude air from fluid samples where possible. Fluid may be collected in a syringe or plain sterile tube if the syringe is evacuated or the tube is filled to exclude air. Seal the syringe or tube with tape.
- Immerse swabs in transport medium immediately after inoculation.

- Hold samples in a cool place but do not refrigerate. Refrigeration (<4°C) kills anaerobes (oxygen absorption is greater at lower temperatures) while higher temperatures (>27°C) favour overgrowth of aerobic bacteria.
- Culture tissue and fluid samples not protected by bacterial transport medium within 24 hours.
- Transport devices are available to maintain anaerobic conditions in aspirated fluids, fresh tissue and swabs. Examples are BBL™ Port-A-Cul™ tubes, jars and vials (Figure 27.2). The viability of anaerobic, aerobic and microaerophilic bacteria is maintained for 72 hours at 20–25°C, making these devices suitable for postal or courier submission to a reference laboratory.

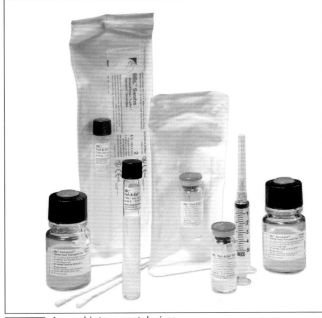

27.2 Anaerobic transport devices.
(Courtesy and © Becton, Dickinson and Company, reprinted with permission)

Sample collection: blood cultures

Blood cultures are indicated for animals suspected of having a bacteraemia (e.g. bacterial endocarditis or pyrexia of unknown origin), and must be taken prior to treatment with antimicrobials.

- Take three samples over a 24-hour period, except for acutely septic patients when three samples may be taken over a 30-minute period, prior to starting antimicrobial treatment.
- Prepare the skin aseptically to prevent bacterial contamination.
- Collect 1 ml of blood per 10 ml blood culture medium using a sterile syringe and needle (or newly inserted jugular intravenous catheter). Small-volume blood culture medium bottles facilitate multiple collections from smaller animals.
- Disinfect the culture medium bottle diaphragm with 70% alcohol and allow to dry.
- Use a new sterile needle to transfer blood to the blood culture medium bottle and mix by inverting several times.
- Store inoculated blood culture medium bottles at room temperature before dispatching to the reference laboratory for incubation and culture.

Sample collection: fluid cultures

Abscess material

- Aerobic and anaerobic cultures are indicated; therefore collect abscess fluid as for anaerobic cultures (above).
- Bacterial culture results from abscess fluid may be unrewarding; this is assumed to be due to the accumulation of neutrophil lysosomes and localization of viable bacteria on the inner wall of the abscess capsule.
- When an abscess is opened for drainage, use a swab to collect material from the lining of the abscess capsule, immersing the swab immediately in transport medium to preserve anaerobic bacterial viability.
- When an abscess is removed surgically, submit tissue samples including the abscess wall, collected aseptically and presented as for anaerobic cultures (above).

Cerebrospinal fluid

- Transfer cerebrospinal fluid (CSF) into a sterile tube for aerobic and anaerobic cultures.
- Consider inoculating CSF into blood culture medium or nutrient broth to maximize recovery of bacteria if bacterial meningitis is suspected.

Peritoneal and pleural fluids

- Collect fluid aseptically, ideally from the unopened body cavity. Occasionally fluid will be collected intraoperatively.
- Aerobic and anaerobic cultures are indicated; therefore, collect fluid as for anaerobic cultures (above).

Synovial fluid

- Approaches to arthrocentesis are illustrated in Chapter 23.
- Collect synovial fluid aseptically into a sterile container or absorb fluid on to a swab for direct culture.
- Ideally, inoculate synovial fluid into blood culture medium to maximize recovery of bacteria (Montgomery et al., 1989). Using this technique, positive cultures were obtained from 50% of cases of septic arthritis in dogs (Clements et al., 2005).

Tracheal, bronchial and prostatic washes

- Collect wash fluid in a sterile container for aerobic bacterial and fungal cultures from respiratory washes, and for aerobic and anaerobic bacterial cultures from prostatic washes.
- Isotonic saline is the most common respiratory wash fluid but better culture results are obtained if a buffered solution, such as lactated Ringer's, is used.

Urine

- Collect urine by cystocentesis, midstream voided urine or catheterization (see Chapter 10). Cystocentesis is the preferred method of collection for urine cultures.
- Culture fresh urine within 2 hours where possible.
- Where urine culture is delayed, urine may be refrigerated for up to 24 hours (Weese et al., 2011). Otherwise, place the sample in boric acid preservative, being careful to maintain the ratio of urine to boric acid.

A fill line is indicated on the side of the tube; decant boric acid preservative from the tube for lower volumes of urine. Boric acid urine samples held at room temperature give culture results comparable to fresh urine for up to 48 hours. Similar results can be obtained by using dip-slide urine culture and transport tubes (Perrin and Nicolet, 1992).
- A recent study in dogs and cats indicated that cystocentesis urine samples maintained at room temperature should be submitted overnight in plain tubes for culture (rather than boric acid tubes) to minimize false negative culture results (Rowlands et al., 2011).

Sample collection: fungal cultures

Sampling techniques for dermatophytes are detailed in Chapter 26. Sampling techniques for yeasts and other pathogenic fungi depend upon the site of infection.

Deep skin and tissue mycoses

- Surgical biopsy samples are preferred for deep skin and tissue mycoses. Submit tissue samples unfixed and without preservative in a sealed sterile leak-proof container. Add a small volume of sterile saline or wrap in saline-soaked sterile surgical swabs if sample desiccation is a concern.
- Absorb discharge from sinus tracts or fistulae on to a swab and submit in transport medium. Such samples are often contaminated with bacterial skin commensals and occasionally with environmental fungi.
- Submit fine-needle aspirates, collected after aseptic skin preparation, absorbed on to a swab and placed in transport medium. However, such samples may contain too little material for effective culture.

Nasal mycoses

- If a mycotic rhinitis is suspected in a dog then collect nasal discharge on a swab. If nasal biopsy samples are taken, submit one for culture.
- Submit nasal wash fluid in a sterile container.
- A culture positive for Aspergillus species or Penicillium species in dogs is not proof of pathogenicity because both species are saprophytes prevalent in the environment. Diagnosis can be supported by cytology of the nasal discharge or wash fluid, rhinoscopy (for fungal plaques), radiology (for radiolucency due to turbinate destruction) and serology (see later section on polymerase chain reaction (PCR) testing, antigen detection and serology). Definitive diagnosis requires demonstration of tissue invasion in biopsy material.
- If Cryptococcus neoformans or Cryptococcus gattii infection is suspected in a cat then collect nasal discharge on a swab placed in transport medium. CSF or tissue biopsy samples may also be submitted for culture depending on the clinical presentation. Cryptococcosis is a potential zoonosis and suspected infected tissues should be handled with care (ideally in a microbiological safety cabinet).
- Diagnosis of cryptococcal infection can be supported by cytology of the nasal discharge or fine-needle aspirates of affected tissues, PCR testing or serology for circulating antigen (see later section on PCR testing, antigen detection and serology).

Skin, ear, eye and nail disease

- Gently roll or rub a swab over an area of skin to be sampled. If the skin surface is dry then moisten the swab with sterile saline or water for injection first, to increase the amount of material collected.
- Collect ear swabs either through an otoscope (minitip swabs) or from the vertical ear canal.
- Collect conjunctival swabs by gently passing a swab back and forth over the surface of the lower palpebral conjunctiva.
- Culture corneal scrapings patient-side if possible, submitting inoculated plates to the reference laboratory for incubation.
- If mycotic nail disease is suspected then submit either a cast nail or shavings from the proximal intact nail in a sterile pot for fungal culture including dermatophytes. Include discharge from the nailbed on a swab, or swab into the claw fold adjacent to the claw if bacterial cultures are also required.

Sample collection: mycobacteria

Specialized culture techniques and containment facilities are required to culture and identify mycobacterial species. Details of UK mycobacterial reference laboratories are given in the Resources section at the end of this chapter, but samples may also be submitted through a veterinary reference laboratory. Some laboratories also offer PCR testing.

- Submit fresh surgical biopsy specimens for culture from skin lesions or intestinal tubercles, lymph nodes, pulmonary tubercles, bone and tonsils in the case of suspected systemic infection. Submit in a sterile universal tube. If the sample is small then a small volume (drops) of sterile saline or sterile water for injection may be added.
- The diagnosis can be supported by cytology (air-dried fine-needle aspirate smears, fluid smears, impression smears from biopsy samples) or histology (biopsy material in 10% neutral buffered formal saline). Request acid-fast staining where mycobacterial infection is suspected.
- *Mycobacterium tuberculosis* was transmitted accidentally to veterinary personnel during the post-mortem examination of a dog (Posthaus *et al.*, 2010). Care must be exercised in obtaining and handling tissues from animals suspected of having mycobacterial infections. Aerosol infection is a particular hazard.

Sample collection: *Mycoplasma*, *Ureaplasma* and *Acholeplasma* species

Haemotropic mycoplasmas are discussed in Chapter 29. Non-haemotropic mycoplasmas are commensals of the respiratory and urogenital mucosal membranes. Often the pathological significance of *Mycoplasma* isolates is not proven. Mycoplasmas may be isolated in association with:

- Bite wound abscesses in cats
- Conjunctivitis in cats (*Mycoplasma felis* is considered to be a significant pathogen)
- Genital tract infections in cats and dogs
- Lower respiratory tract infection in cats and dogs
- Urinary tract infection (UTI) in dogs.

Sample submission:

- Submit swabs in liquid-phase *Mycoplasma* transport medium where available and request specific cultures for *Mycoplasma*
- Submit plain swabs in sterile tubes for PCR testing for *Mycoplasma* spp. or *M. felis* (see later section on PCR testing, antigen detection and serology).

Sample storage

There is contradictory evidence regarding the effects of refrigeration on the survival of bacterial pathogens of veterinary significance. Bacterial survival is, however, likely to be optimized when samples are held at room temperature; refrigeration is harmful to some species of bacteria, especially anaerobes. If samples are sent to a reference laboratory then same-day or overnight courier services or Royal Mail special delivery should be used to ensure that bacterial cultures are inoculated within 24 hours of collection where possible.

Microscopy and staining

The goals of microscopy are:

- To identify a host inflammatory response
- To detect bacteria and other microorganisms and to determine their morphology
- To assist interpretation of culture results.

Suitable samples for microscopy include:

- Impression smears from superficial cutaneous lesions or tissue biopsy specimens
- Fine-needle aspirate smears from deeper lesions including lymph nodes, subcutaneous lesions, and internal mass and organ aspirates
- Smears from swabs of aural, conjunctival, vaginal or nasal discharges
- Direct smears from turbid peritoneal or pleural fluids and abscess material
- Concentrated sediment smears from urine, respiratory washes, prostatic washes and cellular CSF
- Tissue sections fixed in 10% neutral buffered formalin (for histopathological examination).

Microscopy is usually performed alongside bacterial and fungal cultures. Bright-field microscopy using an oil immersion lens at X1000 magnification allows resolution of bacteria down to 0.2 μm in size. The stains of choice for initial microscopy for bacteria and other microorganisms are Romanowsky stains, including Leishman's and modified Wright–Giemsa. Bacteria are readily visualized with Romanowsky stains as both Gram-negative and Gram-positive bacteria stain uniformly dark blue (Figures 27.3, 27.4 and 27.5). Rapid Romanowsky stains, such as Diff-Quik®, are a useful practice tool but there is reduced contrast between microorganisms and background material. Stain precipitate, which is more common with this type of stain, can be mistaken for bacteria. Bacteria may also be stained by other cytological stains including Papanicolaou stain (Figure 27.6).

A Gram stain provides additional information on bacterial structure. Gram-positive and Gram-negative bacteria have differing cell wall composition and therefore also

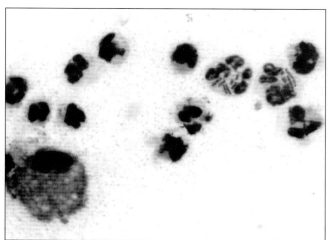

27.3　Prostatic wash from a dog containing *Pasteurella multocida*, a macrophage and neutrophils, two with phagocytosed bacterial bacilli. Phagocytosis of bacteria by neutrophils supports bacterial infection. (Modified Wright–Giemsa stain; original magnification X1000)

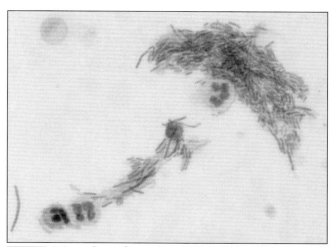

27.6　Urine sediment from a dog with *Escherichia coli* infection; bacterial bacilli and neutrophils with one crenated erythrocyte are visible. (Papanicolaou stain; original magnification X1000)

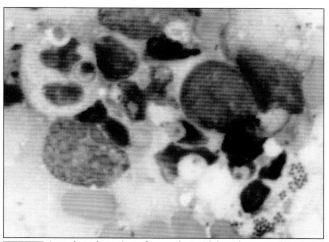

27.4　Lymph node aspirate from a dog with lymphoma and bacterial lymphadenitis. The image shows neutrophils, one lower right with phagocytosed bacterial cocci, degenerate cells, a small lymphocyte and a neoplastic lymphoid cell. (Modified Wright–Giemsa stain; original magnification X1000)

differ in their susceptibility to enzymes, disinfectants and antimicrobials. Gram-positive bacteria and fungi (yeasts) stain blue or purple. Gram-negative bacteria stain red and may be difficult to visualize against proteinaceous or mucinaceous backgrounds, which often also stain red. The Gram stain is routinely employed in microbiology laboratories and for histopathology sections.

Acid-fast stains are used in suspected mycobacterial infection; most mycobacteria do not stain with Romanowsky stains due to lipids and waxy material in their cell walls (Figure 27.7). Ziehl–Neelsen stain, a common acid-fast stain, stains mycobacteria pink against a blue background (Figure 27.8).

Mycotic elements and yeasts may stain adequately with Romanowsky stains (Figures 27.9 and 27.10) but fungal cell walls remain unstained (Figure 27.11). Gram stain has a similar utility. Periodic acid–Schiff (PAS) stain can be used to identify fungal elements in direct smears and histopathology sections. Routine haematoxylin and eosin stain will detect some fungal elements in tissue sections (Figure 27.12).

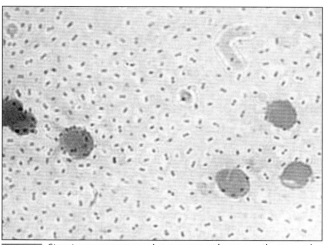

27.5　*Streptococcus pneumoniae*, a common human pathogen and occasional pathogen in cats. Degenerate erythrocytes and characteristic paired bacterial cocci with non-staining capsules are visible. (Modified Wright–Giemsa stain; original magnification X1000)

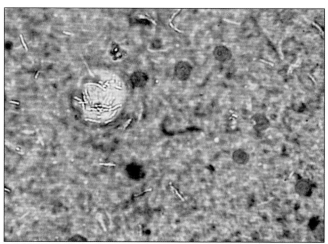

27.7　Discharge from a cat spay wound. Probable *Mycobacterium* species; non-staining bacterial bacilli and a macrophage left of centre with intracellular bacteria are visible. (Modified Wright–Giemsa stain; original magnification X1000)
(Courtesy of M Dunlop)

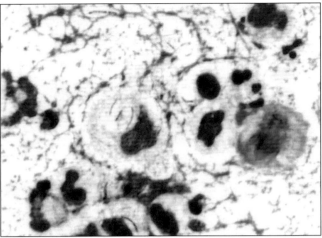

27.8 Discharge from a cat spay wound (same case as Figure 27.7). Probable *Mycobacterium* species; acid-fast bacilli stain pink/red against a blue background and the macrophage left of centre contains intracellular bacteria. (Ziehl–Neelsen stain; original magnification X1000)
(Courtesy of M Dunlop)

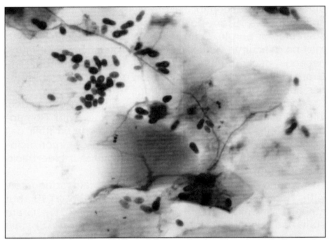

27.9 Smear of ear discharge from a dog. *Malassezia pachydermatis*; characteristic broad-based apical budding yeasts and anucleate superficial squamous epithelial cells are seen. (Modified Wright–Giemsa stain; original magnification X1000)

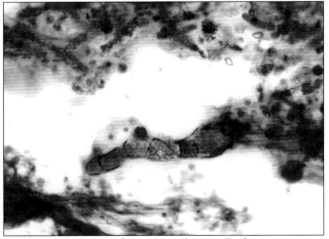

27.10 Nasal discharge from a dog with *Aspergillus fumigatus* infection. Fungal elements (hyphae) are seen, with numerous free conidia (spores). (Modified Wright–Giemsa stain; original magnification X1000)
(Courtesy of M Serra)

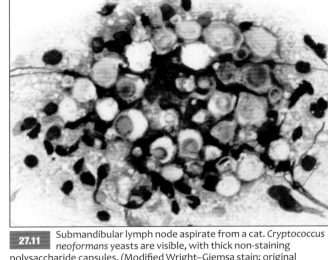

27.11 Submandibular lymph node aspirate from a cat. *Cryptococcus neoformans* yeasts are visible, with thick non-staining polysaccharide capsules. (Modified Wright–Giemsa stain; original magnification X1000)
(Courtesy of M Serra)

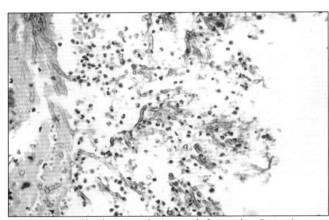

27.12 Fungal hyphae in a splenic capsule from a dog. Systemic mycosis in this 5-year old Whippet occurred secondary to azathioprine therapy. (Haematoxylin and eosin stain; original magnification X400)
(Courtesy of J Hargreaves)

Bacterial and fungal identification

Bacterial and fungal identification techniques all involve a comparison between the characteristics of an unknown organism and those of known organisms.

Colonial morphology, microscopy and confirmatory tests

Colonial morphology refers to the appearance of individual bacterial or fungal colonies, usually on solid media. Solid media are described as non-selective, selective or differential depending on their chemical composition and function.

- **Blood agar:** a non-selective, differential medium; aerobic bacteria can be differentiated on the basis of haemolysin production. Used for samples from all common sample sites.
- **MacConkey agar:** a selective, differential medium for the isolation of enterobacteria and other aerobic

Gram-negative bacteria; aerobic bacteria are differentiated on the basis of lactose fermentation. Used for all common sample sites except nasal/respiratory.

- **Sabouraud's dextrose agar:** a selective medium for the isolation of dermatophytes, other fungi and yeasts; the acidic pH inhibits bacterial growth. The medium usually contains chloramphenicol to reduce the growth of non-target species. Used for most common sample sites except bile, other fluids and urine.
- **Chromogenic media:** contain enzyme substrates linked to a chromogen (colour reaction) with specificity for particular organisms. *Brilliance*™ MRSA 2 Agar allows for rapid screening of clinical samples for meticillin-resistant bacteria, producing blue or lilac colonies against an opaque background (Figure 27.13).

Microscopy involves the preparation and examination of Gram-stained smears of bacterial colonies and stained wet preparations taken from fungal colonies.

Combinations of simple confirmatory tests are employed to identify many bacterial isolates to genus or species level. For example, identification of Gram-positive coccoid bacteria utilizes a combination of simple biochemical tests, antimicrobial susceptibility, growth characteristics on specific media and serological grouping (Figure 27.14). *Staphyloccus* spp. are divided into **coagulase-negative** and **coagulase-positive** species, based on their ability to coagulate rabbit serum in the coagulase tube test (Figure 27.15).

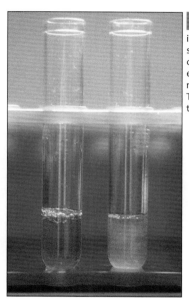

27.15 The tube coagulase test: rabbit plasma is incubated with a bacterial suspension. Fibrinogen is converted to fibrin by coagulase enzyme to give a clot in the right-hand tube, a positive test. The left-hand tube is clear and therefore negative.

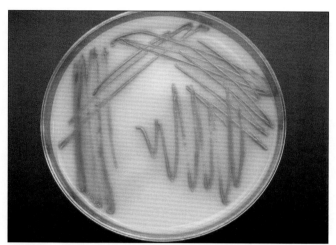

27.13 Meticillin-resistant *Staphylococcus aureus* growth on a selective chromogenic agar. Blue colonies are presumed positive for meticillin-resistant *Staphylococcus* spp.

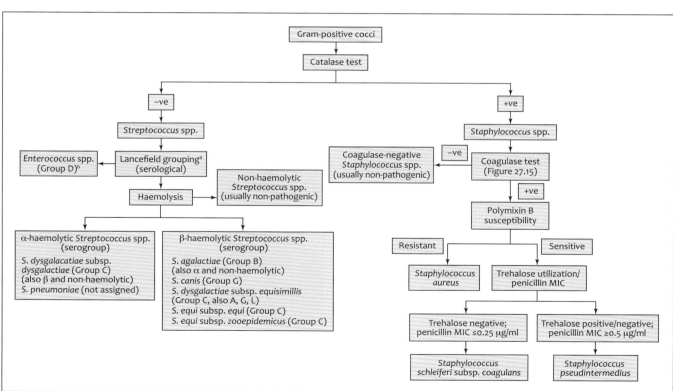

27.14 Identification of Gram-positive coccoid bacteria. [a] Lancefield grouping is a method of grouping catalase-negative, coagulase-negative bacteria based on the carbohydrate composition of bacterial antigens found on the cell walls. [b] *Enterococcus* was believed to be a member of the genus *Streptococcus* at the time the Lancefield grouping was devised. MIC = minimum inhibitory concentration.

Biochemical identification

Manual systems are available to identify bacteria to genus or species level through detection of enzymatic activity and/or fermentation of sugars. The API® system is one example. The results are read as colour changes and are converted to a numerical profile that is compared to an online database to identify the isolate (Figure 27.16).

Automated analysers utilize similar biochemical tests with additional substrates measuring carbon source utilization, nitrogen source utilization, enzymatic activities and resistance. In the VITEK® 2 analyser, a bacterial (or yeast) suspension is prepared and is inoculated into a card specific for the type of organism under investigation (e.g. anaerobes, corynebacteria, Gram-negatives, Gram-positives, yeasts). Test results are compared to a database and the probability of a match with a named microorganism is reported.

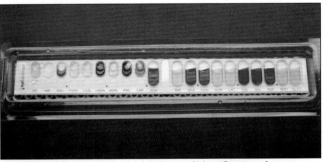

27.16 API® test strip for the biochemical identification of *Streptococcus* spp.

Staphylococcus pseudintermedius

Bacteria previously classified as *Staphylococcus intermedius* are now divided into three species: *Staphylococcus intermedius*, *Staphylococcus pseudintermedius* and *Staphylococcus delphini*.
S. pseudintermedius is the species that colonizes and infects dogs and cats. This species was first described in 2005; laboratory reports and literature predating this will refer to *S. intermedius* infections

---

Molecular identification

Molecular techniques are not routinely used for the identification of cultured bacteria and fungi in veterinary microbiology laboratories. However, they have an important role in the detection of some bacterial infections (see later section on PCR testing, antigen detection and serology). Molecular techniques are important for epidemiological investigations, for identifying genes encoding virulence mechanisms and in defining the taxonomy of bacterial species. There has been much modification of phenotypic taxonomy of bacteria in recent years.

MALDI-TOF-MS

Matrix-assisted laser desorption/ionization time-of-flight mass spectrometry (MALDI-TOF-MS) is an example of the next generation of technology to be employed by veterinary laboratories for the identification of microorganisms. Single colonies are transferred from solid media to target plates. This technique identifies bacterial and fungal ribosomal proteins through a process of ionization. Ions are accelerated in a magnetic field and separated on the basis of mass to generate a sample spectrum. The spectrum is compared to reference spectra in a database and a probable identification is returned. This technique can be used to identify yeasts, dermatophytes and anaerobic bacteria in addition to aerobic bacteria. MALDI-TOF-MS offers increased speed of identification, a comprehensive database of organisms and the facility to improve organism identification by adding new isolates to the database. Systems like MALDI-TOF-MS are likely to replace many of the biochemical/phenotypic bacterial identification techniques currently in use in larger laboratories.

Significance of bacterial isolates

Most bacteria are harmless *saprophytes*, organisms that feed or grow on dead or decaying organic material. Bacteria have also evolved to colonize mucous membranes and other epithelial surfaces in animals. Where this does not cause disease, these bacteria are called *commensals* and form part of the *normal bacterial flora*.

Bacteria that cause disease are called *pathogens*. These may live in permanent association with animals or may be saprophytes. *Opportunist pathogens* are commensals or saprophytes that do not cause disease under normal circumstances. An impaired host immune response, introduction to new sites or tissues and disturbed normal flora all predispose to opportunist infection.

Samples collected from sites that are not sterile are often contaminated with non-pathogenic bacteria. These *contaminants* may originate either from the environment or from an animal's normal bacterial flora. Voided urine samples, for example, frequently contain bacterial contaminants originating from the terminal urethra, genital tract and external genitalia. Care must be taken when accessing normally sterile sites, usually through needle puncture, not to introduce contaminants from the skin surface into the sample (Figures 27.17 and 27.18).

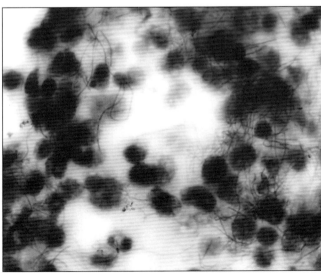

27.17 Direct smear of a cystocentesis urine sample from a dog. Transitional epithelial cells, neutrophils and filamentous bacterial bacilli are visible. (Modified Wright–Giemsa stain; original magnification X1000)

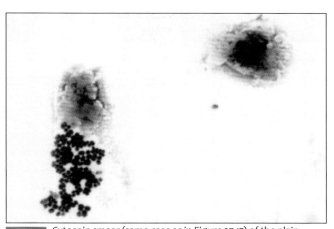

27.18 Cytospin smear (same case as in Figure 27.17) of the plain cystocentesis urine sample viewed 24 hours later. Degenerate nucleated cells with bacterial cocci are present. *Staphylococcus pseudintermedius* was isolated. This is likely to represent overgrowth in the plain urine sample by a skin surface contaminant introduced during cystocentesis. (Modified Wright–Giemsa stain; original magnification X1000)

The isolation of a bacterial species from diseased tissue is not proof of pathogenicity. Features to consider when assessing the significance of a bacterial isolate include:

- Was the bacterium isolated in pure and profuse growth or as part of a mixed bacterial culture?
- Is the bacterium part of the normal microbial flora at this site?
- Does the clinical presentation match the likely pathogenicity of the bacterial species?
- Is there clinical or other evidence of infection, including evidence of a host response? (See sections on Microscopy and PCR testing, antigen detection and serology.)

Normal microbial flora of cats and dogs

There is limited information regarding normal microbial flora of cats and dogs compared with humans (and mice). The following information on the normal microbial flora of dogs and cats is drawn from a series of original studies. The composition of the normal flora is influenced by the microenvironment (including pH, temperature and nutrients), sampling technique, culture techniques, the age of the patient, geographical location, nutrition, breed, climate and seasonality. There are limited temporal studies to distinguish between resident and transient microbial flora. There is more information available on canine (Figure 27.19) than on feline (Figure 27.20) normal flora.

Bacteria are identified to species or genus level, or are grouped according to haemolysin or coagulase production. Anaerobic bacteria, yeasts, saprophytic fungi and mycoplasmas are not further classified.

Microbe	Conjunctiva	Ear	Nasal cavity	Prepuce	Skin	Urine contaminants	Vagina
(Number of references)	(6)	(4)	(3)	(3)	(5)	(1)	(5)
Achromobacter spp.	O						
Acinetobacter baumannii	O						
Acinetobacter calcoaceticus subsp. *anitratus*	O		O				
Acinetobacter lwoffii	O		O				
Acinetobacter spp.	O	O		O	X		O
Actinomyces spp.		O					
Aeromonas hydrophila			O				
Aggregatibacter aphrophilus			O				
Alcaligenes spp.	O		O				
Bacillus spp.	X	O	X	O	O		O
Bordetella bronchiseptica			O				
Branhamella catarrhalis	O		O				
Brucella canis			O				
Burkholderia cepacia			O				
Citrobacter spp.	O						O
Corynebacterium spp.	X	O	O	X	X		X
Eikenella corrodens			O				
Enterobacter aerogenes			NS				
Enterobacter agglomerans	O		O				
Enterobacter cloacae			O				
Enterobacter spp.	O						O
Enterobacteriaceae (other)		O					

27.19 Canine normal microbial flora. NS = frequency not specified; O = infrequent isolate (<10% of isolates); X = frequent isolate (≥10% of isolates). (continues)

Microbe	Conjunctiva	Ear	Nasal cavity	Prepuce	Skin	Urine contaminants	Vagina
Enterococcus spp.	O		NS	O			O
Escherichia coli	O	O	O	X	O	X	X
Flavobacterium spp.	O		O	O			O
Haemophilus spp.	O		O	O			O
Klebsiella pneumoniae	O		O	O			O
Klebsiella spp.	O						
Lactobacillus spp.	O		O				O
Micrococcus spp.	O	X	O		X	O	O
Moraxella spp.	O		O	O			O
Mycobacterium spp.	O						
Neisseria spp.	X	O	O				O
Nocardia spp.	O				O		
Pasteurella multocida			O	X			X
Pasteurella spp.	O		O	O			X
Pediococcus spp.		O					
Proteus mirabilis			O	O	O	X	X
Proteus spp.	O			O		O	X
Pseudomonas aeruginosa	O	O	O				O
Pseudomonas spp.	O		O	O			O
Simonsiella spp.	NS		O				
Staphylococcus pseudintermedius	X			O			O
Staphylococcus xylosus		X					
Staphylococcus spp. – coagulase-negative	X	X	X	X	O	O	O
Staphylococcus spp. – coagulase-positive	X	X	X	X	X	X	X
Staphylococcus spp.	X	X					
Streptobacillus spp.			O				
Streptococcus bovis							O
Streptococcus canis	O			O		X	X
Streptococcus durans			O				
Streptococcus equi subsp. *equi*			O				
Streptococcus equi subsp. *equisimilis*				O			
Streptococcus equi subsp. *zooepidemicus*							O
Streptococcus faecalis			O	O			O
Streptococcus faecium			O				
Streptococcus lactis			NS				
Streptococcus mitis			O				
Streptococcus pneumoniae	O						
α-haemolytic *Streptococcus* spp.	X	O		O	X		X
β-haemolytic *Streptococcus* spp.	O	O		X			X
Non-haemolytic *Streptococcus* spp.	X	O		O			O
Streptococcus spp.		O	X		X		
Streptomyces spp.	O	O	O	O			
Veillonella spp.	O						
Anaerobes	O	O	X		X		
Yeasts	O	X					
Mycoplasma spp.		O		X			X
Saprophytic fungi	O	O		O			

27.19 (continued) Canine normal microbial flora. NS = frequency not specified; O = infrequent isolate (<10% of isolates); X = frequent isolate (≥10% of isolates).

Microbe	Conjunctiva	Prepuce	Skin	Urine contaminants	Vagina
(Number of references)	(5)	(1)	(1)	(1)	(2)
Acinetobacter spp.			X		O
Actinomyces pyogenes					O
Aerococcus spp.					O
Alcaligenes spp.			O		
Bacillus spp.	O		O		
Corynebacterium spp.	O	O		X	O
Escherichia coli		X	O	X	X
Flavobacterium spp.				O	O
Haemophilus spp.					X
Klebsiella ozaenae					O
Lactobacillus spp.					O
Micrococcus spp.			X		
Moraxella spp.		O			O
Pasteurella haemolytica					O
Pasteurella multocida		X			
Pasteurella spp.		X		O	O
Proteus mirabilis			O		
Pseudomonas aeruginosa	O				
Pseudomonas spp.			O		O
Simonsiella spp.		O			O
Staphylococcus felis		O			O
Staphylococcus pseudintermedius					O
Staphylococcus spp. – coagulase-negative	X	O	X		X
Staphylococcus spp. – coagulase-positive	O		O		
Staphylococcus spp.	X			X	
Streptococcus agalactiae					O
Streptococcus canis		O			X
Streptococcus dysgalactiae					O
Streptococcus mitis					O
Streptococcus uberis					O
α-haemolytic *Streptococcus* spp.	O	O	X		O
β-haemolytic *Streptococcus* spp.			O		
Non-haemolytic *Streptococcus* spp.	O				
Streptococcus spp.				X	O
Streptomyces spp.	O				
Anaerobes		X			O
Yeasts	O				
Mycoplasma spp.	X				
Saprophytic fungi	X				

27.20 Feline normal microbial flora. O = infrequent isolate (<10% of isolates); X = frequent isolate (≥10% of isolates).

Clinical presentations

Samples from a limited number of clinical conditions give rise to the majority of submissions to veterinary microbiology laboratories for bacterial and fungal cultures; these conditions are considered below.

Anaerobic infection

Anaerobic bacteria associated with disease in dogs and cats are most commonly isolated in mixed growths of two (or more) anaerobic species. Mixed infections with aerobes are also common. Commonly isolated anaerobic bacterial pathogens (≥10% of isolates) include *Bacteroides melaninogenicus*, other *Bacteroides* spp., *Clostridium perfringens* and other *Clostridium* spp. Less common isolates (<10% of isolates) include *Actinomyces* spp., *Bacteroides fragilis*, *Eubacterium* spp., *Peptostreptococcus anaerobius*, *Propionibacterium acnes* and other *Propionobacterium* spp., *Fusobacterium necrophorum* and other *Fusobacterium* spp.

Bacteraemia

Significant isolates from blood cultures in bacteraemic cats and dogs include *Bacteroides* spp., *Bartonella* spp., *Clostridium perfringens*, Enterobacteriaceae, *Fusobacterium* spp., *Pseudomonas* spp., *Staphylococcus pseudintermedius*, β-haemolytic streptococci, non-β-haemolytic streptococci and *Enterococcus* spp. Contaminants include *Corynebacterium* spp., *Bacillus* spp., coagulase-negative *Staphylococcus* spp. and other skin commensals. Multiple blood cultures assist distinction between pathogens and contaminants. The results must be correlated with the patient's clinical status, and potential sources for a bacteraemia should be identified (Calvert and Thomason, 2012).

Bacterial enteritis

Faecal cultures reflect the microbial flora of the caecum and colon. Anaerobes predominate but most laboratories do not routinely inoculate anaerobic cultures from faecal samples. The composition and distribution of the aerobic faecal flora are altered in enteric disease, but faecal cultures are usually not quantitative and subtle changes in faecal flora may not be detected (see also Chapter 13).

Aerobic faecal flora include *Escherichia coli*, other Enterobacteriaceae and *Enterococcus* spp. *Campylobacter* spp. have been isolated from 0–87% of faecal samples from asymptomatic dogs and from 0–75% of faecal samples from asymptomatic cats (Marks *et al.*, 2011). *Salmonella* spp. have been isolated from 0–3.6% of faeces from healthy dogs (Marks *et al.*, 2011) and 1–18% of faeces from healthy or hospitalized cats (Greene, 2012a).

Established enteric pathogens include *E. coli*, *Campylobacter* spp., *Clostridium perfringens*, *Salmonella* spp., *Shigella* spp. (rare) and *Yersinia* spp. (rare). Enteric bacterial infection is most common in neonates but has been reported in dogs over 3 months of age.

Most *E. coli* isolated from faeces are likely to be normal faecal flora. Seven distinct pathotypes of *E. coli* are recognized to cause diarrhoea in humans and have been isolated from dogs with and without diarrhoea. The role of these strains in enteric disease in dogs and cats remains poorly characterized and typing of strains is not routinely available.

There is limited information on the incidence of *C. perfringens*-associated diarrhoea in dogs and cats. Reported clinical signs range from mild self-limiting diarrhoea to haemorrhagic gastroenteritis. There is poor correlation between faecal endospore counts (on stained faecal smears) and diarrhoea. Combined faecal toxin detection and PCR identification of enterotoxigenic strains is recommended for reliable diagnosis (Marks *et al.*, 2011; see later section on PCR testing, antigen detection and serology).

Clostridium difficile is an important cause of hospital-associated infections in humans and is seen with increasing incidence in community-associated disease. Its significance in dogs and cats is less clear. There are multiple reports linking *C. difficile* toxin production and disease in dogs and one report of disease in cats. Infection has not, however, been reproduced experimentally in dogs. Colonization is relatively common and likely to be transient. A combination of toxin testing by enzyme-linked immunosorbent assay (ELISA) and organism detection (culture, antigen ELISA, real-time PCR) is recommended for the diagnosis of infection (Marks *et al.*, 2011).

Conjunctivitis

Conjunctivitis is the most common feline ophthalmic disorder and is often associated with feline herpesvirus-1, *Chlamydophila felis* and *Mycoplasma felis* infections. Bacteria isolated from cases of feline and canine conjunctivitis are similar to the normal conjunctival bacterial flora (Figure 27.21).

Otitis externa

Bacterial and fungal organisms are not considered to be primary causes of otitis externa. Secondary infections, often by more than one pathogen, are common. Cats have similar pathogenic bacteria to dogs (Figure 27.21; see also Chapter 26).

Septic arthritis

Direct inoculation is the most common route of bacterial joint infection (surgery or penetrating wounds) (see also Chapter 23). Haematogenous spread is much less common but may be seen in neonates.

Common bacterial isolates from infected joints in dogs include *Staphylococcus pseudintermedius* and β-haemolytic streptococci. Less common isolates include Enterobacteriaceae, anaerobes, *Pasteurella multocida*, *Pseudomonas aeruginosa*, *Proteus* spp. and *Nocardia*

Bacterium	Canine				Feline	
	Conjunctivitis/ external ocular disease	Otitis externa	Urinary tract infection	Vaginitis	Conjunctivitis	Urinary tract infection
(Number of references)	(3)	(5)	(7)	(2)	(2)	(4)
Achromobacter spp.						O
Acinetobacter spp.	O	O	O			
Actinobacillus spp.				O		
Actinomyces spp.			O	O		
Alcaligenes spp.			O			O
Bacillus spp.	O	O	O	O		
Bordetella spp.			O			
Brucella spp.			O			
Caryophanon spp.	O					

27.21 Aerobic bacteria associated with canine and feline bacterial infections. NS = frequency not specified; O = infrequent isolate (<10% of isolates); X = frequent isolate (≥10% of isolates); (Isolates include fungi, yeasts, anaerobic bacteria and *Mycoplasma* species where surveyed.) (continues)

Bacterium	Canine				Feline	
	Conjunctivitis/ external ocular disease	Otitis externa	Urinary tract infection	Vaginitis	Conjunctivitis	Urinary tract infection
Citrobacter spp.	O	O	O	O		
Corynebacterium pseudotuberculosis		O				
Corynebacterium urealyticum			NS			NS
Corynebacterium spp.	O	O	O	O		O
Edwardsiella spp.			O			
Enterobacter spp.		O	O			O
Enterococcus spp.	O	O	O	O		X
Enterobacteriaceae (other)		O				
Erysipelas spp.			O			
Escherichia coli	X	O	X	X		X
Haemophilus spp.	O		O	O		
Hafnia spp.			O			
Klebsiella pneumoniae			O			
Klebsiella spp.	O	O	O	O		O
Lactobacillus spp.			O		O	O
Micrococcus spp.		O	O	O		O
Moraxella spp.	O	O	O			
Morganella spp.			O			
Mycobacterium spp.	O					
Neisseria spp.		O				
Oligella spp.			O			
Pasteurella multocida	X	O		X	O	X
Pasteurella spp.	O	O	O	O		O
Prevotella spp.			O			
Proteus mirabilis	O	O	X	O		O
Proteus vulgaris						O
Proteus spp.	O	X	X			X
Providencia spp.		O	O			
Pseudomonas aeruginosa	O	X	O	O		O
Pseudomonas spp.	O	O	O			O
Salmonella spp.			O			O
Serratia spp.	O	O	O			
Staphylococcus aureus		O				O
Staphylococcus felis						X
Staphylococcus pseudintermedius	X	X	NS	X		O
Staphylococcus spp. – coagulase-negative	X	X	O	O	X	
Staphylococcus spp. – coagulase-positive	X	X	X	X		X
Staphylococcus spp.	X		X		X	X
Streptococcus bovis						O
Streptococcus canis	X			X		
Streptococcus epidermidis		O				
Streptococcus equi subsp. equisimilis				O		
Streptococcus faecalis				O		
α-haemolytic Streptococcus spp.	X	O	X	O		
β-haemolytic Streptococcus spp.	X	O	O	X	X	
Non-haemolytic Streptococcus spp.		O			X	
Streptococcus spp.	O	X	O		X	X

27.21 (continued) Aerobic bacteria associated with canine and feline bacterial infections. NS = frequency not specified; O = infrequent isolate (<10% of isolates); X = frequent isolate (≥10% of isolates); (Isolates include fungi, yeasts, anaerobic bacteria and *Mycoplasma* species where surveyed.)

asteroides. Joint infections in cats are uncommon and usually due to penetrating bite wounds. Oropharyngeal flora, including *Pasteurella multocida*, *Bacteroides* spp., *Streptococcus* spp. and spirochaetes predominate.

Cytological examination of synovial fluid will identify an inflammatory arthritis but will not reliably distinguish between septic arthritis and immune-mediated arthritis. Bacteria tend to localize on the synovial membrane and are not visualized in cytology smears. Polyarthritis in cats and dogs is most often immune mediated; septic arthritis is more likely when a single joint is affected.

Skin wounds and infections

Skin infections, particularly pyoderma, are very common in dogs but uncommon in cats, with the exception of subcutaneous bite wound abscesses (see also Chapter 26). Underlying conditions, such as seborrhoeic skin disease, modify the microenvironment so that normal skin flora multiply, increasing the supply of potentially pathogenic bacteria.

Most cases of pyoderma are associated with coagulase-positive staphylococci, predominantly *Staphylococcus pseudintermedius*, which is resident on the mucous membranes of dogs and forms part of the transient flora of the skin and hair coat. Opportunist Gram-negative pathogens tend to be isolated from chronic and deep pyodermas (Figure 27.22). Mycobacteria are an occasional cause of cutaneous lesions, especially in cats (Figure 27.23).

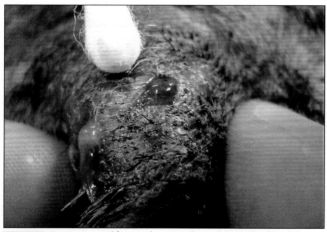

27.22 Pus expressed from a deep pyoderma lesion in a dog with concurrent demodicosis.
(Courtesy of R Wilkinson)

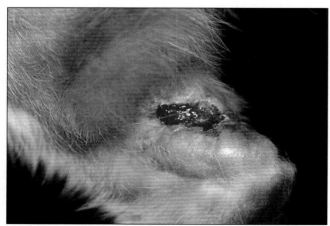

27.23 *Mycobacterium microti*-like cutaneous lesion in a cat.
(Courtesy of D Gunn-Moore)

Urinary tract infection

A UTI is defined as continuing bacterial multiplication within the urinary system detected by the presence of a bacteriuria (see also Chapter 10). UTIs are sometimes asymptomatic.

Urine in the bladder is normally sterile. Voided and catheterized urine samples are contaminated by resident bacterial flora from the mid-urethra to the external genitalia (vagina, vestibule and prepuce). In dogs, bacterial contamination occurs in up to 85% of voided midstream samples and up to 26% of catheterized samples. Contamination is greater in samples from bitches than from male dogs. Contamination is uncommon in cystocentesis samples but has been reported in up to 12% of samples, presumed to originate from the skin, inadvertent enterocentesis, transport or microbiological processing.

Differentiation between urine contaminants and pathogens is assisted by urine sediment microscopy and quantitative bacterial culture.

Urine sediment microscopy

- Midstream voided urine: >8 WBCs per hpf associated with UTI
- Catheterized urine: >8 WBCs per hpf associated with UTI
- Cystocentesis urine: >3 WBCs per hpf associated with UTI

(WBC = white blood cell; hpf = X400 high-power microscope field; sediment prepared from 5 ml urine)

These are guidelines only. Factors that affect the number of white blood cells (WBCs) in urine sediment include the method of urine collection, cell lysis on storage, the volume centrifuged (only small volumes may be possible with centrifuges in practice), the speed and time of centrifugation, concurrent prostatic or vaginal inflammation (free-catch samples), suppression of inflammation by endogenous or exogenous glucocorticoids, the ability of a pathogen to induce inflammation and the administration of antimicrobials. The absence of WBCs does not rule out UTI.

Bacteriuria is quantified on culture and expressed as the number of colony-forming units (cfu) per ml of urine. Interpretation depends upon the collection method. Also, the antibacterial properties of feline urine mean that different levels of significance are used from those for canine urine (Figure 27.24).

Bacterial species associated with UTIs in dogs and cats are detailed in Figure 27.21.

Method of urine collection	Dog			Cat		
	UTI	Equivocal	No UTI	UTI	Equivocal	No UTI
Cystocentesis	>10^3		<10^3	>10^3		<10^3
Catheterized	>10^5	10^3–10^5	<10^3	>10^3	10^2–10^3	<10^2
Voided	>10^6	10^5–10^6	<10^5	>10^5	10^4–10^5	<10^4

27.24 Urine bacterial counts (colony-forming units/ml) associated with urinary tract infection (UTI).

Vaginitis and infertility

Vaginal swabs are commonly submitted from bitches for the investigation of vaginitis and infertility, and also prior to mating in healthy bitches, despite the fact that there are no known sexually transmitted bacterial diseases of dogs in the UK. The relationship between vaginitis and infertility is not a simple one (see Chapter 19), but vaginal bacteriological sampling of infertile bitches without clinical signs of genital infection is usually not indicated.

Juvenile vaginitis is commonly seen in prepubertal bitches and usually resolves at the first 'heat'. Concurrent UTIs are seen in 20% of older bitches with vaginitis. Bacteria prevalent in vaginitis in bitches (see Figure 27.21) are also prevalent in the normal vaginal flora. Usually only one or two bacterial species are isolated from cases of vaginitis, but up to 18% of normal dogs also have only one bacterial species cultured from vaginal swabs.

PCR testing, antigen detection and serology

The principles of PCR testing are reviewed in Chapter 28. Antigen detection techniques have largely been superseded by PCR techniques that offer superior sensitivity and often specificity of detection (Figure 27.25). Limitations of PCR testing are that there is no differentiation between live and dead organisms and that antimicrobial susceptibility testing cannot be performed in the absence of a viable isolate. Serology refers to the evaluation of antigen–antibody reactions *in vitro* and is used in this section to describe the detection and quantification of specific antibodies in serum. These techniques are often used to detect infections with bacterial or fungal organisms that are difficult or hazardous to culture. Detection of protozoal and arthropod-borne infections and detection and identification of haemotropic mycoplasmas are reviewed in Chapter 29.

Commercially available tests

These include, but are not limited to, those discussed below.

Aspergillus fumigatus

* Serology: serum; agar gel immunodiffusion (AGID) test, can detect antibodies specific to *A. fumigatus*.

Pomrantz *et al.* (2007) reported moderate sensitivity (67%) and high specificity (98%) for the diagnosis of nasal aspergillosis in dogs.

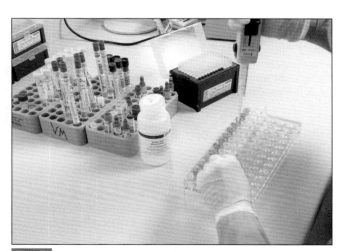

27.25 Manual nucleic acid extraction for PCR testing.

Bartonella henselae

* PCR: ethylenediamine tetra-acetic acid (EDTA) blood, lymph node aspirate, conjunctival swab; identified to genus level (*Bartonella* spp.).
* Serology: serum; ELISA, quantitative.

Bordetella bronchiseptica

* PCR: bronchoalveolar lavage (BAL) samples, or tracheal, nasal or conjunctival swabs.

Borrelia burgdorferi (Lyme disease)

* PCR: synovial fluid, synovial membrane biopsy, CSF, tick; identified to genus level (i.e. *Borrelia burgdorferi sensu lato*).
* PCR tests on blood and synovial fluid are often negative in symptomatic infected animals. PCR on synovial membrane biopsy samples and other affected tissue, such as skin, are likely to be more sensitive. There is little evidence that PCR examination of CSF is indicated in dogs.
* Serology: serum; ELISAs for qualitative and quantitative detection of antibody to C6 peptide, ELISA for quantitative detection of antibody to surface antigens, indirect fluorescent antibody (IFA) test.

C6 is a peptide produced during infection and multiplication in the mammalian host, but not in the arthropod vector. Tests that detect antibody to C6 are relatively specific for active *Borrelia* spp. infection. Quantitative tests are used to monitor response to treatment.

Brucella canis

* PCR: cervical or preputial swab, semen, EDTA blood, urine, tissue, bone marrow; identified to genus level (*Brucella* spp.).
* Serology: serum; rapid slide agglutination (RSA) test or serum agglutination test (SAT).

Serological tests occasionally give false positive results, because antibodies to lipopolysaccharide antigens of several bacterial species cross-react with *B. canis*. False negative reactions are less common.

Campylobacter jejuni and C. coli

* PCR: faeces.

Chlamydophila felis

* PCR: conjunctival or tracheal swabs.
* Antigen detection: conjunctival swab; immunodiffusion or ELISA; qualitative tests; identified to genus level.

Clostridium difficile

* PCR: faeces; *C. difficile* toxin A and toxin B genes.
* Antigen detection: faeces; *C. difficile* toxin; ELISA.

C. difficile toxin ELISAs, designed for human use, perform poorly in dogs, with false negative and false positive results. Currently, a combination of toxin testing by ELISA and organism detection (e.g. by selective culture) is recommended for the diagnosis of infection. PCR tests for toxigenic strains are in use in human medicine, with reported high sensitivity. These assays are now available in commercial veterinary laboratories.

Clostridium perfringens

- PCR: faeces; *C. perfringens* alpha toxin and *C. perfringens* enterotoxin (*cpe*) genes; quantitative.
- Antigen detection: faeces; *C. perfringens* enterotoxin (CPE); ELISA or reverse passive latex agglutination assay (RPLA).

Combined PCR detection of toxin-producing strains of *C. perfringens* (especially *cpe*) and antigen detection of CPE are recommended to improve specificity.

Cryptococcus neoformans and C. gattii

- PCR: CSF, conjunctival or nasal swabs, BAL, faeces; identified to genus level.
- Antigen detection: serum or CSF; latex agglutination test (LAT); semiquantitative; detects cryptococcal capsular antigen.

Antigen detection in serum or CSF is highly specific and sensitive for tissue invasion. There are occasional false positive results. Correlation with nasal cultures maximizes specificity.

Helicobacter species

- PCR: gastric biopsy or faeces.

Leptospira species

- PCR: EDTA blood, CSF, urine; identified as *Leptospira interrogans* (contains all pathogenic serovars).
- Serology: serum; microscopic agglutination test (MAT); quantitative, titres to individual leptospiral serovars; also IFA test.

MAT titres may not rise significantly in acute infection; acute and convalescent sera may be required to identify active infection (4-fold increase in titre in 2–4 weeks). Titres in field infection are usually greater than vaccinal titres but may be reduced by early effective antibiotic treatment.

Mycobacterium species

- PCR: fresh tissue or formalin-fixed tissue.

Initially identified as *M. tuberculosis* complex or *Mycobacterium* spp. Further differentiation of *Mycobacterium* spp. or *M. tuberculosis* complex also available by PCR.

Mycoplasma felis

- PCR: conjunctival, nasal mucosa or genital swabs, nasal or tracheal secretion.

Mycoplasma species

- PCR: conjunctival, nasal mucosa or genital swabs, nasal or tracheal secretion; identified to genus level.

The *Mycoplasma* spp. PCR will also detect *Ureaplasma* spp.

Pneumocystis carinii

- PCR: lung tissue.

Salmonella species

- PCR: faeces; identified to genus level.

Antimicrobial susceptibility testing

Principles of *in vitro* testing

In vitro antimicrobial susceptibility testing is indicated for any bacterial pathogen when the susceptibility cannot be reliably predicted and/or when the organism is capable of developing resistance to antimicrobial drugs. The goal of *in vitro* antimicrobial susceptibility testing is to accurately predict *in vivo* therapeutic efficacy. 'Antimicrobial' is the preferred term when describing susceptibility testing.

Antibiotics *versus* antimicrobials

An antibiotic is a low molecular weight substance produced by a microorganism that inhibits or kills other microorganisms at low concentrations.

An antimicrobial is any natural, semi-synthetic or synthetic substance that kills or inhibits the growth of microorganisms while causing little or no damage to the host

---

Veterinary diagnostic laboratories are likely to use either agar gel disc diffusion or a variant of the broth dilution technique for *in vitro* susceptibility testing. These techniques have several important characteristics in common.

- They are usually performed on aerobic bacteria. Most veterinary reference laboratories do not offer susceptibility testing for slow-growing aerobic bacteria, anaerobic bacteria, bacteria growing in a microaerophilic (low oxygen) environment (e.g. *Campylobacter* species) or fungi.
- They predominantly test antimicrobials intended for systemic use. The pharmacokinetics of oral or parenteral dosing and subsequent plasma concentrations are predictable and measurable. Those of topical dosing are less predictable, with variables including how many drops are given and the presence or absence of organic material.

Agar gel disc diffusion

An agar gel plate is 'seeded' with a standardized suspension of the bacterium to be tested. Discs impregnated with antimicrobials at known concentrations are added to the surface of the plate and the plate is incubated. The antimicrobial agents diffuse out of the discs into the agar until a zone of inhibition is established around each disc. Zones of inhibition are measured and compared with published data. The bacterium is reported as Susceptible, Intermediate or Resistant to a particular antimicrobial depending on the diameter of the zone of inhibition (Figure 27.26). Results have been shown to be 95% reproducible

---

Antimicrobial susceptibility interpretation: agar gel diffusion

'S' means SUSCEPTIBLE: an infection can be treated with a standard dose of the antimicrobial.

'I' means INTERMEDIATE SUSCEPTIBILITY: an infection may still be successfully treated, but only if the agent is concentrated at the site of infection or if higher than normal doses are given.

'R' means RESISTANT: unlikely to respond to therapy

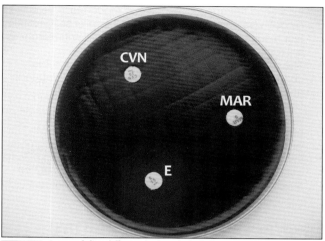

27.26 Agar gel disc diffusion: α-haemolytic *Streptococcus* species from canine urine grown on Mueller–Hinton agar with 5% sheep blood. Susceptible *in vitro* to cefavecin (CVN) and erythromycin (E). Intermediate susceptibility to marbofloxacin (MAR).

Minimum inhibitory concentration

The MIC of an antimicrobial is the lowest concentration required to inhibit growth of a microorganism *in vitro*. If this concentration can be achieved at the site of infection then it is anticipated that a microorganism will be killed outright or its growth slowed sufficiently for host defence mechanisms to eliminate the infection

Automated MIC testing

Automated analysers facilitate the rapid throughput of MIC testing. An example is the VITEK® 2 analyser. This analyser employs repetitive turbidimetric monitoring of bacterial growth at a limited number of antimicrobial concentrations. Growth is significantly inhibited at concentrations greater than the MIC value. The incubation time is reduced to an average of 9 hours (compared with 18–24 hours for disc diffusion and broth dilution techniques).

Interpretation of results

Agar gel diffusion and broth dilution MIC results are compared in Figure 27.27.

- The list of antimicrobials selected for testing is appropriate for the bacterial species and follows recommendations from the Clinical and Laboratory Standards Institute (CLSI), the European Committee on Antimicrobial Susceptibility Testing (EUCAST) and the British Society for Antimicrobial Chemotherapy (BSAC).
- Both techniques classify the bacterial isolate as resistant (R), susceptible (S) or of intermediate resistance (I) *in vitro* to each antimicrobial.

Interpretation of the MIC test results in Figure 27.27 follows a logical sequence:

- Each letter s, i and r corresponds to a test well on a plate. There are 10 test wells for penicillin and three test wells for amoxicillin/clavulanate (co-amoxiclav)
- Antimicrobial is added to each test well in doubling concentrations reading from left to right. The lowest and highest concentrations are given. For penicillin the concentration series is from 0.03 μg/ml in the first well on the left to 16 μg/ml in the final well on the right
- A suspension of the bacterium is added to each test well and the plate is incubated

between laboratories when standardized procedures are used. Disc diffusion is a low-cost, flexible, qualitative method of antimicrobial susceptibility testing. However, the exact concentration of an antimicrobial that inhibits bacterial growth is not determined.

Broth dilution MIC testing

Broth dilution is used to determine the minimum inhibitory concentration (MIC) of an antimicrobial against a bacterial isolate *in vitro*. Tubes, or wells in microtitre plates, contain antimicrobial agents titrated in 2-fold increases in concentration. The range of concentrations approximates to the range of antimicrobial concentrations that can be achieved in plasma. A bacterial suspension is prepared to a standard turbidity and is inoculated into each tube or well before incubation. The MIC is the antimicrobial concentration in the first well in which there is inhibition of growth (the lowest antimicrobial concentration that inhibits growth). The bacterium is reported as susceptible (S), of intermediate susceptibility (I) or resistant (R) to the antimicrobial. Broth dilution testing is relatively expensive to perform and often lacks the flexibility of agar gel disc diffusion testing. Broth dilution testing results are, however, highly reproducible and, critically, present the clinician with quantitative MIC data.

Agar gel disc diffusion		Broth dilution MIC					
Antibiotic	**Result**	**Antibiotic**	**Result**	**MIC**	**Antibiotic concentration range (μg/ml)**		
Penicillin	R	Penicillin	Resistant	≥16	0.03	sssrrrrrR	16
Ampicillin	R	Ampicillin	Resistant	≥16	0.12	ssrrrrrR	16
Amoxicillin/clavulanate	S	Amoxicillin/clavulanate	Sensitive	≤2	2	Ssr	8
Cefalexin	S	Cefalexin	Sensitive	≤2	2	Sssir	32
Erythromycin	S	Erythromycin	Sensitive	≤0.5	0.5	Siiir	8
Clindamycin	S	Clindamycin	Sensitive	≤0.5	0.5	Siirr	8
Enrofloxacin	S	Enrofloxacin	Sensitive	≤0.25	0.25	Ssir	2
Marbofloxacin	S	Marbofloxacin	Sensitive	≤0.25	0.25	Ssir	2
Trimethoprim/sulphonamide	S	Trimethoprim/sulphonamide	Sensitive	≤10	10	Sssrrr	320
Tetracycline	S	Tetracycline	Sensitive	2	1	sSsrr	16

27.27 Agar gel disc diffusion and broth dilution MIC test results for a *Staphylococcus pseudintermedius* isolate. Agar gel diffusion: I = intermediate; R = resistant; S = sensitive. Broth dilution MIC: r = resistant; i = intermediate; s = sensitive.

- Reading from left to right, the MIC is the antimicrobial concentration in the first well in which there is inhibition of growth. This is indicated by a capital letter on the s–i–r scale. In the case of tetracycline this falls in the second well, giving an MIC of 2 μg/ml
- If growth of the bacterium is inhibited at the lowest antimicrobial concentration tested, the MIC is given as less than or equal to the lowest concentration tested; in the case of cefalexin, growth is inhibited in the first well, giving an MIC of ≤2 μg/ml (the lowest concentration of antimicrobial tested)
- If growth is not inhibited at the highest antimicrobial concentration tested, the MIC is given as more than or equal to the highest concentration. By convention, a capital letter is placed in the last well
- The key to interpreting the results of MIC testing concerns the positions of the letters s, i and r. These letters indicate the interpretation of what an endpoint in each well would mean. In the case of cefalexin, an endpoint in any of the first three wells would be considered susceptible, in the fourth well intermediate resistance and in the fifth well resistant
- The 'breakpoint' is the concentration at which the interpretation switches from susceptible or intermediate to resistant.

Antimicrobial susceptibility interpretation: MIC broth dilution

Taking cefalexin as an example (MIC figures in brackets), the following general rules are applicable to the interpretation of MIC broth dilution antimicrobial susceptibility results.

SUSCEPTIBLE (cefalexin MIC ≤2 μg/ml): the antimicrobial is effective at the lowest concentration tested and should be effective *in vivo*.

SUSCEPTIBLE (cefalexin MIC 4–8 μg/ml): the antimicrobial is effective, but not at the lowest concentration tested. Refer to the MIC range to determine where in the range it fell. The closer the MIC is to the breakpoint, the less likely it is that the bacterium will be susceptible *in vivo* to this antimicrobial.

INTERMEDIATE SUSCEPTIBILITY (cefalexin MIC 16 μg/ml): the antimicrobial may be effective in high doses, or if it concentrates at the site.

RESISTANT (cefalexin MIC ≥32 μg/ml): the antimicrobial will be unlikely to reach effective plasma levels. Choose an antimicrobial to which the organism is susceptible

The following additional points should be considered when selecting an antimicrobial:

- The prescribing cascade
- Safety, ease of use and cost
- MIC testing uses concentration series based on plasma levels but antimicrobials show variable tissue penetration (usually low in CSF and high in urine compared with plasma levels)
- If an organism shows resistance to all the antimicrobials selected then this may be overcome by selecting one that reaches high tissue concentrations or by increasing the dose and/or frequency of administration
- Animals with compromised immune systems will require a higher drug concentration than the MIC to achieve bactericidal concentrations of the antimicrobial in tissues
- Generally, *in vitro* antimicrobial susceptibility testing is most successful at predicting failure of a drug to clear infection *in vivo*. The predictive value of *in vitro* testing

for a good therapeutic response is moderate. A veterinary surgeon (veterinarian) must always interpret susceptibility test results against a knowledge of which antimicrobials are most effective at which anatomical sites
- The relationship between the optimal antimicrobial concentration in plasma and the *in vitro* MIC depends upon the mode of activity of the antimicrobial. Concentration-dependent antimicrobials (fluoroquinolones and aminoglycosides) require a high peak plasma concentration compared with the MIC for the infecting bacterium. Time-dependent antimicrobials (most other groups) achieve optimal activity when plasma concentrations are maintained at 4 times the MIC for 50–80% of the dosage interval (Green and Boothe, 2012).

In-practice bacterial culture and antimicrobial susceptibility testing

A survey administered through the Veterinary Information Network investigated biosafety and quality aspects of in-practice bacterial culture (Weese and Prescott, 2009). Most respondents were from North America, with <1% of respondents from the UK. No equivalent data are available for UK practices.

Of those clinics performing bacterial cultures, 96% performed aerobic bacterial cultures only (no anaerobic or microaerophilic cultures); 41% of clinics also performed some form of antimicrobial susceptibility testing, most commonly disc diffusion testing.

The advantages and challenges highlighted by the survey are summarized in Figure 27.28.

Advantages
- Reduced cost to clients
- Reduced turnaround time for results from specimens that yield no growth
- More rapid availability of antimicrobial susceptibility testing results
- Increased numbers of urine cultures with more appropriate treatment decisions
- Perception that results are more accurate because shipping of specimens is not required
- Desire to provide an integrated full service
- Career satisfaction for individual employees with an interest in microbiology
- Alternative service where there is lack of access to a good diagnostic laboratory
- Increased practice profitability

Challenges
- Methodological errors, e.g. failure to use quality control strains in performing antimicrobial susceptibility testing
- Unsuitable equipment in a minority of clinics, e.g. the use of insulated containers without thermostat-controlled heating for incubating cultures
- Antimicrobial susceptibility testing often performed with little or no identification of the organism. Identification is important in respect of intrinsic resistance to antimicrobials
- Failure to provide biosafety level (BSL)-2 containment, consistent with the risk group classification of common veterinary pathogens
- Handling of culture specimens in a non-dedicated laboratory
- Storage and consumption of food in the laboratory area
- Failure to have appropriate protective clothing requirements
- Lack of guidelines, lack of a biosafety manual and lack of supervision by a person with training in microbiology
- Involvement in microbiological procedures of untrained personnel such as lay staff, students and volunteers
- Direct disposal of culture plates into non-clinical waste in contravention of biosafety regulations

27.28 Advantages and challenges of in-practice bacterial culture and antimicrobial susceptibility testing.
(Weese and Prescott, 2009)

Multidrug-resistant bacterial pathogens

The emergence of bacterial species exhibiting multiple mechanisms of drug resistance is a challenge to veterinary practitioners and laboratories.

- Multidrug-resistant bacteria must be isolated, accurately identified and their *in vitro* antimicrobial susceptibility determined.
- Drug choice is likely to be limited.
- Responsible use of systemic and topical antimicrobials must include consideration of the implications for public health.
- Practices may need to introduce barrier nursing and other precautions to prevent direct and indirect transmission of multidrug-resistant bacteria in veterinary premises.
- There is often potential for zoonotic transmission.

Multidrug-resistant bacteria most commonly encountered in veterinary practice include *Pseudomonas aeruginosa*, *Enterococcus* species, meticillin-resistant *Staphylococcus* species and extended spectrum beta-lactamase-producing coliforms (ESBLPCs).

Meticillin-resistant *Staphylococcus* species

Resistance to meticillin (previously known as methicillin) is historically a marker for resistance to beta-lactam antimicrobials (penicillins and cephalosporins) through expression of the *mecA* gene. This encodes a modified penicillin-binding protein, which has a low affinity for beta-lactam antimicrobials. Oxacillin susceptibility usually substitutes for meticillin susceptibility for *in vitro* antimicrobial susceptibility testing.

Both coagulase-negative and coagulase-positive staphylococci may carry the *mecA* gene, but generally only coagulase-positive meticillin-resistant species are considered to be clinically significant. The emergence of meticillin-resistant, coagulase-negative *Staphylococcus felis* and *Staphylococcus schleiferi* subsp. *schleiferi* strains may, however, challenge this assumption.

Enrichment broths and selective media enhance recovery from clinical specimens (see Figure 27.13).

Meticillin-resistant *Staphylococcus aureus*

Meticillin-resistant *Staphylococcus aureus* (MRSA) is an important source of infection for hospitalized human patients and has emerged as an important community-associated human infection. The emergence of MRSA in dogs and cats is a reflection of MRSA in the human population.

MRSA carriage (colonization) in dogs and cats is not common and arises through contact with humans infected with or carrying the organism. Risk factors for MRSA infection in small animals include ownership by a human healthcare worker or hospital visitor. MRSA infection should be suspected with wound infections, surgical site infections, pyoderma, otitis and UTIs that are refractory to treatment. Risk factors include skin damage or disease, immunosuppression, long-term hospitalization, multiple courses of antimicrobial therapy, surgery, surgical implants and the use of catheters.

MRSA (and meticillin-resistant *Staphylococcus pseudintermedius;* MRSP) are commonly isolated from the nares and perineum of infected or colonized animals. There is little data on effective decolonization of animals, but colonization is likely to be transient (1–6 months).

MRSA isolates tend to be susceptible to one or more systemic antimicrobials including clindamycin, tetracycline (doxycycline) and trimethoprim sulpha. Topical antimicrobials, including gentamicin, silver sulfadiazine, mupirocin and fusidic acid, should be considered in all cases of MRSA infection where topical application would be practical.

Antimicrobials used to treat MRSA and other serious infections in humans should be avoided where possible to limit development of resistance to these antimicrobials. These include vancomycin, linezolid and teicoplanin. The use of imipenem and rifampicin should also ideally be restricted. In all MRSA (and MRSP) infections, any underlying condition must be identified and managed.

Meticillin-resistant *Staphylococcus pseudintermedius*

> ### MRSA *versus* MRSP
> - MRSA is primarily a human pathogen; strains infecting animals are likely to be of human origin. MRSP is primarily an animal pathogen; strains infecting animals are likely to have originated from an animal reservoir
> - MRSA transfers both ways between in-contact humans and other animals. MRSP colonization of humans is less common and probably transient
> - Human infection with MRSA is a major medical concern. Reports of MRSP infections in humans are rare

Staphylococcus pseudintermedius is part of the normal flora of healthy dogs and cats. It is also an opportunist pathogen causing infections of the skin and other tissues, ear, body cavity infections and surgical wound infections. Since 2006, meticillin-resistant strains of *S. pseudintermedius* have emerged as an important cause of infections in dogs and cats.

MRSP isolates commonly express multiple drug resistance, often to more classes of antimicrobials than MRSA isolates. This may leave no options for systemic treatment with veterinary authorized antimicrobials. Non-antimicrobial control options should be considered in all cases of MRSP infection. These include wound cleaning, surgical debridement and the use of topical antiseptics (chlorhexidine). Topical and systemic antimicrobial treatment should be based on patient need and the results of *in vitro* susceptibility testing.

Meticillin-resistant *Staphylococcus schleiferi*

Both coagulase-negative *Staphylococcus schleiferi* subsp. *schleiferi* and coagulase-positive *Staphylococcus schleiferi* subsp. *coagulans* are emerging as important veterinary pathogens. Meticillin-resistant strains (MRSS) are prevalent and have been associated with inflammatory skin disease in dogs and cats and with carriage in asymptomatic dogs and cats. 'Methicillin-resistant staphylococci in companion animals' and 'BSAVA practice guidelines – reducing the risk from MRSA and MRSP' can be accessed at www.bsava.com.

Extended-spectrum beta-lactamase-producing coliforms

Extended-spectrum beta-lactamases (ESBLs) are variants of the beta-lactamase enzyme (predominantly AmpA-type) produced by bacteria, which confer resistance to third-generation cephalosporins in addition to other penicillins and cephalosporins. This resistance is plasmid mediated and transferable between strains and species of Gram-negative bacteria (coliforms). Initially, strains of ESBL-producing coliforms (ESBLPCs) caused hospital-acquired infections in human medicine and were probably selected for by the clinical use of third-generation cephalosporins. ESBLPCs, especially *Escherichia coli*, have since emerged and spread in the community, presenting a serious threat to effective therapy for infections caused by Gram-negative bacteria.

Before reporting a strain as an ESBL producer, a confirmatory test must be performed. This requires that synergy is demonstrated between selected oxyimino (second- and third-generation) cephalosporins and clavulanic acid. Manual techniques commonly utilize combination antibiotic-impregnated discs (Mast Group or Becton Dickinson and Company) containing cephalosporin with or without clavulanic acid, on agar gel media. Automated analysers run confirmatory tests in parallel with routine antimicrobial susceptibility tests (e.g. the VITEK® 2 ESBL test utilizes cefepime, cefotaxime and ceftazidime, with or without clavulanic acid) to generate a positive or negative ESBL result.

ESBLPCs have been slow to emerge in veterinary medicine but have been isolated from dogs, cattle, horses, poultry (and other birds), pigs and rabbits. In most cases they are part of the normal gut flora and are not associated with clinical disease. The dynamics of ESBLPC carriage in animals remain largely unknown, but individually kept pets may present an increased risk for direct spread to and from human contacts.

Antimicrobial therapy is not indicated unless there is clear evidence that an ESBLPC isolate is causing clinical disease. In selecting antimicrobials, care must be taken to test all appropriate veterinary authorized antimicrobials before considering those authorized only for human use. The Animal and Plant Health Agency can be contacted via the nearest Regional Laboratory by veterinary surgeons requiring specific advice on managing a case involving ESBLPCs.

AmpC beta-lactamase-producing Enterobacteriaceae

AmpC-type beta-lactamases differ from ESBLs in that they are poorly inhibited by clavulanic acid. They confer resistance to penicillins, cephalosporins (including third-generation cephalosporins) and monobactams (aztreonam). Their frequency remains far below that of ESBLs. Resistance is usually plasmid mediated, as for ESBLs. Plasmids carrying genes for ESBLs and AmpC beta-lactamases often also carry genes encoding resistance to other drug classes, such as fluoroquinolones, aminoglycosides, sulpha-derivatives and trimethoprim. Therefore, treatment options for infections caused by ESBL- and/or AmpC-producing organisms are often limited.

Case examples

CASE 1

SIGNALMENT

10-year-old male neutered German Wirehaired Pointer.

HISTORY

Known to have prostatic carcinoma. Now developed dysuria suspicious for a concurrent urinary tract infection (UTI). Urine was collected by catheterization.

URINALYSIS, BACTERIAL CULTURE AND ANTIMICROBIAL SUSCEPTIBILITY TESTING

- 10–50 WBCs per high power field (hpf) (reference interval <8 WBCs/hpf), 20–30 red blood cells (RBCs)/hpf, moderate numbers of rods
- Swab in bacterial transport medium: moderate growth of *Escherichia coli*.
- Boric acid urine quantitative culture: 6000 cfu/ml of *E. coli*.

Antimicrobial	Result	MIC	Sensitivity range	
Ampicillin	Resistant	≥32	2	sssiR	32
Amoxicillin/clavulanic acid	Resistant	≥32	2	sssiR	32
Cefalexin	Resistant	≥64	4	ssssR	64
Cefovecin	Resistant	≥8	0.5	sssiR	8 ▶

Antimicrobial *continued*	Result	MIC	Sensitivity range	
Gentamicin	Resistant	≥16	1	sssiR	16
Enrofloxacin	Resistant	≥4	0.12	sssiiR	4
Marbofloxacin	Resistant	≥4	0.5	ssiR	4
Tetracycline	Resistant	≥16	1	sssiR	16
Potentiated sulphonamides	Resistant	≥320	20	ssrrR	320

HOW WOULD YOU INTERPRET THESE RESULTS?

Increased numbers of WBCs in the urine sediment are consistent with urogenital tract inflammation (see earlier section on Urinary tract infection).

A bacterial count of 6 x 10³ cfu/ml of *E. coli* in a catheterized urine sample from a dog is considered equivocal in respect of urinary tract infection (see Figure 27.24).

The *E. coli* isolate is multidrug resistant. This includes resistance to a third-generation cephalosporin (cefovecin) and fluoroquinolones (enrofloxacin and marbofloxacin), raising suspicion that this could be an extended-spectrum beta-lactamase-producing coliform (ESBLPC). This was confirmed by the VITEK® 2 analyser ESBL test.

WHAT FURTHER TESTS WOULD YOU PERFORM?

Antimicrobial treatment was indicated by the clinical presentation.

→ CASE 1 CONTINUED

Many antimicrobials concentrate in urine, including amoxicillin/clavulanic acid and cefalexin. An alternative manual system of determining the MIC, the E-test, was employed for these two antimicrobials. The E-test covers a wider range of antimicrobial concentrations than the VITEK® 2 analyser.

MICs for additional antimicrobials, not authorized for veterinary use, were determined by the VITEK® 2 analyser.

E-test MIC results

Cefalexin (Figure 27.29a) fails to inhibit growth at concentrations up to 256 µg/ml. Amoxicillin/clavulanic acid (Figure 27.29b) inhibits growth from 128 µg/ml, the MIC for this ESBLPC isolate.

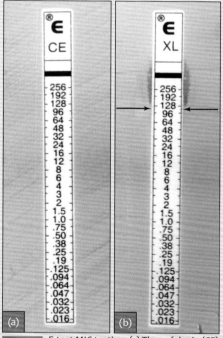

27.29 E-test MIC testing. (a) The cefalexin (CE) strip does not inhibit bacterial growth (bacteria have grown around the whole length of the strip); the MIC is given as >256 µg/ml. (b) The amoxicillin/clavulanic acid strip (XL) shows a narrow elliptical zone of inhibition that intersects the MIC scale where the concentration of the antimicrobial inhibits bacterial growth (arrowed); the MIC is given as 128 µg/ml.

Amoxicillin/clavulanic acid MIC: 128 µg/ml
Predicted mean concentration of amoxicillin/clavulanic acid in urine (dosage 25 mg/kg orally q8h) (Dowling, 2012): 201 µg/ml

Cefalexin MIC: >256 µg/ml
Predicted mean concentration of cefalexin in urine (dosage 30 mg/kg orally q8h) (Dowling, 2012): 500 µg/ml

There was concern over the likely efficacy of cefalexin and amoxicillin–clavulanic acid because of the high MIC relative to the predicted concentration of the antimicrobial in urine. For a 90–95% probability of efficacy, the mean urine concentration of an antimicrobial should be greater than four times the MIC concentration. This was not satisfied for either antimicrobial.

Further MIC testing: VITEK® 2 analyser

Antimicrobial	Result	MIC
Imipenem	Sensitive	≤1
Chloramphenicol	Sensitive	4
Nitrofurantoin	Sensitive	≤16

Imipenem was not selected owing to the lack of an oral preparation and reservation of this antimicrobial for human use where possible. Chloramphenicol was considered but there were issues of cost, likely efficacy and a risk of myelosuppression in both the patient and the human administering the treatment. The use of nitrofurantoin for UTIs caused by resistant *E. coli* is supported in the literature (Maaland and Guardabassi, 2011). Nitrofurantoin was prescribed for use in this patient.

CASE OUTCOME

The patient developed gastrointestinal tract signs on the nitrofurantoin and this was discontinued after 1 week. Amoxicillin/clavulanic acid treatment was substituted at twice the normal therapeutic dose. The urinary tract infection resolved, but the dog was subsequently euthanased because of progressing clinical signs associated with the prostatic carcinoma.

CASE 2

SIGNALMENT

9-year-old female neutered Domestic Shorthair cat.

HISTORY

The cat was missing for 6 months and returned with swelling of the right hindlimb. The right hindfoot was distorted and seeping pus. The right popliteal lymph node was enlarged and there were discrete subcutaneous swellings over the right tarsus with fistulae discharging pus.

RADIOGRAPHY (FIGURE 27.30) AND CYTOLOGY (FIGURE 27.31)

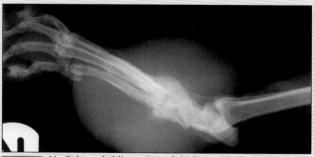

27.30 Mediolateral oblique view of the lower hindlimb of the cat. (Courtesy of K Alexander)

→ **CASE 2 CONTINUED**

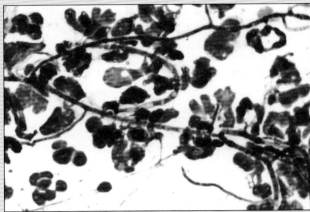

27.31 Impression smear of a sample obtained from a discharging sinus. (Diff Quik® stain; original magnification X1000)

(Courtesy of K Alexander)

WHAT ABNORMALITIES ARE PRESENT?

Radiograph (see Figure 27.30): there is gross soft tissue swelling around the tarsal and tarsometatarsal joints and the proximal metatarsal region with extensive smooth new bone formation. Aspects of the contour of this new bone are irregular, with some hazy mineralization of the adjacent soft tissues.

Photomicrograph (see Figure 27.31): there are large numbers of degenerate neutrophils with a branching filamentous microorganism.

WHAT FURTHER TESTS WOULD YOU PERFORM?

Bacterial and fungal cultures were indicated.

Bacterial cultures isolated *Dermatophilus congolensis*. No antimicrobial susceptibility testing was performed because the isolate is slow growing and no procedural or interpretive standards exist for this bacterium. Ampicillin, amoxicillin and tetracyclines have, however, been used successfully to treat dermatophilosis in cats.

Dermatophilosis is an uncommon infection in cats and tends to be associated with deep abscesses in muscle, lymph nodes and subcutaneous tissues, sometimes with draining fistulae. Fever and anorexia are common, as is a regional lymphadenopathy. Infection through a contaminated puncture wound is likely.

CASE OUTCOME

Therapy was initiated with cefalexin and metronidazole pending culture results. After 1 week the soft tissue swelling had reduced. The patient was then lost to follow-up.

References and further reading

Calvert CA and Thomason JD (2012) Cardiovascular infections. In: *Infectious Diseases of the Dog and Cat, 4th edn*, ed. CE Greene, pp. 912–936. Elsevier Saunders, St. Louis

Carter GR and Wise DJ (2004) *Essentials of Veterinary Bacteriology and Mycology, 6th edn*. Iowa State Press, Ames

Clements DN, Owen MR, Mosley JR *et al.* (2005) Retrospective study of bacterial infective arthritis in 31 dogs. *Journal of Small Animal Practice* **46**, 171–176

Defra (2013) ESBLs – A threat to human and animal health. *Report by the Joint Working Group of Defra Antimicrobial Resistance Coordination and Advisory Committee on Antimicrobial Resistance.* Available at: http://www.vmd.defra.gov.uk/pdf/ESBL_report.pdf

Dowling PM (2012) Bacterial urinary tract infections. Available at: http://www.merckmanuals.com/vet/pharmacology/systemic_pharmacotherapeutics_of_the_urinary_system/bacterial_urinary_tract_infections.html

Greene CE (2012a) Salmonellosis. In: *Infectious Diseases of the Dog and Cat, 4th edn*, ed. CE Greene, p. 385. Elsevier Saunders, St. Louis

Greene CE (2012b) *Infectious Diseases of the Dog and Cat, 4th edn*. Elsevier Saunders, St. Louis

Greene CE and Boothe DM (2012) Antibacterial chemotherapy. In: *Infectious Diseases of the Dog and Cat, 4th edn*, ed. CE Greene, pp. 283–309. Elsevier Saunders, St. Louis

Maaland M and Guardabassi L (2011) *In vitro* antimicrobial activity of nitrofurantoin against *Escherichia coli* and *Staphylococcus pseudintermedius* isolated from dogs and cats. *Veterinary Microbiology* **151**, 396–399

Marks SL, Rankin SC, Byrne BA *et al.* (2011) Enteropathogenic bacteria in dogs and cats: diagnosis, epidemiology, treatment, and control. *Journal of Veterinary Internal Medicine* **25**, 1195–1208

Montgomery RD, Long IR, Milton JL *et al.* (1989) Comparison of aerobic culturette, synovial membrane biopsy and blood culture medium in detection of canine bacterial arthritis. *Veterinary Surgery* **18**, 300–303

Perrin J and Nicolet J (1992) Influence of the transport on the outcome of the bacteriological analysis of dog urine comparison of three transport tubes. *Journal of Veterinary Medicine* **39**, 662–667

Pomrantz JS, Johnson LR, Nelson RW *et al.* (2007) Comparison of serology and fungal culture for the diagnosis of nasal aspergillosis in dogs. *Journal of the American Veterinary Medical Association* **230**, 1319–1323

Posthaus H, Bodmer T, Alves L *et al.* (2010) Accidental infection of veterinary personnel with *Mycobacterium tuberculosis* at necropsy: a case study. *Veterinary Microbiology* **149**, 374–380

Quinn PJ, Markey BK, Leonard FC *et al.* (2011) *Veterinary Microbiology and Microbial Disease, 2nd edn.* Wiley-Blackwell, Oxford

Rowlands M, Blackwood L, Mas A *et al.* (2011) The effect of boric acid on bacterial culture of canine and feline urine. *Journal of Small Animal Medicine* **52**, 510–514

Van Duijkeren E, Catry B, Greko C *et al.* (2011) Review on methicillin-resistant *Staphylococcus pseudintermedius*. *Journal of Antimicrobial Chemotherapy* **66**, 2705–2714

Weese JS, Blondeau JM, Boothe D *et al.* (2011) Antimicrobial use guidelines for treatment of urinary tract disease in dogs and cats; Antimicrobial Guidelines Working Group of the International Society for Companion Animal Infectious Diseases. *Veterinary Medicine International* **2011**, 1–9

Weese JS and Prescott JF (2009) Assessment of laboratory and biosafety practices associated with bacterial culture in veterinary clinics. *Journal of the American Veterinary Medical Association* **234**, 352–358

Weese JS and van Duijkeren E (2010) Methicillin-resistant *Staphylococcus aureus* and *Staphylococcus pseudintermedius* in veterinary medicine. *Veterinary Microbiology* **140**, 418–429

Resources

Mycobacterial reference laboratories in the UK:

Diagnostic Microbiology Service
School of Veterinary Science,
University of Liverpool, Leahurst,
Chester High Road, Neston CH64 7TE
(offers PCR for mycobacteria)

HPA National *Mycobacterium*
Reference Laboratory (NMRL), London

HPA Regional Centres for Mycobacteriology,
Birmingham and Newcastle

Northern Ireland Public Health Laboratory,
City Hospital, Belfast

Royal Brompton Hospital
Microbiology Department, London

Scottish Mycobacterial Reference Laboratory,
Edinburgh Royal Infirmary, Edinburgh

Wales Centre for Mycobacteriology,
Llandough Hospital, Cardiff

Chapter 28

Diagnosis of viral infections

Alan Radford and Susan Dawson

Viral infections of small animals are common and frequently represent an important cause of disease. Although precise diagnosis is not always necessary, it may be required to determine appropriate therapy and prognosis, and to give advice about the potential for disease in other susceptible animals sharing the same environment. In many cases, a presumptive diagnosis may be made without recourse to specific diagnostic tests, based on the signalment, history, clinical signs and more routine diagnostic assays, such as haematology and biochemistry. For example, lack of vaccination and panleucopenia in an acutely ill dog with haemorrhagic diarrhoea suggests canine parvovirus (CPV); mouth ulcers and upper respiratory tract disease suggest feline calicivirus (FCV). However, a more definitive diagnosis may be facilitated by using one or more of a wide range of specific diagnostic tests.

This chapter covers the most common diagnostic tests available for small animal viruses. In order to interpret any given result correctly, it is critical to understand both the biology of the virus in question and the principles of the test used. For a more detailed discussion of virus biology, readers are referred to other texts (e.g. Greene, 2012).

Viral diagnostic tests can be divided into two categories:

* Tests that detect either all or a part of the virus, such as isolation, antigen detection, polymerase chain reaction (PCR) and both light and electron microscopy (EM)
* Tests that detect antibodies produced by the immune response to the virus, following either infection or vaccination.

Virus detection

These tests include historically well established tests, such as virus isolation (VI) and haemagglutination (HA), and newer ones, such as those based on PCR. Some rely on the presence of the whole virus (e.g. isolation, EM) whereas others detect specific components or fractions of the virus (e.g. antigen or nucleic acid). Currently, no one test consistently outperforms the others in all cases, and all methodologies are still used in routine diagnosis.

Virus isolation

Virus isolation (VI) relies on the ability of some viruses to replicate in cell cultures in the laboratory. Clinical samples are taken and usually placed into specialized

virus transport medium (VTM), which restricts the growth of bacterial contaminants in the sample during transit to the laboratory. The VTM is available as a liquid medium in a bottle, which can be stored frozen until required, or in a swab case similar to a bacteriology swab. VI relies on having both functional virus particles and a cell line that supports the replication of the virus in the laboratory. It works best for viruses that are stable outside the host (e.g. CPV, FCV, cowpox virus), but works poorly for very fragile viruses that rapidly lose infectivity outside the host (e.g. feline coronavirus). The cell cultures used are generally semi-permanent cell lines grown as a monolayer on plastic. However, primary cell lines, organ explants, eggs and even whole animals may be used, although the latter is now very uncommon.

In cell culture, virus replication is usually associated with cellular toxicity that is manifested as a cytopathic effect (cpe). Common cpes include cell lysis, syncytium formation and inclusion body formation (Figure 28.1). Usually the combination of the cell type that supports virus growth and the nature or pattern of the cpe is sufficient to achieve a diagnosis. In some cases, the virus may be further characterized by fixing the cells and staining the viral antigens with virus-specific antisera.

The principal disadvantage of VI is the requirement for dedicated facilities to maintain the growth of cells in culture, limiting such tests to specialist laboratories. It is advisable to use the correct VTM supplied by the laboratory, as this medium will have been tested to ensure it is not harmful to the cell culture system being used. Despite the use of VTM, viruses can still be inactivated in transport or the VTM can become contaminated with bacteria from the sample, and this can render the sample unusable. Arguably, the major drawback of VI is the time taken to report samples as 'no virus isolated', which may be as long as 2–3 weeks, and may be too late to inform clinical decision making.

Viral antigen detection in clinical specimens

Antigen detection relies on the ability of viral antigens present within clinical samples (e.g. blood and tissue sections) to react specifically with antibodies raised to that particular antigen. There are two common sources of these antigen-specific antibodies:

* Polyclonal antisera contain a range of antibodies to different epitopes from the virus and usually come from infected animals, such as recovered naturally infected

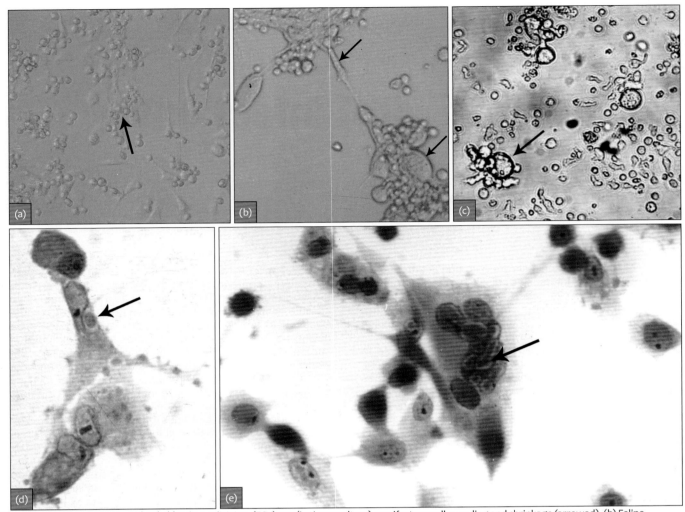

28.1 Cytopathic effects (cpe). (a) Feline calicivirus (FCV) cpe (in tissue culture) manifests as cell rounding and shrinkage (arrowed). (b) Feline herpesvirus (FHV) cpe (in tissue culture) manifests as ballooning of cells and long strands of cellular material (arrowed). (c) Feline immunodeficiency virus (FIV) cpe (in lymphocytes in liquid co-culture) manifests as ballooning of infected cells (arrowed). (d) Cowpox virus causes intracytoplasmic inclusion bodies (arrowed). (Haematoxylin and eosin stain). (e) FHV cpe induces syncytium formation and intranuclear inclusion bodies (arrow shows inclusion body within a syncytium) (Haematoxylin and eosin stain).
(a, © Susan Dawson; c, Courtesy of O Jarrett; d, Courtesy of M Bennett; e, Courtesy of RM Gaskell)

animals, or more commonly larger experimental animals such as rabbits
- Monoclonal antibodies almost always come from experimental mice; they are produced from a single clone of B cells and therefore are specific for a single epitope.

In the first stage of antigen detection assays, the antigen in question needs to be immobilized on a solid surface. In some clinical specimens, the viral antigen may already be immobilized on a glass slide within infected cells, such as in a tissue smear (feline leukaemia virus (FeLV), canine distemper virus) or tissue section (immunohistology) (Figure 28.2ab). In other cases, where the antigen is free in a biological suspension, such as in blood or serum, the antigen must first be captured. This can be achieved with a specific antibody which itself is bound to a solid surface (antigen capture or 'sandwich') (Figure 28.2cd).

Once the antigen has been immobilized, it can be detected by incubation with a specific antibody. Sometimes this antibody has a coloured molecule directly attached to it, such as fluorescein or colloidal gold particles, to allow the direct visualization of bound antibody; immunofluorescence (Figure 28.3) and rapid immunomigration (RIM). Alternatively, the antibody may have an enzyme attached to it; commonly phosphatase or peroxidase (Figure 28.4) that catalyses the subsequent synthesis of a coloured product. However, more commonly, this antibody is unlabelled and its specific binding is detected with a second antibody that is labelled (Figure 28.2bd). In such a two-antibody system the antibodies are referred to as the primary and secondary antibodies.

The best example of viral antigen detection from clinical specimens in small animals is probably FeLV, in which p27 is detected in the blood. This viral protein is produced in abundance within infected cells in FeLV-infected animals and spills out into the serum. The p27 protein may be detected directly on blood smears where antigen is present, particularly within white blood cells and platelets; immunofluorescence (Figure 28.3). Alternatively, it can be detected by antigen capture using either an enzyme-linked immunosorbent assay (ELISA) in a laboratory, or the RIM kits most frequently used in general practice (Figure 28.5). Note that the term 'ELISA' refers to a wide range of tests that take place on a plastic surface and can be used for the detection of either antigen or antibody (see below). The principal advantage of direct viral antigen detection within infected cells is the ability to localize viral

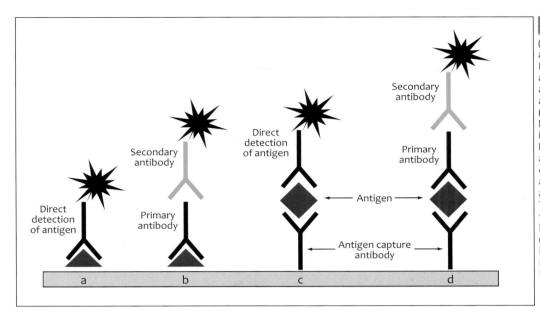

28.2 Viral antigen detection by (a–b) direct and (c–d) indirect methods. The antigen to be detected is in red. In direct antigen detection, the antigen is already immobilized and can be detected either (a) by a labelled laboratory antibody or (b) by an unlabelled primary laboratory antibody which itself is detected by a secondary labelled antibody. In indirect antigen detection (sometimes called antigen capture), the antigen is first immobilized using an antibody to a solid surface. This immobilized antigen can then be detected either by (c) a labelled laboratory antibody or (d) by an unlabelled primary laboratory antibody which itself is detected by a secondary labelled antibody.

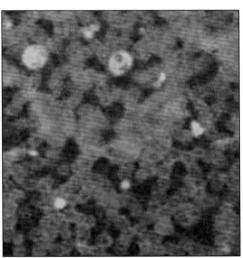

28.3 Immunofluorescence of FeLV antigens in a peripheral blood smear, showing green positive fluorescence in leucocytes and platelets.
(Courtesy of O Jarrett)

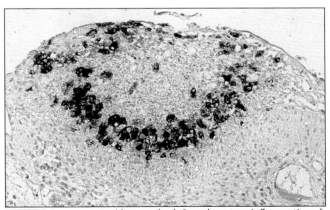

28.4 Immunoperoxidase method. Granulomatous inflammation of the intestinal serosa in a cat with feline infectious peritonitis, showing a central area of necrosis surrounded by macrophages expressing viral antigen.
(Courtesy of A Kipar)

antigen expression to the appropriate cellular compartment, thereby reducing the number of false positives. This does not apply to RIM practice kits and may explain some of the false positives obtained with such tests.

Polymerase chain reaction

Unlike other methods for detecting virus, PCR is unique in detecting the viral genetic information rather than viral protein. PCR allows the specific multiplication (amplification) of small amounts of DNA to a level that can be readily detected. The amplification is specific, being limited to a particular region of DNA (target) by the use of short molecules of single-stranded DNA (primers) that are complementary to the DNA on either side of the target. While the specifics of any given PCR may vary, the principles of each remain the same and consist of denaturation, annealing and extension phases, which are repeated multiple times in the same order.

- In the first stage of the PCR, the DNA double helix (template) is heated to around 94°C to separate (denature) the two strands of DNA (Figure 28.6a).
- In the second stage of the PCR, the DNA is cooled down to allow the single-stranded primers to bind (anneal) specifically to their target sequence in the single-stranded template. The annealing temperature is one of the most critical factors in any PCR and depends on the sequence of the primer (Figure 28.6b; primers in red).
- In the third round of the PCR, the DNA is heated to approximately 72°C. At this temperature, the DNA polymerase extends the primers in the 5' to 3' direction (Figure 28.6c).

At the end of the extension phase, the DNA is again double-stranded and one cycle has been completed. An individual PCR will typically repeat this cycle 35–40 times, with the number of target molecules, in theory, doubling in each cycle. Amplified DNA molecules are detected by running them on an agarose gel, where an electric current separates them on the basis of their size (Figure 28.6d).

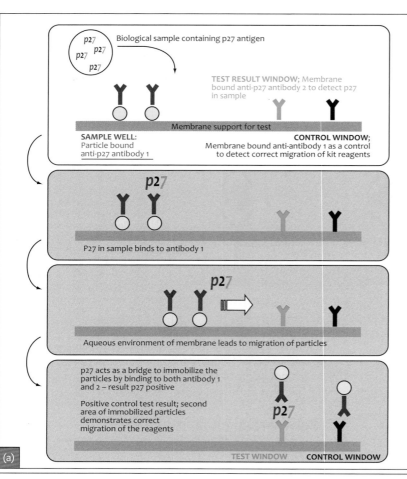

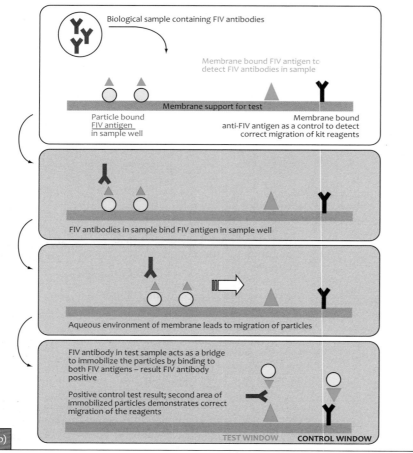

28.5 Examples of rapid immunomigration technology used for the detection of (a) FeLV p27 antigen and (b) FIV antibodies.
(Based on pictures kindly provided by Synbiotics Europe)

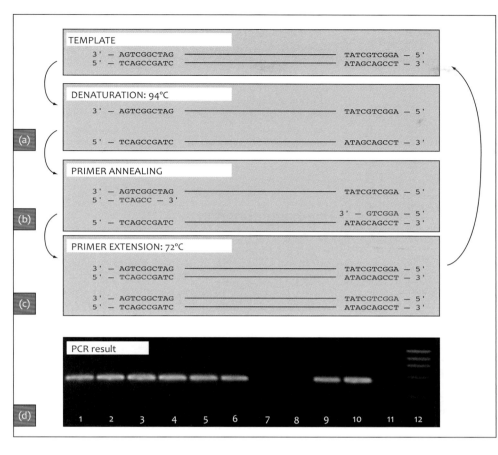

28.6 Polymerase chain reaction. Reactions occur in a solution containing the template DNA, the DNA polymerase enzyme and nucleotides. The template is double-stranded DNA, shown as two black lines with the nucleotides at each end specified; 3' and 5' refer to the different chemical ends of the DNA, and are shown because DNA polymerase extends the sequence only in the 5' to 3' direction. (a) Denaturation: the DNA template is heated, so the two strands separate, allowing access by the primers and enzyme. (b) Primer annealing: at a lower temperature, specifically designed primers (short sequences of DNA, shown in red) complementary to the DNA sequence flanking the area of interest bind (anneal) to their target sequence on the new single-stranded template DNA. (c) Primer extension: DNA polymerase creates a complementary DNA strand (shown in blue) from the primer in a 5' to 3' direction. The result is double-stranded DNA that is a copy of the template DNA. These cycles are repeated and the number of DNA copies increases exponentially. (d) Results of a typical PCR (there is one sample present in each lane): lanes 1–6 are positive; lanes 7 and 8 are negative; lanes 9 and 10 are positive controls; lane 11 is the negative control; lane 12 contains a molecular weight marker to identify the size of the amplified DNA product.

Given that the DNA polymerases used in the reaction only replicate DNA and not RNA, the PCR must be modified for RNA viruses. In this case, the viral RNA must first be converted to DNA by incubation with a reverse transcriptase enzyme; this DNA can then be amplified by PCR. The whole protocol is referred to as a reverse transcriptase PCR (RT-PCR).

The principal advantage of PCR is its speed (a result may be attainable within 1 working day, whereas VI may take up to 2–3 weeks). In addition, PCRs may be set up to detect more than one pathogen, saving on cost and time (e.g. feline herpesvirus (FHV) and *Chlamydophila felis*; Sykes *et al.*, 1999; Helps *et al.*, 2003). Some companies now offer extensive panels of PCR-based tests covering many potential viral as well as non-viral pathogens (e.g. respiratory and gastrointestinal panels).

As well as its speed, a well designed PCR is extremely sensitive, being capable of detecting very small quantities of DNA. Clearly, being very sensitive is generally advantageous. However, the ability to detect even tiny levels of fragmented viral DNA can sometimes bring into question the clinical and epidemiological significance of a positive PCR result. For example, cats that have stopped shedding detectable levels of infectious FHV, as measured by VI, continue to test positive by PCR. In some cases, PCR sensitivity can be increased further by using a nested PCR, where the products of the PCR are re-amplified in a second reaction. With such high sensitivity, PCR may give a positive result when other tests, such as VI or EM, are negative (Mochizuki *et al.*, 1993; Schunck *et al.*, 1995). Nested PCRs are not commonly used because their sensitivity and complexity make them more prone to contamination.

An exciting development in PCR technology was so-called 'real-time' PCR. This system is even more rapid than conventional PCR and also allows the quantification of specific DNA in the original sample. Two types of real-time PCR are generally described. In the first, a non-specific molecule binds to double-stranded (amplified) DNA and fluoresces; the level of fluorescence is proportional to the amount of PCR product. In the second type, a probe molecule binds specifically to the DNA template, between the two primers. Amplification of the primers leads to the degradation of the probe, thereby releasing a fluorescing marker molecule, which again can be measured. Fluorescence can be measured during each cycle of the PCR, giving results in real time, without having to open the tube or run a gel. The cycle threshold (Ct) is the number of cycles when fluorescence significantly rises above background. The smaller this number, the greater the viral load in the original sample. Most new assays are based on these real-time technologies. Real-time PCR and reverse transcriptase PCR are both often referred to as RT-PCR: it is sometimes necessary to clarify which one is being talked about.

In human medicine, real-time PCR is being used to quantify viral load in many viral infections, most notably to stage human immunodeficiency virus infection and monitor the response to antiviral therapy. Quantification of proviral load is important in FeLV to identify those cats likely to develop FeLV-related disease. Ct values are also often reported for other assays such as feline immunodeficiency virus (FIV), and in the future this may aid clinical staging of infection.

Once viral DNA has been amplified in a PCR, its nucleotide sequence can also be determined. This allows confirmation that the DNA amplified by the PCR is indeed the target DNA, and this is important for assay validation. In addition, by sequencing a variable region of a virus genome, strains of virus can be compared and differentiated. This is particularly useful for typing studies, often allowing the source of infections to be identified. While this is not always clinically necessary, it can prove useful in investigating the potential ability of live vaccines to cause disease (e.g. feline calicivirus; Radford *et al.*, 2000). In the future, it may be possible to design PCRs that identify virulent forms of virus and distinguish them from less harmful types. In small animal virology such a test would be of great use in the diagnosis of feline infectious peritonitis (FIP).

The principal drawbacks of PCR are the requirement for specialist facilities (although most laboratories now have these available) and its sensitivity. There have been attempts to manufacture kits that would be used in general practice, but to the author's knowledge these are not yet available for companion animal infections. Because it is so sensitive, PCR is extremely prone to false positives unless carried out in specially designed laboratories by highly trained staff.

Histopathology

Apart from the largest viruses, the vast majority of viruses are generally too small to allow direct visualization of individual virus particles by light microscopy. However, for some viruses, the pattern of the histopathological changes associated with the virus is so specific that it can allow a definitive diagnosis to be made (Figure 28.7). Another common diagnostic feature of some viruses are inclusion bodies, which represent aggregates of virus proteins within the cell. These may be intranuclear (herpesviruses, canine adenovirus) or intracytoplasmic (cowpox virus, rabies Negri bodies, canine distemper virus). In many cases, the presence of viral antigen within histological sections may be confirmed by immunohistology (see above). Such tests are fairly labour intensive and require specialist pathological interpretation. However, they still have their use in those cases where more definitive diagnosis cannot be achieved by other means (e.g. FIP).

Electron microscopy

Perhaps the purest example of virus antigen detection is direct visualization of the virus in clinical samples by electron microscopy (EM). However, virus particles are very small and can easily be missed, even with the electron microscope. EM is particularly suited to those cases where large amounts of virus are present within clinical samples. Visualization of virus particles can be enhanced by first clumping them together with specific antisera (immune EM). Once seen, most viruses have a fairly distinctive appearance to the trained eye, allowing them to be identified on the basis of their morphology and size (Figure 28.8). The use of EM is limited because of its expense, associated with the need for highly specialized equipment, and the availability of cheaper, more sensitive, assays for most viruses. It may still be used for the demonstration of poxvirus particles in clinical specimens (e.g. cowpox virus), or for the demonstration of virus particles in faeces. It also remains a valuable tool in research for the investigation of outbreaks of disease caused by new viruses, where, by definition, specific tests will not be available.

Haemagglutination

For many years it has been recognized that some viruses have the seemingly peculiar ability to agglutinate (clump) red blood cells; this is termed haemagglutination (HA). Although the mechanism by which this occurs may not be known, HA can be used for diagnosis. The result can be confirmed by inhibiting the HA with specific antiserum raised against the virus: haemagglutination inhibition (HAI; Figure 28.9). The best examples of viruses in small animal virology that cause HA are the parvoviruses of cats and dogs, and influenza viruses.

A look to the future

Diagnosing known pathogens can be tricky, but working out the cause of new diseases can be much more challenging: a bit like looking for something small in a haystack, when you don't even know what the 'something small' looks like! Recent advances in sequencing technology have revolutionized our ability to detect new as well as existing pathogens. Collectively called 'next-generation sequencing', these technologies allow a single experiment to generate 1 billion bases of DNA in a few days. As such, the DNA in samples can now be sequenced without the need for primers of known sequence and prior amplification. The resulting DNA can then be compared to published databases to identify any potential pathogens they contain. A recent veterinary example was Schmallenberg virus (Hoffmann *et al.*, 2012). One vision of the not-too-distant future is that all diagnostics aimed at detecting a pathogen will be done in this way.

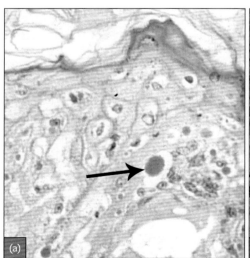

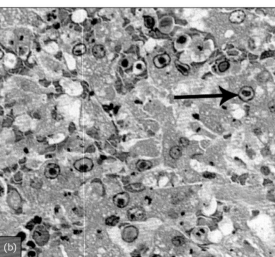

28.7 Histopathology. Lesions can sometimes be used to provide a diagnosis for viral infections. (a) Cowpox lesion in a cat. The arrow indicates an intracytoplasmic inclusion. (Haematoxylin and eosin stain; original magnification X400). (b) Infectious canine hepatitis, showing adenoviral inclusions (arrowed) in infected hepatocytes. (Haematoxylin and eosin stain; original magnification X1000) (a, Courtesy of M Bennett; b, Courtesy of A Kipar)

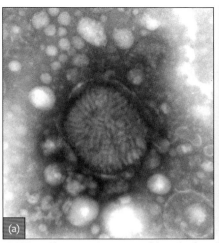
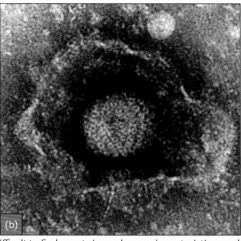
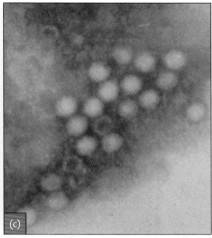

28.8 Electron microscopy. Although often difficult to find, most viruses have a characteristic morphology that can allow a diagnosis to be made. (a) Cowpox virus with typical orthopoxvirus morphology. (b) Feline herpesvirus particle showing capsid morphology and envelope. (c) Canine parvovirus particles in a faecal sample.
(a, Courtesy of M Bennett; b, Courtesy of RM Gaskell; c, ©Alan Radford)

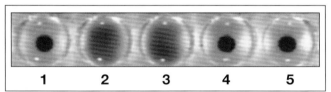

| 1 | 2 | 3 | 4 | 5 |

28.9 Haemagglutination inhibition. The presence of specific antibodies to a virus is detected by the inhibition of red cell agglutination. Where agglutination occurs, cells are clumped and remain in suspension; where agglutination is inhibited, cells settle to form a pellet. Wells 1, 4 and 5 are positive (agglutination is inhibited). Wells 2 and 3 are negative (no inhibition of agglutination). If this were a haemagglutination test, the opposite results would be reported.
(Courtesy of DD Addie)

Antibody detection

In contrast to those tests that directly demonstrate part or the whole of a specific virus to diagnose infection, antibody tests detect the host's immune response to viral antigens, and this is used to infer exposure to that particular virus. For all antibody tests there are some factors that must be considered.

- Antibodies may persist for a long time after acute viral infection and therefore detection of antibodies indicates previous as well as current infection. Where animals are able to mount an immune response but antibodies are unable to eliminate the virus, as with FIV infection, the presence of antibodies can indicate current infection.
- As well as determining the simple presence or absence of a particular antibody, with many antibody tests (ELISA, immunofluorescence, virus neutralization, HAI) it is also possible to determine the amount (titre) of antibody to a particular virus. The test antiserum is serially diluted until it no longer produces a positive reaction in a given test. This point is called the endpoint, and the antibody titre is usually given as the amount of times the test antiserum needs to be diluted to reach this endpoint. Thus, the higher the level of antibodies present in the test sample, the more the serum can be diluted before reaching the endpoint. Although not routine in clinical practice, measurement of antibody levels is being used more commonly to demonstrate a satisfactory response to vaccination (see section below), and it remains an important part of the diagnostic panel for feline coronavirus infection and suspect cases of FIP.

- A rise in antibody levels can also be used to suggest recent infection. This usually means comparing the antibody titre in a sample during acute disease with that in a convalescent sample.
- If comparing antibody titres, it is important to use the same diagnostic method and laboratory for all titre comparisons. This is because there can be marked differences in titres between the same samples tested using different methodologies. Even with the same method in a single laboratory, differences in the titres may be observed for a given sample run on different days. Therefore, an allowance has to be made for experimental error. For many tests, up to 4-fold differences in titre are generally acceptable as experimental error, whereas differences of >4-fold are taken as significant.
- Another method of differentiating acute and previous infection is to look for immunoglobulin (Ig) M class antibodies, which are present early in infection. These IgM tests are not always available for individual viral infections. Examples of such tests include those available for distemper and parvoviruses.
- Antibodies do not develop immediately after viral infection, so there is a lag phase where infection is present but antibodies cannot be detected. This may be the period of time when clinical signs are present and, therefore, diagnosis is required.
- Antibodies are also likely to be present following vaccination and these can make the interpretation of test results difficult. For some viruses, antibody titres would be expected to be higher after acute infection than following vaccination. However, in most cases it is not possible to differentiate between infection and vaccination based on antibody titres alone. Therefore, detection of antibody for diagnosing infection in animals that have been previously vaccinated is not appropriate. Novel marker or DIVA (Differentiating Infected from Vaccinated Animals) vaccines allow the immune response in a vaccinated animal to be differentiated from that in an infected animal. Although no such vaccines are available currently for use in dogs and cats, these may become available in the future.

- The presence of maternally derived antibody (MDA) may interfere with antibody tests for diagnosis. The age of the animal may indicate whether the antibodies found are from the dam. However, some antibodies last longer than others, dependent on the levels acquired from the dam, and there are 'grey' areas where interpretation can be difficult. MDAs cause most problems when screening kittens for FIV infection. In this case, kittens can be tested at 12 weeks of age. However, there is some evidence that MDAs may last longer, for up to 6 months in occasional animals.
- The purpose of an antibody is to bind to its antigen. In circumstances where high levels of antigen are present in the animal, antibody can be bound or 'mopped up', and may then lose its ability to bind antigens used in a test. These can lead to false negatives, and may explain why some animals with end-stage FIV infection test negative for antibody.

Broadly speaking, antibody tests can be divided into two groups:

- Detection using bound antigen (Figure 28.10); tests incorporating this methodology include antibody ELISA, immunofluorecense, Western blotting and rapid immunomigration
- Detection by inhibition of a detectable feature; such methods include virus neutralization tests and HAI.

Antibody ELISA

Commercial ELISAs are most commonly carried out in plastic plates with small wells for each sample. In the general practice setting they are often carried out on membranes. The most commonly used antibody ELISA test for small animal viruses is for anti-FIV antibodies. The

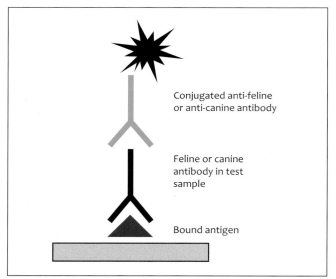

Conjugated anti-feline or anti-canine antibody

Feline or canine antibody in test sample

Bound antigen

28.10 Detection of antibody using bound antigen. Antigen from the virus is immobilized on a solid surface to bind or 'capture' any virus-specific antibodies present in the test sample. Unbound, non-specific antibodies are removed by washing. Subsequently, the presence of bound specific antibody is detected with a second, species-specific, antibody that reacts with any antibody from that species, i.e. anti-dog IgG or anti-cat IgG. This second antibody incorporates a marker system that allows its binding to be detected. This may be a directly visible product (e.g. fluorescein or colloidal gold particles) or, more commonly, an enzyme that catalyses a colour reaction with its substrate (e.g. peroxidase and alkaline phosphatase). The same format is essentially used for ELISA, immunofluorescence, Western blot and RIM tests.

ELISA format is particularly appropriate for processing large numbers of samples and also for measuring antibody titres, and is also used for some in-house test kits.

Immunofluorescence

In immunofluorescence, the test serum (antiserum) is incubated on infected cell cultures. If specific antibody is present, it will bind to the specific viral antigens, and is detected using a further species-specific antibody with a fluorescent molecule attached. The infected cells with the antibodies attached are then examined under a fluorescent microscope and fluorescence is seen where the antibody is present (Figure 28.11). The antibody only attaches to areas of the cell where virus is present; this localization within the cell helps to ensure the specificity of the test. The cell cultures should contain both infected and uninfected cells to improve the specificity of the test; in a true positive reaction only infected cells should fluoresce. The titre of antibodies can be determined by serially diluting the antiserum. Immunofluorescence is used commonly to determine anti-feline coronavirus antibody titres.

Western blotting

In Western blotting, the virus against which antibodies are to be detected is first disrupted into its individual proteins (Figure 28.12). These proteins are then separated by size on a gel using an electric current, transferred (blotted) on to a membrane, and used to detect specific antibodies present in the test antiserum. If specific anti-virus antibodies are present they bind to the individual viral proteins on the membrane and are detected by a secondary antibody system. Positive results are seen as a series of bands on the membrane, corresponding to the individual viral proteins recognized by the immune response. This banding pattern is highly specific for each virus and makes the Western blot a highly specific test. Western blotting is used by some laboratories for the detection of anti-FIV antibodies. It is a fairly time-consuming and expensive test, so is not routinely used for the majority of viral diagnostics. It can be used to confirm positive FIV RIM tests. Because it detects antibodies to several viral proteins it may also be of use in 'end-stage' FIV infection where RIM tests may be falsely negative (see later section on FIV).

Rapid immunomigration

In this RIM test the antigen–antibody complexes are captured on colloidal gold particles and they then diffuse along a membrane to be captured by the secondary antigen (see Figure 28.5b). Where they are captured, a colour change develops which indicates a positive test result. There is also a positive control band to confirm that the complexes have migrated sufficiently along the membrane. If this control reaction does not develop, the test should be repeated, because a false negative result is possible if the complexes did not migrate as far as the test window.

The best examples of antibody RIM tests in small animal virology are for the detection of specific anti-FIV antibodies. These tests are commonly used in the practice situation and have the advantage of being easy to use and rapid. They are usually combined with FeLV antigen detection. They do, however, have limitations and in some cases positive results should be confirmed by other tests, particularly in low prevalence populations and where a positive result is unexpected (see below).

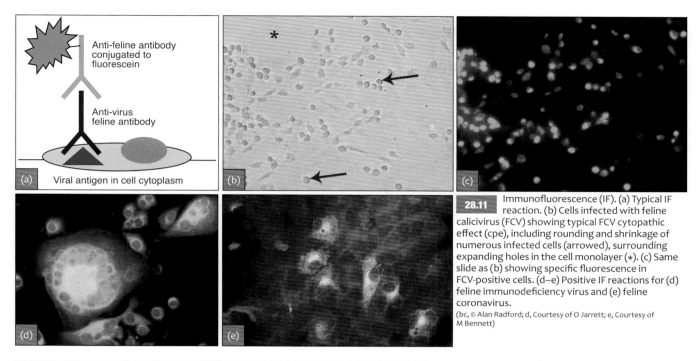

28.11 Immunofluorescence (IF). (a) Typical IF reaction. (b) Cells infected with feline calicivirus (FCV) showing typical FCV cytopathic effect (cpe), including rounding and shrinkage of numerous infected cells (arrowed), surrounding expanding holes in the cell monolayer (*). (c) Same slide as (b) showing specific fluorescence in FCV-positive cells. (d–e) Positive IF reactions for (d) feline immunodeficiency virus and (e) feline coronavirus.
(bc, © Alan Radford; d, Courtesy of O Jarrett; e, Courtesy of M Bennett)

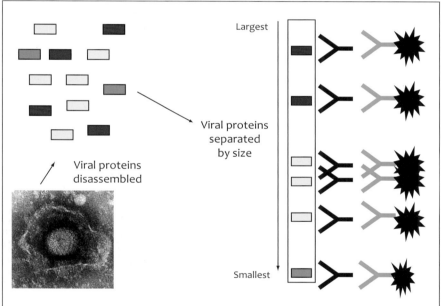

28.12 A typical Western blot reaction. The viral proteins are disassembled and separated on a gel according to their molecular weight. Specific anti-viral antibodies from the patient's serum (black) are used as a target for subsequent antibody detection by the secondary antibody system (blue with black spiked star).

Virus neutralization

Specific antibody in the test sample is used to neutralize a set amount of a laboratory virus. Neutralization of the virus is detected by the lack of development of cpe in cell culture. Virus neutralization tests are relatively laborious and, for many viral infections, have been superseded by newer and quicker methods. A good example of their remaining use is the measurement of anti-rabies antibody titres following vaccination as part of the PETS travel scheme, where the antibody titre has to reach a certain level for the animal to be classified as responding to vaccination, thus allowing travel from certain non-EU countries.

Haemagglutination inhibition

Where viruses are capable of HA, the presence of specific antibodies to these viruses can be detected by the inhibition of this agglutination (see Figure 28.9). Again, the test antiserum can be diluted until no further HAI occurs, giving a titre for the antibodies present. This methodology is relatively labour-intensive and is carried out only at specialist laboratories. HAI is only applicable for viruses that have HA activity (e.g. canine and feline parvoviruses, influenza viruses).

Pre-vaccination screening of antibodies

An oft-quoted principle of medical intervention is 'do no harm'. Reports linking vaccination to what seem to be rare possible side effects (e.g. injection site sarcoma in cats and immune-mediated haemolytic anaemia in dogs) have driven a move to vaccinate individual animals only as often as is necessary (Day, 2011; Horzinek et al., 2013). These guidelines generally enshrine the principle of core and non-core vaccines, and promote the use of less frequent vaccination, particularly for animals at low risk of infection. Antibody testing can be used to give greater confidence to the decision not to vaccinate an animal. Any of the quantifiable tests for antibody described above are appropriate for this purpose and the reference laboratory performing the test will give guidelines for titre interpretation. In addition, in-house assays are available that can give rapid results in the veterinary surgery. Such tests may be used by veterinary surgeons (veterinarians) to help owners decide on the most appropriate vaccination schedule for their pets, and some have suggested they become an accepted part of an annual pet health check. They may also detect genetic non-responders, as well as inform about levels of protection in animals with an unknown vaccination status.

Feline viruses

Diagnosis and interpretation of test results for feline virus infections is often complicated. This reflects complex carrier states, and the frequent use of vaccines that often do not protect against infection. It is essential to understand this biology when interpreting any given test.

Feline calicivirus

Feline calicivirus (FCV) is one of the viruses involved in upper respiratory tract disease. In addition, owing to the large number of different strains of the virus, there can be variable clinical signs ranging from subclinical infection to a severe systemic disease with high mortality.

Until quite recently, the diagnosis of FCV was routinely made by VI from oropharyngeal swabs or other affected tissues (cpe shown in Figure 28.1a). A plain sterile cotton-tipped swab is used to collect saliva from inside the cat's mouth and this is placed in VTM. The VTM is best supplied by the laboratory that is carrying out the isolation. As FCV can be isolated from clinically normal carrier animals, care must be taken when interpreting positive virus isolations. VI does not necessarily equate to disease. FCV usually survives well in transport (providing appropriate sampling has been performed, the sample is in appropriate VTM and it is processed as soon as possible) and grows relatively well in culture so false negatives are not generally believed to be a problem. In addition to VI, some laboratories offer RT-PCRs to detect the viral RNA genome. These have the potential advantage of being quick. However, because FCV is so genetically variable, there is a potential for individual strains to be less efficiently amplified, which may lead to false negative results. Those relying on this test may want to contact their laboratory and discuss the evidence for the strain cross-reactivity of the assay used (i.e. has the laboratory shown that their assay can detect a wide range of FCV strains?)

Tests based on detection of antibody titres (virus neutralization) are generally not used because of vaccination and the high prevalence of infection in the population. They have some use in determining whether a vaccine response is likely to neutralize a particular strain of virus. They also form part of some in-house vaccine check assays. However, interpretation is difficult, because animals with an antibody response to the antigens used in the assay may not have antibodies to locally circulating field strains. Clinicians intending to use these tests for this purpose should discuss this with the manufacturer.

Sequencing of portions of the FCV genome can be used as a method of molecular typing of FCV, although this technique is only carried out in certain specialist laboratories and is expensive. For this test, the viral genome must first be amplified by RT-PCR, either from virus in a swab or, more usually, from virus first grown in cell culture. This typing method has been used in the investigation of adverse vaccine reactions (Radford et al., 2000).

Feline herpesvirus

Feline herpesvirus (FHV-1) is also associated with upper respiratory tract disease and, similarly to FCV, clinically recovered cats can become carriers. It is also frequently associated with ocular disease.

Diagnosis of FHV-1 is most commonly made by VI from oropharyngeal or conjunctival swabs (cpe shown in Figure 28.1b) or PCR, which is quicker than VI, and may allow the detection of higher numbers of shedding cats. Some laboratories offer a combined PCR to detect FHV-1 and another feline ocular/respiratory pathogen, Chlamydophila felis (so-called multiplex PCR). PCR-based assays are generally more sensitive than FHV-1 isolation, and cats that have stopped shedding detectable levels of infectious virus continue to test positive by PCR. A positive PCR result may therefore indicate low-level shedding or viral latency and does not necessarily mean that the virus is responsible for the observed clinical signs. It does, however, suggest latent infection and the possibility of recurring signs in the future. Quantitative real-time PCR gets around some of these problems, with high viral loads suggestive of active replication and involvement of the virus in the clinical signs. The DNA is usually amplified directly from oropharyngeal swab material. It is advisable to contact the laboratory prior to sample collection.

Once infected with FHV-1, it is likely that all cats become latently infected carriers. Shedding becomes intermittent and often follows a period of stress, so latently infected carriers may not be detected by single diagnostic tests, especially with VI.

As with FCV, tests based on detecting antibody titres (virus neutralization) are generally not used because of vaccination and the high prevalence of infection in the population. Some advocate their regular use to determine the need for vaccination.

Feline leukaemia virus

Historically, most FeLV infections were diagnosed using antigen detection, most commonly by RIM. Following infection, cats develop antigenaemia, testing positive for live virus and antigen in the blood. However, most cats appear to clear circulating infectious virus and become negative for circulating antigen. These cats seem to have no elevated risk of FeLV-related diseases such as lymphoma, leukaemia and anaemia and have been considered free of infection.

A minority of cats fail to clear the virus, becoming persistently antigenaemic and going on to develop FeLV-related disease. This is the basis of retesting positive animals 12 weeks later to see if they have cleared antigen.

Recently, following the advent of reliable diagnostic PCRs, our understanding of the biology of FeLV has changed, with important implications for diagnosis. Using PCR-based tests that detect integrated provirus in the blood, it appears that most cats that have been infected remain persistently infected with low levels of provirus detectable in the blood, even though they have cleared circulating antigen (Gomes-Keller et al., 2006). These antigen-negative, PCR-positive cats (sometimes referred to as those with latent or regressive infections) are generally considered to be healthy and to pose little risk for transmission. However, experimentally, virus can sometimes be isolated from peripheral tissues such as the bone marrow of such cats and, in rare instances, chronic stress, immune suppression, lactation or infection with other viruses may lead to reactivation and virus shedding. Therefore, these cats may be considered to pose a small risk of transmission.

The results of such quantitative PCR assays should be discussed carefully with the originating laboratory, in association with antigen results. The mean proviral load in cats that have overcome antigenaemia is several hundred times lower than in cats with persistent antigenaemia. If one is considering sampling a cat to determine whether it is latently infected with FeLV, it is advisable first to contact the laboratory to discuss the optimal sample collection procedure.

Initial screening tests available for FeLV usually rely on detection of free p27 antigen in heparinized blood by RIM or ELISA (see Figure 28.5a). FeLV antigen can also be detected in white blood cells by immunofluorescence, usually on smears of heparinized blood (see Figure 28.3). The sensitivity and specificity of these tests varies, and is likely to be reasonably high for the commercially available kits. However, because of the low prevalence of FeLV in some populations (approximately 1% of healthy cats), the positive predictive value (PPV) of in-house testing is low and more than half the positive results may be false positives (see Chapter 2). This is most important if a positive result is found in a healthy cat, and as a general recommendation positive results should be confirmed by an alternative test. Vaccination does not interfere with FeLV antigen detection tests because a different antigen is involved. It is similarly unlikely that a diagnostic PCR would detect any FeLV vaccine components, because in most cases vaccines are protein based. However, if there remains some uncertainty, the laboratory offering the PCR should be asked to comment on whether its PCR could pick up those recombinant vaccines that contain replicating nucleic acid.

VI is sometimes used to confirm positive results from p27 screening tests, and can be carried out using the same heparinized sample. VI is expected to be 100% specific but may give negative results if the cat is undergoing recent infection or recovery from infection.

As well as diagnosing infection, PCR can also be used to detect FeLV viral genes, for example integrated retroviral elements in the DNA of some lymphoid tumours. The presence of these DNA fragments confirms that the animal has been exposed to FeLV but does not imply persistent infection. These are specialized techniques requiring cell or tissue samples.

Virus neutralizing (VN) antibodies can be detected in feline serum, and the presence of VN antibodies in the absence of viral antigen is an excellent indicator of a protected cat that has previously been exposed to natural infection. Cats positive for VN antibodies do not require FeLV vaccination. Conversely, because the current vaccines may not induce VN antibodies, the virus neutralization test does not give any indication of whether a cat has been previously vaccinated or whether vaccination has been protective. Finally, cats with persistent FeLV infection become immunotolerant to FeLV antigens and do not make antibodies.

Feline immunodeficiency virus

Infection with this retrovirus is characterized by a prolonged incubation period before the development of clinical signs. Once clinical signs develop, they are associated with immunosuppression and accompanying secondary infections, so are very variable. Therefore, cats with a range of clinical signs may be tested for FIV infection, along with many healthy cats as part of routine testing.

Most diagnostic tests for FIV infection detect antibody. For FIV, the presence of antibody is indicative of persistent infection, as the immune response is not able to eliminate the virus. Most samples are tested with in-house RIM or ELISA kits (see Figure 28.5b), but antibodies can also be detected in laboratories with immunofluorescence (see Figure 28.11a), ELISA tests or Western blotting (see Figure 28.12).

Where diagnosis relies on detection of antibody it is important to be aware that:

- Maternally derived antibody (MDA) may last up to 6 months in some individuals
- The time to seroconversion means that infected animals will be antibody negative early in disease. Seroconversion typically takes around 8 weeks but may be longer (up to 6 months) in some cats
- Loss of antibody may occur in terminal disease owing to a combination of immunosuppression and antigen excess. If there is a high clinical suspicion that a cat has terminal FIV-related disease and it is antibody negative by RIM, it should be retested using a different method, such as Western blotting, VI or PCR
- An FIV vaccine is available in the USA. Vaccinated cats will test positive for antibody.

Because of these limitations with antibody tests, it may be appropriate to use VI (cpe is shown in Figure 28.1c) or PCR in certain circumstances.

Feline coronavirus

Feline enteric coronavirus (FCoV) infection is common in cats, especially where they are grouped together in larger colonies. Infection is most commonly subclinical or associated with mild diarrhoea. However, in occasional cats, infection leads to FIP, which is usually a fatal disease. It is not completely understood why some cats develop FIP, although the immune status and genetics of the cat, the strain of the coronavirus and mutation of the virus within the cat are all thought to play a role.

It is extremely challenging categorically to obtain an ante-mortem diagnosis of FIP. High circulating coronavirus antibody levels are often present and are easily measured, but lack sensitivity and specificity for FIP diagnosis. Definitive diagnosis is based on histopathology and immunohistopathology of affected tissues; however, lesions are not always easy to identify or biopsy (see Figure 28.4). In its absence, there are no definitive diagnostic tests available for FIP, and diagnosis is often based on a combination of laboratory tests and clinical examinations. Demonstration of viral nucleic acid by PCR in effusions and cerebrospinal fluid in cats with neurological disease is highly suggestive of FIP, although still may not be completely specific. Positive immunofluorescence of macrophages in effusions is thought to be more diagnostic, but it can be less sensitive where macrophages are rare (Ives et al., 2013). It is beneficial to identify such effusions even if they are not apparent clinically by using, for example, ultrasonography.

Other more routine tests can be helpful as an aid to the diagnosis of FIP; these tests make a diagnosis of FIP more likely when combined with consistent clinical signs, but none provide conclusive evidence. They include:

- Routine haematology: lymphopenia, neutrophilic leucocytosis, non-regenerative anaemia
- Routine biochemistry: hyperproteinaemia (hypergammaglobulinaemia which is moderate to marked, typically polyclonal but may appear monocloncal), low albumin:globulin ratio (<0.8, and if <0.5 increased likelihood)
- Acute phase proteins: elevated alpha-1 acid glycoprotein (AGP) and haptoglobin
- Examination of effusions: high protein content (>35 g/l or as evaluated by Rivalta test (Hartmann et al., 2003)) (see Chapter 22), low albumin:globulin ratio of <0.8 (and if <0.4 increased likelihood), low total cell count (see Chapter 21).

The final step that ultimately allows FCoV to cause FIP is believed to be a mutation in the individual cat. There is increasing evidence that mutations in one particular gene are very commonly found in viruses associated with FIP, and not those restricted to the intestine (Chang et al., 2012). This opens the exciting possibility of a PCR-based test to detect these mutations, and such a test has recently been made available.

Diagnosis of FCoV infection is easier, although the results still have to be interpreted with care. Antibody titres can be measured by immunofluorescence (see Figure 28.11e) or ELISA, and viral genome can be detected by PCR. Several in-house RIM assays are also available. If antibody or viral antigen is present in blood samples, this may indicate infection with FCoV but does not diagnose FIP. Cats should never be euthanased on the grounds of a positive FCoV test result alone. Many healthy cats have positive FCoV test results and never go on to develop FIP. Although not routinely performed, PCR has also been used to monitor FCoV shedding patterns in faeces and may help identify carriers (Addie and Jarrett, 2001).

Cowpox virus

Cowpox virus circulates in wild rodents and can occasionally infect cats, causing skin lesions. It is a zoonotic infection and more severe disease is seen in both human and feline immunocompromised patients. Therefore, care should be taken when handling infected cats and samples.

The virus survives for long periods in the environment and samples of scab material can be transported to the laboratory without specialist transport media. PCR is now probably the preferred method to detect the virus, but VI (see Figure 28.1d) or EM (see Figure 28.8a) may also be used. If tissue samples have been fixed, eosinophilic intracytoplasmic inclusion bodies can be seen histopathologically (see Figure 28.7a).

Feline panleucopenia virus

Feline panleucopenia virus (FPV; also called feline parvovirus) multiplies in rapidly dividing cells and the clinical signs reflect this propensity. The clinical signs range in severity from subclinical to sudden death, with enteritis and panleucopenia. Cerebellar hypoplasia may be seen in kittens infected in utero or the first 2–3 weeks of life.

Where cerebellar hypoplasia is present in kittens, the diagnosis may be based on clinical signs. However, diagnostic tests are required where enteritis or sudden death is the main clinical sign. Commonly used tests include VI or detection (HA or ELISA/RIM tests) of antigen in faecal samples. However, false negatives may occur, as many animals will have ceased to shed detectable viral antigen

by the time overt clinical disease develops. PCR is likely to be a more sensitive method of viral detection in faecal and tissue samples. In-house tests intended primarily for CPV are generally suitable for use in cats but the reader should check their particular kit.

Antibody titres can be measured, although many cats will have antibodies present as a result of vaccination or previous infection. Rising antibody titres may be difficult to demonstrate over the course of infection.

As the name of the virus suggests, affected cats are usually severely panleucopenic and this can help diagnosis. A recent study has suggested that many clinically normal cats may be shedding detectable levels of the virus in their faeces (Clegg et al., 2012). This should be considered when interpreting a positive result, especially in cats with less than typical clinical signs.

Canine viruses

Diagnosis of disease associated with viral infections is generally more straightforward in the dog than in the cat because canine viruses tend not have complex carrier states, and canine vaccines appear to be much more efficient in blocking infection and disease. As such, vaccination history is an important part of the diagnostic workup for canine viral infections.

Canine distemper virus

The clinical signs of acute distemper are varied and depend on the epithelial surface most infected. Possible clinical signs include nasal discharge, conjunctivitis, coughing, dyspnoea, vomiting, diarrhoea and hyperkeratosis. Some dogs go on to develop acute and/or chronic neurological signs.

Ante-mortem diagnosis of canine distemper virus (CDV)-associated disease is not always straightforward. Sensitive RT-PCRs have been developed to detect the viral genome in a variety of samples (conjunctival/nasal/rectal swabs, cerebrospinal fluid (CSF)) and are now becoming more widely available, replacing the more traditional tests.

VI can be difficult but may be possible, and is most likely to succeed from the buffy coat. Some laboratories may use immunofluorescence to demonstrate viral antigen directly in acetone-fixed cytological smears. Suitable samples include conjunctiva, tonsil, buffy coat, respiratory epithelium, CSF, bone marrow or urine sediment. As these tests are not routinely performed, it is recommended to contact the diagnostic laboratory to discuss the most suitable samples for collection.

Paired VN tests (carried out using serum samples) may demonstrate rising antibody titres, but often antibody levels have already peaked by the time clinical samples are first taken. Antibody levels may also be measured in the CSF and this may be more specific in cases of neurological disease. Anti-CDV antibodies are produced locally in the central nervous system (CNS) in animals with neurological disease and are not usually present in vaccinated dogs or dogs with distemper but without CNS signs. In order to rule out iatrogenic contamination of CSF with blood-derived antibodies, a serum:CSF antibody ratio can be calculated and compared to that for another infectious agent. Some laboratories offer assays for CDV specific IgG and IgM and these may aid in the diagnosis of acute disease.

Characteristic histopathological changes found on post-mortem examination include eosinophilic intracytoplasmic inclusion bodies and detection of viral antigen in infected cells by immunohistology.

Laboratory-based VN tests and in-house immuno-chromatography assays to measure serum antibody can be used to characterize the immune response to vaccination and inform the decision on the requirement for booster vaccinations.

Canine parvovirus

Canine parvovirus-1 (CPV-1) (also called minute virus) has been suggested to be a rare cause of diarrhoea. The clinical signs associated with CPV-2 are variable and range from inapparent to severe gastrointestinal disease with vomiting and diarrhoea; severely affected puppies may die within 72 hours of the onset of clinical signs.

In a suspected case the clinician should initially collect a faecal sample for virus testing. CPV-2 can be detected in the faeces of clinically affected animals by isolation, EM (see Figure 28.8c), HA, antigen capture assays, including in-house RIM assays, and PCR. The latter is likely to be most sensitive and now is widely used, with EM and HA being the least sensitive. In-house ELISA/RIM tests have the advantage of an immediate result which is not only important for the patient, but also for in-contact animals and also to inform decisions on whether the animal needs to be nursed in isolation. In all cases, the amount of virus shed in faeces has often severely declined by the time clinical signs develop and so false negatives are a possibility, especially where sampling is delayed. This is less of a significant issue where PCR is used.

Animals that have received a live CPV-2 vaccine within the previous 2 weeks may also have false positive results on some faecal virus tests. The precise duration of these positive tests in vaccinated animals is not yet known. Some molecular assays can differentiate vaccine and field strains of virus, but these are not widely available.

Antibody levels can be measured against CPV-2 but may be difficult to interpret, and are complicated by MDA and vaccination. High antibody titres in unvaccinated animals that have been sick for ≥3 days are highly suggestive of CPV infection. Since antibody levels are often high by the time clinical signs develop, it is often not possible to demonstrate rising antibody titres. Measurement of IgM levels may be offered by some laboratories and is likely to be more useful in cases of acute disease.

HAI (see Figure 28.9) as well as in-house assays can be used to characterize the immune response to vaccination and inform the decision on the requirement for booster vaccinations.

Canine coronavirus

Canine enteric coronavirus infection is generally associated with only mild diarrhoea. Virus can be isolated from fresh faecal samples providing they arrive at the laboratory quickly, although not all strains can be isolated this way. PCR tests are now available and are probably more reliable.

Canine respiratory coronavirus is a relatively recently identified addition to the potential causes of 'kennel cough'. Diagnostic PCR assays are available, often in combination with other pathogens associated with this syndrome.

Canine herpesvirus

The clinical signs associated with canine herpesvirus are varied and depend on the age of the dog when infected. They range from abortion and stillbirth to fading puppy syndrome and mild respiratory disease in puppies; more rarely, canine herpesvirus causes vesicular genital lesions in adults.

Virus can be isolated from many tissues in cases of fading puppy syndrome, including the kidneys and adrenal glands, lungs, spleen, liver and lymph nodes. In adult dogs, the virus can normally only be isolated from the oral mucosa and the respiratory and genital tracts. PCR tests are also now available and appear to be sensitive. On post-mortem examination, intranuclear inclusion bodies are evident in affected organs. Some dogs may be vaccinated against canine herpesvirus. Since these vaccines are inactived they should not interfere with tests that look for the virus itself. Serology for antibodies may be commercially available and can be useful in dogs that have not been vaccinated.

Canine adenovirus

The clinical signs associated with canine adenovirus (CAV) type 1 infection are variable and range from mild pyrexia to acute abdominal catastrophe and death. CAV-2 is one of the pathogens associated with the 'kennel cough' complex.

In the more severe cases of CAV-1-associated disease, hepatic necrosis leads to marked biochemical changes and disseminated intravascular coagulopathy are suggestive of infection.

VI from throat swabs in laboratory VTM can be used to demonstrate infection; the virus grows readily. PCR tests are also now available that can differentiate the types. On post-mortem examination, liver changes are often quite specific for CAV-1 infection and include intranuclear inclusion bodies (see Figure 28.7b). Similar inclusion bodies are evident in the respiratory epithelium of dogs with CAV-2-associated kennel cough. Immunohistology may also be available at some laboratories, and may be performed on acetone-fixed impressions for rapid diagnosis.

Laboratory-based VN tests and in-house immuno-chromatography assays are available to measure anti-CAV-1 serum antibody and can be used to characterize the immune response to vaccination and assess the need for booster vaccination.

Canine parainfluenza virus

Like CAV-2, canine parainfluenza virus is one of the pathogens associated with the 'kennel cough' complex. Diagnosis is by virus isolation from an oropharyngeal swab in VTM, virus neutralization test or by PCR.

Canine influenza virus

Influenza viruses are being increasingly recognized as a potential cause of 'kennel cough' syndrome. In the USA, influenza H3N8 of equine origin has adapted to the canine host, causing widespread infection, and vaccines are now marketed. PCR-based assays are now available, and should be considered, especially in outbreaks of disease that lack another cause, where there is a history of travel to the USA, where there is close contact with horses, and possibly where there is contact with humans with confirmed influenza.

Rabies virus

Rabies virus is a neurotropic virus capable of infecting many animal species worldwide, including humans. Although clinical signs can be variable, a progression is often described through prodromal (behavioural changes), excitative (nervousness, aggression, tremors, spasms, vocalization) and paralytic (incoordination, convulsions, paralysis, coma) phases. Infection is usually fatal in the absence of specific post-exposure immune therapy. Rabies is a notifiable disease.

Veterinary surgeons suspecting a case of rabies based on history and clinical signs should detain the animal and notify the local veterinary officer. Specific diagnosis is coordinated by government agencies (Defra in the UK) and carried out by a specialist laboratory. Possible tests used to detect virus include VI (initially in mice but mostly now replaced by cell culture) or PCR. Histopathological examination shows characteristic Negri inclusion bodies in the brain. Immunological techniques can be used to confirm the specificity of antigen in cell cultures or fixed tissues.

While it is hoped that veterinary surgeons in the UK are unlikely to be involved in diagnosing rabies infection, it is now common for owners to request vaccination under the UK PETS Travel Scheme. Until recently, in order to be certified, all animals had to show an adequate response to vaccination. More recently, following changes to the relevant legislation, only animals entering the EU from certain non-listed countries still need to be tested to confirm vaccine response. Serum samples for this purpose must be sent to an approved laboratory where a fluorescent antibody virus neutralization test is usually carried out.

Case examples

CASE 1

SIGNALMENT

10-week-old male Siamese kitten.

HISTORY

Recently purchased from the breeder and received first vaccine (live attenuated) against FCV, FHV-1 and FPV four days ago. The kitten presented with clinical signs of inappetence, mild lethargy, mouth ulcers and slight ocular discharge.

WHAT ARE YOUR DIFFERENTIAL DIAGNOSES?

FCV is the most likely differential. FHV-1 could cause an ocular discharge and lethargy but not usually mouth ulcers.

WHICH TESTS WOULD YOU PERFORM?

Sampling for FCV and FHV-1, by either PCR or VI.

VIRUS RESULTS

A plain swab in VTM is submitted for FCV/FHV-1 PCR. The cat tests positive for FCV but negative for FHV-1.

HOW WOULD YOU INTERPRET THESE RESULTS?

The mouth ulcers in conjunction with the other clinical signs are consistent with acute FCV infection. This is confirmed by the positive PCR. FCV infection does cause a carrier state and is shed by ~10% of clinically normal cats. However, the positive test with the range of clinical signs is strong evidence that this is a clinical case of acute FCV infection. The recent history of live vaccination may lead some to ask if the vaccine is involved in the disease. In very rare cases there is some evidence that vaccine virus may play such a role. However, published evidence suggests such cases are rare, with field virus much more frequently implicated, being picked up either at the breeder's premises, at the veterinary clinic, or in the new home (Radford *et al.*, 1997). Whether field virus or vaccine virus is involved can be determined by RT-PCR and sequencing. This is a non-standard assay offered by some laboratories. Veterinary surgeons could contact their vaccine manufacturer to discuss options further.

CASE 2

SIGNALMENT

17-week-old male British Shorthair cat.

HISTORY

5-day history of vague inappetence, lethargy and possible mild faecal tenesmus. The cat was thin and lethargic, hypothermic (34°C) but ambulatory on presentation. There was a mildly distended abdomen with a small palpable bladder. The intestines felt empty.

WHAT ARE YOUR DIFFERENTIAL DIAGNOSES?

The mildly distended abdomen could be due to free fluid, gas or a mass. Poor body condition, hypothermia and lethargy are non-specific findings.

WHAT INVESTIGATIONS WOULD YOU PERFORM?

Haematology, biochemistry and abdominal imaging would be useful to investigate possible causes for the abdominal distention and more general clinical signs.

CLINICAL PATHOLOGY DATA

Haematology	Results	Reference interval
RBC (x 10^{12}/l)	**6.99**	7.00–11.6
Haematocrit (l/l)	**0.24**	0.29–0.46
Haemoglobin (g/dl)	**7.6**	9.0–14.0
MCV (fl)	38.0	37.0–47.6
MCHC (g/dl)	31.7	26.2–35.9
MCH (pg)	**10.9**	11.3–17.2
Reticulocytes (x 10^9/l)	10	<60

Abnormal results are in **bold.**

→ CASE 2 CONTINUED

Haematology *continued*	Results	Reference interval
WBC (x 10⁹/l)	18.49	5.5–19.5
Neutrophils (band) (x 10⁹/l)	0.37	0.0–0.5
Neutrophils (segmented) (x 10⁹/l)	**13.1**	2.5–12.5
Lymphocytes (x 10⁹/l)	2.96	1.5–7.0
Monocytes (x 10⁹/l)	**2.03**	0.0–1.0
Eosinophils (x 10⁹/l)	0.0	0.0–1.5
Basophils (x 10⁹/l)	0.0	0.0–0.1
Platelets (x 10⁹/l)	456	250–800

Abnormal results are in **bold**.

Film comment: red and white cell morphology normal.

Biochemistry	Results	Reference interval
Total protein (g/l)	57	54–78
Albumin (g/l)	**20**	24–39
Globulin (g/l)	37	20–45
ALP (IU/l)	**3**	4–62
ALT (IU/l)	**12**	30–85
Sodium (mmol/l)	**135**	138–155
Potassium (mmol/l)	5.0	3.6–5.6
Chloride (mmol/l)	**103**	112–129
Calcium (mmol/l)	2.2	2.1–2.6
Inorganic phosphate (mmol/l)	**2.4**	1.0–1.9
Glucose (mmol/l)	**4.0**	4.3–6.6
Urea (mmol/l)	8.1	6.0–10.0
Creatinine (µmol/l)	42	40–150
Cholesterol (mmol/l)	**5.1**	1.9–3.9
Bilirubin (µmol/l)	**29**	0–10

Abnormal results are in **bold**.

WHAT ARE THE SIGNIFICANT ABNORMALITIES AND THE POSSIBLE CAUSES OF THESE?

The mild hypoalbuminaemia could be secondary to third-space loss into an effusion, but is not low enough to cause an effusion. It could also be due to intestinal or renal loss, or decreased hepatic production. Third-space loss is the most likely cause for the low sodium and chloride. There is a mild increase in bilirubin, without significant anaemia. Prehepatic causes are excluded and there are no elevations in liver enzymes to support hepatic or posthepatic causes. Bilirubin can increase in FIP, though the mechanisms are not fully understood.

There is a mild non-regenerative anaemia, which could be secondary to chronic inflammatory disease or possibly acute blood loss. The leucogram is consistent with an established inflammatory response.

RADIOGRAPHY AND ULTRASONOGRAPHY

The abdomen is moderately distended, with poor overall serosal detail. Ultrasonography shows small pockets of ascites, which can be sampled under ultrasound guidance.

WHAT FURTHER TESTS WOULD YOU PERFORM?

As the cause of the abdominal distension has been confirmed as an effusion, obtaining a sample of the fluid is the next priority. Initially, tests to categorize the type of effusion are most appropriate.

ASCITIC FLUID ANALYSIS

Parameter	Results
Appearance	Clear, bright yellow
Nucleated cell count	12.3 x 10⁹/l
Total protein	46 g/l
Albumin	19 g/l
Globulin	27 g/l
Albumin:globulin ratio	0.7
Cytology	85% neutrophils, 10% macrophages, 5% small lymphocytes. No organisms seen

HOW WOULD YOU CLASSIFY THIS EFFUSION AND WHICH FURTHER TESTS WOULD YOU PERFORM?

The effusion is an exudate with a moderately high cellularity and a high protein content with a predominance of globulin and a low albumin:globulin (A:G) ratio. This raises suspicion for FIP and so an alpha-1 acid glycoprotein (AGP) and a coronavirus antibody titre on the serum and coronavirus PCR on the fluid would be helpful.

FURTHER RESULTS

Parameter	Results
Coronavirus antibody (serum)	1280
Alpha-1 AGP (µg/ml) (serum) (reference interval 0–500)	**3360**
Coronavirus PCR (ascitic fluid)	**Positive with high viral load at 258 x 10⁵**

Abnormal results are in **bold**.

INTERPRETATION

The coronavirus antibody titre in the serum is high (>640 is considered high). Antibodies in young kittens can be maternally derived but not normally after 14 weeks, and are not likely to be so high, together suggesting they are endogenously derived in this case.

Several factors consistently point to a diagnosis of FIP, including the high FCoV serum antibody, high AGP and a sterile exudate with an A:G ratio less than 0.81. Most definitive is the high viral load in the ascitic fluid. The key to diagnosis in this case was recognizing and obtaining a sample of the ascitic fluid.

OUTCOME

The cat deteriorated acutely, becoming collapsed and non-responsive, and was euthanased. Post-mortem examination revealed diffuse marked acute fibrinous and exudative serositis, peritonitis and phlebitis consistent with FIP.

References and further reading

Addie DD and Jarrett O (2001) Use of a reverse-transcriptase polymerase chain reaction for monitoring the shedding of feline coronavirus by healthy cats. *Veterinary Record* **148**, 649–653

Chang HW, Egberink HF, Halpin R, Spiro DJ and Rottier PJ (2012) Spike protein fusion peptide and feline coronavirus virulence. *Emerging Infectious Diseases* **18**, 1089–1095

Clegg SR, Coyne KP, Dawson S, Spibey N, Gaskell RM and Radford AD (2012) Canine parvovirus in asymptomatic feline carriers. *Veterinary Microbiology* **157**, 78–85

Day MJ (2011) Vaccination of dogs and cats: no longer so controversial? *Veterinary Record* **168**, 480–482

Gomes-Keller MA, Gonczi E, Tandon R et al. (2006) Detection of feline leukemia virus RNA in saliva from naturally infected cats and correlation of PCR results with those of current diagnostic methods. *Journal of Clinical Microbiology* **44**, 916–922

Greene CE (2012) *Infectious Diseases of the Dog and Cat, 4th edn.* WB Saunders, Philadelphia

Hartmann K, Binder C, Hirschberger J et al. (2003) Comparison of different tests to diagnose feline infectious peritonitis. *Journal of Veterinary Internal Medicine* **17**, 781–790

Hartmann K, Werner RM, Egberink H and Jarrett O (2001) Comparison of six in-house diagnostic tests for the rapid diagnosis of feline immunodeficiency virus and feline leukaemia virus infections. *Veterinary Record* **149**, 317–320

Helps C, Reeves N, Egan K, Howard P and Harbour D (2003) Detection of *Chlamydophila felis* and feline herpesvirus by multiplex real-time PCR analysis. *Journal of Clinical Microbiology* **41**, 2734–2736

Hoffmann B, Scheuch M, Höper D et al. (2012) Novel orthobunyavirus in Cattle, Europe, 2011. *Emerging Infectious Diseases* **18**, 469–472

Horzinek MC, Addie D, Belák S et al. (2013) ABCD: Update of the 2009 Guidelines on Prevention and Management of Feline Infectious Diseases. *Journal of Feline Medicine and Surgery* **15**, 530–539

Ives EJ, Vanhaesebrouck AE and Cian F (2013) Immunocytochemical demonstration of feline infectious peritonitis virus within cerebrospinal fluid macrophages. *Journal of Feline Medicine and Surgery* **15**, 1149–1153

Mochizuki M, San Gabriel MC, Nakatani H, Yoshida M and Harasawa R (1993) Comparison of polymerase chain reaction with virus isolation and haemagglutination assays for the detection of canine parvoviruses in faecal specimens. *Research in Veterinary Science* **55**, 60–63

Radford AD, Bennett M, McArdle F et al. (1997) The use of sequence analysis of a feline calicivirus (FCV) hypervariable region in the epidemiological investigation of FCV related disease and vaccine failures. *Vaccine* **15**, 1451–1458

Radford AD, Dawson S, Wharmby C, Ryvar R and Gaskell RM (2000) Comparison of serological and sequence-based methods for typing feline calicivirus isolates from vaccine failures. *Veterinary Record* **146**, 117–123

Schunck B, Kraft W and Truyen U (1995) A simple touch-down polymerase chain reaction for the detection of canine parvovirus and feline panleukopenia virus in feces. *Journal of Virology Methods* **55**, 427–433

Sykes JE, Anderson GA, Studdert VP and Browning GF (1999) Prevalence of feline *Chlamydia psittaci* and feline herpesvirus 1 in cats with upper respiratory tract disease. *Journal of Veterinary Internal Medicine* **13**, 153–162

Chapter 29

Diagnosis of protozoal and arthropod-borne diseases

Laia Solano-Gallego and Gad Baneth

Protozoal and arthropod-borne infections cause important diseases in dogs and cats. Some diseases, particularly arthropod-borne, are endemic to some areas because they are transmitted by vectors restricted by geographical boundaries. However, these diseases are frequently also presented in non-endemic areas as a result of the travel and importation of animals. In addition, some of these diseases are zoonotic and, therefore, of public health concern. Arthropod-borne diseases are common in the Mediterranean countries of Europe and some of them are endemic in Central and Northern Europe. The importance of arthropod-borne diseases is increasing in non-endemic areas because of climate change and the spread northwards of infections, and owing to the increasing number of animals travelling abroad or imported. The main protozoal and arthropod-borne diseases of small domestic animals that are currently endemic in the UK include neosporosis, toxoplasmosis, anaplasmosis, bartonellosis, borreliosis, haemoplasmosis and also gastrointestinal parasitic infections such as giardiasis and cryptosporidiosis (see Chapter 13, and the *BSAVA Manual of Canine and Feline Haematology and Transfusion Medicine*). This chapter describes the diagnosis of protozoal and arthropod-borne diseases of dogs and cats, with an overview of geographical distribution, main transmission modes, chief clinical signs, clinicopathological abnormalities and diagnostic methods.

General laboratory diagnosis of protozoal and arthropod-borne diseases

The classical concept of an infectious disease as a process which includes three consecutive stages; infection, an incubation period and acute clinical disease, is not always followed in the diseases described in this chapter. Infection may occur without evidence of disease, and animals may be carriers of infection, or disease may be chronic without a clear acute stage. Subclinical carriers are common in persistent insidious chronic arthropod-borne infections such as *Leishmania infantum* infection. This has important diagnostic implications because animals may be infected without detectable seroconversion, and persistent infections may be present simultaneously with other disease conditions and not necessarily be responsible for the clinical signs observed.

Diagnosis is usually performed to confirm disease in a dog or cat with clinical signs or clinicopathological abnormalities compatible with protozoal or arthropod-borne disease. However, detection of infection may also be pursued for research studies, for screening clinically healthy animals living in endemic regions, to prevent transmission by blood transfusion, to avoid importation of infected dogs and cats to non-endemic countries, and to monitor response to treatment for the detection of the pathogen. Different diagnostic procedures can be used, depending on the purpose of the diagnostic investigation, e.g. for the confirmation of a disease in a dog with compatible clinical signs, or for the detection of a subclinically infected blood donor, and most likely to be affecting the dog or cat, based on the differential diagnosis list. Test result interpretation will be influenced by the type of pathogen and the clinical status of the animal.

Accurate diagnosis of these diseases requires an integrated approach consisting of thorough clinical history, physical examination, pertinent routine laboratory tests such as complete blood count (CBC), complete biochemical profile, urinalysis and specific pathogen diagnostic assays. Correct diagnosis is most likely to be obtained when multiple pathogen diagnostic assays are used, including microscopic examination, serology and molecular assays. Moreover, the presence of co-infections or concomitant diseases might complicate the diagnosis.

Main diagnostic techniques

The main techniques for the diagnosis of protozoal and arthropod-borne infections employed in clinical practice are microscopic examination of microorganisms in cytological preparations or histopathological specimens, serology, polymerase chain reaction (PCR) and culture of the organism in appropriate medium. The advantages and disadvantages of these diagnostic techniques are listed in Figure 29.1.

Microscopic examination

Diagnosis can be based on cytological or histological detection of pathogens, either contained inside cells or free in routinely stained smears. Detection by light microscopy may be difficult, depending on the type of microorganisms causing infection. Cytology is a more rapid and simple technique than histopathology for the detection of some microorganisms. Histopathology commonly requires special staining to detect bacterial, mycobacterial, fungal

Diagnostic technique	Advantages	Disadvantages
Serology (antibody detection)	• Detection of antibodies formed against the pathogen causing infection • Permits evaluation of seroconversion to confirm recent infection	• Does not detect the actual presence of pathogen • Does not differentiate between vaccinated and naturally infected animals or those with maternally derived antibodies • Serological cross-reactivity between related organisms is possible
Qualitative	• Rapid in-clinic test • Cheap to run	• Provides only positive or negative results • Variable sensitivities and performance with risk of false negative results due to conservative cut-off level and use of recombinant proteins • A positive result will benefit from additional validation by quantitative serology
Quantitative (IFAT, ELISA)	• Determines the antibody level, which is of major importance in some diseases such as leishmaniosis where high antibody levels in the presence of compatible clinical signs and/or clinicopathological abnormalities are diagnostic for clinical leishmaniosis	• Performance and accuracy of cut-off vary among laboratories • Frequent lack of sufficient standardization of techniques among laboratories • Low antibody levels frequently require further testing
Microscopic examination (cytology/histopathology)	• Permits direct detection of the pathogen and nature of the host response ○ Findings could be suspicious of infection or allow exclusion of other differential diagnoses • Cytology is rapid and less invasive than obtaining tissues for histopathology by biopsy • Cytology usually permits easier visualization of pathogens compared with histopathology	• Relatively low sensitivity for the detection of pathogens in tissues or body fluids • Requires further diagnostic tests such as immunohistochemistry and/or PCR when pathogens are not visualized • Does not differentiate morphologically similar organisms • Requires experience
PCR	• Allows the detection of pathogen DNA • High sensitivity and specificity for target loci • Allows pathogen load quantification (by real-time PCR)	• False positive results possible owing to DNA contamination or to amplification of erroneous targets including host DNA • Different techniques used by diagnostic laboratories and lack of standardization • Often more expensive
Culture	• Permits isolation of pathogens and their maintenance for further comparisons and analysis • Facilitates in-depth identification of pathogens	• Time-consuming and laborious • Requires special equipment and biohazard conditions and therefore restricted to specialized laboratories • May take up to 1 month to provide a result

29.1 Advantages and disadvantages of common diagnostic methods for the detection of protozoal and arthropod-borne pathogens in dogs and cats. ELISA = enzyme-linked immunosorbent assay; IFAT = indirect fluorescent antibody test; PCR = polymerase chain reaction.

or protozoal infections. Standard Romanowsky stains such as Giemsa are used for cytological detection of the majority of organisms. Special stains can also be used in cytology for enhancing the visualization of microorganisms but are less frequently needed. Exceptions do exist; for instance, *Bartonella* is difficult to detect in cytology and easier to observe when Warthin–Starry silver stain is employed on histopathological specimens.

The specificity of these methods is high; however, it is important to highlight that identification of species based solely on morphology is often not possible and molecular analysis is required for speciation. Sensitivity will depend on the time spent searching for microorganisms, type of pathogen, tissue sampled, amount of organism in the tissue (parasite load), experience/degree of suspicion of the microscopist and clinical status of the patient. Generally speaking, higher diagnostic sensitivity is found in sick animals when compared with subclinically infected dogs or cats. The detection of chronically infected and carrier animals remains a diagnostic challenge owing to low and often intermittent bacteraemia or parasitaemia, or low tissue pathogen load, which frequently make pathogen observation by microscopic evaluation difficult. Therefore, the use of molecular diagnostic assays is strongly recommended in these cases. In addition, identification of microorganisms in formalin-fixed, paraffin-embedded sections of different tissues may be facilitated by immunohistochemical methods such as immunoperoxidase staining (Figure 29.2) or *in situ* hybridization techniques.

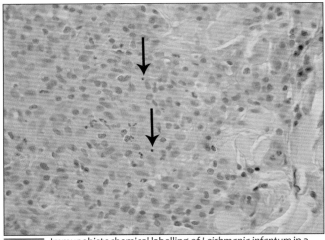

29.2 Immunohistochemical labelling of *Leishmania infantum* in a skin section from a dog with leishmaniosis. Note the *Leishmania* amastigotes stained brown within the cytoplasm of macrophages (arrowed). (Original magnification X200)
(Courtesy of Laura Ordeix, Universitat Autònoma de Barcelona, Spain)

The optimal tissue or body fluid for sampling will depend on the pathogen involved and the lesions found on physical examination. Blood-borne organisms such as *Babesia*, *Ehrlichia*/*Anaplasma* or haemoplasmas can be found in blood smears (Figures 29.3 to 29.5), concentrated and stained buffy coat or splenic specimens. Other

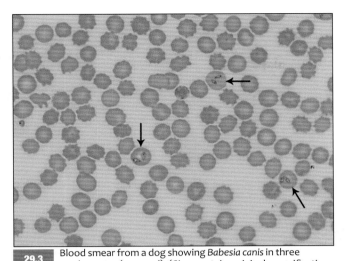

29.3 Blood smear from a dog showing *Babesia canis* in three erythrocytes (arrowed). (Giemsa stain; original magnification X400)
(Courtesy of Drs Caldin and Furlanello, San Marco Veterinary Laboratory, Padua, Italy)

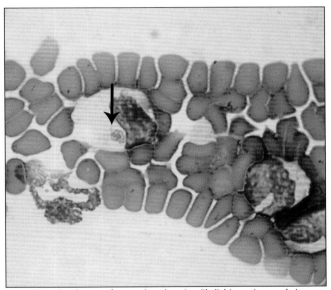

29.4 Blood smear from a dog showing *Ehrlichia canis* morula in a monocyte (arrowed). (Giemsa stain; original magnification X1000)

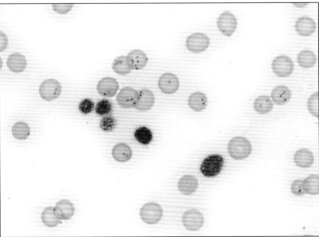

29.5 Blood smear from a cat showing *Mycoplasma haemofelis* on the surface of erythrocytes. (Giemsa stain; original magnification X200)
(Courtesy of Drs Caldin and Furlanello, San Marco Veterinary Laboratory, Padua, Italy)

important tissue samples used for the detection of arthropod-borne pathogens are lymph node aspirates, skin touch impressions, bone marrow, joint fluid, cerebrospinal fluid (CSF) or other body fluids and tissues.

Serology (antibody and antigen detection)

Antibody detection: Several serological methods can be used to detect specific serum antibodies directed against protozoal and arthropod-borne pathogens. Methods include the indirect fluorescent antibody (IFA) test, the enzyme-linked immunosorbent assay (ELISA), immuno-chromatographic rapid in-house devices, direct agglutination assays and Western blotting. The most common serological tests employed in clinical practice are quantitative assays (IFA and ELISA) and qualitative tests (rapid in-house devices). In general, most of these methods have good sensitivities and specificities; however, sensitivity and specificity greatly depend on the antigens employed. Whole-parasite extracts are sensitive for the detection of subclinical or clinical canine or feline infections but provide lower specificity. On the other hand, assays that employ recombinant protein antigens are very specific but may lack sensitivity for the detection of infection, depending on the antigen employed and the level of serum antibodies. The majority of serological assays detect immunoglobulin (Ig)G or total immunoglobulins and IgM is rarely measured for both acute and convalescent antibody levels in these infectious diseases, except in the case of toxoplasmosis.

Serological cross-reactivity is common with pathogens of the same genus or otherwise closely related organisms. Therefore, cross-reactivity between antibodies directed at different pathogens is possible with some serological tests, especially those based on whole-parasite antigen, and are less likely to occur when using recombinant protein antigens. It is important to note that the use of antigens of similar species will frequently result in cross-reaction at a high level. For example, antibodies to *Bartonella quintana* will cross-react with *Bartonella henselae* antigen. Pathogens of closely related but different genera are more likely to cross-react at low levels, for example the cross-reactivity between antibodies to *Trypanosoma cruzi* and *Leishmania infantum*.

Antibody detection can indicate past exposure or current acute or persistent infection. Acute diseases may be difficult to diagnose owing to the lack of detectable antibody production and low pathogen load in blood or other tissues. Therefore, false negative results are possible in peracute or acute disease. Evidence of seroconversion is fundamental in the diagnosis of some acute diseases. In these cases, the measurement of acute and convalescent antibody levels (paired samples) is confirmatory of acute infection. Antibody level determination may vary between different laboratories, and, therefore, it is recommended to use the same laboratory and assay for comparison of antibody levels. Furthermore, variations are also likely between assays carried out on different days. Therefore, ideally, paired samples should be tested at the same time. Seroconversion is considered when a 4-fold or greater increase in antibody titre is demonstrated in paired samples over a 2–4-week period (e.g. an IFA titre increase from 1:80 to 1:320 or greater).

In addition, antibodies induced by vaccination may be detected by serological assays, making it impossible to discriminate between vaccinated and naturally infected animals. Examples of this include vaccination against *Borrelia burgdorferi* and *Leishmania infantum*.

High antibody levels are associated with high tissue parasite loads and disease in some protozoal and arthropod-borne chronic diseases. In contrast, cases with suspected clinical signs and compatible clinicopathological abnormalities and low antibody levels require the use of additional detection methods to exclude or confirm the disease, because low antibody levels may also be detected in subclinical carriers suffering from a different clinical disease. Canine leishmaniosis is a good example of a disease in which moderate to severe clinical disease is usually manifested by medium to high antibody levels, whereas subclinical infection is more often associated with lower antibody levels or seronegativity (Solano-Gallego et al., 2009).

Antigen detection: The detection of circulating plasma or blood antigen specific for a pathogen is an additional and usually very specific serological technique. For example, the most common detection technique for canine heartworm infection caused by Dirofilaria immitis is based on the detection of a circulating secretory antigen of the female adult worm.

Polymerase chain reaction

PCR is a sensitive and specific diagnostic technique which is frequently employed for the diagnosis of protozoal and arthropod-borne diseases (see also Chapter 28). This technique is used for diagnostic purposes, monitoring during and after treatment, research studies and for screening of blood donors. Moreover, it is particularly useful for detection of infection in animals with low levels of parasitaemia and for speciation of pathogens. PCR can be carried out on DNA extracted from tissues, blood, body fluids, conjunctival and oral swabs, or even cytological preparations or histopathological specimens.

A large number of PCR assays and protocols using a variety of gene targets have been described for the detection of protozoal and arthropod-borne infections of dogs and cats. It is important to highlight that, for diagnostic purposes, the best DNA target will be the locus or gene with the largest number of copies per organism. For instance, the kinetoplast DNA (kDNA) of L. infantum is an excellent target as it has about 10,000 copies in each Leishmania amastigote. Other targets are more useful to differentiate between species, such as the leishmanial ribosomal internal transcribed spacer 1 (ITS1). Owing to the fact that, in some endemic areas, several species coexist and infect animals, and may have differing pathogenicities, e.g. Mycoplasma haemofelis and Candidatus Mycoplasma haemominutum, molecular techniques have been developed to discriminate DNA from different species of the same genus or related genera. These techniques include semi-nested PCR, reverse line blotting, PCR–restriction fragment length polymorphism (RFLP) and high-resolution melting curve quantitative fluorescence resonance energy transfer–PCR. Sequencing may also reveal infections with novel organisms that have not been described before.

It is important to highlight that negative results obtained by molecular techniques only indicate that specific DNA was not detected under the assay conditions and should not be interpreted as absolute evidence for the absence of infection. In addition, false positive results are possible due to DNA contamination or the amplification of DNA from other sources which may not be noticed if sequencing is not performed. Controls should be included in each step of the assay to ensure that DNA contamination has not occurred.

Culture

Diagnosis may also be established by culture of the infectious agent. As this technique is usually tedious and time consuming, sometimes requiring special conditions and a long duration for obtaining results, it is less commonly used in clinical practice for parasites and arthropod-borne pathogens. This technique is employed in research studies as it permits identification and maintenance of pathogens. It is important to highlight that some blood-borne pathogens such as the haemotropic haemoplasmas and Anaplasma platys have, to date, not been successfully cultured in vitro. Other organisms such as Babesia and Ehrlichia spp. are difficult to culture. The culture method is pathogen specific and usually requires special media and temperature conditions. Special culture medium is used for the isolation of some protozoal pathogens such as Leishmania infantum, whereas cell culture is required for isolation of Ehrlichia canis, Anaplasma phagocytophilum or Rickettsia spp., restricting their isolation to research laboratories with expertise (Allison and Little, 2013).

Monitoring after diagnosis

Appropriate diagnostic techniques are required for monitoring dogs and cats during or after treatment. In some diseases, such as canine leishmaniosis, monitoring is also performed to check that a subclinically infected animal is not developing disease (Solano-Gallego et al., 2009). The main diagnostic assays used for monitoring are quantitative serology and PCR.

Diagnostic screening of blood donors

With the advance of small animal medicine, blood product transfusions are commonly used in clinical practice as a lifesaving measure. However, as immune-mediated reactions can occur and infectious agents may be transmitted by transfusion, diagnostic screening of blood donors for blood-borne pathogens is essential (Wardrop et al., 2005). A consensus statement recommends that canine blood donors should be screened for leishmaniosis, babesiosis, ehrlichiosis, anaplasmosis, bartonellosis, brucellosis, trypanosomiasis and neorickettsiosis. Feline blood donors should be screened for haemoplasmosis, cytauxzoonosis, ehrlichiosis, anaplasmosis and neorickettsiosis, and also feline leukaemia virus (FeLV) and feline immunodeficiency virus (FIV) infections (Wardrop et al., 2005). Notably, not all diseases are present in every geographical location; trypanosomiasis, neorickettsiosis and cytauxzoonosis caused by Cytauxzoon felis are not endemic in Europe. Thus, screening for these infections may not be necessary unless the donors have travelled to endemic areas. The main diagnostic techniques recommended for screening are PCR and quantitative antibody detection assays such as IFA and ELISA (Wardrop et al., 2005). A diagnostic protocol for screening blood donors for canine leishmaniosis has been described elsewhere (Solano-Gallego et al., 2011). Blood-borne pathogens can remain viable and infective in blood products for long durations. It has been shown that Leishmania present as intracellular amastigotes in monocytes in blood products was infective after 30 days of storage under blood bank conditions (Grogl et al., 1993). Furthermore, transmission of haemoplasmas to naïve cats occurred after the administration of infected feline blood that has been stored in citrate-dextrose-adenine solution after 1 week for Candidatus Mycoplasma haemominutum, and after 1 hour for Mycoplasma haemofelis (Gary et al., 2006). This highlights the risk of using blood products from donors that have not been screened for pathogens, even after weeks of storage.

Diagnostic tests for specific disease

Arthropod-borne bacteria

Ehrlichia

Ehrlichia canis is an intracellular rickettsial pathogen which causes canine monocytic ehrlichiosis worldwide (Harrus and Waner, 2011). It infects dogs in Africa, Asia, America and Europe, where autochthonous (non-imported) cases have been reported mostly from Spain, Portugal, southern France, Italy, the Balkans, Turkey and Greece. *Ehrlichia canis* morulae found in monocytes and macrophages are a 'microcolony' of bacteria surrounded by a membranous vacuole.

Ehrlichia canis is transmitted by the tick *Rhipicephalus sanguineus*. The pathogenesis of the disease involves an incubation period of about 8–20 days, followed by three consecutive phases: an acute phase which lasts 1–4 weeks; a subclinical phase which may last from months to years; and a chronic phase. Not all infected dogs progress through all of the stages to develop the severe chronic form of the disease, and some experience the acute phase without this being noticed and may carry infection subclinically thereafter for long periods. *Ehrlichia canis* is not considered zoonotic, except for a strain described only in Venezuela.

The clinical manifestations most frequently reported in canine ehrlichiosis are lethargy, anorexia, fever, lymphadenomegaly, splenomegaly and bleeding tendencies, with haemorrhage seen mainly as cutaneous petechiae, ecchymoses and epistaxis. Ocular manifestations include scleral haemorrhages, anterior uveitis, keratoconjuctivitis, hyphaema, glaucoma, chorioretinitis and retinal detachment (Harrus and Waner, 2011). Polyarthritis and polymyositis have also been described in *E. canis* infection. Neurological abnormalities found in some cases are associated with lymphocytic infiltration of the central and peripheral nervous system or nervous system haemorrhages.

Thrombocytopenia is the most frequent haematological abnormality, occurring in >90% of cases of canine monocytic ehrlichiosis. Anaemia, usually non-regenerative normocytic and normochromic, and mild to severe leucopenia are frequent. Dogs in the chronic severe stage of the disease may develop severe pancytopenia as their bone marrow becomes hypocellular. Hyperglobulinaemia, hypoalbuminaemia and mild elevation of alkaline phosphatase (ALP) and alanine aminotransferase (ALT) activities are also frequently reported in ehrlichiosis.

Immune-mediated responses play a major role in *E. canis* infection and anti-platelet antibodies have been demonstrated less than a week after experimental infection of dogs. Platelet aggregation abnormalities, antinuclear antibodies, red blood cell (RBC) autoagglutination with positive Coombs' test, and circulating immune complexes have been shown in infected dogs and are associated with the disease process. The decrease in platelets during canine ehrlichiosis is a result of several mechanisms, which include: increased consumption with vascular endothelial changes; platelet sequestration and pooling in the spleen; thrombophagocytosis with immunological destruction; a decrease in the half-life of circulating platelets due to opsonization with antibodies; and production impairment due to bone marrow destruction with hypocellularity. In addition to the decrease in circulating platelet number, platelet dysfunction (thrombocytopathy) is another factor contributing to abnormalities of primary haemostasis in the disease.

The detection of morulae in monocytes in stained blood smears is rare (see Figure 29.4) and reported in only 4% of clinical cases. It cannot serve as the main diagnostic option; however, large activated monocytes are frequently present at the feathered edge of the blood smear. Detection of *E. canis* DNA by PCR is highly sensitive and specific and has become the most useful diagnostic test for the confirmation of canine ehrlichiosis, but pathogen DNA disappears rapidly from the blood after beginning treatment and samples must be taken before treatment (Baneth *et al.*, 2009). Several conventional and real-time PCR protocols are used in commercial laboratories. PCR assays can be performed on blood or tissue aspirates from the spleen, lymph node or bone marrow.

Serology is indicative of exposure to *E. canis* but not necessarily of active infection because seropositive dogs with previous exposure to the pathogen may also present with other disease conditions. Anti-*E. canis* antibodies may not be detectable during the very early stage of infection; however, they persist long after recovery from the disease following medical treatment. Several qualitative point-of-care kits for *E. canis* serology are available from different manufacturers. Serology by commercial IFA or a semi-quantitative kit is preferable because it is sensitive and allows comparison of antibody titres before and after treatment.

Anaplasma phagocytophilum and A. platys

Anaplasma phagocytophilum is an intracellular Gram-negative rickettsial bacterium transmitted by ticks of the genus *Ixodes*. It infects a wide spectrum of mammals including dogs, cats, domestic and wild ruminants, horses and humans. Infection is endemic worldwide where ticks of the genus *Ixodes*, such as *I. ricinus* (Europe), *I. pacificus* and *I. scapularis* (North America), are prevalent. *Anaplasma phagocytophilum* infects granulocytes, predominantly neutrophils, and rarely eosinophils, where it forms cytoplasmic morulae (Carrade *et al.*, 2009).

Clinical manifestations of this infection vary from inapparent infection to mild or moderate acute disease. The main clinical signs are lethargy and fever, which occur after an incubation period of 1–2 weeks. Uncommon clinical signs include diarrhoea, vomiting, cough and respiratory distress, polydipsia, pale mucous membranes, lymphadenomegaly, splenomegaly and neurological signs. Bleeding tendencies are very rarely documented in this disease (Carrade *et al.*, 2009). Sporadic feline clinical cases are documented, with similar clinical signs to those reported in dogs (Lappin *et al.*, 2004).

Anaplasma platys is a Gram-negative rickettsial bacterium that infects canine platelets. This infection has a wide distribution in temperate climates in the Mediterranean Basin, South-eastern USA, South America and Australia. It is suspected to be transmitted by *R. sanguineus* ticks. Bacteraemia and thrombocytopenia are cyclic, at approximately 10–14-day intervals, and most dogs are infected subclinically unless co-infected with additional pathogens. The main clinical signs, clinicopathological abnormalities and diagnostic methods for both infections are described in Figure 29.6.

Similar diagnostic methods are used for both infections. Morulae of *A. phagocytophilum* may be visualized within the cytoplasm of neutrophils (Figure 29.7) and *A. platys* may be detected in platelets (Figure 29.8) during cytological examination of stained peripheral blood smears. Morulae of *A. phagocytophilum* are more commonly noted on examination of blood smears from sick dogs with this disease

Pathogen	Main vector or mode of transmission	Main clinical signs	Main clinicopathological abnormalities	Chief diagnostic methods
Ehrlichia canis	The tick Rhipicephalus sanguineus	Bleeding tendencies: cutaneous and mucous membrane petechiae, ecchymoses, epistaxis. Lethargy, anorexia, fever, lymphadenomegaly, splenomegaly, keratoconjunctivitis, scleral hemorrhage and uveitis	Thrombocytopenia, non-regenerative normocytic, normochromic anaemia, mild to severe leucopenia. Pancytopenia in the chronic severe form with hypocellular bone marrow, hyperglobulinaemia (polyclonal and rarely oligoclonal), hypoalbuminaemia, mild elevation of ALP and ALT	PCR is best for confirmation of infection Serology is indicative of exposure to E. canis but not necessarily of active infection Morulae are rarely detected in blood smears
Anaplasma phagocytophilum	The tick Ixodes ricinus	Dog: fever, lethargy, anorexia, weakness, reluctance to move and lameness	Dog: thrombocytopenia, non-regenerative mild to moderate normocytic, normochromic anaemia, lymphopenia, neutropenia, neutrophilia or normal concentration of neutrophils Hyperglobulinaemia, hypoalbuminaemia, increased ALP activity Neutrophilic inflammation in synovial fluid	Microscopic examination of stained blood smears: morulae observed in cytoplasm of neutrophils in 17–56% of cases and rarely in eosinophils PCR is very sensitive and useful for confirming infection Sampling: blood and buffy coat before treatment serology: high cross-reactivity with A. platys and lesser cross-reactivity with E. canis. Detects past exposure and active infection. Consider using paired samples to detect seroconversion and confirm recent infection
Anaplasma platys	The tick R. sanguineus (suspected)	Usually considered subclinical. Fever, lethargy, lymphadenomegaly and pallor reported in some cases. Co-infection with other pathogens is frequent	Thrombocytopenia, mild non-regenerative anaemia, hyperglobulinaemia and hypoalbuminaemia	Microscopic examination of stained blood smears: morulae are commonly observed within platelets PCR: useful technique with high sensitivity Sampling: blood before treatment
Borrelia burgdorferi	The tick Ixodes spp.	Lameness with arthritis and joint swelling, fever, lymphadenomegaly, anorexia and malaise, kidney disease	Non-regenerative anaemia, thrombocytopenia and hypoalbuminaemia may be present. Azotaemia with proteinuria is found in Lyme-associated kidney disease Synovial fluid: increased cell counts and protein concentration	Positive serology with compatible clinical signs using the C6 peptide assay or whole-cell-based IFAT or ELISA Western blotting can be used as a confirmatory assay The C6 peptide assay is not reactive with antibodies produced by the commonly used Lyme disease dog vaccines
Feline and canine haemotropic Mycoplasma spp.	Dog: The tick R. sanguineus (M. haemocanis) Cat: suspected arthropod-borne (most likely by fleas)	Pale mucous membranes, lethargy, anorexia, tachycardia, tachypnoea, weight loss, depression, dehydration, fever, splenomegaly and jaundice	Regenerative anaemia, autoagglutination, positive Coombs' test, hyperbilirubinaemia, hyperproteinaemia, increased liver enzyme activities	PCR assay: the test of choice. Highly sensitive Microscopic examination of stained blood smears: low sensitivity. A negative result does not exclude infection. False positives might occur due to stain precipitate artefacts. PCR is frequently needed for confirmation Specific serology is not available
Bartonella spp.	Arthropod-borne transmission is highly suspected for the majority of Bartonella species. Fleas are responsible for the transmission of B. henselae and B. claridgiae among cats	Dog: endocarditis, myocarditis, cardiac arrhythmias, polyarthritis, anterior uveitis, chorioretinitis, pyogranulomatous rhinitis and lymphadenitis, and peliosis hepatis Cat: endocarditis, uveitis, mild fever presented as pyrexia of unknown origin, pyogranulomatous myocarditis, lymphadenomegaly, diaphragmatic myositis and reproductive disorders	Usually non-specific clinicopathological abnormalities	Dog: Bartonella pre-enrichment culture (BAPGM) before PCR with a highly sensitive PCR assay targeting the 12s–23s ITS region Cat: serology, blood culture on blood agar medium plates or by using Bartonella alpha Proteobacteria growth medium and PCR assays

29.6 The main mode of transmission, clinical signs, clinicopathological abnormalities and diagnostic methods for major protozoal and arthropod-borne pathogens infecting dogs and cats in Europe. ALP = alkaline phosphatase; ALT = alanine aminotransferase; AST = aspartate aminotransferase; CK = creatine kinase; CSF = cerebrospinal fluid; ELISA = enzyme-linked immunosorbent assay; IFAT = indirect fluorescent antibody test; PCR = polymerase chain reaction. (continues) ▶

Pathogen	Main vector or mode of transmission	Main clinical signs	Main clinicopathological abnormalities	Chief diagnostic methods
Leishmania infantum	Sandflies of the genus *Phlebotomus* (Old World) or *Lutzomyia* (New World)	Dog: lymphadenomegaly, weight loss, decreased appetite, lethargy, skin and ocular lesions, splenomegaly, polyuria and polydipsia, more rarely vomiting and diarrhoea	Dog: polyclonal or very rarely oligoclonal hypergammaglobulinaemia, hypoalbuminaemia, mild non-regenerative anaemia, proteinuria, renal azotaemia and elevated liver enzyme activities Pyogranulomatous, granulomatous or lymphoplasmacytic inflammation in different tissues Reactive hyperplasia in lymphoid organs	Dog: cytology and histopathology ± immunohistochemistry Quantitative antibody detection by ELISA or IFAT. Antibodies at various levels may also be detectable post-vaccination Kinetoplast DNA PCR assay of lymph node, bone marrow, spleen, skin and conjunctival swabs. Blood PCR is less sensitive than PCR of haemolymphoid tissues Quantitative real-time PCR is preferable over conventional PCR, if well designed and optimized
Babesia canis	The tick *Dermacentor* spp.	Fever, lethargy, anorexia, jaundice	Thrombocytopenia, mild to moderate non-regenerative normocytic, normochromic anaemia, infrequent regenerative anaemia, neutropenia, hyper-bilirubinaemia, pigmenturia, bilirubinuria (due to haemolysis)	PCR assays: most useful technique with high sensitivity; permits species differentiation Microscopic examination of stained blood smears Serology is not very useful. It detects past exposure and not necessarily current infection, and there is also cross-reactivity with other species of *Babesia*
Babesia vogeli	The tick *R. sanguineus*	Fever, lethargy, anorexia, jaundice	Haemolytic regenerative immune-mediated anaemia, non-regenerative anaemia, leucocytosis, leucopenia, thrombocytopenia	As for *B. canis*
Babesia gibsoni	The ticks: *Haemophysalis longicornis* *H. bispinosa?* *R. sanguineus?* Dog-to-dog transmission via bite wounds	Fever, lethargy, pallor, jaundice, lymphadenomegaly, splenomegaly, weight loss	Haemolytic regenerative anaemia, thrombocytopenia, hyperbilirubinaemia, pigmenturia, bilirubinuria	As for *B. canis*
Babesia vulpes (synonym *Babesia microti*-like and *Theileria annae*)	The ticks: *I. hexagonus?* *I. ricinus?* *R. sanguineus?*	Fever and lethargy, haemoglobinuria, tachycardia, tachypnoea	Moderate to severe regenerative anaemia, thrombocytopenia, azotaemia, proteinuria, urinary casts	As for *B. canis*
Hepatozoon canis	The ticks: *R. sanguineus*, *Amblyomma ovale* in South America	Lethargy, fever, cachexia and pallor	Mild to moderate non-regenerative anaemia, neutrophilia in cases of high parasitaemia	Microscopic detection of *H. canis* gamonts in blood neutrophils and monocytes PCR is sensitive and helpful in the detection of low parasitaemia
Hepatozoon americanum	The tick *A.maculatum*	Fever, lameness, muscular pain induced by myositis, generalized muscle atrophy, mucopurulent ocular discharge	Mild to moderate non-regenerative anaemia, extreme neutrophilia, increased ALP, hypoalbuminaemia	PCR of blood Muscle biopsy demonstrating typical parasitic cysts and pyogranulomas Detection of blood gamonts by microscopy is difficult because of very low parasitaemia
Hepatozoon felis	Unknown arthropod vector; transplacental in cats	No clinical signs known	Elevated serum muscle enzyme concentrations may be detected	PCR of blood Detection of blood gamonts by microscopy is difficult because of very low parasitaemia
Toxoplasma gondii	Cats are infected by ingestion of infected tissues (prey) or sporulated oocysts from faeces. Intermediate hosts are infected by the same routes or transplacentally (some host species)	Systemic infection in cats: fever, anorexia, abdominal pain, dyspnoea, ocular inflammation and central nervous disorders Acute disease in dogs: fever, neuromuscular, respiratory, gastrointestinal, hepatic and more rarely ocular manifestations	Non-regenerative anaemia, leucopenia with lymphopenia, or neutrophilic leucocytosis, monocytosis and eosinophilia Hypoproteinaemia, hypoalbuminaemia Increased ALT and AST	Serology showing seroconversion IgM suggesting recent infection in cases of clinical toxoplasmosis Cytology of ascitic and pleural fluids, CSF, aqueous humour and tissue aspirates demonstrating tachyzoites PCR of the above fluids and tissues

29.6 (continued) The main mode of transmission, clinical signs, clinicopathological abnormalities and diagnostic methods for major protozoal and arthropod-borne pathogens infecting dogs and cats in Europe. ALP = alkaline phosphatase; ALT = alanine aminotransferase; AST = aspartate aminotransferase; CK = creatine kinase; CSF = cerebrospinal fluid; ELISA = enzyme-linked immunosorbent assay; IFAT = indirect fluorescent antibody test; PCR = polymerase chain reaction. (continues) ▶

Pathogen	Main vector or mode of transmission	Main clinical signs	Main clinicopathological abnormalities	Chief diagnostic methods
Neospora caninum	Dogs are infected by ingestion of parasite cysts from tissues of intermediate hosts (cattle) and transplacentally	Puppies: ascending hindlimb paresis and ataxia, muscle atrophy, muscular back pain, head tilt, ocular abnormalities and dysphagia Infected adult dogs: encephalomyelitis, focal cutaneous nodules or ulcers, pneumonia, peritonitis or myocarditis	Increased CK and AST CSF: mild increase in protein and nucleated cell counts with predominantly mononuclear cells	Serology by ELISA or IFAT PCR of CSF or muscle biopsy samples *N. caninum* tachyzoites can occasionally be detected in the CSF
Dirofilaria immitis	Different mosquito vectors	Dog: exercise intolerance, chronic right heart failure with ascites, hepatomegaly and syncope, respiratory distress with dyspnoea, tachypnoea, cough and haemoptysis Cat: cough, dyspnoea, intermittent vomiting	Non-regenerative anaemia, thrombocytopenia, neutrophilia and eosinophilia Elevated liver enzymes, azotaemia, hyperbilirubinaemia and proteinuria may be present	Dog: circulating antigen tests in combination with detection of microfilaraemia by the concentration Knott's test or directly by blood microscopy. Occult infection with no microfilaraemia is common Cat: serology for anti-*D. immitis* antibodies in combination with circulating antigen tests. Microfilaraemia is rare so the Knott's test is not recommended

29.6 (continued) The main mode of transmission, clinical signs, clinicopathological abnormalities and diagnostic methods for major protozoal and arthropod-borne pathogens infecting dogs and cats in Europe. ALP = alkaline phosphatase; ALT = alanine aminotransferase; AST = aspartate aminotransferase; CK = creatine kinase; CSF = cerebrospinal fluid; ELISA = enzyme-linked immunosorbent assay; IFAT = indirect fluorescent antibody test; PCR = polymerase chain reaction.

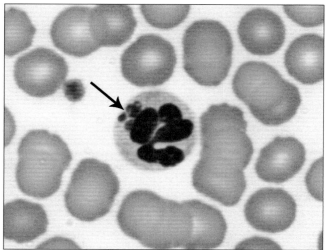

29.7 Blood smear from a dog showing *Anaplasma phagocytophilum* in a neutrophil (arrowed). (Giemsa stain; original magnification X1000)
(Courtesy of Drs Caldin and Furlanello, San Marco Veterinary Laboratory, Padua, Italy)

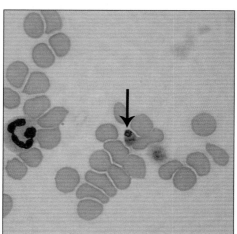

29.8 Blood smear from a dog showing *Anaplasma platys* in a platelet (arrowed). (Giemsa stain; original magnification X1000)

prior to treatment (17–56% of cases), which is high when compared with canine *E. canis* cases (4%) (Allison and Little, 2013). *Anaplasma platys* is also commonly observed in blood films from infected dogs but PCR for *Anaplasma* spp. in blood taken before treatment is far more sensitive than blood smear examination for the detection of infection. The available PCR assays can be specific for *A. phago-cytophilum* or *A. platys.* However, commercial laboratories frequently use broad PCR primers to detect DNA from *Ehrlichia/Anaplasma*; DNA sequencing may be required to determine the final identity of the pathogen. Target genes include the 16s RNA and major surface protein 2 (msp2). Serology is less specific because of cross-reactivity at high levels between *A. phagocytophilum* and *A. platys.* Acute and convalescent samples (paired samples) are employed to confirm active infection. *Anaplasma platys* has not been cultured *in vitro* and, therefore, antibody detection relies on production of recombinant antigens and not on whole bacterial antigen assays. To date, specific serology for *Anaplasma platys* is not available in the clinical setting (Carrade *et al.*, 2009; Allison and Little, 2013).

Haemoplasma

Haemoplasmas are small (0.2–0.8 µm) epierythrocytic bacteria that can cause severe haemolytic anaemia in some domestic mammals including cats and dogs (Sykes, 2010). Feline haemoplasmosis is caused by several species of haemotropic *Mycoplasma* including *Mycoplasma haemofelis, Candidatus* Mycoplasma haemominutum and *Candidatus* Mycoplasma turicensis. The three species are distributed worldwide with varying prevalence of infection. *Candidatus* M. haemominutum is the most prevalent species, found worldwide, while *M. haemofelis* is the least prevalent. However, the most pathogenic species is *M. haemofelis*, and acute infection can result in severe haemolytic anaemia. In contrast, *Candidatus* M. haemominutum and *Candidatus* M. turicensis commonly cause a chronic subclinical infection. Haemolytic anaemia with these species is associated with FIV or FeLV infections or concurrent diseases. Another species, *Candidatus* M. haematoparvum-like, appears to infect cats but has only been documented in one study from the USA (Sykes *et al.*, 2007). The feline haemoplasmas are suspected to be transmitted by arthropods such as fleas or ticks but confirmation is still lacking. Other possible routes of transmission include bites and vertical transmission. Blood transfusion is a proven route of transmission (Sykes, 2010).

Mycoplasma haemocanis and *Candidatus* M. haematoparvum have been described in dogs and associated with haemolytic anaemia, which has mainly been described in splenectomized or immunocompromised patients.

Blood smear examination using routine Romanowsky stains including Diff-Quik® permits the visualization of *M. haemofelis* (see Figure 29.5) and rarely *Candidatus* M. haemominutum because this haemoplasma is smaller. *Candidatus* M. turicensis has only been observed by electron microscopy and not on blood films owing to its small size. Canine haemoplasmas are easier to visualize by microscopic examination as they are larger. Fresh smears are essential to visualize the microorganisms in the membrane of erythrocytes because they detach in stored blood.

Several PCR assays are available to differentiate among canine and feline haemoplasmas and are considered the diagnostic test of choice for these infections. A positive result does not equate with clinical illness and, therefore, PCR results should be interpreted in conjunction with clinical findings and the species identified. These microorganisms have not been cultured *in vitro*. Therefore, antibody detection relies on production of recombinant antigens. So far, serology is not available in clinical practice and is only used in research studies.

The main clinical signs, clinicopathological abnormalities and diagnostic methods are described in Figure 29.6.

Bartonella

Bartonella spp. are fastidious Gram-negative bacteria which are well adapted to specific mammalian reservoir hosts, in which the bacteria usually cause a long-lasting intraerythrocytic bacteraemia. Multiple species of *Bartonella* infect a wide range of hosts, including humans, with worldwide distribution (Breitschwerdt *et al.*, 2010).

Infections with *Bartonella* spp. are being recognized in dogs and cats with increasing frequency as a result of the availability of more accurate and sensitive diagnostic techniques. Many *Bartonella* species infect dogs and cats as primary reservoirs or accidental hosts. The most prevalent *Bartonella* species in dogs are *B. henselae*, *B. vinsonii* subsp. *berkhoffii* (primary reservoir), *B. koehlerae*, *B. volans*-like and *B. bovis*, while cats can be infected with *B. henselae*, *B. clarridgeiae*, *B. koehlerae*, *B. quintana* and *B. bovis*. Arthropod-borne transmission is highly suspected for the majority of these *Bartonella* species and fleas are responsible for the transmission of *B. henselae* and *B. clarridgeiae* among cats, which serve as their primary reservoirs (Breitschwerdt *et al.*, 2010).

The majority of *Bartonella* species infect cats but do not cause clinical illness. Clinical abnormalities are described with *B. henselae* infection and include endocarditis, uveitis, mild fever presented as pyrexia of unknown origin, pyogranulomatous myocarditis, lymphadenomegaly, diaphragmatic myositis and reproductive disorders (Brunt *et al.*, 2006). Some of the clinical abnormalities reported in dogs are endocarditis, myocarditis, cardiac arrhythmias, polyarthritis, anterior uveitis, chorioretinitis, pyogranulomatous rhinitis and lymphadenitis, and peliosis hepatis. The most commonly reported abnormality caused by several *Bartonella* species in dogs is endocarditis (Breitschwerdt *et al.*, 2010).

In cats, good sensitivities are found with serology, blood culture on blood agar medium plates or using a specialized growth medium (*Bartonella* alpha-Proteobacteria growth medium) and PCR assays. However, positive serology, culture and PCR can be detected in healthy as well as sick cats. Therefore, in sick cats, the combination of positive diagnostic assay results with clinical parameters and response to therapy is used to make a presumptive diagnosis (Brunt *et al.*, 2006).

In dogs, the most sensitive diagnostic technique is the use of *Bartonella* pre-enrichment culture (insect-based liquid culture medium (BAPGM)) before PCR with a highly sensitive PCR assay targeting the 12s–23s ITS region. Poorer sensitivities are associated with culture in conventional blood culture medium or PCR amplification following direct DNA extraction from blood, fluid samples or tissues. *B. henselae* or *B. vinsonii* subsp. *berkhoffii* serology is positive in only approximately half of infected dogs. Detection of antibodies might indicate past exposure or current infection, and although serology has limitations, including cross-reactivity with other *Bartonella* species and low sensitivity, it remains an important diagnostic test. The use of a combination of diagnostic techniques is recommended in suspected canine *Bartonella* infections (Breitschwerdt *et al.*, 2010).

Borrelia

Canine Lyme borreliosis is caused by the bacterial spirochaete *Borrelia burgdorferi* sensu stricto, and outside the USA also by other *Borrelia* species including *Borrelia garinii* and *Borrelia afzelii* in Europe (Krupka and Straubinger, 2010).

Lyme disease borreliae are transmitted by *Ixodes* spp. ticks, including *I. ricinus* in Europe, and mainly by *I. scapularis* and *I. pacificus* in North America, and *I. persulcatus* in Eurasia. The spirochaetes circulate among sylvatic rodent and wild bird hosts but may also infect dogs and humans as end-stage hosts.

Clinical disease usually appears after a long incubation period and the main clinical manifestations of canine Lyme disease include shifting lameness with arthritis and joint swelling, fever, lymphadenomegaly, anorexia and malaise. Membranoproliferative glomerulonephritis, termed 'Lyme nephritis' has been associated with Lyme borreliosis and is reported more frequently in Labrador Retrievers, Golden Retrievers and Bernese Mountain Dogs. Dogs are often infected subclinically and do not exhibit disease despite being seropositive. The clinical manifestations of infection with *B. afzelii* and *B. garinii* appear to be less severe than those found in dogs with *B. burgdorferii* sensu stricto.

Laboratory abnormalities may include non-regenerative anaemia, thrombocytopenia and hypoalbuminaemia. Renal azotaemia with proteinuria is found in Lyme-associated kidney disease. Synovial fluid from swollen joints may show inflammatory changes with increased neutrophil and protein concentrations.

Positive serology with compatible clinical signs is the current basis for the diagnosis of canine Lyme borreliosis. Dogs with clinical Lyme disease are almost always seropositive following a prolonged incubation period. However, the presence of seropositive subclinically infected dogs in endemic areas complicates the diagnosis, as does vaccination.

Whole-cell-based IFA or ELISA serological tests are available and frequently used as screening assays. Positive results on these tests may require follow-up by Western blot for more accurate evaluation of the antibody response. Previous vaccination or exposure may result in false positive serology with whole cell antigen. The C6-based assay (Idexx Laboratories) targets antibodies to a gene that is only expressed in active infection of mammalian hosts. Antibodies reactive with the C6 assay decrease more rapidly following successful treatment of infection than antibodies detected by whole-cell assays, and the assay is also not reactive with antibodies produced by the commonly used canine vaccines against Lyme disease. The serological response with the commercially available tests to Lyme borreliae other than *B. burgdorferii* sensu stricto may be variable and less consistent.

Lyme spirochaetes are not detectable by conventional blood smear microscopy and may be found in synovial fluid using dark-field microscopy, but low numbers preclude direct visualization. PCR of affected tissues is available but its sensitivity is limited owing to the low spirochaete load in clinical samples.

Arthropod-borne nematodes

Dirofilaria

Filariosis is an arthropod-borne nematode infection caused in dogs and cats by a number of species, of which some are highly pathogenic and inflict severe disease whereas others are associated with subclinical infection. *Dirofilaria immitis* infects domestic and wild canine and feline species in warm and temperate regions and causes heartworm disease. It is present in southern Europe, North and South America, Africa, Asia and Australia (Simon *et al.*, 2012).

Microfilariae, the first stage larvae of *D.immitis*, are present in the circulation of the host. When a mosquito vector takes a blood meal it ingests these larvae, they develop into L3 larvae which are subsequently injected into the skin of a new host by the mosquito bite. The immature worm migrates through the skin and muscles to the lung blood vessels, reaching the pulmonary arteries. Adult worms are found in dogs primarily in the pulmonary artery and the right heart chambers. The mosquito vectors of *D. immitis* vary in different geographical regions and include species belonging to the genera *Culex*, *Anopheles* and *Aedes*.

Heartworm disease results from progressive proliferative endarteritis and thromboembolism of the pulmonary artery caused by adult worms. Progressive vascular changes lead to pulmonary hypertension, right ventricular hypertrophy or dilatation and cor pulmonale. The first clinical signs typically include exercise intolerance and cough. This is followed by chronic right heart failure with ascites, hepatomegaly, syncope and respiratory distress with dyspnoea, tachypnoea, cough and haemoptysis. A heavy worm burden may cause vena cava syndrome with a haemolytic crisis. The most common signs in feline heartworm disease are coughing, dyspnoea and intermittent vomiting.

Haematological abnormalities may include non-regenerative anaemia, thrombocytopenia, neutrophilia and eosinophilia. Elevated liver enzyme concentrations, azotaemia and hyperbilirubinaemia may be present and urinalysis may show proteinuria.

Detection of microfilaraemia by microscopic examination of anticoagulated blood is possible when there are large numbers of microfilariae (Figure 29.9). The Knott's test allows detection of low numbers of circulating microfilariae

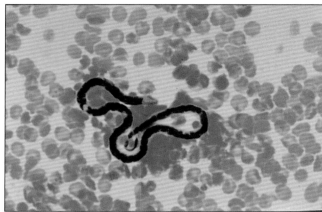

29.9 Microfilaria of *Dirofilaria immitis* in canine blood. (Giemsa stain; original magnification X400)

concentrated from a larger volume of blood. One millilitre of anticoagulated blood is mixed with 9 ml of 2% formalin, which haemolyses the blood cells, in a conical centrifuge tube and centrifuged for 5 minutes. The supernatant is discarded, the sediment is stained with methylene blue and a drop of stained sediment is coverslipped and examined by microscopy for the presence of microfilariae, which stain blue. About 20% of canine infections are occult with no shedding of detectable microfilariae by adult worms. Other common filariae that produce circulating microfilariae which represent a differential diagnosis for *D. immitis* in Europe include *D. repens* and *Acanthocheilonema reconditum*.

Antigen detection, available as commercial point-of-care or laboratory kits, is a sensitive screening method for detection of heartworm that is commonly used in dogs. It is based on the detection of a glycoprotein secreted into the blood circulation by adult female worms and may be negative in the rare occasion of absence of adult female worms or if they are present in very small numbers. Although antigen testing is the most sensitive, current recommendations from the American Heartworm Society are that the antigen test and microfilaria test are performed in tandem to have the best chance of making a diagnosis.

Cats are considered less well adapted to *D. immitis* infection than dogs, harbour a smaller number of mature adults than dogs and develop shorter durations of microfilaraemia. In cats, more than in dogs, immature heartworms which reach the lungs cause disease even if they do not mature to adult worms or result in infections that produce microfilariae. Antigen detection tests are therefore less sensitive in cats but may be used with serology to detect feline anti-*D.immitis* antibodies in conjunction with thoracic radiography and echocardiography in order to make a diagnosis.

Arthropod-borne protozoa

Leishmania infantum

Leishmania infantum is the causative agent of canine leishmaniosis, which is a major zoonotic disease endemic in more than 70 countries. It is present in regions of southern Europe, Africa, Asia and South and Central America and is also an important concern in non-endemic countries where imported disease constitutes a veterinary and public health problem (Shaw *et al.*, 2003). *L. infantum* is a diphasic protozoan that completes its life cycle in two hosts, a sandfly which harbours the flagellated extracellular promastigotes and a mammal where the intracellular amastigote parasite forms develop. Dogs are the main reservoir of this infection and sandflies are the only arthropods that are adapted to its biological transmission. However, other proven non-sandfly routes of transmission include blood transfusion, vertical and venereal transmission (Solano-Gallego *et al.* 2009, 2011; Baneth and Solano-Gallego, 2012).

Canine leishmaniosis is a good example of a disease in which infection does not always lead to clinical illness; there is a high prevalence of persistent subclinical infection. Clinical illness varies from self-limiting disease to very severe fatal disease. Clinical staging of canine leishmaniosis includes four stages of severity based on clinical signs, clinicopathological abnormalities and serology. The main clinical signs, clinicopathological abnormalities and diagnostic methods of this disease are described in Figure 29.6 (Solano-Gallego *et al.* 2009, 2011; Baneth and Solano-Gallego, 2012).

The methods used for diagnosis in dogs with suspected clinical leishmaniosis include the detection of amastigotes in stained cytological smears of aspirates (Figure 29.10) obtained from: cutaneous lesions (Figure 29.11); lymph nodes; bone marrow and spleen; or other tissues or body fluids. Histopathology and immunohisto-

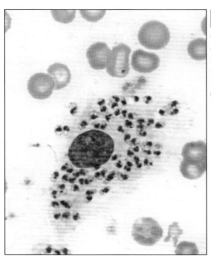

29.10 Bone marrow smear from a dog showing *Leishmania* amastigotes within a macrophage. (Giemsa stain; original magnification X1000) (Courtesy of Drs Caldin and Furlanello, San Marco Veterinary Laboratory, Padua, Italy)

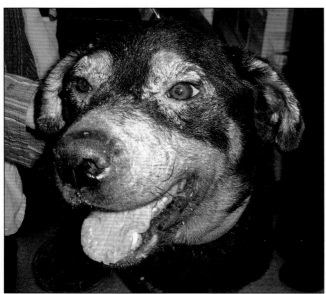

29.11 A dog with leishmaniosis manifesting typical facial exfoliative dermatitis.

chemical staining of tissue sections (see Figure 29.2) are employed to detect the presence of *L. infantum* in the tissue. The isolation in culture of parasites from infected tissues is not suitable for rapid diagnosis.

The most useful diagnostic approaches for investigation of infection in sick and healthy subclinically infected dogs include: first, the detection of specific serum anti-leishmanial antibodies by quantitative serological techniques; and, second, the demonstration of the parasite DNA in tissues by applying molecular techniques (PCR). Since it has been shown that many dogs in endemic areas are infected with *L. infantum*, as indicated by PCR, but may never develop clinical leishmaniosis, quantitative serology demonstrating a high antibody titre is better correlated with the presence of clinical disease, and therefore quantitative serology should be used as the first test for dogs with suspected clinical leishmaniosis. Serological cross-reactivity exists between different species of *Leishmania* and *Trypanosoma*. High antibody levels considerably above the cut-off titre are usually associated with disease and a high parasite density and, for this reason, they are conclusive of a diagnosis of leishmaniosis. However, the presence of lower antibody levels is not necessarily indicative of patent disease and needs to be confirmed by other diagnostic methods such as PCR, cytology or histology (Solano-Gallego *et al.*, 2009). Antibodies at various levels may also be detectable post vaccination and, therefore, a careful history must be obtained from the owners when testing dogs that may have been vaccinated against leishmaniosis. The best specimens for PCR diagnosis of *Leishmania* infection are lymph node, bone marrow, spleen, skin and conjunctival swabs.

In cats, clinical illness due to *L. infantum* is less commonly reported. However, as in dogs, feline infection is more widespread than clinical disease. The most common abnormalities on physical examination are cutaneous lesions affecting the face and ears. Visceral involvement is less commonly described, and is thought to be associated with immunosuppression caused by FeLV or FIV infection, or other concomitant diseases. Diagnosis is made in the majority of cases by serology, cytology, histopathology or PCR. Serological techniques are poorly standardized (Solano-Gallego and Baneth, 2012).

Piroplasms: *Babesia*, *Theileria* and *Cytauxozoon*

Piroplasms are protozoal parasites that infect red blood cells. Canine babesiosis, caused by different *Babesia* species, is a protozoal tick-borne disease with worldwide distribution and global significance. The natural transmission of *Babesia* to vertebrate hosts occurs through the bite of a vector tick. Other routes of transmission include blood transfusion, transplacental transfer and dog-to-dog transfer via bite wounds in some babesial species (Solano-Gallego and Baneth, 2011).

Historically, *Babesia* infection in dogs was identified in erythrocytes on the basis of morphological characteristics on blood smears. *Babesia* occurs in large and small forms; in the past all large-form *Babesia* were designated *B. canis*, whereas all small forms of *Babesia* were thought to be *B. gibsoni*. However, the development of molecular methods has demonstrated that other *Babesia* species such as *B. conradae*, a *B. microti*-like piroplasm, *Theileria* spp. (small forms) and an as yet unnamed large-form *Babesia* species, infect dogs and cause distinct diseases. *Babesia rossi*, *B. canis* and *B. vogeli*, previously considered as subspecies, are identical morphologically but differ in the severity of clinical manifestations which they induce, their tick vectors, genetic characteristics and geographical distributions, and are therefore currently considered separate species (Solano-Gallego and Baneth, 2011).

The geographical distribution of *B. rossi* and *Theileria* spp. are to date restricted to Africa, and *B. canis* has mostly been reported from central and northern Europe, whereas *B. vogeli* has a wide distribution in both the Old and New World continents. *Babesia vulpes* (synonym B. microti-like) has been described in Europe and North America in dogs and feral foxes (Baneth *et al.*, 2015). *B. gibsoni* is found in Asia, North America and Australia and sporadically reported in Europe. *B. conradae* and an unnamed large-form *Babesia* sp. have only been described in North America. Therefore, in Europe, the species that can infect dogs are *B. vogeli*, *B. canis*, *B. vulpes* and *B. gibsoni* (Solano-Gallego and Baneth, 2011).

In general, small-form *Babesia* causes a more severe disease than large-form *Babesia* (see Figure 29.3), with the exception of *B. rossi,* which can cause a very severe fatal disease. In addition, small-form *Babesia* infection is more difficult to treat with the available drugs. Therefore, the prognosis in small-form *Babesia* infection is guarded to poor while, in general, patients with large-form *Babesia* have a better prognosis after treatment. Subclinical *B. gibsoni* infection has been reported, mainly in the Pit Bull Terrier.

The main clinical signs, clinicopathological abnormalities and diagnostic methods for the piroplasmid species that infect dogs in Europe are described in Figure 29.6. The clinicopathological abnormalities found in infections with different *Babesia* spp. differ according to the infecting species and the host characteristics. Thrombocytopenia is a common abnormality found in infections with many species of *Babesia*, in particular with *B. canis* infection, where 100% of clinical cases develop thrombocytopenia, while regenerative anaemia is much less frequently encountered. In infection with other babesial species, regenerative anaemia is frequently present.

Detection of *Babesia* in stained blood smears has been the standard test for diagnosis for many years (see Figure 29.3). This method is reliable when a moderate to high parasitaemia is present; however, correlation between the level of parasitaemia and the magnitude of clinical signs is not always established. It also provides a rapid and cost-effective means of diagnosis in endemic areas. Smears made from capillary blood (from ear tip or toenail) may be better for exhibiting large-form *Babesia* parasites than blood from a central vein. Serology is not helpful in diagnosing the infection because it can indicate a past exposure. Serological cross-reactivity exists among different species of *Babesia*. False negative results are likely in peracute or acute infection and therefore convalescent antibody levels are needed to prove acute infection. PCR is particularly useful in the diagnosis of babesiosis in dogs with a low parasitaemia or for speciation of parasites. Several molecular assays have been developed to detect and discriminate DNA from different species of large- and small-form piroplasms (Solano-Gallego and Baneth, 2011).

Babesia infection in cats is associated with anorexia, lethargy, anaemia and icterus. Information on the clinical manifestations of domestic feline babesiosis is limited mostly to publications on *B. felis* infection in South Africa, in which most infected cats were anorexic and lethargic and showed macrocytic hypochromic regenerative anaemia and hyperbilirubinaemia (Schoeman *et al.*, 2001). *Babesia lengau* has been reported from two cats in South Africa, of which one had cerebral babesiosis (Bosman

et al., 2013), and *B. canis presentii* infection in a cat from Israel, which was co-infected with FIV and *Candidatus* M. haemominutum, was accompanied by fever, icterus, moderate anaemia and thrombocytopenia, which resolved following anti-babesial therapy (Baneth *et al.*, 2004).

Cytauxzoonosis is another infection caused by piroplasms in domestic and wild felids; it infects red blood cells and also has an earlier stage which infects macrophages. *Cytauxzoon felis*, which infects the bobcat (*Lynx rufus*) and domestic cats in some parts of the USA, is transmitted by *Dermacentor variabilis* and *Amblyomma americanum* ticks. In domestic cats, clinical manifestation of this infection varies from inapparent infection to severe fatal disease due to the occlusion of small blood vessels by large macrophages containing the schizont stage of the parasite. The bobcat commonly shows a subclinical parasitaemia (Holman and Snowden, 2009). In Europe, *Cytauxzoon* species other than *C. felis* have been reported to infect domestic cats (Carli *et al.*, 2012) and Iberian lynx (Millan *et al.*, 2007), but information on the epidemiological and clinicopathological aspects of this infection is limited and it is not as virulent as *C. felis* infection. Diagnosis is made by microscopic observation of organisms in erythrocytes on blood smears (Figure 29.12) or in macrophages in tissues. PCR assays are also available and have good sensitivity.

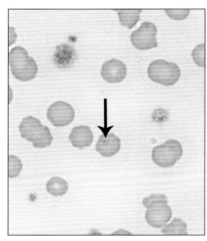

29.12 Feline blood smear; note the small-form piroplasms within the erythrocytes (*Cytauxzoon* spp., arrowed). (Modified Wright's stain; original magnification X1000) (Courtesy of Drs Carli, Caldin and Furlanello, Veterinary San Marco Laboratory, Padua, Italy)

Hepatozoon canis, *H. americanum* and *H. felis*

Hepatozoonosis is an arthropod-borne infection caused by an apicomplexan protozoa. Two different species of *Hepatozoon* infect dogs, *H. canis* globally, and *H. americanum* in southern USA (Baneth, 2011). Canine *H. canis* infection has also been reported as a rare infection in the UK which may have originated from importation. Feline hepatozoonosis is caused by *H. felis*, which is prevalent in the Mediterranean Basin, Asia, Africa and South America (Baneth *et al.*, 2013).

In contrast to most tick-borne pathogens that are transmitted via the tick salivary glands, *Hepatozoon* spp. infect vertebrates when they ingest arthropod hosts containing infective sporozoites. The main vectors of *H. canis* are the ticks *Rhipicephalus sanguineus* worldwide and *Amblyomma ovale* in South America. The Gulf Coast tick *A. maculatum* is the vector of *H. americanum* in North America. The vector of *H. felis* has not been identified to date but intrauterine transmission is evident.

Infection with *H. canis* generally causes mild clinical signs but can vary from being subclinical in apparently healthy dogs to a severe disease in dogs presenting with lethargy, fever, cachexia and pale mucous membranes due to anaemia. In contrast to the mild disease usually found in *H. canis* infection, *H. americanum* infection is frequently a severe disease with fever, gait abnormalities, muscular pain induced by myositis, generalized muscular atrophy and mucopurulent ocular discharge. *Hepatozoon felis* infection has not been associated directly with overt clinical manifestations.

A subclinical to mild disease is the most common presentation of *H. canis* infection and it is usually associated with a low level of parasitaemia (1–5% of neutrophils and monocytes), while a severe illness is found in dogs with a high parasitaemia, often approaching 100% of the peripheral blood neutrophils. High parasitaemia rates are sometimes accompanied by extreme neutrophilia, reaching as high as 150 x 10^9 leucocytes per litre of blood. A marked neutrophilia is also one of the consistent haematological findings in *H. americanum* infection, with leucocyte counts of 30–200 x 10^9/l; however, the level of parasitaemia is typically very low. Serum biochemical abnormalities include increased ALP and hypoalbuminaemia.

Hepatozoon canis infection is usually diagnosed by microscopic detection of intracellular *H. canis* gamonts in stained blood smears (Figure 29.13). The gamonts are found in the cytoplasm of neutrophils and monocytes, have an ellipsoidal shape and are about 11 x 4 μm. In contrast, *H. americanum* parasitaemia usually does not exceed 0.1% of the leucocytes, and confirmation of infection can be achieved by muscle biopsy and demonstration of typical parasite cysts and granulomas. PCR on blood for *H. canis* or *H. americanum* is a sensitive and specific diagnostic option. *H. felis* infection (Figure 29.14) is usually associated with a low parasitaemia and is best detected by blood PCR.

Protozoal pathogens

Toxoplasma

Toxoplasma gondii is a tissue cyst-forming coccidian with a sexual life cycle in the intestines of felids, the definitive hosts, and an asexual phase in intermediate hosts. The

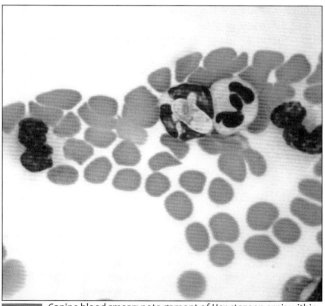

29.13 Canine blood smear; note gamont of *Hepatozoon canis* within a neutrophil in the feathered edge. (Giemsa stain; original magnification X1000)

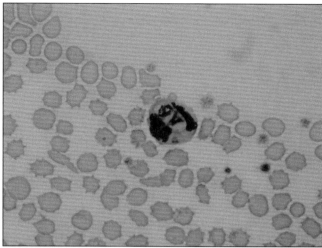

29.14 Feline blood smear; note gamont of *Hepatozoon felis* within a neutrophil. (Giemsa stain; original magnification X1000)

parasite can invade the gut, become systemic and localize in organs such as muscles and nervous system tissues. In most cases infection is subclinical and parasites are eventually encysted as tachyzoites in tissue cysts, but severe and fatal disease can occur as a result of acute infection or reactivation of parasites in cysts (Lappin, 2010).

All warm-blooded vertebrates including humans may serve as intermediate hosts and be infected by *T. gondii* bradyzoites in meat, by sporulated oocysts from cat faeces, or by intrauterine transmission of tachyzoites (proven in some hosts).

Clinical signs in cats are rare and seldom related to the gastrointestinal stage of development, which is usually subclinical. Affected cats may show signs of systemic infection including fever, anorexia, abdominal pain, dyspnoea, ocular inflammation and central nervous system disorders. Acute disease in dogs may be accompanied by neuromuscular, respiratory, gastrointestinal, hepatic and, more rarely, ocular manifestations. Cats and dogs with toxoplasmosis may develop pancreatitis.

Cats and dogs with acute systemic toxoplasmosis may develop non-regenerative anaemia, leucopenia with lymphopenia, or neutrophilic leucocytosis, monocytosis and eosinophilia. Serum biochemistry abnormalities during acute toxoplasmosis may include hypoproteinaemia with hypoalbuminaemia. Increased concentrations of ALT and aspartate aminotransferase (AST) are found in animals with hepatic and muscle necrosis.

Excretion of oocysts by cats can be detected by faecal examination or PCR. Oocysts are relatively small and, although they are shed in large numbers following infection of young kittens, shedding usually lasts <2 weeks. Diagnosis in clinically ill cats and dogs is based on clinical signs and the detection of specific serum antibodies in the blood, demonstration of parasite DNA by PCR, or visualization of tachyzoites in clinical samples (see below). Subclinically infected animals may display antibody titres, and therefore positive serological results may only indicate previous infection, which is not necessarily acute. Serology is carried out by ELISA, IFA, agglutination assays and immunochromatographic kits. The demonstration of increased IgG titres (by at least 4-fold) in paired sera taken at least 2 weeks apart suggests acute infection; however, this is often not observed.

Immunoblotting assays and ELISAs have been developed for the measurement of IgM, IgG and IgA antibody classes in an effort to follow some typical kinetic pattern of antibody formation in feline infection. About 80% of healthy cats experimentally infected with *T. gondii* develop detectable specific IgM antibodies within 2–4 weeks post infection, and most become seronegative by 16 weeks (Lappin, 2014). However some cats, particularly those with FIV or ocular toxoplasmosis, may have persistent IgM titres. Given that some cats never develop a detectable IgM response and others have persistent IgM antibodies, it is not possible to use IgM serology to predict recent infection accurately, although a positive titre can be suggestive. Furthermore, *T. gondii*-specific IgG can be detected by serum ELISA in healthy cats from 3–4 weeks after experimental infection (Lappin, 1996). By this time, oocyst shedding has usually been completed and therefore IgG-seropositive cats are usually considered to be of low risk to public health. However, *T. gondii* IgG antibodies usually persist in the sera of infected cats for years or even for their lifetime, owing to the persistence of tissue infection.

In a study of clinical feline toxoplasmosis, 93% of the cats had positive *T. gondii* IgM titres, whereas only 60% had positive IgG titres, indicating that measuring IgM antibodies could be more useful than IgG when clinical feline toxoplasmosis is suspected (Lappin, 2014). In addition, anti-*T. gondii* antibodies can be measured in the CSF and aqueous humour to demonstrate local production of antibodies as an indication of organ infection. These local titres can be compared with the serum antibody concentration using an antibody coefficient to determine whether local production of antibodies is present or antibodies have just diffused from the blood circulation.

Toxoplasma gondii tachyzoites may be detected in peritoneal and ascitic fluids by cytology during acute toxoplasmosis, and more rarely in CSF, blood and bronchoalveolar lavage washings or other tissues (Figure 29.15). PCR performed on CSF, aqueous humour or any other body fluid or internal organ tissue can be used for confirmation of infection with *T. gondii*.

Neospora caninum

Neospora caninum is a coccidian parasite which is an important cause of abortion in livestock worldwide and can also cause neurological disease in dogs. Several domestic (e.g. dogs, cattle, sheep, goats, horses, chickens) and wild animal species (deer, rodents, rabbits, coyotes, wolves, foxes, birds) can be infected with *N. caninum* (Dubey and Schares, 2011).

The sexually reproductive stage of the parasite's life cycle occurs in the intestine of a canine definitive host which passes oocysts in the faeces that can be ingested, following sporulation in the environment, by intermediate

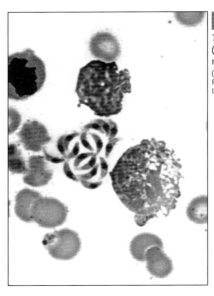

29.15 Bone marrow smear showing *Toxoplasma* tachyzoites. (Giemsa stain; original magnification X1000) (Courtesy of Drs Caldin and Furlanello, Veterinary ISan Marco Laboratory, Padua, Italy)

hosts such as cattle. Dogs acquire the infection mainly by ingesting parasite cysts from tissues of infected intermediate hosts, in particular cattle. In addition, transplacental transmission during pregnancy has been shown to occur in dogs, sheep and cattle.

In dogs, *N. caninum* can cause neurological disease, especially in congenitally infected puppies, where it forms cysts in the central nervous system. Typical signs in puppies include ascending hindlimb paresis and ataxia which becomes progressively severe, muscle atrophy, muscular back pain, head tilt, ocular abnormalities, urinary incontinence and dysphagia. Infected adult dogs may suffer from encephalomyelitis, focal cutaneous nodules or ulcers, pneumonia, peritonitis or myocarditis (Lyon, 2010).

Muscle enzyme concentrations such as creatine kinase (CK) and AST may be increased. CSF abnormalities include mild increases in protein concentrations and nucleated cell counts with predominantly mononuclear cells.

The diagnosis of canine neosporosis can be based on clinical signs and positive serology by ELISA or IFA. Puppies usually seroconvert 2–3 weeks after infection and antibody levels are frequently high in clinically sick dogs. A 4-fold increase in titre is associated with recent infection, and titres of ≥1:800 in conjunction with compatible clinical signs suggest clinical neosporosis. Suspicion of canine neosporosis can be confirmed by demonstrating the presence of the parasite's DNA by PCR on CSF or muscle biopsy samples. *Neospora caninum* tachyzoites can occasionally be detected in the CSF.

Case examples

CASE 1

SIGNALMENT

4-year-old entire female mixed-breed dog.

HISTORY

2-month history of cutaneous lesions and progressive loss of bodyweight with normal appetite. The dog lives in London but travels to Malta for 2 months every year. Cutaneous lesions are present, characterized by exfoliative dermatitis, mainly on the face and tips of the ears (Figure 29.16).

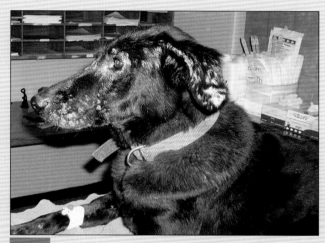

29.16 Cutaneous lesions in a 4-year-old mixed breed dog.

Mild to moderate generalized peripheral lymphadenomegaly is noted.

CLINICAL PATHOLOGY DATA

CBC was within normal limits.

Biochemistry	Result	Reference interval
Total protein (g/l)	72	54–77
Albumin (g/l)	**22**	25–40
Globulin (g/l)	**50**	23–45
Urea (mmol/l)	6.5	2.5–7.4
Creatinine (μmol/l)	130	40–145
Potassium (mmol/l)	5.1	3.4–5.6
Sodium (mmol/l)	144	139–154
Chloride (mmol/l)	107	105–122
Calcium (mmol/l)	2.8	2.3–3.0
Inorganic phosphate (mmol/l)	1.28	0.60–1.40
Glucose (mmol/l)	4.8	3.3–5.8
ALT (IU/l)	50	0–55
AST (IU/l)	27	0–49 ▶

Abnormal results are in **bold**.

Biochemistry *continued*	Result	Reference interval
ALP (IU/l)	48	0–50
Bilirubin (μmol/l)	1	0–16
Cholesterol (mmol/l)	4.1	3.8–7.0
Triglyceride (mmol/l)	1.1	0.56–1.14
Creatine kinase (IU/l)	53	0–190

Abnormal results are in **bold**.

Sample quality: clear.

Urinalysis	Result
Gross appearance	Yellow, clear
Specific gravity	1.035
Dipstick	pH 6.5 Negative for bilirubin, ketones, glucose and urobilinogen Positive for protein (3+, 300 mg/dl)
Sediment examination	WBC/hpf=1, RBC/hpf=1 No epithelial cells, casts or crystals seen
Urine protein:creatinine ratio	4.7 (normal <0.2)

Cytology of the fine-needle aspirate from the right popliteal lymph node is shown in Figure 29.17.

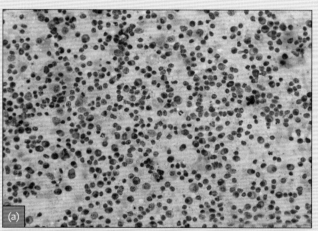

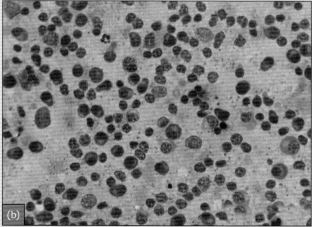

29.17 (a–b) Cytology of the fine-needle aspirate from the right popliteal lymph node. (Diff-Quik® stain; original magnification (a) X20, (b) X40)

(Courtesy of Antonio Melendez, Universitat Autonoma de Barcelona, Spain)

→ **CASE 1 CONTINUED**

Biochemical profile

Hypoalbuminaemia and hyperglobulinaemia are present with normal concentration of total protein.

Urinalysis

Proteinuria with an inactive sediment is present, based on urinalysis and urine protein:creatinine ratio.

Lymph node cytology

The majority of lymphocytes are small, with lower numbers of intermediate lymphocytes. Plasma cells are increased, including Mott cells. There are rare non-degenerate neutrophils but no microorganisms.

HOW WOULD YOU INTERPRET THESE RESULTS AND WHAT ARE THE DIFFERENTIAL DIAGNOSES?

Hypoalbuminaemia with evidence of proteinuria suggests an ongoing protein-losing nephropathy in this patient. In the presence of hyperglobulinaemia an inflammatory process (infectious or immune-mediated diseases) would be the principal consideration, but other less likely differentials include neoplastic lymphoproliferative disorders.

The cytological findings are compatible with a marked reactive lymph node hyperplasia.

Canine leishmaniosis is the main consideration in this case owing to the presence of classical cutaneous lesions and lymphadenomegaly with a reactive lymph node and classical clinicopathological abnormalities (hypoalbuminaemia, hyperglobulinaemia and proteinuria). However, other less likely differentials cannot be completely ruled out, such as an immune-mediated disease (e.g. systemic lupus erythematosus) or lymphoproliferative disorder.

WHAT FURTHER TESTS WOULD YOU RECOMMEND?

Serum electrophoresis is recommended to characterize the hyperglobulinaemia further. Ultrasonography of the kidneys may be helpful. Renal biopsy may be considered, but only after very careful analysis of the risk/clinical benefit balance inherent in this procedure.

The most common test employed for the diagnosis of canine leishmaniosis is a quantitative serological test to detect specific *Leishmania* antibody levels. PCR on the lymph node aspirate could also be employed as a complementary test.

CASE OUTCOME

In this case, serum electrophoresis was performed and was abnormal, with evidence of hypoalbuminaemia and polyclonal gammaglobulinaemia supporting (in the presence of compatible clinical signs and clinical laboratory data) a diagnosis of leishmaniosis.

Abdominal ultrasonography revealed slightly small kidneys with preservation of normal renal architecture. These findings are compatible with protein-losing nephropathy.

Quantitative serological testing was also performed by ELISA to detect specific *Leishmania infantum* antibody levels, resulting in a high positive antibody level (300% of positivity by ELISA; cut-off: 35%). In addition, real-time *Leishmania* PCR from the lymph node sample was carried out as a complementary test with a positive result. A high positive antibody level in the presence of compatible clinicopathological findings and no previous history of *Leishmania* vaccination confirms a diagnosis of canine leishmaniosis. However, the presence of lower antibody levels is not necessarily indicative of patent disease and needs to be confirmed by another diagnostic method such as PCR, cytology or histology. Serology and PCR confirmed the diagnosis of leishmaniosis in this patient. It is important to highlight that PCR should not be employed alone because, in endemic areas, clinically healthy infected dogs might be PCR positive and never develop clinical disease. Whereas a high anti-leishmanial antibody level is better correlated with clinical disease and found in dogs with clinical leishmaniosis, or often in dogs progressing towards clinical disease. Therefore, PCR results should be interpreted in conjunction with the clinical history, clinicopathological findings and a quantitative serological test.

The dog recovered well with specific treatment (meglumine antimoniate for 1 month and long-term treatment with allopurinol for >1 year).

CASE 2

SIGNALMENT

5-year-old entire female German Shepherd Dog.

HISTORY

The dog lives in a village in a Mediterranean country and roams freely. She gave birth 2 weeks previously and the puppies died. The owners' main complaint is that the dog is bleeding from the nose and sneezing, and has shown decreased food and water intake that started 5 days before admission. The physical examination on presentation revealed:

- Temperature: 39.2°C, heart rate: 152 bpm, respiratory rate: panting
- Pale mucous membranes
- Unilateral epistaxis (right nostril); later the epistaxis became bilateral
- No other remarkable findings were noted.

→ CASE 2 CONTINUED

CLINICAL PATHOLOGY DATA

Haematology	Result	Reference interval
WBC (x 10⁹/l)	**0.1**	6–17
RBC (x 10¹²/l)	**1.61**	5.5–8.5
PCV (%)	**10**	37–55
MCV (fl)	62	60–77
MCHC (g/dl)	33.7	31–44
Platelets (x 10⁹/l)	**0**	150–500

Abnormal results are in **bold**.

Blood smear examination revealed no evidence of poly-chromasia, rare white blood cells (WBCs), no evidence of platelet aggregates or macroplatelets or clot in the whole blood. Rare platelets were seen with <1–2 platelets per field (X1000).

Biochemistry	Result	Reference interval
Total protein (g/l)	70	54–77
Albumin (g/l)	25	25–40
Globulin (g/l)	**45**	23–40
Urea (mmol/l)	7.1	2.5–7.4
Creatinine (μmol/l)	120	40–145
Potassium (mmol/l)	3.5	3.4–5.6
Sodium (mmol/l)	145	139–154
Chloride (mmol/l)	106	105–122
Calcium (mmol/l)	2.5	2.3–3.0
Inorganic phosphate (mmol/l)	1.1	0.60–1.40
Glucose (mmol/l)	4.9	3.3–5.8
ALT (IU/l)	50	0–55
AST (IU/l)	23	0–49
ALP (IU/l)	45	0–50
Bilirubin (μmol/l)	2	0–16
Creatine kinase (IU/l)	105	0–190

Abnormal results are in **bold**.

Coagulation profile

Prothrombin time (PT): 6.45 seconds (6–8).
Activated partial thromboplastin time (aPTT): 11 seconds (11–17).

WHAT ABNORMALITIES ARE PRESENT AND WHAT ARE THE POSSIBLE DIFFERENTIALS?

Haematology

The CBC shows a marked pancytopenia. There is a marked anaemia with no evidence of regeneration and marked leucopenia and thrombocytopenia. This suggests a generalized decrease in haemopoiesis in the bone marrow. Causes of decreased haemopoiesis include bone marrow hypoplasia or aplasia, bone marrow necrosis/fibrosis/sclerosis, myelophthisis and myelodysplastic syndrome. Many infectious, neoplastic, inflammatory, toxic or immune-mediated diseases can result in decreased cellular production by various mechanisms.

Biochemical profile

Hyperglobulinaemia is present with a normal concentration of total protein. Hyperglobulinaemia suggests an inflammatory process (infectious or immune-mediated diseases) but other less likely differentials include neoplastic lymphoproliferative disorders.

Coagulation profile

PT and aPTT are within normal limits.

WHAT FURTHER TESTS WOULD YOU PERFORM?

Bone marrow aspiration was attempted but this gave a non-diagnostic 'dry tap'. A biopsy was performed and histopathological evaluation of the bone marrow is shown in Figure 29.18.

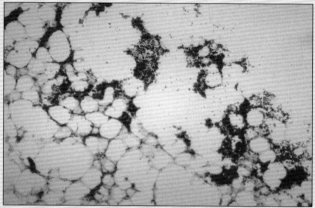

29.18 Histopathological appearance of bone marrow. (Haematoxylin and eosin stain; original magnification X40)

Bone marrow histopathological evaluation

Cellularity is extremely decreased. No evidence of megakaryocytic precursors and very rare erythroid and myeloid precursors are noted. No aetiological agents or neoplastic cells are observed.

HOW WOULD YOU INTERPRET THESE RESULTS AND WHAT ARE THE DIFFERENTIAL DIAGNOSES?

The histopathological findings are compatible with aplasia of the megakaryocytic, myeloid and erythroid cell lines.

The most likely differential diagnoses for pancytopenia in this case, based on the clinical history, clinical findings and clinicopathological abnormalities, are infectious causes (ehrlichiosis due to *Ehrlichia canis*, histoplasmosis or, less likely, leishmaniosis) or aplastic anaemia (e.g. due to oestrogen toxicity, an oestrogen-producing tumour or drug-induced toxicity).

WHAT FURTHER TESTS WOULD YOU RECOMMEND?

Serum protein electrophoresis is recommended to characterize the hyperglobulinaemia further.

The most common tests employed for the diagnosis of canine ehrlichiosis are a quantitative serological test to detect specific *E. canis* antibody levels and PCR on blood or splenic specimens.

→ **CASE 2 CONTINUED**

The most common test employed for the diagnosis of canine leishmaniosis is a quantitative serological test to detect specific *Leishmania* antibody levels and rule out co-infection.

CASE OUTCOME

In this case, serum electrophoresis was performed and was abnormal, with evidence of polyclonal gamma-globulinaemia supporting (in the presence of compatible clinical signs and clinical laboratory data) a diagnosis of an infectious disease as a cause for the pancytopenia.

Quantitative serological testing was also performed by ELISA to detect specific *L. infantum* and *E. canis* antibodies, resulting in negative (optical density of 0.05) and high positive (1:1280) antibody levels, respectively. In addition, *Leishmania* and *Ehrlichia* PCRs were carried out on blood samples with negative and positive results, respectively. Serology and PCR confirmed the diagnosis of ehrlichiosis due to *E. canis* in the patient.

The dog did not recover despite treatment with doxycycline, amoxicillin-clavulanic acid (co-amoxiclav) (broad-spectrum antibiotics were used because of the severe leucopenia), an immunosuppressive dose of prednisone and famotidine, and the owners elected euthanasia.

References and further reading

Allison RW and Little SE (2013) Diagnosis of rickettsial diseases in dogs and cats. *Veterinary Clinical Pathology* **42**, 127–144

Baneth G (2011) Perspectives on canine and feline hepatozoonosis. *Veterinary Parasitology* **181**, 3–11

Baneth G, Florin-Christensen M, Cardoso L, *et al.* (2015) Reclassification of *Theileria annae* as *Babesia vulpes* sp. nov. *Parasite and Vectors* **8**, 207

Baneth G, Harrus S, Ohnona FS *et al.* (2009) Longitudinal quantification of *Ehrlichia canis* in experimental infection with comparison to natural infection. *Veterinary Microbiology* **136**, 321–325

Baneth G, Kenny MJ, Tasker S *et al.* (2004) Infection with a proposed new subspecies of *Babesia canis*, *Babesia canis* subsp. *presentii*, in domestic cats. *Journal of Clinical Microbiology* **42**, 99–105

Baneth G, Sheiner A, Eyal O *et al.* (2013) Redescription of *Hepatozoon felis* (Apicomplexa: Hepatozoidae) based on phylogenetic analysis, tissue and blood form morphology, and possible transplacental transmission. *Parasites and Vectors* **6**, 102

Baneth G and Solano-Gallego L (2012) Global aspects of leishmaniosis: canine leishmaniosis. In: *Infectious Diseases of Dogs and Cats, 4th edn*, ed. CE Greene, pp. 734–746. Saunders Elsevier, Philadelphia

Bosman AM, Oosthuizen MC, Venter EH, Steyl JC, Gous TA and Penzhorn BL (2013) *Babesia lengau* associated with cerebral and haemolytic babesiosis in two domestic cats. *Parasites and Vectors* **6**, 128

Breitschwerdt EB, Maggi RG, Chomel BB *et al.* (2010) Bartonellosis: an emerging infectious disease of zoonotic importance to animals and human beings. *Journal of Veterinary Emergency and Critical Care* **20**, 8–30

Brunt J, Guptill L, Kordick DL, *et al.* (2006) American Association of Feline Practitioners 2006 Panel report on diagnosis, treatment, and prevention of *Bartonella* spp. infections. *Journal of Feline Medicine and Surgery* **8**, 213–226

Carli E, Trotta M, Chinelli R *et al.* (2012) *Cytauxzoon* sp. infection in the first endemic focus described in domestic cats in Europe. *Veterinary Parasitology* **183**, 343–352

Carrade DD, Foley JE, Borjesson DL *et al.* (2009) Canine granulocytic anaplasmosis: a review. *Journal of Veterinary Internal Medicine* **23**, 1129–1141

Day M and Kohn B (2012) *BSAVA Manual of Canine and Feline Haematology and Transfusion Medicine, 2nd edn*. BSAVA Publications, Gloucester

Dubey JP and Schares G (2011) Neosporosis in animals – the last five years. *Veterinary Parasitology* **180**, 90–108

Gary AT, Richmond HL, Tasker S *et al.* (2006) Survival of *Mycoplasma haemofelis* and 'Candidatus Mycoplasma haemominutum' in blood of cats used for transfusions. *Journal of Feline Medicine and Surgery* **8**, 321–326

Grogl M, Daugirda JL, Hoover DL *et al.* (1993) Survivability and infectivity of viscerotropic *Leishmania tropica* from Operation Desert Storm participants in human blood products maintained under blood bank conditions. *American Journal of Tropical Medicine and Hygiene* **49**, 308–315

Harrus S and Waner T (2011) Diagnosis of canine monocytotropic ehrlichiosis (*Ehrlichia canis*): an overview. *Veterinary Journal* **187**, 292–296

Holman PJ and Snowden KF (2009) Canine hepatozoonosis and babesiosis, and feline cytauxzoonosis. *Veterinary Clinics of North America: Small Animal Practice* **39**, 1035–1053

Krupka I and Straubinger RK (2010) Lyme borreliosis in dogs and cats: background, diagnosis, treatment and prevention of infections with *Borrelia burgdorferi* sensu stricto. *Veterinary Clinics of North America: Small Animal Practice* **40**, 1103–1119

Lappin MR (1996) Feline toxoplasmosis: interpretation of diagnostic test results. *Seminars in Veterinary Medicine and Surgery (Small Animal)* **11**, 154–160

Lappin MR (2010) Update on the diagnosis and management of *Toxoplasma gondii* infection in cats. *Topics in Companion Animal Medicine* **25**, 136–141

Lappin MR (2014) Toxoplasmosis. In: *Canine and Feline Infectious Diseases*, ed. JE Sykes, pp. 693–703. Elsevier, St. Louis

Lappin MR, Breitschwerdt EB, Jensen WA *et al.* (2004) Molecular and serologic evidence of *Anaplasma phagocytophilum* infection in cats in North America. *Journal of the American Veterinary Medical Association* **225**, 893–896

Lyon C (2010) Update on the diagnosis and management of *Neospora caninum* infections in dogs. *Topics in Companion Animal Medicine* **25**, 170–175

Millan J, Naranjo V, Rodriguez A *et al.* (2007) Prevalence of infection and 18S rRNA gene sequences of *Cytauxzoon* species in Iberian lynx (*Lynx pardinus*) in Spain. *Parasitology* **134**, 995–1001

Schoeman T, Lobetti RG, Jacobson LS *et al.* (2001) Feline babesiosis: signalment, clinical pathology and concurrent infections. *Journal of the South African Veterinary Association* **72**, 4–11

Shaw SE, Lerga AI, Williams S *et al.* (2003) Review of exotic infectious diseases in small animals entering the United Kingdom from abroad diagnosed by PCR. *Veterinary Record* **152**, 176–177

Simon F, Siles-Lucas M, Morchon R *et al.* (2012) Human and animal dirofilariasis: the emergence of a zoonotic mosaic. *Clinical Microbiology Reviews* **25**, 507–544

Solano-Gallego L and Baneth G (2011) Babesiosis in dogs and cats: Expanding parasitological and clinical spectra. *Veterinary Parasitology* **181**, 48–60

Solano-Gallego L and Baneth G (2012) Feline leishmaniosis. In: *Infectious Diseases of Dogs and Cats, 4th edn*, ed. CE Greene, pp. 748–749. Saunders Elsevier, Philadelphia

Solano-Gallego L, Koutinas A, Miro G, *et al.* (2009) Directions for the diagnosis, clinical staging, treatment and prevention of canine leishmaniosis. *Veterinary Parasitology* **165**, 1–18

Solano-Gallego L, Miro G, Koutinas A, *et al.* (2011) LeishVet guidelines for the practical management of canine leishmaniosis. *Parasite Vectors* **4**, 86

Sykes JE, Drazenovich NL, Ball LM, *et al.* (2007) Use of conventional and real-time polymerase chain reaction to determine the epidemiology of hemoplasma infections in anemic and nonanemic cats. *Journal of Veterinary Internal Medicine* **21**, 685–693

Sykes JE (2010) Feline hemotropic mycoplasmas. *Veterinary Clinics of North America: Small Animal Practice* **40**, 1157–1170

Wardrop KJ, Reine N, Birkenheuer A, *et al.* (2005) Canine and feline blood donor screening for infectious disease. *Journal of Veterinary Internal Medicine* **19**, 135–142

Useful websites

Maps showing the occurrence of canine vector-borne diseases are available at: http://www.cvbd.org/en/occurrence-maps/world-map/

Chapter 30

Diagnosis of inherited diseases

Alex Gough

It has long been recognized that some diseases in domestic animals are due wholly or partly to inheritance, with Darwin himself describing inherited conditions such as polydactyly in the dog and cat, and noting that there is a 'unanimity of belief among veterinaries of all nations in the transmission of various morbid tendencies' (Darwin, 1865). Since Darwin's time, numerous inherited diseases have been described in companion animals. Inherited diseases in dogs and cats can be divided into those related and those unrelated to breed standards. In one recent review of the top 50 UK Kennel Club registered breeds, each breed was found to have at least one aspect of its conformation that predisposed it to a disorder. In total, 84 disorders were identified that were associated with conformation. Many of these were associated with the brachycephalic head shape, such as brachycephalic obstructive airway syndrome and Chiari-like malformation/syringomyelia. Other common conditions related to conformation included degenerative disc disease associated with chondrodystrophic breeds, skin disorders due to excessive skin folds and dermoid sinus associated with the hair ridge of Rhodesian Ridgebacks (Asher *et al.*, 2009). In a further review, 213 inherited disorders not linked to conformation were identified in the top 50 breeds, with the Golden Retriever and German Shepherd Dog having the largest number of disorders. The four non-conformational disorders affecting the largest number of breeds were hypothyroidism, adult-onset cataract, progressive retinal atrophy and von Willebrand's disease. Of the conditions identified, 71% had an autosomal recessive mode of inheritance (Summers *et al.*, 2010).

A great deal of public and media attention in recent years has been focused on inherited diseases of pedigree animals. An independent inquiry by Professor Sir Patrick Bateson (Bateson, 2010) identified welfare costs of current breeding practices to individual dogs, including 'use of breeding pairs carrying inherited disorders' and 'artificial selection for extreme characteristics'. He recommended that 'the best available science and advice should be provided to breeders to guide their efforts.' For veterinary surgeons (veterinarians) to fulfil this role, they need an understanding of basic genetics, and of the variety and extent to which genetic diseases affect their patients, as well as methods of diagnosing these conditions. This chapter offers an introduction to this subject, but those wanting more in-depth information should consult the References and further reading section below. A glossary of terms used in this chapter is found in Figure 30.1.

Term	Definition
Allele	Any of the different forms of a gene that are found at a particular position or locus on a chromosome
Autosomes	Any of the chromosomes, not including the sex chromosomes
Base	A unit of DNA – adenine, cytosine, guanine or thymine
Base pair	Two complementary bases that join together to form the DNA double helix. Guanine always pairs with cytosine, and adenine with thymine
Chromosomes	Microscopic structures within the cell nucleus that contain DNA, and carry the majority of the genetic information found within the cell
Congenital	Present at or before birth. Congenital conditions are often, but not necessarily, inherited
DNA	Deoxyribonucleic acid, the famous helical compound which stores an organism's genetic code
Dominant	A dominant gene will be expressed in the organism's phenotype, regardless of whether the gene found at the same location on the chromosome which forms its homologous pair is identical. This means it will mask the expression of a recessive gene
Exon	A sequence of DNA that codes for synthesis of a protein. Exons are separated by introns
Gene	The basic unit of inheritance, found at a particular locus on a chromosome
Genome	The totality of the genetic information in an organism
Genotype	The genetic make-up of an individual organism
Heterozygous	Having different alleles at a particular location on homologous chromosomes
Homologous pair	A pair of chromosomes that match up during cell division. They code for similar but not necessarily identical genes
Homozygous	Having the same allele at a particular location on homologous chromosomes
Inheritance	The transmission of characteristics from parents to offspring
Intron	A sequence of DNA situated between exons that does not code for protein synthesis
Locus	A position on a chromosome

30.1 Definitions of terminology used in this chapter. (continues) ▶

Term	Definition
Nucleotide	A monomer or subunit of nucleic acids such as DNA and RNA. They contain the sugar deoxyribose (DNA) or ribose (RNA), a base (cytosine, thymine, uracil, guanine or adenine) and a phosphate group
Penetrance	The frequency with which a trait is expressed in a population carrying the gene that codes for the trait. This can be expressed as a percentage, or can be termed complete or incomplete
Phenotype	The observable characteristics of an organism resulting from the interaction of its genotype with the environment
Recessive	An allele that is not expressed if present with a dominant allele, but only if another recessive allele is present, i.e. it will only be expressed if the organism is homozygous for the recessive allele
Single nucleotide polymorphism	Variation between individuals of a single base in the DNA code

30.1 (continued) Definitions of terminology used in this chapter.

The canine and feline genome

Dogs have an enormous variation in phenotype: in conformation, coat and other attributes. It is generally accepted that dogs are descended from wolves, although there are various estimates regarding the time at which dogs genetically diverged from their ancestors, ranging from 15,000 to 100,000 years ago. It may be that there was more than one domestication event, and interbreeding with wolves may have continued after this time. Wolf pups taken as pets would have been artificially selected for sociability and decreased flight behaviour (Driscoll et al., 2009). Most of the several hundred currently existing dog breeds were developed in the last few hundred years (Wayne and Ostrander, 1999), although the oldest known breed, the Tibetan Mastiff, has been estimated to have diverged from wolves 58,000 years ago (Li et al., 2008). Dogs had two genetic bottlenecks in their history; one, thousands of years ago when they diverged from wolves, and one more recently with the creation of modern dog breeds.

As most dog breeds are young in evolutionary terms, there has been little time, for new mutations to occur in the genome. It is therefore thought that most genetic mutations causing disease occurred prior to the foundation of the breeds. This means that related breeds of dogs are more likely to share inherited diseases and predispositions to disease. It has also been shown that there is more variation in non-silent (i.e. functional) genes in domestic dogs than in wolves. In many cases, an alteration of the function of the gene will be deleterious. It may be that population bottlenecks and selective breeding have reduced selection against these genes. The consequence is that modern dog breeds may be more prone to genetic diseases than their wild ancestors (Cruz et al., 2008).

By contrast, cats have a much more limited variation in phenotype than dogs. They are thought to have become domesticated later than dogs, when their wildcat ancestors exploited human environments. However, being solitary, obligate carnivores, unable to perform directed tasks, they were of limited utility to early humans. Consequently, there was less deliberate breeding and artificial selection of cats. Domestic cats do not have reduced genetic diversity when compared with wildcats. The wildcat, *Felis silvestris*, has five wild subspecies, and the domestic cat is considered to be a sixth subspecies, *Felis silvestris catus* (Driscoll et al., 2009).

A high-quality canine genome sequence was published in *Nature* in 2005 (Lindblad-Toh et al., 2005). The canine genome comprises 2.4 billion base pairs, with an estimate of just under 20,000 genes. A 'first draft' feline genome was initially sequenced in 2007 (Pontius et al., 2007), with further research building on this work since. The feline genome is estimated to comprise 2.7 billion base pairs.

Basic genetics

Genetics is the study of the hereditary transmission of characteristics and of the variation in inherited characteristics. The material that stores the genetic code is deoxyribonucleic acid (DNA), found predominantly in the cell nucleus but also in the mitochondria. DNA is composed of matching pairs of bases, guanine–cytosine and adenine–thymine, arranged into the well-known double helix. A DNA nucleotide contains the sugar deoxyribose, a base (cytosine, thymine, guanine or adenine) and a phosphate group. A length of DNA that carries the code for a particular protein is known as a gene. Chromosomes are long strands of DNA comprising genes plus long regions that do not code for specific proteins. Previously, these non-coding regions of DNA were thought to be of no importance and were termed 'junk DNA'. It is now recognized that at least some of these regions do have important functions, for example in transcription and translation of protein-encoding sequences.

When a somatic cell divides, the chromosomes in the cell nucleus shorten and thicken. They then replicate, and one copy of each chromosome ends up in each new cell. However, when a gamete is produced, the chromosomes line up with a companion, the two being termed a homologous pair. Chromosomes always match up with the same companion. Cell division here leads to cells with half the normal number of chromosomes, so that when two gametes combine in the process of fertilization, the zygote has the correct number of chromosomes. Most of the chromosomes that make up a homologous pair code for similar, although not necessarily identical, genes. These chromosomes are called autosomes. However, the sex chromosomes are markedly different, with the X chromosome coding for many more genes than the Y chromosome. An animal with an XX genotype will be female and one with an XY chromosome arrangement will be male.

One animal may carry up to two different versions of each gene, one on each chromosome of a homologous pair. However, more versions of a gene may exist in a population. These different versions of a gene are called alleles. When two different alleles are present on the two homologous chromosomes, they may be expressed in different ways. One allele may be dominant, and the other recessive. In this case, the phenotype for the characteristic encoded by the gene will be that of the dominant type. The recessive phenotype will only be expressed if the animal has two recessive alleles for that characteristic. Sometimes, alleles are co-dominant, and both will play a role in the expression of the phenotype. However, the presence of a dominant gene does not always mean that the gene's phenotype will be expressed. Some genes have incomplete penetrance, meaning that they are not fully expressed in every individual. Penetrance is the proportion of individuals carrying a particular allele that express the associated trait. An example of this is polycystic kidney disease in Persian cats, which is inherited in an autosomal dominant fashion with incomplete penetrance (Biller *et al.*, 1996).

Given that, in the process of gamete production, alleles separate randomly, the inheritance of different genetic traits is independent. However, genes on the same chromosome, especially ones located close to each other, will often be passed on together. This means that two traits controlled by different genes will often be found together in the same individual, a process known as linkage.

Simple Mendelian inheritance

Where conditions are inherited in a simple way, i.e. a single gene with an autosomal dominant or recessive mode of inheritance, it is possible to predict likely outcomes of matings if the parents' genetic make-up is known. This is known as Mendelian genetics after Gregor Mendel, the monk who discovered many of the rules of heredity. One example is the determination of coat colour in the Labrador Retriever. Black or brown coat coloration is determined by the expression of a gene coding for tyrosine-related protein 1, which is found in melanosomes, the cellular organelles that produce and store pigments. Mutations in this gene lead to a reduction in enzyme activity. As the dog has inherited two copies of the gene, one from each parent, provided at least one copy is functional (in this example referred to as B), black pigment will be produced and the coat colour will be black. If the dog has inherited two mutated copies (referred to as b), enzyme production will be reduced and the coat colour will be brown. Therefore, the black coat colour is dominant because one B allele and one b allele will result in a black coat. It requires two copies of the b allele for the brown coat colour to be expressed. Thus, a black Labrador could have the genotype BB or Bb, while a chocolate Labrador would have the genotype bb. Note that the yellow coat type involves a different gene. Animals carrying two identical copies of a gene are known as homozygotes and animals carrying two different copies of a gene are known as heterozygotes.

To understand the likely outcomes of matings, a matrix can be produced to help visualize the results. For example, if a BB black male is crossed with a bb brown bitch, each of the male's spermatozoa carries a single B gene, and each female ovum carries a single b gene, producing the following mating matrix:

		Male	
		B	B
Female	b	Bb	Bb
	b	Bb	Bb

All offspring would have the genotype Bb and would be phenotypically black. However, if two Bb genotype black Labradors were crossed, the matrix would look like this:

		Male	
		B	b
Female	B	BB	Bb
	b	Bb	bb

Thus, one in four offspring would have the BB genotype, two in four the Bb genotype and one in four the bb genotype. This means three would be phenotypically black

and one phenotypically chocolate. In reality, because the process of fertilization is random, these are only probabilities, and may not reflect the situation in a small litter.

Sex-linked inheritance

The situation is different for characteristics encoded by genes situated on the X chromosome because generally there is no equivalent copy on the Y chromosome. Therefore, males with an affected copy of the gene will express the phenotype of the gene regardless of its dominant or recessive nature, whereas in females the phenotype will be expressed in accordance with dominance, in the manner of autosomes. To understand this, consider X-linked muscular dystrophy in the Golden Retriever. The allele for muscular dystrophy (here referred to as M) resides on the X chromosome, as does the normal version of the gene (here referred to as N). M is recessive to N, so a female carrying a single copy of the gene would not be phenotypically affected. However, if this female carrier was mated to an unaffected male, the matrix for their offspring would appear as follows:

		Male	
		X^N	Y
Female	X^M	$X^M X^N$	$X^M Y$
	X^N	$X^N X^N$	$X^N Y$

From the matrix it can be seen that in this cross, all of the females will be phenotypically unaffected, since they all carry a normal copy of the gene, although 50% will be carriers. However, 50% of males will carry the abnormal gene and be affected because they carry no normal gene. The other 50% of the males will neither carry the gene nor exhibit the phenotype.

It can be seen that, for sex-linked diseases, most affected individuals will be male (unless an affected male breeds with a female carrying the gene, making it possible for a female to have two faulty copies of the gene). Furthermore, males cannot normally be asymptomatic carriers.

Complex modes of inheritance

A more complicated situation occurs when there is more than one gene responsible for the expression of a disease. Some conditions also arise as a result of the interaction between genotype and environment. For example, hip dysplasia, the most common hereditary skeletal disorder in dogs, has been shown to have a polygenic mode of inheritance. Recently, nine single nucleotide polymorphisms (SNPs: variations between individuals of a single base in the DNA code) found on five different chromosomes have been found to have a significant association with canine hip dysplasia (Fels *et al.*, 2014). The genotypic effects of these nine SNPs were estimated to be responsible for between 22 and 34% of the phenotypic variance of hip dysplasia in German Shepherd Dogs. It has been estimated that roughly between a quarter and a half of the variability in the development of hip dysplasia is due to genetic factors. This means that there are also significant environmental factors involved in the aetiopathogenesis of canine hip dysplasia, such as nutritional factors and over-exercise during immaturity (Wilson *et al.*, 2011).

Some diseases are inherited not via the DNA of the nucleus at all, but through the DNA of the mitochondria. Mitochondria are always passed down from the mother and so diseases and characteristics associated with mito-chondrial DNA can only be inherited from the mother. One example of this is sensory ataxic neuropathy of the Golden Retriever (Baranowska *et al.*, 2009). In diseases due to mitochondrial inheritance, breeding from affected females is not recommended.

Diagnosis of genetic disease

The index of suspicion that a condition in an individual presenting to a clinician is genetic in origin may be raised in certain circumstances, including the following situations.

- More than one individual in a litter is affected. However, hereditary diseases tend to involve only a few individuals in a litter, because most of the genetic diseases of companion animals are recessive, or dominant with incomplete penetrance. If the entire litter is affected, then toxic, infectious and nutritional causes should be considered.
- Clinical signs arise early in life. Many genetic defects will lead to resorption, abortion or stillbirth, and many others will lead to death in the first few weeks of life when the maternal system can no longer support a fetus with a serious defect. Failure to thrive, or fading puppy or kitten syndrome, may be related to a genetic defect. Many of these cases will never have the exact condition diagnosed, and in fact many will not even be presented to veterinary surgeons, being considered normal losses by breeders. In cases where the genetic condition is not rapidly fatal, clinical signs will still often be apparent early in life. However, there are many genetic conditions that do not manifest until adulthood, such as many of the hereditary ocular and neurological diseases. Note that the term congenital disease means present at birth, and does not necessarily mean that the condition is hereditary. Nevertheless, many congenital diseases will have a genetic component.
- The disease is recognized as a breed predisposition in that patient's breed.
- The condition is chronic and progressive. Some genetic diseases, however, can have intermittent signs, for example von Willebrand's disease.

A disease in a population may be suspected to be genetic in origin if it meets some or all of the above criteria. It may also be recognized as genetic in origin by analysing pedigree lines, and identifying affected individuals. Diseases with breed predispositions will often have a genetic component, although not all breed predispositions are genetic. Some breed predispositions relate to the use to which the breed is put, or to its behaviour. For example, Springer Spaniels are prone to grass awn migration because of their behaviour on exercise (although it could be argued that their behaviour has a genetic component). Greyhounds are prone to musculoskeletal injuries related to their use in racing.

The heritability of a disease in a population can be estimated using statistical methods, especially if a large enough sample of the population is studied. The heritability is the proportion of phenotypic variance due to genetic variance, i.e. the extent to which the variance in phenotype is due to the effect of alleles which can be inherited. Heritability of 0 means there is no genetic cause, and 1 means that the trait is entirely due to genetic factors. For example, the heritability of hip dysplasia in the Labrador Retriever has been estimated at between 0.15 and 0.38 (Lewis *et al.*, 2010). This means that there is a large environmental component in the development of hip dysplasia, making the control of the disease by breed schemes challenging.

Diagnosis of suspected genetic disease

Information and tests useful in identifying genetic diseases include:

- Signalment
- History and physical examination
- Clinical pathology: haematology, biochemistry, urinalysis, endocrine testing, coagulation testing
- Imaging: radiography, ultrasonography, computed tomography (CT), magnetic resonance imaging (MRI)
- Tests for inborn errors of metabolism, e.g. urine metabolic screening
- Genetic tests.

When the clinician is presented with a patient with a suspected genetic disease, the diagnostic steps followed are generally the same as for the diagnosis of any medical disease. First, a detailed history should be taken, with particular reference in the case of suspected genetic diseases to the prevalence of similar signs in related individuals, as well as the age of onset. It can be useful to ask the client to contact their pet's breeder to request this information, although the veterinary surgeon should be aware of the potential repercussions, in which a client may seek recompense from a breeder for an animal with a genetic disease, and the breeder may resist the suggestion that they are breeding animals with genetic diseases.

A physical examination should be undertaken, assessing all body systems, but with particular attention paid to the system known to be affected. For example, an ataxic patient should undergo a full neurological examination.

At this stage, a problem list comprising all the abnormal findings should be formulated, and a differential diagnosis list can then be constructed for each problem. From here, diagnostic tests that can help determine or narrow the diagnosis can be selected. This might involve clinicopathological testing such as haematology, biochemistry, urinalysis and cytology. It may also involve imaging, such as radiography and ultrasonography, or even advanced imaging in some cases, for example MRI for the detection of syringomyelia. The choice of tests should be selected on a cost or risk:benefit basis, taking into account diagnostic yield, invasiveness and financial costs.

The results of these tests may lead to a definitive diagnosis. If a definitive diagnosis is not made, a presumptive diagnosis may be sufficient for the client. In some cases only a presumptive diagnosis can be made ante-mortem. In other cases, further testing may be required to make a definitive diagnosis. In the case of genetic diseases, definitive diagnosis can often be achieved by non-DNA testing methods. For example, a definitive diagnosis of syringomyelia can be achieved with MRI, von Willebrand's disease can be diagnosed by measuring von Willebrand factor (vWF; see Chapter 6), chronic hepatitis by histology and hypothyroidism from thyroid hormone panels (see Chapter 17). However, these tests do not prove that the disease in an individual has a genetic origin.

Note that, in some cases, clinicopathological testing can help to identify asymptomatic carriers of a disease. For example, vWF is deficient in von Willebrand's disease. It is measured in comparison to the concentration in a pooled canine sample, which is defined as 100%. A value of >70% is considered normal, whereas a value of <35% is often associated with clinical bleeding. Those with intermediate values may be asymptomatic carriers of the disease. In a normal dog, each allele contributes 50% of the normal total production of vWF. In type I von Willebrand's disease, the abnormal allele produces <15% of the normal production. Therefore, a heterozygote will produce around 65% of the normal level of vWF, and will probably be asymptomatic, while a homozygote for the abnormal allele will produce <30% of normal vWF, and is likely to be symptomatic. A prolonged buccal mucosal bleeding time may also raise the index of suspicion for von Willebrand's disease in dogs of the appropriate signalment. Other examples of clinicopathological tests that can aid in the diagnosis of genetic disease include low trypsin-like immunoreactivity (TLI) in congenital pancreatic insufficiency, low total thyroxine (T4) in congenital hypothyroidism and cystine crystals in the urine in cystinuria.

Other tests that are useful in achieving a definitive diagnosis in suspected genetic diseases include blood smear examination, coagulation tests, urinalysis, metabolic screening tests and DNA tests.

Blood smear examination

A number of hereditary diseases can be diagnosed or suspected from examination of a blood smear. Some of these are not necessarily clinically significant.

- Macrothrombocytopenia in the Cavalier King Charles Spaniel can be diagnosed by finding abnormally large platelets on a blood smear, together with reduced platelet numbers on both manual and automated counts. However, this is an asymptomatic condition (Brown *et al.*, 1994).
- Pelger–Huet anomaly can be diagnosed from abnormalities in the shape of the nucleus of neutrophils, which are band shaped but with mature clumped chromatin (Figure 30.2; Bowles *et al.*, 1979).
- Hereditary stomatocytosis can also be identified on a blood smear, and can be associated with haemolytic anaemia.
- Storage disorders can be suspected from the presence of granulation or storage vacuoles within white blood cells (Sewell *et al.*, 2007).

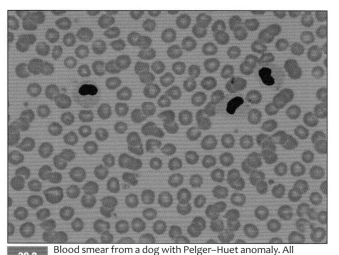

30.2 Blood smear from a dog with Pelger–Huet anomaly. All neutrophils have a band-shaped nucleus with mature chromatin. (Wright–Giemsa stain; original magnification X500)
(Courtesy of S D'Agorne of Axiom Veterinary Laboratories)

Coagulation tests

Measurement of prothrombin time (PT), activated partial thromboplastin time (aPTT), vWF and individual clotting factors can assist with the diagnosis of genetic disorders causing coagulopathies (see Chapter 6).

Urinalysis

Urine can be assessed for the presence of glucosuria, and the sediment can be examined for the presence of crystalluria.

Metabolic screening

Inborn errors of metabolism are a group of diseases attributable to a genetically determined specific defect in the structure and/or function of a protein. These include enzyme deficiencies such as pyruvate kinase and phosphofructokinase deficiencies, as well as disorders affecting protein receptors, membrane transporters and other proteins. Some genetic disorders lead to a block in a biochemical pathway, which can lead to a deficiency in a protein, e.g. von Willebrand's disease, while in other cases there may be accumulation of a protein (a storage disease) e.g. fucosidosis, or production of an abnormal substance, e.g. L-2-hydroxyglutaric aciduria. Inborn errors of metabolism lead to a variety of signs including neonatal death, growth retardation, neurological signs and skeletal abnormalities.

Urine testing is often performed for metabolic screening because abnormal metabolites do not undergo selective reuptake in the kidneys, and excessive levels of normal metabolites can overwhelm the tubular reuptake systems. Examples of genetically determined metabolic diseases for which urine tests can be useful or diagnostic include:

- Fanconi syndrome (testing for glucosuria in the presence of normal blood glucose concentrations, metabolic screening for aminoaciduria, fractional excretion tests for abnormal electrolyte excretion; see also Chapter 11)
- Cystinuria (cystine crystals or uroliths)
- Selective cobalamin malabsorption (methylmalonic aciduria)
- L-2-hydroxyglutaric aciduria (L-2 hydroxyglutaric acid)
- Mucopolysaccharidosis (excessive mucopolysaccharides in the urine).

DNA testing

Although the above techniques may be strongly indicative or definitively diagnostic for a genetic disease, they do not directly examine the patient's genetic make-up. DNA testing provides information about the presence of a specific genotype that is associated with disease, and so can help with both the diagnosis and the development of breeding strategies. DNA tests are developed using research studies that compare the genomes of affected and unaffected animals in order to identify a mutation that correlates with the presence of the disease. From this, a DNA test can be created that can be offered commercially.

Development of a DNA test

The first step in developing a DNA test for a disease that is known to be inherited is to identify the locus, or preferably a specific mutation, that is associated with the disease.

Generally, this is most practical for diseases attributable to a single gene mutation. It is more complicated to identify the mutations involved in diseases inherited in a polygenic manner. To identify the gene mutation responsible, the genomes of affected animals are compared to the genomes of a healthy population sample, usually by assessing polymorphic markers, such as SNPs or microsatellites, to identify areas that are associated with the disease (i.e. genome-wide association study; GWAS). Following this process, fine mapping or candidate gene analysis can be used to identify specific mutation(s). Often, polymerase chain reaction (PCR) technology is used to amplify the DNA, prior to sequencing it, allowing specific nucleotides to be compared between the diseased and healthy populations. The method for performing PCR is outlined in Chapter 28.

Researchers can narrow the region of the genome they need to examine by already having knowledge of the area likely to be involved. For example, the region of DNA that codes for factor IX is known from the sequencing of the entire dog genome. Therefore, when researchers wished to identify which mutation was responsible for factor IX deficiency (haemophilia B) in the Rhodesian Ridgeback, they were able to concentrate only on this area. In this case, blood samples were taken from six phenotypically affected dogs of this breed, four carriers and 12 healthy controls. Oligonucleotide primers were used to amplify the coding region and intron–exon boundaries, which were then purified and sequenced in an automatic sequencer. The sequences of the different groups were compared, allowing identification of a G–A missense mutation at nucleotide 752 in exon 7 of the factor IX gene. This allowed the development of a rapid screening test for this specific mutation using fluorescent probes specific for the normal and mutated versions of the sequence (Mischke et al., 2011).

In other situations, where the pathophysiology is more poorly understood, a GWAS is necessary as the first step. For example, Awano et al. (2009) performed genome-wide SNP genotyping on 38 Welsh Corgis with degenerative myelopathy and compared them with 17 clinically normal controls, allowing identification of the superoxide dismutase (SOD)-1 gene as a candidate gene for the disease; mutations in this area were already known to cause amyotrophic lateral sclerosis in humans. Once the gene had been identified as a candidate, resequencing of the genes from affected and healthy dogs allowed the identification of the specific mutation, which in turn allowed a DNA test to be developed.

Different laboratories and different tests vary in their sample requirements for genetic testing, and it is always sensible to contact the laboratory providing the test to check submission requirements. Commonly a blood sample or a cheek swab is required.

Most DNA tests currently available are for diseases attributable to single gene mutations, and many of these will be recessive. Given that a DNA test will be able to identify whether an animal possesses none, one or two copies of the faulty gene, in the cases of diseases inherited in a recessive manner, it will be possible to distinguish unaffected animals (homozygous wild-type) from carriers (heterozygous), as well as those animals likely to be clinically affected (homozygous mutant). Animals carrying a dominant mutation will usually express the disease, and genetic testing will help to confirm the diagnosis, but there are also occasions where testing is useful prior to disease onset, for example where clinical signs are of late onset or there is incomplete penetrance.

It is important to interpret the results of DNA testing with caution, because what appears to be a clear-cut result may be misleading. The SOD-1 mutation (Figure 30.3) that was discovered to be associated with degenerative myelopathy in a number of dog breeds is a useful illustration. Degenerative myelopathy is a progressive, incurable degenerative spinal cord disease of older dogs, causing clinical signs of ascending hindlimb neurological dysfunction, progressing from ataxia and paraparesis to paraplegia and tetraplegia. In cases that are homozygous for the normal version of the gene, degenerative myelopathy seems never to occur. Animals that are heterozygous are carriers, and also seem not to develop the disease. Animals that are homozygous for the SOD-1 mutation are deemed at risk of developing the disease. However, this does not mean that the animal will inevitably develop the disease; because it is such a late-onset disease, some animals will never show clinical signs of the condition during their lifetimes. There may also be environmental and other genetic factors associated with the expression of the condition. Moreover, there are a number of other conditions that can cause similar clinical signs, such as degenerative disc disease and neoplasia. When a 'positive' DNA test is obtained in an asymptomatic animal, the clinician should counsel the owner on whether this will inevitably lead to disease, and when a 'positive' DNA test is obtained in a symptomatic animal, the clinician should consider whether all other likely differentials have been excluded.

Another factor to consider when interpreting DNA test results is the selection of the test itself. Some apparently similar diseases are caused by different genetic mutations in different breeds. The DNA test for muscular dystrophy in

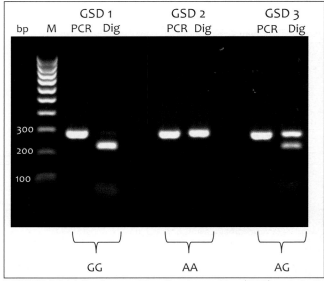

30.3 Restriction fragment length polymorphism (RFLP) analysis of the canine SOD-1:c.118G>A mutation in three German Shepherd Dogs (GSDs). DNA was extracted from ethylenediamine tetra-acetic acid (EDTA) blood and PCR used to amplify a specific product, using primers designed to flank the site of the mutation. Digestion (Dig) was then performed, in which an enzyme was used to digest the PCR product, and the results analysed by agarose gel electrophoresis. In an animal carrying normal genes, digestion occurs and the original PCR product of 292 base pairs (bp) is cut into two fragments, one of 230 bp and one of 62 bp. However, if the mutation is present, digestion does not occur. In the example shown here, a PCR product is seen in all three dogs at 292 bp. GSD 1 is unaffected (homozygous wild-type), so after digestion two fragments (230 bp and 62 bp) are seen; GSD 2 is affected (homozygous mutant) so bands are only seen at 292 bp, i.e. digestion has not occurred; and GSD 3 is a carrier (heterozygous), showing three bands after digestion at 292 bp (uncut), 230 bp and 62 bp (digestion fragments).
(Courtesy of B Catchpole, Royal Veterinary College)

the Golden Retriever (which is due to a mutation in intron 6 of the dystrophin gene on the X chromosome) would not be suitable to diagnose muscular dystrophy in the Cavalier King Charles Spaniel (which is due to a mutation in exon 50) (Walmsley *et al.*, 2010; Kornegay *et al.*, 2012). It is important to check that the test is available for the breed in question. In some cases, the same test is used for closely related breeds. For example the test for phosphofructo-kinase deficiency is available from PennGen (see below) for English Springer Spaniels and Cocker Spaniels.

Most DNA tests are designed to identify a specific mutation associated with a disease. These have essentially 100% accuracy in identifying carriers of a mutation. Some tests, however, are linkage based: rather than identifying the mutation itself, the test identifies markers close to the mutation. In a small number of cases where chromosomal recombination has occurred in the region between the marker and the mutation, these tests will be inaccurate. A laboratory providing DNA testing should be able to provide information on whether their test is mutation or linkage based, as well as general information about the condition, such as penetrance, mode of inheritance and the presence of any genetically distinct forms of the same disease within the breed (to prevent an owner thinking a pet cannot get a disease, when in fact it is only clear of one genetic variant of the disease).

Examples of genetic tests are listed in Figure 30.4. However, many more are currently available, and new genetic mutations are being identified and turned into DNA tests all the time. At the time of writing, the most recent genetic mutation associated with a companion animal disease to be discovered a CHRNE frameshift mutation found in Jack Russell Terriers with congenital myasthenic syndrome (Rinz *et al.*, 2015).

Condition	Examples of breeds affected
Eye disorders	
Canine multifocal retinopathy	Australian Shepherd, Bullmastiff, Dogue de Bordeaux, Pyrenean Mountain Dog
Collie eye anomaly	Australian Shepherd, Bearded Collie, Border Collie, Lancashire Heeler, Nova Scotia Duck Tolling Retriever, Shetland Sheepdog, Whippet
Cone degeneration	Alaskan Malamute, Australian Shepherd, German Shorthaired Pointer
Cone–rod dystrophy	American Pit Bull Terrier
Primary lens luxation	Chinese Crested, Jack Russell Terrier, Yorkshire Terrier
Progressive retinal atrophy	American Eskimo Dog, Australian Cattle Dog, Australian Shepherd, Gordon Setter, Spanish Water Dog, Swedish Lapphund
Stationary night blindness	Briard
Haematological/immunological disorders	
Canine cyclic neutropenia	Border Collie
Canine leucocyte adhesion deficiency	Irish Red and White Setter, Irish Setter,
Factor VII deficiency	Airedale Terrier, Beagle, Deerhound, Giant Schnauzer
Glanzmann's thrombasthenia	Otterhound, Pyrenean Mountain Dog
Globoid cell leukodystrophy	Cairn Terrier, Irish Setter, West Highland White Terrier
Haemophilia A (factor VIII deficiency)	German Shepherd Dog
Haemophilia B (factor IX deficiency)	Airedale, Bull Terrier, Cairn Terrier, German Wirehaired Pointer, Lhasa Apso, Rhodesian Ridgeback
Phosphofructokinase deficiency	American Cocker Spaniel, Cocker Spaniel, Springer Spaniel, Wachtelhund, Whippet
Pyruvate kinase deficiency	Basenji, Beagle, Cairn Terrier, Chihuahua, Labrador Retriever, Pug, West Highland White Terrier
von Willebrand's disease	Boxer, Dobermann, German Pinscher, German Shorthaired Pointer and Wirehaired Pointer, Kerry Blue Terrier, Papillon, Scottish Terrier, Standard Poodle, Toy Poodle, Welsh Corgi, West Highland White Terrier
X-linked severe combined immunodeficiency	Basset Hound, Welsh Corgi
Neurological/neuromuscular disorders	
Cerebellar ataxia	American Pit Bull Terrier, American Staffordshire Terrier, Coton de Tulear, Spinone
Ceroid lipofuscinosis	American Bulldog, American Pit Bull Terrier, American Staffordshire Terrier, Australian Shepherd, Border Collie, Dachshund, English Setter, Gordon Setter, Irish Setter
Degenerative myelopathy	Boxer, German Shepherd Dog, Rhodesian Ridgeback, Standard Poodle, Wirehaired Fox Terrier
Episodic falling	Cavalier King Charles Spaniel
Exercise-induced collapse	American Cocker Spaniel, Boykin Spaniel, Chesapeake Bay Retriever, Labrador Retriever
Fucosidosis	English Springer Spaniel
Hereditary ataxia	Jack Russell Terrier
Juvenile epilepsy	Lagotto Romagnolo
Labrador myopathy	Labrador Retriever
L-2-hydroxyglutaric aciduria	Staffordshire Bull Terrier, Yorkshire Terrier
Muscular dystrophy	Golden Retriever, Japanese Spitz

30.4 Examples of available DNA tests. (continues) ▶

Condition	Examples of breeds affected
Neurological/neuromuscular disorders (cont)	
Myotonia	Australian Cattle Dog, Miniature Schnauzer
Narcolepsy	Dachshund, Dobermann, Labrador Retriever
Pyruvate dehydrogenase phosphatase deficiency	Clumber Spaniel, Sussex Spaniel
Hepatic diseases	
Copper toxicosis	Bedlington Terrier
Renal/urinary diseases	
Cystinuria	English and French Bulldog, Labrador Retriever, Miniature Pinscher, Newfoundland
Fanconi syndrome	Basenji
Hyperuricosuria	Bulldog, Dachshund, Dalmation, German Shepherd Dog, Giant Schnauzer, Labrador Retriever, Pomeranian, Russian Black Terrier, Weimaraner
Polycystic kidney disease	British Longhair, British Shorthair, Himalayan, Maine Coon, Persian cat, Ragdoll, Siamese
Renal dysplasia	Bernese Mountain Dog, Bichon Frise, Boxer, English Cocker Spaniel, Lhasa Apso, Shih Tzu, Soft Coated Wheaten Terrier, Tibetan Terrier, Weimeraner
X-linked nephritis/glomerulopathy	Samoyed
Miscellaneous diseases	
Anal furunculosis	German Shepherd Dog
Cobalamin malabsorption	Australian Shepherd, Beagle, Border Collie, Giant Schnauzer

30.4 (continued) Examples of available DNA tests.

DNA testing for breed identification

In 2004, Parker *et al.* used molecular markers to study the genetic relationships among a large number of dog breeds. Since then, a number of commercial tests have been used to help identify the ancestry of mixed-breed dogs. These tests have been criticized for variable accuracy, with some discordant results being found (http://news.vin.com/VINNews.aspx?articleId=23206).

One study of 20 dogs with mixed-breed ancestry and unknown parentage found that 87.5% of the dogs identified by visual inspection by an adoption agency as having specific breeds in their ancestry did not have all of those breeds detected by DNA analysis (Voith *et al.*, 2009). This may be due to inaccuracy in the DNA testing, or inaccuracy in the adoption agencies' presumption of breed make-up. DNA testing for ancestry may be of use in appropriate homing of mixed-breed dogs, may inform behavioural and training advice, and may alert a clinician and owner to certain breed predispositions.

Animal forensics

Some laboratories offer animal forensic DNA testing services. These include identification of an animal involved in an attack on a person or another animal, animal theft, and linking a suspect with a crime scene through animal DNA.

Finding a genetic test provider

Figure 30.5 lists the major institutions providing genetic tests for dogs and cats. Useful websites to search for an up-to-date list of currently available tests worldwide include those of the Orthopaedic Foundation for Animals and PennGen. The Inherited Diseases in Dogs Database compiled by David Sargan at Cambridge University gives comprehensive information on a range of genetic diseases, including whether a DNA test is available and, if so, at what institution.

Institution	Websites
Animal Genetics	www.animalgenetics.us
Animal Health Trust	www.aht.org.uk
Animal Network	www.animalnetwork.com.au
Antagene	www.antagene.com/en
Auburn University	www.vetmed.auburn.edu/
Cornell University	https://ahdc.vet.cornell.edu/sects/Molec/
DDC Veterinary	www.vetdnacenter.com
Ecole Veterinaire Alfort	www.labradorcnm.com
Genefast	www.genefast.com
Genindexe	www.genindexe.com
Genomia	www.genomia.cz
Genoscoper	www.genoscoper.com
GenSol	www.gensoldx.com
HealthGene	www.healthgene.com
Laboklin	www.laboklin.co.uk
Michigan State University	https://cvm.msu.edu/
North Carolina State University	www.ncstatevets.org/genetics/
OptiGen	www.optigen.com
Orivet	http://orivet.com.au/
Orthopedic Foundation for Animals	www.offa.org
Paw Print Genetics	www.pawprintgenetics.com
PennGen	http://research.vet.upenn.edu/Penngen
Project Dog	https://projectdog.org/
University of California, Davis	www.vgl.ucdavis.edu/services/index.php
University of Kentucky	www2.ca.uky.edu/gluck/AGTRL.asp
University of Missouri	www.caninegeneticdiseases.net
Utrecht University	e-mail:P.A.J.Leegwater@uu.nl
Vetgen	www.vetgen.com
Vetnostic Laboratories	www.vetnostic.com

30.5 Major institutions providing genetic tests for dogs and cats. (Data from: Mellersh and Sargan, 2011; Orthopaedic Foundation for Animals) (www.offa.org)

Ethical aspects of genetic testing

Genetic testing in human medicine is fraught with legal and ethical problems. The results of genetic testing can cause problems with insurance as well as long-term anxiety. Although the problem of inducing anxiety about the prognosis in veterinary patients does not exist, owners may worry about the results of screening tests of healthy animals, and positive results may also affect veterinary insurance. The main reasons for genetic testing in veterinary medicine are the diagnosis of disease and screening for genetic disease in healthy animals. There are generally no ethical problems with genetic testing for diagnosis of disease in suspected cases, but there are ethical considerations when screening healthy animals, for example for breeding selection.

At an individual level, situations in which ethical problems may arise include:

- Genetic testing for non-health reasons. Cheek swabs may be acceptable for parentage analysis but consideration should be given to whether a more invasive test such as a blood test is acceptable if there is no health benefit to the individual or population
- Cosmetic genetic testing is becoming very common, with nearly half of all feline genetic tests requested at the University of California, Davis Veterinary Genetics Laboratory in 2011–2012 being for hair length or colour (Lyons, 2012). As well as the potential invasiveness of the test, which is of no benefit to the animal, there may be a linkage between some coat colours and disease (e.g. cyclic neutropenia in Blue Merle Collies)
- Prognostication for asymptomatic animals. A positive test for a genetic disease does not inevitably mean that all positive animals will show signs of the disease. False positives and incomplete penetrance are two possible reasons why an animal with a positive test for a genetic disease may never develop the disease. Furthermore, some diseases, such as degenerative myelopathy caused by the SOD-1 mutation, are late-onset disorders, with affected dogs often living long, healthy lives before clinical signs arise. Early

identification of the mutation in an individual may lead to anxiety in the owner and even premature euthanasia.

For breeders, and at a population level, situations in which ethical problems may arise include:

- Test matings. For conditions in which a genetic test is not available, test matings may be necessary to identify carriers of an inherited disease. This has ethical implications because it is likely to lead to affected individuals being born, which many deem unacceptable
- Genetic diversity and breed screening schemes. Many breed screening schemes exist to attempt to reduce the incidence of specific diseases in a population, for example, the British Veterinary Association hip, elbow and eye schemes. In schemes based on phenotype rather than a genetic test, there is often a subjective element to the grading, or an arbitrary cut-off point between affected and unaffected individuals. This can lead to breeder dissatisfaction with these schemes, reducing uptake. Furthermore, it is possible that strict adherence to breeding policies eliminating affected animals from the gene pool may reduce genetic diversity in a breed, and possibly increase the incidence of other genetic disorders
- Client confidentiality. A diagnosis of a genetic disorder in a line may have significant financial implications for a breeder. The clinician who diagnoses this condition may find a conflict between client confidentiality and the desire to inform the owners of affected relatives, as well as breed clubs. For screening as part of an official breed scheme, the terms and conditions of participation may include publication of results of individual tests, as in, for example, the British Veterinary Association Chiari Malformation/Syringomyelia scheme. However, for testing outside a specific scheme, a breeder may wish the results of testing to remain confidential. The clinician who feels that the welfare of patients would be compromised by keeping the results confidential should seek advice from their governing body, such as the Royal College of Veterinary Surgeons.

Case examples

CASE 1

SIGNALMENT

3-year-old neutered female Staffordshire Bull Terrier cross.

HISTORY

Sudden-onset ataxia with mild proprioceptive deficits in all four limbs, following a general anaesthetic. Prior to this she had been well, although the owners thought she had been a slow learner. The ataxia improved over a few days but the dog had ongoing behavioural abnormalities.

CLINICAL PATHOLOGY DATA

Routine haematology, biochemistry and electrolytes were within normal limits.

USING THE DAMNIT-V CLASSIFICATION, WHAT ARE THE MOST LIKELY DIFFERENTIAL DIAGNOSES FOR THIS CONDITION AND WHAT FURTHER TESTS WOULD YOU REQUEST?

- Degenerative: genetic metabolic disease.
- Anomalous: hydrocephalus, other congenital intracranial malformations, portosystemic shunt.
- Metabolic: portosystemic shunt.
- Neoplastic: brain tumour, spinal cord tumour.
- Idiopathic/inflammatory/infectious: toxoplasmosis, neosporosis, meningoencephalomyelitis of unknown origin.
- Toxic: organophosphate, lead.
- Vascular: cerebrovascular accident, hypoxic episode during anaesthesia.

Further testing could include a bile acid stimulation test, serology for *Toxoplasma* and *Neospora*, cerebrospinal fluid analysis and advanced imaging.

→ CASE 1 CONTINUED

Results of further blood tests

Dynamic bile acids were within normal limits. *Toxoplasma* and *Neospora* serology was negative.

Results of cerebrospinal fluid analysis

Parameter	Description
Physical appearance	Watery, clear
Protein	Insufficient volume for analysis
Red cells	**250**/μl (reference range <2 cells/μl)
Nucleated cells	4/μl (reference range <5 cells/μl)
Cytological comment	Occasional small lymphocytes seen. No infectious agents detected. The red cells most likely represent iatrogenic blood contamination.
Culture	No growth

Abnormal results are in **bold**.

Results of magnetic resonance imaging

Bilaterally symmetrical regions of hyperintensity on T2-weighted MR images of the brain are suggestive of a metabolic disease (Figure 30.6).

WHAT GENETIC TEST WOULD YOU REQUEST TO MAKE A DEFINITIVE DIAGNOSIS IN THIS CASE?

A DNA test was performed for L-2-hydroxyglutaric aciduria (L-2HGA). This confirmed that the patient was homozygous for the L-2HGA genotype. An alternative test would be a urine test to look for elevated L-2HGA levels (although this is not widely available).

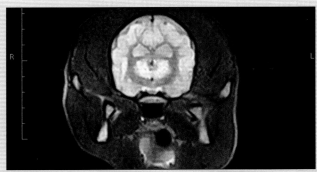

30.6 T2-weighted transverse MR image of the brain, showing bilaterally symmetrical regions of hyperintensity.

L-2HGA is a neurometabolic disorder which is particularly common in the Staffordshire Bull Terrier breed. It presents with a spectrum of neurological signs including ataxia, seizures, tremors and behavioural abnormalities. The usual age of onset is between 6 and 12 months of age, but can be as late as 7 years. It tends to progress over a number of years, and there is no cure, although symptomatic treatment may be helpful in maintaining quality of life. The condition is inherited as an autosomal recessive trait. This case is interesting in that it involved a crossbreed, which was nevertheless homozygous for the mutation. Being a recessive condition, crossing a carrier to an unaffected breed should have produced clinically unaffected offspring. One copy of the mutation in this case will have been inherited from the Staffordshire Bull Terrier parent, but the other was inherited from a non-Staffordshire of unknown breed. This other parent may have had Staffordshire Bull Terrier ancestry, or may have belonged to one of the other breeds reported to be affected by the condition, such as the West Highland White Terrier.

CASE 2

SIGNALMENT

18-month-old entire male Labrador Retriever.

HISTORY

Progressive lethargy with extreme tiredness after short bursts of activity for several months. Chronic coughing had also been noted. No neurological deficits or orthopaedic disease on examination. Gait normal. Thoracic auscultation unremarkable. Cough elicited on tracheal palpation.

WHAT IS YOUR PROBLEM LIST AND DIFFERENTIAL DIAGNOSES?

Cough:

- Infectious, e.g. angiostrongylosis, bordetellosis, *Mycoplasma* infection, pneumonia
- Inflammatory, e.g. chronic bronchitis
- Neoplasia
- Pulmonary oedema, e.g. cardiogenic
- Left atrial enlargement
- Upper or lower airway collapse
- Inhaled foreign body.

Exercise intolerance:

- Cardiovascular disease, e.g. structural heart disease, arrhythmia
- Genetic disease, e.g. exercise-induced collapse of the Labrador Retriever
- Metabolic disease, e.g. anaemia, hypoglycaemia
- Endocrine disease, e.g. hypothyroidism, hypoadrenocorticism
- Neuromuscular disease, e.g. myasthenia gravis, polymyositis
- Musculoskeletal disease, e.g. osteoarthritis, polyarthritis
- Respiratory disease, e.g. upper respiratory obstruction, pleural effusion, pulmonary oedema.

WHAT WOULD YOUR INITIAL TESTS BE TO NARROW THE DIFFERENTIAL DIAGNOSIS LIST?

Routine haematology and biochemistry were performed to rule out haematological and metabolic causes of exercise intolerance. Echocardiography was within normal limits. Thoracic radiography showed a mild increase in bronchial pattern. Electrocardiography showed a sinus arrhythmia.

→ **CASE 2 CONTINUED**

WHAT FURTHER TESTS WOULD YOU PERFORM TO INVESTIGATE THE REMAINING DIFFERENTIALS?

- Adrenocorticotropic hormone (ACTH) stimulation test:
  - Pre-ACTH 41.4 nmol/l (25–125 nmol/l)
  - Post ACTH 163.0 nmol/l (125–520 nmol/l).
- T4: 23.4 nmol/l (13–51 nmol/l).
- TSH: 0.06 ng/ml (0–0.5 ng/ml).
- Acetylcholine receptor antibody: 0.18 nmol/l (range <0.60 nmol/l).

HOW WOULD YOU INTERPRET THESE TESTS AND WHAT TESTS WOULD YOU PERFORM NEXT?

No metabolic, endocrine, cardiac or neuromuscular disease has yet been identified as a cause of the signs. Given the presence of a cough and the changes on radiography, bronchoscopy is a reasonable next step.

Assessment of the larynx under a light plane of anaesthesia showed normal motion. Bronchoscopy was performed, which showed increased mucus in the main and small airways plus some dynamic collapse of the lower airways. Bronchoalveolar lavage showed minimal inflammation on cytology but PCR on the lavage fluid was positive for *Mycoplasma*.

HOW WOULD YOU TREAT THESE FINDINGS, AND DO YOU THINK THEY ARE SUFFICIENT TO EXPLAIN THE CLINICAL SIGNS? IF NOT, WHAT OTHER TEST COULD BE CONSIDERED?

Treatment was instituted with doxycycline and theophylline. However, while it was considered that the findings of lower airway collapse and mycoplasmosis could explain the cough, it was not considered sufficiently severe to explain the level of exercise intolerance. A genetic test was therefore performed for exercise-induced collapse of the Labrador Retriever. It was found that this patient was homozygous for the abnormal gene. The dog showed a good response to treatment in terms of the cough, but remained significantly exercise intolerant.

Exercise-induced collapse of the Labrador Retriever causes signs of episodic limb weakness and collapse brought on by extreme exercise or excitement, usually noticed for the first time in young adults. It is caused by a mutation in the gene encoding the dynamin 1 protein, which is required for neurotransmission during strenuous exercise. It is inherited in an autosomal recessive mode. There is no specific treatment other than to avoid triggers for the collapse. Clinical signs tend to stabilize or improve with age, although some dogs have died during episodes of collapse.

References and further reading

Asher L, Diesel G, Summers JF et al. (2009) Inherited defects in pedigree dogs. Part 1: Disorders related to breed standards. The Veterinary Journal 182, 402–411

Awano T, Johnson GS, Wade CM et al. (2009) Genome-wide association analysis reveals a SOD1 mutation in canine degenerative myelopathy that resembles amyotrophic lateral sclerosis. Proceedings of the National Academy of Sciences of the United States of America 106, 2795–2799

Baranoswka I, Jaderlund KH and Nennesmo I (2009) Sensory ataxic neuropathy in golden retriever dogs is caused by a deletion in the mitochondrial tRNATyr gene. PloS Genetics 5(5), e1000499

Bateson P (2010) Independent Inquiry into Dog Breeding. Published privately by Patrick Bateson in 2010, and printed by Micropress Ltd, Halesworth, Suffolk. Also available at: http://www.breedinginquiry.files.wordpress.com/2010/01/final-dog-inquiry-120110.pdf

Biller DS, DiBartola SP, Eaton KA et al. (1996) Inheritance of polycystic kidney disease in Persian cats. Journal of Heredity 87, 1–5

Bowles CA, Alsaker RD and Wolfle TL (1979) Studies of the Pelger–Huet anomaly in foxhounds. American Journal of Pathology 96, 237–247

Brown SJ, Simpson KW, Baker S et al. (1994) Macrothrombocytosis in the Cavalier King Charles Spaniel. Veterinary Record 135, 281–283

Cruz F, Vila C and Webster MT (2008) The legacy of domestication: accumulation of deleterious mutations in the dog genome. Molecular Biology and Evolution 25, 2331–2336

Darwin C (1865) The Variation of Animals and Plants under Domestication, vol. 2. J. Murray, London.

Driscoll CA, Macdonald DW, O'Brien SJ et al. (2009) From wild animals to domestic pets, an evolutionary view of domestication. Proceedings of the National Academy of Sciences of the United States of America 106(Suppl. 1), 9971–9978

Fels L, Marschall Y, Philipp U et al. (2014) Multiple loci associated with canine hip dysplasia (CHD) in German shepherd dogs. Mammalian Genome 25, 262–269

Gilliam D, O'Brien DP, Coates JR, et al. (2014) A homozygous KCNJ10 mutation in Jack Russell terriers and related breeds with spinocerebellar ataxia with myokymia, seizures, or both. Journal of Veterinary Internal Medicine 28, 871–877

Gough A and Thomas A (2010) Breed Predispositions to Disease in Dogs and Cats, 2nd edn. Wiley-Blackwell, Oxford

Kornegay JN, Bogan JR, Bogan DJ, et al. (2012) Canine models of Duchenne muscular dystrophy and their use in therapeutic strategies. Mammalian Genome 23, 85–108

Lewis TW, Woolliams JA and Blott SC (2010) Genetic evaluation of the nine component features of hip score in UK Labrador Retrievers. PLoS One 5, e13610

Li Z, Liu Z and Li Y (2008) Origin and phylogenetic analysis of Tibetan Mastiff based on the mitochondrial DNA sequence. Journal of Genetics and Genomics 35, 335–340

Linblad-Toh K, Wade CM, Mikkelsen TS et al. (2005) Genome sequence, comparative analysis and haplotype structure of the domestic dog. Nature 438, 803–819

Lyons LA (2012) Genetic testing in domestic cats. Molecular and Cellular Probes 26, 224–230

Mellersh C and Sargan D (2011) DNA testing in companion animals – what is it and why do it? In Practice 33, 442–453

Mischke R, Kuhnlein P, Kehl A et al. (2011) G244E in the canine factor IX gene leads to severe haemophilia B in Rhodesian Ridgebacks. The Veterinary Journal 187, 113–118

Nicholas FW (2013) Introduction to Veterinary Genetics, 3rd edn. Wiley-Blackwell, Oxford

Ostrander E and Ruvinsky A (2012) The Genetics of the Dog, 2nd edn. CABI Publishing, Wallingford

Parker HG, Ki LV, Sutter NB et al. (2004) Genetic structure of the purebred domestic dog. Science 304, 1160–1164

Pontius JU, Mullikin JC, Smith DR, et al. (2007) Initial sequence and comparative analysis of the cat genome. Genome Research 17, 1675–1689

Rinz CJ, Lennon VA, James F, Thoreson JB et al. (2015) A CHRNE frameshift mutation causes congenital myasthenic syndrome in young Jack Russell Terriers. Neuromuscular Disorders doi: 10.1016/j.nmd.2015.09.005

Sewell AC, Haskins ME and Giger U (2007) Inherited metabolic disease in companion animals: searching for nature's mistakes. The Veterinary Journal 174, 252–259

Summers JF, Diesel G, Asher L et al. (2010) Inherited defects in pedigree dogs. Part 2: Disorders that are not related to breed standards. The Veterinary Journal 183, 39–45

Voith VL, Ingram E, Mitsouras K et al. (2009) Comparison of adoption agency breed identification and DNA breed identification of dogs. Journal of Applied Animal Welfare Science 12, 253–262

Walmsley GL, Arechavala-Gomez V, Fernandez-Fuente M et al. (2010) A Duchenne muscular dystrophy gene hot spot mutation in dystrophin-deficient Cavalier King Charles spaniels is amenable to exon 51 skipping. PLoS One 5(1), e8647

Wayne RK and Ostrander EA (1999) Origin, genetic diversity, and genome structure of the domestic dog. BioEssays 21, 247–257

Wilson B, Nicholas FW and Thomson PC (2011) Selection against canine hip dysplasia: success or failure? The Veterinary Journal 189, 160–168

Useful websites

Canine Inherited Disorders Database: www.upei.ca/cidd
Inherited Diseases in Dogs Database: http://idid.vet.cam.ac.uk
Online Mendelian Inheritance in Animals: http://omia.angis.org.au/home
Orthopaedic Foundation for Animals: www.offa.org
PennGen: http://research.vet.upenn.edu/Penngen

Use and abuse of microscopes

Tim Nuttall

- The ideal microscope should have binocular eyepieces, an integral light source, a focusing condenser, a mechanical stage and four lenses: X4, X10, X40 and X100 oil-immersion (eyepieces are usually X10, giving a final magnification of X40 to X1000).
- Adjust the eyepieces by focusing on a slide with one eye and then use the eyepiece to correct the focus for your other eye.
- Close the light diaphragm and focus the condenser until there is a sharp image of the diaphragm. If there is no diaphragm, focus on a piece of card held against the light source. Open the light source diaphragm fully once it is focused.
- Adjust the condenser iris diaphragm to give the clearest image for each lens.

- For parasites, it is useful to close the condenser iris diaphragm; the image is poorer but the increased contrast makes the parasites stand out better. For cytology, open the diaphragm to reduce contrast and give a more detailed image.
- Always use coverslips. They give a better image, a defined search area, and protect the lenses. You do not need to use glass coverslips to examine adhesive tape strips because the acetate backing acts as the coverslip.
- Use the oil-immersion lens last of all to avoid getting oil on the other lenses.
- Clean the lenses and stage with lens cleaner and fine tissue or lens cloths immediately after use.

BSAVA Manual of Canine and Feline Clinical Pathology, 3rd edition. Edited by Elizabeth Villiers and Jelena Ristić. ©BSAVA 2016

Test sample requirements

Haematology

Test	Sample requirements
Complete blood count	EDTA blood Air-dried blood smears
Erythropoietin	Serum
Blood typing	EDTA blood

Haemostasis

Test	Sample requirements
Platelet count	EDTA blood
von Willebrand factor antigen	Sodium citrate–plasma (fill tube exactly to line; mix gently but thoroughly, separate plasma within 15 minutes and submit frozen)
Prothrombin time Activated partial thromboplastin time Fibrin(ogen) degradation products	Sodium citrate–plasma (fill tube exactly to line; mix gently but thoroughly, separate plasma within 15 minutes)
D-dimer	EDTA or sodium citrate–plasma (fill tube exactly to line; mix gently but thoroughly, separate plasma within 15 minutes)

Bone marrow

Test	Sample requirements
Bone marrow cytology/histology	Air-dried bone marrow smears EDTA blood Air-dried blood smears ± Core biopsy in formalin
Flow cytometry (for immunophenotyping leukaemia)	EDTA blood ± ACD-anticoagulated bone marrow Fix in Streck preservative if >24-hour delay

Immunology (general)

Test	Sample requirements
Coombs' test	EDTA blood
Antinuclear antibody	Serum
Rheumatoid factor	Serum
Acetylcholine receptor antibodies	Serum
2M antibodies (masticatory muscle myositis)	Serum

Biochemistry and endocrinology

Test	Sample requirements
Routine analytes (enzymes, proteins, electrolytes)	Serum (preferably) or heparinized plasma
Glucose	Separated serum or fluoride oxalate plasma
Fructosamine	Serum
Iron	Serum
Bile acids	Serum
Drug levels (phenobarbital, digoxin, potassium bromide)	Serum (gel tubes interfere with analysis of many drug concentrations)
Adrenocorticotropic hormone (ACTH)	Sample into cooled plastic EDTA tube and separate plasma immediately. Transfer plasma into cooled plastic plain tube on ice. Freeze and send in freezer transport pack
Aldosterone	Heparinized plasma or serum
Cortisol	Heparinized plasma or serum
17-Hydroxyprogesterone	Heparinized plasma or serum
Insulin-like growth factor (IGF)-1	Heparinized plasma or serum
Insulin	Serum – sometimes frozen, check with laboratory (requires concurrent glucose measurement)
Insulin antibodies	Serum
Parathyroid hormone (PTH) PTH related protein	Sample into cooled plastic EDTA tube and separate plasma immediately. Transfer plasma into cooled plastic plain tube on ice. Freeze and send in freezer transport pack
Thyroxine (T4)	Heparinized plasma or serum
Thyroid-stimulating hormone (TSH)	Heparinized plasma or serum
Free T4 by equilibrium dialysis	Serum
Thyroglobulin autoantibody	Serum
Reproductive hormones (oestradiol, progesterone, testosterone)	Either heparinized plasma or serum, but not gel tubes for testosterone and progesterone
Canine relaxin	Heparinized plasma

Miscellaneous tests

Test	Sample requirements
Genetic testing (DNA)	EDTA blood or mucosal swab
Blood gas analysis	Fresh or heparinized blood that has not been in contact with air
Cerebrospinal fluid (CSF): • Cell counts, culture, serology • Cytology	Plain CSF CSF in EDTA plus one drop of serum or formalin (contact laboratory)
Effusions: • Cell counts, cytology, polymerase chain reaction (PCR) • Biochemistry • Culture	EDTA effusion Plain effusion Plain sterile effusion
PCR for antigen receptor rearrangement (PARR)	EDTA blood, bone marrow, lymph node aspirate or smears (stained smears can be used)

Tests for gastrointestinal disease

Test	Sample requirements
Trypsin-like immunoreactivity (cTLI, fTLI)	Serum
Folate	Serum
Cobalamin (vitamin B12)	Serum
Canine or feline pancreatic lipase immunoreactivity (canine PLI/Spec cPL®/SNAP®; feline PLI/Spec fPL®/SNAP®)	Serum
Faecal α1-proteinase inhibitor	Three fresh faecal samples, pooled and shipped on ice

Tests for cardiac disease

Test	Sample requirements
Amino-terminal fragment of proBNP (NT-proBNP)	EDTA plasma (check with individual laboratory)
Cardiac troponin I (cTnI)	Serum (not gel tubes)
Taurine	Dog: heparinized plasma Cat: heparinized plasma or blood

Tests for skin disease

Test	Sample requirements
Sarcoptes immunoglobulin (Ig)G	Serum
Canine or feline flea IgE	Serum
Allergy tests for allergen-specific IgE or IgG/IgE food allergen serology	Serum

Urinalysis

Test	Sample requirements
Urine culture	Boric acid/borate–urine (plain if fresh, especially cystocentesis)
Dipstick analysis and sediment examination	Plain urine
Urine protein:creatinine ratio	Plain urine
Urine cortisol:creatinine ratio	Plain urine

Tests for infectious diseases

Infectious agent	Test or method	Sample requirements
Anaplasma phagocytophilum	Polymerase chain reaction (PCR)	EDTA blood
	ELISA	Serum
Angiostrongylus vasorum	ELISA	Heparinized plasma or serum
	Polymerase chain reaction (PCR)	EDTA blood
Aspergillus spp.	Agar gel double diffusion	Serum
Babesia canis	Polymerase chain reaction (PCR)	EDTA blood
Bartonella spp.	Polymerase chain reaction (PCR)	EDTA blood; lesional tissue (fresh/frozen)
Bordetella bronchiseptica	Polymerase chain reaction (PCR)	Deep pharyngeal dry swab or bronchoalveolar lavage (BAL)
Borrelia spp.	ELISA	Serum
	Immunofluorescence	
	Polymerase chain reaction (PCR)	EDTA fluid, e.g. synovial fluid or fresh tissue are preferable, can use whole blood but less sensitive
Canine adenovirus	ELISA	Heparinized blood or serum
	Polymerase chain reaction (PCR)	Dry throat swab
	Virus isolation	Throat swab in VTM
	Virus neutralization test	Serum
Canine distemper virus	ELISA	Heparinized plasma, serum or CSF
	Polymerase chain reaction (PCR)	Fresh tissue; CSF; aqueous humour
	Virus neutralization test	Serum

continues ▶

Tests for infectious diseases *continued*

Infectious agent	Test or method	Sample requirements
Canine herpesvirus	Virus neutralization test	Serum
	Polymerase chain reaction (PCR)	Dry throat swab
Canine parainfluenza virus	Virus isolation	Throat swab in VTM
	Virus neutralization test	Serum
	Polymerase chain reaction (PCR)	Dry throat swab
Canine parvovirus	Polymerase chain reaction (PCR)	Faeces or gut contents
	Virus isolation	
Canine parvovirus (antibody)	ELISA	Heparinized plasma or serum
	Haemagglutination inhibition test	Serum
Canine parvovirus (antigen)	ELISA	Faeces or gut contents
	Haemagglutination test	
	Rapid immunomigration (RIM)	
Chlamydophila felis	Polymerase chain reaction (PCR)	Deep pharyngeal dry swab or bronchoalveolar lavage (BAL)
Cowpox virus	Electron microscopy	Scab or skin biopsy material
	Virus isolation	Scab material
Cryptococcus (antigen)	Latex agglutination	Serum or CSF
Dirofilaria immitis (antigen)	ELISA	Serum
Ehrlichia spp.	ELISA Immunofluorescence	Serum
	Polymerase chain reaction (PCR)	EDTA blood
Feline calicivirus	Polymerase chain reaction (PCR)	Oropharyngeal swab into VTM
	Virus isolation	
	Virus neutralization test	Serum
Feline coronavirus	Immunofluorescence	Heparinized blood or effusion
	Polymerase chain reaction (PCR)	EDTA–CSF or whole blood; dry swab of discharge or fresh tissue; heparinized blood or effusion
Feline coronavirus (antibody)	ELISA	Heparinized blood, serum or effusion
Feline herpesvirus	Polymerase chain reaction (PCR)	Oropharyngeal swab into VTM
	Virus isolation	
	Virus neutralization test	Serum
Feline parvovirus	Polymerase chain reaction (PCR)	Faeces or gut contents
	Virus isolation	
Feline parvovirus (antibody)	ELISA	Heparinized or EDTA plasma/serum
	Haemagglutination inhibition test	Serum
Feline parvovirus (antigen)	ELISA	Faeces or gut contents
	Haemagglutination	
	Rapid immunomigration (RIM)	
FeLV	Immunofluorescence	Smear of whole blood (heparin or EDTA)
	Polymerase chain reaction (PCR)	EDTA blood or bone marrow
	Virus isolation	Heparinized blood or bone marrow
FeLV (p27 antigen)	ELISA	Heparinized blood or serum
	Rapid immunomigration (RIM)	Heparinized blood
FIV	Polymerase chain reaction (PCR)	EDTA blood
FIV (antibody)	Immunofluorescence	Serum
	ELISA	Heparinized blood or serum
	Rapid immunomigration (RIM)	
	Western blot	
Leishmania	Immunofluorescence	Serum

continues ▶

Tests for infectious diseases *continued*

Infectious agent	Test or method	Sample requirements
Leishmania spp.	Polymerase chain reaction (PCR)	EDTA blood, fresh bone marrow, lymph node or skin biopsy tissue, conjunctival swab
Leptospira spp.	ELISA	Serum
	Microscopic agglutination test	
	Polymerase chain reaction (PCR)	Urine or tissue
Mycoplasma	Polymerase chain reaction (PCR)	Deep pharyngeal dry swab or bronchoalveolar lavage (BAL)
Mycoplasma haemofelis and *Candidatus* M. haemominutum	Polymerase chain reaction (PCR)	EDTA blood
Neospora caninum	ELISA	Serum
	Immunofluorescence	
Parainfluenza	Virus neutralization test	Serum
Rabies	ELISA	Serum
	Virus neutralization test	
Toxoplasma gondii	ELISA	Serum
	Latex agglutination	Serum
	Polymerase chain reaction (PCR)	Fresh tissue; CSF; aqueous humour
Tritrichomonas	Polymerase chain reaction (PCR)	Faeces or gut contents

Abbreviations: ACD = acid citrate dextrose; EDTA = ethylenediamine tetra-acetic acid; ELISA = enzyme-linked immunosorbent assay; FeLV = feline leukaemia virus; FIP = feline infectious peritonitis; FIV = feline immunodeficiency virus; VTM = virus transport medium.

Common laboratory abnormalities and differential diagnoses

These tables indicate the **major** differential diagnoses for abnormalities of parameters discussed throughout the Manual. Square brackets denote rare causes.

Haematology

Abnormality	Differential diagnoses
Erythrocytosis	Dehydration Splenic contraction Primary erythrocytosis (polycythaemia rubra vera) Secondary to renal neoplasia, extrarenal neoplasia, other renal diseases Secondary to hypoxia, e.g. respiratory disease, right to left cardiac shunts Hyperthyroidism
Anaemia (regenerative)	Immune-mediated haemolytic anaemia (dogs > cats; often secondary in cats) Haemotrophic *Mycoplasma* infection Babesiosis FeLV (may have other mechanisms concurrently) Onion toxicity Zinc toxicity Acute or chronic haemorrhage Microangiopathic haemolytic anaemia associated with, for example, neoplasia, disseminated intravascular coagulation, splenic torsion Haemophagocytic histiocytic sarcoma PK deficiency, PFK deficiency
Anaemia (non-regenerative)	Anaemia of chronic/inflammatory disease Anaemia of renal failure Liver disease, e.g. portosystemic shunt Iron deficiency Aplastic anaemia (aplastic pancytopenia) Pure red cell aplasia Immune-mediated non-regenerative anaemia Myelofibrosis Myelo/lymphoproliferative disease Myelodysplasia FeLV-related Infectious agents, e.g. ehrlichiosis Endocrine disease, e.g. hypothyroidism, hypoadrenocorticism, hyperoestrogenism Drug toxicity, e.g. oestrogens, chemotherapy Severe malnutrition
Neutrophilia	Physiological response to exercise, fear, pain Stress/corticosteroid-induced Acute inflammatory response: • Bacterial infection (localized or general) • Immune-mediated disease, e.g. IMHA, polyarthritis • Tissue necrosis, e.g. pancreatitis • Neoplasia, especially tumour necrosis ▶

Abnormality	Differential diagnoses
Neutrophilia *continued*	[Neutrophil dysfunction] [Chronic granulocytic leukaemia] [Paraneoplastic syndromes]
Neutropenia	Overwhelming demand (e.g. sepsis) Reduced granulopoiesis: • Myeloproliferative and lymphoproliferative disease • Myelofibrosis • Cytotoxic drug-related myelosuppression • Idiosyncratic drug reactions, e.g. phenobarbital in dogs, chloramphenicol and azathioprine in cats • Endogenous or exogenous oestrogens (NB neutrophilia early) • Some infections (e.g. canine parvovirus, feline panleucopenia virus, FeLV, FIV, *Ehrlichia*) Ineffective granulopoiesis: • Myeloproliferative and myelodysplastic diseases [• Cyclic haemopoiesis] [Immune-mediated neutropenia] Cobalamin deficiency
Monocytosis	Acute, in trauma Stress/corticosteroids (especially dogs) Chronic inflammation: • Infection • Malignancy • Internal haemorrhage • Pyogranulomatous inflammation • Necrosis Immune-mediated disease Compensatory, secondary to neutropenia Haemolysis [Monocytic or myelomonocytic leukaemia]
Lymphocytosis	Physiological: stress (especially cats), excitement, exercise Reactive: • Chronic infection • Transient post-vaccination • Young animals Lymphoproliferative disease Hypoadrenocorticism Immune-mediated disease
Lymphopenia	Corticosteroids: • Endogenous (hyperadrenocorticism) • Exogenous *continues* ▶

Haematology *continued*

Abnormality	Differential diagnoses
Lymphopenia *continued*	Acute inflammation, e.g. bacterial or viral infection Loss: • Chylothorax • Lymphangiectasia Decreased production: • Immunosuppressive drug therapy • Destruction of lymphoid tissue, e.g. multicentric lymphoma [Inherited immunodeficiency]
Eosinophilia	Parasitic infection (endo- and ectoparasites) Allergy/hypersensitivity: • Allergic skin disease, eosinophillic granuloma complex in cats • Eosinophilic enteritis • Eosinophilic bronchopneumopathy (pulmonary infiltrate with eosinophils (PIE)) • Feline asthma Inflammatory: • Panosteitis • Eosinophillic myositis Paraneoplastic: • Mast cell tumours • T cell lymphoma Inconsistently in hypoadrenocorticism Feline hypereosinophilic syndrome [Eosinophilic leukaemia]
Eosinopenia	Corticosteroids: • Endogenous (hyperadrenocorticism) • Exogenous Acute infection/inflammation Bone marrow aplasia/hypoplasia ▶

Abnormality	Differential diagnoses
Thrombocytosis	Stress/corticosteroids Rebound following acute haemorrhage or thombocytopenia Chronic gastrointestinal (GI) bleeding/iron deficiency Secondary to inflammation (e.g. infection, immune-mediated) Secondary to neoplasia Following vincristine Primary (essential) thrombocythaemia Acute megakaryoblastic leukaemia
Thrombocytopenia	Sequestration: splenomegaly Decreased production: • Drug toxicity: oestrogens, TMS • Myelofibrosis • Myelo/lymphoproliferative disease • Aplastic anaemia (aplastic pancytopenia) Increased destruction: • Immune-mediated thrombocytopenia (primary and secondary) • Disseminated intravascular coagulation (DIC) • Vasculitis/endocarditis Loss: acute blood loss Mixed aetiology: • Infectious (ehrlichiosis/anaplasmosis, babesiosis, FeLV, FIV, CPV) • Neoplasia Breed-related: Cavalier King Charles Spaniel, Norfolk Terrier, Greyhound, Lurcher, Whippet

Assessment of clotting times

NB Not affected by thrombocytopenia because platelet-poor plasma is used for testing.

Coagulation test	Possible causes
Prolonged PT, normal aPTT	Early rodenticide toxicity or vitamin K deficiency (PT usually increases before aPTT) Factor VII deficiency *Angiostrongylus vasorum* Occasionally in liver disease
Prolonged aPTT, normal PT	Deficiency of factor XII, XI, IX or VIII Early DIC *Angiostrongylus vasorum* Occasionally in liver disease
Prolonged PT and aPTT	Rodenticide toxicity Vitamin K deficiency, e.g. due to cholestasis Deficiency of factors X, V, II or fibrinogen *Angiostrongylus vasorum* DIC Liver disease Drug therapy: heparin

Biochemistry

Electrolytes

Analyte	Increased	Decreased
Bicarbonate	**Alkalosis** Metabolic alkalosis due to 'gastric' vomiting Hypokalaemia Drug therapy: bicarbonate, loop or thiazide diuretics Compensatory response to respiratory acidosis	**Acidosis** Metabolic acidosis: • Loss of bicarbonate in diarrhoea, renal tubular acidosis • Accumulation of unmeasured anions (e.g. lactate, phosphate, sulphate, citrate (renal failure), ketone bodies (ketoacidosis) • Toxins (e.g. ethylene glycol) • Decreased renal excretion of H$^+$ in renal failure, uroabdomen, hypoadrenocorticism • Rapid infusion of saline Compensatory response to respiratory alkalosis Spurious: delay in analysis/sample exposed to air
Calcium	**Hypercalcaemia** Growing animals Malignancy-associated (e.g. lymphoma, anal sac adenocarcinoma, multiple myeloma) Hyperparathyroidism Hypoadrenocorticism Chronic renal failure Acute renal failure – diuretic phase Osteolytic bone lesions Vitamin D intoxication Granulomatous disease Excessive calcium supplementation [Chronic dietary phosphate restriction]	**Hypocalcaemia** Low albumin (hypocalcaemia not clinically significant) Eclampsia (lactation tetany) Acute pancreatitis Hypoparathyroidism following thyroidectomy (common) or lymphocytic parathyroiditis (rare) Acute renal failure Chronic renal failure Malabsorption, protein-losing enteropathy Ethylene glycol toxicity Post-transfusion (excess anticoagulant) [Furosemide treatment] Spurious: EDTA contamination
Chloride	**Hyperchloraemia** In parallel with hypernatraemia (e.g. due to dehydration, diabetes insipidus) Hyperchloraemic metabolic acidosis (e.g. due to alimentary loss of bicarbonate, renal tubular acidosis) Hyperaldosteronism Potassium chloride (KCl) in fluid therapy Respiratory alkalosis Spurious: bromide therapy (interferes with assay)	**Hypochloraemia** In association with hyponatraemia (see sodium) Hypoadrenocorticism Metabolic alkalosis due to loss of hydrogen chloride (HCl) in gastric vomiting High anion gap metabolic acidosis (e.g. ketoacidosis, lactic acidosis) Chronic respiratory acidosis Furosemide and thiazides
Magnesium	**Hypermagnesaemia** Renal failure (prerenal, renal or postrenal azotaemia) Intravascular haemolysis	**Hypomagnesaemia** Hypoproteinaemia Acute or chronic diarrhoea Diabetes mellitus, especially with ketoacidosis
Phosphate	**Hyperphosphataemia** Young animals Reduced glomerular filtration rate (due to prerenal, renal or postrenal causes) Ruptured urinary bladder Vitamin D toxicity Diabetic ketoacidosis Tumour lysis syndrome Acute severe myopathy Osteolytic bone lesions Hyperthyroidism (cats) Phosphate-containing enemas Ischaemic intestinal lesions [High phosphate:calcium diet]	**Hypophosphataemia** Hyperparathyroidism Malignancy-associated hypercalcaemia with release of PTHrP Hypovitaminosis D (e.g. intestinal malabsorption, dietary deficiency) Following insulin therapy Re-feeding syndrome (cats) Anorexia/decreased intake Phosphate binders Vomiting and diarrhoea Fanconi syndrome Eclampsia
Potassium	**Hyperkalaemia** Acute oliguric or anuric renal failure Urinary tract obstruction or rupture Hypoadrenocorticism Severe diarrhoea, e.g. due to trichuriasis (pseudohypoadrenocorticism) Metabolic acidosis Tumour lysis syndrome Rhabdomyolysis or tissue necrosis Drug therapy: • Spironolactone • ACE inhibitors • Heparin • Mitotane • KCl in intravenous fluids • Transfusions [Hypoaldosteronism] [Repeated drainage of chylous thoracic effusions] [Peritoneal effusions in cats] Spurious: marked thrombocytosis or leucocytosis; haemolysis (Japanese Akitas); EDTA contamination of sample	**Hypokalaemia** Anorexia Fluid therapy using low potassium fluids Vomiting and/or diarrhoea Chronic renal failure Diabetic ketoacidosis Initial insulin therapy of diabetes mellitus (especially ketoacidotic) Hyperaldosteronism (Conn's syndrome) Acute hyperventilation (respiratory alkalosis) Hypokalaemic myopathy of Burmese cats Drug therapy: • Furosemide • Thiazides [Fanconi syndrome]

continues ▶

Electrolytes *continued*

Analyte	Increased		Decreased
Sodium	**Hypernatraemia** Osmotic diarrhoea Diabetes mellitus Central diabetes insipidus Nephrogenic diabetes insipidus Primary adipsia Heatstroke Burns or extensive degloving injury Water deprivation Hypertonic intravenous fluid therapy/increased salt intake Hyperaldosteronism Sodium bicarbonate therapy		**Hyponatraemia** Hypoadrenocorticism Vomiting or diarrhoea Third-space loss of fluid: pleural effusion or peritoneal effusion Volume overload associated with congestive heart failure, liver disease, nephrotic syndrome, hypotonic fluid administration Diuretics (e.g. thiazide) Diabetes mellitus with marked hyperglycaemia and/or ketoacidosis Mannitol infusion [Fanconi syndrome] [Syndrome of inappropriate antidiuretic hormone secretion (SIADH)] Psychogenic polydipsia Spurious: lipaemia

Enzymes

Enzyme	Increased
Alanine aminotransferase (ALT)	Hepatocyte damage in primary liver disease: • Inflammatory hepatic disease (e.g. chronic active hepatitis, cholangiohepatitis, FIP, infectious canine hepatitis) • Drug-related, due to phenobarbital, carprofen, glucocorticoids, methimazole/carbimazole in cats • Trauma • Toxic damage • Hepatic neoplasia Hepatocyte damage secondary to extrahepatic disease. Examples include: • Pancreatitis • GI disease • Periodontal disease • Endocrine disease (e.g. diabetes mellitus, hyperadrenocorticism, hyperthyroidism) • Hypoxia due to anaemia or reduced blood flow (e.g. in thromboembolism) • Congestive heart failure
Alkaline phosphatase (ALP)	Cholestasis: • Intrahepatic (e.g. cholangiohepatitis, hepatic lipidosis, chronic hepatitis, nodular hyperplasia, neoplasia) • Posthepatic (e.g. pancreatitis, cholangitis, cholelithiasis, ruptured gallbladder) Steroid induction – dogs only: • Hyperadrenocorticism • Steroid therapy Drug induction: • Phenobarbital Bone remodelling: • Young animal • Fracture • Neoplasia • Osteomyelitis • Hyperthyroidism ▶

Enzyme	Increased
Alkaline phosphatase (ALP) *continued*	Secondary to extrahepatic disease. Examples include: • GI disease • Periodontal disease • Endocrine disease (e.g. diabetes mellitus, hyperadrenocorticism, hyperthyroidism) • Congestive heart failure
Amylase	Pancreatitis Pancreatic neoplasia Azotaemia (2–3 times upper reference limit) Intestinal disease
Aspartate aminotransferase (AST)	Hepatocyte damage: see ALT Muscle damage Haemolysis
Creatine kinase (CK)	Myopathies Myositis Muscle ischaemia, e.g. aortic thromboembolism Trauma Intramuscular injections Haemolysis
Gamma-glutamyl transferase (GGT)	Cholestasis: • Intrahepatic (e.g cholangiohepatitis, neoplasia) • Posthepatic (e.g. pancreatitis, cholangitis, cholelithiasis) Drug-induced: • Corticosteroids • Phenobarbital
Lipase	Pancreatitis Pancreatic neoplasia Azotaemia Glucocorticoids Hepatic disease (especially neoplasia) Enteritis (?)

Other

Analyte	Increased	Decreased
Bile acids	Biliary obstruction/cholestasis Reduced hepatic function (e.g. chronic active hepatitis, cirrhosis) Portosystemic shunt Microvascular dysplasia Reactive/secondary hepatopathy, e.g. due to hyperadrenocorticism	
Bilirubin	**Hyperbilirubinaemia** Prehepatic: haemolysis (e.g. immune-mediated haemolytic anaemia, oxidant toxicity, haemotrophic mycoplasmosis, babesiosis) Intrahepatic (e.g. cirrhosis, hepatic lipidosis, cholangiohepatitis, neoplasia, FIP) Posthepatic (e.g. pancreatitis, cholangitis, cholelithiasis, biliary neoplasia)	
Cholesterol	**Hypercholesterolaemia** Postprandial Diabetes mellitus Hypothyroidism Hyperadrenocorticism Pancreatitis Cholestasis (many liver diseases) Protein-losing nephropathy with nephrotic syndrome Drug therapy: glucocorticoids, methimazole Primary hyperlipidaemia	**Hypocholesterolaemia** Severe liver disease Portosystemic shunt Protein-losing enteropathy (especially lymphangiectasia) Hypoadrenocorticism Severe malnutrition
Triglycerides	**Hypertriglyceridaemia** Postprandial Diabetes mellitus Hypothyroidism Hyperadrenocorticism Oestrogens Acute pancreatitis Idiopathic/familial hyperlipoproteinaemia	**Hypotriglyceridaemia** Drug therapy: heparin
Creatinine	Prerenal causes (though less affected than urea): hypovolaemia, decreased cardiac output, shock Renal disease Postrenal conditions: urinary tract obstruction, urinary tract rupture Increased production: high protein diet, protein catabolism, intestinal haemorrhage Dogs with high muscle mass, e.g. sighthounds	Decreased muscle mass
Glucose	**Hyperglycaemia** Stress (especially cats) Diabetes mellitus Hyperadrenocorticism Growth hormone excess Dioestrus Pancreatitis Neuroendocrine tumour, e.g. glucagonoma Drugs: intravenous glucose; alpha-2 agonists (e.g. medetomidine); ketamine, propofol, progestagens Ethylene glycol toxicity Postprandial (mild) Spurious: lipaemia	**Hypoglycaemia** Toy breeds Neonates Starvation Bacteraemia/septicaemia Parvovirus and other severe GI infections Hypoadrenocorticism Insulinoma Hepatic and GI smooth muscle tumours Renal failure Liver failure (severe) Portosystemic shunt Cachexia (cardiac or neoplastic) Seizure activity Glycogen storage disease Drugs: insulin overdose, ethanol, salicylates, propanolol Xylitol ingestion Artefact: delay in processing Polycythaemia and leucocytosis (may only be relevant in cases of delayed sample separation)
Protein (A = albumin; G = globulin)	**Hyperproteinaemia** Dehydration (A and G) Inflammation, particularly of liver (G) Infectious diseases e.g. FIP, *Leishmania*, *Ehrlichia*, *Anaplasma* Neoplasia (G) Plasma cell myeloma (monoclonal G) Spurious: lipaemia (A and G)	*Hypoproteinaemia* Haemorrhage (A and G) Protein-losing nephropathy (A) Protein-losing enteropathy (A and G) Third-space loss of fluid (A>G) Severe liver disease (A) Young animals Starvation Diuresis Acute phase response (A) (mild)
Urea	High-protein diet GI bleeding Renal failure (acute or chronic) Prerenal azotaemia Urinary obstruction Rupture of ureter, bladder or urethra	Severe starvation Diuresis Portosystemic shunts Hepatic disease/insufficiency Diabetes insipidus

Urinalysis

Specific gravity

Increased (>1.030 in dog, >1.035 in cat)
- Hypovolaemia
- Marked increase in glucose or protein content

Mildly decreased (1.015–1.030 in dog, 1.015–1.035 in cat)
- Early renal failure
- Diabetes mellitus
- Hyperadrenocorticism
- May be normal (dog)

Isosthenuria (I) (1.007–1.015) or hyposthenuria (H) (<1.007)
- Renal failure (I)
- Hyperadrenocorticism (I, H)
- Steroid therapy (I, H)
- Hypercalcaemia (I, H)
- Pyometra (I, H)
- Pyelonephritis (I, H)
- Renal medullary washout (e.g. post-obstruction) (I, H)
- Hyperthyroidism (I, rarely H)
- Psychogenic polydipsia (I, H)
- Fluid therapy (I, H)
- Liver disease (I, H)
- Partial central diabetes insipidus (I, H)
- Central or nephrogenic diabetes insipidus (usually H)

pH (normal 6.0–7.5)

Increased: alkaluria
- Urease-producing bacteria
- Aged sample
- Transient (postprandial)
- Renal tubular acidosis
- Metabolic alkalosis
- Diet rich in vegetable protein

Decreased: aciduria
- Acidifying diet
- Metabolic acidosis
- Hypochloraemic metabolic alkalosis (gastric vomiting)
- Hypokalaemia
- Furosemide therapy
- Artefactual – run-off of buffer from protein test pad

Dipstick

Glucose
Positive: glucosuria
Diabetes mellitus
- Stress hyperglycaemia (cats)
- Renal tubular disease:
  - Fanconi syndrome
  - Primary renal glucosuria
- [• Aminoglycosides]
- [• Hyperadrenocorticism]
- Artefactual – contamination of collection pot

Ketones
Positive: ketonuria
- Diabetes mellitus
- Very young animals
- [• Starvation]
- Hyperthyroidism in cats
- Pregnancy ketosis
- [• Very concentrated and acidic urine can give false positive]

Protein
Increased (>trace): proteinuria
- Pyuria
- Protein-losing nephropathy
- Haemorrhage
- [• Genital tract secretions if voided]

Bilirubin
Increased (>trace in cats, >2+ in dogs): bilirubinuria
- Haemolytic anaemia
- Hepatobiliary disease (especially cats)
- Obstructive cholestasis
- [• Very concentrated urine can give false increase]

Blood
Positive: haematuria (a speckled or uniform colour change)
- Urolithiasis
- Inflammation (any cause including urinary tract infection)
- Trauma
- Coagulopathy
- Neoplasia
- Iatrogenic

Haemoglobin
Positive: haemoglobinuria (a uniform colour change of the blood test pad)
- Intravascular haemolysis, e.g. with IMHA
- *In vitro* lysis of red blood cells from haematuria
- NB Myoglobinuria, e.g. due to muscle damage also causes a uniform colour change on the blood test pad

Myoglobin:
Positive: myoglobinuria
- Muscle damage

Sediment

White blood cell count
Increased: leucocytosis >5 per x400 hpf
- Urinary tract inflammation
- Urinary tract infection
- NB Absence of WBCs does not rule out urinary tract infection

Red blood cells
Increased >5 per x400 hpf
- Traumatic catheterization or cystocentesis
- Haemorrhage anywhere in the urogenital tract
- Inflammation (e.g. infection, crystalluria, obstruction)
- Neoplasia
- Trauma
- Coagulopathy
- Oestrus in entire females (voided samples)

Epithelial cells
Increased >2 per x100 lpf
- Traumatic catheterization
- Mucosal inflammation
- Mucosal hyperplasia
- Neoplasia

Abbreviations: ACE = angiotensin converting enzyme; aPTT = activated partial thromboplastin time; CPV = canine parvovirus; DIC = disseminated intravascular coagulation; EDTA = ethylenediamine tetra-acetic acid; FeLV = feline leukaemia virus; FIP = feline infectious peritonitis; FIV = feline immunodeficiency virus; GI = gastrointestinal; hpf = high power field; IMHA = immune-mediated haemolytic anaemia; lpf = low power field; PFK = phosphofructokinase; PK = pyruvate kinase; PSS = portosystemic shunt; PT = prothrombin time; PTH = parathyroid hormone; PTHrP = parathyroid hormone related protein; TMS = trimethoprim–sulphonamide; WBC = white blood cell.

Age-related changes on haematology and biochemistry profiles

Parameter	Change	Magnitude	Reason
Red blood cells	Low HCT/RBC/Hb in puppies <8 weeks	HCT: In dogs generally >0.30 l/l by 8 weeks and >0.40 l/l by 16 weeks (Harper *et al.*, 2003) Mean HCT 0.48 l/l at 24 weeks In cats mean HCT 0.30 l/l at 8 weeks, 0.35 l/l at 16 weeks, 0.37 l/l at 30 weeks	Destruction of fetal red cells, expansion of blood volume with growth without sufficient erythropoiesis, also may be iron deficient at weaning
	Higher reticulocyte counts	Absolute reticulocyte count >70 × 10^9/l for first 8 weeks in dogs	Reticulocytosis develops to compensate
Lymphocyte count	Young animals have higher counts	<6 months lymphocyte count: Dogs: 2–10 x 10^9/l Cats: 4–10 x 10^9/l	Maturation of the immune system
Total protein (TP)	Lower in young animals until about 6 months Albumin declines and TP/globulin increase with old age (Batamuzi *et al.*, 1996)	Mean TP 49 g/l in Beagles and 48 g/l in Labrador Retrievers at 3–8 weeks of age, rising to 55 g/l and 50 g/l, respectively, at 8–16 weeks (Harper *et al.*, 2003)	Physiological low globulin, low IgG
Calcium	Dogs (especially large breeds) increased levels until approximately 12 months	Approximately 10% change from the RI	Bone growth
Phosphate	Increased in dogs <12 months (especially large breeds), cats <6 months	Dogs: ≤2.9 mmol/l Cats: ≤2.6 mmol/l	Bone growth
Alkaline phosphatase	Increased in young animals, adult levels reached once growth slows, typically by 1 year	Typically 2–3x adult concentrations	Bone isoenzyme increased during growth
Creatine kinase	Higher for first 8 weeks in puppies	2–5x adult concentrations, sometimes higher	Birth trauma in very young

Abbreviations: Hb = haemoglobin; HCT = haematocrit; Ig = immunoglobulin; RBC = red blood cell; RI = reference interval.

References and further reading

Batamuzi EK, Kristensen E and Jensen AL (1996) Serum protein electrophoresis: potential test for use in geriatric companion animal health programmes. *Zentralblatt für Veterinarmedizin A* 43, 501–508

Clinkenbeard KD, Cowell RL, Meinkoth JH *et al.* (2001) The haemopoietic and lymphoid systems. In: *Veterinary Paediatrics, 3rd edn*, ed. JD Hoskins, pp. 300–322. Saunders, Philadelphia

Harper EJ, Hackett RM, Wilkinson J and Heaton PR (2003) Age-related variations in hematologic and plasma biochemical test results in Beagles and Labrador Retrievers. *Journal of the American Veterinary Medical Association* **223**, 1436–1442

Lowseth LA, Gillett NA, Gerlach RF and Muggenburg BA (1990) The effects of aging on hematology and serum chemistry values in the beagle dog. *Veterinary Clinical Pathology* **19**, 13–19

Rosset E, Rannou B, Casseleux G, Chalvet-Monfray K and Buff S (2012) Age-related changes in biochemical and hematologic variables in Borzoi and Beagle puppies from birth to 8 weeks. *Veterinary Clinical Pathology* **41**, 272–282

Breed variations in haematological and biochemical parameters

Parameter	Change	Breed
PCV, RBC count, Hb	Higher	Greyhound, Lurcher, Saluki
MCV	Higher	Greyhound, Miniature and Toy Poodles
	Lower	Akita, Chow Chow, Shar Pei, Shiba Inu
WBC count	Lower	Greyhound, Whippet
Neutrophil, lymphocyte and monocyte counts	Lower	Greyhound, possibly Tervuren
Platelet count	Lower	Cavalier King Charles Spaniel, Greyhound, Lurcher, Norfolk Terrier, Whippet
Eosinophil count	Higher	Brittany Spaniel, GSD, Rottweiler
Globulin	Lower	Greyhound
Creatinine	Higher	Well muscled dogs, e.g. GSD, sighthounds
Urea and creatinine	Higher	80% of Birman kittens >6 months old, 35% of adult Birmans
ALT	Higher	Greyhound and other sighthounds. Possibly of muscle origin
TT4 ± FT4	Lower	Greyhound

Abbreviations: ALT = alanine aminotransferase; FT4 = free thyroxine; GSD = German Shepherd Dog; Hb = haemoglobin; MCV = mean corpuscular volume; PCV = packed cell volume; RBC = red blood cell; TT4 = total thyroxine; WBC = white blood cell.

References and further reading

Bourgès-Abella N, Geffré A, Concordet D, Braun JP and Trumel C (2011) Canine reference intervals for the Sysmex XT-2000iV hematology analyzer. *Veterinary Clinical Pathology* **40(3)**, 303–315

Campora C, Freeman KP, Lewis FI, Gibson G, Sacchini F and Sanchez-Vazquez MJ (2011) Determination of haematological reference intervals in healthy adult Greyhounds. *Journal of Small Animal Practice* **52**, 301–309

Campora C, Freeman KP, Serra M and Sacchini F (2011) Reference intervals for Greyhounds and Lurchers using the Sysmex XT-2000iV hematology analyzer. *Veterinary Clinical Pathology* **44**, 467–474

Uhríková I, Lačňáková A, Tandlerová K *et al.* (2013) Haematological and biochemical variations among eight sighthound breeds. *Australian Veterinary Journal* **91**, 452–459

Zaldívar-López S, Marín LM, Iazbik MC, Westendorf-Stingle N, Hensley S and Couto CG (2011) Clinical pathology of Greyhounds and other sighthounds. *Veterinary Clinical Pathology* **40**, 414–425

Therapeutic drug monitoring

The type of assay used to measure concentrations of drugs varies from one laboratory to another. High-performance liquid chromatography (HPLC) is considered the gold standard but is rarely used owing to the cost entailed and the slow turnaround time. Most laboratories use immunoassays such as chemiluminescence or radioimmunoassay.

Collection tubes containing separators, e.g. serum gel tubes, have been shown to adsorb some drugs, e.g. phenobarbital, resulting in artefactually lower serum concentrations. Therefore, it is best not to use these tubes for samples intended for therapeutic drug monitoring. The frequency of monitoring will depend on the individual case; in many cases checking levels every 6–12 months is reasonable and also after any alteration of the dose or change in the clinical condition of the animal.

Drug	Time to steady state	Trough	Peak	Suggested time for sampling	Sample type	Therapeutic/target range when sampling at suggested time	Toxic level	Notes
Ciclosporin	N/A: short half-life compared with dosing interval	12 hours post pill	Approximately 2 hours	12 hours post pill 7 days after starting treatment or changing dose	EDTA blood	300–600 ng/ml (may vary depending on disease)	Risk of nephrotoxicity in cats with levels >700–800 ng/ml	NB Some animals respond when levels are below the suggested range. No correlation between drug concentration and therapeutic efficacy
Digoxin	7 days	Pre pill	2–5 hours	6–8 hours post pill 7 days after starting treatment or changing dose	Serum	0.65–2.55 nmol/l when on monotherapy Some suggest ≤1.28 nmol/l	>2.55 nmol/l, sometimes seen lower	Toxic dose close to therapeutic dose
Levetiracetam	N/A: short half-life compared with dosing interval	Pre pill	Approximately 2 hours for standard preparations. Longer for extended release preparations	Trough 7 days after starting treatment or changing dose	Serum	Unknown In humans 5–45 µg/ml	Unknown	No correlation between drug concentration and therapeutic efficacy
Phenobarbital	1–2 weeks	Pre pill	4–6 hours	Any time 2 weeks after starting therapy or changing dose	Serum	15–35 µg/ml in dogs (65–150 µmol/l) 10–30 µg/ml in cats (43–129 µmol/l)	>35 µg/ml >150 µmol/l	Can use peak and trough in cases that are difficult to stabilize. Peak for suspected toxicity. If used in combination with bromide aim for approximately 25 µg/ml

continues ▶

Drug	Time to steady state	Trough	Peak	Suggested time for sampling	Sample type	Therapeutic/ target range when sampling at suggested time	Toxic level	Notes
Potassium bromide	2–4 months	N/A	N/A: long half-life	Any time 3 months after starting treatment, or 1–24 hours after completing loading dose	Serum	1000–2500 mg/l	2000–3000 mg/l when used with phenobarbital	If sole therapy can go slightly higher, up to 3000 mg/l If with phenobarbital usually 1000–2000 mg/l sufficient
Thyroxine	2–3 days	Pre pill	3 hours	4–6 hours post pill 2 weeks after commencing therapy or changing dose NB Check data sheet for specific advice on individual products	Serum	>35 nmol/l	100 nmol/l	Aim for high end of RI for q24h dosing, slightly lower for q12h dosing. Trough levels low normal or just below RI

Abbreviations: EDTA = ethylenediamine tetra-acetic acid; N/A= not applicable; RI = reference interval; TSH = thyroid-stimulating hormone.

Drug	Clinical pharmacology				Therapeutic range	Major possible adverse effects
	$T_{1/2}$ (hr)	Tss (d)	Vd (l/kg)	Protein binding (%)		
Bromide	20–46 days	100–200	0.45	0	Monotherapy: 1000–3000 mg/l With phenobarbital: 1500–2500 mg/l	Sedation; weakness; polydipsia; possible pancreatitis; possible behavioural disorders
Clorazepate	5–6	1–2	1.6	85	20–75 µg/ml (nordiazepam)	Sedation; withdrawal seizures
Felbamate	5–6	1–2	1.0	25	25–100 mg/l	Blood dyscrasia; liver toxicity; induces p450 system
Gabapentin	2–4	1	0.2	0	4–16 mg/l	Sedation; ataxia
Levetiracetam	2–4	2–3	0.5	<10	Variable	Not greater than placebo; sedation; ataxia
Phenobarbital	24–40	10–14	0.8	40	[a]20–40 mg/dl	Sedation; polydipsia; liver toxicity; induces p450 system; blood dyscrasias
Zonisamide	15–20	3–4	1.5	50	10–40 µg/ml	Sedation; ataxia; loss of appetite; keraconjunctivitis sicca; vomiting

Antiepileptic drugs available for treating epilepsy in dogs. $T_{1/2}$ = elimination half-life; Tss = approximate time to steady state; Vd = volume of distribution.
[a] There may be an increased risk of drug-induced liver dysfunction with levels over 35 µg/ml so careful monitoring is advised, ± bile acid measurement.
(Reproduced from the BSAVA Manual of Canine and Feline Neurology, 4th edition)

Conversion tables

Temperature

SI unit	Conversion factor	Conventional unit
°C	(x 9/5) + 32	°F

Hypodermic needles

	Metric	Non-metric
Needle gauge	0.8 mm	21 G
	0.6 mm	23 G
	0.5 mm	25 G
	0.4 mm	27 G
Needle length	12 mm	$^1/_2$ inch
	16 mm	$^5/_8$ inch
	25 mm	1 inch
	30 mm	1.25 inch
	40 mm	1.5 inch

Haematology

Parameter	SI unit	Conversion factor	Conventional unit
RBC	$10^{12}/l$	1	$10^6/\mu l$
Haemoglobin	g/l	0.1	g/dl
MCH	pg/cell	1	pg/cell
MCHC	g/l	0.1	g/dl
MCV	fl	1	μm^3
Platelet count	$10^9/l$	1	$10^3/\mu l$
WBC	$10^9/l$	1	$10^3/\mu l$

To convert from SI units to conventional units, multiply by the conversion factor; to convert from conventional units to SI units, divide by the conversion factor.

Biochemistry

Parameter	SI unit	Conversion factor	Conventional unit
Alanine aminotransferase	IU/l	1	IU/l
Albumin	g/l	0.1	g/dl
Alkaline phosphatase	IU/l	1	IU/l
Aspartate aminotransferase	IU/l	1	IU/l
Bilirubin	μmol/l	0.0584	mg/dl
BUN	mmol/l	2.8	mg/dl
Calcium	mmol/l	4	mg/dl
Carbon dioxide (total)	mmol/l	1	mEq/l
Cholesterol	mmol/l	38.61	mg/dl
Chloride	mmol/l	1	mEq/l
Cortisol	nmol/l	0.0362	ng/dl
Creatine kinase	IU/l	1	IU/l
Creatinine	μmol/l	0.0113	mg/dl
Glucose	mmol/l	18.02	mg/dl
Insulin	pmol/l	0.1394	μIU/ml
Iron	μmol/l	5.587	μg/dl
Magnesium	mmol/l	2	mEq/l
Phosphorus	mmol/l	3.1	mg/dl
Potassium	mmol/l	1	mEq/l
Sodium	mmol/l	1	mEq/l
Total protein	g/l	0.1	g/dl
Oestradiol	pmol/l	0.273	pg/ml
Progesterone	nmol/l	0.315	ng/ml
Testosterone	nmol/l	0.288	ng/ml
Thyroxine (T4) (free)	pmol/l	0.0775	ng/dl
Thyroxine (T4) (total)	nmol/l	0.0775	μg/dl
Triiodothyronine (T3)	nmol/l	65.1	ng/dl
Triglycerides	mmol/l	88.5	mg/dl

Abbreviations: BUN = blood urea nitrogen; MCH = mean corpuscular haemoglobin; MCHC = mean corpuscular haemoglobin concentration; MCV = mean corpuscular volume; RBC = red blood cells; WBC = white blood cells.

Index